Psychiatric Mental Health Nursing

Fifth Edition

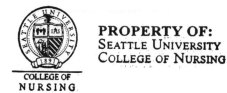

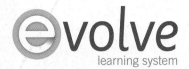
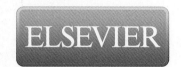
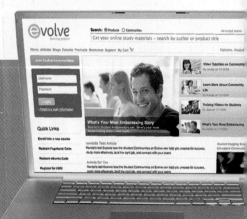

Psychiatric Mental Health Nursing

Fifth Edition

KATHERINE M. FORTINASH, MSN, APRN, PMHCNS

Advanced Practice Clinical Specialist
Psychiatric Mental Health Nursing
Formerly:
Clinical Specialist
Sharp Hospital Behavioral Health Services
Professor, Psychiatric Nursing
Department of Nursing Education
Grossmont College
San Diego, California

PATRICIA A. HOLODAY WORRET, MSN, APRN, PMHCNS

Advanced Practice Clinical Specialist
Psychiatric Mental Health Nursing
Professor Emerita
Department of Nursing Education
Palomar College
San Marcos, California

ELSEVIER

3251 Riverport Lane
St. Louis, MO 63043

NOTICE

Knowledge and best practice in this field are constantly changing. As new research and experience broaden our knowledge, changes in practice, treatment, and drug therapy may become necessary or appropriate. Readers are advised to check the most current information provided (i) on procedures featured or (ii) by the manufacturer of each product to be administered, to verify the recommended dose or formula, the method and duration of administration, and contraindications. It is the responsibility of the practitioner, relying on their own experience and knowledge of the patient, to make diagnoses, to determine dosages and the best treatment for each individual patient, and to take all appropriate safety precautions. To the fullest extent of the law, neither the Publisher nor the Authors assume any liability for any injury and/or damage to persons or property arising out of or related to any use of the material contained in this book.

The Publisher

Library of Congress Cataloging-in-Publication Data
Psychiatric mental health nursing / [edited by] Katherine M. Fortinash, Patricia A. Holoday Worret.—5th ed.
   p. ; cm.
Includes bibliographical references and index.
ISBN 978-0-323-07572-5
1. Psychiatric nursing. I. Fortinash, Katherine M. II. Holoday-Worret, Patricia A.
[DNLM: 1. Mental Disorders—nursing. 2. Psychiatric Nursing. WY 160]
RC440.P7338 2012
616.89′0231—dc22

       2011003988

Senior Editor: Yvonne Alexopoulos
Senior Developmental Editor: Lisa P. Newton
Publishing Services Manager: Deborah L. Vogel
Project Manager: John W. Gabbert
Designer: Paula Catalano

Printed in China

Last digit is the print number: 9 8 7 6 5 4 3 2 1

DEDICATION

*We continue to dedicate this book to all those who live with mental
illness every day, and to their families, their friends,
and the nurses who care for them.*

ACKNOWLEDGMENTS

We want to thank our readers who selected this fifth edition of *Psychiatric Mental Health Nursing*—the students on their journey into psychiatric mental-health nursing theory and practice, the instructors who guide and mold the path to learning, and the practitioners who role model best practice patient care with skill and compassion. We sincerely hope this textbook fulfills your professional needs, answers and satisfies many questions, and heightens your life-long interest in the fascinating specialty of mental health nursing.

We are grateful to those who worked diligently and traveled closely with us on this textbook's course to completion and publication. We especially thank each of our talented contributors, several of whom have been with us since the beginning of the first edition, and also those who joined us for the first time.

Special thanks to Pam Marcus and Ruth Grendell for their extra efforts and contributions to this edition of our textbook, and to all past contributors whose work continues to positively influence our readers.

The success of this book is due to the dedicated efforts of many people working together; the authors, the contributors, the editors, and the entire Elsevier team. We especially thank Yvonne Alexopoulos, Lisa Newton, Johnny Gabbert, Paula Catalano, and Eloise DeHaan as well as the staff who worked behind the scenes, paying careful attention to all those details that tied the book together and made it come to life.

We also thank our families and friends for patience and understanding while this book was being written, and we especially thank each other for our continuing united vision for nursing and the undeniable importance it plays in the lives of millions of patients and their families.

Kathi Fortinash and Pat Holoday Worret

CONTRIBUTORS

Merry A. Armstrong, DNSc, ARNP, BC
Associate Professor
Washington State University College of
    Nursing
Spokane, Washington
    *Chapter 15 Substance-Related Disorders
        and Addictive Behaviors*

**Ann Wolbert Burgess, DNSc, APRN,
BC, FAAN**
Professor of Psychiatric Nursing
William F. Connell School of Nursing
Boston College
Chestnut Hill, Massachusetts
    *Chapter 23 Violence: Anger, Abuse, and
        Aggression*
    *Chapter 24 Forensic Nursing in Clinical
        Practice*

**Pauline Chan, RPh, MBA, BCPP,
FCSHP, FASHP**
Senior Pharmaceutical Consultant
Medi-Cal Pharmacy Policy Unit
California Department of Health Services
Sacramento, California
    Chapter 25 Psychopharmacology

Anna Clarkin, MSW, LCSW
Private Practice
San Diego, California
    *Chapter 18 Eating Disorders: Anorexia
        Nervosa and Bulimia Nervosa*

**Nancy A. Coffin-Romig, DNSc,
PMHCNS-BC**
Assistant Professor
California State University San Marcos
School of Nursing
San Marcos, California
    *Chapter 26 Therapies: Theory and
        Clinical Practice*

Judy A. Malone Cole, RN, PhD
Clinical Director
Richmond State Hospital
Richmond, VA
    *Chapter 13 Schizophrenia and Other
        Psychotic Disorders*

Robert L. Erb, Jr., PhD, RN, CS, CLNC
Advanced Clinician
Sharp HealthCare
San Diego, California
    *Chapter 9 Legal and Ethical Aspects in
        Clinical Practice*

Chantal M. Flanagan, RN, MS, CNS
Associate Professor
Palomar College
San Marcos, California
    *Chapter 17 Disorders of Infancy,
        Childhood, and Adolescence*

Candice A. Francis, EdD
Professor Emerita
Palomar College
San Marcos, California
    *Chapter 6 Neurobiology in Mental
        Health and Mental Disorder*

Ruth N. Grendell, DNSc, RN
Nursing Professor Emerita
Point Loma Nazarene University
San Diego, California
Faculty
University of Phoenix
    *Chapter 8 Culture, Ethnicity, and
        Spirituality: A Global Perspective*
    *Chapter 27 Complementary and
        Alternative Therapies*
    *Chapter 29 Mental and Emotional
        Responses to Medical Illness*

Bonnie M. Hagerty, PhD, RN
Assistant Dean, Undergraduate Programs
Associate Professor
School of Nursing
University of Michigan
Ann Arbor, Michigan
    *Chapter 12 Mood Disorders: Depression,
        Bipolar, and Adjustment Disorders*

Linda Hollinger-Smith, PhD, RN, FAAN
Vice President
Mather LifeWays Institute on Aging
Evanston, Illinois
    *Chapter 7 Human Development Across
        the Life Span*

Russell A. Kelley, MN, ARNP, BC
Instructor
Intercollegiate College of Nursing
Washington State University College of
    Nursing
Private Practice
Spokane, Washington
    *Chapter 16 Cognitive Disorders: Delirium,
        Dementia, and Amnestic Disorders*

Deborah Eimer King, RN, MS, PhD
Columbia, Maryland
    *Chapter 21 Crisis: Theory and
        Intervention*

**Shelly F. Lurie-Akman, MS, APRN/
PMH-BC, CTHY**
Associate Director of Nursing
Perkins Hospital Center
Jessup, Maryland
Associate Faculty
Johns Hopkins School of Nursing
Baltimore, Maryland
Associate Staff
The Institute for the Study, Prevention and
    Treatment of Sexual Traumas
Baltimore, Maryland
    *Chapter 20 Sexual Disorders: Sexual
        Dysfunctions and Paraphilias*

Pamela E. Marcus, RN, APRN/PMH-BC
Associate Professor of Nursing
Prince George's Community College
Largo, Maryland
Advanced Practice Nurse Psychotherapist
Private Practice
Upper Marlboro, Maryland
    Chapter 5 Adaptation to Stress
    *Chapter 10 Anxiety and Related
        Disorders*
    *Chapter 11 Somatoform, Factitious, and
        Dissociative Disorders*
    Chapter 14 Personality Disorders
    *Chapter 22 Suicide: Prevention and
        Intervention*

Susan Fertig McDonald, DNP, PMHCNS-BC
Clinical Nurse Specialist
Inpatient Psychiatry & Alcohol Drug
 Treatment
VA San Diego Healthcare System
San Diego, California
 Chapter 4 Therapeutic Communication:
 Interviews and Interventions

Nancy Stark Napolitano, EdD, MSN, RN
Professor of Psychiatric Nursing and
 Health Science
Mt. San Jacinto College
Menifee, California
Nursing Education Consultant
 Chapter 19 Sleep Disorders: Dyssomnias
 and Parasomnias

Kathleen L. Patusky, PhD, APRN-BC
Assistant Professor
School of Nursing
University of Medicine and Dentistry of
 New Jersey
Newark, New Jersey
 Chapter 12 Mood Disorders: Depression,
 Biopolar, and Adjustment Disorders

Dona Petrozzi, RN, MSN
PhD Candidate
William F. Connell School of Nursing
Boston College
Chestnut Hill, Massachusetts
Psychiatric Liaison
Boston Medical Center
Boston, Massachusetts
 Chapter 23 Violence: Anger, Abuse, and
 Aggression
 Chapter 24 Forensic Nursing in Clinical
 Practice

Alwilda Scholler-Jaquish, RN, PhD
Associate Professor
Nursing Program
Graduate and Professional Studies
Stevenson University
Owings Mills, Maryland
 Chapter 30 Community Mental Health
 Nursing for Patients with Severe and
 Persistent Mental Illness

Kate Thomas, PhD
Faculty
Johns Hopkins University School of
 Medicine
Education Director
The Sexual Behaviors Consultation Unit
Johns Hopkins University
Adjunct Professor
Stevenson University
Loyola University
Baltimore, Maryland
 Chapter 20 Sexual Disorders: Sexual
 Dysfunctions and Paraphilias

FEATURE CONTRIBUTORS

Diane Fischer Hickman, RN, PHD, PMHCNS-BC
Psychiatric-Mental Health Clinician
Mental Health Intensive Case Management
 Program
VA San Diego Healthcare System
San Diego, California
 Medication Key Facts boxes

REVIEWERS

Patricia Becker, MSN, BSN
Instructor, Nursing
Walla Walla Community College
Walla Walla, Washington

Sue S. Butell, RN, MS
Professor of Nursing
Linfield-Good Samaritan School of Nursing
Portland, Oregon

Harvey "Skip" Davis, RN, PhD, CARN
Associate Professor, San Francisco State University
School of Nursing
Adjunct Researcher, University of California
San Francisco, California

M. Paulette Humphries, MS, MA, RN
Senior Lecturer
Indiana University East School of Nursing
Richmond, Indiana

Diane M. Sandhoff, MS, RN
Associate Professor of Nursing
Dakota Wesleyan University
Mitchell, South Dakota

PREFACE

ABOUT THIS BOOK

We, the authors, thank you for selecting the fifth edition of Psychiatric Mental Health Nursing. This edition of our textbook publishes at a significant time in the health care industry. State-of-the-art information and current issues and trends in scientific research are shared with our readers, while we also maintain the primary focus of this text, which is to present current theoretic and clinical content that teach the elements of Psychiatric Mental Health (PMH) nursing practice, and guide our readers toward successful, rewarding careers.

CURRENT HEALTH CARE

While the future of mental health care in this country is uncertain, we know that the entire health care industry is poised on the threshold of extraordinary actual and proposed advances and changes, unprecedented in our history. These include several significant changes within the psychiatric mental health arena. Controversy always surrounds major shifts in policy, such as the national Health Care Reform bill signed in 2010, and the costs that accompany those shifts. Portions of that legislation may remain in transition for years because of different political views; however, this textbook identifies salient proposed changes in health care that may directly impact our clients as well as the psychiatric mental health nurses who care and advocate for them. Now, as in the past and in the future, psychiatric mental health nurses will meet the challenges of change and deliver best practice mental health care for clients, their families, and the community.

RESEARCH AND TREATMENT

Advances rapidly continue in the neurosciences that encompass multiple areas such as psychobiology, psychopharmacology, and innovative diagnostic and treatment approaches for psychiatric disorders. Particularly exciting are those areas of research and current treatments that target some of the more serious and resistant psychiatric disorders such as the schizophrenias, mood disorders, Alzheimer's disease, and the spectrum disorders to name a few. This edition thoroughly reflects the importance of PMH research and treatment throughout the book, in the body of chapter text, and in features such as Evidence-Based Research boxes.

INTEGRATED NURSING AND MEDICAL MODELS

In actual clinical settings, the patient's psychiatric diagnoses are correlated with nursing diagnoses, resulting in care derived from effectively combining both medical and nursing classifications and models that culminate in total patient care. From our first edition, we purposefully integrate nursing and medical care throughout our textbooks, which is one of its major strengths. The contents of this edition continue to reflect a blend of the most current nursing and psychiatric assessments, diagnoses, interventions, and outcomes. Also incorporated are information and interventions from several other PMH related disciplines that come together to form a comprehensive, multidimensional text. Best practice methods are emphasized. Evidence-based practice (EBP), Integrated Care, and recent use of Recovery Models are also described and discussed.

PMH NURSING FOCUS

PMH nursing is a dynamic professional career choice and is given full recognition within the contents of this fifth edition. PMH nurses use all aspects of their nursing education with an emphasis on those principles related to the PMH specialty. Practical application of theory and clinical skills is emphasized in these chapters. In addition, the time honored nursing process enables critical thinking that results in total patient care. Nursing process is widely represented in several forms and models to facilitate the application of the nursing process in the clinical practice setting. These include NANDA-I (North American Nursing Diagnosis Association International); NOC (Nursing Outcomes Classification); and NIC (Nursing Interventions Classification).

INTERDISCIPLINARY CARE PLANNING TOOLS

We offer the reader multiple tools to plan patient care, such as standard care plans and comprehensive concept maps, to facilitate the reader's critical thinking and learning, and assist in decision making that ultimately affects patient outcomes. All care planning tools incorporate the nursing classifications and models of NANDA-I, NOC, and NIC, described above, as well as the DSM, the medical classification. The DSM can be located on the Evolve site http://evolve.elsevier.com/Fortinash/.

We believe that this interdisciplinary approach to planning care reflects what actually occurs in the practice setting. The various care planning tools are interspersed throughout the text and all of them include patient scenarios that reflect real life situations, and the steps of the nursing process. Numerous additional care plans can be found on our Evolve site.

LANGUAGE AND TERMINOLOGY

Now as in past editions, we recognize and respect the contributions of both men and women in the nursing profession. Whenever possible, plural nouns are used in place of the singular *him* or *her*. While the terms *client* and *patient* are both used by nurses and nursing organizations, we have opted to use the term *patient* throughout the text.

We recognize that though the term *family* is often used to designate blood relatives, many people call friends and significant others their family. We continue to maintain an objective and nonjudgmental view of all individuals depicted in this text.

FEATURES

Chapter consistency fosters learning. We strive to facilitate this in various ways. Appearance: The full color format is highlighted in print, illustrations, figures, tables, boxes, and graphs with topic-specific color consistency demonstrated from chapter to chapter; Organization and Format: Chapters are organized under one of seven distinct parts that are arranged by content; Prioritization: Students, instructors, and practitioners know the importance of prioritization during every step in the total care of patients, including the assessment, diagnosis, expected outcomes, planning, interventions, and evaluation of patients. We strive to demonstrate this principle whenever possible, keeping in mind that the nursing process is fluid and interactive, and the nurse may assess the patient at any given time according to the patient's needs and responses.

SPECIAL FEATURES

A new, exciting fifth edition featuring the Latest Content in Research and Practice, a Bold, Concise Format with Easy-to-Learn Critical Concepts, and Objectives!

1. Disorder Chapter (Schizophrenia)

Every chapter begins with a famous quote reflecting chapter content, chapter objectives, a list of key terms bolded throughout the text for easy access to key concepts, and an opening statement that introduces the reader to the chapter content.

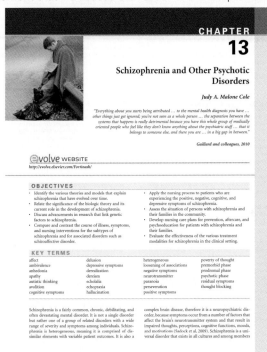

2. Concept Map

Newly designed concept maps with concept map case studies add another dimension to student care planning and combine medical and nursing principles in a user-friendly format.

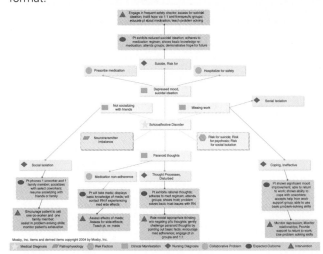

3. Research for Evidence-Based Practice Box

Research for Evidence-Based Practice is featured throughout the text to empower the reader with the most current research and treatment, and to encourage best practice psychiatric mental health nursing care.

RESEARCH FOR EVIDENCE-BASED PRACTICE

Swanson JW, et al: Comparing antipsychotic medication effects on reducing violence in persons with schizophrenia. *Br J Psychiatry* 193:37-43, 2008.

Clinical Antipsychotic Trials of Intervention Effectiveness (CATIE) compared the newer atypical medications quetiapine (Seroquel), olanzapine (Zyprexa), risperidone (Risperdal) and ziprasidone (Geodon) with the older antipsychotic perphenazine (Trilafon). Results that were previously reported showed that perphenazine was just as effective in treating symptoms of schizophrenia symptoms than the newer atypical types. This new analysis examined whether any of the medication reduced the frequency of violence, a rare symptom associated with the disorder. Researchers from Duke University examined data from the 1445 CATIE participants for which baseline information on violent behaviors was available. They found that among the 653 participants who completed six months of treatment on their initially assigned medication, the frequency of violent acts declined from 16% to 9% overall. None of the atypical medications performed better than perphenazine, and quetiapine particularly appeared to be less effective than perphenazine. Those who took the medication as directed were less likely to be violent, except for those who had a history of childhood conduct problems. Those who lived with others, had substance use problems, had been victimized in the past, and were of lower socioeconomic status, were more likely to have problems with violent behavior regardless of the medication usage. The researchers concluded that contrary to some previous studies, the atypical antipsychotics have no advantage over the older medication in reducing violence. Also, violence associated with situations unrelated to the disorder, such as a history of conduct problems, are unlikely to be treated effectively with antipsychotics alone. Participants with these risk factors would require more intensive psychosocial or family-based treatments in order to reduce violent behavior.

4. Patient and Family Teaching Guidelines

Patient and Family Teaching Guidelines are placed throughout the text to provide knowledge, support, and treatment compliance strategies for patients and their families.

PATIENT AND FAMILY TEACHING GUIDELINES
Medications for the Treatment of Schizophrenia

TEACH THE PATIENT AND FAMILY	STRATEGIES	RATIONALE
Right to informed consent and disclosure regarding benefits, side effects, anticipated prognosis with and without medication, and alternatives	Initially and any time that the medication or dosage is changed, written permission is obtained from the patient, and the following points are discussed with the patient about his or her medication: Right to informed consent and disclosure regarding benefits, side effects, anticipated prognosis with and without medications, and alternatives. The nurse consults with the physician regarding disclosure that is beneficial to the patient as compared with disclosure that may be harmful.	The patient has the right to choose how much society intervenes. The patient experiences independence, self-esteem, and self-control. The patient develops trust because of others' regard for his or her concerns.
Correct storage and administration of medications	Explain, demonstrate, and request a return demonstration of the handling and administration of medications. Work with the patient to prepare a check chart for his or her medications, dosages, and times. Take control of the environment: reduce distractions, simplify instructions, teach in small segments, and reinforce teaching often.	The safety of the patient and others is ensured. The patient who is involved develops ownership of the process and adherence to the treatment plan. The patient will be able to better focus, minimize frustration, and feel successful.
Action of the medication as well as the symptoms that are reduced or eliminated by the use of the medication	Encourage the patient's own desire to prevent relapse; explain in a matter-of-fact way that many people have various illnesses and take medication to treat them.	This offers the patient hope and reinforcement and informs him or her of the rationale for treatment.
Side effects that may be experienced	Show the patient how to use a journal to record feelings, thoughts, and behaviors over time.	This helps the patient to assume responsibility for self-care and documents treatment effects.
Food and drug interactions to be avoided	Inform the patient about symptoms and events to report and who to tell.	This keeps side effects from getting out of control and causing complications.
How to use the support of family and friends	Include significant others in teaching sessions. Offer thorough education, answer questions, and engage in discussion.	This elicits the support of significant others, decreases family anxiety, and allows the nurse to be a patient advocate.

5. Case Studies with Critical Thinking Skills

Students can test their knowledge with critical thinking questions and accompanying real life case studies that are featured throughout the text.

CASE STUDY

Lance, a 35-year-old man with chronic schizophrenia, was living in a single room in a downtown hotel that houses people with mental illness. Lance was never able to budget his minimal income to last the whole month. He had a fixed delusion that he owned the hotel where he lived but that the manager and the government were defrauding him of his rent money. When Lance was short of cash at the end of the month, he became abusive and aggressive. When Lance was assaultive, the manager called the police, and Lance was readmitted to the psychiatric hospital involuntarily for dangerousness to others. After about 10 days, he was discharged to the same hotel, where he would live quietly for a while and help the manager with tasks until the next delusional episode. This was a repetitive pattern for Lance, who had no support from relatives or friends.

Critical Thinking

1 What is the significance of Lance's delusion?
2 Lance received good care at the psychiatric hospital, and standard outcome criteria for discharge were always met. If this pattern continued, what would the chances be that Lance would hold onto his delusion?
3 Why might a nurse's attempt to challenge the delusion be risky? What are some teaching strategies that nurses could use with Lance? In what form would they best be implemented? When Lance is stable, can he identify any early warning signs that things are starting to break down for him? Is Lance willing to accept or identify someone as a supporter who can help him?
4 If you were a community mental health nurse, how would you perform follow-up care for Lance? Consider his money-management issues and how these may affect his ability to obtain his medications, food, and other necessities at the end of each month.
5 What signs of escalating anxiety would you look for in Lance's behavior? How would you manage his anxiety?

6. Clinical Alert Boxes

Clinical Alert Boxes placed throughout the text capture the reader's attention to the most critical issues in each chapter that affect the patient's safety and well-being.

❖ CLINICAL ALERT #1

Suicide is the leading cause of premature death among people who have been diagnosed with schizophrenia. Up to 30% attempt suicide and 4% to 10% die as a result of suicide. Suicide is most common within the first 6 years after the initial hospitalization and then again during periods of remission after 5 years of illness (APA, 2004).

Specific risk factors for suicide among individuals with schizophrenia include young age and a high socioeconomic status background. In addition, the person who is experiencing schizophrenia sometimes considers suicide if he or she has a high intelligence level and a high level of achievement and if he or she has set goals high before symptoms occurred and is aware of perceived future losses. Earlier onset and multiple relapses add to suicide risk. People with severe depression who feel hopeless are at risk. People who have expressed suicidal thoughts are also at risk. Despite the identification of these risk factors, it is often difficult to predict whether an individual will attempt suicide. Professionals need to evaluate these patients for suicide risk during all stages of the person's illness (APA, 2004). Overdose of prescribed medications as a method of suicide is not common because antipsychotics have a high therapeutic index and lethal doses are much higher than the doses that produce a therapeutic effect (Schultz et al, 2007).

7. Chapter Summary, Review Questions, and References with Online Resources

All chapters close with our hallmark bulleted Chapter Summary, followed by NCLEX-driven review questions, a list of online resources, and current and classic references.

CHAPTER SUMMARY

- Schizophrenia is one of the most complex and debilitating mental disorders.
- Schizophrenia is a not a single disorder but rather a syndrome (group of diseases) known as *the schizophrenias.*
- The schizophrenias are the largest group of mental disorders.
- Biologic factors are the primary focus of the research regarding the etiology and treatment of schizophrenia.
- The five biologic models that are currently being considered are as follows: (1) heredity/genetic; (2) neuroanatomic/neurochemical; (3) neurotransmitter function (specifically the dopamine hypothesis); (4) immunologic; and (5) stress/disease/trauma/drug abuse.
- Advancements in genetic research hold promise for the more effective treatment of schizophrenia during the next decade.
- The five major subtypes of schizophrenia are paranoid, disorganized, catatonic, undifferentiated, and residual.
- The diagnostic criteria for schizophrenia include two or more of the following symptoms being evident for at least 1 month: hallucinations, delusions, disorganized or catatonic behavior, and disorganized speech.
- Involving the patient with schizophrenia and the patient's family or significant others in the patient's treatment plan, as appropriate, is important and contributes to more effective treatment.
- Many practitioners use psychopharmacology as an intervention for many symptoms of schizophrenia. New medications with fewer side effects offer hope and more effective treatment outcomes for the complex symptoms of schizophrenia.
- Milieu therapy, psychosocial rehabilitation, patient and family education, and behavior modification are some treatments that are used with patients with schizophrenia.
- Community resources are critical for rehabilitating patients with schizophrenia and reintegrating them back into the community.

REVIEW QUESTIONS

1. A nurse plans a series of psychoeducational groups for persons with schizophrenia. Which topic would take priority?
   1. How to complete an application for employment
   2. The importance of taking your medication correctly
   3. The ways to dress and behave when attending community events
   4. How to give and receive compliments
2. A young adult is hospitalized with undifferentiated schizophrenia. The parents are distraught and filled with guilt. Which of the following would be an appropriate nursing response?
   1. "There are many theories about the cause of schizophrenia, but this illness is not your fault."
   2. "Does anyone in your family have mental illness? Schizophrenia is a genetically transmitted disease."
   3. "Look on the bright side. With the right medications and treatment, this disease can be cured."
   4. "I'll recommend some excellent Web sites with information about schizophrenia and other mental illnesses."
3. A person with disorganized schizophrenia participates in a rehabilitative outpatient program. Select the most appropriate initial outcome for this individual.
   1. The individual will identify environmental triggers that produce feelings of fear.
   2. The individual will have increased organization of thought patterns.

Murphy MC: The agitated, psychotic patient: guidelines to ensure staff and patient safety, *J Am Psychiatr Nurses Assoc* 8(Suppl 4):S2-S8, 2002.

National Institute of Mental Health: *Schizophrenia research at the National Institute of Mental Health, 2005* (website): www.nimh.nih.gov/publicat/schizresfact.cfm. Accessed April 5, 2006.

Reeves RR, Torres RA: Medical disorders among psychiatric patients, *Psychiatr Serv* 54:748, 2003.

Rogers CP: *Client-centered therapy,* Boston, 1951, Houghton Mifflin.

Sadock BJ, Sadock VA, Ruiz P: *Kaplan and Sadock's comprehensive textbook of psychiatry,* ed 9, Philadelphia, 2009, Lippincott Williams & Wilkins.

Schultz H et al: Schizophrenia: A Review. *Am Fam Physician* 75(12):1821-1829.

Selye H: *Stress of life,* ed 2, New York, 1978, McGraw-Hill.

Sullivan H: *The interpersonal theory of psychiatry,* New York, 1953, WW Norton. (classic)

Sullivan PF: The genetics of schizophrenia, *PLoS Medicine,* 2(7):e12, 2005. doi:10.1371/journal.pmed.00202212.

Swanson JW et al: Newer antipsychotics no better than older medications in reducing schizophrenia-related violence. *Science Update of the National Institutes of Mental Health,* 2008 (1 page).

Swartz MS et al: Substance use in persons with schizophrenia: baseline prevalence and correlates from the NIMH CATIE study, *Journal of Nerv Ment Dis* 194(3) 2006.

Thirthalli J, Benegal V: Psychosis among substance users, *Curr Opin Psychiatry* 19:239-249, 2006.

Online Resources
Mental Health America (NARSAD): www.nmha.org
NARSAD, the Brain and Behavior Research Fund: www.narsad.org
National Alliance on Mental Illness: www.nami.org
National Institute of Mental Health: www.nimh.nih.gov

TEACHING AND LEARNING PACKAGE

A complete ancillary package to enhance teaching and learning is provided for this text.

The **Evolve Learning Resources** that accompany the fifth edition of *Psychiatric Mental Health Nursing* are available for both students and instructors located at http://evolve.elsevier.com/Fortinash/.

STUDENT RESOURCES

Students will find valuable resources such as:

- Chapter outlines for in-class or independent note-taking
- Rationales for the case study critical thinking questions
- Expanded answers to the textbook end-of-chapter review
- Supplemental review questions
- A concept mapping tool
- A complete listing of psychiatric disorders in the DSM-IV-TR

INSTRUCTOR RESOURCES

In addition to the information available to students, instructors are able to access all of the components of the Instuctor's Resources on the Evolve site, which include the following, each corresponding to the 30 chapters of the textbook:

- An *Instructor's Manual* including a chapter focus, objectives and key terms, critical thinking exercises, and enrichment activities

- *ExamView Test Bank* with more than 800 questions (including alternate item formats) organized by chapter and including objective, nursing process step, cognitive level, NCLEX category of Client Need, correct answer, rationale, and text page reference
- *PowerPoint slide presentations*, with more than 400 text and illustration slides
- *Audience Response Questions*, in PowerPoint format for i>clicker and other systems, with multiple answer questinos designed to stimulate student discussion and survey understanding of key concepts.

A special thank you to the fifth edition Ancillary writers for their valuable time and expertise:

Ruth N. Grendell
Student Resources

Mary Blessing Gilkey
Instructor's Manual and PowerPoint slides

Linda Turchin
Test Bank

Kathleen Slyh
Test Bank Reviewer

Teresa Burckhalter
Audience Response Questions

CONTENTS

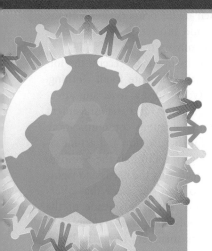

Psychiatric Nursing: Theory, Principles, and Trends

Patricia A. Holoday Worret

"The greatest wealth is health."

Virgil

evolve WEBSITE

http://evolve.elsevier.com/Fortinash/

OBJECTIVES

- List four fundamental objectives that guide psychiatric mental health nurses and their colleagues in the core mental health disciplines.
- Discuss the levels of prevention of mental disorders, and provide an example of each.
- Define *evidence-based practice* and its role in psychiatric mental health nursing.
- Discuss the importance of integrating patient care in the psychiatric setting.
- Describe the reasons for added national interest in the recovery phase of patient treatment.

- Name four main organizations that guide and govern nursing practice.
- State the benefits for the patient and the nurse that are derived from a therapeutic alliance.
- Explain why psychiatric diagnoses are necessary.
- Describe the outcomes of the social stigma of mental disorders.
- List the potential benefits for patients that result from the enactment of health care reform.

KEY TERMS

allopathic	incompetence	patient	sick role
best practice	inextricable	prevalence	stereotype
comorbid	integrated care	psychosis	stigma
evidence-based practice	intrinsic	relational	syndrome
extrinsic	neuroplasticity	resilience	therapeutic alliance
incidence	parity	risk and protective factors	

Psychiatric mental health nursing (PMHN) is one of five core mental health licensed disciplines designated by the U.S. Department of Health and Human Services to professionally serve the nation in the promotion of mental health, the prevention of mental disorders, the treatment of disorders, and the restoration of health. Licensed PMH nurses—in collaboration with other core mental health disciplines, psychiatry, psychology, psychiatric social work, and marriage and family therapy—recognize the fundamental fact that mental health is an integral part of total health. PMHN has traditionally held this conviction, which is now confirmed by empiric evidence and presented in multiple national and international health reports.

UNIVERSAL AGREEMENT

It is widely accepted and agreed upon in the United States and other developed nations that mental health is an inextricable or inseparable component of overall human health, welfare, and safety (New Freedom Commission, 2003;

National Institutes of Medicine, 2006). Quality of life, effective daily functioning, and overall perception of well-being are closely linked to sound mental health. The core PMH disciplines practice within this framework and are mindful of its principles and fundamental objectives during interactions.

FUNDAMENTAL OBJECTIVES

Standard objectives guide PMH nurses and members of related disciplines in the care of patients (individuals, families, communities, and organizations). The objectives and criteria are as follows:

(1) The promotion and protection of mental health
(2) The prevention of mental disorders
(3) The treatment of mental disorders
(4) Recovery and rehabilitation

Promotion and Protection

The first fundamental objective is the promotion and protection of mental health are primary functions within the health care system, but they are equally important in all systems. Health care provider involvement is essential to achieve intended outcomes, but often socioeconomic and cultural factors have a strong influence over the success or failure of this objective (USDHHS, 2010). The following activities are associated with the attainment of this goal:

- Disseminating information to increase public knowledge and awareness of mental health and mental disorders
- Ensuring access to health care
- Encouraging and providing support for individuals, families, communities, and organizations that value principles and activities that promote mental health
- Supporting organizations that assist others with meeting the many demands of daily living and that facilitate healthy socialization
- Providing ongoing education
- Providing mentoring
- Supporting patients with defining their personal life goals and in their efforts to achieve those goals
- Reducing the stigma associated with mental disorders

Nursing functions that have been identified as meeting these first-line objectives include but are not limited to initial and ongoing assessments; therapeutic communication; facilitating family, group, and community seminars; teaching; advocating; role modeling; mentoring; collaborating with patients and colleagues; and monitoring outcomes.

Sites for Health Promotion

PMH nurses promote and protect mental health in a wide variety of settings. Homes, schools, community agencies, and organizations are primary resources for educating young people and their families. Health promotion begins by learning about and living the importance of early life experiences, especially in the home. This is a major objective for mental health care providers everywhere. Nurses engage and interact with family members to provide assistance and support to strengthen intact homes, which are the primary sites with the potential for the promotion and protection of the mental health and well-being of the family unit.

Ideally, a home ensures that its members receive the following: physical sustenance, with adequate food, clothing, and shelter; safety and security; nurturing, love, and affection; consideration, attention, support, and encouragement for each member; clear and unambiguous communication; role modeling; opportunities for socialization and actualization; and instructions for navigating through the world to meet one's own needs while considering the needs and rights of others. Home is intended to be a safe place that offers respite from the daily problems that arise outside of the home. A healthy home is a school of life and an open, supportive laboratory for all of its members to learn, build, practice skills, and reap rewards. When families function effectively, demonstrate understanding, and meet their responsibilities to each other and to the world outside of their homes, everyone benefits directly and indirectly; this includes each member within the home and, ultimately, in the surrounding community and the world at large. Abraham Maslow expressed this clearly and succinctly when he diagramed a hierarchy of human needs; see the adapted diagram in Figure 1-1.

Promotion Inhibitors

Practicing PMH nurses learn the reality that some individuals, for a variety of reasons, fail to meet the standards of care that ensure healthy homes for their families. Sound mental health cannot flourish in neglectful or noxious environments in which one or more members are unable or unwilling to fulfill their roles. For example, when families live with a dominant member who has a persistent and severe mental disorder (e.g., ongoing substance abuse, paranoid schizophrenia, antisocial personality disorder) or when the family dynamic is dysfunctional (e.g., the ongoing mental, physical, emotional, or sexual abuse of any member), the outcomes are often expressed as disrupted homes, family members who are at increased risk for physical and mental illnesses or early deaths, or consequential legal or ethical problems that inevitably spill out into the community. In all cases, the earliest possible detection of and intervention with mental disorders is imperative.

Expanded Involvement

Although homes provide an initial basis for overall health or illness, it is agreed that more than the home must be involved in health promotion. Societal, economic, cultural and environmental factors also play a large part in the nation's health. Responsibility is broadened beyond the family and includes schools; places of employment, worship, recreation and entertainment; community agencies and organizations; plus governments and their agencies.

Additionally, our current media industry is a major influence on health in both positive and negative ways. That high profile giant has a responsibility for shaping and molding ideas about healthy living. The protection and promotion of

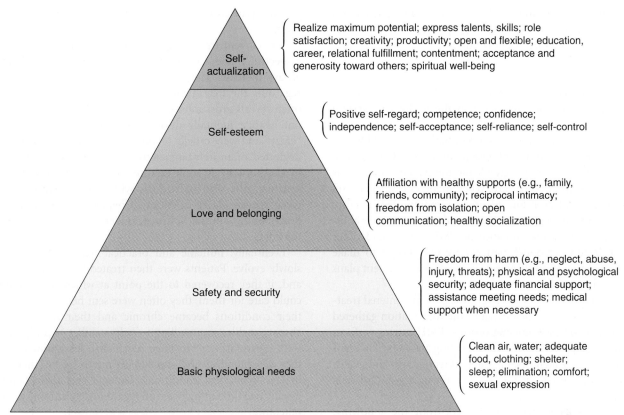

FIGURE 1-1. Maslow's hierarchy of needs. Basic human needs must be met before patients can begin to self-actualize. (Adapted in 2008.)

sound mental health is a multifocal, interrelated endeavor that also requires an active interest on the part of world health organizations.

Prevention

The second fundamental objective is the prevention of mental disorders and occurs on several levels.

Primary Prevention

Primary prevention helps to reduce the incidence (occurrence) of mental disorders. Proactive involvement by care providers is necessary. Initiating and staying involved, promoting awareness, and providing information are key PMHN activities at this stage. Examples include the following:

- Offering stress-reduction techniques and mindful meditation to high-risk adolescents in a program that promotes drug-free environments
- Teaching the normal stages of child development and effective parenting skills to high-risk single women who are pregnant for the first time
- Holding seminars for recently widowed and potentially isolated seniors to discuss strategies for accessing community resources and activities for staying physically, cognitively, and socially active and involved

Secondary Prevention

Secondary prevention helps to reduce the prevalence (existing number at a given time) of mental disorders. This type of prevention includes early identification and treatment to prevent increased disability. Examples include the following:

- Providing comfort and arranging for the safety of a child who comes to school with multiple bruises and cigarette burns on his or her body
- Interacting with a woman who was just admitted to the psychiatric intensive care unit because of her attempted suicide

Tertiary Prevention

Tertiary prevention objectives are twofold:

(1) To reduce the residual effects of a disorder
- Examples include organizing and facilitating an outpatient group of people who share the same diagnosis (e.g., young adults with schizophrenia) or the same situational problem (e.g., parents whose children have died; caregivers of patients with Alzheimer's disease) to offer support, to provide information and resources, or to evaluate members' progress or to monitor their medications

(2) To promote rehabilitation
- Examples include holding seminars for families to gain insight by learning more about a member's mental disorder and how to effectively interact with the member; learning about prescribed medications and how families help to monitor symptoms; learning skills to modify troublesome behaviors; teaching

interviewing and job skills to recovering patients; and arranging job fairs that align patients and industries for employment opportunities

Treatment

The third fundamental objective is the treatment of mental disorders. Treatment approaches in the health care system have undergone transformation during the past several decades and evolved into the current patient-centered health care model. The course of treatment is based on several factors, with a primary factor being the patient's intentions regarding his or her own care. When mental disorders occur, professional intervention is often required. Patients are central to the process that determines their care as their abilities allow. Under the guidance of PMH nurses and other mental health personnel, patients are encouraged to make decisions and to actively engage in their own treatment plans to meet their needs.

Several other factors determine the patient-centered treatment objectives and include all of the information gathered and used during the nursing process. PMH nurses perform the nursing process when first meeting patients; the steps of assessment, diagnosis, planning, intervention, and evaluation help to determine the best practice treatment for each patient.

Treatment objectives are derived from the following: patient assessment data gathered from all sources; the diagnosis (i.e., the type and severity of the disorder); current observable and reported symptoms and other responses; patient readiness and willingness to participate in treatment; available treatment resources and options; the cost of treatment; and the patient's capacity and ability to regain health and to take responsibility for the maintenance of wellness. Careful consideration is given to each person's unique personal characteristics and the expression of the condition or disorder as well as all relational aspects, situations, and circumstances. Specific treatment is tailored to and outlined for each individual.

Another patient-focused determinant of treatment is whether an episode is considered acute or chronic. Acute episodes and chronic disorders are managed and treated differently. When an acute episode occurs, hospitalization may be required for the alleviation and management of symptoms, the prescribing and monitoring of medications, the stabilization of the immediate condition, and the support or modification of current living situations. Chronic disorders may be treated in a wide variety of settings in the community, and they require the following: ongoing monitoring of the person's symptoms, medications, living conditions, and circumstances; collaboration with families and agencies; and advocating in the community. Detailed treatment options for all major psychiatric conditions are provided throughout this textbook.

Background. The philosopher George Santayana made a statement that is quoted in many circles: "Those who cannot remember the past are condemned to repeat it." It is of utmost importance to remember how mentally ill patients were

treated in the past so that these treatments are never repeated again.

The current treatment of psychiatric patients is humane, respectful, mandated, and monitored. However, this was not always the case. The review of several past eras in history regarding the treatment of those with psychiatric disorders often reveals gross inhumanities and exploitation. Throughout history, mentally disordered people were often called "crazy" and were cruelly tortured, manipulated, imprisoned, neglected, or entirely banned from the societies in which they lived. Alternatively, some cultures viewed mental disorders as spiritual gifts, and individuals with these conditions were given special places in society. Chapter 8 of this textbook describes the cultural, spiritual, and ethical aspects of mental disorders.

Eventually, humane and practical treatments began to slowly evolve. Patients were then treated for acute episodes, and, if they recovered to the point at which their families could care for them, they often were sent home. However, if their conditions became chronic and their families were absent, unable, or unwilling to help stabilize them, patients were invariably sent to huge psychiatric institutions where they were literally warehoused to live out the rest of their lives in less than ideal conditions. Patients and their families usually had little influence with regard to determining patient outcomes.

The discovery of psychotropic medications rapidly and completely changed the way that treatment was delivered. Beginning during the early 1960s, the majority of large long-term care psychiatric facilities called *mental institutions* were closed (i.e., deinstitutionalization). Very few of these chronic-care facilities remain open today. Some large prisons still house the mentally ill who have broken the law. Many do not respond to treatment (have intractable mental disorders) and cannot live in society.

During the past several decades, the primary site for the long-term treatment of mental disorders has shifted from the hospital to community outpatient settings. Hospitalization may be necessary for acute care, but, when patients are stabilized, they move into community-based, patient-centered settings or are discharged home with continued outpatient treatment in the community. Concentrated efforts are made to reduce the patient's sick role by providing opportunities for the development of a purposeful life and instilling hope for each patient's future.

Treatment Plan. Patients are encouraged to take responsibility for their own care. Patients' participation in their own care is a primary objective of all treatment plans. From their first meetings with patients and throughout the acute phases of treatment, nurses work collaboratively with the treatment team to involve patients, families, and others who will provide ongoing care after discharge. Together these individuals establish patient objectives that are directed toward learning skills and techniques that will assist patients to restore and maintain health.

Patients' Rights in Treatment. Within their capacities and abilities, patients are encouraged to make important decisions that affect their lives. Each patient's decisions about his or her care and his or her willingness to receive treatment are important considerations for care providers. However, sometimes a patient's symptoms are very severe and interfere with his or her ability to act on his or her own behalf.

A patient's health and safety may become jeopardized by his or her severely impaired judgment and result in the loss of a patient's right to make choices about treatment. Two examples illustrate this: (1) when a person is unable to cognitively process information or to make decisions about his or her own welfare as a result of mental incompetence or severe psychosis; and (2) when a person is so severely depressed that he or she is intent on committing suicide. At such times, it often becomes necessary to prescribe treatment that is contrary to the patient's will to preserve the patient's health, safety, and security until symptoms abate. In addition, if threats of violence toward the self or others become a factor, then the patient's rights are suspended to protect the family or the public and also to protect the patient from his or her own poor judgment and acting out of dangerous behaviors. Additional information about patient's rights in relation to mental disorders is found in Chapter 9 of this textbook.

During treatment, individual patients and their families benefit in many ways when they gain insight, form realistic expectations about their situations, and are able to maintain healthy optimism. PMH nurses, in collaboration with interprofessional teams, assist families with the achievement of these goals. A family member's realism often increases in direct proportion to his or her perception of the patient's condition and situation; level of knowledge; attitudes about the patient's disorder; and personal experiences with mental disorders. Time and the willing involvement of the patient and family members often result in successful outcomes. Support and guidance from skilled nurses and other health care professionals is often necessary as well.

Evidence-Based Practice

The current standard of practice for all health care institutions and health care providers is evidence-based practice (EBP), which includes the identification and application of empiric research evidence to solve clinical problems (Rice, 2008a). EBP is a departure from the therapist–patient interactions that are based on intuition or the repetition of interventions merely because they were always done that way before or because techniques were agreed upon and approved by experts or colleagues over decades of use (Melnyk, 2005; French, 2002). EBP requires a shift in thinking and in the approach to therapy as well as the commitment to make use of empirically supported interventions. EBP is the current goal for all disciplines and for the mental health care industry. Many facilities promote research studies in the interest of providing quality EBP for patients.

The transition to EBP in nursing is steadily growing as PMH nurses collaborate with other disciplines to identify and apply research evidence to clinical situations and problems when caring for patients. As evidence-based research is completed and specific interventions are identified, the resulting practice outcomes will be reflected in patient care and published in the literature (Rice, 2008b; Cohen, 2005).

Integrated Care: The Mind and the Body

The majority of health disciplines now recognize that mental disorders and physical illnesses are closely linked. The presence of a mental disorder increases the risk for the development of physical illnesses and vice versa (Weiss, 2009). The mind–body connection is undeniable. As a result of the prevalence of combined medical and behavioral or psychiatric problems, patients are often receiving integrated care as a preferred form of treatment.

Hippocrates (400-377 BC), who is often referred to as the "father of medicine," was one of the first to recognize and teach his followers that health depended on the harmony and balance of the mind, the body, and the environment. After that time, Cartesian mind–body dualism was popularized and flourished for centuries, thus forming the basis for modern Western (allopathic) medicine (Grendell, 2010). The emphasis shifted from treating the whole person. A clear dichotomy occurred between the diagnosis and treatment of physical diseases or ailments and the diagnosis and treatment of mental and emotional problems.

That belief shifted again and the pendulum has swung back to current thinking that links mind and body etiologies and approaches to treatment as health care providers from all disciplines become familiar with growing evidence that the mind and the body are not separable. After accepting the premise that mental health problems and mental disorders are often exacerbated by physical problems and that the opposite is also true, integrated care that addresses both the mental and physical aspects of any illness or disorder is found to be the most efficient and effective treatment method (Hine, 2008).

Nursing Implications. One of nursing's primary strengths lies in its long-held belief that every human, regardless of his or her diversity, is more than the sum of many parts and is instead a uniquely blended biologic, psychologic, social, and spiritual being who is deeply rooted in and influenced by culture and environment (Figure 1-2). Traditional nursing theory is based on a holistic view of each person as an integrated being. With this conceptual and theoretic background coupled with experience in the clinical setting, nurses find it natural to integrate patient care.

The application of these concepts to practice is necessary. In the psychiatric setting, the PMH nurse primarily focuses on psychiatric nursing and patient problems but integrates care by incorporating theory, principles, skills, and nursing practices from all areas of nursing. When nurses first enter a PMHN specialty and begin to work with patients in psychiatric settings, they may be distracted and need to remind themselves of the whole-person concept during assessment, treatment, and interactions with their patients. Distractions come in the form of both content and process in this setting.

Psychiatric content regarding mental disorders often seems fascinating when it is first encountered in textbooks and lectures. Interesting descriptions of symptoms and

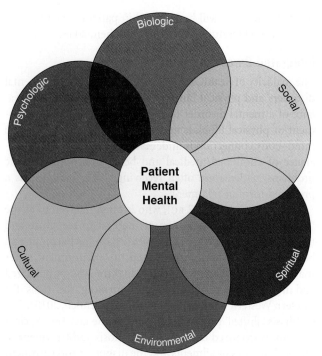

FIGURE 1-2. Comprehensive care model for psychiatric mental health nursing.

behaviors take on new importance and may eclipse previous information. In addition, when a nurse begins to practice in psychiatric clinical settings, actual patients' symptoms and responses to their disorders may seem dramatic and capture the nurse's attention. Nurses strive to associate actual patient responses with what they learned when reading, and, at the same time, they try to recall the best nursing practice interactions or interventions for the situation. Nurses often focus solely on the mental, emotional, and behavioral content as well as their own next best response. As a result, the patient's other problems slide into secondary position. Nurses and their mentors need patience during this transition. With time, increased familiarity with content, and adequate clinical experience, nurses are able to provide integrated care to their patients (Weiss, 2009).

The following two clinical examples help to illustrate nurses' responsibilities for integrating care in a clinical setting:

A 17-year-old girl is admitted to the psychiatric facility after she was found wandering in her neighborhood in the middle of the night. She is pregnant and close to term. She is also delusional, and she has superficially stabbed herself multiple times in the abdomen with a sharp stick. The nurse quickly determines that the patient's problems must be prioritized and treated and that several areas of nursing care are involved, including obstetrics, medical/surgical, and psychiatric.

A 78-year-old man who does not speak English is admitted to the senior unit. His wife died 2 weeks ago, and today he was found alone in his home depressed, disoriented, disheveled, and dehydrated. He wears a bracelet that shows that he has type 1 diabetes. His feet are bare, with multiple cuts, and two of his toes appear to be necrotic.

It becomes apparent from these examples that psychiatric nurses must be prepared to address several types of nursing care. The patients in these two vignettes require immediate medical attention and a variety of diagnostic tests in addition to psychiatric interventions that include health and safety issues plus caring and empathic responses. Educated and experienced nurses are well positioned and prepared to address and intervene effectively with these complex health problems and to provide integrated care.

In many medical centers and facilities, psychiatric patients are admitted to units on the basis of problems and diagnoses other than their psychiatric diagnoses (e.g., cardiology, neurology, obstetrics, orthopedics). Nurses who choose employment in these nursing specialties need to be prepared to integrate patient care when the admitted medical patient also exhibits a mental disorder.

Recovery and Rehabilitation

The fourth fundamental objective is patient recovery and rehabilitation. The recovery phase of health care is currently recognized as being very important for patients, their families, and the community. In the past, acute treatment phases consistently overshadowed the importance of recovery-oriented treatment. Care providers' time, effort, and resources plus payment for psychiatric services were primarily allocated to acute care. However, that approach was insufficient to prevent repeated and unnecessary episodes of symptom recurrence and subsequent hospitalizations.

Multiple "revolving door" episodes and their consequences were personally and painfully experienced by individual patients and their families, and they also took an economic toll on the budgets of treatment facilities and local, state, and federal agencies. Personal and financial costs were unnecessarily high. The trend shifted, which increased the focus of attention and resources on keeping patients out of the hospital.

The recovery and rehabilitation phase of mental health care is currently receiving necessary recognition, and it has become a model for the treatment of mental disorders and relapse prevention. For decades, reports from national mental health organizations cited insufficient funding for psychiatric patient treatment and rehabilitation, especially for the severely mentally ill. One program to address this issue is proposed by the Substance Abuse and Mental Health Services Administration (SAMHSA), a national organization within the U.S. Department of Health and Human Services.

This program, which is entitled "Illness Management and Recovery," facilitates and advocates for those who have mental illnesses (SAMHSA, 2009). It is designed to reintegrate patients into the community and to support them as they more actively participate in their own treatment. The program focuses on EBP, and it provides a set of strategies that enables patients to take responsibility for their care and that empowers them to become their own change agents as they learn to identify and define personal recovery goals.

PMH staff teaches strategies while supporting patients and families as they learn and use techniques to effectively manage and cope with their symptoms, stress, and the challenges of daily living; to strengthen their resilience (the ability to bounce back after stressful situations or events); and to collaborate with the mental health professionals who assist them with their recovery. Communicating with others, building social networks, and establishing a meaningful role and purpose in life are also important objectives for patients who are functioning within this model.

The emphasis is on symptom management, restoration, rehabilitation, a return to the pre-illness level of function or better, and reconnection with family, significant others, and the community. Patients aim for independence that enables them to live life more fully, to learn, to work, and to participate in their communities. They strive to reestablish meaningful, healthy, supportive relationships with the use of learned effective techniques to maintain these connections. The goal is to engage again in purposeful activities and meaningful social relationships.

PSYCHIATRIC MENTAL HEALTH NURSING TODAY

As a nationally designated health care discipline, PMHN plays a significant role in fulfilling the previously mentioned objectives in the interest of promoting mental health, preventing and treating mental disorders, and facilitating the restoration of health in the nation. The role of the professional psychiatric nurse is guided, determined, and governed at national, state, and local levels.

In their publication about the scope and standards of practice of psychiatric nursing, the American Nurses Association—in collaboration with the International Society of Psychiatric Mental Health Nurses, the American Psychiatric Nurses Association, and other colleagues—describes PMHN as follows:

"… a specialized area of nursing practice committed to promoting mental health through the assessment, diagnosis, and treatment of human responses to mental health problems and psychiatric disorders. Psychiatric mental health nursing, as a core mental health profession, employs a purposeful use of self as its art, and a wide variety of nursing, psychosocial, and neurobiological theories and research evidence as its science." (American Nurses Association, 2008)

The role of the nurse is described in conjunction with current issues, trends, and the responsibilities for which professional nurses are accountable at defined levels of practice. The American Nurses Association provides certification for registered nurses at both the entry level (i.e., the RN-PMH, which requires a bachelor's degree) and advanced levels of education and practice (i.e., the APRN-PMH requires a master's or doctoral degree). Certification recognizes and validates the nurse's competence, which is derived from the completion of specified levels of education and is achieved with additional advanced clinical experience and the mastery of practice complexities. PMH nurses select from careers that focus on clinical practice, education, research, administration, or a combination of those roles.

Each state in the country determines nursing titles (these vary by state) and mandates in their individual state practice acts the nurses' functions and limitations of function. Licensing for nurses is achieved by passing an individual state's licensure examinations. Additional factors that guide and govern nursing practice include the extent of education, nurses' professional code of ethics (American Nurses Association, 2001), and the position description and other standards and limitations set by the employer or the practice setting.

Current Issues and Trends

The Recovery Initiative. On the forefront of nursing and all other areas of the health care delivery system is the position of the patient (individual, family, community) at the center of care. In response to the final report of the President's New Freedom Commission on Mental Health, the American Psychiatric Nurses Association and four other national organizations from various psychiatric disciplines were selected in 2010 to participate in a SAMHSA project to address the continuing transformation of recovery practice. The overall goal of this initiative is to improve both access to care and the quality of mental health services (American Psychiatric Nurses Association, 2010).

Nowhere is a recovery-based treatment plan more important than in psychiatric and community settings, where patients are encouraged to and assisted with taking a meaningful, active role in their own care (SAMHSA, 2005). PMH nurses and other care providers will continue to include individual patients and significant others in all aspects of their care, including taking responsibility for decision-making, engaging in their own treatment plans and interventions, completing collaborative evaluations, and setting long-term goals under the guidance of the interdisciplinary team.

In this person-centered model of recovery, patients are no longer passive recipients of treatment that renders people helpless and unable to duplicate necessary behaviors when they are released from the direct care of the nurse, the physician, or the facility. Independence within the patient's capacity is a valuable characteristic to encourage. Patient recovery is faster and more effective when the team includes the patient. PMH nurses are and will be a major force for this program's success.

Nursing and Evidence-Based Practice. "The movement of psychiatric nursing from traditional practices and expert opinions to evidence based practice (EBP) is driven by the most cost effective and efficacious treatment" (Rice, 2008b). As discussed previously and as described throughout this text, PMHN joins in the continued transformation of clinical practice that is based on empiric outcomes.

Other Salient Issues

- Funding for necessary implementations and changes remains of special interest to nurses and all others involved in the transformational process of the mental health care delivery system.
- Safety issues in psychiatric treatment centers—particularly the use of patient restraints and the necessity of effective nurse–patient ratios—remains a high priority and an ongoing issue for PMHN and the entire industry.
- Quality-of-care issues and access to health care for minority populations continue to be issues.
- The social stigma related to mental disorders and its devastating outcomes for patients and families remain constant issues for PMH nurses at all levels as well as for their colleagues from all mental health professions.
- The standardization of advanced practice nurse roles needs to be addressed; currently, the scopes of practice of these nurses vary widely from state to state.

THE ART AND SCIENCE OF PMHN

Nursing is both an art and a science. It is derived from a broad-based educational foundation, with an added emphasis on the nursing curriculum and its specialties. PMHN is a specialized area of practice that further makes use of a wide range of theories and research regarding human behavior as its science and the purposeful use of the self as its art. The knowledge base and the application of skills in this discipline focus on mental health issues, problems, and disorders.

The science of nursing serves as a foundation and ensures patients' health and safety. Both the patient and the nurse rely on the nurse's mastery of all of the science-based aspects of the profession. The science of nursing is also evidenced in the nursing process. This reliable, long-standing, problem-solving method organizes information and provides guidelines and a framework for delivering nursing care to patients in any setting. The six-step nursing process (i.e., assessment, diagnosis, outcome identification, planning, intervention, and evaluation) is based on the scientific method of problem solving, but it has its own distinctive language and unifying themes. Nurses routinely use the nursing process during all interactions with patients. The nursing process is described in depth in Chapter 3 of this book.

Although the mastery of science is crucial in nursing, the importance of the art of PMHN cannot be overemphasized. A primary aspect of working with patients in any setting and particularly in the psychiatric setting is the development of a therapeutic alliance with the patient. Such an alliance is established on trust. It is a professional bond between the nurse and the patient that serves as a vehicle for patients to freely discuss their needs and problems in the absence of the nurse's criticism or judgment. The relationship that is formed between the nurse and the patient is not to be confused with an ordinary friendship; rather, it is based on certain principles, and it is a valuable tool as patients engage in the process of healing. The therapeutic alliance is described and discussed in several chapters of this book.

MENTAL HEALTH AND MENTAL DISORDER

Mentally healthy people are prone to recover relatively quickly from illnesses, thus making it important for nurses to identify, reinforce, support, and promote health when interacting and working with patients. Conversely, mental disorders interfere with overall health (Kessler, 2005). People who have these disorders are more vulnerable and have a greater incidence of other diseases and earlier deaths (National Council for Community Behavioral Health Care, recovered 6/20/10). The early recognition of symptoms and early treatment of mental disorders is a primary objective.

It is necessary for psychiatric nurses as well as the nurses who work with patients in any specialty area to be skilled at discerning healthy responses from disordered ones. Symptoms that are associated with mental disorders may manifest and be demonstrated in any type of setting, including homes, schools, workplaces, neighborhoods, public places, hospitals (all units), clinics, places of worship, organizational meetings, battlefields, and correctional facilities, to name but a few. For the benefit of both their patients and themselves, nurses must be prepared by being able to identify symptoms of mental disorders when they occur and then to intervene. Such skills begin with a knowledge base related to mental health and disorders.

Attempts to define *mental health* and *mental disorder* in simple terms fall short of the depth and breadth of the meanings of both terms. Various definitions and descriptions are available from multiple reliable sources, but no single definition of either term is considered to be official.

Mental Health

It is often written that mental health is more than the absence of mental illness. This statement is true, but it only begins to address this complex subject. An encompassing attempt to identify or explain ideal mental health might be that healthy individuals live productive, creative, and satisfying lives; experience relatively low internal and external stress; are cognitively, emotionally, physically, and behaviorally stable; have realistic perceptions, ordered thought patterns, and feelings of overall well-being; are able to function autonomously and in harmonious relationships with others; and maintain the capacity, abilities, and motivation to meet life's daily needs, demands, inevitable changes, and challenges. Any expectation for "ideal" mental health is somewhat unrealistic, but this description begins to explain mental health and subsumes multiple factors that must be intact and in play for a person to experience the fulfillment of this objective.

Factors and Indicators

Several indicators of mental health are illustrated in Box 1-1, and Box 1-2 lists factors that may influence mental health or mental disorder. Note that some of the factors and indicators in Boxes 1-1 and 1-2 are considered to be intrinsic (internal

---

BOX 1-1   INDICATORS OF MENTAL HEALTH

Intact anatomy and physiology of the brain and central nervous system

Absence of signs and symptoms of mental disorder

Freedom from excessive mental and emotional disability and pain

Demonstrates mental and physical competence and skills

Perceives self, others, and events correctly and realistically

Recognizes own strengths, weaknesses, capabilities, and limitations

Separates fantasy from reality

Thinks clearly

    Solves problems

    Uses good judgment

    Reasons logically

    Reaches insightful conclusions

Negotiates each developmental stage

Attains and maintains a positive self-system

    Self-concept

    Self-image

    Self-esteem

Accepts self and others as uniquely different but humanly similar

Appreciates life

Finds beauty, joy, and goodness in self, others, and the environment

Is creative

Is optimistic but realistic

Is resilient

Is autonomous

Uses talents to the fullest

Involves self in purposeful and meaningful life work

Engages in play

Develops and demonstrates an appropriate sense of humor

Expresses emotions

Exhibits congruent thoughts, feelings, and behaviors

Accepts responsibility for actions

Controls impulses and behavior

Is accountable for own behaviors

Respects societal rules and sanctions

Learns from experiences

Maintains wholesome values and belief system

Copes with internal and external stressors in constructive and adaptive ways

Returns to usual or higher function after crises

Delays gratification

Functions independently

Maintains reasonable expectations of self and others

Adapts to social environment

Relates to others

    Forms relationships

    Maintains close, meaningful, loving, and adaptive relationships

    Works and plays well with others

    Is appropriately and selectively intimate

    Responds to others in need

    Feels and exhibits compassion and empathy toward others

    Demonstrates culturally and socially acceptable interpersonal interactions

    Manages interpersonal conflict constructively

    Gives and receives gracefully

    Learns from and teaches others

    Functions interdependently

Seeks self-actualization

Attains self-defined spirituality

BOX 1-2   INFLUENCING FACTORS FOR MENTAL HEALTH OR DISORDER

Inherited factors (i.e., genetic or familial)

    Predisposition

    Capacities

    Limitations

Pregnancy environment and experience, from conception to birth

Psychoneuroimmunologic factors

Biochemical influences

Hormonal influences

Family

    Composition

    Birth position

    Bonding

    Members' mental health

Developmental events

    Completion of clearly defined stages

    Resolution of developmental crises

Cultures

Subcultures

Values

Belief systems

Perception of self

Cognitive abilities

    Capacity

Volition

Personality traits and states

    Competence

    Resilience

    Motivation

Goals and aspirations

Worldview

Internal stressors

External stressors

Support system

    Choice

    Availability

    Quality

Demographic factors

Geographic location

Health practices and beliefs

Spirituality or religion

Negative influences

    Internal and external

    Mental disorders

    Crime

    Drugs

    Psychosocial stressors

    Poverty

or intrapersonal; or occurring within the individual), whereas other factors and indicators are extrinsic (external or interpersonal) and refer to influences that exist or occur outside of the individual. Interpersonal factors are said to be relational, which refers to a person's relationships with others and the environment. Identifying these internal and external factors and influences is a helpful step as nurses assess and treat their patients.

These lists provide a beginning framework for thoughtful consideration about the meaning of mental health. Nurses begin to identify the presence or absence of these factors, characteristics, and influences in their patients and in their patients' lives and are able to assess unique manifestations and expressions of mental health. These lists are meant to stimulate thinking about the multiple factors related to mental health. They are a starting point that leads to the more thorough knowledge and understanding gained by nurses when they interact with patients and their families.

Risk Factors and Protective Factors

Risk factors are internal predisposing characteristics and external influences that increase a person's vulnerability and potential for developing mental disorders. Types of risk factors and examples include the following:

- Biologic (i.e., genetic predisposition for a specific disorder; age; gender)
- Psychologic (i.e., a mentally disordered family member in the home; difficult personality style; pessimistic or suspicious worldview; negative attitudes; lower level of intelligence; threatening belief systems)
- Sociocultural (i.e., absence of parents; abusive or neglectful home; poverty; inadequate social skills; rejection by ethnic or religious group; punitive gangs; school bullies)
- Environmental (i.e., exposure to toxins, illegal drugs, or pollution)

Some risk factors are fixed and unchanging, whereas others may change over time to positively or negatively influence mental health. Protective factors are characteristics that guard against risks and that may decrease an individual's potential for developing the risk for mental disorders. They are either internal or external.

Some examples of internal protective factors are resilience; good overall health; high stress tolerance; average or higher intelligence; optimism; high motivation; competence in several areas; flexibility; healthy curiosity and interest in life; and useful skills.

Examples of external protective factors include healthy, skilled, and caring parents, family, and friends; supportive teachers, bosses, cultures, and subcultures; sufficient income; and available and appropriate resources, recreation, and hobbies.

Altered factors may influence patient responses and affect the outcome toward mental health or mental disorder. Lives of individuals, their families, and their communities are all affected by the emergence or recurrence of mental disorder.

MENTAL DISORDER

Not all mental, emotional, or behavioral disturbances are mental disorders. People who experience great losses (e.g., the death or disappearance of a loved one, divorce), traumatic crises, and other events (e.g., war, hurricane, earthquake, rape) may demonstrate dramatic withdrawal or explosive acting out behaviors that are determined to be normal responses. Nurses and other health professionals learn these distinctions and respond with certain principles in mind.

The term *mental disorder* defies simple definitions. A mental disorder is identified by the patient's responses to the disorder, and manifestations are specific for each disorder. One symptom or trait alone is not considered a disorder. Rather, a syndrome (a cluster of symptoms) that express impaired perception, cognition, mood, affect, behavior, or a combination of these must be present. The syndrome may cause distress to the individual in some cases, and this distress varies with the type of disorder. The person's ability to function and their relationships are usually impaired at some level. Symptoms vary depending on the type of disorder, and more than one disorder may occur at the same time (comorbid).

Acute episodes that signal the emergence or recurrence of a mental disorder usually occur rapidly, are intense, and have a relatively brief course (e.g., brief reactive psychosis). There also may be acute episodes of a chronic disorder (e.g., an acute psychotic episode in an individual with paranoid schizophrenia). Chronic mental disorders are marked by symptoms that remain more constant, and the course is longer in duration (e.g., autism, disorganized schizophrenia, Alzheimer's disorder). Symptoms of both acute episodes and chronic conditions are also considered on a continuum from mild to moderate to severe.

Mental disorders are sometimes referred to as "mental illness." There were times when that term was strongly contested as a result of theoretic and conceptual differences regarding the etiology (the source or origin) of mental disorders. Patients, families, students of psychiatric nursing, and others want to know what causes the symptoms that they witness during disruptive episodes of mental disorders.

The Etiology Argument

At the turn of the twentieth century, psychiatrists trained in Western medicine were almost solely responsible for diagnosing and managing the treatment of what was called mental illness. As medical doctors, they determined that the etiology for mental disorders was biologic. Theoretic polarization occurred over the next several decades as biologic theories were challenged by nonmedical theoreticians and practitioners (e.g., psychologists and other proponents of psychosocial and behavioral interventions). These individuals stated and wrote that biology was not the sole cause of mental disorders and that other causes must be considered.

It was simultaneously noted that funding for biologic research and treatment had not significantly reduced the actual numbers of individuals reported to have mental disorders. As a result of these outcomes, other approaches to treatment were supported in the effort to reduce the incidence and prevalence of mental disorders. Many new theories in psychology and its many subsets, sociology, and other fields emerged throughout the 20th century and were supported by research studies. Papers, journals, and books were presented and published, and schools sprung up on university and college campuses to teach the new theories and treatment approaches for mental disorders. However, despite these efforts and new approaches to treatment, it became disappointing to find that the numbers of mentally disordered individuals remained fairly constant.

At the turn of the 21st century, the impetus toward brain-based, neuroscientific research burgeoned again. In July 2000, a presidential proclamation was the impetus for the National Institutes of Mental Health and other agencies to establish the Project on the Decade of the Brain. The entire first decade of the century was designated "The Decade of The Brain" (www.loc.gov/loc/brain/. Accessed June 15, 2010). An explosion of research and information occurred, and more was learned about brain biology during that decade than during the entire time that preceded it. That window of time became a conduit for an ongoing stream of information that still continues to reveal the brain as an incredible human organ, as well as for the emergence of innovative neuroscientific technologies that are now being used in this field.

Multiple discoveries began to blur the polarization of etiologic theories that existed between biomedical and nonmedical theoreticians and practitioners. Research findings not only increased knowledge about the brain's complexities but also served to calm the age-old argument of nature (i.e., a person's biologic makeup) versus nurture (i.e., all other influences) by demonstrating how the environment influences neurobiologic expression (i.e., the effects of an individual's environment on gene expression and the neuroplasticity of the brain).

To conclude, most researchers and professional organizations currently agree that mental disorders result from a combination of multiple sources that invariably include neurobiologic elements (e.g., genetics, neurotransmitter activity) as well as psychologic, social, cultural, and other environmental factors that are uniquely aligned and that converge uniquely in each individual. Several chapters about mental disorders within this textbook offer detailed and scientifically researched descriptions of theories regarding the etiology of mental disorders.

Statistics for Mental Disorders

Despite the illuminating research about this subject and all of the information that is now available, current statistics reveal that the number of people with mental disorders remains fairly constant in the United States and throughout the world (Kessler, 2005). Approximately 26% of the adult population (i.e., 1 in 4 adults 18 years old or older) currently has a diagnosable mental disorder during any given year. Of that group, the seriously mentally ill comprise approximately

6%. The prevalence of mental disorders is widespread throughout the entire population (Figure 1-3).

In the United States, Canada, and Western Europe, mental disorders are the leading cause of disability (World Health Organization, 2004). Nearly half of those who are diagnosed with mental disorders also have two or more disorders (Kessler, 2005). Depression is the most prevalent psychiatric disorder. All together, mental disorders take a huge toll both in the United States and worldwide.

Great efforts are made to help people with mental disorders and their families. Hope-inspiring research continually evolves into the identification and development of new treatments for subsequent use by patients. When it comes to caring for these patients, there is an abundance of educated, empathic, benevolent individuals with positive intentions. Often the missing component in patient care is adequate funding, which may be earmarked for other economic and political priorities.

Classification of Mental Disorders

Mental disorders continue to occur in all areas of the world and require identification and diagnosis before treatment begins. To facilitate this process, standardized diagnostic classifications have been developed and are widely used by mental health practitioners of all disciplines in the United States and beyond. The diagnostic manuals describe specific symptoms to identify each mental disorder, and they are seen by some as valuable tools for that reason. Alternatively, some clinicians think that these diagnoses are based on description only, which allows room for subjective errors. Disagreement is inherent in diagnosis methodology as a result of differing philosophies, but the existence of these manuals that specify diagnoses provides for a workable classification.

Two classifications, *The Diagnostic and Statistical Manual of Mental Disorders* (DSM-IV-TR; American Psychiatric

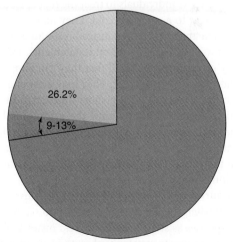

FIGURE 1-3. Approximately 26.2% of the adult population of the United States has a diagnosable mental disorder; 9% to 13% of the those are seriously mentally ill (SMI). (From Kessler R et al: Prevalence, severity, comorbidity of 12 month DSM-IV disorders in the National Comorbidity Survey Replication (NCS-R), *Arch Gen Psychiatry* 62(6):617-627, 2005.)

Association, 2000) and *The International Classification of Diseases* (ICD-10; World Health Organization, 1992) list categories for all mental disorders and include each diagnosis with its symptoms. Both manuals are widely used in psychiatric facilities and other settings. This textbook's companion Evolve website offers the DSM-IV-TR list of diagnoses and their categories in its Appendix.

The DSM is currently in revisions for its fifth edition with a planned publication date of 2013. Psychiatric diagnoses in these textbooks have been fairly consistent to this point, which may change in 2013. The DSM writers continue to carefully consider several changes.

At this writing, the plan for the DSM calls for some diagnoses to be renamed (e.g., "mental retardation" will be changed to "intellectual disability"; "substance abuse and dependence disorders" will be changed to "addiction and related disorders"). Some diagnoses that do not appear in the current edition will be added (e.g., gambling disorder, binge-eating disorder). The plan specifies a combination of other diagnoses for a reduction in the total number of diagnoses that will appear (e.g., all four autism disorders will become autism spectrum disorders). Some categories will be eliminated, and, for the first time, a category may be created for relational diagnoses (American Psychiatric Association, 2010).

Patient Diagnoses and Nursing

Regardless of the cause or course of a mental disorder, the first time that one is diagnosed is often frightening, and it can be devastating for the individual and the family, especially when the diagnosis is one that runs a chronic course. Nurses are prepared to respond to this situation.

Because they may be scared, anxious, and feeling overwhelmed, patients and their families are frequently in denial about the actual impact that some disorders will have on their lives, especially disorders that have a chronic course. It is common for these individuals to treat the first episode or two as if it is similar to a common cold. They may refuse to hear and assimilate the message and instead respond by overreacting with unrealistic optimism and statements about *cures*. They may go online to learn all that they can about the disorder and then try to self-treat. They may even engage in all the prescribed treatments for a short time, attending therapies and taking medications until the symptoms begin to clear, but then they stop, and symptoms return. This cycle may continue until patients allow themselves to realistically appraise the actual condition and situation and then begin making long-range plans, one step at a time.

PMH nurses remain patient and guard against their own frustration when this happens. They learn to see patient and family responses as steps toward progress instead of failures, and they remember to stay focused on the patient and family needs. Nurses' role modeling of patience is valuable for families who will return home with their family members.

The patient and family frequently become discouraged because of the many disruptions that mental, emotional, and behavioral episodes cause in their lives. Nurses remain hopeful and use all opportunities to instill hope and to support a more optimistic yet realistic outlook. Nurses help patients to realize that they are not defined by their diagnoses; that they do indeed have mental disorders but that these conditions are always treatable although they may not be curable; and that new treatments and interventions are constantly being developed.

Nurses remain realistic at all times, but they show empathy and understanding when interacting with patients. They avoid giving false reassurances to soothe patients. Reassurances that cannot be realized are major obstacles for a patient's journey to wellness and only serve to stall their progress. Nurses' realism stems from the reasons that diagnoses are necessary. Box 1-3 illustrates the purposes of diagnoses.

BOX 1-3   PURPOSES OF DIAGNOSES

Communication: Diagnoses define disorders and the manifestations that accompany them. Naming a diagnosis facilitates communication and avoids unnecessary repetitive explanations of diagnosis-specific symptoms.

Treatment: Diagnoses direct treatment approaches and guide staff to interact and intervene accordingly. For example, the treatment plan and approach for a depressed, withdrawn patient who is threatening suicide will be different from that for a patient who is admitted for drug-induced hallucinations.

Prognosis: A diagnosis often carries an initial prognosis. For example, paranoid schizophrenia has a long-term chronic prognosis, whereas adjustment disorders have a more favorable prognosis. The outcome from any diagnosis may change or vary with time and circumstances, but prognoses are guides that direct the delivery of care.

Funding: Diagnostic criteria dictate payment for treatments and services in the health care setting. In addition, the allocation of research funds in both the public and private sectors is designated for specifically named diagnoses.

Social Stigma

Few things rival the pain caused by social stigma in the lives of patients and their families. Patients with chronic mental disorders often suffer deeply from stigma, which, in this respect, is defined as a mark of disgrace or the shame of mental illness. The public who may be uneducated about or unaware of the true nature of mental disorders frequently react as a result of negative connotations of the term *mental illness.* People act out of fear or concern for their own safety when they hear the term. Most patients with mental disorders are nonviolent, but the public does not know that because of common misconceptions or beliefs in myths about people who are thought to be "crazy." In addition, there is constant bombardment by films, television, and other forms of media that portray the mentally ill as people to be feared, used, or ignored (Benbow, 2007). As a result, mentally disordered individuals who are already compromised by their symptoms are also forced to experience painful exclusion, rejection, alienation, overt and covert ridicule, exploitation, and sometimes even violence. They receive labels, and they become victims of bias and negative stereotypes.

Stigma is a definite obstacle on their road to recovery. It creates barriers to community integration and for accessing basic necessities such as safe housing and employment (Perese, 2007). Patients may be temporarily sheltered from stigmatizing societal gestures and behaviors when they are hospitalized for acute episodes of their disorder, but they often need assistance when they are discharged. PMH nurses are instrumental as advocates for reducing stigma and discrimination against patients and their families by working directly with patients, especially in community mental health treatment centers. These nurses also provide assistance by being involved in organizations that advocate for change. Psychiatric nursing organizations continually act on behalf of this cause at local and national levels in support of the humane treatment of the mentally ill.

Another major advocate for the reduction of stigma is the National Alliance on Mental Illness (NAMI). This organization and several others continually work an all levels, lobbying for legislative changes that will increase the respect and acceptance of patients and that will ensure that the practical needs of this population are met. The Alliance and members of other associations provide families and the public with educational materials to increase awareness of these problems. It is most important for nurses and other advocates to stay connected with patients, to teach and encourage the use of skills, to support successes, and to encourage families to be involved in patient care and to help patients to be responsible for their lives.

GLOBAL MENTAL HEALTH AND DISORDERS

Mental health status is monitored throughout the world by the World Health Organization and its several partners that track and report diseases and disorders due to all causes in all countries. The Organization's *Global Burden of Disease* report is a comprehensive statistical assessment of the health of the world population. It provides information about mortality, disability, and loss of health among people of all ages and from all causes. Mental disorders are common and occur in all nations. At the turn of the century, the *Global Burden of Disease* report stated that neuropsychiatric disorders would increase significantly during the next two decades.

Unipolar depression was predicted to rank second among all other noninfectious health-related causes by the year 2020. However, some sources say that major depression is already a leading cause of disability in 2010 (WHO, 2004). The *Global Burden of Disease* report that was updated in 2004 demonstrated a significant increase in substance use disorders as a major factor in worldwide disability, disease, disorder, and death. Several other neuropsychiatric disorders are also cited in these reports. The burden of mental disorders is significant in terms of human suffering in addition to taking economic and social tolls, which are illustrated in part by the following categories:

Human suffering: There is an alarmingly high annual loss of life from suicide and other injuries as a result of mental disorders all over the world. In addition, there is loss of purpose for living, a lack of any enjoyment of life, and the loss of support from family members and friends who no longer can live with the problems caused by these disorders. In other words, the consequences of one person's disorder are experienced by many.

Economic costs: Treatment costs may reach catastrophic amounts for some families. Wages are lost and productivity is decreased as a result of the patient's inability to work. A downward spiral leads to poverty and results in the patient's inability to contribute money, time, or talents back to society because of the limitations of the disorder.

Social costs: Homelessness, unemployment, poverty, welfare, incarceration, and degradation from limited choices for employment may lead to drug involvement or prostitution.

MENTAL HEALTH CARE REFORM

Standards of care for psychiatric patients in the United States are generally high as compared with those other nations, but access to care and funding remain persistent issues in PMH health care. Patients, families, organizations, communities, and practitioners share the frustration when required treatments and services fail to meet or match health care needs. According to some reports, fewer than half of the adults who require treatment and fewer than one third of the children who need it actually receive it (President's New Freedom Commission on Mental Health, 2003). These statistics remain constant across time.

National health care reform laws were recently passed with provisions to increase services and treatment for the underserved. March 30, 2010, marked a potential major milestone for mental health care and other areas of health care. The Patient Protection and Affordable Care Act became law, and it was followed a few days later by The Health Care and Education Reconciliation Act. Together these two laws definitively address several issues related to mental health, and they clearly state that mental health is an "essential health benefit" for all. Current health care reform is very controversial, but if important items stand as written, this legislation will provide improved access to previously unavailable health care for many underserved patients, individuals, families, and communities. For more information, see www.opencongress.org/bill/111-h3590/text and www.opencongress.org/bill/111-h4872/text. Patients, PMH professionals, and other mental health care advocates eagerly anticipate the changes that would address these issues.

The plan calls for specific items within the law to be activated over several years. Because of strong political differences regarding the operating costs for implementing these health laws, many revisions are expected before the provisions are finally in place. Four significant benefits for psychiatric patients are addressed in the current health care reform plans:

- There will be inclusion of care for patients who are diagnosed with psychiatric disorders, substance use disorders, or both; currently not all diagnoses are covered.
- Care cannot be refused to patients with preexisting mental health conditions or disorders. Currently many patients are refused insurance if they have been diagnosed with mental disorders.
- Increased funding will be provided to grow the current number of community mental health care centers. Numerous community centers will have to be established to meet the needs of patients who may be treated only a few days in a mental health care facility before being discharged.
- Parity will be in place for mental health and substance use disorder diagnoses. The term *parity* as used here refers to payments for mental health services that equal payment schedules for medical or surgical conditions. Parity for mental health diagnoses was previously written into law, but it was often bypassed through legal loopholes, which resulted in many psychiatric patients not having access to care.

Several items within the health care reform laws are not scheduled to take effect until 2014, leaving room for modification or denial of some provisions; however, as they stand, these laws offer long awaited hope for mental health patients and their families who often are left untreated or underserved in the current health care system.

The impact that these changes will have on nursing and other mental health professions remains to be seen. The Institutes of Medicine (IOM) issued a report in October, 2010, on the Future of Nursing. The report, prepared by the Robert Wood Johnson Foundation Initiative states that nursing is the largest segment of the health care work force and, as such, will be instrumental in meeting the demands of the new health care reform laws. To accomplish this, it is recommended that nursing expand its scope of practice in the following ways: (1) nurses will practice to "the full extent of their education and training"; (2) seek and achieve higher levels of education in improved systems; (3) partner fully with physicians and other health care professionals to redesign health care where needed; and (4) function within effective information infrastructures and data collecting processes (IOM, 2010). This is a hopeful and challenging time for nurses.

CHAPTER SUMMARY

- PMHN is a nationally designated core discipline that has been assigned to provide mental health care and to monitor the nation's mental health. PMHN engages actively in fulfilling the fundamental objectives of promoting mental health, preventing and treating mental disorders, supporting recovery, and restoring health. Every person's quality of life is based on sound mental health.
- The role of the PMH nurse is determined at local, state, and national levels. Among current issues and trends in psychiatric nursing are the recovery initiative; the growing influence of EBP in nursing; safety issues for patients and nurses in the psychiatric setting; and long-standing issues of social stigma and its outcomes. PMHN is an art and a science that involves the use of principles and theories from many sources. Nurses engage with patients to establish and use the therapeutic alliance, which is a valuable tool in total patient care.

- Mental health and disorders are thoroughly described in addition to the need for diagnoses and their classifications. Global mental health and the burden of psychiatric disorders take an enormous personal and economic toll. National health care reform laws were passed in 2010, and implementation will occur over several years. Nurses' active participation in the demands of health care reform will be significant in the coming decade.

REVIEW QUESTIONS

1. Which activity of the core PMH disciplines is considered to be the most important for national mental health care?
   1. The promotion and protection of mental health
   2. The prevention and treatment of mental disorders
   3. Recovery and rehabilitation
   4. All of the above
2. Select the statement that best describes the successful treatment of mental disorders in the United States.
   1. Treatment outcomes were most successful when they focused on biologic interventions.
   2. The treatment of mental disorders has greatly improved during the 21st century, and this is reflected in the reduction of the number of mental disorders.
   3. Statistics regarding the prevalence of mental disorders in the United States remain static.

4. The combination of medications with interactive and biologic therapies has been the most successful for reducing the prevalence of mental disorders.
3. Which of the following scenarios identifies a mental disorder?
   1. A 67-year-old woman says that she has not spent one day without crying several hours a day since her husband died last month.
   2. A mother says that her 15-year-old child spends all of his spare hours in his room with the computer and even misses meals.
   3. A 19-year-old man begins to hear voices that no one else hears during lectures in his college math course.
   4. All of the above

REVIEW QUESTIONS—cont'd

4. Risk factors for the development of physical and mental disorders include which of the following?
   1. A parent who gets drunk every night after work and says that it is relaxing
   2. A school in which students either ignore or bully the new students
   3. A higher-than-average intelligence level and many satisfying hobbies
   4. A large circle of friends who play sports together

5. Which of the following statements about PMHN are true?
   1. Nurses may be certified in their specialty at the entry level or at the advanced practice level.
   2. The art of PMHN is more important than the science of nursing.
   3. Integrated care is reserved for psychiatrists and is not for nurses.
   4. None of the above

REFERENCES

American Nurses Association: *Code of ethics for nurses with interpretive statements*, Washington, DC, 2001, American Nurses Association Publishing.

American Nurses Association: *Psychiatric mental health nursing: scope and standards of practice*, Silver Spring, Md, 2008, American Nurses Association Publishing.

American Psychiatric Association: *Diagnostic and statistical manual of mental disorders*, ed 4, text revision, Washington, DC, 2000, American Psychiatric Association.

Benbow A: Mental illness, stigma, and the media, *J Clin Psychiatry* 68(Suppl 2):31-35, 2007.

Cohen A: A collaborative approach to primary mental health care, *Primary Care Mental Health* (3):3-4, 2005.

French P: What is the evidence on evidence based nursing? An epistemological concern, *J Adv Nurs* 37(3):250-257, 2002.

Grendell R: Complementary and alternative therapies. In Fortinash K, Holoday Worret P, editors: *Psychiatric mental health nursing*, ed 4, St. Louis, 2010, Elsevier.

Hine C et al: Integration of medical and psychological treatment within the primary care setting, *Soc Work Health Care* 47(2):122-134, 2008.

Institutes of Medicine Report: The Future of Nursing: Leading Change, Advancing Health. 2010 (website): www.iom.edu/reports/2010/the-future-of-nursing-heading-advancing-health.aspx. Accessed October 13, 2010.

Kessler RC et al: Prevalence, severity and comorbidity of 12 month DSM-IV disorders in the National Comorbidity Survey Replication (NCS-R), *Arch Gen Psychiatry* 62(6):617-627, 2005.

Melnyk BM, Fineout-Overholt E: *Making the case for evidence-based practice*, Philadelphia, 2005, Williams & Wilkins.

New Freedom Commission on Mental Health: *Achieving the promise: transforming mental health in America—final report*. U.S. Department of Health and Human Services Publication No. SMA-03-3832. Rockville, Md, 2003, U.S. Department of Health and Human Services.

Perese E: Stigma, poverty and victimization: roadblocks to recovery for individuals with severe mental illness, *J Am Psychiatr Nurses Assoc* 13:285, 2007.

Rice MJ: Evidence-based practice in psychiatric care: defining levels of evidence, *J Am Psychiatr Nurses Assoc* 14(3):183-187, 2008a.

Rice MJ: Psychiatric mental health evidence based practice, *J Am Psychiatr Nurses Assoc* 14:107-111, 2008b.

Substance Abuse and Mental Health Services Administration: *Illness management and recovery: how to use the evidence-based practice KITs*. U.S. Department of Health and Human Services Publication No. SMA-09-4462. Rockville, Md, 2009, Center for Mental Health Services, Substance Abuse and Mental Health Services Administration, U.S. Department of Health and Human Services.

Substance Abuse and Mental Health Services Administration: *Transforming mental health care in America. The federal action agenda: first steps*. U.S. Department of Health and Human Services Publication No. SMA-054060. Rockville, Md, 2005, Substance Abuse and Mental Health Services Administration.

Weiss SJ et al: The inextricable nature of mental health and physical health: implications for integrative care, *J Am Nurses Assoc* 15(6):371-382, 2009.

World Health Organization: *International classification of mental disorders*, revision 9, Geneva, Switzerland, 1992, World Health Organization.

World Health Organization: *The global burden of disease: 2004 update* (website): www.who.int/healthinfo/global_burden_disease/2004_report_update/en/index.html. Accessed September 29, 2010.

Online Resources

American Psychiatric Nurses Association: *Recovery to Practice Task Force* (website): www.apna.org/recovery. Accessed September 29, 2010.

American Psychiatric Association: *DSM-5: the future of psychiatric diagnosis* (website): www.dsm5.org. Accessed September 29, 2010.

Library of Congress: *Project on the Decade of the Brain* (website): www.loc.gov/loc/brain. Accessed September 29, 2010.

National Council for Community Behavioral Healthcare: *An avoidable tragedy—the relationship of premature death and serious mental illness* (website): www.thenationalcouncil.org/galleries/policy-file/premature%20death.pdf. Accessed September 29, 2010.

2

Nursing Practice in the Clinical Setting

Patricia A. Holoday Worret

"You must be the change you wish to see in the world."

Gandhi

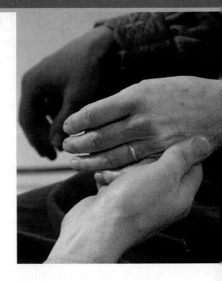

evolve WEBSITE

http://evolve.elsevier.com/Fortinash/

OBJECTIVES

- Discuss major contributions to psychiatric mental health nursing made by three outstanding psychiatric mental health nurse leaders.
- Discuss the impact of evidence-based practice and integrated care in the psychiatric clinical setting.
- Name the patient-centered reasons for establishing a therapeutic alliance.
- Explain the benefits to patients and nurses that result from the nurse's autodiagnosis.
- Discuss the concepts of power and control and their significance for patients and nurses.
- Describe in detail five principles of the therapeutic nurse–patient relationship.
- Identify the stages of the therapeutic nurse–patient relationship.

- Explain the working phase of the nurse–patient relationship and how nurses identify that phase.
- Discuss the effect that a nurse's indifference has on patients by listing patient responses.
- Describe the sources of a nurse's fear when first entering a psychiatric setting and ways to manage that fear.
- Explain reasons for avoiding the promise to keep a patient's secrets in the psychiatric setting.
- List the additional principles that guide nursing practice in the clinical setting.
- Explain the benefits for patients and families of identifying their strengths early during the patient's care and treatment.
- Describe five rewards of interacting with patients and their families in the psychiatric mental health setting.

KEY TERMS

altruism	indifference	motives	subjective
autodiagnosis	insight	objective	sympathy
boundaries	integrated patient care	patient-centered care	therapeutic alliance
empathy	interpersonal	power	therapeutic relationship
evidence-based practice	intrapersonal	rapport	vicarious learning
helping	nurse–patient relationship	resistance	

Psychiatric mental health nursing (PMHN) is an active and dynamic specialty within the nursing profession. A noteworthy evolution of psychiatric nursing clinical practice occurred during the past century. Despite all of these advances, direct patient care remains at the forefront of PMHN involvement. This is true for nurses who work at the patient's side as well

as for nurses who teach, mentor, or hold administrative positions.

The PMH nurse's role in the clinical setting has steadily expanded during the past several decades. Nursing autonomy has greatly increased, as have PMHN contributions to health care delivery on all levels, from the patient to the industry and beyond. Advanced-practice PMH nurses now hold primary-care privileges, and some are involved at the national level, where they set policies for the delivery of care to patients and their families (Institute of Medicine, 2010). However, PMHN continues to maintain its focus on patient-centered care. This chapter discusses salient clinical issues for PMHN practice and highlights several aspects of nurse–patient interactions that are useful in any health care setting.

Practice as we know it today began with the vision, determination, interest, and actions of preeminent nursing leaders whose foresight spearheaded advances in the PMHN discipline. Current PMHN practice has its roots in a notable past. What follows is a tribute to three distinguished nurses and their contributions to the profession.

PSYCHIATRIC MENTAL HEALTH NURSING LEADERS

The life of Florence Nightingale (1820–1910), the founder of modern nursing, was honored and celebrated in 2010, which marked the hundredth anniversary of her death. She made many contributions as a supervising nurse during the Crimean war (1853–1856). Nightingale assessed, recorded, and reported that the soldiers' trauma and illnesses were affecting far more than their bodies. She noted that many of these patients were depressed and dying even though some injuries and diagnoses seemed not to be life threatening.

Nightingale acted to make changes; she was instrumental in mitigating the squalid conditions that existed in hospital environments, and she helped nurses to modify their interactions with patients. Patients responded with noticeably improved physical and mental health. She mentored and taught nurses to care for the whole person rather than just their obvious physical injuries, and her approach proved invaluable. Nightingale's ideas and actions helped to identify many issues that led to improved health care (Vickers, 2000; Dossey, 2000). Her concepts helped to form a basis for nursing's current holistic view of each person as a human functional integration of body, mind, and spirit that is inextricably influenced by culture and the environment.

Throughout history, many nurse leaders who had a specific interest in mental health contributed to the practice of administering humane care to psychiatric patients. Linda Richards (1841–1930) graduated from the New England Hospital for Women and Children as the first trained nurse in the United States. She is also considered the first psychiatric nurse because of her dedicated work with patients in state mental institutions and with the nurses who were assigned to care for them. During her lifetime, she established several health care institutions in the nation, and, in 1882, she opened the first school for psychiatric nurses.

One of the most notable 20th century nurses was Hildegard Peplau (1909–1999), who is often referred to as the "mother of psychiatric nursing" (Haber, 2000). She is credited with molding the theory and practice of PMHN. The PMHN framework is effective in concept, theory, and practice, and it is enriched by its assimilation of elements from other

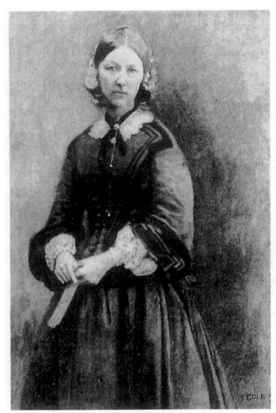

Florence Nightengale (1820-1910) is honored for her many contributions to the nursing profession and for establishing a basis for psychiatric mental health nursing.

disciplines, such as psychiatry, psychology, social science, and neuroscience. Peplau's pioneering endeavors and contributions were largely influenced by interpersonal psychotherapy as practiced by psychiatrist Harry Stack Sullivan. Unlike the ideas of contemporary psychiatrist Sigmund Freud, who thought that mental disorders were a product of intrapersonal characteristics (i.e., the unconscious mind, instinctual drives, and what transpired inside people), Sullivan theorized that disorders evolved in the social context of interpersonal interactions. His interest was in social relationships (i.e., what went on between people).

Peplau agreed with the interpersonal premise. She used these principles and processes in her own nursing practice with patients, and then formalized the principles for use by other nurses. She is most recognized in psychiatric nursing for her textbook *Interpersonal Relations in Nursing* (1952), in which she outlined theoretic concepts and instructions for practice. This work became the foundation for psychiatric nursing practice, which to that point was not clearly defined. Her theoretic framework provided the first systematic template and guide for nurses to interact with patients in the clinical setting. Some of Peplau's suggestions for interacting with patients are included in this chapter and also chapters 4 and 10.

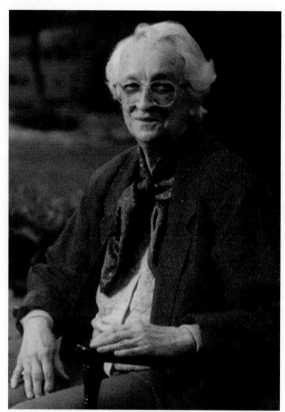

Hildegard Peplau (1909-1999) is one of the most notable pioneers of psychiatric mental health nursing. She established and recorded theory and practice principles that still guide clinical practice today.

PSYCHIATRIC MENTAL HEALTH NURSING: A PRACTICE-ORIENTED PROFESSION

PMHN is a practice profession with an emphasis on interpersonal interactions that take place between the patient and the nurse in the clinical setting. Today's patient is considered a partner in his or her own health care by all nursing disciplines. In PMHN, this partnership takes the form of an active relationship that is referred to as the *therapeutic alliance*. Other names that are sometimes used interchangeably for this alliance are the therapeutic relationship and the *nurse–patient relationship*. The patient and the nurse collaboratively use the therapeutic alliance as a vehicle for the patient's change and growth. Herein lies the art of psychiatric nursing, which is described in more detail below.

In addition to interpersonal interactions, which are an important element of successful patient outcomes in any PMH setting, nurses also focus on the science of their profession. They correlate and use multiple principles, policies, and treatments that guide and govern their time with patients in clinical practice. In keeping with the health care industry's trend toward combining treatment for medical and behavioral health, nurses in any setting find themselves practicing integrated patient care. The interplay between physical and mental health is clearly recognized. In integrated care, these disorders are not treated as separate illnesses; rather, they are treated together (Weiss, 2009).

Evidence-based practice (EBP) is currently at the center of all health care delivery, and PMH nurses continue to identify and apply empiric research evidence to solve clinical problems (Rice, 2008). At this point, the paradigm shift to EBP is gaining momentum (Fineout-Overholt, 2006; Rice, 2008). Health care systems are participating in the shift in nursing practice by encouraging research in their facilities and by implementing interventions that increase nurses' knowledge about EBP. Nurses are participating to make evidence-based nursing practices available for their use, and they are helping to determine the outcomes that will benefit patients. Specific evidence-based nursing practices continue to emerge. As EBP evolves, it will be written into teaching manuals and treatment plans and used by nurses in psychiatric settings within this dynamic specialty.

The Therapeutic Alliance: Definition and Description

A major objective for nurses when interacting with patents in any clinical psychiatric setting is to establish a therapeutic alliance. This alliance is a professional bond that exists between the nurse and the patient, and it often plays a significant role in the patient's well-being. The therapeutic alliance is at the heart of the nurse–patient relationship, and it is the cornerstone of nursing interventions in any psychiatric setting. The nurse–patient relationship is not an ordinary social friendship; rather, it is guided by standards and objectives.

Although a therapeutic alliance benefits the nurse by facilitating the interpersonal process, the alliance primarily focuses on patient-centered needs, issues, and short- and long-term goals.

The alliance serves as a vehicle for patients to accomplish the following:

(1) Freely discussing their needs and problems in the absence of judgment and criticism
(2) Gaining insight into their problems, expectations, abilities, and support systems
(3) Learning and practicing new skills
(4) Effecting life changes
(5) Healing mental and emotional wounds
(6) Promoting growth

The nurse provides a safe environment for this relationship to occur and grow.

The alliance begins when the nurse demonstrates the following:

- Knowledge of principles that guide the formation and maintenance of the nurse–patient relationship and its inherent responsibilities
- Understanding of the relational aspects of all nursing interventions and interactions
- Knowledge of, understanding of, and commitment to maintaining healthy boundaries

- Willingness to engage and interact with patients and to guide them on their return to wellness
- Commitment to practice nursing interventions and interactions within prescribed reliable guidelines and to integrate time-tested EBP interpersonal skills
- Inclusion of the patient in a therapeutic process that focuses on the patient's health
- Encouragement of the patient's responsibility for his or her own health within the patient's capacity

Those who choose the nursing profession for a career genuinely care about people, enjoy interacting with them, care about what people experience in their lives, and sincerely want to help them when needed. These altruistic characteristics of kindness and concern are important for anyone who works with patients, and they are essential to PMHN. However, in order to be effective, altruism and its affective components must be accompanied by objectives, learned skills, motivation, intention, and a planned direction. Examples of altruism are described later in this chapter.

Nurses who enter helping relationships learn that intentions and motives for helping others are complex. This chapter clarifies these issues, guides the reader with regard to the art of helping others, and offers suggestions for incorporating skills into PMHN practice while maintaining a healthy therapeutic alliance with the patient.

The nurse's commitment is also necessary to actively and skillfully engage with patients when assisting them to meet their needs and solve their problems. The term *active* signifies the nurse's balanced participation in the patient's process of overcoming obstacles to mental health. This includes giving assistance to patients who are unable to manage their own present situation because of the severity of their symptoms or a crisis event. However, it does not imply taking charge of the patients' lives and leaving them as passive nonparticipants in their own care.

A significant objective for nurses is to assist patients with maintaining their independence within their capacity while achieving their goals. This is especially important today, when therapy and treatment time are shortened. New nurses sometimes miss the significance and importance of encouraging patients to manage as many aspects of their own lives as possible, even when the outcomes do not appear perfect to the nurse. In their enthusiastic need to help others, nurses sometimes find it easier to do things and complete projects *for* the patient rather than doing things *with* the patient or waiting until the patient acts on his or her own behalf. This encourages the patient's dependence on others. The patient's achievement of independence is a main goal for both the patient and the nurse, and ensures higher functioning when the patient is on his or her own.

For several reasons, some patients will not be able to achieve total independence, and nurses provide more assistance where needed. Balance is the key. This begins with the nurse's careful and continual assessment of each situation, and it is maintained within the nurse–patient relationship. Regardless of a patient's abilities, the skill-based therapeutic alliance becomes a working partnership, with both parties

focusing on the patient and his or her goals. Several principles guide this process.

Principles of the Nurse–Patient Relationship

The therapeutic interpersonal relationship that develops between the nurse and the patient is an important factor for effecting patient change and growth. The following principles focus on the development and maintenance of a healthy alliance:

- The relationship is therapeutic rather than social.
- The focus remains on the patient's needs and problems rather than on the nurse or other issues. Interactions are patient centered.
- The relationship is purposeful and goal directed.
- The relationship is objective rather than subjective in quality.
- The relationship is time limited rather than open ended.

Therapeutic Versus Social. The therapeutic alliance is formed to help patients solve problems, make decisions, achieve growth, learn coping strategies, let go of unwanted behaviors, reinforce self-worth, and examine current relationships. The meetings between the nurse and the patient are not for mutual satisfaction. Although the nurse can be friendly with the patient, the nurse is not there to be the patient's friend. Table 2-1 clarifies this point with a comparison of therapeutic and social interactions.

Healthy **boundaries** help to define the nurse's role. They are important in any relationship, but especially in the therapeutic alliance. Trying to be a patient's friend blurs boundaries and confuses roles. The nurse must not confuse maintaining healthy boundaries with acting cold or distant toward patients. Warmth and genuineness are important qualities in any nurse. The nurse helps patients to increase their awareness and knowledge of the presence or absence of their own boundaries, as well as understanding the purposes that others have for maintaining boundaries. The nurse also helps patients to practice boundary setting. Box 2-1 illustrates some examples that the nurse may use to assist patients with the recognition of boundary violations.

Some social conversation usually occurs at the beginning of meetings and helps to establish or maintain rapport. Occasionally during meetings, superficial or social conversations briefly reappear. The nurse then returns to the preferred topic and keeps the conversation focused and therapeutic.

Patient Centered. Frequently during a session, a patient redirects the focus away from himself or herself by changing the subject; talking about the weather; focusing on the nurse, the nurse's appearance, the nurse's personal problems, problems in the environment; or other issues that do not pertain to the patient. The nurse recognizes that such diversion tactics are commonly a form of **resistance**. Patients divert the topic for one or more of several reasons: a fear of being judged; a resistance to discussing anxiety-producing material; boredom; avoiding the repetition of material that has been previously discussed with other therapists; or the inability to stay cognitively focused as a result of a mental disorder. The nurse

TABLE 2-1	THERAPEUTIC VERSUS SOCIAL INTERACTIONS: COMPARISONS	
THERAPEUTIC	**SOCIAL**	
Offer the patient therapeutic assistance	Give and receive friendship equally	
Focus on the patient's needs	Meet both individuals' needs	
Discuss the patient's perceptions, thoughts, feelings, and behaviors	Share mutual ideas and experiences	
Actively listen to the patient with the use of therapeutic communication skills	Give personal opinions and advice	
Encourage the patient to choose the topic for discussion	Randomly discuss topics at will or whim	
Encourage the patient to problem solve toward independence	Insist on helping; tolerate dependence	
Keep no secrets; some may be harmful to the patient	Promise to keep secrets at any cost	
Assist the patient with setting objectives and goals	Goals are not relevant	
Remain objective	Become subjectively involved	
Maintain healthy boundaries	Accept blurred boundaries	
Evaluate interactions and objectives with the patient	Avoid relational evaluations	

BOX 2-1   SIGNS OF UNHEALTHY BOUNDARIES

- Going against personal values or rights to please another
- Not noticing when someone displays inappropriate boundaries
- Not noticing when someone invades your boundaries
- Talking at an intimate level during the first meeting with someone
- Falling in love with a new acquaintance
- Falling in love with anyone who reaches out
- Being overwhelmed by or preoccupied with a person
- Acting on first sexual impulse
- Being sexual for your partner rather than for yourself
- Accepting food, gifts, touch, or sex that you do not want
- Touching a person without asking
- Taking as much as you can for the sake of getting
- Giving as much as you can for the sake of giving
- Allowing someone to take as much as they can from you
- Letting others direct your life
- Letting others describe your reality
- Letting others define you
- Believing others can anticipate your needs
- Expecting others to fill your needs automatically
- Falling apart so someone will take care of you
- Self-abuse
- Sexual and physical abuse
- Food and drug abuse
- Loaning money you do not have
- Flirting or sending mixed sexual messages
- Telling all

recognizes the diversion in a matter-of-fact way and refocuses the topic.

Goal Directed. A primary purpose for establishing the therapeutic alliance is to help patients to reach their adaptive goals. Together the patient and nurse determine problematic issues and collaboratively decide and identify the patient needs and what is realistically achievable. After goals are established, the nurse and the patient agree to work toward those goals and to put intentions into action, modifying strategies when necessary until the identified goals are achieved. The activities involved vary according to the patient's needs, but each activity is purposefully planned with the patient's individual treatment plan in mind.

Objective Versus Subjective. Nurses are therapeutic only when they remain objective. The term *objective* refers to remaining free from bias, prejudice, and personal identification during interactions with the patient and being able to process information that is based on facts. Alternatively, the term *subjective* refers to emphasis on one's own feelings, attitudes, and opinions when interacting with the patient. When nurses act subjectively in relation to the patient's problems or situations, they lose effectiveness in the relationship. With a conscious intent to remain objective, the nurse will see situations and events realistically rather than

identifying with the patient or becoming overly and personally involved with the patient's problems, needs, or life. Of course, this approach does not imply that the nurse withdraws from feelings or constructs barriers to protect himself or herself by intellectualizing or avoiding responses. With knowledge, awareness, practice, and experience, the nurse will be both objective and fully attentive to patients' situations and needs.

An example of objectivity versus subjectivity involves the nurse's ability to remain empathic instead of becoming sympathetic when interacting with a patient, even when the nurse has experienced a similar painful situation. For example, consider a nurse who has lost a child in an accident and then encounters a patient who is depressed and grieving the recent death of his or her own child. With empathy, the nurse is genuinely aware of the patient's emotions; however, with sympathy, the nurse loses objectivity and moves into his or her own personal feelings.

The nurse demonstrates objectivity by allowing and facilitating the patient's full expression of thoughts and feelings and then responding in a warm, empathic way that remains patient-centered. This approach helps the patient to relieve suppressed feelings as part of the normal grieving process, allows the patient to feel understood, and helps the patient to process and organize thoughts that are directed toward the solving of his or her own problems.

An example of a nontherapeutic response is a nurse in the same situation who hears the patient's expression of feelings and responds with excessive self-disclosure about his or her own similar experience. This approach represents a loss of therapeutic boundaries by identifying with the patient's problem and becoming enmeshed in the situation by personalizing it. The patient's response to the nurse who is unable to be objective will most likely be negative. The patient will probably stop sharing information because he or she feels unimportant and negated; because he or she worries that the nurse is fragile and does not want to cause the nurse any more emotional pain; or because he or she thinks that the nurse is inept and unable to manage his or her own problems, much less the patient's problems. Patients who are compromised by their own conditions and situations cannot be burdened by the nurse's problems. Healthy nurses seek supervision or private therapy when personal problems arise, and they maintain fulfilling personal relationships outside of the work setting.

Time-Limited Interactions. Before establishing the relationship, the nurse sets necessary parameters by agreeing with the patient about specific days and times that they will meet and the numbers of times that meetings will take place. Such structure helps the patient to realize that this relationship has limits and that it is not open ended (i.e., the patient cannot meet with the nurse whenever he or she wants and for as long as he or she wants). The principle of time-limited interaction is important for several reasons.

Sometimes patients have not learned as part of their formative relationships that limits are important for all relationships and that, when limits are absent, problems will occur. When basic rules are set at the beginning of the relationship, participants define the amount of time that they are willing and able to give, thus eliminating anxiety-provoking guesswork. Individuals then decide how to make appropriate use of the time that they have together. In addition, all relationships have inevitable endings. Much grief is avoided if both the nurse and the patient are certain of the limits and boundaries of the relationship and enforce them together. The nurse–patient relationship demonstrates how the patient can appropriately begin and end future alliances.

Stages of the Nurse–Patient Relationship

The nurse–patient relationship progresses through distinct stages. The nurse's knowledge and recognition of each stage facilitates the patient's therapeutic progress.

Preorientation Stage. During this initial phase, before the nurse and the patient ever meet, the nurse will accomplish several tasks. The first is to gather data about the patient, his or her condition, and the present situation. Information is taken from all available sources, including the patient, the patient's chart, staff reports, physician's reports, the patient's family, and other reliable sources such as the police and ambulance attendants.

From the information gathered, the nurse engages in a period of autodiagnosis that involves addressing his or her thoughts, feelings, perceptions, and attitudes about this particular patient and the surrounding circumstances. Judgmentalism, biases, and stereotyping sometimes arise that could influence the contact between the nurse and the patient in a nontherapeutic way. For example, if the nurse learns information about a patient that reminds him or her of a personal loved one or of someone who is feared, then the nurse's response to the patient may be subjective, nontherapeutic, and ineffective if he or she does not recognize and examine the facts.

The following is a critical thinking example that illustrates the importance of the nurse's autodiagnosis:

Consider Nurse A, whose father was alcohol dependent and who verbally abused her mother when he drank. What are some possible responses that Nurse A may demonstrate in the following situations if she fails to engage in autodiagnosis?

- **A male patient is admitted to the unit because of alcohol intoxication and spousal abuse.**
- **A matronly female is admitted to the unit with major depression. Her husband drinks and abuses her, both physically and emotionally.**

Conscious efforts to examine each situation and to see it from an objective perspective are important so that the nurse will avoid overidentification, judgmentalism, and stereotyping.

Orientation Stage. After the introduction of the nurse to the patient, the relationship begins to grow. During this stage, the participants become acquainted, build trust and rapport, and demonstrate an acceptance of the process that develops when the patient begins to work on his or her own important life issues. A contract or agreement is also established during the orientation phase of the relationship.

The Contract. The contract is either formal or informal, and it may be written or verbal. Nurses most frequently use verbal and informal contracts with patients in acute-care settings in which the patient and nurse meet on a regular basis. It may become necessary for the nurse to write a more specific and formalized contract for patients who seek therapy outside of an acute-care setting and when there is an expectation that a patient behavior will continue (e.g., a "no self-harm" contract) after discharge.

Some contracts are short but still effective and efficient. To prepare, the nurse looks over the patient's schedule and then meets with the patient. Here is an example of what the nurse on an inpatient unit may say to a patient:

"My name is _____, and I will be your contact person while you are here. I will be here Monday through Friday from 8 AM to 4 PM. Because of your schedule on this unit, it seems that the best time for us to meet is 9 AM. If that is a good time for you, we can plan on meeting again tomorrow."

The nurse validates plans with the patient. If the patient agrees, then the contract is established. The patient always maintains the right to refuse to enter into a contract, and the nurse does not take that personally. There are several reasons that a patient may not be ready to meet and work with another person on a regular basis.

In a community setting (e.g., home care, partial day treatment program, halfway house), some nurses write a contract for the patient that specifies dates, days, and times of meetings and that includes phone numbers where the patient can reach the nurse if he or she has questions between appointments. Some contracts specifically identify behaviors (i.e., expected outcomes) for the patient to practice between meetings in addition to goals to be achieved.

Regardless of the type of contract, the nurse will explain the purpose of the meetings, what is expected during the meetings, and the roles for both the nurse and the patient. Together, the nurse and the patient will determine long-term goals as well as the short-term objectives for reaching those goals.

Dependability is important, and nurses must keep all agreed-upon appointments with their patients. When circumstances prevent this, the nurse will take the initiative to let the patient know and then set a new meeting time. Patient dependability is also expected.

During the orientation stage, the nurse and the patient together identify the patient's strengths, limitations, and problem areas. Outcome criteria are established, and a plan of care is formulated. Patients' responses to this phase vary widely.

Working Stage. The orientation stage ends and the working stage begins when the patient takes responsibility and actively engages in his or her own plan of care. This requires the patient's commitment to reinforcing positive aspects of his or her life as well as working on problems and concerns that cause disruptions in life. It also requires making behavioral changes. Until the patient actually participates in making changes, the working stage is not reached. Patients are not in the working stage merely because they keep repeating their "story." As nurses gain experience, they are able to recognize when patients are actually in the working phase and when they are no longer resisting changes. Nurses help patients to gain insight, independence, and mastery over their lives as they encourage and reinforce patients' participation in their own growth processes.

Prioritizing patients' needs and problems helps to determine which ones require immediate attention and promotes an organized way to manage treatment. A general principle to keep in mind is that safety and health problems are a main priority above all others. For example, the nurse first determines whether patients are free from danger to themselves or others and then addresses pertinent physical needs before other interactions begins. Within the established relationship, the nurse proceeds to help the patient examine cognitive, affective, and behavioral problems. Patients trust the relationship, and they begin to explore thoughts and feelings and change problematic behaviors in a safe environment where they can practice new skills; the nurse is able to reinforce positive outcomes and patient achievements.

Termination Stage. During this stage, the relationship comes to a close. Termination actually begins during the orientation phase, when the nurse first sets meeting times. This lets the patient know that the relationship is about to begin but also that it has limits and will end. It avoids confusion on the part of the patient, who may be unable or unwilling to recognize relationship boundaries and who may want to contact the nurse outside of the facility or after discharge. The nurse must be clear and clarify with the patient that the professional relationship exists only within the context of the current treatment plan and time.

Termination naturally occurs when the patient has improved and is discharged, but it also occurs if the patient or nurse is transferred. When termination is anticipated, the nurse uses strategies to prepare for the event to avoid an abrupt closure. Ending treatment is sometimes traumatic for patients who have come to value the relationship as well as the nurse's attention and assistance. Some methods that the nurse may use when preparing for termination include the following:

- Reduce the amount of time spent with the patient during each session and increase the amount of time between sessions as the patient's condition improves.
- Prepare for the patient's postdischarge situation (i.e., plans for future) rather than focusing on new or past problems.
- Identify with the patient the individuals who will help with future therapy.
- Have the patient identify the changes that he or she has made toward growth; share the nurse's perceptions of the patient's growth.
- Help the patient express feelings about ending the relationship; tell the patient if the relationship has been pleasant.
- Tell the patient in advance when and if the nurse will no longer be able to meet with the patient.

When nurses identify relationship stages and know and use effective strategies and responses during each stage, the course of the therapeutic process runs more smoothly. The nurse is not caught off guard or shocked by unexpected negative or dismissive responses. When nurses are unaware of potential patient responses, they may erroneously take responsibility for what can seem like a relationship failure; however, this is often a result of the patient's fears or unresolved pathology. When nurses lack insight into the patient's needs or problems, they may even abandon the relationship because it is unrewarding or unfulfilling. Alternatively, when the nurse has insight into patient responses, he or she remains focused on patient-centered care during all stages of the relationship and continues to use strategies to facilitate positive treatment outcomes and patient growth. See Table 4-3 for more examples of the stages of the nurse-patient relationship.

Clinical Concepts and Techniques
Helping: The Concept and the Activity

The act of **helping** other people is a fundamental element in nursing, but it is not a simple one. Nurses and patients benefit when nurses understand this complex concept before they enter any nursing discipline, and this is particularly important in psychiatric mental health settings.

Nurses need insight regarding their own motives and behaviors associated with helping others. Insight coupled with knowledge and necessary skills for interacting with patients leads to the fulfillment of expected patient outcomes.

Nurses frequently identify the desire to help others as a core motivator for entering and maintaining employment in their profession. Patients in the psychiatric setting are often vulnerable because of altered thoughts or emotions due to a mental disorder. This makes it essential for the nurses who work in PMH settings to be mentally and emotionally healthy as well as skillfully prepared for therapeutic interactions. This includes the nurse's awareness of his or her own reasons for choosing a helping profession. Frequent autodiagnosis by nurses and other health care providers will promote self-awareness and improve the quality of their interactions. Figure 4-2, the Johari window, reinforces this topic.

Nurses have various reasons for working with patients within the helping professions. A nurse's motives directly or indirectly influence interactions between the nurse and the patient, and they may affect patient outcomes. Some motives and reasons will promote health and benefit both the patient and the nurse, but others are not productive. The following sections present examples of motives and reasons for helping others in addition to describing nursing opportunities for meeting challenges that may arise while helping patients.

Altruism

The term *altruism*, which is defined as having and showing compassion, generosity, goodwill, charity, kindness and benevolence toward others, is a desirable and useful quality in the psychiatric setting, and it is a common reason for why nurses help others. Often the world outside of the therapeutic environment shuns, alienates, and abuses patients with mental disorders. Patients who are healing from mental and emotional wounds welcome the nurse's genuine altruism and unconditional positive regard. These qualities also promote patient wellness.

Astute nurses continually examine their own actions and motives when interacting with patients. What seems like a kind gesture by the unskilled nurse is sometimes an obstacle or barrier to the patient's improvement. A challenge occurs when nurses allow their feelings of kindness toward a patient cloud their judgment. For example, a nurse who is new to a unit and somewhat unsure of her role may tell a patient that he does not have to attend one of his scheduled activities after the patient states he is "too tired to think today" and wants to "go back to bed." However, the scheduled activity is a priority in this patient's individual treatment plan. In this case, the nurse's misplaced kindness is inappropriate. This is a nursing opportunity in which the patient should be encouraged to attend the meeting and engage in his own treatment.

Nursing Opportunity. Recognize the patient's avoidance, and focus on the patient and his established treatment plan of care. The nurse's generosity in wanting to help the patient

resulted in a nontherapeutic response. The next step for the nurse in the preceding situation is autodiagnosis, which involves questioning why the treatment plan was manipulated. The answer may result in nurse-centered rather than patient-centered reasons. Altruism is an excellent quality for nurses to have when it is understood and coupled with critical thinking and a solid knowledge of specific therapeutic interventions and their rationales.

Satisfaction From Helping Patients

Nurses and all other professionals seek satisfaction from their life work. Satisfaction is usually a sign that the nurse engages in purposeful therapeutic activities with the patients and that both the nurse and the patient are benefiting from their professional relationship. Without job satisfaction, nurses frequently change their location or type of employment, describe burnout, or leave the profession entirely. Gaining satisfaction is one positive outcome that results from using educated efforts for the purpose of helping others.

However, a challenge occurs if a nurse requires more than job satisfaction and is helping others to fulfill his or her own personal needs for affiliation. At that point, there is a risk that the nurse–patient relationship could become nontherapeutic. To ensure that the professional relationship is not for the purpose of filling an emotional deficit in the nurse's personal life, the nurse's sources of support, attention, and affiliation must exist outside of the nurse–patient relationships.

Nursing Opportunity. First, a thorough understanding of boundaries as described in Chapters 2 and 4 will help to prevent this problem. Second, recognizing and identifying the problem if it occurs is also beneficial. The nurse may personally become aware of the problem, or coworkers will recognize it. A work environment that fosters open, honest, and professional interpersonal critiques among skilled nurses is a preventive factor for avoiding this and other problems. In addition, each nurse who works closely with patients consciously makes the effort to form and maintain healthy interpersonal relationships, personal supports, and sources of affection and affiliation in his or her personal life outside of the workplace.

Desire to Protect Others

Wanting to protect others can be an incentive and generate a nurse's desire to help patients. There are times in the PMH setting when patients are at risk and require various levels of protection because of poor judgment and other symptoms related to their mental disorder or current life crisis. For example, a depressed patient with suicidal thoughts and gestures definitely requires close observation and protection from self-harm; a patient with dementia who wanders and gets lost needs the protection of a closed unit, and the staff needs to be alert to prevent the patient from coming to any harm. In these situations, the nurse makes decisions that protect the patient in accordance with individual needs and situations.

A challenge may arise if the nurse fails to recognize when external protection is necessary and when to modify or remove it. With knowledge and experience, the nurse knows when patients are able to safely make their own choices and decisions. Inexperienced nurses may think that making all decisions for patients is helpful and that this will prevent patients from experiencing negative consequences. However, this can be counterproductive. Overprotection encourages dependence on the nurse and the health care system and robs patients of opportunities to succeed in the management of their own lives.

Nursing Opportunity. Assess each individual condition, event, and situation, and allow patients to make their own decisions when it is safe and they are able. Protect patients when they are not able to remain safe because of symptoms of their disorders or because of their response to a current life crisis situation. Continually assess patients' readiness and willingness, and encourage them to make their own decisions, remembering that some minor mistakes can also be learning tools. This helps patients to gain or regain independence, to use learned skills, and to negotiate their own way in the world. Increased self-esteem and self-confidence are frequent outcomes for patients who succeed in making their own successful decisions.

Power and Control

Nurses and other health care professionals recognize the imbalance of power and control between the nurse and the patient in some psychiatric settings. Patients often perceive caregivers as being more knowledgeable or believe that they themselves have little power or control over their own situations. This may manifest as patient submission, compliance, or aggression.

Nursing Opportunity. Avoid taking unnecessary control over situations and events, and avoid seeking importance or power from working with patients. Recognize and respect the potential imbalance of power and control in nurse–patient interactions and relationships, and do not take advantage of it. Patients surrender various levels of control when they are admitted to any psychiatric setting, so nurses will act purposefully to preserve the dignity of all patients, regardless of their situation. This includes making sure that patients maintain control of areas of their lives that do not interfere with their treatment.

When the nurse is perceived as being knowledgeable, this often has a positive influence on the patient's compliance with necessary treatments. Nurses never take advantage of this position. However, if patients refuse treatment, nurses encourage but do not insist that the patients comply. If a patient's life is in danger because of noncompliance, procedures will change to ensure patient safety.

In addition, the registered nurse (RN) supervises his or her treatment team and is responsible for reminding other members about the dignity and rights of patients admitted to the health care setting. In the interest of safety, the use of chemical or physical restraints is necessary in some situations, and this often involves control issues. Nursing actions are guided by standards of nursing practice and the policies and procedures of the facility. The RN also acts as a role model in all situations, sharing power and control with team members and with patients, when appropriate. With few exceptions, most patients show improved function and report satisfaction when they are able to make decisions and have sufficient control over their own lives.

Insight From Helping

Throughout clinical practice, PMH nurses learn that increased insight and vicarious learning are frequent outcomes of interacting with patients. In the psychiatric setting, insight comes from various sources, which include the following:

- Therapeutic interactions with the patient
- Reading patient records
- Being involved in patient therapies
- Interdisciplinary team meetings
- Specific patient-focused interactions with other professionals
- Educational classes

Insight into patients' disorders, problems, needs, and outcomes is beneficial to both patients and nurses, and it is essential for growth. A potential challenge arises when nurses discover similarities between a patient's problem and their own or that of their own family member or acquaintance. When this occurs, the focus may shift from the patient to the nurse unless the nurse identifies the dynamic.

Increased insight often occurs in patients as they engage in their own treatment plan. They also gain insight during group activities when they have an opportunity to listen and vicariously learn ways that other people manage their problems and relationships. Increased family insight is valuable if patients will live at home. The more that family members understand about the patient's disorder, symptoms, behaviors, medications, and treatments and accept the situation, the healthier the living environment will be.

Nursing Opportunity. Patient outcomes may become distorted when the nurse identifies with patients' problems. Therefore, maintain focus on the patient and the patient's care and treatment plan. Clearly distinguish between the patients' and the nurse's issues at all times. Nurses avoid manipulating situations to get answers to their own problems. To ensure that this does not happen, seek and maintain supervision over your practice, and discuss both successes and problems that arise. If a personal problem persists and interferes with nurse–patient interactions, seek professional advice or therapy outside of the practice setting.

Various factors influence the decision to enter and remain in a helping profession. Psychiatric nursing is based on sound knowledge and practice, healthy self-awareness, an understanding of personal motivation, and open critiques with colleagues regarding interpersonal relationships and the art, science, and act of helping patients. Primary objectives for the entire interdisciplinary team include the maintenance of therapeutic interactions, interventions, and relationships that are beneficial for patients and their care. A therapeutic environment is maintained when nurses are able to collaborate with the treatment team and to openly discuss ideas about all topics that are relevant to the clinical setting.

Fear in the Psychiatric Setting

Fear of entering a psychiatric setting for the first time is a common response that stems from one or more sources. One source is *fear of the patients* or what they will do. Another source is *fear of failure* and doubt about the nurse's own performance. A third source is the nurse's past or present *personal* experiences with someone who is mentally disordered or fear of the nurse's own stability. The challenge for nurses is to identify their fear, to overcome it through increased insight and understanding, and to take action toward becoming effective communicators.

Fear of the Patients

Often a fear of patients comes from the nurse's preconceived thoughts and distorted images of people who have mental disorders. Frequent exposure to stories that have been dramatized in television, films, news, literature, or video games designed to shock the viewer may influence a nurse's perception of mentally ill patients. Mentally disordered individuals are stereotypically portrayed as frightening individuals who are out of touch with reality and dangerous. Unfortunately, these thoughts and stereotyped images result in a nurse's fear of being injured by such patients. Stereotyping not only creates a major problem for mentally disordered patients, their families, and the community, but it often creates negative expectations in the nurse who lacks experience in the psychiatric setting. Unrealistic preconceived images, stereotyping, and biases have an effect on nurses. Their fear is often observable when student nurses first enter the psychiatric mental health rotation or when graduate nurses find out that a psychiatric patient has been admitted to their medical-surgical unit.

Fear of Failure

When nurses have strong doubts about their own ability to interact with patients, often the result is anxiety and avoidance. The most common doubt among nurses first entering the psychiatric setting is not knowing what to say or do. New nurses fear embarrassment or that patients will reject them. Imagined failure, rejection, or embarrassment is difficult to tolerate in any situation, but it is magnified in this setting, because nurses want to appear competent when interacting with patients. For example, when fearful, the nurse may avoid approaching patients who require the nurse to initiate communication. As a result, both the nurse and the patient fail to benefit from interactions. The nurse misses two opportunities in this case: the first is providing an empathic ear for the patient and the second is in increasing his or her own experience to practice communication skills.

Fear Based on Personal Experience

Some nurses have had negative experiences with relatives or people in their neighborhood who have mental disorders, and they enter nursing with a conditioned fear of patients who have psychiatric disorders. Alternatively, some nurses have gained skills and learned acceptance from the opportunity to interact with a mentally disordered person before coming into the nursing profession.

Thinking about past experiences before experiencing the present situation promotes a barrier to therapeutic communication. The nurse has yet to learn that no two patients are the same, even when they have the same diagnosis. Nurses grow personally and improve professionally when they see each patient as an individual with individual needs, problems, and strengths and then interact with each patient accordingly.

Some apprehension is expected before entering a new and dynamic area such as the psychiatric setting for the first time. Occasionally a nurse may worry excessively about his or her own stability in this area. This may be generated from an exaggerated lack of confidence in his or her own abilities or a personal experience of having a psychiatric disorder. In either case, the nurse is encouraged to seek professional assessment and assistance before entering the PMH area rather than to conceal these facts and fears. Patients in this setting have a right to healthy responses and behaviors by nurses that are reflected in the nursing care provided. Patient progress will likely be interrupted if the nurse focuses on personal distractions rather than assisting patients with their needs and opportunities for change and growth. In most cases, nurses facing these problems will meet their professional and personal objectives if they engage in facilitative supervision before and during a psychiatric clinical rotation.

Nursing Opportunities. Enter the psychiatric setting with positive but realistic expectations for interacting with patients. Perfect performance is not a requirement. Being able to tolerate mistakes and to rethink situations to determine successful alternatives is important. New nurses are frequently surprised when patients welcome them or when patients make efforts to help the nurse feel more at ease. Being honest and open with patients about the nurse's level of experience during the initial meeting often gains the patients' trust and cooperation. This does not mean that the nurse overemphasizes personal shortcomings or divulges excessive personal information, but when appropriate information is expressed openly, patients know that this is a new rotation and that the nurse is willing to learn.

Fear appears in many unintended ways, and sometimes a patient perceives the nurse's fear as rejection. A relaxed facial expression and an unimposing, open stance show interest and concern for the patient. Learning skills from this chapter and reviewing the basic communication skills discussed in Chapter 4 will be helpful for many situations.

Fear breeds avoidance, but knowledge and preparation diminish fear and bring confidence. Being prepared before entering the psychiatric setting includes having knowledge and understanding of mental disorders. It is equally important to have knowledge of specific nursing interventions and the rationales for each intervention. Take time to learn specific theories and to practice therapeutic communication skills before entering the psychiatric setting. Role-playing is often helpful, and valid clinical media aids can be useful as well. However, it is unreasonable to think that the nurse will know everything during his or her first encounter with the psychiatric setting.

Time and experience will increase the nurse's knowledge and help to improve his or her skills, but it is necessary to take the first step toward gaining experience. This means taking some risks and seeking multiple opportunities to practice skills in interactions with patients in a variety of situations. Nurses who purposefully practice mastering these skills while focusing on the patient and not on the self will succeed. Studies repeatedly reveal that patients improve in facilitative, genuinely caring, therapeutic environments, regardless of the therapist's educational degrees or preparation.

Additional suggestions for minimizing fear include the following:

- Initiate interactions. Approach patients for conversation, and do not wait for them to come to you. Patients have the right and sometimes refuse to talk to the nurse for many reasons. It is important that the nurse avoids taking this personally and avoids focusing on oneself or one's own performance. The patient may have another appointment or may be worried about disclosing information to someone that he or she does not know. Regardless of the reason, continue on and talk to other patients. Make a concerted effort at another time to seek interaction with the patients who refused to talk initially.
- Approach each patient on the unit with the use of therapeutic communication techniques and open-ended questions and statements whenever possible.
- Make a conscious effort to avoid stereotyping and to omit biases. If this is a planned objective, it is easier to accomplish.
- Focus on the patient rather than on the self and one's own performance. When thinking about what the patient is saying and showing genuine concern, the nurse is less likely to worry about his or her own appearance or performance. The patient senses your intention and is less interested in your skills than in honest connection. The outcome is usually rewarding for both the patient and the nurse. The patient becomes less threatening when the nurse interacts with him or her and sees the patient as a human being instead of a psychiatric label to be feared.
- Learn basic communication techniques and skills, and practice them at every opportunity.
- Challenge yourself by taking the initiative to interact with patients with various diagnoses. Learn about the symptoms that are associated with each psychiatric diagnosis, and learn specific interventions intended for these symptoms and responses. The outcome of doing this is effective nursing care. Perfecting skills brings a sense of control in each situation and further reduces fear.
- Keep expectations about performance realistic. Nurses are not expected to be therapists by the end of their first few clinical experiences. Nurses become more skilled

and confident each day as they practice and continue to learn about this specialty. Increased skill will be its own reward.

- Use positive self-affirmations, such as "I am doing well" and "I am exactly where I should be in the level of my performance."
- Review theory and policies that address safety, confidentiality, and boundaries.
- Write specific personal objectives before each clinical day. These objectives will become the nursing plan, and they will function as rehearsal tools for the actual clinical experience. An increase in confidence follows. Here are some examples of personal objectives:
  - Interact with a patient who has major depression and use the following interventions:
    - Ensure patient safety by following the unit procedures (e.g., suicide assessment and precautions).
    - Interact with the patient and allow time for answers; sit quietly while the patient collects his or her thoughts.
    - Create a safe, nonjudgmental environment in which the patient can interact.
    - Encourage the patient to express his or her thoughts and feelings.
    - When the patient is able, help him or her to join groups and activities by accompanying him or her.
    - Remember that the patient with depression does not always want to socialize, but continue to initiate brief, frequent, unobtrusive contacts.
  - Use the following therapeutic communication techniques with a depressed patient:
    - Silence
    - Reflection
    - Giving recognition
    - Offering self
    - Encouraging comparisons

Safety is always the first and foremost nursing intervention to keep in mind, and it is the primary objective of the entire staff, the instructor, and the student nurse. The assigned unit environment should also be safe for new nurses to practice their skills, or the inexperienced nurses will be reassigned to other units. Learning agency policies and procedures is also necessary.

Manage Stress

Our fast-paced world is stressful for individuals, both young and old. It is doubly stressful for patients who live with mental disorders, their families, and their caregivers. Mentally disordered patients and their families have difficulty meeting the daily demands of managing symptoms and medications, caring for other family members' needs, negotiating with agencies, and maintaining healthy social contacts outside of the family.

Nurses also experience stress because of internal and external demands and circumstances related to helping patients in a health care environment. Professional nursing practice carries great responsibility. Patients, physicians, administrators, and colleagues depend on the nurse's educated decisions and actions, and they expect positive outcomes. Financial and other constraints that change over time may also be a source of stress in the work setting. The challenge for nurses is to realize and also to teach patients the two main truths about stress. One is that some stress is inevitable in the real world: there is no sustained stress-free place when participating in life. The second is to learn healthy ways to manage stress or else it manages us and reduces our quality of life.

Nursing Opportunities. Some stressors are motivating and lead to positive activity, growth, or change. Other stressors interfere with health. The nurse must first recognize and identify stressors when they occur. The next steps are to modify, decrease, or eliminate harmful stressors when possible; accept those that cannot be changed; and manage the effects of stress. Nurses and other healthcare professionals realize the importance of learning and practicing techniques for relieving stress. Nurses practice the techniques themselves and teach techniques to patients in all PMH settings. Many techniques are available for patients of all ages and states of health. Stress relief measures and stress management techniques appear in several chapters of this textbook.

Increase and Synthesize Knowledge and Skills

One challenge for nurses is to continually seek new ideas and skills to improve their practice. State nursing boards require that nurses stay current in education for the purpose of ongoing licensure, but most nurses exceed this requirement. Learning continues throughout a dynamic career. In addition, content that is learned in basic nursing courses is not forgotten; rather, it is synthesized and incorporated into the nurse's specialty. This is particularly true today, with the trend toward integrated care. Nurses continually draw from knowledge that was gained in several specialties. The following example illustrates how an RN synthesized prior knowledge with data from a current clinical crisis to benefit both the patient and the staff.

Cindy, an emaciated and pregnant young woman, was admitted to the obstetric unit from the emergency department of a large and busy health care facility. Workers found her screaming on the cold tile floor of the ladies' bathroom in a fast-food restaurant. They determined that she was homeless and that she had been living on the street. Paramedics reported that she was in active labor, and she was unable to contain her loud outbursts. She seemed very frightened, she fought staff who tried to help her, and she cursed at everyone around her during each contraction. In addition to the cursing, she gave loud commands to demons and witches who she said were all around her bed and who were telling her that they were going to take her baby to the devil. Laboratory results revealed no illicit drugs in Cindy's body.

Darlene, the admitting RN, realized that the patient was psychotic and began to use therapeutic interactive skills that she learned during a psychiatric affiliation. Cindy responded positively with decreased outbursts and soon stated that she was less frightened when Darlene stayed in the room and talked with her. Cindy said that she wanted her mother; she gave Darlene the phone number, and Darlene helped Cindy place the call. Cindy's mother was very relieved to learn that Cindy was safe. Cindy had run away from home after becoming pregnant and never contacted her mother until now. The mother later reported to the staff that Cindy was diagnosed as being mildly mentally retarded but that she had also demonstrated periodic delusions and hallucinations since she was a child. She had been able to live at home and function in the care of her family until she ran away.

The nurse and staff managed Cindy's physical and obstetric needs, but they also promoted a therapeutic environment by using learned psychiatric nursing interventions to address the patient's psychotic symptoms, thus averting a crisis. Cindy calmed down considerably when she felt accepted. She responded positively when the staff used simple and specific psychiatric nursing interventions, and she cooperated with their instructions for labor and delivery. The staff modified their instructions so that Cindy would understand them. In addition, Cindy's sense of security increased when her mother was encouraged to stay with her during labor. A psychiatric evaluation was ordered, and a postdelivery plan of care that included psychiatric follow-up was prescribed.

Psychiatric nursing skills can be used in any health care setting, and nurses quickly learn that these valuable skills will enhance practice in all fields of nursing. This example of integrated care represents a successful synthesis of skills from various nursing theory and practice areas. Cindy benefited from the nurse's ability to use information from many sources and to modify the patient's care on the basis of her immediate needs rather than continuing with the scripted obstetric protocol. All patients benefit from a nurse's abilities and willingness to be flexible and to synthesize theory and practice.

Nursing Opportunities. Maintain an open cognitive approach to each situation in the clinical setting. Follow safe standards, procedures, and policies, and continually be aware of opportunities to improve your patients' experiences in the health care system. Strive to use all relevant nursing knowledge in the clinical setting, and be willing to synthesize information and practice components from several nursing specialties to integrate patient care. Nurses' efforts are reflected in patients' outcomes.

Set Priorities

Among the most important skills that the nurse learns and practices is prioritizing. Identifying and determining priorities is essential in any psychiatric setting. The astute nurse begins to set priorities even before entering the psychiatric setting; he or she then uses data from the work environment and continues to modify priorities throughout each day. This is an open-ended activity that does not end until the patient is discharged, or when other caregivers or agencies take up the prioritizing.

In relation to patient care, the nurse prioritizes nursing diagnoses, expected patient outcomes, and nursing interventions while being prepared to change each of these in accordance with patient responses and nursing evaluations. The following example illustrates a challenge and one nurse's choice of priorities:

Albert, a 65-year-old man, was admitted to the unit with a diagnosis of severe major depression. His wife died 5 months earlier, and he then completely ended his social life, refusing all invitations from friends. Albert has three grown children who care for him, but they all have their own families and jobs.

For the past 2 weeks, Albert has eaten very little food, he has stayed in his pajamas all day, he has not bathed, and he has refused to go out of the house at all. His family called his physician, and he was admitted to the psychiatric facility for evaluation and treatment. During the intake assessment, it was clear that Albert was not an imminent suicide risk, but he made vague statements that resulted in the staff closely watching him during each shift. He began a regimen of antidepressants plus daily scheduled activities and therapy, and he received a copy of the unit introduction and guidelines. Staff explained guidelines to Albert, that he was not allowed to go outside of the building for walks by himself at this time to ensure his safety.

Albert continued to isolate himself for more than a week, and he did not attend any activities. Staff watched him closely on every shift. He began to dress himself in the morning without being asked. He came to scheduled groups and participated occasionally, but he was still guarded when he talked about himself and his situation. After a few days, his privileges were increased so that he was able to dine in the main dining room, but he still could not go outside alone.

One day, Sam, who was Albert's assigned RN for the day, kept his scheduled appointment to interact with Albert, who told Sam that he felt "much better today." Albert was wearing a bright plaid shirt that one of his daughters brought in, and Sam commented about the colors. Albert responded, "That is exactly how I feel today: bright and cheerful." Sam told Albert that Albert was saying the words he thought Sam wanted to hear but that they didn't seem genuine. Sam stayed with Albert for a long time, and he then told the unit manager and charted that Albert appeared even more depressed, although he was trying to mask it with forced cheerfulness.

Sam prepared for an important scheduled meeting that was to focus on Sam's promotion to another position. Sam reported off the unit, but as he walked down the hall, he caught a glimpse of Albert's plaid shirt outside a window as Albert headed quickly for a busy intersection. Sam changed directions, told the receptionist at the front desk as he passed her to send more help, and ran after Albert. Sam caught up with Albert, who resisted and seemed angry at first but who then held on to Sam tightly and started to cry, saying that he had snuck outside and was going to step into traffic in front of the first large speeding vehicle that he saw. He wanted to die. Sam and Albert walked back to the unit, and Sam stayed with Albert, who was put on suicide precautions with close staff attendance.

In the preceding vignette, the RN's ability to place his personal agenda secondary to the patient's acute need is a pointed example of the importance of prioritizing.

Nursing Opportunities. It cannot be overstated that safety is always the first consideration when setting priorities. An established and organized plan is necessary for the efficient functioning of any system. However, a set prioritized plan often requires modification, depending on circumstances, and this is true in the psychiatric setting. Nurses set priorities and assess them continually, and they must be ready to respond when the situation demands changes. Often, making a change will interfere with the nurse's well-thought-out plan for the day; however, patient needs come first, and when the situation demands it, necessary changes occur. Clear thinking and the ability to organize and manage are valued qualities, but flexibility is also a valued characteristic in the psychiatric setting, where the unpredictable usually does happen. Prioritizing includes these steps:

- Obtain all relevant data.
- Analyze and organize the information.
- Identify immediate problems and needs before prioritizing.
- Intervene in order of importance, as follows:
  - Safety
  - Health
  - Intrapersonal patient needs and problems
  - Interpersonal patient needs and problems
  - Be flexible in the approach to patient care.

With this sequence in mind, nurses continually reassess individual patient responses to treatment, and they then set and modify priorities during each step of the dynamic nursing process.

Secrets and Promises

Keeping confidences is important in any meaningful relationship. In families and friendships, members often share private information and secrets. As stated previously, an important principle for nurses to learn and maintain is that the nurse–patient relationship is a professional one rather than a personal one. In other words, it is not a friendship. Nurses and other healthcare professionals do not keep secrets or make promises to patients when the secret may interfere with the patient's treatment. Challenges occur when nurses fail to understand this principle and do not distinguish between professional and personal relationships. The following example illustrates this principle:

Sarah was in her fifth week of the psychiatric rotation in an RN program. She felt comfortable on the psychiatric unit, having diligently studied the theory and practiced skills each day that she was assigned to the clinical setting. Sarah established a contract with Kimberly, a 15-year-old female patient on the locked adolescent unit, and met with her each clinical day. Kim's parents had admitted her because of her out-of-control behaviors that included polysubstance abuse, running away from home for weeks at a time, not attending school, and hanging out with friends who were many years older and who had histories of drug use. Kim said that they were good friends because they gave her what she needed. She said she didn't get what she needed at home.

One day, Sarah was preparing to leave the unit to attend a scheduled adjunctive therapy session. Kim stopped her and quietly said that she had a secret. Sarah explained to Kim that she was scheduled to attend a meeting and that she had 20 minutes to talk. Kim continued to say she wanted to tell Sarah her secret but that she had to promise not to tell anyone else. Sarah was surprised that Kim chose to confide in her but she maintained her composure and remembered from class discussions and reading what she had to do. Sarah told Kim that she couldn't keep any secret that might affect her care and that the physician and the staff who work as a team would need to know. Then Sarah continued with the next step. She told Kim that her secret probably was very important or she wouldn't have brought it up, and then he offered to talk with her about it for the next 15 minutes.

Kim cried as she told Sarah that she had been sexually abused for 3 years by an uncle who came to her home often and who frequently offered to stay with her and her younger sister when her parents went out for the evening. She said the uncle threatened to abuse her little sister if she told and that her parents would not believe her and that they would blame her if they found out.

Sarah listened and responded therapeutically, and she used many of the communication skills that she had recently learned to encourage Kim to talk more about her situation. She empathized with what Kim had been through. Kim said that her recent "craziness" and acting out had made her scared for her life, and she was worried about her sister. Sarah commented on Kim's bravery for telling what had to be told, and Kim said that she felt relieved.

Sarah reminded Kim that she had to leave for the meeting but that she would be back the next clinical day and would get another nurse to be with her now. Sarah reported the incident to the RN unit manager, who assigned another RN to respond to the Kim's needs. Sarah discussed this incident with her instructor, and the classmates processed this important learning experience in postconference, learning vicariously and gaining insight from Sarah's experience.

Nursing Opportunities. This example illustrates why it is important for nurses to explain to patients the rationale for not keeping secrets before the patient discloses information. Patients want to relieve themselves of the burden of their secret, and they will usually reveal information in the hope of getting help in a safe environment. The nurse's honesty often increases the patient's trust and subsequent disclosure. When nurses forget or ignore this principle and encourage patients to tell secret information that the nurse then shares with the staff, the patient feels betrayed and stops trusting the nurse and others. More importantly, the patient stops discussing problems. This causes a stall in the nurse–patient relationship, and trust is often difficult to recover. Ultimately, the patient is cheated of valuable ongoing therapeutic interactions.

The following steps will assist with this process:
- Describe the theory and rationale for avoiding making promises and keeping secrets with patients.
- Practice and role-play a situation in which a patient asks the nurse to keep a secret.
- Tell the patient the rationale for not keeping secrets.
- Keep communication open by recognizing the importance and meaning that the secret holds for the patient and by offering to discuss its content with the patient.
- Share the content of all therapeutically significant information with the treatment team.
- Make a list of several potential topics of significant secrets that patients typically reveal. This rehearsal list will help nurses to avoid being caught off guard.

Recognize Variations of Change

Unlike most physical sciences that are predictable and exact, psychiatry and psychology may seem elusive and ambiguous to the nurse. The definition, description, and categorization of psychiatric diagnoses in the *Diagnostic and Statistical Manual of Mental Disorders* appear to be exact. However, because of the complex nature of human beings, each patient will express his or her symptoms in unique ways.

Initially, a new nurse will think in absolutes, seeing symptoms as being totally present or totally absent (i.e., "all or none"). In reality, the patient's symptoms may change slightly or dramatically over hours or days (i.e., "more or less"). Because psychiatric symptoms are not always measured by laboratory values, charts, and graphs, beginning nurses sometimes overlook or miss them completely. Subtle changes are sometimes clues that more dramatic changes are coming, so the nurse will need to carefully note any increases or decreases in symptoms. The following clinical situation demonstrates this.

> *Gloria was admitted to the psychiatric acute care unit because she was jogging down the center of a busy boulevard with two-way traffic and taunting motorists. She was wearing multiple layers of brightly colored clothes, high heels, and excessive jewelry. On admission, she shouted about the indignity of having to be in this facility against her will, which she called a "violation of her personal, important rights." Gloria was diagnosed with bipolar disorder, mania type.*
>
> *After several days of quiet surroundings, consistent unit routines, staff interventions, and medication (which she had stopped taking before admission), Gloria calmed down. Staff reports and charting stated that she seemed ready to return home.*
>
> *However, just before discharge, Gloria's contact staff person noted that Gloria began to change her clothes every few hours and that the content of her conversation centered on "very important" things that she was planning to accomplish when she got home. The nurse asked her if she had been taking her medication. Gloria admitted that she had been flushing all of her medications down the toilet because she was getting "too normal to accomplish her plans." Her discharge was postponed.*

Nursing Opportunities. Be prepared to routinely assess the patient's behaviors and responses to treatment and the environment. Observing and interacting with the patient throughout the day, careful listening during shift reports, and conferring with other staff members are important. Also consider the following:

- Be aware of even subtle changes in the patient's symptom pattern.
- Avoid absolute (i.e., black-and-white) thinking.

- Be prepared for and accept an unpredictable course toward wellness.
- Avoid predicting outcomes regarding patient progress.
- Keep patients' expected outcomes hopeful but realistic.

Symptoms are dynamic and are often more like changing shades of gray than black and white. Observe for the fluctuation of symptoms rather than static, set patterns of behaviors and responses. For example, a patient who is paranoid demonstrates mistrust by being loud and accusatory on admission. He then quiets down but remains guarded, suspicious, and controlled on subsequent days. The symptom of paranoia is the same, but the manifestations change depending on the patient's internal stimuli, the unit environment, the present situation or events, and the patient's personality style.

In addition, have care plans that reflect a realistic appraisal of the patient's symptoms with expected outcomes that indicate a reduction in symptoms (i.e., "more or less") rather than a total absence of symptoms (i.e., "all or none"). Interdisciplinary treatment plans aim at symptom reduction within reasonable time limits, with the expectation that patients will achieve these objectives with assistance. Symptom "cure" is an unreasonable expectation for some patients.

Avoid Evaluative Responses

Patients respond more favorably to interpersonal communication and treatment when they do not feel that they are under a microscope, that they are constantly being evaluated, or that they have to perform in a specific way to be accepted. For this reason, nurses avoid making evaluative responses of approval or disapproval that indicate that the patient is good, bad, right, or wrong. Neutral recognition of the patient's appearance, behavior, and progress is more effective. The following example illustrates this principle.

> *Maria, a 47-year-old unmarried woman, was the primary caregiver for her chronically ill mother in their home, and she had devoted her entire life to her mother for the past decade. The mother's condition finally required admission to a nursing home. Maria was hospitalized soon after that time for major depression. She acted shy on the unit and demonstrated low self-esteem in her posture, dress, and interactions. She continually said that her life was meaningless and that she had nothing to live for.*
>
> *Maria's married sister visited and brought Maria clothes from home. Maria chose and wore only drab-colored clothing, she failed to care for her hygiene unless she was encouraged to do so, and she refused to attend most group therapies or activities.*
>
> *One morning, 2 weeks after admission, Maria showered voluntarily and came out of her room in a pale yellow dress, ready for breakfast. Brian, an enthusiastic nursing student, saw her and replied*

loudly so that everyone turned toward her, "Wow, Maria, you sure look better today in that yellow dress than any day since I've been on this unit." Her face flushed, and she turned around. With her head and shoulders drooping, she went back to her room, changed back into her drab clothes, and stayed in her room for the rest of the day, refusing meals and meetings

Withdrawn or depressed patients reject praise for several reasons. One reason is these things do not fit their present feeling and thinking states or their negative self-image. Praise is an evaluative comment of approval, and it conflicts with a depressed person's mindset of "I am unlovable," "No one cares about me," or "I am unworthy." There is also evidence in that clinical example that Maria experiences anxiety in social situations. The student nurse's praise that drew attention to her from others in the room had an additional negative impact on her.

Another reason why some depressed patients recoil from praise about their progress is because they fear external support may be withdrawn when they are still feeling vulnerable and in need of help. They often sabotage their own progress and revert to old behaviors to cling to support. In addition, sometimes patients are not well enough to maintain the new expected behaviors. When they fail, they may feel even more unworthy, as if they let the staff down in addition to failing themselves.

Evaluative comments of disapproval are equally nontherapeutic and may reinforce pathology. Patients may perceive either strong approval or disapproval as parental or authoritarian and reject such statements for that reason.

The nurse faces two challenges with regard to this principle. The first comes with awareness and the conscious decision to avoid using strong evaluative comments and statements and to instead learn and practice using neutral statements. Neutral interactions show recognition, acceptance, and respect for the patient without attaching requirements or qualifications. An example of a neutral statement that could be made to Maria is presented below.

The second challenge comes with overcorrecting and making the mistake of acting or being indifferent. Giving neutral statements of recognition to the patient is far from being indifferent.

Indifference toward a patient who is mentally or emotionally compromised is on the top 10 list of the worst characteristics of a nurse or therapist. Indifference quickly dampens or completely deflates a patient's spirit, and it decreases the patient's motivation and will to engage in his or her own process of getting well. It is the antithesis of effective psychiatric nursing practice.

Nursing Opportunities. The following suggestions will guide nurses when they are making responses:
- Give neutral recognition.
- Avoid evaluative statements.

- Be neutral but not indifferent.
- Comment about the patient's behaviors and not about the patient.

With these principles in mind, one example of a therapeutic response to the patient in the previous scenario would be as follows: "Good morning, Maria. You are already showered and dressed. I'll walk down to breakfast with you."

The neutral statement implies neither approval nor disapproval by the nurse, but it does offer recognition. The patient is not negated as she would be if the nurse avoided interaction. In addition, the nurse offers her or his presence. The nurse's willingness to be with the patient helps the patient to feel unconditionally accepted as she is, rather than for her appearance or performance. An evaluative statement usually closes communication. Patients withdraw or become defensive, or they may feel unaccepted because they do not meet certain criteria or act in a prescribed way.

There are exceptions to this principle. Well-timed and appropriately placed praise acts as an incentive for patients to repeat or continue a desired behavior. Behavior modification programs make specific use of praise, and, with experience, nurses learn when and how to praise. The nurse will also distinguish between cold indifference toward patients and the effective intervention of *extinguishing* that is used in behavior modification.

Identify and Reinforce Strengths

When nurses first encounter patients and their families in the PMH setting, they invariably focus on patients' disorders and the dysfunctional aspects of human behavior and its causes. The theoretic content and clinical experiences in this specialty are interesting, engaging, and sometimes dramatic. For that reason, nurses sometimes forget or overlook the healthy aspects and strengths of these patients and their families. Nurses may occasionally fail to identify and reinforce strengths, which are the keys to patient wellness and relative independence from the systems that treat them.

Nurses and all other members of the health care team help the patient, the patient's family, and staff to identify patient strengths and work with patients to help them build strengths, increase competence, and develop or regain a purpose for being healthy and staying alive. Unless the patient and his or her family become invested in this pattern, the patient is at risk for failing to overcome life crises or for having trouble learning to live with a recurrent or chronic mental disorder (Figure 2-1).

For many reasons, patients and their families may not be able to identify strengths at the beginning of an acute psychiatric episode. Family members sometimes are in shock or denial, are overwhelmed by the patient's behavior, or are angry about the circumstances that surround the episode. When patients are psychotic, severely depressed, under the influence of substances, or have low self-esteem, they are frequently unable to identify strengths. The family is often able to focus only on one detail at a time, and it is not always the patient's strengths at that point. The nurse assesses patient and family readiness for moving toward any

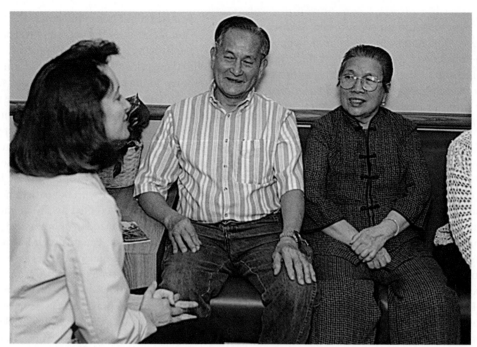

FIGURE 2-1. The nurse interacts with family members as they identify strengths and other positive aspects of their family unit. (From Wilson SF: *Health assessment for nursing practice,* ed 3, St. Louis, 2005, Elsevier.)

positive aspects of the current disruptive event and gives these individuals time to understand and accept what has occurred.

At a time like this, nurses can review the Maslow hierarchy of needs (see Figure 1-1). Patients are not ready or able to self-actualize when their basic needs are unmet as a result of a disruptive episode of a severe mental disorder. However, when the time is right, the nurse will help patients and their families to identify and reinforce their strengths. When strengths are discussed and family members can see some hope for the situation, negative aspects of the situation decrease, and the patient's courage, self-esteem, and motivation begin to increase.

The amount of time that a nurse has available to help patients can be short because of the care model and early discharges. Patients are often discharged well before the staff has time to intervene in all of the areas that they know are important for patients to address to maintain wellness. By discussing patient and family strengths much earlier during the treatment plan, the nurse hopes to grasp the opportunity to help make a difference in the patient's future.

Nursing Opportunities
- Assess patient and family readiness for the identification of strengths.
- Give objective input, and encourage the patient.
- Help the patient to name specific reasons for and benefits of recovering and staying well.
- If the patient is unable to verbalize strengths, modify the plan, or use other methods:

(1) Have the patient make a list of these things after the meeting, and assign it as homework for him or her to think about and complete before next meeting.
(2) Allow more time for the patient to process information.
(3) Have the patient draw the "reasons" in art therapy or express his or her strengths in recreational therapy or in other types of alternative therapy.
- Ask the patient what a valued member of the family, a member of the clergy, or a friend would say about his or her strengths.
- Have the patient attend an interdisciplinary team meeting and hear what the physician and other staff members say are his or her strengths.
- Assign the task of discussing each other's strengths to patients in a process group.

Make Observations Versus Inferences

It is sometimes difficult for the nurse who is new to the psychiatric setting to avoid making inferences about a patient's behavior. An *inference* is an interpretation of a response or behavior; the inference is made by finding motives and forming conclusions without having all of the information. When a nurse makes inferences, she or he interprets the patient's behavior, makes a decision about the behavior's cause, assigns a motive, and forms a conclusion. There is great potential for error and unfairness during this process.

Sometimes while drawing inferences, the nurse is operating from his or her own perceptions, experiences, and frame of reference, which have little or no connection to the patient's actual behavior. In addition, when the nurse makes an inference and forms a conclusion, this removes the patient's opportunity to solve problems and share thoughts and ideas about important issues. A false conclusion can also misdirect treatment objectives.

Experienced nurses often interpret patient behaviors and make correct inferences that lead to therapeutic conclusions. The difference is that experienced nurses take additional steps before reaching their final conclusions, as illustrated in the following paragraphs.

Nursing Opportunities. Solutions to avoid making inferences include the following:

- Respond through observation rather than inference.
- Validate interpretations with the patient to reach mutual conclusions.
- Explore conclusions with the patient.

To avoid making inferences, the nurse strives to understand the patient's viewpoint with regard to situations and events that affect the patient's own life rather than forming a personal opinion. In addition, the nurse draws conclusions by responding to patient behaviors but omits the interpretation. This means that the nurse simply observes behaviors. For example, the nurse might say any of the following:

- "I saw your wife leave, Don, and now you're crying."
- "Yesterday you sat alone, Amber, but today you joined the other children."
- "Jose, what you just said received a major reaction from the group."

Notice that the nurse does not assign motives or reasons or offer any conclusions regarding these obviously significant situations. It may be difficult to withhold opinions, but it is necessary.

The patient usually responds to the nurse's statement, and then communication, reasoning, and problem solving can begin. The experienced nurse continues beyond observation to interpretation. The critical difference is that the nurse immediately validates the interpretation with the patient, and both form a mutual conclusion or at least are aware of the situation for future discussion. Here is an example of the entire process:

(1) "I saw your wife leave, Don, and now you're crying." *(Observation)*
(2) "You said earlier that she was coming in today to discuss a divorce." *(Interpretation)*
(3) "Is that the reason you're crying?" *(Seeking validation)*
(4) "This might be a good time for us to discuss your marriage relationship." *(Offer to explore the situation)*

Notice that the nurse is not guessing but rather is reasoning on the basis of prior information. In addition, the patient now has an opportunity to validate. The last important step is the nurse's willingness to be available to the patient for processing this event with the use of therapeutic communication.

Offer Alternatives Versus Resolutions

Nurses sometimes feel inadequate when they begin to work in the psychiatric setting, because they worry that they do not have answers for patients' problems. They sometimes make the mistake of thinking that they are responsible for resolving problems. However, nurses are not responsible for solving patient problems. Nurses actively listen and guide the patient's process while the patients solve their own problems and find answers that fit their circumstances and situations.

Nursing Opportunities. The nurse considers the following in the interest of helping patients form their own conclusions:

- Assist the patient with expressing his or her concerns and problems.
- Encourage the patient to express his or her feelings.
- Assist the patient to problem solve toward solutions.
- Avoid giving advice.
- Offer multiple alternatives or options only when the patient is unable to come up with them himself or herself.
- Facilitate the patient's ability to making choices.

The nurse engages in therapeutic communication with the patient and facilitates the expression of thoughts and feelings. When the patient is able to listen to his or her own words, the problem-solving process begins, and the patient starts to form his or her own solutions.

Patients will ask the nurse what he or she would do in the same situation. The patient probably does not want the nurse's opinion as much as he or she wants the nurse to stay in the conversation. There is a relief that accompanies expressing problems openly to a willing listener. If the patient asks, "What would you do?" or "What do you think I should do?," the nurse should reply, "I think it is more important for you to decide what works best for you. Let's talk about your ideas."

Telling the patient what to do or how to do it negates the patient's experience. This makes the patient feel less worthy and childlike, as if the nurse is the parent telling her or him how to conduct life. In addition, the nurse's solutions may not fit the patient's situation or lifestyle.

If for any reason the patient is unable to find answers (e.g., depression, cognitive impairment or deficit, shock during crisis), then the nurse may then offer alternatives or options. This means offering assistance and giving some prompting without providing answers or advising. For example, the nurse might say the following:

- "Some things that have worked for other people in similar situations are … [*name several options*]. Do any of these seem reasonable for you?"
- "Have you considered … [*give several choices*]?"
- "What are some of the options that you have for placement when you're discharged?" If the patient has no answer, the nurse may say, "Some that come to mind are … [*give several relevant and appropriate choices*]."

Sometimes the nurse will need to be more direct when helping the patient if the patient does not see any solutions. For example, "You said that you are a workaholic and that you can't relax since you started your own business. What leisure activities have you enjoyed in the past? Which ones would you enjoy now if you had the time? What did you like most about [*whatever activities the patient named*]? Who do you trust to run the business while you are away? Since the business is open Monday through Friday, when could you find time to [*participate in leisure activities that the patient talked about*]?"

Most patients know the solutions, they may just need some assistance to organize their thoughts, bring these solutions into awareness, and take action toward change.

Manage Your Own Frustration

Frustration may occur when expectations are unmet or when a plan fails. Frustration is difficult to experience and tolerate. Nurses enter the PMH setting ready to interact with patients. They have diligently studied theory, practiced communication skills, and written specific and organized care plans, with the expectation that the patient will achieve certain outcomes.

However, interventions are not always successful, and patients may respond in unexpected ways. Some patients who originally consent to a plan of care will change their minds about parts of the plan or later choose not to cooperate. Nurses may experience varying degrees of frustration with these types of responses. In addition, some nurses lose confidence; think they that have failed, or they may feel embarrassed by, rejected by, or even angry with patients who do not cooperate. When this occurs, the nurse must manage his or own responses, find meaning in the patient's responses, discuss the plan of care with the patient, and seek supervision.

Nursing Opportunities. When frustration occurs in an exaggerated way as a result of a clinical incident, the nurse will step back, put the situation into a realistic perspective, and review some basic principles of PMHN. This will involve the nurse examining his or her own reactions and then validating and discussing the situation with appropriate staff, the instructor, or another knowledgeable therapist. In addition, the nurse should review principles of care planning and recall that care plans must have the following characteristics:

- Be patient focused rather than nurse focused: The nurse requires patient input to develop a realistic plan.
- Be goal directed and address the patient's goals rather than the nurse's goals: If the nurse ignores the patient's needs or goals when making the plan, the completion of the objective usually fails.
- Be objective versus subjective in approach: The nurse must keep an appropriate perspective and maintain boundaries regarding the patients, their problems, and their own plans.

An inappropriate reaction to frustration for some beginning nurses is to abandon the plan or, in extreme cases, to abandon the patient. When the nurse has insight and understands that people want and need some control over their lives (even though it may be limited in many cases because of symptoms), the nurse begins to come closer to working *with* the patient rather than *on* the patient. When patients believe that they have sufficient input into their plan of care, cooperation usually increases relative to the patient's capacity to engage. The nurse's collaboration with the patient on a mutually formulated plan of care reduces frustration for both parties.

Some specific patient-focused objectives for the nurse to use as guidelines are as follows:

- Maintain an awareness of the patient's ability and capacity to engage in his or her own care.
- Collaborate with the patient regarding the plan of care.
- Assist the patient with understanding the positive aspects of self-help.
- Encourage the patient to engage in behaviors and activities that are directed toward reducing or eliminating problems and maintaining health and well-being.
- Teach and rehearse with the patient skills that will assist him or her with making change possible.
- Encourage the patient's attempts to improve.
- Continually evaluate the patient's progress and reassess changes.

The nurse benefits from incorporating personal goals that involve helping patients to meet their needs. These include the following:

- Being respectful of the patient's need to maintain some control over his or her own life
- Refraining from the need to complete your own agenda
- Refraining from abandoning the patient if frustration occurs (i.e., look for alternatives)
- Remaining objectively involved in the problem-solving process
- Lightening up and using appropriate humor and relaxation techniques when needed to ease tension
- Reviewing principles frequently
- Getting supervision (i.e., staff, instructor) to validate your own and the patient's progress

ADDITIONAL CLINICAL PRINCIPLES

Clinical experience is enhanced when the nurse integrates basic principles into practice. The previous sets of principles will be useful when interacting with patients in the PMH setting. The following is a list of additional principles that will facilitate the nurse–patient relationship.

1. *Accept the patient's feelings; however, it is not necessary to accept all of the patient's behaviors.* Assist the patient by setting limits on patient behaviors that are self-defeating or that threaten the patient or others in any way. Limits are not punishment; rather, they are external controls that are available when the patient is unaware or unable to use his or her own internal controls. Patients learn that their actions have consequences. Allowing them to do anything that is socially unacceptable not only impedes their progress and insight while under treatment, but it also interferes with their acceptance by society when they are discharged. Set limits, and then follow through by discussing the incident with the patient for the purpose of assessing the patient's understanding, by reinforcing the patient's positive attempts to control behaviors, and by

encouraging and helping the patient to continue the effective behaviors.

2. *Avoid false reassurances, clichés, and global statements.* Give hope, but do not provide false reassurance. New nurses are sometimes uncomfortable with the patient's strong emotions and want to fix the situation or see the patient cured. They say things like, "Don't worry, I bet your wife will come back to help you," "You'll be better in just a few weeks as soon as the medications take effect," "Everyone gets sick some time, and you'll get through this," or "There is a light at the end of every tunnel!" Statements with superficial content and clichés only serve to deny the patient's concern about the severe problems that he or she is facing. Learn to tolerate the fact that all patients in the psychiatric setting are not cured of their mental disorders. Remember to remain hopeful but realistic and willing to assist the patient with his or her process and progress.

3. *Avoid giving advice.* Advice often seems to be the perfect solution, but it does not always fit the patient's situation as he or she perceives it or his or her way of addressing a problem. If patients are not able to assess their own situations, they will not be ready to make changes. Instead, help a patient to identify and formulate alternatives and options and to select what the patient believes will work in his or her unique situation. If the patient is completely blocked and cannot think of any solutions, offer several options. When it is evident that a patient is struggling for answers, some helpful statements are, "Have you ever tried … [*offer two or three choices*]" or "In the past I knew some people with similar situations, and they were successful by doing … [*name two or three solutions for the patient to try*]."

4. *Avoid rescue fantasy.* When a nurse thinks that he or she is the only one who can help a specific patient, it is time to talk with a supervisor. Members of the health care team collectively assist patients with making changes toward wellness. No one staff member does this alone. Nurses who form the idea that they are special in a patient's life may act outside or even against the treatment plan, or they may do the patient favors that are actually nontherapeutic. Stay with the collective treatment plan that has been prepared for the patient, or discuss ideas with the entire health care team before acting on your own.

5. *Use simple, concrete, and direct language with patients.* Avoid psychiatric jargon and language. Patients in the acute-care setting in particular respond better to plainly spoken conversation than they do to language that they do not understand. Patients with low self-esteem are embarrassed or ashamed and sometimes believe that they are not smart enough to understand what the nurse or physician is telling them when medical terminology is used. The patient who is cognitively impaired cannot track long or complex sentences, particularly when they contain psychiatric terms or are abstract in content. Patients who have delusions often misinterpret content. Speaking plainly is most therapeutic.

6. *Avoid heroics.* When a nurse notices that a patient's behavior is starting to get out of control or aggressive, then that nurse should get help. Failing to act soon enough often leads to a patient's loss of control over his or her own behavior, which could lead to unnecessary injury to the patient or others. Use good judgment and be safe in all cases by getting help from other staff members instead of trying to intervene alone or to change the patient's behavior by yourself.

7. *Consider the clinical setting the patient's laboratory.* Create a physically and emotionally safe and supportive environment for patients to practice their newly learned skills. Encourage patients to discuss and role-play situations and events with the nurse, in individual therapy, or in supportive group therapy sessions. Often patients are able to solve many of their own problems when nurses make themselves available to discuss patients' ideas and to let them practice new behaviors with the nurse's guidance.

8. *Encourage patients to take responsibility for their own actions, decisions, choices, and lives whenever they are capable.* Avoid fostering dependence. This may occur in stages, with a healthy mixture of nurturing, encouragement, limit setting, teaching, coaching, releasing control, and role modeling. There is no one perfect recipe, and the ingredients vary with each patient. With genuine support from staff, most patients learn to structure their own lives within the parameters of their abilities and support systems.

REWARDS

Nurses who actively engage in the clinical practice of PMHN for an extended time give multiple reasons why they choose the discipline. PMH nurses describe their professional involvement with patients as meaningful, purposeful, and amply rewarding. Nurses in this field will often plainly say that their role "fits" them.

Skilled and experienced RNs gave the following responses about the intrinsic rewards that they receive while working with patients and their families in the psychiatric setting:
• "In other clinical settings, there was never time to talk to patients or their families. I enjoyed the work, but the patient load and lack of time forced me to focus 90% on the person's physical problems or illness and I never really get to learn the human side of the patients or help with those needs. I felt that my job was only partially done and that somehow I cheated the patient. The PMH setting allows time for the human being."
• "It's a privilege to be paid for doing what I love to do, which is talking and working with patients in what I consider a purposeful, professional way, with a strong emphasis on interpersonal interactions. No other setting gives me so much opportunity to do just that."
• "Psychiatric nursing calls on all of my educational background. I thought I was going to only have conversations with patients all day long, but that's not so. My knowledge and skills from every area of nursing are constantly being

challenged, causing me to integrate information and data. For example, people are admitted with psychiatric diagnoses, but in addition may have a variety of medical problems, or are pregnant, or dying, or need surgical attention and are unable to communicate symptoms. Critical thinking is definitely necessary here. It is stimulating and satisfying."

- "Nurses frequently work with patients in other health care settings who have physical pain, but patients in the psychiatric setting often live with agonizing mental and emotional pain. I am glad to be part of the team that helps them find ways to ease the pain or to help patients just find meaning for it."

- "Intervening with a suicidal patient who voluntarily stares death in the face is a constant challenge. Then, with watchful intervention a patient will turn that corner and return from hopelessness. It is a very humbling experience to see life revisited and embraced, and is only one important reason why I stay."

- "Working with the patients often means working with their families. Frequently in this setting, a family member's mental disorder seriously disrupts the family's functioning. It's wonderful to see them change with intervention and education and time. It is especially rewarding to see them unite again."

- "Never a dull day! Each day brings unexpected events. Keeps me on my toes like no other position I ever held."

- "With experience, psychiatric nurses learn to see immense progress in even the smallest changes made by patients who struggle with severe and persistent mental disorders. To the untrained eye, or the uncaring individual, these changes seem insignificant, or worse are completely overlooked. But the experienced and astute nurses know that common daily routines are often difficult for these patients to meet. They recognize patients' efforts as sometimes being heroic for them, and we encourage them. What is more rewarding than to take part in a patient's conquests in their daily personal struggles?"

- "To see patients reach the point where they identify their own solutions to problems, and gain insight that has potential for changing their lives, is very rewarding. When they stop defending themselves or blaming others for all their problems and begin to take appropriate responsibility, then their existence often takes on new meaning. I am glad to be a witness, especially knowing that my colleagues and I have played some small role in facilitating their progress."

- "It is good to observe a calm patient who was admitted the previous day for violent behavior that was dramatically out of control. It's difficult for patients in turmoil over their disorders, but it's rewarding to see them gain control and take actions toward managing their own wellness. Nurses help them do that."

Rewards are a natural consequence of interacting with patients on their journey to wellness. As in all other nursing disciplines, not all events in the psychiatric setting are rewarding, but many in fact are just that. Nurses are amply rewarded as they help patients to manage their symptoms and to become more resourceful and hopeful. With the focus on human behavior, each unpredictable day presents a unique set of challenges and satisfactions for nurses who are providing care for people in psychiatric mental health settings.

CHAPTER SUMMARY

- PMHN is a dynamic profession that has seen dramatic clinical advances and role changes over the past several decades. However, it remains steadily focused on its core: patient-centered care.
- Notable nurse leaders were pioneers that molded and set a foundation for the current PMH conceptual, theoretic, and clinical frameworks.
- PMH nurses follow the trend toward EBP and integrated patient care.
- The therapeutic alliance is an invaluable vehicle that is collaboratively used by the nurse and the patient in the PMH clinical setting to affect patient change and growth.
- Establishing and maintaining a therapeutic nurse–patient relationship requires the nurse's knowledge and awareness of personal and affective characteristics that are additionally reinforced by learned principles and techniques.
- Helping others is a complex concept and activity in the treatment of patients in the PMH clinical context. Nurses must clarify their motives for helping others.
- Clinical PMH principles provide nurses with opportunities to increase their knowledge and skills for interacting with patients in any clinical setting.
- Establishing and modifying priorities are essential skills for nurses in all nursing disciplines. However, they are critical skills in the PMH setting, where unpredictability is the norm.
- Several examples set into clinical vignettes will assist the nurse with clarifying clinical situations.
- Experienced nurses state that they gain many rewards from working with patients in the PMH setting.

REVIEW QUESTIONS

1. A beginning psychiatric nurse grew up with a mother who had schizophrenia. The nurse recalls feelings of embarrassment and anger about her mother's behavior in the community. Select the best ways for this nurse to cope with her memories. You may select more than one answer.
   1. Recognize that the memories are unhealthy. The nurse should try to forget them while working with patients.
   2. Reexamine the choice of psychiatric nursing as an appropriate area of practice. Explore other specialties.
   3. Begin each new patient relationship with the statement, "My mother had mental illness, so I know what you're going through."
   4. Recognize that early experiences have the potential to positively influence the nurse's practice.
   5. Seek ways to use the information and experience gained from childhood to help patients cope with their own illnesses.

2. Prioritize these outcomes for a patient with mental illness.
   1. The patient will consume at least 50% of every meal within 3 days.
   2. The patient will identify his or her assets and strengths within 1 week.
   3. The patient will describe characteristics of healthy relationships with others within 1 week.
   4. The patient will have a contract with the team to report the incidence of suicidal thoughts within 24 hours.

3. A psychiatric nurse designs an hour-by-hour plan for working with patients for the day. Select the best analysis of this nurse's action.
   1. The nurse has demonstrated goal-directed behavior.
   2. The nurse is likely to feel rewarded at the end of the day.
   3. The plan is likely to result in feelings of frustration for the nurse.
   4. The plan will support the development of the nurse's organizational skills.

4. The therapeutic alliance is a vehicle for patients to accomplish which of the following?
   1. Identifying other patient's problems in group therapy
   2. Gaining insight into their own problems
   3. Forgetting about past emotional abuse
   4. Gaining courage to eliminate support systems after discharge

5. A nurse is assigned to the following four patients. Which patient should receive the nurse's priority attention?
   1. A newly admitted patient who has been diagnosed with major depression whose assessment is incomplete
   2. A patient with schizophrenia who is having auditory hallucinations of someone crying
   3. A patient who recently became unemployed and who has a 10-year history of daily alcohol use
   4. A patient with disorganized schizophrenia who has difficulty completing activities of daily living

REFERENCES

Dossey BM: *Florence Nightingale: mystic, visionary, healer,* Philadelphia, 2000, Springhouse.

Fineout-Overholt E, Johnston L: Teaching EBP: implementation of evidence: moving from evidence to action, *Worldviews Evidence Based Nurs* 3(4):194-200, 2006.

Fortinash K, Holoday Worret P: *Psychiatric mental health care plans,* ed 5, St. Louis, 2007, Mosby Elsevier.

Haber J, Peplau HE: The psychiatric nursing legacy of a legend, *J Am Psychiatr Nurses Assoc* 6(2):56-62, 2000.

Institute of Medicine Report 2010 (website): www.IOM.edu/reports/2010/the-future-of-nursing-leading-change-advancing-health.aspx. Accessed October 18, 2010.

Peplau HE: *Interpersonal relations in nursing: a conceptual frame of reference for psychodynamic nursing,* New York, 1952, Putnam.

Rice MJ: Psychiatric mental health evidence based practice, *J Am Psychiatr Nurses Assoc* 14:107-111, 2008.

Vickers R, Weiss SJ: *Florence Nightingale,* Chicago, 2000, Heineman Library.

Weiss SJ et al: The inextricable nature of mental and physical health: implications for integrative care, *J Am Psychiatr Nurses Assoc* 15(6):571-382, 2009.

3

The Nursing Process and Standards of Practice

Katherine M. Fortinash

"Nursing is a significant, therapeutic interpersonal process. It functions cooperatively with other human processes that make health possible for individuals."

Hildegard Peplau

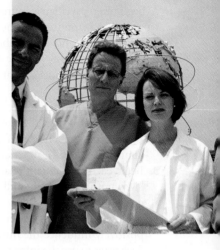

evolve WEBSITE

http://evolve.elsevier.com/Fortinash/

OBJECTIVES

- Analyze the six steps of the nursing process, and list the nursing actions for each step.
- Discuss the roles of critical thinking, expertise, and intuitiveness, and apply them to the nursing process.
- Describe the mental status examination, and discuss its role in physical assessment findings.
- Conduct a nursing assessment on a classmate with the use of the mental status examination and the psychosocial assessment.
- Explain how standardized rating scales help nurses assess patients' functioning and status.
- Describe the North American Nursing Diagnosis Association International taxonomy, and compare an actual diagnosis with a risk diagnosis.
- Develop outcomes that accurately measure patients' achievable behaviors on the basis of their nursing diagnoses.
- Explain the interchangeable role of patient outcomes and behavioral goals for measuring patient achievements.
- Define evidence-based practice, and describe how its critical elements apply to nursing research and scientific reasoning.

- Formulate nursing interventions that describe a course of action or therapeutic activity that mobilizes the patient toward a more functional state.
- Describe the Nursing Interventions Classification and its complementary relationship with Nursing Outcomes Classification and the North American Nursing Diagnosis Association International taxonomy.
- Construct rationale statements that explain the reasons for each nursing intervention in words that improve understanding and ensure nurses' accountability.
- Evaluate patients' progress and achieved outcomes at various intervals along the continuum to ensure accountability for nurses' standards of practice.
- Document patients' progress and responses to treatment with the use of problem-oriented recording (i.e., SOAP notes) that adhere to charting standards.
- Describe the electronic method of documentation in the behavioral health setting, and explain its benefits to patients and personnel.
- Explain the role of the Health Insurance Portability and Accountability Act with regard to patient confidentiality.

KEY TERMS

assessment rating scales
clinical pathway
concept map
critical thinking

cyclic and interactive nature of the nursing process
evidence-based practice
intuitive reasoning
mental status examination

NANDA-I diagnoses
Nursing Interventions Classification
Nursing Outcomes Classification

psychosocial assessment
Rapport
SOAP note
standards of practice

The nursing process is an organized problem-solving method that is unique to nursing and is designed to meet the needs of the patient, the family, the community, and the environment. Its universal language acts as a common thread that unites nurses in delivering quality care to patients in all settings. The relationship between the nurse and the patient gives life and meaning to the nursing process. Although it may be challenging to engage patients with mental illnesses, their participation in the nursing process is vital to its success, because patients are the focus of care. The partnership between the nurse and the patient transforms the nursing process from a conceptual framework to a dynamic problem-solving collaboration in which the patient plays a critical role. This chapter analyzes the six steps of the nursing process according to the American Nurses Association Standards of Practice as they relate to psychiatric mental health nursing (American Nurses Association, 2007).

The Standards of Practice and the Steps of the Nursing Process

Standard I. Assessment
Standard II. Nursing diagnosis
Standard III. Outcome identification
Standard IV. Planning
Standard V. Implementation
Standard VI. Evaluation

HISTORY AND THEORY OF THE NURSING PROCESS

Nurses have accepted the nursing process theory since 1967, when it was described as a four-part process of assessment, planning, implementation, and evaluation. Six years later, in an effort to interpret all of the data that had been collected, a group of nurses from the United States and Canada gathered for the first conference that addressed nursing diagnosis, and they formulated the first selection of nursing diagnoses. Since then, the list of nursing diagnoses has steadily grown, and it continues to be refined as nurses research diagnoses and submit them for approval by the members of the nursing diagnosis association, which is known as the North American Nursing Diagnosis Association International (NANDA-I; see the Nursing Diagnosis section later in this chapter). Today, nurses everywhere agree that the nursing process is a systematic, patient-centered method that is used by nurses in all areas of practice to identify, diagnose, treat, and resolve problems.

Cyclic Nature of the Nursing Process

Nurses believe in the cyclic and interactive nature of the nursing process (Figure 3-1) in which the nurse continuously collects data, critically analyzes it, and then incorporates it into the treatment plan in accordance with the patient's changing responses to health and illness. In 1978, Kritek (2001) recognized that the steps of the nursing process overlap and influence each other and the patient at the same time. She realized that nurses do not always perform the steps of the nursing process in order (i.e., they do not always start with assessment and end with evaluation). Nurses may go back and forth between the steps as the patient's needs change. For example, nurses may continue to assess their patients while also planning interventions, and they may discover new problems to diagnose while constructing outcomes. The nurse needs to closely observe the patient throughout this fluctuating process, knowing that the steps can merge at any given time. The dynamic nature of the nursing process continues to guide and challenge both the new graduate and the seasoned nurse with regard to making reliable clinical judgments and decisions.

Nursing Process as a Scientific Method

Nursing theorists and practicing nurses agree that the nursing process embodies the qualities of a scientific method that is unique to the nursing profession. Some of these qualities include the following (NANDA-I, 2009):

- A systematic, analytic approach to health care that encompasses critical thinking, specific actions, and decision making (see "Critical Thinking in the Nursing Process" later in this chapter)
- Research methods that promote evidence-based standards of practice (see "Evidence-Based Practice in Mental Health Nursing" later in this chapter)
- Standards, principles, and problem-solving methods that have been effective and reliable over time
- A common language and body of knowledge that is universally accepted by medical, nursing, and other health care professionals

STANDARDS OF PRACTICE IN MENTAL HEALTH NURSING

The standards of practice developed by the American Nurses Association, the American Psychiatric Nurses Association, and the International Society of Psychiatric-Mental Health Nurses (American Nurses Association, 2007a) describe the professional activities that the nurse performs during the steps of the nursing process. The standards of practice are listed in the Appendix on the Evolve website, and they are presented here as they apply to mental health nursing. They are the basis for the following:

- Certification criteria
- Nursing's legal definition, which is noted in the Nurse Practice Act in many states
- The National Council of State Boards of Nursing Licensure Examination (i.e., the NCLEX-RN)

Nurses who work in the mental health setting use these standards as guidelines to help them make clinical decisions that provide quality psychiatric mental health care to all patients.

Standard I. Assessment

The nurse assesses the patient's mental status, psychosocial state, physical health, pain level, and nonverbal behaviors with the use of various methods of data collection.

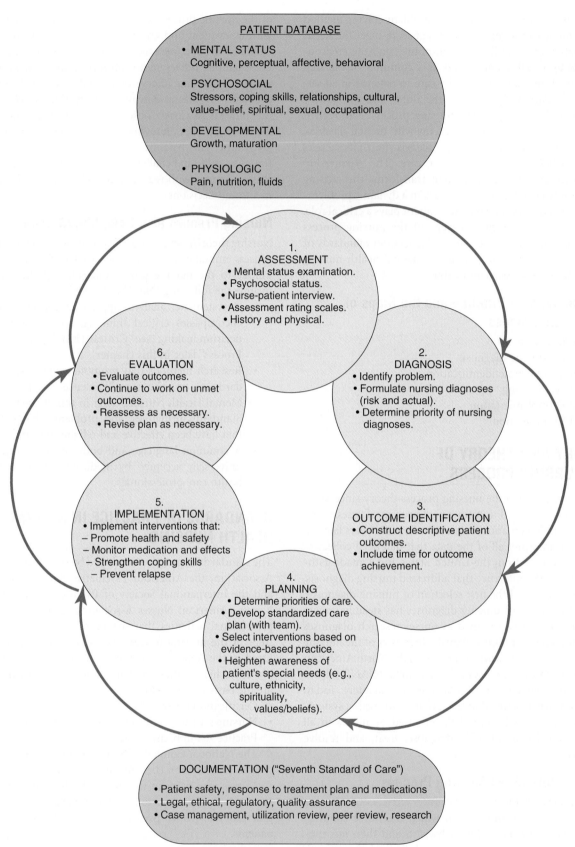

FIGURE 3-1. The cyclic nature of the nursing process and standards of care.

The mental status examination (MSE) and the psychosocial assessment are essential parts of every nursing assessment, and they include the assessment of the patient's physical health and pain level. The MSE is as important to psychiatry as the physical examination is to general medicine. The MSE helps the nurse to collect objective data about the patient's appearance, behavior, activity, attitude, speech, mood, affect, perceptions, thoughts, sensorium, cognition, insight, and reliability. Psychosocial criteria include the patient's stressors; coping skills; relationships; and cultural, spiritual, and work-related issues. The completion of the MSE sometimes involves several interviews, because the patient is not always immediately responsive to all parts of the examination during the acute phase of illness; therefore, patience and persistence are important.

The MSE may be administered to patients who are acutely ill on a daily basis, with the nurse being careful to not overwhelm the patient. Nurses conduct the MSE in a variety of settings other than the mental health unit (see "Assessment Settings" later in the chapter). Box 3-1 describes elements of the MSE and psychosocial criteria. Important steps of the nursing assessment include the following:

- Assess for behaviors or risk factors that threaten the safety of the patient or others (e.g., suicide, self-harm, assault/violence, withdrawal from alcohol or other substances, allergic reactions, command hallucinations).
- Assess for physical pain on a scale of 1 to 10 and for medical problems that may affect patient functioning, mood state, or overall well-being.
- Establish trust, rapport, and respect throughout patient contact. Rapport can be defined as feelings of warmth, acceptance, trust, and non-judgmental attitude between the patient and the nurse that ideally takes place at the beginning of a therapeutic relationship.
- Maintain a calm, empathetic, and nonjudgmental attitude.
- Identify the current problem, and explain it clearly to the patient and his or her family with the use of language that is basic but not condescending; consider the age, ethnicity, culture, sexuality, and language of patient and the family.
- Determine the patient's current level of mental, emotional, and psychosocial functioning; include cognition, mood, affect, coping, relatedness, recent stress or trauma, hygiene, and posture.
- Recognize aspects of the patient's behaviors, vulnerabilities, beliefs, or other areas that require attention to affect a positive outcome. In addition, determine the importance of religion to the patient.
- Conduct an MSE (see Box 3-1).
- Ask the patient and his or her family what outcomes they expect to obtain from treatment; family expectations may differ from realistic outcomes.
- Develop a patient-centered treatment plan, and prioritize problems to be addressed to meet the patient's needs.

The Nurse as the Primary Communicator

The nurse is the primary tool that is used for communication with the patient. Although assessment is the first step in the nursing process, the nurse never stops assessing the patient until the day of discharge, and he or she may even continue assessment throughout follow-up care. Nurses collect a large amount of data through interviewing, observing verbal and nonverbal behaviors, distinguishing between functional and dysfunctional behaviors, and recognizing the patient's adaptation or maladaptation to life stressors. The nurse's broad background and insight into the psychodynamics and psychopathology of human behavior ensure the effective assessment of the patient's overall (holistic) health state. Although a broad base of knowledge is important, the success of the interview relies heavily on the development of trust, rapport, and respect between the nurse and the patient and the nurse and the family. The nurse recognizes the effects of mental illness on the patient's relationships with his or her family and significant others; the nurse treats each patient as an individual and avoids stereotyping or biases that compromise quality care. The nurse is aware of each patient's unique qualities and situations and understands how these qualities and situations influence the patient's response to illness, his or her treatment, and the return to stabilization. The nurse–patient interview allows the nurse to use the senses of sight, hearing, touch, and smell as well as knowledge and experience to explore key topics and concerns that the patient expresses while conducting a thorough (holistic) nursing history and assessment (Box 3-2). It is important to recognize that physical issues sometime present as impairment in mental functioning. Therefore, the nurse always conducts a complete physical and mental assessment of the patient.

Managed Care and Nursing Assessment

Because of managed care regulations and payment issues, a holistic and thorough nursing assessment ensures that the nurse is less likely to miss critical symptoms, such as risk for suicide, risk for violence, other safety issues, or relapse potential. A comprehensive nursing assessment often takes longer than the number of days that the patient has for care; however, a complete assessment is necessary for recovery and to prevent relapse.

The Health Insurance Portability and Accountability Act and the American Nurses Association Code of Ethics for Nursing Assessment

The Health Insurance Portability and Accountability Act (HIPAA) of 1996 guarantees the security and privacy of health information. The final HIPAA Privacy Rule became effective on April 14, 2003, for all health care providers. All patient information that a facility keeps, files, uses, or shares in an oral, written, or electronic form is protected under the privacy rule that defines protected health information. The American Nurses Association Code of Ethics (American Nurses Association, 2007b) also defines the importance of the

BOX 3-1   COMPONENTS OF ASSESSMENT: MENTAL STATUS EXAMINATION AND PSYCHOSOCIAL CRITERIA

Mental Status Examination

Appearance
Dress, grooming, hygiene, cosmetics, age, posture, and facial expression

Behavior/Activity
Hypoactivity or hyperactivity; rigid, relaxed, restless, or agitated motor movements; gait (way of walking) and coordination; facial grimacing; gestures or mannerisms that are passive, combative, or bizarre (e.g., odd repetitive gestures, abnormal movements)

Attitude
Interactions with the interviewer: cooperative, resistive, friendly, hostile, or ingratiating

Speech
Quantity: poverty of speech (few words), poverty of content (lack of content), or voluminous (too many words)
Quality: articulate (well spoken), congruent (makes sense), monotonous (monotone), talkative, repetitious, spontaneous, circumlocutory (circular), confabulation (fabrication), tangential (superficial), pressured (rapid, urgent), stereotypic (repetitive), disorganized (unstructured), or fragmented (broken speech)
Rate: Slowed, rapid, or normal

Mood and Affect
Mood (intensity, depth, and duration): sad, fearful, depressed, angry, anxious, ambivalent (opposing feelings), happy, ecstatic, or grandiose (feeling of greatness)
Affect (intensity, depth, and duration): appropriate, sad, apathetic (indifferent), constricted (narrowed), blunted (little expression), flat (no expression), labile (changing expressions), euphoric (exaggerated happiness), or bizarre (odd or abnormal)

Perceptions
Hallucinations (experiences an unreal presence; can be auditory, visual, tactile, or olfactory), illusions (misinterprets reality; can be auditory, visual, tactile, or olfactory), depersonalization (detachment), derealization (disconnects from reality), or distortions (views objects out of proportion)

Thoughts
Form and content: logical versus illogical, loose associations (fragmented), flight of ideas (rapid thoughts), autistic (internally stimulated thoughts), blocking, broadcasting, neologisms (new words), word salad (mixed-up words), obsessions (persistent thoughts), ruminations (rethinking the same thought), delusions (fixed beliefs), or abstract (conceptual) versus concrete (literal)

Sensorium/Cognition
Levels of consciousness, orientation (awareness of person, place, time, and situation), attention span, recent and remote memory (can recall current and past events), and concentration; ability to comprehend and process information; intelligence, fund of knowledge (sufficient amount of knowledge), judgment (makes rational decisions), and insight (awareness of situation, such as of own illness and reason for hospitalization); and ability to abstract and use proverbs (understands meanings of common sayings and expressions)

Judgment
Ability to assess and evaluate situations, make rational decisions, understand consequences of behavior, and take responsibility for actions

Insight
Ability to perceive and understand the cause and nature of own and others' situations; aware of his or her mental illness and its effects and symptoms

Reliability
Interviewer's impression that individual reported information accurately and completely

Psychosocial Criteria

Stressors
Internal: psychiatric or medical illness, including pain and perceived loss (e.g., loss of self-concept or self-esteem)
External: actual loss (e.g., death of a loved one, divorce, lack of support system, job or financial loss, retirement, dysfunctional family system)

Coping Skills
Adaptation to internal and external stressors, the use of functional and adaptive coping mechanisms and techniques, the management of activities of daily living, and the ability to solve problems associated with daily life

Relationships
Attainment and maintenance of satisfying interpersonal relationships congruent with developmental stage, including sexual relationships as appropriate for age and status

Cultural
Ability to adapt and conform to prescribed norms, rules, ethics, and mores of an identified group

Spiritual (Value Belief)
Presence of a self-satisfying value-belief system that the individual regards as right, desirable, worthwhile, and comforting

Occupational
Engagement in useful and rewarding activity that is congruent with developmental stage and societal standards (i.e., work, school, and recreation)

Modified from Fortinash KM, Holoday Worret PA: *Psychiatric nursing care plans,* ed 5, St. Louis, 2007, Mosby.

BOX 3-2   THE NURSE–PATIENT INTERVIEW: SAMPLE GENERAL QUESTIONS

Presenting Problem

Tell me the reason that you are here in treatment.

Present Illness

When did you first notice the problem?

What changes have you noticed in yourself?

What do you think is causing the problem?

Have you had any troubling feelings or thoughts? If yes, describe them.

Family History

How would you describe your relationship with your parents? If it was troubling, what do you think was the cause?

Did either of your parents have emotional or mental problems? If yes, describe the problems.

Were either of your parents treated by a psychiatrist or a therapist?

Did their treatment include medication or electroconvulsive therapy?

Did the treatment help them? Minimally? Moderately? Greatly?

How was your relationship with them after their treatment?

Childhood and Premorbid History

How did you get along with your family and friends? If you think that there were problems, what do you think contributed to them?

How would you describe yourself as a child? Quiet? Outgoing? Happy? Sad? Angry? Fearful?

If your childhood was troubled, what do you think may have caused it?

Medical History

Do you have any serious medical problems? If yes, describe them.

Are you taking any illegal substances?

Do you drink alcohol? If yes, how often and how much?

How have these conditions affected your current problem?

Are you experiencing pain? (If yes, complete a pain history and assessment.)

Psychosocial and Psychiatric History

Have you ever been treated for an emotional or psychiatric problem? Have you been diagnosed with a mental illness? Substance abuse? Alcoholism?

Have you ever been a patient in a psychiatric hospital or in an alcohol or drug rehabilitation facility?

Have you ever been in counseling or therapy for an emotional or psychiatric problem?

Have you ever taken prescribed medications for an emotional problem or a mental illness? Did you ever have electroconvulsive therapy? If so, did the treatment help your symptoms or problem?

How frequently do your symptoms occur? About every 6 months? Once a year? Every 5 years? Or is this your first episode?

How long are you generally able to function well in between the onset of symptoms? Weeks? Months? Years?

What if anything do you feel may have contributed to your symptoms? Nothing? Stopping taking medications? Beginning to use alcohol or street drugs?

Recent Stressors and Losses

Have you had any recent stressors or losses in your life? If yes, describe them and the effects that they had on you.

What are your relationships like? Poor? Fair? Good?

How do you get along with people at work? Well? Not well? If not well, what do you think is the reason for this?

Education

How did you do in school?

What were your grades like? Poor? Fair? Good?

Did you get along well with your teachers? With other students? If not, what do you think was the reason?

How did you feel about school?

Were you active in school activities? If not, what do you think prevented you from being involved?

Did you drink or use drugs while in school?

Did you get into trouble while in school? If yes, what happened, and how was it resolved?

Legal

Have you ever been in trouble with the law? If yes, describe the problem and how it was resolved.

Martial History

How do you feel about your marriage? (If patient is married)

How would you describe your relationship with your spouse? Poor? Fair? Good?

How would you describe your relationship with your children? (If patient has children)

How involved are you in your children's lives? Minimally? Moderately? Greatly?

What kinds of things do you do as a family?

Social History

Tell me about your friends and your social activities.

How would you describe your relationship with your friends? Poor? Fair? Good?

Do you and your friends support each other equally?

Support Systems

Who would you turn to if you were in trouble?

Do you feel you that need someone to turn to right now?

Insight

Do you consider yourself different now from the way you were before your problem began? In what ways?

Do you think that you have an emotional problem or a mental illness?

Do you think you need help for your problem?

What are your goals for yourself?

Value-Belief System, Including Spiritual

What kinds of things give you comfort and peace of mind?

Will those things be helpful to you now?

Continued

BOX 3-2   THE NURSE–PATIENT INTERVIEW: SAMPLE GENERAL QUESTIONS—cont'd

Special Needs, Including Cultural
How can staff help you during your treatment?
What kinds of things will be most helpful to you now?

Discharge Goals
How do you want to feel by the time you're ready for discharge?
What do you think you can do to help yourself reach that goal?
What things will you do differently from the way you did them before?
What things can you do to help prevent your symptoms from recurring and stay out of the hospital?
What are your goals for taking your medication each day as prescribed?

How will you manage your leisure time?
What activities do you plan to do each day (e.g., swimming, exercise, sports)?
Are there community centers in your area that can help you with these activities?

Patient Participation
Would you like to add anything to the topics that we have covered?
Contact the staff at any time with questions or concerns that you may have.
Thank you for your contributions to this interview.

---

confidentiality of patient information. At the time of admission to a mental health facility, patients often sign a release of information document that specifies what information will be released, for what purpose, to whom, and over what period of time. In compliance with HIPAA and the American Nurses Association Code of Ethics, patient assessment data are shared only with authorized health care personnel who are caring for the patient, and only the information related to the care and safety of that patient is discussed. Nurses must conduct patient assessment in a private area to ensure confidentiality and never discuss the assessment, even with other caregivers, in open areas such as elevators, stairways, hallways, or the hospital cafeteria, where others can hear it. Written patient information must never leave the designated charting area, and the information is placed in the patient's medical record and not anywhere else. When nursing students or other health caregivers take notes during a report, they should shred the notes in the nursing station before leaving the area and make sure that the notes do not contain the patient's name (see Chapter 9 for more information about legal and ethical issues).

Intuitive Reasoning and Expertise in the Nursing Process

Intuitive reasoning is when a nurse applies insight into a situation without first performing a critical analysis. A "strong hunch" or a "gut feeling" is an example of intuitive reasoning, which most nurses agree is compatible with scientific reasoning, because both are likely linked to practice and experience. A nurse learns intuitive reasoning through clinical practice rather than from school or books. Benner's significant work, *From Novice to Expert: Excellence and Power in Clinical Nursing Practice* (2001), described the role of intuition among critical care nurses. She concluded that the nurses' reasoning that was based on both intuitiveness and science often reflected superior insight and sensible judgment when delivering nursing care. Fidaleo (2008)—a clinical psychiatrist, author, and educator specializing in suicidality—stated that

"a gut feeling does not come out of nowhere." He noted that it generally comes from a patient who transfers his or her pain to a nurse who approaches the patient in a "neutral state," which means that the nurse is open and accessible to the patient's feelings and emotions. This type of intuitive reasoning is especially important when assessing patients who are suicidal, as in the following example:

A patient tells a nurse that a staff member told her that she is no longer suicidal and that she has no need for close supervision. The patient says that she is looking forward to some privacy, and she proceeds to enter her room. Although the patient appears calm and self-assured, the nurse decides to follow her into the room. As the nurse quietly stands in the room, the patient sits on her bed and begins to cry. The nurse sits on a chair next to the patient, and the patient confesses that she was thinking about taking a whole bottle of medication that she had been saving. When the nurse was later questioned about his nursing actions, he stated that he had a gut feeling that made him stay with the patient at this particular time and that he did not feel the patient should be alone. The patient admitted that it was the nurse's caring and concern that made her express her suicidal feelings and intentions at that moment.

The critical analysis and skills that come from a broad background of knowledge and clinical practice reflect the level of expertise that a nurse has. Both expertise and intuitive reasoning are necessary for making reliable clinical judgments, and both influence phases the nursing process. Expertise and intuition are worthwhile goals that nurses continue to pursue and develop throughout their professional lives.

Critical Thinking in the Nursing Process

Critical thinking is a concept that includes judgment, intuition, and expertise. Critical thinking skills develop over time and increase the nurse's expanding knowledge base. Like the nursing process, it is a circular rather than a linear method. The nurse generally selects a course of action that is based on knowledge, experience, and scientific principles. This requires hypothesizing many possible reasons for a problem so that the nurse doesn't make rapid or hasty diagnoses.

Critical thinking skills include the following:

- The nurse hypothesizes alternative problem-solving methods for assessing patients when the usual methods fail.

Example: A patient is unable to speak, but his cognition is intact, so the nurse consults with a speech therapist, who suggests an alphabet board with words and pictures to help the patient to communicate.

- The nurse distinguishes meaningful data from irrelevant data, validates critical data through observations and communication, and retrieves the data when necessary.

Example: A nurse discovers that a patient who was initially viewed as independent has real concerns that her suicidal thoughts will return when she is discharged home. The nurse validates this critical data through more intense observations and communication.

- The nurse combines knowledge, experience, and judgment from nursing courses and other disciplines and applies her broad background to all aspects of the nursing process.

Example: A nurse is concerned that the nurses' notes do not provide a complete picture of a certain patient, so she reviews physician and laboratory notes and discovers that abnormal glucose levels may be contributing to the patient's agitation (Table 3-1).

Assessment Settings

Psychiatric nurses often conduct mental status examinations with patients in a variety of settings other than a mental health unit. This includes the emergency department, the intensive care unit, the medical-surgical unit, the home environment, a school, a correctional facility, a community center, a homeless shelter, or in private practice. Examples include the following:

- A senior citizen with chronic depression who is living at home
- A teenager with multiple injuries who is brought to the emergency department
- A critically ill and grieving father in the intensive care unit
- A homeless mother and child staying at a local community shelter
- A child with mental and emotional problems in a school health clinic
- A family's anxiety about a parent's forgetfulness, brought up during a routine doctor's visit
- A juvenile who attempts suicide while staying in a correctional facility

TABLE 3-1	EXAMPLES OF MOOD CHANGES ASSOCIATED WITH ABNORMAL BODY CHEMISTRY
LABORATORY RESULTS	**ASSOCIATED BEHAVIORS**
Abnormal blood urea nitrogen or electrolyte levels (related to kidney disease); abnormal liver enzymes	Agitation, depression, and lethargy (sluggishness)
Abnormal glucose and insulin levels (related to diabetes)	Changes in mood and sensorium; possible agitation
Positive toxicology screen (i.e., the presence of prescription or illicit drugs)	Possible violence (see Chapters 15 and 23)

NOTE: Paradoxically, with elderly patients, behaviors such as agitation and irritability are also associated with such conditions as difficulty with urination, dehydration, fecal impaction, and pneumonia. These conditions must be thoroughly explored before they become life threatening.

The nurse has many opportunities to observe the patient and to adjust assessment data according to the patient's continued responses to the environment, the treatment regimen, and the progress made during hospitalization or in the outpatient setting.

Assessment Sources

Ideally, the patient is the primary source of information. If the patient is too ill to offer a complete or accurate health history, a reliable source such as a family member or a friend may be interviewed on the patient's behalf. For example, patients who are extremely confused, delusional, hallucinating, unable to speak, or unconscious cannot be interviewed, so the nurse will rely on others. However, as soon as the patient is able to respond, the nurse can approach the patient for information. Information given by anyone other than the patient needs to be evaluated in terms of that person's relationship with the patient. For example, a person who is not familiar with the patient's behavior or who is not on good terms with the patient may not provide accurate information about the patient's problem. It is useful to check the information with other sources as much as possible. The medical record is also a source of information if the patient has a written history. It is important to review the most current patient information as soon as it is available, because past records, although helpful, do not always completely describe the patient's current response to mental illness. Many hospitals provide electronic charting, so nurses are able to access recent patient information in a quick, efficient manner. Laboratory studies also provide useful information about the patient's body chemistry, abnormal liver enzymes, and drug levels in the blood. Abnormal body chemistry sometimes

TABLE 3-2	STANDARDIZED RATING SCALES*	
SCALE	**ASSESSMENT PURPOSE**
Hamilton Anxiety Scale	Anxiety
Beck Inventory	Depression
Geriatric Depression Scale	
Hamilton Depression Scale	
Mania Rating Scale	Mania
Brief Psychiatric Rating Scale	Schizophrenia
	General psychiatric assessment
Abnormal Involuntary Movement Scale	Extrapyramidal side effects
Mini-Mental State Examination	Cognitive disorders
Alzheimer's Disease Rating Scale	
Eating Disorders Inventory	Eating disorders
Body Attitude Test	
Brief Drug Abuse Screen Test	Substance use disorders
Global Assessment of Functioning Scale	Level of overall functioning

*Nurses and other mental health professionals can use these scales to help assess patient status and to plan patient care. It is important to note that patient responses may be subjective.

results in personality and mood changes as well as violent behaviors (Table 3-1).

Consultation with the patient's physician will also help to clarify information found in the medical record. Other health care team members will also have observations about patients. Usually the staff is careful to not allow past negative experiences with a patient to influence the current assessment. Student nurses are a significant help to staff, instructors, and psychiatrists for expanding the patient's database. Police officers who transport patients with psychiatric problems to the emergency department have information about the patient's behavior as well. Regardless of the source of information, it is critical to confirm the database as much as possible. If the nurse cannot confirm that the information is true and correct, he or she should make sure to document that the information is unverified. An assessment that is based on good and verifiable data is the foundation for logical clinical judgments and the framework for the patient's treatment plan.

Assessment Rating Scales

Several standardized assessment rating scales are used to assess and monitor a patient's psychiatric diagnosis, mental functioning, and abnormal behaviors (Table 3-2). Usually a clinical nurse specialist, a psychiatric nurse practitioner, a psychologist, a licensed social worker, or a psychiatrist administers these rating scales. Some scales are self-administered with guidance.

Standard II. Nursing Diagnosis

The nurse diagnoses the patient with the use of subjective and objective data that are analyzed during the assessment phase.

Nursing diagnoses are statements that describe a person's health state and responses to actual or potential health problems. They are based on reliable clinical judgments made by the nurse after an extensive nursing assessment as described in the previous section.

It is critical for the nurse to select nursing diagnoses that are based on an accurate assessment of the patient's immediate needs, because these diagnoses are the basis for the selection of therapeutic outcomes and interventions that will move the patient toward wellness.

History of Nursing Diagnosis

Throughout history, nurses attempted to identify patient responses to illness and performed specific tasks within their scope of responsibility under the auspices of the physician. The word *diagnosis* as it applied to nursing first emerged in the literature during the 1950s. During the 1970s, the American Nurses Association began writing its standards of practice and correlating those standards with the nursing process, of which nursing diagnosis is a critical part. The term *nursing diagnosis* has therefore been integral to the nursing process and the standards of practice since the 1970s.

The formalization of the nursing diagnosis concept began in 1973, when the First Task Force to Name and Classify Nursing Diagnoses convened. The North American Nursing Diagnosis Association International (NANDA-I) has defined the term *nursing diagnosis* as "a clinical judgment about an individual, family or community response to actual or potential health problems/life processes which provide the basis for definitive therapy toward achievement of outcomes for which the nurse is accountable" (NANDA-I, 2009, page 41) This text uses NANDA-I diagnoses and terminology to unite nurses with a common language that defines nursing diagnoses and treatments.

Nursing Diagnoses: Actual and Potential

A nursing diagnosis is either an actual problem that the individual is currently experiencing or a potential problem that is called a *risk diagnosis*. An obvious example of a risk diagnosis is the risk for suicide, in which there are risk factors that indicate that an individual is at risk for suicide, such as a history of suicide attempts or verbal threats of suicide. Risk factors replace the etiology and defining characteristics that accompany an actual diagnosis, because, with a risk diagnosis, the actual problem has not happened, so there are no defining characteristics. In addition, the etiology usually refers to the probable cause; because there cannot be a cause without an effect, there is no etiology or cause with a risk diagnosis. NANDA-I states that a nurse is able to change any actual diagnosis on the NANDA-I list to a risk diagnosis if the problem has not occurred yet. A risk diagnosis becomes an actual diagnosis if the problem happens. Box 3-3 lists examples of actual diagnoses and risk diagnoses. Figure 3-2 describes risk and actual diagnoses in the context of the nursing process. NANDA-I also includes health promotion and wellness diagnoses as categories that are less commonly used in acute care settings. See a complete list of NANDA-I approved diagnoses on the inside back cover of this text.

Mental Disorders as Defined by the *Diagnostic and Statistical Manual of Mental Disorders*

In the medical model of psychiatry, "health problems" are the mental disorders in the *Diagnostic and Statistical Manual of Mental Disorders* (DSM). The first DSM edition was published in 1952, and the fifth edition is scheduled for release in 2013. The patient's diagnosis consists of five parts or axes according to the current DSM, which is the fourth edition, text revision, that was published in 2000 (DSM-IV-TR):

Axis I   Psychiatric diagnosis
Axis II   Personality disorder or mental retardation
Axis III   Medical diagnosis
Axis IV   Psychosocial stressors
Axis V   Global assessment of functioning

The Global Assessment of Functioning (GAF) Scale measures a patient's overall functional state at the time of admission and within the past year. The GAF Scale is one of the tools that nurses use to assess patient functioning and possible prognosis. It is coded on a numerical continuum, with 91 to 100 indicating superior functioning and absent

---

BOX 3-3   **FORMAT FOR NURSING DIAGNOSES: RISK AND ACTUAL**

Risk Diagnosis (Two Parts)
Part 1: Nursing Diagnosis (Potential Problem)
Risk for suicide

Part 2: Risk Factors (Predictors of Risk Problem)
History of suicide attempts
Verbal remarks about possibly harming the self ("I just want to end it all"; "I think I'd be better off dead")
Low impulse control

Actual Diagnosis (Three Parts)
Part 1: Nursing Diagnosis
Posttrauma syndrome

Part 2: Etiology (Probable Cause)
Overwhelming anxiety as a result of the following:
   Rape or other assault
   Catastrophic illness
   War or disaster

Part 3: Defining Characteristics
Reexperiencing of traumatic event (i.e., flashbacks)
Repetitive dreams or nightmares
Intrusive thoughts about a traumatic event
Excessive verbalization about a traumatic event

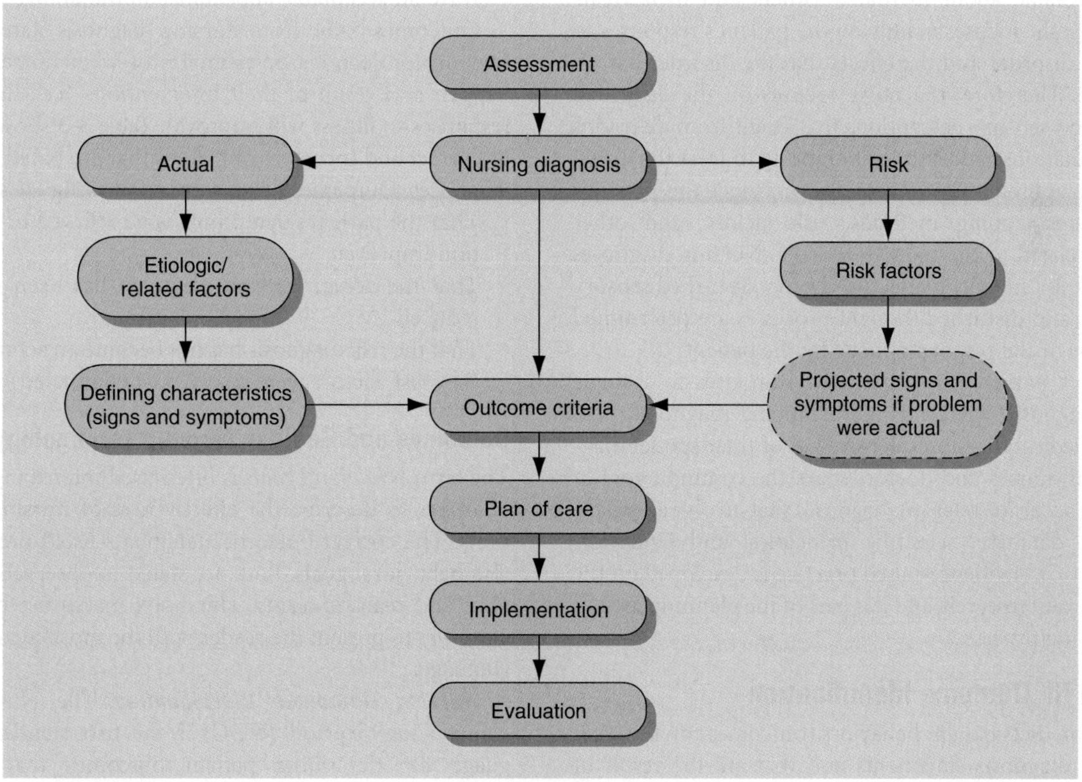

FIGURE 3-2. The nursing process, depicting the actual and risk diagnosis format of the six-step process.

symptomatology, and 1 to 10 indicating severe or persistent danger, and possible suicidality. Most GAF scores are comprised of the numbers in between these two extremes. Patients with severe and persistent mental illness have low GAF scores usually in the 30s that remain virtually unchanged at the time of admission and within the past year. Patients with acute disorders that are more amenable to treatment, may have a low GAF score on admission, but a noticeably higher one within the past year; that is, because these patients often function well until they encounter a stressor that tends to lower their score dramatically. GAF scores are shown in the Axis V section of the DSM-IV-TR Diagnoses boxes in the nursing care plan and concept map sections throughout this text. The DSM-V is due to be published in 2013 and may modify or change the GAF and other parts of its manual to reflect current research.

Nursing diagnoses come from the medical diagnoses; their relationships with each other are discussed in the next section. The complete DSM-IV-TR classification is shown in the Appendix on the Evolve website.

The Relationship of Nursing Diagnoses and Medical Diagnoses

Nursing diagnoses are based on patient responses and needs that the nurse is able to treat. They differ from medical diagnoses in that the medical diagnosis names the disease.

In psychiatry, the medical diagnosis is a mental disorder such as schizophrenia. The psychiatrist focuses mainly on the disease state of the diagnosis and works to find the cause, treatment, and cure, if a cure is possible. Although the nurse is knowledgeable about mental disorders and their treatments, he or she focuses mainly on the patient's responses to the mental disorder and the effects that the disorder has on the patient. Therefore, the nurse focuses on the disturbed thoughts and sensory perceptions that result from delusions and hallucinations rather than attempting to treat the disorder of schizophrenia. The nurse also manages the patient's vulnerabilities, coping methods, risk factors, and other responses related to the mental disorder. Nursing diagnoses such as risk for suicide, ineffective coping, disturbed sensory perception, and disturbed thought processes are determined on the basis of the responses made by the patient.

Because a patient can have many responses to a single medical diagnosis, there are more nursing diagnoses than there are medical diagnoses. Regardless of their special diagnostic focus, nurses and doctors share the common goal of developing accurate, relevant diagnoses that involve a sensible assessment database, scientific principles, and evidence-based practice. (Evidence-based practice is developed on the basis of relevant research, and it is part of the planning section of the nursing process.)

Standard III. Outcome Identification

The nurse predicts patient behaviors (outcomes) on the basis of nursing diagnosis statements and that are the result of nursing interventions.

Outcome statements are specific, measurable indicators that nurses use to evaluate the results of their interventions. They are measured along a continuum, and they describe the best health state that the patient can realistically achieve. The nurse states outcomes in descriptive, measurable terms that begin with action verbs instead of using vague, nonspecific terms. Timelines are most accurate in actual patient situations rather than in hypothetical cases; they are thoroughly discussed in the outcomes sections later in this chapter.

The following are examples of correct outcomes (i.e., outcomes that are descriptive, with measurable timelines):

The patient will:
- Verbalize the absence of suicidal thoughts and plans in 24 hours.
- Display an absence of self-mutilating behaviors in 24 hours.
- Interpret environmental stimuli accurately in 36 hours.
- Contact staff when experiencing troubling thoughts and feelings in 24 hours.
- Interact socially with patients and staff in 36 hours.
- Bathe and dress self by 8:00 AM each day in 72 hours.

The following are examples of incorrect outcomes (i.e., outcomes that are not descriptive and that do not include timelines):

The patient will:
- Not be overwhelmed by suicidal feelings.
- Have no self-destructive tendencies.
- Not hear voices.
- Talk to other people on the unit.
- Have an acceptable appearance in the dining room.

Outcomes come from nursing diagnosis statements, and they are projections or estimates of what nurses expect to happen as a result of their interventions (i.e., that patient's responses to illness will improve). Table 3-3 shows examples of correct and incorrect outcomes that are based on nursing diagnoses. Outcomes illustrate the following:
- That the patient's symptoms were relieved or their function improved
- That the actual nursing diagnosis has been resolved or reduced
- That the risk diagnosis has not become an actual diagnosis (i.e., risk factors were resolved or eliminated)

Outcomes and Goals in Nursing Terminology

The term *behavioral goals* is often used interchangeably with *outcomes* to describe the effectiveness of nursing interventions. The correct outcome statements listed previously are also behavioral goals. Both are stated in observable, measurable, and realistic terms. This book makes use of the term *outcomes* to present the reader with the most current nursing language.

Nursing Outcomes Classification. The Nursing Outcomes Classification (NOC) is the first standardized language for describing patient outcomes that are most responsive to nursing care or that are most influenced by the

TABLE 3-3	CORRECT AND INCORRECT OUTCOME STATEMENTS	
NURSING DIAGNOSIS	**INCORRECT OUTCOME STATEMENT**	**CORRECT OUTCOME STATEMENT**
Anxiety	Exhibits decreased anxiety; engages in stress reduction	Verbalizes feeling calm and relaxed, with an absence of muscle tension and diaphoresis; practices deep breathing
Ineffective coping	Demonstrates effective coping abilities	Makes own decisions to attend groups; seeks staff for interactions rather than remaining isolated in room
Hopelessness	Expresses increased feelings of hope	Makes plans for the future (e.g., to continue therapy after discharge); states "My kids need me to be well"

actions or interventions of nurses. NOC outcomes contain indicators that are rated on a five-point continuum, which allows the nurse to measure a patient's mental or physical state in relation to an outcome (Moorhead et al, 2008).

The Nursing Outcomes Classification's Outcomes Continuum. Unlike goal statements, NOC does not use short-term and long-term outcomes in its classification system. The outcomes that are used throughout this text comply with NOC outcomes that are "variable concepts that reflect patient states (e.g., mobility, hydration, coping) that can be measured on a continuum rather than as discrete goals that are met or unmet" (Moorhead et al, 2008, p. 15). Outcomes reflect the patient's actual health state at the time of achievement and are met at any place along the continuum. Some outcomes are achieved in less time than others, and the nurse continues to intervene with the patient until the patient reaches all outcomes at the highest possible level.

The Nursing Outcomes Classification's Relationship With the North American Nursing Diagnosis Association International and the Nursing Interventions Classification. NOC outcomes appear appropriately in each care plan throughout this text to reflect how NOC outcomes are related to the language of NANDA-I diagnoses and the Nursing Interventions Classification (NIC) (Bulechek et al, 2008). The interventions sections of the care plans include NIC, and the implementation section of this chapter further describes NIC.

Table 3-4 provides a comparison of NANDA-I diagnoses and NOC outcomes.

Outcome statements are the opposite of defining characteristics or risk factors. This helps the nurse to establish areas that require improvement. Examples are listed below, followed by NOC statements:

Defining characteristics: Body odor, soiled clothing, disheveled appearance

Outcomes: Displays clean body and clothing and a neat physical appearance

NOC: Self-care: activities of daily living

Risk factors: History of suicide attempts, verbalizes intent to commit suicide

Outcomes: Verbalizes absence of suicidal thoughts and plans as well as an absence of suicidal gestures

NOC: Risk control, suicide self-restraint

Outcomes and Timeline Projections. Nurses often rely on their background of knowledge and practice, the information

TABLE 3-4	COMPARISON OF NANDA-I DIAGNOSES AND NOC OUTCOMES
NANDA-I DIAGNOSIS	**NOC OUTCOME**
Impaired physical mobility	Mobility
Hopelessness	Hope
Deficient knowledge	Knowledge: disease process
	Knowledge: medication
	Knowledge: health behavior
	Knowledge: treatment regimen
Constipation	Bowel continence
Diarrhea	Bowel elimination
Stress urinary incontinence	Urinary continence
Reflex urinary incontinence	Tissue integrity: skin and mucous membranes
	Urinary elimination
Interrupted family processes	Family functioning
	Family physical environment
	Family coping

Data from North American Nursing Diagnosis Association International: *NANDA nursing diagnoses, 2009-2011, Definitions and Classification,* Ames, Iowa, 2009, Wiley-Blackwell.

that they have about the patient, and the patient's usual response to treatment to predict timelines for outcomes. Although it is useful to suggest a measurable timeline, in actual patient situations, outcomes do not always occur when they are expected. Sometimes other factors influence the outcomes, such as when the patient misses a dose of medication, receives a troubling phone call, or has a discussion with a visitor or when the discharge date is changed. In addition, concepts such as anxiety, hopelessness, powerlessness, or ineffective coping require the patient's subjective perceptions and often resist measurability. Outcome statements such as "patient appears less anxious," "patient seems more hopeful," or "patient copes effectively" do not give measurable criteria for patient achievement. Outcomes should be stated so that they clearly describe patient behaviors and use the patient's own words to describe his or her feelings and thoughts, as appropriate. It is important to include some type of measurement tool or limits for predicting patient progress or problem resolution (see the outcome examples listed previously in this section).

Standard IV. Planning

The nurse plans and prioritizes patient care with the patient, the physician, and the interdisciplinary team.

The planning of patient care builds on the previous three phases of the nursing process, and it is crucial to the ultimate selection of nursing interventions that will help to provide successful patient outcomes. The planning phase consists of the total planning of the patient's treatment to achieve quality outcomes in a safe, effective, and timely manner. Nursing interventions with rationales are selected during the planning phase on the basis of the patient's identified risk factors and defining characteristics. The nurse's planning process includes the following:

- Meeting and working with patients, family members, and treatment team members
- Identifying priorities of care
- Coordinating and delegating responsibilities according to the treatment team's expertise as it relates to patient needs
- Making clinical decisions about the use of psychotherapeutic scientific principles with the use of evidence-based practice

Evidence-Based Practice in Mental Health Nursing

Evidence-based practice is a frequently used term in the psychiatric literature. It refers to practice that is based on evidence and scientific principles that have been developed through research. The more closely clinical practice reflects relevant research, the more likely it is that patients will receive the best available care. A review of the evidence-based practice literature stresses the importance of including empiric methods in clinical practice when relevant rather than using only intuitiveness, experience, fashion, or ideology, because many research findings conflict with public beliefs about mental health. Many health care facilities regularly promote research studies as part of their goal to provide quality, evidence-based practice for their patients. Advanced-practice mental health nurses play a critical role in the development of performance improvement projects for their discipline and then include these findings when planning patient care.

The Research for Evidence Based practice box describes a therapeutic staff's effect on patient outcomes. The information was taken from a longitudinal study.

Clinical Pathways

A clinical pathway (also called a *critical pathway* or a *care map*) is a standardized multidisciplinary planning tool that monitors patient care through projected caregiver interventions and expected patient outcomes and that is based on the patient's DSM mental disorder. The pathway is mapped along a continuum of chronologic targets, and it usually includes an estimate of the patient's length of stay which is based on the designated related group of mental illnesses and the patient's need for continued treatment.

The pathway projects the patient's entire length of treatment from the day of admission through discharge. Figure 3-3 shows a pathway for a patient with bipolar disorder

RESEARCH FOR EVIDENCE-BASED PRACTICE

Pulido R et al: Institutional therapeutic alliance and its relationship with outcomes in a psychiatric day hospital program, *Arch Psychiatr Nurs* 22(5):277-287, 2008.

A study was conducted to explore the institutional therapeutic alliance (ITA), which is the alliance formed by a patient and the entire therapeutic staff acting as a single therapeutic entity that interacts with patients as a whole, and its relationship to patient outcomes. The authors contrast this with Peplau's landmark Interpersonal Relationship Nursing Theory, in which the patient interacts with a single therapist (the nurse) at any given time vs. an entire team. The overall functional level of 55 patients with psychiatric disorders in a partial hospitalization setting, were evaluated on admission, at discharge, and after 3 months. They all gave their consent to participate in the study, and were informed of the purpose. A variety of measurement instruments were used, with a 90-item self-report symptom check list measured on a 5-point Likert scale (0 = no symptoms and 4 = extreme symptoms). The emergence of the alliance relied upon the quality of the relationship between the patient and the therapist(s). The authors noted that the effectiveness of the relationship depended on the patient's ability to form strong alliances. Many patients with severe mental illness have weak capacities for forming real relationships; therefore, more time was spent on alliance-building for these patients. Eight patients left the study prematurely. The institutional therapeutic alliance was assessed after one week of treatment and at discharge from both the patients' and the staff's perspectives. Preliminary findings suggest that the institutional therapeutic alliance represents a specific phenomenon that is different from the classical therapeutic alliance (i.e., patient and therapist), which would be particularly relevant for the treatment of patients with serious mental illness. In terms of treatment outcomes, the authors noted that the therapeutic alliance itself (the first, middle, or final phase of treatment) would be a factor influencing the outcomes only for patients who possessed an optimal interpersonal ability. As for patients with severe disturbances, it could be the development of the alliance itself that helps the patient's improvement, as these patients have difficulty in establishing interpersonal relationships with a single therapist. Future studies are recommended for further confirmation of these findings.

(mania) with an 8-day length of stay. The upper columns list patient outcomes, and the lower columns are categories of care (processes). The evaluation of patient progress is measured daily along the pathway timelines. Nurses primarily initiate pathways, and they involve other disciplines in planning and implementation. A pathway may be extended to include the patient's transfer to home care or to another treatment facility. A pathway that begins in a patient's home or in a home-care situation is developed by the home-care team.

Pathway Variances. Variances are actions that occur when a patient's response "falls off" the pathway, which

Clinical Pathway: Mania
DRG #430 - LOS - 8 Days

	Interval	Day of Admit	Day 2	Day 3	Day 4
	Location				
O U T C O M E S	Physiologic	*Absence of pain *Takes adequate nutrition, fluids with assistance *Complies with lithium level evaluation	*Absence of pain *Demonstrates increased sleep/rest time *Demonstrates adequate elimination	*Absence of pain *Takes adequate nutrition/fluid with reminders *Demonstrates adequate elimination	*Absence of pain *Sleeping 4–6 hours *Demonstrates adequate elimination
	Psychologic	*Involved in stimulation-reducing activities with staff supervision	*Oriented to person and place	*Demonstrates reduction in: movement racing thoughts grandiosity/euphoria irritability	*Demonstrates increased attention span *Reality tests with staff *Oriented to person, place, time, and situation
	Functional Status/Role	*Tolerated orientation to the unit *Refrains from harming self/others with assistance	*Interacting with staff as told *Attends to hygiene/grooming needs with assistance *Refrains from harming self/others with assistance	*Engages in unit activities with staff supervision	*Maintains impulses with reminders *Complies with meds with reminders
	Family/Community Reintegration		*Identifies significant others to staff	*Attends community meetings with staff supervision	*Significant others involved in treatment/discharge planning
P R O C E S S E S	Discharge Planning	*SW Assessment *Identify DC Placement *ELOS, contact family/SO *Nursing Assessment *Identify H/O chronicity *Med compliance, strengths, needs, knowledge deficit	*Team: Involved in DC Planning Discuss with MD *UR notify managed care ( )	*SW eval completed *Treatment Team meeting #1 ( ) *Specific DC plans, placement facility identified ( )	*Involve family/SO in DC plans *Review DC plans with patient
	Education	*Orient to unit *Inform of client's rights *Assess client's and family's/SO knowledge of disorder/meds	*Assist with symptom recognition and importance of compliance *Teach family/SO as needed	*Continue with symptom recognition *Continue assessing patient and family/SO learning needs	*Assist in linking symptoms with precipitating events
	Psychosocial/Spiritual	*Assess: Safety ( ) *Mental status ( ) Spirituality ( ) *Legal status: Vol ( ) 72 hour hold ( ) *Revise Writ ( ) Payor ( ) Conservator ( )	*Continue to assess: Safety issues Mental status Spiritual needs Legal status	*Continue to assess: Safety issues Mental status (e.g. racing thoughts, grandiosity, euphoria, irritability) Spiritual/Legal needs	*Continue to assess: Safety issues Mental status (e.g. racing thoughts, grandiosity, euphoria, irritability) Spiritual/Legal needs
	Consults	*Physical exam within 24 hours	*Other consults as needed	*Other consults as needed	*Other consults as needed
	Tests/Procedures	*Lithium level ( ) *Tegretol level ( ) *Drug screen ( ) *Thyroid function ( ) *CBC/SMAC ( ) *Other ( )	*Tests/Procedures as ordered	*Tests/Procedures as ordered	*Tests/Procedures as ordered
	Treatment	*Monitor: I&O *Sleep/Rest patterns *Level A ( ) *Reduce milieu stimulation *S&R yes( ) no( ) *Other	*Monitor: I&O *Sleep/Rest patterns *Level A ( ) *Reduce milieu stimulation *S&R yes( ) no( ) *Other	*Move to level B ( ) *Continue with treatment plan: Monitor: I&O Sleep/Rest Other	*Move to level B ( ) *Continue with treatment plan: Monitor: I&O Sleep/Rest Other
	Medications (IV & Others)	*Medications as ordered *See relevant protocols: Lithium *Other *Monitor side effects *Toxicity	*Medications as ordered *Continue to monitor side effects/toxicity	*Medications as ordered *Continue to monitor side effects/toxicity	*Medications as ordered *Continue to monitor side effects/toxicity
	Activity	*OT assessment *1:1 brief contacts *Reality orientation *Intervene to manage impulses: prevent harm to self/others	*Engage in stimulation-reducing activities as tolerated *Assist with hygiene, grooming, ADLs *Prevent harm to self/others during activities	*OT eval completed *Encourage hygiene, grooming, ADLs with reminders *Prevent harm to self/others during activities	*Engage in 2 groups per day *Increase group stimulation as tolerated *Prevent harm to self/others during activities
	Diet/Nutrition	*Offer adequate nutrition and fluids; normal salt intake	*Provide simple meals, finger foods, easy to carry drinks	*Encourage meals in client community as tolerated with staff supervision	*Encourage meals in client community as tolerated with staff supervision

FIGURE 3-3. An example of a clinical pathway for a patient with bipolar disorder (mania). *ADLs,* Activities of daily living; *DC,* discharge; *DRG,* diagnosis-related group; *ELOS,* estimated length of stay; *I&O,* intake and output; *OT,* occupational therapist; *SO,* significant other; *SR,* seclusion and restraint; *SW,* social worker; *UR,* utilization review. (Courtesy of Sharp Behavioral Health Services, Sharp HealthCare, San Diego, Calif.)

Continued

Interval		Day 5	Day 6	Day 7	Day 8
Location					
O U T C O M E S	Physiologic	*Absence of pain *Takes adequate nutrition/fluid *Sleeps 4-6 hours *Lithium level in therapeutic range *Other drug level in therapeutic range	*Absence of pain *Sleeps 5-8 hours *Absence of drug toxicity	*Absence of pain *Sleeps 5-8 hours	*Absence of pain *Sleeps 5-8 hours *Able to manage food and activity requirements independently
	Psychologic	*Demonstrates more reality based thoughts *Able to focus on one topic x5-10 minutes	*Demonstrates euthymic mood *Able to focus on one topic x5-10 minutes	*Able to complete activities and unit assignments	*Able to complete activities and unit assignments independently *Able to plan and structure day
	Functional Status/Role	*Demonstrates less intrusive behaviors	*Able to interact with peers *Able to make simple decisions	*Demonstrates safe appropriate activities/behaviors *Independently complies with medical regimen	*Verbalizes need for ongoing medication compliance
	Family/Community Reintegration	*Identifies discharge needs	*Identifies discharge needs	*Identifies discharge needs *Able to identify supports and their appropriate use	*Able to utilize supports and lists ways to access them *States specific plans to manage symptoms, comply with medications, and aftercare
P R O C E S S E S	Discharge Planning	*Assist client/family/SO to identify discharge needs *UR contact managed care as needed ( )	*Continue to problem-solve discharge needs with client, family/SO	*Treatment team meeting #2 ( ) *Transition to Day Treatment if indicated *Assist client, family/SO in finalizing discharge plans	*Discharge to least restrictive environment completed *UR inform managed care as needed ( )
	Education	*Teach client/family/SO about medication effects on symptom management *Instruct in medication, diet, exercise regimen	*Emphasize importance of compliance with meds after discharge *Teach about drug-to-drug effects on symptom management	*Develop aftercare plan to manage symptoms and contact supports	*Reinforce aftercare teaching plan with client, family/SO as needed
	Psychosocial/ Spiritual	*Continue to assess: Safety issues Mental status Spirituality Voluntary status	*Continue to assess: Safety issues Mental status Spirituality Voluntary status	*Continue to assess: Safety issues Mental status Spirituality Voluntary status	*Complete assessments confirm: Safety Mental status Spirituality Legal status
	Consults	*Complete consults as ordered *Arrange for aftercare consults as ordered	*Complete consults as ordered *Arrange for aftercare consults as ordered	*Complete consults as ordered *Arrange for aftercare consults as ordered	*Complete consults as ordered *Arrange for aftercare consults as ordered
	Tests/ Procedures	*Check lithium level for therapeutic range *Check other drug levels for therapeutic range as needed *Tests/Procedures as needed	*Check lithium level for therapeutic range *Check other drug levels within therapeutic range as needed *Tests/Procedures as needed	*Check lithium level for therapeutic range *Check other drug levels within therapeutic range as needed *Tests/Procedures as needed	*Confirm lithium level for therapeutic range *Confirm other drug levels within therapeutic range as needed *Tests/Procedures as ordered aftercare
	Treatment	*Move to level C ( ) *Continue with treatment plan I&O Sleep/Rest Other	*Move to level C ( ) *Continue with treatment plan I&O Sleep/Rest Other	*Transfer to open unit ( ) *Aftercare treatment instructions reviewed with client, family/SO as needed	*DC with aftercare treatment instructions
	Medications (IV & Others)	*Medications as ordered *Contact managed care if any change in medication regimen	*Medications as ordered *Contact managed care if any change in medication regimen	*Medications as ordered *Review of medications with client, family/SO as needed	*DC with medications and instructions as ordered
	Activity	*Encourage: Independent hygiene and grooming Independent ADLs Increased participation in groups	*Engage in all unit activities and groups *Encourage independent decision-making	*Reinforce active participation in all unit activities and groups; independent decision-making	*Confirm: Ability to complete activity assignments independently Ability to make decisions independently
	Diet/Nutrition	*Teach family/SO importance of adequate foods/fluids/salt intake	*Teach family/SO importance of adequate foods/fluids/salt intake	*Reinforce adequate nutrition fluids and normal salt intake	*Confirm client/SO/family knowledge of adequate foods/fluids/salt intake

FIGURE 3-3, cont'd

means that the patient did not respond to the interventions in the typical way. Examples include the following:

Positive variance: A patient responds more rapidly to treatment than expected and leaves the hospital before the estimated length of stay.

Negative variance: A patient fails to achieve the desired state or condition on the projected timeline or by the anticipated date of discharge, so the length of stay is prolonged.

Clinical pathways are tools that promote cost-effectiveness, interdisciplinary care, and accessible patient status reports among staff.

Concept Mapping

A concept map is a problem-solving plan that includes all of the relevant elements of the patient's database (i.e., medical diagnosis, nursing diagnosis, pathophysiology, risk factors, clinical manifestations, collaborative problems, expected outcomes, and interventions.) Interventions include medication, administration, therapeutic modalities, laboratory tests and other procedures, social skills, and teaching and learning needs. This broad profile promotes an understanding of the relationships among concepts, and topics, much like an algorithm. However, unlike an algorithm, the concept map is more interactive than linear in configuration. The patient is the focus of care and data are arranged in a logical structure that show the relationships among the elements via lines or arrows. There is generally a brief case history or case study of the patient's status (i.e., diagnosis, objective data, subjective data, orders) and a summary statement at the end. Students may develop concept maps in place of lengthy written care plans and then present them as PowerPoint programs. Hospitals can use them as efficient reference tools for planning patient care. The structure of concept maps provides the following benefits for students, nurses, and instructors:

- It breaks down complex relevant data into manageable pieces that can be quickly absorbed.
- It promotes an understanding of the patient situation as a whole rather than requiring the nurse to rely on memory or lengthy notes.
- It helps to clarify connections among concepts.

Some nursing programs use concept maps as care plans, and others use them as adjuncts to care plans. Concept maps provide a unique visual framework for the planning of patient care.

(See chapters 10, 11, 12, 13, 14 and 22 for concept maps and associated case studies, nursing diagnoses and NIC and NOC concepts.)

Standard V. Implementation

The nurse sets in motion the interventions prescribed during the planning phase and implements them as meaningful actions.

Some general nursing considerations directed toward patients and families during this phase include the following:

- Promoting health and safety
- Monitoring medication schedules and effects
- Providing adequate nutrition and hydration

- Creating a nurturing and therapeutic environment
- Continuing to build trust, self-esteem, and dignity
- Participating in therapeutic groups and activities
- Developing patient strengths and coping methods
- Improving communication and social skills
- Connecting family and community support systems
- Preventing relapse with the use of effective discharge planning

Nursing Interventions

Nursing interventions, which are also known as *nursing orders* or *nursing prescriptions,* are critical action components of the implementation phase and the most powerful pieces of the nursing process. They make up the management and treatment approach to an identified health problem, and they are selected for the achievement of patient outcomes and to prevent or reduce problems. Nursing interventions describe a specific course of action or a therapeutic activity that helps the patient to move toward a more functional state; they do not simply respond to physician orders.

The following are examples of descriptive, action-oriented interventions:

- Engage the patient gradually in interactions with other patients, beginning with individual contacts and progressing to informal gatherings and eventually to structured group activities.
- Teach the patient and the patient's family that the therapeutic effects of antidepressants sometimes take up to 2 weeks to appear but that side effects often begin immediately.
- Praise the patient for attempts to seek out staff and other patients for interactions and activities and for responding positively to others' attempts at socialization.

The following are examples of nondescriptive, weak, or vague interactions:

- Assist the patient with talking to others.
- Teach the patient and the patient's family about medications.
- Praise the patient for socializing.

The following are examples of interventions that repeat physician orders and that lack definition:

- Monitor the patient's progress.
- Check lithium levels.
- Notify social services.

Nursing Interventions Classification. In NIC, the authors define nursing interventions as "any treatment based upon clinical judgment and knowledge that a nurse performs to enhance patient/patient outcomes" (Bulechek et al, 2008, p. 3). The Nursing Interventions Classification is the first comprehensive standardized classification of interventions for nurses. The NIC states that one should not change intervention labels and definitions so that there is not confusion across settings. However, one is permitted to modify activities to provide individualized care. Box 3-4 lists the NIC definition and accompanying activities for delusion management. NIC interventions are linked to NOC outcomes, NANDA-I diagnoses, and other organizing structures to ensure clear and consistent language for nurses in all practice settings and locations. The NANDA, NOC, and NIC systems are the results of many studies conducted over time by groups of expert nurses who have made use multiple research methods, including clinical field testing. Research continues to define and redefine evidence-based diagnoses, outcomes, and interventions.

Impact of Interventions on Etiologies and Risk Factors. Interventions have the greatest influence when they are focused toward etiologies (related factors) that accompany an actual diagnosis or when the nurse aims them at the risk factors of a risk diagnosis. Etiologies and risk factors change from patient to patient, even when the diagnosis is the same, so it is important to select interventions that target each patient's specific etiologies, risk factors, and defining characteristics (signs and symptoms) (NANDA-I, 2009). The following examples illustrate the effect of interventions on two patients with the same nursing diagnosis of powerlessness but different etiologies:

1. Powerlessness related to a loss of control over mental illness

   As evidenced by: Patient states "Nothing will change my mental condition."

   Outcome: Patient will gain some power and control over his or her mental illness.

Interventions: Teach the patient that mental illness is treatable with medication and therapies.

2. Powerlessness related to an inability to engage in social interactions

   As evidenced by: Patient says "I feel powerless and incompetent in social interactions."

   Outcome: Patient will demonstrate more control and competence in social interactions.

   Interventions: Discuss and role-model competent social interactions with the patient.

Rationale Statements. A rationale statement is the reason for the nursing intervention. Rationales are not always part of the written care plan in clinical practice, yet they are generally part of the overall discussion of treatment in team meetings. Rationales reflect nurses' accountability for their actions. Clear and descriptive rationale statements (shown in italics) follow the interventions in each chapter about disorders to help explain the selected interventions. Consider the following examples:

- Listen actively to the patient's expressed feelings *to show the patient respect and dignity.*
- Engage the patient in brief interactions during the day *to acknowledge the patient's self-worth.*
- Praise the patient for participating in activities *to reinforce healthy and functional behaviors.*

BOX 3-4 DELUSION MANAGEMENT

Definition: Promoting the Comfort, Safety, and Reality Orientation of a Patient Who is Experiencing False Fixed Beliefs That Have Little or No Basis in Reality

Activities

Establish a trusting interpersonal relationship with the patient

Provide the patient with opportunities to discuss delusions with caregivers

Avoid arguing about false beliefs; state doubt matter-of-factly

Avoid reinforcing delusional ideas

Focus the discussion on underlying feelings rather than the content of the delusion (e.g., "It appears that you may be feeling frightened.")

Provide comfort and reassurance

Encourage the patient to validate delusional beliefs with trusted others (e.g., reality testing)

Encourage the patient to verbalize delusions to caregivers before acting on them

Assist the patient with identifying situations in which it is socially unacceptable to discuss delusions

Provide recreational and diversional activities that require attention or skill

Monitor the patient's self-care ability

Assist the patient with self-care as needed

Monitor the physical status of the patient

Provide for adequate rest and nutrition for the patient

Monitor the patient's delusions for the presence of content that is self-harmful or violent

Protect the patient and others from delusion-based behaviors that might be harmful

Maintain a safe environment for the patient

Provide an appropriate level of surveillance or supervision to monitor the patient

Reassure the patient of his or her safety

Provide for the safety and comfort of the patient and others when the patient is unable to control his or her behavior (e.g., limit setting, area restriction, physical restraint, seclusion)

Decrease excessive environmental stimuli for the patient, as needed

Assist the patient with avoiding or eliminating stressors that precipitate delusions

Maintain a consistent daily routine for the patient

Assign consistent caregivers for the patient on a daily basis

Administer antipsychotic and antianxiety medications to the patient on a routine and as-needed basis

Provide medication teaching to the patient and significant others

Monitor the patient for medication side effects and desired therapeutic effects

Educate the family and significant others about ways to deal with a patient who is experiencing delusions

Provide illness teaching to the patient and significant others if delusions are illness-based (e.g., delirium, schizophrenia, depression)

Bulechek M et al: *Nursing Interventions Classification (NIC)*, ed 5, St. Louis, 2008, Mosby, page 254.

Standard VI. Evaluation

The nurse evaluates the patient's outcomes, which reflect the success of nursing interventions.

Evaluation of the patient's progress and the nursing activities involved are critical because nurses are accountable for the standards of care in each discipline. The evaluation of achieved outcomes occurs at various times during treatment as stated in the outcomes section, with the patient's health state and capabilities being the primary considerations. There are two steps in the evaluation phase:

1. *The nurse compares the patient's current mental health state or condition with the outcome statement.* For example, is the patient's anxiety reduced to a tolerable level? Can he or she sit calmly for 10 minutes, attend to an activity for 15 minutes, or socialize with the staff for 5 minutes without distractions? Is there a significant reduction in pacing, fidgeting, or scanning? Did the patient achieve these outcomes within the times that were initially projected? In addition, the degree to which the patient achieves outcomes is an evaluation of the effectiveness of nursing, although other factors influence outcomes as well.

2. *The nurse considers all of the possible reasons that the patient did not achieve outcomes.* For example, sometimes it is too soon to evaluate outcomes, and the plan of action needs to continue for a longer period of time, or the patient may need another 2 days of one-to-one interactions before attending group activities. Occasionally the interventions are too strong and frequent, or they may be too weak and infrequent. Some outcomes are unattainable, impractical, or just not possible for a patient, or sometimes they are not within the patient's capabilities on a developmental or sociocultural level. What about the validity of the nursing diagnosis? Did the nurse develop it with a questionable or faulty database? Does he or she need more data? What were the conditions during the assessment phase? Was the assessment hurried? Did the nurse draw conclusions too quickly? Were there any language, cultural, or other barriers to communication? The nurse will make recommendations on the basis of the conclusions drawn from these questions, and this often includes a review of the previous steps of the nursing process. An informal evaluation of the patient's progress takes place continually.

Documentation: The Seventh Standard of Care

It is mandatory for the nurse to record an evaluation of the patient's changing condition, informed consents (for medication and treatment), response to medication, ability to engage in treatment programs, signs and symptoms (with suicidal and homicidal tendencies being the most critical), concerns (in the patient's words, as appropriate), and any other critical incidents that occur. The nurse performs this documentation in accordance with facility standards. This can be in a narrative, a checklist, or an electronic (computerized) form. Although the entire mental health team is responsible for relating patient progress, the nurse in charge is generally accountable for accurate record keeping. This is critical because documentation involves more than communicating patient progress among team members. Documentation is important for legal issues such as confidentiality and privacy acts, insurance reimbursement, accreditation, quality assurance, case management, utilization review, peer review, and research (see the HIPAA information in the assessment section of this chapter and Chapter 9, and see the managed care information in the assessment and planning sections of this chapter and Chapter 30).

Problem-Oriented SOAP Charting

In an effort to reduce ineffective documentation, Dr. Lawrence Weed, a physician, developed the problem-oriented medical record in 1968. The SOAP note evolved from the problem-oriented medical record in 1969 (Fitz, 2005; Weed, 1969). The SOAP note is a problem-solving method that nurses commonly use in all health care settings to analyze relevant patient problems and to prevent long text. It is a form of *charting by exception,* because the identified problem is an exception to the patient's usual behavior.

SOAP is an acronym for *s*ubjective data (patient statement), *o*bjective data (nurse's observations), *a*ssessment (nurse's analysis of S and O, which is often a problem statement or nursing diagnosis), and *p*lan (nurse's proposed actions). SOAP notes are generally based on problems or diagnoses that are formulated by the multidisciplinary team. SOAP notes then become part of the patient's care plan. Although this promotes consistency during problem solving, it also restricts entries to only identified problems; therefore, recorders need to be aware of other patient issues that happen and to report them as well. Two other letters were added later to the SOAP note: *I* (*i*nterventions, or nurse's response to problem) and *E* (*e*valuation of patient outcomes). There are a number of similar problem-oriented methods, such as DAR (for *d*ata, *a*nalysis, and *r*esponse) and PIE (for *p*roblem, *i*ntervention, and *e*valuation). Table 3-5 is an example of a SOAPIE note.

THE NURSING PROCESS IN COMMUNITY AND HOME SETTINGS

As trends in health care delivery continue to shift to community and home-care settings, psychiatric nurses continue to rely on the nursing process to treat patients outside of traditional inpatient facilities. Areas of assessment include patient safety, the ability to manage symptoms, how patients use effective coping skills, how patients follow their medication regimen, and patients' use of support systems. The psychiatric home health nurse leads the team in identifying outcomes and developing treatment plans and interventions on the basis of problems that are identified during the assessment phase. Community and home care are primary alternatives to hospitalization, and the nursing process plays a major role in helping nurses to deliver effective care wherever it is needed (see Chapter 30).

TABLE 3-5   EXAMPLE OF A SOAPIE DOCUMENTATION NOTE

Admitting diagnosis: Bipolar disorder, mania with psychotic features (persecutory delusions)
Identified problem: Cognitive impairment (patient believes that people are planning to harm him)

S—Subjective data (patient statement)	"I'm sure there are people here who are planning to hurt me; I see them talking and whispering together whenever I'm around."
O—Objective data (nurse's observation)	Patient is hyperverbal; scans the environment; demonstrates worried affect (facial expression); is unable to attend activities for more than 5 minutes; cannot engage in one-to-one conversation for more than 2 minutes
A—Assessment (nurse's analysis)	Disturbed thought processes (delusions of persecution) related to worsening of manic symptoms Moderate anxiety because of belief that staff and other patients are planning to hurt him
P—Plan (proposed action plan)	Reinforce patient safety. Orient patient to reality. Offer medications as needed, and explain reason. Redirect patient and remain with him as necessary. Alert staff of patient's condition.
I—Interventions (response to problem)	Reassured the patient that he will not be harmed on the unit: "You are safe on this unit. No one here will hurt you." Oriented patient in a nonthreatening way: "I know that you think this way now, but those people are staff as I am, and the others are patients." Administered 2 mg of haloperidol (Haldol) by mouth as needed, as ordered Informed the patient that the medication will help to clear his thoughts and reduce his anxious feelings in time Redirected patient to other unit activities and remained with him until his symptoms were reduced and he felt safe on the unit Alerted staff of patient's delusions of persecution and anxious feelings Continued to monitor patient's response to treatment
E—Evaluation (of patient outcome)	Patient's speech has slowed down to a normal pace; he no longer has a worried affect; he is able to attend activities for 10 minutes; he is able to engage in one-to-one conversation for 5 minutes; and he states that his "thoughts are more subdued and less troubling, but still occur off and on." He believes that the medication has helped to reduce his anxiety about his thoughts, and he feels safe as long as staff members are close by and talk to him now and then. He no longer says others are talking about him and planning to harm him; he is spending more time on the unit arranging magazines and watching TV.

Psychiatric Case Management System

Psychiatric case management is a system that identifies candidates who are eligible for home care. A multidisciplinary team led by a registered nurse treats the patients on a health care continuum. The team relies on all available resources to meet treatment goals and to achieve patient outcomes in a quality and cost-effective manner. At one end of the continuum is the highest degree of wellness within the patient's capacity, and at the other end of the continuum is death, with varying levels of wellness and illness in between. The accurate placement of the patient at the entry point on the continuum and a clear understanding of the team's best estimate for the final date of home-care services are critical to the success of case management (see Chapter 30).

CHAPTER SUMMARY

- The nursing process is a six-step problem-solving method that is used by nurses to deliver care in all settings. The six steps are assessment, diagnosis, outcome identification, planning, implementation (interventions), and evaluation. The nursing process was once a four-step method.
- The nursing process is a dynamic and cyclic approach to care in which data are continually analyzed and incorporated into a treatment plan. It is not a linear method. The

patient and the nurse are partners in the process, with the patient as the focus of care.
- The MSE and the psychosocial assessment are the foundations of the psychiatric nursing assessment. The patient's history and the physical examination, including a pain assessment, are also relevant.
- HIPAA mandates the protection and privacy of a patient's health information.

CHAPTER SUMMARY—cont'd

- Evidence-based research, critical thinking, expertise, and intuitiveness are all elements that are used in the nursing process.
- Assessment includes collecting data that are subjective (i.e., the patient's history) and objective (i.e., the patient's mental state and behavior).
- Assessment rating scales are tools that help nurses to evaluate and monitor patient functioning and progress (e.g., the GAF Scale).
- NANDA-I provides nurses with research-based diagnoses, a common language that distinguishes the profession and defines the practice, and a way to ensure accountability for care.
- A nursing diagnosis consists of a problem or need, an etiology (i.e., related factors or probable cause), and defining characteristics (i.e., signs, symptoms, and supporting data). A risk diagnosis consists of risk factors as supporting data and has no etiology.
- NOC and NIC are two nursing classification systems that present taxonomies for outcomes (NOC) and interventions (NIC) that complement the NANDA-I taxonomy and language.
- Outcome statements are highly specific, measurable, achievable indicators that come from nursing diagnoses. Outcomes evaluate patient progress anywhere along a continuum. Outcomes are also known as *behavioral goals.*
- The planning phase consists of the total planning of the patient's treatment approach and the nurse's selection of nursing interventions.
- A concept map is a problem solving plan of care that includes all of the relevant elements of the patient's data base (i.e., medical diagnosis, nursing diagnosis, pathophysiology, risk factors, clinical manifestations, collaborative problems, expected outcomes, and interventions). It promotes an understanding of the relationships among concepts and topics effectively because of its visual pattern that uses lines or arrows to connect the elements related to patient care.
- A clinical pathway is an interdisciplinary standardized format that is used to provide and monitor patient care and progress. The pathway is a projection of the patient's entire length of treatment that begins on the day of admission and continues through discharge.
- The implementation phase involves the actual application of the interventions and the rationale (i.e., the reasons for the interventions) developed during the planning phase.
- Evaluation of the patient's expected outcomes as designated by the outcome criteria occurs at various levels along the health continuum.
- Documentation is often called the "seventh step of the nursing process." The patient's chart is a legal document that effectively communicates patient outcomes, medications, treatments, responses, and unusual incidents. Insurance companies often use these data to justify the patient's hospital stay, so documentation needs to be accurate, timely, and specific.
- A SOAP note is a problem-oriented recording that is based on problems or diagnoses that have been developed by the interdisciplinary team. SOAP notes become part of the patient's care plan, and they promote consistency during problem solving. The nurse should not restrict SOAP notes to only identified problems. *SOAP* is an acronym for *s*ubjective, *o*bjective, *a*ssessment, and *p*lanning. Other types of problem oriented recording methods are DAR (for data, analysis and response) and PIE (for problem, Intervention and evaluation).

REVIEW QUESTIONS

1. The nurse completes a thorough nursing assessment of a new patient. What is the nurse's next action?
   1. Implementing the plan of care
   2. Developing behavioral goals and outcomes
   3. Formulating the nursing diagnoses
   4. Constructing interventions with rationale statements
2. The nurse uses which question to assess the patient's judgment?
   1. What situations in your life have caused you the most anxiety?
   2. What does the saying "People in glass houses shouldn't throw stones" mean to you?
   3. If you had a high fever and were vomiting for 3 days, what would you do?
   4. How would you rate your anxiety level on a scale of 1 to 10, where 10 means panic?
3. Select the nursing diagnosis that best matches the following etiology and defining characteristics. _____

related to lack of approval and perceived lack of respect from others as evidenced by exaggerated or rejected negative feedback about self.
   1. Chronic low self-esteem
   2. Social isolation
   3. Disturbed personal identity
   4. Powerlessness
4. Which of the following diagnostic documentation formats would the nurse expect to see in a psychiatric acute care setting?
   1. I.   Congestive heart failure
      II. 30/60
      III. Schizophrenia, undifferentiated type
      IV. Ran away from board and care home 3 days ago
      V.   Paranoid personality disorder
   2. I.   Substance abuse, alcohol
      II. Antisocial personality disorder
      III. 65/85

IV. Chronic renal failure

V. Arrested for domestic violence 5 days ago

3. I. Generalized anxiety disorder

II. Hypertension

III. 65/75

IV. No personality disorder

V. Loss of employment 1 month ago

4. I. Major depression

II. Dependent personality disorder

III. Diabetes, type 2

IV. Home foreclosed on 2 weeks ago

V. 60/80

5. A patient with bipolar disorder who has been taking lithium is admitted to the mental health unit. In what part of the nursing care plan would the nurse record the following item?

"Monitor the patient closely for nausea and vomiting, muscle weakness, lack of coordination, drowsiness, confusion, and seizures."

1. Assessment

2. Diagnosis

3. Outcomes

4. Planning

5. Implementation

6. Evaluation

REFERENCES

American Nurses Association: *Code for nurses, psychiatric mental health nursing scope and standards of practice*, Silver Spring, Md, 2007a, American Nurses Association.

American Nurses Association: *Standards of practice, psychiatric mental health nursing scope and standards of practice*, Silver Spring, Md, 2007b, American Nurses Association.

Benner P: *From novice to expert: excellence and power in clinical nursing practice*, Menlo Park, Calif, 2001, Addison-Wesley.

Bulechek GM et al: *Nursing interventions classifications (NIC)*, ed 5, St. Louis, 2008, Mosby.

Fidaleo RA: *Suicide assessment and interventions: a videotaped program for nurses and physicians*, San Diego, Calif, 2008, Sharp HealthCare.

Fitz M: *The POMR (problem oriented medical record)*, Loyola University Chicago, Strich School of Medicine, *update*, Oct 2005.

Moorhead S et al: *Nursing outcomes classification (NOC)*, ed 4, St. Louis, 2008, Mosby.

North American Nursing Diagnosis Association International: *Nursing diagnoses: definitions & classification, 2009-2011*, Ames, Iowa, 2009, Wiley-Blackwell.

Pulido R et al: Institutional therapeutic alliance and its relationship with outcomes in a psychiatric day hospital program, *Arch Psychiatr Nurs* 22(5):277-287, 2008.

Weed LL: *Medical records, medical education, and patient care: the problem-oriented record as a basic tool*, Cleveland, Ohio, 1969, Case Western Reserve University Press.

Therapeutic Communication
Interviews and Interventions

Susan Fertig McDonald

"It is the province of knowledge to speak and it is the privilege of wisdom to listen."

Oliver Wendell Holmes

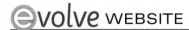 WEBSITE

http://evolve.elsevier.com/Fortinash/

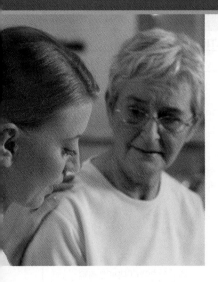

OBJECTIVES

- Analyze the components of communication.
- Discuss factors that influence communication.
- Differentiate among social, intimate, collegial, and therapeutic communication.
- Describe the characteristics of effective helpers.
- Discuss the core qualities of the nurse and the various roles that the nurse plays when interacting therapeutically with patients.
- Explain the principles of therapeutic communication.

- Compare and contrast the communication techniques that enhance and block therapeutic communication.
- Examine therapeutic communication in the context of the nursing process.
- Discuss three special communication challenges and their implications for the future.
- Discuss communication challenges that arise with patients and coworkers.

KEY TERMS

boundary violations
communication
confidentiality
congruent
countertransference
cultural competence
empathy

feedback
genuineness
interpersonal
    communication
intrapersonal
    communication
medium

message
nonverbal communication
positive regard
receiver
resistance
self-disclosure
sender

stimulus
therapeutic communication
transference
verbal communication

Communication is the most powerful tool in psychiatric nursing, and it is the method that is used to activate the nursing process. Communication is the foundation of the nurse–patient relationship in the domain of psychiatric nursing. Hildegard E. Peplau, who was a pioneer and educator in mental health nursing, first identified this concept in 1952. Peplau believed that the therapeutic interaction between the nurse and the patient occurs in the environment of the nurse–patient relationship and passes through distinct but overlapping phases from orientation (admission) to resolution (discharge). As a way to educate nurses about the effects

of therapeutic interaction, Peplau developed process recording, which is a time-proven method that helps nurses to examine the relationship between the nurse and the patient through a written account of the interaction that the nurse records privately directly after the interaction occurs (Table 4-1). Peplau (1991) believed that both the nurse and the patient are equal participants in the therapeutic process and that the overall goal is to improve the patient's health and wellness.

Communication is a dynamic process in which two or more people share all types of information. Because we learn

TABLE 4-1   **PROCESS RECORDING**

NURSE'S COMMUNICATION (VERBAL AND NONVERBAL)	PATIENT'S COMMUNICATION (VERBAL AND NONVERBAL)	COMMUNICATION TECHNIQUES	
		PATIENT	**NURSE**
1. *Verbal:* "Good afternoon, Janet. I'm Heather, a student nurse. I'll be here two evenings a week for about 8 weeks. I'd like to spend some time talking with you about your hospital stay. How does that sound?" *Nonverbal:* open posture, eye contact, moderate voice tone, calm manner, and good spatial boundaries	1. *Verbal:* "It sounds OK to me, I guess, as long as we don't have to talk when I'm scheduled for my cigarette breaks and group activities. I'm making a picture for my daughter. I really miss her." *Nonverbal:* Closed posture, worried facial expression, shaky voice, restless, and fidgeting in chair	1. Agreeing to interact with the condition that the patient's own needs are met; revealing regard for the patient's schedule and her need to bring her daughter something positive from her hospital stay; may be anxious because of the effects of medications or may be nervous about revealing herself to a stranger	1. Offering self and giving information; setting limits and boundaries; open-ended questioning (i.e., therapeutic techniques that build trust and rapport)
2. *Verbal:* "I understand your need to participate in the activities and will not interrupt your schedule. How have things been going for you in the hospital?" *Nonverbal:* Same as in #1	2. *Verbal:* "Oh, not so good. I'm not sure I really belong here with the other patients. Their problems seem really serious. I just want to finish my daughter's picture and then go home." *Nonverbal:* Same as in #1	2. Expresses slightly negative feelings (i.e., "not so good"), which indicates that she has not yet completely regained her mental health; Uses defense mechanism of denial and lack of insight (i.e., "I'm not sure I belong here with the other patients")	2. Acknowledging and respecting the patient's expressed needs; using open-ended questioning and listening skills to elicit patient's perceptions and feelings about her hospital stay and progress
3. *Verbal:* "You don't think you need to be in the hospital? What brought you here?" *Nonverbal:* Leaning slightly toward the patient to show interest, moderate voice tone, and concerned facial expression	3. *Verbal:* "Oh, I guess I just had too much energy and too many thoughts all at one time. I liked it when I had lots of energy, but all of those thoughts were too much for me, and I was confused. I feel better now, and I just want to go home!" *Nonverbal:* Gesturing with arms in the air to show lots of energy, and uses a tone that seems to indicate that she feels the episode was not serious	3. Still denying the problem; appears to minimize the seriousness of her mental illness episode and repeats her desire to go home	3. Using reflectional restatement to repeat the patient's response, so that she can think more about the content of her words; using open-ended questions to elicit the source of the patient's hospitalization
4. *Verbal:* "Tell me about the energy and the thoughts you were having." *Nonverbal:* Eye contact, concerned facial expression, and a tone of voice that indicates interest	4. *Verbal:* "Well, my doctor told me that I had a manic episode, so I must have skipped a few doses of my medication." *Nonverbal:* No eye contact and gesturing with her hands as if to dismiss the seriousness of these actions	4. Patient admits to having episode of mania, which is part of her bipolar disorder; also admits to skipping her medication; body language indicates that actions were not significant	4. Using exploration to determine more fully the patient's experiences; showing interest with nonverbal expressions
5. *Verbal:* "I see. So you're saying your manic episode happened because you stopped taking your medication?" *Nonverbal:* Leaning forward to show interest and slightly frowning to show concern and a desire to understand the patient's admission	5. *Verbal:* "Yeah, I guess I shouldn't have stopped taking my meds, but the side effects were bothering me." *Nonverbal:* Slight eye contact and fidgeting in her chair	5. Admits to experiencing a manic episode and links it to stopping her medications; shows some insight into why she stopped taking her medication and seems to understand the cause and effect of her illness and symptoms	5. Using consensual validation to determine the congruence of nurse and patient understanding

TABLE 4-1   PROCESS RECORDING—cont'd

NURSE'S COMMUNICATION (VERBAL AND NONVERBAL)	PATIENT'S COMMUNICATION (VERBAL AND NONVERBAL)	COMMUNICATION TECHNIQUES	
		PATIENT	NURSE
6. *Verbal:* "Janet, stopping medications because of side effects is very common, but it can also cause your symptoms to return. Perhaps we can talk about the side effects that you were experiencing." Nonverbal: Same As #5	6. *Verbal:* "Yeah, that would be OK. I know it was really dumb of me to stop them." *Nonverbal:* Taking her face in her hands and shaking her head from side to side	6. Seems upset with herself because of her behavior (i.e., stopping her mediations); acting out her frustration by shaking her head and referring to herself as "dumb" when she actually is feeling inadequate	6. Providing information; acknowledging patient's stated reasons for stopping medication; using refocusing to concentrate on a single important point; suggesting collaboration to solve the problems that the patient is having with her medication
7. *Verbal:* "It sounds as if you recognize that stopping your medication may have resulted in your manic episode." *Nonverbal:* Eye contact and empathetic tone and body language *(Moment of silence)* *Verbal:* "Janet, it's OK to question your actions. That is one way we all learn." *Nonverbal:* Eye contact, sitting quietly next to the patient, and having an empathetic demeanor	7. *Verbal:* "I guess so. It's just that I keep making the same mistake and then I end up in this stupid hospital, where I don't belong." *Nonverbal:* Hanging her head low toward her chest and shaking her head from side to side	7. Seems to understand how stopping her medication worsens the symptoms of her mental illness, although she lacks insight as to how her thoughts and behaviors result in hospitalization	7. Acknowledges insight and shows empathy for patient's distress; gives patient permission to express her feelings; makes self available to the patient by sitting quietly and not attempting to leave patient during her time of need
8. *Verbal:* "Today we talked about the connection between the medication you take, your symptoms, and the problems you run into that prevent you from taking your medication. This may be a good point to end our time together today. The next time we meet, let's talk about the ways you might be able to handle the same situation differently in the future." *Nonverbal:* Sitting back with an open posture and offering eye contact 9. *Verbal:* "OK, Janet, I understand. I'll talk to you in a couple of days. Thanks for talking with me." *Nonverbal:* Begins to stand slowly	8. *Verbal:* "OK, that's good, because I need a cigarette now. Thanks for listening. I'll see you next time you're here." *Nonverbal:* Gets up to begin her patio break and makes very brief eye contact with the nurse	8. Patient did well to remain throughout the entire interaction; still has a need to downplay her problems; Uses smoking to help herself cope; agreed to talk to the nurse again; thanked the nurse for listening, which shows maturity and respect	8. Summarized what was discussed and terminated conversation by encouraging the formulation of a plan of action that suggests collaboration

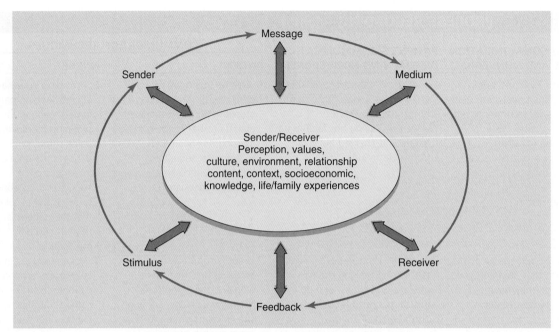

FIGURE 4-1. A model of the communication process.

how to communicate at an early age, this seems like a relatively simple task. However, communication is a complex process that consists of a combination of verbal and nonverbal behaviors that are used in various ways for the sharing of information. Thus, communication requires much practice to be effective.

Effective communication is critical to the successful outcome of nursing interventions, and it is a major factor in the determination of patient satisfaction, treatment compliance, and recovery. Without effective communication, a therapeutic nurse–patient relationship is unlikely to happen. Therefore, the nurse needs to understand and master the general principles of communication as well as the specific principles and benefits of therapeutic communication.

COMMUNICATION PROCESS

Communication consists of several structural components: the stimulus, the sender, the message, the medium, the receiver, and feedback. Usually there is a stimulus or a reason for the communication to occur. The individual who initiates the transmission of information is the sender. Each transmission is both verbal and nonverbal. The information that is being sent and received, such as feelings or ideas, is the message. The method by which the message is sent is the medium. The medium can be seen (visual), heard (verbal), felt (tactile), or smelled (scent). For example, a note or a letter is seen; a shout, a scream, or a whisper is heard; body odor or the scent of perfume is smelled; and a hug or a pat on the back is felt.

The receiver both receives and interprets the message. In an ideal situation, the receiver will interpret the message exactly as the sender intends it, thus resulting in effective communication. The feedback that the receiver provides to

the sender is a means of measuring the effectiveness of the message. Feedback is a continual process, because it is a response to the message, and it provides a new stimulus to the sender, thus causing the original sender to become the receiver. In any interaction, the sender and the receiver continually reverse roles. Figure 4-1 shows a model of the communication process (Berlo, 1960).

FACTORS THAT INFLUENCE COMMUNICATION

Communication is a learned process that is influenced by several factors, including the environment, the relationship between the sender and the receiver, the content of the message, and the context in which the message takes place. Other factors include attitude, values, ethnic background, socioeconomic status, family dynamics, life experience, knowledge level, and the ability to relate to others.

Environmental factors that control the effectiveness of communication include time, location, noise, privacy, comfort, and temperature. The timing of the interaction is also important. The idea of "counting to 10" describes a waiting or cooling off period that is necessary for some individuals to ensure that they are able to rationally discuss a hot topic or understand a critical concept. For example, the nurse chooses to wait for a better time to begin teaching a patient about medications if the patient has just experienced an emotional outburst in the hallway and is unable to concentrate in that environment. A carefully chosen time will mean the difference between successful and unsuccessful patient learning.

The location of the interaction is also instrumental to conveying the sincerity or importance of communication. For example, a man wishes to propose marriage to a woman and chooses a mutually predetermined and romantic place in which to do it. A carefully chosen location means the difference between a "yes," a "maybe," and a "no." If the location is noisy and other people are present, messages in the conversation may not be heard, thereby resulting in ineffective communication. Therefore, the type, quality, and perceived importance of the specific message conveyed depend in part on the general comfort of the environment.

The relationship between the two people in a conversation greatly influences the communication. For example, a casual friend can give the same message to an individual as an intimate friend, but the receiver may react quite differently to each person according to the nature of each relationship.

The context as well as the content of the message also influences the receiver's response. The context or circumstances need to be appropriate to the type of interaction. Individuals need to feel safe in their environment before they disclose highly personal information.

Attitude also affects interaction. It determines how a person responds to another person and includes the person's biases, past experiences, and levels of openness and acceptance. In addition, people from one socioeconomic class, ethnic background, or family background sometimes have difficulty communicating with individuals from a different background or class, possibly as a result of language, differing values, or knowledge barriers. For example, both eye contact and personal space vary greatly from one culture to another.

How a person is raised greatly influences communication as well. Each person's background encourages, models, and discourages different aspects of communication. For instance, if a traditional household teaches that boys are tough and do not cry, this discourages the boys in the family from expressing sad emotions. Another example is a teenager who is continually told to "shut up" because he talks "too much"; this child will develop a quiet or nonassertive style of communication as an adult because of the way that he was raised.

Knowledge differences often create a problem of understanding during communication. If the sender has greater knowledge of the subject matter than the receiver, it is the responsibility of the sender to make sure that the receiver understands the message. This is always one of the challenges when teaching important concepts to students or patients. Some people have an ability to relate to a variety of people and are able to explain complex information in simple, understandable terms. Some have a great deal of difficulty doing this and are easily intimidated by others. Everyone has the ability to learn to communicate more easily and clearly with the use of communication techniques, practice, and feedback regarding their efforts.

Perception is an individual's subjective experience that influences his or her interpretation of the message. Because misperceptions create problems in communication, the sender needs to be certain that the receiver has a clear understanding of the message. Effective communication depends on understanding the message, interpreting the message, and providing feedback that supports the correct interpretation.

MODES OF COMMUNICATION

Written Communication

Written communication is primarily used to share information. The reader reads for knowledge, pleasure, and understanding. It is important that the nurse clearly expresses ideas in written form, whether it is documentation in the medical record or in the form of statistical reports. Because more and more documentation is in the form of a computerized patient record, the ability to navigate through and document within electronic records and templates is essential. The ability to write legibly, spell correctly, use proper grammar, and organize ideas clearly is critical for the nurse. As part of conducting an assessment and providing interventions, the nurse must have the ability to document a patient's behavior in objective, descriptive, clear, and concise terms.

Verbal Communication

Verbal communication is composed of the spoken words that encompass the symbols of language. Precise verbal communication is important, because spoken words often mean different things to different people. Many words or phrases have slang meanings or have developed new meanings. Some words and phrases also have different meanings for different groups. Figures of speech, jokes, clichés, colloquialisms, and other terms or special phrases carry a variety of meanings. For example, the term *blue Monday* means it is a sad day to a person who has the ability to think on an abstract level, but, to a patient with schizophrenia who interprets concretely and literally, it could mean that the sky is blue. *Don't rain on my parade* means "don't spoil my fun" to one person, but, to the patient with psychosis who has loose associations, it prompts a question about whether a parade is actually occurring or the question, "Why would I rain on a parade?"

Cultural Considerations

Individuals from different cultures or generations often misunderstand and misinterpret slang phrases and idioms such as *double dipping, my bad, sick, right on,* and *let's go clubbing.* It is easy to assume that other people understand intended meanings. However, it is necessary to periodically check their interpretation. This includes examining cues that result from nonverbal responses.

It is increasingly important for nurses to develop a greater sensitivity to the cultural aspects of communication. It is clearly a challenge to learn how to communicate effectively with psychiatric patients who not only have difficulty communicating in a clear, logical, or reasonable manner because of their mental disorder but who are also from other cultures and who use English as a second language. Chapter 8 further discusses issues of communication with those from cultural groups that are different from one's own.

Nonverbal Communication

Many communication theorists believe that nonverbal communication is the most important part of any message and that it composes about 93% of any communication. It includes elements that do not involve actual words. Nonverbal cues involve all five senses. They add to the meaning of verbal messages by performing several functions, such as the expression of feelings, the contradiction or validation of verbal messages, and the preservation of both the ego and the relationship. As a general rule, nonverbal behavior is more revealing and truthful than verbal communication. Actions really do speak louder than words. Therefore, it is important for the nurse to observe and consider the patient's entire message—in other words, both the verbal and the nonverbal messages—before arriving at a conclusion.

To be an effective communicator, nonverbal cues need to be congruent or consistent with the verbal message. An example of congruent communication is as follows:

Verbal: "I became very worried when you did not arrive at 4:00 PM."

Nonverbal: Concerned facial expression, warm, friendly, and outstretched welcoming hand

Here is an example of incongruent or inconsistent communication:

Verbal: "I would like to get to know you better."

Nonverbal: Eyes looking away, detached, and arms folded across chest

Nonverbal communication includes facial expressions; eye movements; body movements such as posture, gestures, and touch; appearance; and the use of space, which is also known as *proxemics* (Arnold and Boggs, 2007).

Body Language

Body language includes facial expressions, reflexes, body posture, hand gestures, eye movement, mannerisms, touch, and other body motions. Body posture and facial expressions, including eye movements, are two of the most important cues to determine how a person is responding to the message. When a patient who is frowning with clenched teeth and fists, narrowed eyes, and a red face, says, "I am always glad to see my mother," there is a contradiction between the verbal and nonverbal cues that the nurse needs to address. A slumped or stooped posture sometimes means that a patient is depressed or, at the very least, feeling sad or dejected. A closed posture with arms folded often indicates that a patient is withdrawing or possibly feeling some anger. An erect posture with the shoulders back means that the patient feels more confident or is trying to appear confident. The gait or way that an individual walks also indicates the patient's self-concept. The person who bounces along with shoulders back and head up high usually seems more upbeat than the individual who walks at a slow-moving pace with a slumped posture.

Nurses need to carefully observe hand gestures, because they also signal anger, restlessness, frustration, hopelessness, relaxation, or apathy. For example, the nurse needs to be aware of impending anger so that early interventions can be implemented to prevent a situation from getting quickly out of control. The old saying "when in doubt, observe what people do, not only what they say" is especially important when dealing with psychiatric patients, because what they say and what they do are often dissimilar.

Paralinguistics

Paralinguistic (paralanguage) behavior includes any sound that is not a spoken word. It includes voice tone, inflection, word spacing, rate, emphasis, intensity, groaning, coughing, laughing, crying, grunting, moaning, and other audible sounds. Along with the silent cues, these audible nonverbal cues are important when assessing patients.

Space (Proxemics)

The use of space is another nonverbal cue. Each person has a comfort zone or space boundary that invisibly surrounds him or her during interactions with others. The boundary becomes larger or smaller depending on the nature of the relationship. *Intimate space* is the closest distance between two individuals. *Personal space* is for close relationships within touching distance. *Consultative space* is farther apart than personal space, thus requiring louder speech. *Public space* is for public gatherings, such as when speeches are presented; it usually applies to individuals in a large hall or auditorium.

Space as a concept of boundaries and safety is important to understand, because the nurse and the patient need to respect the distance that each one needs. For example, if a patient has a recent history of assault, the nurse is advised to stay a reasonable physical distance from the patient for obvious safety reasons (Fox et al, 2010). For successful communication to occur, both parties need to feel safe. Some patients have problems with their boundaries and invade other patients' own safe zones; patients who perceive this as threatening react aggressively to such boundary violations. At such times, the nurse may need to help the patient understand the appropriate distance by stating the boundary for the patient in inches or feet, as needed. When the patient violates the nurse's own comfortable space, the nurse will need to set a limit for the patient after the initial intrusion. For example, the nurse can hold out an arm as a way to help the patient to assess boundaries.

Touch

Touch is a nonverbal message that involves both action and personal space. Touch typically conveys a message to the receiver that the sender wants to connect with him or her. Nurses have used touch to send messages of concern and empathy. You must be careful when deciding whether to touch a patient with a psychiatric disorder. Not all patients want to be touched. Some perceive it as a threat and respond with aggression, or they may interpret it as an intimate move and respond with withdrawal or an inappropriate sexual response. Touch as communication is detailed later in this chapter.

Appearance

Appearance nonverbally communicates a particular image as well as a clue to one's mental status. Appearance refers to the way an individual uses clothing, makeup, hairstyle, jewelry, and other items such as hats, purses, or eyeglasses as well as grooming and hygiene. These nonverbal cues often show how the person wishes to be viewed by others.

For example, a female nurse who comes to work wearing a revealing blouse, tight slacks, and high-heeled shoes looks more suitable for a social situation than a work situation. This image does not represent the nursing profession very well, and it may also confuse patients regarding the nurse's role. Another example is an individual who comes in for a professional job interview wearing jeans, a wrinkled knit shirt, and sandals with his hair uncombed and his beard untrimmed. On first glance, the employer wonders if the candidate is serious about employment, because his appearance is too casual and sloppy, thus giving him an unfavorable image; this individual has forgotten the familiar saying, "dress for success." A third example is an elderly woman who is admitted to the hospital wearing dirty, wrinkled clothing. A home health nurse finds her in a filthy apartment, and she has not bathed in several weeks. On further assessment, she reveals that her husband died 2 months ago, and she was subsequently diagnosed with depression. Therefore, her appearance is one result of her obvious unresolved grief response, which has caused her to stop taking care of herself. Try to interpret a patient's nonverbal behavior while evaluating the verbal content, and incorporate this evaluation into the assessment of the patient and the plan of care.

Finally, nurses need to be aware of their own nonverbal cues. For effective communication to occur, make sure that nonverbal messages are congruent with verbal messages, and communicate genuine interest and respect.

TYPES OF COMMUNICATION

Intrapersonal Communication

Intrapersonal communication is essentially talking to yourself or self-talk. During intrapersonal communication, individuals give themselves all types of positive and negative messages. Self-talk is useful if the messages are helpful or positive. Intrapersonal communication is either functional or dysfunctional.

For example, during a session with the nurse, the patient identifies several problems that she needs to work on as well as realistic goals for her hospital stay. The patient then tells herself that she is happy that she has finally accomplished a useful task and is now clear about what she needs to do before she leaves the hospital. In this situation, the patient gives herself positive messages that assist in her recovery.

An example of dysfunctional self-talk occurs if this same individual persists in giving herself negative, self-defeating messages, such as "I can never do anything right" or "I will never meet this deadline." This type of self-talk stops or delays the recovery process.

In another example, a patient with a diagnosis of schizophrenia continually hears many internal voices that tell him he is a "bad person" and that he must kill himself to "cleanse his soul." These internal voices, which are displays of auditory hallucinations, constitute dysfunctional self-talk and may require medication (see Chapter 13).

Interpersonal Communication

Interpersonal communication occurs between two or more individuals and contains both verbal and nonverbal messages. As stated previously, it is a complex process that consists of a variety of factors that affect its outcome. The nurse communicates on an interpersonal level with a variety of individuals and groups throughout the day. The emphasis is on therapeutic communication and collegial communication when the nurse is at work. This chapter briefly discusses social communication, which is a form of communication that is used primarily when one is away from work. The characteristics of social, collegial, and therapeutic communication are presented in Table 4-2.

Social Communication

Social communication occurs in everyday situations, usually away from the work setting. This type of interaction includes discussions about family relationships, social activities, vacations, school, and church. Much of this interaction is superficial and light, and it usually does not have a goal. The purpose of most social communication is to maintain relationships and for the enjoyment and mutual benefit of those involved.

Varying levels of intimacy exist among those who participate in social communication. Communication between a parent and a child carries a level of intimacy that is different from communication between a parent and a teacher. Self-disclosure is common and occurs at varying levels, but superficiality is usually the standard, because there are no real expectations of help. When an individual expects help as the outcome of social communication, friends and family typically give help in the form of suggestions and advice. This type of help differs dramatically from the help that a nurse gives to a patient in a therapeutic relationship.

Collegial Communication

The purpose of collegial communication is professional collaboration. Collegial communication occurs among colleagues in the professional work setting. In professional nursing groups within the work setting and in the community, this type of collegial communication is called *interdisciplinary communication*.

When psychiatric nurses interact with members of the unit's treatment team, it is called *interdisciplinary collegial communication*. The interdisciplinary team has regularly scheduled treatment team meetings that have been designed to develop, review, and revise the patient's treatment plan. It is important that all members involved in the patient's treatment attend and actively participate in the meeting. Members have roles that are critical to the success of the treatment team process. Sometimes the nurse is the designated leader of the meeting and has to clearly communicate with all members of the team. Sometimes the nurse is the recorder or the person who is responsible for documenting the significant

TABLE 4-2	CHARACTERISTICS OF SOCIAL, COLLEGIAL, AND THERAPEUTIC COMMUNICATION		
	SOCIAL	**COLLEGIAL**	**THERAPEUTIC**
Who	Friends, family, and acquaintances	Coworkers and colleagues in community	Nurse and patient
Setting	Home, away from work; any type of setting	Work, away from patients; professional community	Clinical setting; private, quiet, confidential, and safe environment
Purpose	Maintain relationships; mutual sharing of information, thoughts, beliefs, ideas, and feelings	Communicate to other professionals about patients, professional issues, and ideas	Promote growth and change in patients
Content	Social talk; focus on children, vacations, family, leisure, church, doing favors, and giving advice	Patient's treatment plan; professional practices in work area, sharing observations, and best practices	Therapeutic talk; patient expresses thoughts, beliefs, feelings, anxieties, fears, and problems; patient identifies needs
Characteristics	Superficial and light; not necessarily goal directed; spontaneous and enjoyable; two-way conversation that focuses on both sender and receiver; involves giving suggestions or advice; personal or intimate relationship occurs	Collaborative, collegial, interdisciplinary, and patient or issue focused	Learned skills; purposeful and patient focused; patient sets goals; planned, difficult, and intense; patient discloses personal information; meaningful and personal (but not intimate) relationship occurs
Skills	Uses a variety of resources during socialization	Uses collaborative responses, effective interactions in groups, and assertive interpersonal communication skills	Uses specialized professional skills and primarily therapeutic interpersonal communication

information discussed as part of the patient's treatment plan. This role requires skillful written communication techniques. Within a nursing professional group, the intent of the communication is to share knowledge, collaborate on a project, or in other ways enhance or improve the profession.

Effective cooperation has the advantage of breaking through the power issues and competition that occur when teams of professionals are together. During the collaborative process, no member is more important than another member or than the group as a whole. Each member's contribution is equally important to the success of the project, purpose, or goal.

Therefore, the nurse communicates in the collegial arena with supervisors, coworkers, physicians, consultants, members of the treatment team, and the professional community. Simultaneously, the psychiatric nurse communicates on a therapeutic level with patients and their family members or significant others.

Therapeutic Communication

Therapeutic communication is the foundation of psychiatric nursing, and it is the psychiatric nurse's single most important tool. This type of communication is an interactive process that occurs between the nurse (helper) and the patient (recipient) in any health care setting. The art of interacting therapeutically is a learned skill that involves both nonverbal and verbal communication. One purpose of therapeutic communication is to enhance patient growth. Health-promoting interventions also occur with the use of therapeutic communication.

Therapeutic communication is patient focused, whereas social communication consists of sharing information equally between two or more individuals. Although the nurse will engage in some social interaction with the patient, such as greeting the patient at the beginning of the shift, the progress toward a greater level of health occurs via the therapeutic interactions between the nurse and the patient.

This therapeutic interaction involves the patient disclosing personal information, which sometimes includes hurtful memories and situations that bring up painful emotions. Sharing such feelings is extremely beneficial for the patient, because it allows him or her to identify and discuss experiences and accompanying feelings in a safe, therapeutic setting. The nurse provides a confidential and quiet setting in which the interaction takes place, encourages the patient to openly discuss thoughts and feelings, and practices active listening, acceptance, and empathy.

Therapeutic communication is sometimes intimidating not only for the patient but also for the nurse. Intense negative feelings are not easy to discuss. Many patients have not previously discussed them for fear of undesired responses, such as a lack of understanding on the part of the listener, retaliation, feelings of being unworthy, and inadequacy when explaining them. The intensity of the patient's feelings or verbal responses often frightens or surprises the new nurse; this is especially true when a patient openly discusses such issues as wanting to die because life is not worth living. A nurse may also feel uneasy when a patient discusses an emotion or feeling similar to the nurse's personal experience.

If the nurse has not dealt with the personal problem effectively, this may cause anxiety.

In summary, therapeutic communication has three essential purposes: (1) to allow the patient to express thoughts, feelings, behaviors, and life experiences in a meaningful way to promote healthy growth; (2) to understand the significance of the patient's problems and the roles that the patient and the significant people in his or her life play in perpetuating those problems; and (3) to assist with the identification and resolution processes of the patient's health-related behaviors. Therapeutic communication is the nurse's primary tool to help patients attain successful outcomes to the problems that are currently preventing them from achieving optimum health.

PRINCIPLES OF THERAPEUTIC COMMUNICATION

Personal Attributes

Nurses use their own characteristics and selves as the primary tools in psychiatric nursing in the same way that singers use their voices as instruments to create music. All of the elements that are essential to helping another individual are within the nurse. This is both exciting and challenging.

The therapeutic use of the self begins with knowing oneself. You will not be able to help others unless you are first able to help yourself. Knowing yourself is a complex and lifelong learning process. It is essential to have self-knowledge before using yourself as a therapeutic tool to help others.

At the core of self-knowledge is the nurse's ability to correctly identify his or her own negative or unresolved issues. Nurses need to know what values and beliefs they hold. It is also important for them to know and understand their own family backgrounds, including dynamic cultural and social issues, values, biases, and prejudices.

Nurses need to be aware of unresolved family life issues and make every effort to resolve them as soon as they are recognized. For example, a female nurse has a long-held belief about women and alcohol dependency. She believes that others are able to stop drinking if they really want to stop. Her belief developed because her maternal grandmother died as a result of alcohol-related liver disease. The nurse is perhaps unaware that she holds this belief until she has her first alcohol-dependent female patient. It is only when the nurse understands and resolves her own issues that she can truly succeed in the necessary separation of those issues from those of the patient.

One model of communication that can help the nurse to look at self-awareness is the Johari window, which was developed by Joseph Luft and Harry Ingham during the 1950s (Luft and Ingham, 1955). The Johari window consists of four areas or windowpanes framed in a square box. The four panes—(1) open; (2) blind; (3) hidden; and (4) unknown—represent parts of the whole self (Figure 4-2).

To increase self-awareness, one must strive to increase the open area in pane 1 and to decrease the blind, hidden, and unknown areas in panes 2, 3, and 4. Generally, as the

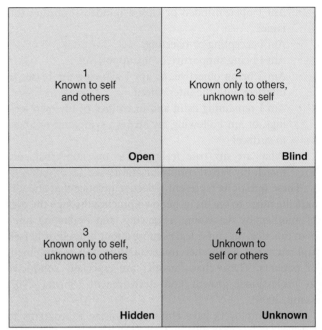

FIGURE 4-2. A Johari window showing the four areas that make up the whole self.

nurse becomes a better communicator, the size of pane 1 increases. As the nurse shares things about himself or herself, pane 3—the hidden area—decreases. In the process of the nurse asking for feedback from others, pane 2 grows smaller. As a result of the nurse becoming more self-aware through interpersonal learning, pane 1, which represents thoughts, feelings, and behaviors that are known to the self and to others, becomes larger as the other three panes decrease in size.

Because therapeutic communication occurs for the purpose of helping others, it is vital that nurses understand what motivates them to help others and recognize their emotional needs so that they do not interfere with the ability to relate therapeutically to patients. Because patients do not take care of nurses' emotional needs, nurses need to meet their own emotional needs outside of work. A well-balanced and multifaceted lifestyle satisfies emotional needs. When your needs are met, you will be able to help the patient through therapeutic communication.

Nurses who are in control of their own lives and emotions engage the patient in effective communication while maintaining therapeutic control of the conversation, especially when a patient is intimidating, manipulative, or threatening.

In addition, nurses who are comfortable with themselves put the patient's needs first by listening attentively and recognizing emotions in the patient that will block a therapeutic exchange. For example, a high level of anxiety produces tunnel vision in a patient, which damages communication.

Finally, a nurse needs to conduct a periodic self-awareness or introspection check with regard to his or her responses to the patient. Questions to ask include the following (Shives, 2007):

- Am I open minded or closed minded regarding this issue?
- Am I accepting or rejecting?
- Am I being supportive or unsupportive?
- Am I being objective, or am I allowing my biases to interfere with the interaction?
- Am I remaining calm and in control of my own feelings, or am I allowing my anxiety, sympathy, or anger to surface?
- What are my true feelings? Do my nonverbal cues match my verbal communication?

These questions represent reflective practice that encourages the nurse to see his or her own practice through the eyes of another. By describing, reviewing, and evaluating one's own practice, the nurse learns more about himself or herself and improves his or her understanding and management of patients. These characteristics are especially conducive to professional growth and development (Shives, 2007; Kemp, 2009).

Many employers have employee assistance programs to help employees with personal issues that occur in the workplace that interfere with their abilities to communicate effectively. Use these employee benefit services to help you deal with personal issues that affect your ability to do your job well.

The Roles of the Nurse in Therapeutic Communication

Nurses assume many roles during therapeutic communication with patients. One is being a professional role model. In the professional role, the nurse acts as teacher, socializer, technician, advocate, parent, counselor, and therapist. As a role model, the nurse is respected by staff, students, and the community. The nurse models therapeutic communication for patients, staff, and students. In the community as well as in the health care setting, the nurse will represent the nursing profession, and others will judge the profession on the basis of the nurse's actions.

Patients learn about their illnesses and treatment methods from the nurse who is acting as a teacher. As a teacher, the nurse uses clear and effective communication to educate other staff and patients. The nurse as a socializer brings patients together for activities to prevent the social isolation of the patient during hospital treatment. In the technician role, the nurse performs a blood glucose level test, administers medications, or takes vital signs. As an advocate, the nurse informs the patient of his or her rights and responsibilities and supports the patient in decision making. The advocate nurse also serves as a protector of the patient by acting as a link between ethics and the law (Arnold and Boggs, 2007). The nurse in the parent role performs traditional nurturing tasks, such as feeding, bathing, and comforting. As a counselor, the nurse assists the patient with personal problems such as a disagreement between the patient and a family member. With advanced education, the nurse can also be a therapist, conducting individual, group, or family therapy sessions in the hospital, clinic, or community setting.

As part of the therapeutic relationship with a patient, the nurse performs some or all of these roles. The number of roles that the nurse assumes varies according to the type and length of the individual nurse–patient relationship as well as the setting of the interactions.

Traits of Therapeutic Communication

The following are traits of effective therapeutic communication: genuineness, positive regard or respect, empathy, trustworthiness, clarity, responsibility, and assertiveness. These characteristics allow the nurse to influence growth and change in others. They incorporate verbal and nonverbal behaviors as well as the attitudes, beliefs, and feelings behind the communication, and they are necessary for therapeutic communication to take place.

Genuineness

Genuineness is demonstrated by being consistent with both verbal and nonverbal behavior. Consistent verbal and nonverbal behaviors show that you are open, honest, and sincere. Genuineness is necessary for patients to develop trust in the nurse. You build trust when you do not appear to just be doing your job but rather when you respond with sincere interest. Genuine interaction does not mean that you have to discuss personal information or relate to the patient in a social manner. Rather, it means that you remain focused on the patient and respond therapeutically with the use of a variety of helpful responses. Do not expect a patient to be open and honest if you do not display these characteristics yourself.

Positive Regard

Positive regard includes respect and acceptance. For example, nurses show that they view their patients as worthy by addressing patients by the names the patients prefer. Nurses accept patients for who and where they are and do not expect them to change except as it relates to their goals in treatment. Positive regard or respect is communicated in a variety of ways. Sitting and listening to a patient, expressing concern about events that affect a patient, validating the patient's feelings, and effectively responding to a patient's negative behavior all communicate respect. For example, a patient who has just been admitted is starting to undress in front of others in the dayroom. After assessing the situation and understanding that this activity is not harmful to others, the nurse explains to the patient that undressing is for the privacy of his or her bathroom. The nurse then closes the door to allow the patient to continue out of the view of others.

Part of positive regard is being nonjudgmental. Avoid harsh judgment of patients' behaviors and feelings, because both are real and cannot be argued with, discounted, or criticized. Do not make patients feel wrong. Labeling behaviors on the basis of your own value system is not useful. Instead, the nurse helps patients to explore their behavior by discussing the thoughts and feelings that determine the behavior. When patients realize that they are not being judged, they will feel free to express their most intimate thoughts and feelings. A nonjudgmental attitude in the nurse relaxes patients by removing patients' fears of being misunderstood or rejected. This open relationship occurs only when nurses identify their own thoughts and feelings about patients' behaviors.

Empathy

Empathy is the foundation of all therapeutic nurse–patient relationships, and it is therefore an essential trait for nurses to have to meet their patient's needs. Empathy or empathic understanding is the nurse's ability to see things from the patient's viewpoint and to communicate this understanding to the patient. The nurse's capacity to be fully and uniquely present with another human being, to be sensitive to that person, and to communicate an understanding of the patient's feelings are essential characteristics of a therapeutic relationship (Carpenito, 2000). Some research implies that empathy is a natural human trait that everyone has in varying degrees and that the trait matures as we grow.

Some researchers suggest that more work is necessary to develop new ways to teach nursing students how to respond empathetically to patients (Walker and Alligood, 2001). Determining levels of empathy in students will help to identify potential problematic levels that are either too low or too high. High levels of natural empathy indicate that the nurse has a tendency to overidentify and thus become too involved with patients' problems. Low levels indicate that the nurse is not able to demonstrate enough genuine concern for patients. Knowing this information will better assist the new nurse with periodic self-assessments.

Empathy should not be confused with sympathy. Sympathy is overinvolvement and sharing your own feelings after hearing about another person's similar experience. It is not objective, and its primary purpose is to decrease your own personal distress.

For example, a patient tells the nurse that his mother died in an automobile accident 2 months before his arrival at the hospital. The nurse responds sympathetically by saying that her own mother died suddenly in an accident and that it had made the nurse feel sad for a year afterward. Here the focus is on the nurse, and the patient does not know how to respond. An empathic response involves an appreciation and awareness of the patient's feelings and keeps the focus on the patient. An empathic response would be the following: "I can understand how difficult that must be for you. Tell me how you are feeling now and how you have been coping with the loss." Now the focus is on the patient, and the patient is better able to reply.

The development of empathy poses a challenge for the psychiatric mental health nurse in the hospital setting, who typically has a brief amount of time with patients and who must primarily use crisis intervention principles. Moderate levels of empathy from the nurse are healthier for patients during the beginning stages of the relationship so the patient will feel understood but not overwhelmed by the nurse's feelings. Research has shown that empathy, especially if it is expressed early during a relationship, is clearly related to positive treatment outcomes, because it is the process that the patient uses to make changes to achieve positive outcomes.

Empathy consists of two stages. When a patient shares important and uncomfortable emotions, the first stage involves the nurse being receptive to and understanding the patient's problem by putting himself or herself in the patient's place. This does not mean that that nurse needs to have had the same problem or associated feeling. One theorist describes this first response as emotional engagement, which may be reflexive or automatic and culturally conditioned. Then, after stepping back into the professional role, the nurse communicates understanding, which demonstrates objectivity and sensitivity to the patient. This second stage is a learned professional response and involves therapeutic empathy (Morse et al, 2006). The following skills help nurses to develop greater empathic responses:

- Attending to the patient physically by sitting in front of the patient at a slight angle and leaning slightly forward with the hands and arms in an open stance
- Attending to the patient emotionally by clearing your mind of other personal or work-related business and focusing your full attention on the patient
- Actively listening by providing a response to each of the patient's verbal and nonverbal communications
- Focusing on the patient's strengths
- Expressing caring, warmth, interest, and concern with the use of nonverbal behaviors
- Determining the most important point of what the patient is trying to say
- Demonstrating consistency between your own nonverbal and verbal communication
- Checking your empathic responses for effectiveness by looking for verbal and nonverbal clues

Active listening, which is considered one of the central elements of understanding (Shattell et al, 2007) is closely associated with empathy, because it incorporates both the nonverbal and verbal behaviors that are necessary for therapeutic communication. Nonverbally, the nurse leans slightly forward and faces the patient, uses eye contact, nods, and uses verbal phrases such as "I see" or "I understand." Active listening is a dynamic and interactive nonjudgmental process. It requires the nurse to listen for facts as well as to try to determine the underlying meaning of the patient's communication, to accurately interpret the meaning, and to provide the patient with feedback regarding the nurse's understanding of the message. The end result of active listening is a full understanding of the meaning of the communication (Arnold and Boggs, 2007). A nurse who listens actively is displaying interest and is engaged. In one study that explored patients' experiences when communicating with nurses, patients reported that the behaviors they valued in nurses were the time that the nurses gave them and the nurses' availability to them (Shattell, 2007). A patient who is trying to work through problems needs to know that the nurse is there to help and that he or she wants to help.

Trustworthiness

Trustworthiness is another essential characteristic of an effective nurse. Trustworthy nurses are responsible and dependable. They keep commitments and promises, and they are consistent in their approach and response to patients. For example, if you tell a patient that you will meet her after breakfast to discuss her treatment goals and then follow through with your promise, you demonstrate dependability and thus increase the patient's trust. Patients need to know that they can rely on the nurse so that trust will be built. Trustworthy nurses respect the patient's privacy, rights, and need for confidentiality. Patients need to be confident that the information they share will not go beyond the members of the health care team.

Clarity

Nurses need to communicate clearly with patients who often have difficulty processing information or thinking clearly as a result of their mental disorders. If the nurse is specific and clear, there will be less miscommunication. Clear communication means selecting simple words when speaking and asking questions to clarify meaning. Although the use of medical vocabulary is part of the nursing profession, remember that patients do not always understand these complex terms. Everyday medical phrases such as *taking your vital signs, NPO after midnight,* and *take these medications at HS* are not common to most patients. Problems will happen if instructions and information are given in a highly technical manner. Patients are often too embarrassed to ask for clarification; they appreciate nurses who not only communicate with them in an open and honest manner but who also use language that is easy to understand. Therefore, the nurse needs to make a conscious effort to speak at a level that the patient will understand. Avoid abstract, lengthy explanations. This is also true for written communication. When using written materials to educate patients, less is more. In addition, make sure that all instructions are written in plain language with the use of the active rather than the passive voice, simple words with one to two syllables, short sentences, clear and straightforward expressions, and a minimum of complex medical terms (Health Literacy Institute, 2010). All written education and instructions should be provided at the patient's level of understanding. If the nurse is not sure about the patient's understanding, ask the patient to teach the material back to you. Examples are as follows:

> *Active, clear, and specific instructions:* "Take your risperidone (Risperdal) 2 mg two times a day with breakfast and dinner as ordered by your doctor." (Be sure to specify the name of the medication and the dosage.)
>
> *Passive, vague, and complex medical terms:* "Make sure that your psychotropic medication regime is strictly adhered to everyday for ultimate efficacy."

Responsibility

Responsible communication involves being accountable for the outcome of professional interactions. When communicating, you are responsible for your part in the interaction, and you need to be sure that your patients receive and interpret your messages correctly. Nurses who communicate responsibly foster growth in others. Responsible language

involves the use of "I" statements when being assertive, as described in the following section.

Assertiveness

Assertive communication involves the ability to express thoughts and feelings comfortably and confidently in a positive, honest, and open manner that demonstrates respect for one's self while respecting others (Balzer Riley, 2007). The nurse who communicates assertively makes a conscious choice about how to communicate with others. Communicating assertively is a style choice that you can apply in any situation at any time. An assertive nurse controls negative feelings, which is important when communicating not only with patients but also with supervisors, employees, physicians, and colleagues. Box 4-1 lists behaviors associated with assertive communication.

BOX 4-1 BEHAVIORS OF ASSERTIVE COMMUNICATION

Assertive
Stands up for own rights and respects those of others; uses expressive, directive, and self-enhancing speech; chooses relevant words and actions

Aggressive
Stands up for own rights but abuses those of others; speaks in demeaning or attacking manner; fails to monitor or control words or actions

Passive
Does not stand up for own rights; accepts the domination and bullying of others; performs unwanted tasks; feels victimized

Examples of Assertive Behaviors
- "I" messages (e.g., "I need," "I feel," "I will")
- Eye contact (e.g., looking directly into the eyes of the person while making or refusing a request)
- Congruent verbal and facial expressions (i.e., making certain that the facial expression matches the intent of the spoken message; a serious message accompanied by laughter negates the credibility of the message)

Example of an Assertive Plan for Change
1. Target the behavior that you want to change (e.g., how to say no and mean it).
2. List approximately 10 situations in which it is difficult to say no, and order them from least to most difficult.
3. Practice saying no by using the least threatening method first, working up to more challenging situations (e.g., imagery, tape recorder, feedback, role-playing), and then practicing in actual situations.
4. Say the word *no* as the first word in the practice response. This is a clear message without excuses or apologies.
5. Follow the *no* with a clear, brief, declarative statement (e.g., "I will not rearrange my schedule; I need my day off").
6. Use eye contact that is appropriate for the intent of the verbal message.

You can practice some basic assertiveness techniques as a nurse. First, use responsibility language by using "I" instead of "you" (e.g., "I am responsible for the medication error" or "I feel unappreciated when you say that to me"). If you blame your behavior on another, you give away your power to make changes. For example, someone who states, "My father made me angry" or "The good Lord told me to hit him" indicates that he has no power or control over his behavior and takes no responsibility for his actions. Being assertive means learning how to say no, expressing opinions and feelings, stating beliefs, and initiating conversations. Nonverbal assertive language includes using good eye contact when speaking.

Assertive messages have the same verbal and nonverbal message. Sometimes, however, patients try to cover up their true sadness by laughing or smiling while relating a painful experience when they do not know how to deal with it in another way.

Responding Techniques That Enhance Therapeutic Communication

Therapeutic responding techniques are methods that encourage patients to interact in ways that promote their growth and that move them toward their treatment goals and to recovery. The nurse needs to be skilled in using these techniques so that the patient can develop a trusting and mutually collaborative relationship that will effectively accomplish mutual goals and objectives (Arnold and Boggs, 2007). These strategies create an atmosphere that promotes communication for problem solving. Table 4-3 provides examples of many of these techniques.

Silence is an important listening skill for psychiatric nurses to develop. It is not the absence of communication; rather, it is a useful and purposeful communication tool that gives patients time to feel comfortable and respond when they are ready. It is best to use silence to serve a particular function and not to frighten or discomfort the already anxious patient. A successful interview is largely dependent on the nurse's ability to remain silent long enough to allow the patient to share relevant information. Silence gives the patient an opportunity to consider the communication, weigh alternatives, and formulate an answer. It also gives the nurse an opportunity to think about what he or she will say to the patient, which will enhance the therapeutic conversation.

Active listening is vital to effective communication. It is not simply the act of hearing. Several techniques are incorporated into this skill, including paraphrasing the patient's thoughts and feelings, understanding the meaning behind the words and phrases, and asking questions. Active listening involves focus and self-discipline, and it engages all of the nurse's senses.

Support and reassurance are provided in a genuine and honest manner. Patients need to be in an atmosphere in which they are able to safely discuss sensitive information. Nurses offer both verbal and nonverbal support so that the patient feels free to share thoughts and feelings, which is necessary for progress toward mental health to occur.

Sharing observations made by the nurse is important to increase the patient's self-understanding. It also demonstrates to the patient that the nurse is actively listening.

Acknowledging feelings is a form of patient support. It is important to let the patient know that his or her feelings are valid and important. There are no right or wrong answers when it comes to feelings; they cannot be taken away, argued with, or discounted.

Broad, open-ended statements allow the patient to assume some control over the topics that you will discuss. However, do not allow the patient to discuss only irrelevant topics or engage in a conversation with superficial or social content. Ask the patient questions that do not produce one-word answers. Open-ended questions result in a fuller, more revealing answer that typically stimulates the asking of more questions.

Information giving is an ongoing process for the nurse who provides information to increase the patient's knowledge about a variety of topics regarding his or her illness and treatment. Information decreases fears and anxiety and increases the patient's fund of resources and support for his or her problem. Examples include information about the patient's disorder and medications, aftercare support groups, structured living options, and treatment alternatives. Information is given in accordance with the patient's level of understanding and his or her willingness to receive it.

The interpretation of what patients are sharing is useful to help them see the real meaning behind their messages. Be careful when using this technique. A patient sometimes disagrees with the nurse's interpretation, which causes obstacles. Helping patients focus to pursue a particular topic allows them to spend their time discussing subjects of most importance. The identification of themes is necessary to help patients see what they repeatedly bring up during the course of the conversation. Placing events in order and in time is also important to help patients develop a greater perspective on events in their lives.

Patients often need encouragement to describe their perceptions regarding their thoughts and feelings. For example, some patients with psychiatric disorders hear imaginary voices that tell them to hurt themselves or others. Ask such patients to tell the staff when this occurs so that you will be able to intervene and to prevent patients' attempts to harm themselves or others. Treatment strategies an then be introduced to reduce this perception and to minimize the patients' dysfunctional behavior (see Chapter 13).

To develop a sense of patients' past and current behaviors, ask patients to compare their present anxiety to that of their last hospitalization, or ask patients if they have ever experienced this behavior before.

Restating what patients say lets them know that you heard and understood them. It is an active listening technique.

Reflecting is a technique that is used to turn around a question to obtain a response from the patient. Coaching patients to answer a question helps them to accept their own ideas and feelings about an important event or behavior.

TABLE 4-3		THERAPEUTIC RESPONDING TECHNIQUES RELATED TO STEPS OF THE NURSING PROCESS AND PHASES OF THE THERAPEUTIC RELATIONSHIP	
THERAPEUTIC RELATIONSHIP PHASE	**NURSING PROCESS STEP**	**TECHNIQUE**	**EXAMPLES**
Orientation	Assessment and nursing diagnosis	*Introducing self.* This occurs when the patient is admitted.	"Hi, my name is Kirsten. I will be your nurse today."
		Offering self. The nurse demonstrates an honest, open posture, and makes himself or herself available to demonstrate concern and interest.	"I have some information to obtain. Let's sit here so that we can begin your admission."
		Active listening. This is practiced by using both verbal and nonverbal skills that show that the nurse is giving full attention to the patient.	The nurse faces the patient, takes an open position, maintains eye contact, and uses verbal and nonverbal messages to demonstrate that the patient has the nurse's full attention: "Go on. I am listening."
		Questioning. The nurse skillfully asks open-ended questions during the initial admission. Interviewing skills are necessary to avoid asking too many personal questions during one session. Direct questions are used to achieve relevance and depth. Closed questions are for gathering factual information.	"How many children do you have?" *(Closed question)* "Has this ever happened before?" *(Closed question)* "How come you have stopped taking your medication?" *(Open-ended question)* "What is that all about?" "Can you tell me how you feel now?" *(Open-ended question)*
		Silence. The nurse uses silence frequently so that the patient has time to verbalize his or her thoughts and feelings. Silence is planned and used to draw out the patient. Silence should be comfortable for both the patient and the nurse.	The nurse sits quietly, maintains comfortable eye contact, and demonstrates interest with the use of nonverbal nods and expressive facial movements.
		Empathizing. The nurse demonstrates warmth and acknowledges the patient's feelings.	"I know how hurt you must have felt. It sounds like it made you sad."
		Reality orienting/providing information. The nurse explains to the patient the type of unit, gives a brief tour, and provides the patient with unit information and admission paperwork.	"Joseph, here is a copy of the unit rules. Let's go over a few important items." "You are on the locked unit now." "Today is Friday. You were admitted yesterday afternoon."
		Restating. The nurse repeats what the patient says to show understanding and to review what was said.	"You say your friend's death makes you sad." "You became depressed soon after the accident?"
		Clarifying. The nurse asks specific questions to help clear up a specific point that the patient makes.	"Did it help when you tried any of the techniques that you mentioned?" "Which technique helped the most?" "So your mother remarried soon after you were born?"
		Offering reality. The nurse presents a realistic view to the patient in a reasonable manner.	"I know you think people are out to get you. I do not think that. You are safe here, and we are here to help you. This medication will help to decrease those thoughts."
		Stating observations. The nurse offers a view of what is seen or heard to increase the patient's verbalization.	"I see that you are quite upset." "I noticed that you had trouble sleeping last night."
		Fostering description of perceptions. The nurse asks the patient to describe the situation.	"Help me to understand how this is affecting you right now." "What is the voice that you hear telling you?" *(to a patient who is hallucinating)*

TABLE 4-3	THERAPEUTIC RESPONDING TECHNIQUES RELATED TO STEPS OF THE NURSING PROCESS AND PHASES OF THE THERAPEUTIC RELATIONSHIP—cont'd		
THERAPEUTIC RELATIONSHIP PHASE	**NURSING PROCESS STEP**	**TECHNIQUE**	**EXAMPLES**
		Placing the event in time and order. The nurse asks questions to determine the relationships of events and helps to put events in perspective.	"Was the birth of your child before or after your mother died?" "Did your alcohol abuse begin immediately after your divorce?"
		Voicing doubt. The nurse discusses any uncertainty regarding the patient's perceptions.	"I find it hard to believe that you felt no joy when you heard that she had survived." "Are you sure that you were in bed for 1 full year after that?"
		Identifying themes. The nurse voices issues that come up repeatedly during the course of conversation.	"It sounds like that is very important to you. You've mentioned it a few times." "When this happens over and over, how do you feel?"
		Encouraging comparisons. The nurse asks for similarities and differences among feelings, thoughts, behaviors, and various life situations.	"Was this the same way that you reacted the last time it happened?"
		Summarizing. The nurse verbalizes a compilation of what has been expressed about a particular subject or event.	"Let me see if I understand your anxiety about _____." "From what you describe, your family seems _____."
		Focusing. The nurse zeroes in on a subject until the important points come into clear view for both the patient and the nurse.	"You talk about loss. Tell me more about the losses you've experienced." "You mentioned his drinking. Tell me more about that."
Working	Outcome identification, planning, and implementation	*Evaluating.* The nurse encourages the patient to express the importance of an event.	"What does this type of behavior mean to you?" "After thinking about it, how does it affect you now?"
		Encouraging plan formulation. The nurse helps the patient to develop steps to make changes and solve problems.	"What steps do you think you'll need to accomplish that?"
		Assisting with goal setting. The nurse encourages the patient to set goals for during hospitalization and after hospitalization.	"I will help you to set some realistic goals during your hospital stay. Do you have some ideas?"
		Providing information. The nurse offers data that will help the patient to set goals and develop a plan of action.	"This list and description of crisis houses will help you to decide which one will be best for you after discharge." "I have a problem-solving guide that helps people go through the necessary steps to follow when solving big problems."
		Offering alternatives. The nurse fosters decision making by encouraging the patient to work on arriving at healthy, growth-producing decisions.	"When you look over the pros and cons, which plan do you think would work best for you?" "What would be your best alternative given this situation?"
		Role-playing. The nurse plays the part of a person the patient needs to say something to in an effort to help the patient practice what he or she wants to say.	"Let's go over what you want to say to him." "I'll play your father, and you play yourself." "Sometimes it helps to say it in the mirror a few times before the real encounter."
		Providing feedback. The nurse provides the patient with supportive comments in response to behaviors or statements that have been made.	"Tell me what you want to say; I'll listen and give you my feedback." "When you walked away, I felt _____." "You will upset some people with behavior like that."

Continued

TABLE 4-3	THERAPEUTIC RESPONDING TECHNIQUES RELATED TO STEPS OF THE NURSING PROCESS AND PHASES OF THE THERAPEUTIC RELATIONSHIP—cont'd		
THERAPEUTIC RELATIONSHIP PHASE	**NURSING PROCESS STEP**	**TECHNIQUE**	**EXAMPLES**
		Confronting. The nurse supports the patient but directly challenges inaction on the part of the patient.	"I know that this is hard to do, but I believe that it will help you to make the right decision." "I understand your concerns; however, you have to take some steps now."
		Setting limits. The nurse provides the patient with external boundaries to an expressed thought, feeling, or behavior.	"You became very angry again. To stay in the dayroom, you'll need to act calmer. You can walk in the hallway if you need to get up."
Termination	Evaluation	*Evaluating actions.* The nurse encourages the patient to look at his or her behaviors and the outcomes that they produce.	"When you tried to do that, how well did it work?" "When you tell her to leave, how do you think she will react?" "Was that useful for you?"
		Reinforcing healthy behaviors. The nurse offers positive responses to the patient who is trying out new growth-producing behaviors and making helpful decisions.	"It sounds like you have made a healthy choice." "Standing up for yourself is new." "You've successfully tried it, so practicing it daily will be important."
		Encouraging posthospital transition. The nurse helps the patient to see that new thoughts and actions can be accomplished after discharge.	"I know you will continue to practice being assertive." "What situations will you run into in which you might try this new behavior?" "How can a relapse prevention plan assist you after you leave the hospital?" "Which coping skills will be useful to you when you return home?"

Clarifying is used to ask patients to elaborate on or restate something that they just said. It increases your understanding and allows patients to rethink and restate their thoughts or feelings.

Confrontation in an accepting manner is necessary for the patient to be more aware of incongruent thoughts, feelings, and behaviors. This helps to bring the issue into focus. However, this technique should only be used when a good relationship has been established between the nurse and the patient (Fortinash and Holoday Worret, 2007).

When a patient is struggling to explore and solve a problem but can only see one or two solutions, offer alternatives. Suggesting to the patient other possible solutions to the problem is not the same as giving advice. Use introductions such as "Have you thought about …?," "Other patients have tried these solutions," and "Other alternatives might be … ." The nurse avoids phrases such as "You should" and "I think you need to solve it the way most people do" (i.e., giving advice).

Voicing doubt is a technique to use when the patient is having difficulty relating in a way that sounds believable. Voicing some doubt helps the patient to be more realistic about perceptions and conclusions regarding events. Use the voicing of doubt cautiously, because doubt sometimes creates barriers between the patient and the nurse.

Summarize the information that the patient provides on a regular basis. Summarizing the main points of what a patient has been discussing helps to put the focus on the most important issues related to the patient's life situation. After the nurse provides the summary, the patient can agree or disagree with any point, and then together the nurse and patient can agree on a final summary.

Role-playing provides a way for the patient to act out a particular event, problem, or situation in a safe environment. The nurse can play the other part or role. The nurse also provides the patient with feedback regarding a variety of issues within the dialog, such as voice tone, use of assertive language, identification of feelings, emotions expressed, and nonverbal behaviors exhibited (Fortinash and Holoday Worret, 2007).

Special Communication Techniques
Self-Disclosure

Self-disclosure involves opening up oneself to another; it is an effective therapeutic skill if it is fully understood and used carefully. Experienced nurses reveal carefully selected thoughts, feelings, and life events to demonstrate to the patient that they understand what the patient is going through.

Disclosing your own personal beliefs, views, and life experiences occurs in social relationships on a continual basis. In intimate relationships, things that you reveal are very personal. Because a professional nurse–patient therapeutic relationship exists for the purpose of helping the patient, carefully think about what you will discuss before you reveal it. Because self-disclosure by the nurse is always for the patient's benefit and never for the nurse's, it is important to explore the what, where, why, and when of self-disclosing to see what purpose it serves (Balzer Riley, 2007).

Make sure that all self-disclosure is brief and relevant to the conversation, and do not imply that your experience is the same as the patient's. Guidelines are available to help the nurse understand when to use self-disclosure. The following are acceptable purposes for self-disclosure (Deering, 1999):

- *To educate.* Will the patient learn more about themselves and be able to deal better with the problems in his or her life?
- *To facilitate the therapeutic relationship.* Will disclosing build rapport and help the patient to open up?
- *To provide concrete reflection that encourages reality testing.* Will this support the patient in his or her natural feelings in response to an event?

The use of self-disclosure requires that the nurse and the patient have a therapeutic relationship. The rationale for the nurse to use self-disclosure comes from the belief that, by doing so, the patient will in turn self-disclose. Both the amount and relevance of your own self-disclosure needs to be monitored. If the self-disclosure is too lengthy, it will decrease the time that the patient has for disclosure and break down the interaction. If the disclosure is irrelevant to the patient's problem, the patient will become distracted and feel alienated from the nurse. Box 4-2 compares an example of therapeutic disclosure with nontherapeutic disclosure.

Both the research and the literature have indicated that self-disclosure is an important tool for patient growth. Realize that not all self-disclosure involves revealing personal information. Rather, it is sometimes as simple as sharing a feeling. Genuine open communication can be used to create a therapeutic relationship without the use of self-disclosure. Self-disclosure enhances the relationship only when you feel comfortable using it and when it will benefit the patient.

Touch

Touch is a powerful nonverbal method of communication that expresses many messages. Shaking hands, holding hands, hugging, and kissing all demonstrate positive regard for another human being. Nonessential touch is purposeful physical contact with the patient that is other than the touch necessary for a procedure. Nonprocedural touches range from a light touch on the arm or a handshake to holding the hand or a full embrace. Touch will only communicate warmth if the nurse is comfortable with it.

Touch carries a different meaning for each person. Several variables influence the intended message of the touch, including the length of the touch, the part of the body touched,

---

BOX 4-2   SELF-DISCLOSURE

Therapeutic

Patient: I'm very upset that I have to leave the hospital today.

Nurse: I have enjoyed working with you. I realize that endings can be sad. It is important for you to use the communication tools that you have learned when you go home.

The nurse is using self-disclosure during the termination phase of the relationship. He is validating the patient's feelings and also validating the relationship with the purpose of encouraging the patient to transfer what she has learned during treatment into life after discharge.

Nontherapeutic

Patient: That lousy husband of mine had to leave me with four children to support.

Nurse: I know how you feel because my husband was just like that. He only cared about himself.

The nurse is using self-disclosure during the admission interview or the beginning phase of the relationship, before there is a rapport or relationship established with the patient. In addition, her comments reveal too much personal information to the patient, which she should not disclose at any time. It seems to serve the nurse's purposes—rather than the patient's—to share the incident.

---

the way in which you touch the patient, and the frequency of the touch.

Use caution when touching patients in a psychiatric setting. The age and gender of the patient, the patient's interpretation of the gesture, the patient's cultural background, and the appropriateness of the touch all influence reactions to touch.

Take potential reactions into consideration when deciding which patients to touch and what type of touch to use, if any. For example, a depressed patient responds positively to touch as a gesture of concern. The nurse comforts an elderly and frail patient or a patient who is dying with the use of touch. However, a paranoid and hostile patient will probably think that touch means confrontation and may hit the nurse. An abused patient may pull away and feel frightened by a hand being placed on his or her shoulder.

Procedural touch includes positioning the arm of a patient when taking a blood pressure or drawing blood for laboratory work, turning a patient to change a dressing or a diaper, assisting a patient from a wheelchair to a bed, or placing restraints on an aggressive patient who is striking out at others (Figure 4-3, *A*). Nonprocedural touch includes holding an older patient's hand as she is expressing sadness about her husband's death, hugging an adolescent patient as he leaves the hospital, shaking hands with new patients, or giving a back rub to patient who has been bedridden for a long time (Figure 4-3, *B*).

The use of nonprocedural touch is a nurse's individual preference, and not all practitioners feel comfortable touching patients. Much depends on the nurse's comfort level, the ability to correctly interpret the situation, and the appropriate use of touch. Using touch is highly beneficial to the patient's

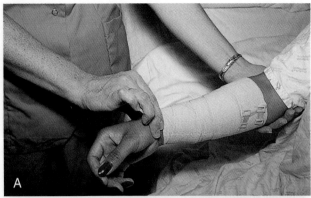

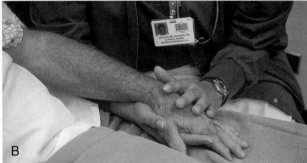

FIGURE 4-3. *A,* The nurse uses procedural touch to evaluate the patient's circulation. *B,* The nurse uses nonprocedural touch to comfort the patient. (From Potter PA, Perry AG: *Fundamentals of nursing,* ed 6, St. Louis, 2005, Mosby.)

progress in that it enhances the nurse–patient relationship and promotes health.

Humor

Humor can be a useful communication tool in psychiatric nursing. When the nurse uses it in a planned way for a specific therapeutic intent, it can be powerful. Humor is a quality that makes things seem funny, amusing, or absurd. Humor also enables us to perceive, appreciate, and express what is funny, amusing, or absurd. A sense of humor, including the ability to laugh with others and to laugh at yourself, has a positive influence on good health. Healthy humor promotes laughter among people; it encourages laughing *with* others and not *at* them. Healthy humor includes others, is appropriate to the situation, respects others, and preserves their dignity. Harmful humor excludes others; it is used to single out people from a group and ridicule them.

A good sense of humor is a mature coping mechanism that helps the nurse to adequately handle difficult situations. It also assists the nurse with gaining a different perspective on the problem by lightening a serious mood for a few moments.

Physiologically, research has linked laughter and an active sense of humor to better health. Laughter can decrease pain sensitivity, increase pain tolerance, and improve the immune response. Many theorize that laughter stimulates the brain to release the brain's natural painkillers (i.e., endorphins), thus creating a natural sense of well-being and promoting the

healing process. In some cases, laughing and having positive social interactions during mealtimes have aided digestion.

There are many psychologic benefits of laughter as well. In two studies, researchers found that humor-based group activities provided to patients with chronic schizophrenia showed that they had a significant reduction in negative symptoms, self-injury, self-reported anger, anxiety, and depression. Although the results may be preliminary, they suggest that humor-based interventions may be beneficial for patients with chronic mental illness (Higueras et al, 2006; Gelkopf et al, 2006).

Assess the degree to which a patient has a sense of humor. In depressed patients, the outward expression of laughter and pleasure is usually missing. Patients with paranoid features are unable to laugh. In fact, they usually view others' laughter as a personal attack. This is important to remember. For example, nurses in the nursing station need to be careful not to laugh and joke behind a glass partition where paranoid patients can see them and interpret the behavior as a personal affront. Alternatively, a manic patient may laugh at everything, whether or not it is actually humorous. This exaggerated sense of well-being demonstrates a lack of judgment on the part of the patient, and it often turns into biting sarcasm that will hurt others. Humor is nontherapeutic when it is used constantly; when rapport has not been established; or when a patient is very ill, fearful, anxious, having a high level of pain, or very depressed (Arnold and Boggs, 2007).

The psychiatric mental health nurse uses humor as a therapeutic tool in a variety of ways. For example, the nurse can use it to teach the patient the difference between hurtful and healthy humor and to encourage healthy humor on the unit by role modeling. The use of humor can help to create a more relaxed, safe, low-key environment that facilitates difficult interactions and enhances the patient's insight.

Obstacles to Therapeutic Communication

Certain obstacles occur in the nurse–patient relationship that affect the nature of communication. Some obstacles are a result of the patient's disorder or lack of knowledge, and some have to do with the nurse's own inability to be effective because of inexperience, lack of knowledge, or personal problems. For the relationship to grow in a healthy manner, these obstacles must be overcome.

Here are four key therapeutic obstacles for discussion: resistance, transference, countertransference, and boundary violations.

Resistance

Resistance occurs in patients who consciously or unconsciously maintain a lack of awareness of their problems to avoid anxiety. It takes the form of a natural and short-lived reservation about accepting a problem or of a long-term and firmly stated denial that there are problems. Resistance to change is part of human nature that both the nurse and the patient need to address and manage so that positive growth will occur. You can help patients overcome resistance by pointing out their progress and strengths.

For example, suppose that a patient resists impending discharge because of a fear of failure, abandonment, or loneliness. The nurse assures the patient that such fears are not uncommon at the time of termination or discharge. The nurse then reminds the patient of progress made (e.g., "You've already achieved some of your goals, and you have made concrete plans to continue treatment after you are discharged; these are accomplishments that you didn't believe were possible when you first arrived at this facility"). Such observations build the patient's confidence and offer hope that will counteract resistance.

Transference

Transference is when a patient unconsciously associates the nurse with someone significant in his or her life. The patient transfers feelings and attitudes about the other person to the nurse. For example, a male patient sees a female nurse as a mother figure because she has a mannerism that reminds him of his own mother. The patient has negative feelings about his mother and, without provocation, becomes angry or bothered by the nurse's interaction with him because of this resemblance. The patient's intense response often does not match the situation or the content of the interaction. The interaction comes to a standstill if the nurse does not address and examine the patient's reasons for transference.

The nurse can deal with both resistance and transference by being prepared to hear a patient's irrational and highly charged responses to the nurse. Listen to the patient and then use the therapeutic techniques of clarifying and reflecting to begin problem solving. The goal is for the patient to be aware and recognize the reason for the resistance.

Countertransference

Countertransference is the nurse's emotional response to a specific patient. The response is irrational, inappropriate, highly charged, and generated by certain qualities of the patient. It is simply the nurse's own transference. Nurses have a natural response to each patient and may like or dislike some patients more than others. Countertransference occurs when the feelings are intense—they may be either positive or negative—and not based in reality. Because countertransference affects your ability to be an effective nurse, always observe for signs of its occurrence.

From time to time, countertransference issues will occur. Even though this is natural, it will be destructive if the nurse ignores it or treats it as insignificant. The nurse most often encounters countertransference when the patient is displaying disruptive, aggressive, irritating, or resistive behaviors. If the nurse remains angry with the patient as a result of these behaviors, he or she will lose the objectivity needed to promote healthy change. Nurses also find themselves attracted positively to patients in excessive ways. Recognize this and take steps to avoid countertransference.

To deal with countertransference, conduct an honest self-appraisal throughout the course of the therapeutic relationship while gaining a good understanding of the patient's background and issues. If the self-appraisal reveals any problems, explore why these feelings are occurring. As soon as you recognize the problem, you need to work on it. If you are not able to handle these feelings alone, seek professional clinical help to deal with these issues.

Boundary Violations

Boundary violations occur when the nurse goes beyond the established therapeutic relationship standards and enters into a social or personal relationship with the patient. Some patients also attempt to violate the boundaries of the nurse–patient relationship. For example, a patient may ask the nurse, "Where do you live?" or "Are you single?," or he or she may try to touch the nurse inappropriately. Violations are more frequent if the nurse spends more time with the patient (thus indicating overinvolvement), treats the patient at odd hours or in a nontreatment setting, or accepts compensation or gifts for treatment. It may also occur if the nurse's language or clothing is nonprofessional or if the nurse's self-disclosure or physical contact lacks therapeutic value. For example, the nurse may disclose too much personal information to the patient in a way that seems to only benefit the nurse.

Violating professional boundaries with patients is also seen as an ethical and legal issue, and it can result in legal and professional sanctions for the nurse. Nurses who are seen as crossing the line by becoming too personally involved with their patients lose therapeutic objectivity in the relationship, and they are not able to provide the desired outcomes for patient growth and recovery. These actions are seen as an abuse of the nurse–patient relationship, and they may cause serious harm to the nurse–patient relationship. Patients who have mental illnesses are vulnerable, and they may become too dependent on the nurse who they trust to guide them in their recovery. Professional nursing ethical standards must be maintained to preserve the therapeutic nature of the nurse–patient relationship and to achieve positive patient treatment outcomes (Arnold and Boggs, 2007; Milton, 2008; Wheeler, 2008).

Responding Techniques That Hinder Therapeutic Communication

Earlier in this chapter, therapeutic skills that have enhanced the communication process were presented. There are also many responses that are counterproductive to healthy outcomes and that are therefore nontherapeutic (Table 4-4).

There are several reasons why nurses fail to interact effectively. The inexperienced nurse's insecurity is one factor. A certain amount of experience and maturity greatly helps the nurse to deal effectively with the difficult and complex behaviors that psychiatric patients often display.

Other explanations for nontherapeutic communication include the following: (1) the nurse has allowed necessary skills to stagnate or diminish; (2) a nurse who has worked with psychiatric patients for several years finds that he or she is on automatic pilot (i.e., repeating the same old strategies) and has lost the ability to begin work each day refreshed and ready to actively be there for the patients; or (3) the nurse has personal problems that have not been dealt with sufficiently

TABLE 4-4	INEFFECTIVE RESPONSES THAT HINDER THERAPEUTIC COMMUNICATION		
RESPONSE	**DISCUSSION**	**NONTHERAPEUTIC RESPONSE**	**THERAPEUTIC RESPONSE**
Offering false reassurances	The nurse, in an effort to be supportive and to make the patient's pain disappear, offers reassuring clichés. This response is not based on fact. It discounts the patient's feelings, and it shuts off communication. Often, it is a result of the nurse's inability to listen to the patient's negative emotions.	"Don't worry, everything will be fine." "Every cloud has a silver lining." "Things will be better soon; you'll see." "God never gives you more than you can handle."	"I know you have a lot going on right now. Let's make a list and begin to discuss your concerns one at a time. Working toward solutions will help you to get through this."
Not listening	The nurse is preoccupied with other work that needs to be done, is distracted by noise in the area, or is thinking about personal problems.	"I'm sorry, what did you say?" "Could you start again? I was listening to another patient."	"That's interesting. Please elaborate." "I really hear what you are saying. It must be difficult."
Offering approval	What is most important is how the patient feels about what he or she said or did. The patient ultimately must approve of his or her own actions.	"That's good." "I agree, I think you should have told him."	"What do you think about what you said to him?" "How do you feel about it?"
Minimizing the problem	The nurse uses this response when it is difficult to hear the importance of a particular problem. This is used in an effort to make the patient feel better, but it cuts off communication.	"That's nothing compared to some other patient's problem." "Everyone feels that way at times; it's not a big deal."	"That seems like a difficult problem for you." "That sounds pretty important for you to deal with."
Offering advice	This response undermines the patient's ability to solve his or her own problems. It renders the patient dependent and helpless. If the solution provided by the nurse does not work, the patient will blame the outcome on the nurse. The patient does not take responsibility for developing outcomes. The nurse maintains control and at the same time devalues the patient.	"I think you should put your mother into a nursing home." "In my opinion, it would be wise to _____." "Why don't you _____?" "The best solution is _____."	"What do *you* think you should do?" "There are several alternatives; let's talk about some. However, the final decision is yours. I will listen to your problem and help you to see it clearly. We can develop a list of pros and cons that will assist you with solving the problem."
Giving literal responses	The nurse feeds into the patient's delusions or hallucinations and denies the patient the opportunity to see reality. This does not provide a healthy response toward growth.	*Patient:* "That TV is talking to me." *Nurse:* "What is it saying to you?" *Patient:* "There is nuclear power coming through the air ducts." *Nurse:* "I'll turn off the air conditioner for a while."	*Nurse:* "The TV is on for everyone." *Nurse:* "There is cool air blowing from the vents. It is the air conditioning system."
Changing the subject	The nurse changes the topic at a crucial time because the discussion is too uncomfortable. It negates what the patient seems interested in discussing. Communication will remain superficial.	*Patient:* "My mother always puts me down." *Nurse:* "That's interesting, but let's talk about _____."	*Nurse:* "Tell me about that."
Belittling	The nurse puts down the patient's expressed feelings to avoid having to deal with his or her own painful feelings.	*Patient:* "I don't want to live anymore now that my child is gone." *Nurse:* "You shouldn't feel that way."	*Nurse:* "Losing a child must be very difficult for you. Tell me more about how you are feeling."

TABLE 4-4	**INEFFECTIVE RESPONSES THAT HINDER THERAPEUTIC COMMUNICATION—cont'd**		
RESPONSE	**DISCUSSION**	**NONTHERAPEUTIC RESPONSE**	**THERAPEUTIC RESPONSE**
Disagreeing	The nurse criticizes the patient who is seeking support.	"I definitely do not agree with your viewpoint." "I really don't support that."	"Let's talk about the way you see that."
Judging	The nurse's responses are filled with his or her own values and judgments. This demonstrates a lack of acceptance of the patient's differences, and it provides a barrier to further disclosures.	"You are not married. Do you think having this baby will solve your problems?" "This is certainly not the Christian thing to do." "You are thinking about divorce when you have three children?"	"It seems hard to believe. Please explain further." "What will having this baby provide for you?" "What do you think about what you are attempting to do?" "Let's discuss this option" or "Let's discuss other options."
Probing excessively	This serves to control the nature of the patient's responses. The nurse asks many questions of the patient before the patient is ready to provide the information. This is self-protective to the nurse by avoiding the anxiety of uncomfortable silences. The patient feels overwhelmed and may withdraw. The use of "why?" questions places the patient in a defensive position and may block further communication.	"Why do you do this?" "What do you think was the real reason?" "Why do you feel this way?" "Why do you think that way?"	"Tell me how this is upsetting to you." "Tell me what you believe to be the reason." "Tell me how you feel when that happens." "Explain your thinking about this if you can."
Challenging	This comes from the nurse's belief that if patients are challenged regarding their unrealistic thoughts, they will be coerced into seeing reality. This patient will feel threatened when challenged and hold onto the beliefs even more strongly.	"You are not a superhero." "If your leg is missing, then why can you walk up and down this hall?"	"You sound like you need to feel important." "It seems to you that you are missing a leg. Tell me more about that."
Offering superficial comments	The nurse gives simple or meaningless responses to the patient. It suggests a lack of understanding of the patient's individuality. The interactions remain superficial, maintaining a distance between the nurse and the patient. No significant communication occurs.	"Great day, huh?" "You should be feeling good; you are being discharged today." "Think positive thoughts; your doctor should be coming to see you anytime now."	"What kind of day are you having?" "How are you feeling about leaving the hospital today?" "You look worried. Your doctor called and said he would be here within the hour."
Defending	The nurse believes that he or she must defend herself or himself, the staff, or the hospital. The nurse does not take the time to listen to the patient's concerns. Effort is necessary to explore the patient's thoughts and feelings.	"Your doctor is one of the best doctors that we have. He would never say that." "We have a very experienced staff here. They would never do that."	"What has you so upset about your doctor?" "Tell me what happened last night."
Self-focusing	The nurse shares his or her own thoughts, feelings, or problems; therefore, focus is taken away from the patient, who is seeking help. The nurse is more interested in what to say next than in actively listening to the patient.	"That may have happened to you last year, but it happened to me just this month, which hurt me a great deal and _____." "Excuse me, but could you say that again? I have a response for you, but I want to be sure about what you just said."	"Tell me about your incident and how it relates to your sadness now." "If I heard you correctly, you said _____."

Continued

TABLE 4-4	INEFFECTIVE RESPONSES THAT HINDER THERAPEUTIC COMMUNICATION—cont'd		
RESPONSE	**DISCUSSION**	**NONTHERAPEUTIC RESPONSE**	**THERAPEUTIC RESPONSE**
Criticizing others	The nurse puts others down in his or her communication with the patient.	*Patient:* "The staff members on the evening shift let me smoke two cigarettes." *Nurse:* "The evening shift is always breaking the rules. On this shift, we follow the one cigarette per break policy." *Patient:* "I know my daughter hates me." *Nurse:* "She sounds just awful to live with."	*Nurse:* "The policy is one cigarette, which we will follow." *Nurse:* "It sounds like you are having a rough time right now with your daughter."
Interpreting or analyzing prematurely	The nurse responds before the patient fully expresses his or her thoughts and feelings about a particular problem. By rushing to a conclusion, the nurse disregards important patient input and misses critical patient concerns.	"I think this is what you really mean." "You think that way consciously, but unconsciously you believe _____."	"What do you think this means?" "So you think _____?"

and that are interfering with his or her ability to focus on the patient and the patient's needs.

It is important that nurses build on the knowledge that they have by continually practicing and perfecting skills and attending skill-building classes and therapeutic communication in-service workshops to refresh and enhance learned strategies. It is also significant that nurses know when to obtain outside help for their own life problems so that high stress levels do not interfere with work. Nurses need to remember that it is important to spend time away from work with friends and family as well as time alone doing the things that they enjoy.

There are other potential instances for a nurse's ineffective responses. Some nurses display anger toward the patient for not behaving in a socially acceptable manner or for not doing what they ask. Alternatively, the nurse may take what the patient says personally. Another instance is when a patient who is angry or delusional and displays out-of-control behavior says something to the nurse that hurts the nurse's feelings. For example, a patient says to the overweight nurse who is placing him in seclusion, "Get out of here, you big fat _____." The nurse, who is upset by the patient's statement, responds angrily or defensively if he or she is not able to detach from the statement and realize that the patient is angry at his or her own behavior and is projecting it onto the nurse in the form of a personal statement.

Communication and the Nursing Process

There are many opportunities to communicate therapeutically throughout the nursing process. Each step of the nursing process—assessment, nursing diagnosis, outcome identification, implementation, planning, and evaluation—corresponds with the three phases of the therapeutic

relationship: beginning (orientation), working, and termination. There are therapeutic responding techniques that are unique to each step and phase.

The nurse's first communication task is to greet the patient on admission. The nurse communicates the nature of his or her role. This orientation or beginning phase starts with the initial contact, continues with the admission interview and assessment, and ends with the formulation of a nursing diagnosis. This phase lasts for one or more sessions, because much highly personal data is collected, and it occurs when the patient is in the most need of help and is displaying highly dysfunctional behavior.

During the working phase of the relationship, when the patient and treatment team are developing the care plan, the nurse will use many therapeutic responding techniques. The therapeutic communication skills used during this phase help patients deal with the issues that brought them into the hospital.

During the termination phase, both evaluation and discharge planning are predominant. The nurse uses communication techniques associated with assisting the patient toward discharge and aftercare. Throughout the nurse–patient relationship, the nurse should avoid responding in ways that block therapeutic communication (see Table 4-4). The stages of the therapeutic relationship are discussed in Chapter 1.

Challenges in Communication
Legal Issues

Confidentiality, legal status, patients' rights, and informed consent are legal issues that affect nurse–patient communication. This chapter briefly discusses these issues as they relate to the therapeutic relationship; Chapter 9 goes into greater detail.

All patient information that the nurse obtains is protected by the patient's right to privacy or confidentiality. The nurse can share information with the health care team to develop the most effective plan of care. However, the nurse must protect the patient's right to privacy and the right to keep that information from individuals outside of the health care team.

Thus, all communication is considered confidential or privileged. During the initial interview, the nurse has the responsibility to inform the patient of the confidential nature of the disclosure. The patient also has the right to know with whom the nurse will share the information. Explain that you will share the information with team members such as the social worker, the physician, and other nursing staff but not with the patient's family members or friends unless the patient has given written permission to reveal specific information. When this happens, the physician is usually the person who informs the family members.

Often patients with mental illness have difficulty trusting others. To encourage the patient to confide in the nurse, the nurse should try to gain the patient's trust through honest, open, and congruent communication and by following through with commitments to the patient when possible. However, it is also the nurse's responsibility to tell the patient that such things as suicidal thoughts or plans are "secrets" that must be shared with the health care team, because this information is critical to the patient's own or others' safety or to the treatment plan. For example, a patient tells a student nurse that he has a sharp object and will cut himself with it when everyone has gone to bed because he is feeling more and more depressed and suicidal. The student explains that she has to share this type of information with the patient's nurse and physician. The patient then begs the student not to share this information. The student replies that she has to communicate attempts at harmful behavior to the patient's physician and to the nursing staff to keep the patient safe.

There is much opportunity for the nurse to communicate with patients about any issues regarding their legal status when necessary. For example, the police bring a patient into the hospital who is on a legal hold. The patient does not understand the term *hold*, which seems confusing, especially to a patient with psychosis. Often the nurse will clarify the exact nature of the patient's legal status and explain the implications and patient rights associated with the status in terms that the patient will understand. Chapter 9 discusses the specific legal rights of patients.

Informed consent is a legal document that outlines a procedure or specific types of medication that the patient will receive. The physician has the responsibility to inform the patient in an understandable manner so that the patient can decide whether to have the procedure or take the specific medication considered helpful to treatment. The nurse often assists the physician with communication regarding informed consent. The nurse works with the physician to verify that the patient has a basic understanding of the informed consent regarding treatment, medication, alternative therapies, or the patient's prognosis with or without treatment.

Effective nurse–patient communication is extremely helpful when processing legal paperwork, especially with patients who have difficulty trusting, understanding legal terms, or knowing their legal rights. Be honest, open, congruent, and clear in all messages given to the patient regarding all communication of a legal nature, thus preparing a patient to be well informed and to consent to treatment.

Length of Stay

Another communication challenge comes with both brief and long-term hospital stays. For the chemically dependent patient, for example, the length of stay is sometimes as short as 1 to 3 days. For the patient with schizophrenia, a stay may last 3 to 7 days. In these cases, communication is delivered in a crisis-intervention mode, so some of the phases of the therapeutic relationship such as assessment gathering and treatment planning have to be completed within hours. Therefore, a relationship should be established with the patient as quickly as possible. If the patient's behavior is not favorable to working within a brief time frame, then the nurse suggests rest and provides medication to calm the patient. The preliminary interview and data gathering can then occur when the patient is better able to respond.

For patients with complex problems, the length of stay may be much longer than the average length of stay. This is often the result of a combination of complex psychiatric and medical problems as well as financial limitations, legal issues, and a lack of viable placement options. Awaiting placement after the active treatment program is concluded can make ongoing therapeutic communication more difficult as a result of the patient and nurse's frustration. The blurring of boundaries can occur if the nurse is not aware of the importance of an ongoing professional therapeutic relationship with the long-term patient (see Chapter 1).

Physical Impairments

Other issues that affect communication involve special patient care needs. For example, consider the patient with a hearing impairment. If the patient reads lips or the nurse knows how to sign (i.e., use sign language), then communication is possible. Sit in a manner that facilitates the communication. Inform the other patients what you are doing and why you are doing it. This is especially helpful in a group setting.

Some patients have both visual and hearing impairments as well as cognitive deficits. Carefully assess each patient to determine his or her special needs when communicating. With patients who have vision problems, the nurse physically assists the patients to and from activities, groups, and their rooms. These actions communicate caring and concern, as does sitting near the patient when speaking. When approaching the visually impaired patient, proceed slowly and speak in soft tones to avoid startling the patient. Communicating with patients with special needs is challenging, but it is effective with the help of the patient and your own sensitivity and knowledge.

Special Populations

Communicating With the Older Patient. Nurses who work with older patients need to use communication that promotes health and successful aging. Because of the physical, sensory, and cognitive deficits listed in the preceding section, sometimes nurses unknowingly communicate messages of dependence and incompetence by using a style of speech that one would use to address a small child, such as addressing older adults as "Honey" or "Cutie pie" or addressing them by their first names without permission. This communication style does not show respect for the older patient. Regardless of the patient's limitations, communicate with the older patient with the use of adult language that shows respect and caring and that maintains the patient's autonomy, independence, and dignity (Arnold and Boggs, 2007)

Communicating With Children and Adolescents. Often the nurse is in a position of caring for infants, children, and adolescents through the age of 18 years. Communicating with these age groups presents unique challenges with regard to adapting the level of communication to the developmental age of the child or adolescent to match the young patient's ability to comprehend.

Generally, several techniques will build rapport with children, including taking a personal interest in them by asking them about school, hobbies, and interests; being a skillful and active listener; using simple language; being nonjudgmental; appearing relaxed; sitting at eye level and establishing good eye contact; communicating directly with the child to demonstrate interest; using broad, open-ended questions; and welcoming the child's thoughts and feelings.

In today's health care environment, the nurse will need to inform children and teenagers about their care and include them in their own health care decisions as much as possible. Including the family in these discussions and observing the interaction between the child and the parent is crucial.

It is important to understand the developmental age of the child with whom you are trying to communicate so that you can modify your language and adapt educational materials to basic concepts that the young patient can easily understand. In addition to using age-appropriate language, the use of stories, pictures, and examples may be needed to convey information. Therefore, it is crucial that you use age-appropriate communication skills and include the family of the child for the communication to be effective.

Because the child's capacity to understand language does not begin until the second year of life, rely on your nonverbal skills when dealing with very young children by using kind and gentle facial expressions, a nurturing and caring attitude, and soothing voice tones. Having the parents participate in the child's care is helpful and will reduce the child's and the parents' anxiety. Between the ages of 2 and 6 years, the child is in the beginning stage of language development, and you are able to communicate verbally with the child by using simple explanations and instructions and by keeping the interactions in the here and now. Use pictures or storybooks to provide information and to help clarify meaning.

The nurse usually experiences less difficulty when communicating with the young school-aged child between the ages of 6 and 10 years, because the child is accustomed to adults other than parents (e.g., teachers, coaches) giving instruction and assistance. By this time, the child has developed a more mature mode of communication and has a need for close relationships, both of which are helpful when interacting with the child. However, rapport and trust should be immediately established with both the child and the parent. Use concrete examples as well as simple videotapes and books that are suitable for the child's age.

During preadolescence, which occurs from the age of 10 years to 12 or 13 years, when the onset of puberty begins, the preadolescent remains receptive to adults and their influence. Use some of the preadolescent's own language to communicate more effectively. Keep explanations relevant, brief, and at an appropriate level for the preteen's understanding.

The adolescent stage begins with puberty, which is ordinarily around the age of 12 or 13 years, and lasts through the age of 18 or 19 years. During the early adolescent years, the child is trying to form a self-identity and feel comfortable with himself or herself. The adolescent is often self-conscious, self-absorbed with his or her body image, and easily embarrassed. Respect the adolescent's privacy, because confidentiality is important in this age group. In addition, you will need to relate more directly with the adolescent and less through his or her parents, because the adolescent is trying to separate emotionally from the parents and become independent. The early-age adolescent begins to develop abstract thinking, and he or she is usually able to understand past and present events and to think about and discuss future events. Use these skills in your interactions with the early-age adolescent. As the adolescent reaches 14 or 15 years old, you will find that joining an activity with the adolescent while communicating allows the adolescent to feel more comfortable with adults. Not being the adolescent's parent is an advantage and assists in the communication process. Regardless of the child's age, present a verbal and nonverbal environment in which the child or teenager feels comfortable. The degree of success that you have when communicating with a child or adolescent greatly depends on your understanding of both the developmental and chronologic age of the child (Arnold and Boggs, 2007) (see Chapter 7).

Culture, Language, and Understanding

The United States is one of the most diverse societies in the world and part of a rapidly changing and growing multicultural world. Therefore, it is imperative that nurses learn to become culturally competent to better deal with the diverse cultures and multicultural patients whom they are likely to encounter. Cultural competence involves a set of values, principles, behaviors, and attitudes that enable the nurse to work effectively across cultures. Cultural competence occurs on a continuum and develops over a long period of time. To become culturally competent, nurses must value and adapt to diversity, conduct self-assessments, manage differences, and obtain cultural knowledge and incorporate it into their clinical practices (National Center of Cultural Competence, 2010).

Communication is one of six areas of cultural uniqueness that the nurse will evaluate during the initial nursing assessment, because communication and culture have an impact on each other. Oral and written language, gestures, facial expressions, and body language are unique to each culture.

Cultural patterns of communication are set early in life and affect the way that a person communicates ideas and feelings and makes decisions. Members within the same culture sometimes respond differently because of their own experience. Cultural competence does not suggest that the nurse needs to know everything about each culture; however, it does suggest that the nurse needs to use communication that respects cultural differences to find a common communication meeting ground. Cultural competence starts with self-awareness, which involves the nurse reflecting on his or her own values, beliefs, and attitudes as well as obtaining some knowledge of another's culture (Leininger, 2000).

Be aware of the potential language barriers to effective intercultural communication. A good nurse–patient relationship depends on your understanding the patient's point of view and frame of reference. First, adopt an attitude of humility when beginning an interview that is not in the patient's native language. Starting the interview by apologizing for not speaking the patient's native language is a good way to begin an interview. Respecting and allowing for a free exchange of the patient's and family's ideas, thoughts, and feelings will promote effective intercultural communication (Aronson Fontes, 2008).

For patients who are not native English speakers, the nurse's use of effective intercultural communication and learned verbal and nonverbal techniques will promote the following:

- An accurate understanding of the patient's diagnosis, progress, and prognosis
- Assurance about what is happening and what procedures will be performed
- Assurance regarding the expertise of the nurse and other health care providers
- The ability of the patient to explain his or her symptoms to the nurse to assist with his or her diagnosis and treatment

Thus, nurses need to make a special effort to provide patients with all of the available resources that will enhance their understanding of the situation. This includes locating an interpreter who can speak the patient's language and translate at the level required. Most hospitals have lists of local interpreters who offer their services and who will communicate technical terminology to the patient. For nontechnical and uncomplicated translations, locate a hospital staff member who communicates in the patient's own language. Peplau (1952, 1991) believed that understanding is an essential component of the nurse–patient relationship and that, as such, it significantly influences nurse–patient interactions in the acute psychiatric setting. An awareness of the importance of and the skills necessary to clarify individual meaning to promote understanding with patients is emphasized in cultural sensitivity and diversity training. Because each culture has varying degrees of diversity within the culture, the nurse needs to avoid cultural stereotyping and to concentrate on the uniqueness of the individual. It is important to note that the nurse will not always fully understand what a patient means. However, it is important for the nurse to not assume an understanding of what a patient means. Avoid asking "why" questions and the use of the phrase "I completely understand." Instead, it is useful to practice learned therapeutic techniques. Here are some examples:

- Demonstrate verbal (e.g., "Continue, please") and nonverbal (e.g., nodding of the head) responses to show interest and to give the patient sufficient opportunity to respond (i.e., active listening).
- Restate (i.e., repeat) what the patient says to ensure understanding and to review what was said.
- Clarify the patient's message by repeating it back in a more specific way to further elicit the specific meaning.
- Ask open-ended questions (e.g., "Please tell me more about this"; "Please describe how you felt") to encourage the patient to respond.
- Explore the patient's verbal and nonverbal expressions regularly throughout the interaction to expand understanding.
- Summarize what the patient has said at regular intervals throughout the interaction and at the end of the interaction to confirm mutual understanding.

Table 4-3 includes additional examples of therapeutic techniques.

Difficult Patients

Most nurses find it difficult to communicate with patients who are aggressive, distressed, unpopular, or resistive to change. Patients who exhibit aggressive behaviors are hostile and often verbally or physically abusive, rejecting, and manipulative. Some have a violent history that includes jail or prison time for violent offenses related to their aggressive behavior. These are unpleasant behaviors that are difficult to be around. This attacking style of behavior demonstrates a general lack of consideration and respect for others, and the natural response is to protect the self and reject the patient. Although your self-esteem and personal safety are under attack, meet the aggression assertively by setting firm limits that do not embarrass the nurse or the patient. A specific behavioral treatment plan and a unified team approach are critical to treatment success. Most facilities offer assault-response training and education to help staff members manage these behaviors.

Distressed patients express their physical or emotional pain both verbally and nonverbally, and they sometimes do so continuously. Becoming too involved with a patient's distress can overwhelm the nurse and interfere with effective communication. Often the nurse feels inadequate when dealing with severe emotional or physical distress. It is important to remain clearheaded and to responsibly communicate

---

BOX 4-3   GENERAL CHARACTERISTICS OF UNPOPULAR PATIENTS

- Claim that they have more problems than what the nurses think they do
- Often express their dislike of the hospital
- Take up much of the nurse's time and attention
- Misuse hospitalization
- Are uncooperative and argumentative
- Are very aggressive or assaultive
- Have severe, complicated problems and a poor prognosis
- Have problems that nurses think are brought on by their own behavior (e.g., alcohol-related disease)
- Have multiple character flaws or social stigmas
- Produce feelings of incompetence in the nurse

---

understanding and concern without becoming judgmental or diminishing the patient's perceptions and related feelings.

Unpopular patients have a variety of characteristics. They are unreasonably demanding, possess unacceptable personal habits, or behave in ways that are sexually inappropriate. When dealing with unpopular patients, nurses often feel frustrated, angry, or fearful. These patients are sometimes ignored or labeled as *troublemakers* or *problem patients*. They are medicated more often, frequently admonished, and generally given less care or attention than other patients. Nurses naturally have likes and dislikes with regard to patient behaviors. One nurse may prefer working with patients who exhibit certain behavioral characteristics, whereas another nurse may dislike those behaviors. Some general characteristics of unpopular patients are listed in Box 4-3.

Resistant patients can delay positive treatment outcomes. When the patient presents resistance, it is important that the nurse employs an empathetic, supportive, and facilitative approach to the patient rather than a preaching or confronting style. Being receptive to resistance and exploring the resistance with the patient in a sensitive, empathetic manner can help to effectively manage it. Viewing resistance as negative and using a confrontation and teaching style may only serve to increase patient noncompliance (Arkowitz et al, 2008).

Difficult Coworkers

Conflicts inevitably arise in the workplace. Not only will you have to deal effectively with patients who are distressed and aggressive, but there are also times when you will deal with health care professionals who exhibit these same types of behaviors. Health care is emotionally and physically demanding, which produces stress and conflict in the health care environment. There are times when colleagues become irritated, angry, argumentative, and occasionally even verbally abusive. Although most health care environments have zero tolerance for workplace violence, conflict invariably occurs.

Lateral violence, which is sometimes referred to as *relational aggression,* consists of intimidating and disruptive behaviors. It has been identified by The Joint Commission (2008) as undermining the culture of safety in hospitals. Not communicating effectively with one's peers in ways that may include gossiping, ignoring, and withholding information creates a hostile work environment, presents safety risks, and can lead to patient errors. Nurses may feel undue anxiety, hurt feelings, and anger that may result in them leaving a certain job or even the profession (Dellasega, 2009).

Conflict in health care settings has to do not only with the level of stress in the work environment but also with varying levels of responsibility, role differences, work status uncertainty, power issues, and cultural and value differences. The best time to deal with conflict between members of the health care team is before it becomes a crisis situation. Effective communication skills are necessary to deal with a variety of conflicting professional relationships. The primary goal when dealing with workplace conflict is to find a high-quality strategy that is acceptable to all and that will result in a growth-producing outcome. The same principles of nurse–patient communication (e.g., empathy, active listening, respect for the dignity of others) are also necessary for successful relationships with other health care professionals.

The skills that are necessary to communicate therapeutically with patients and their families are the same ones that are required to communicate effectively with other health care professionals. In general, it is important to consider the ego of the other person and his or her emotional vulnerability when communicating with colleagues in the work setting. Professional collegial communication also involves collaboration, coordination, networking, and sometimes negotiation and conflict resolution (Arnold and Boggs, 2007).

CHAPTER SUMMARY

- The components of communication are the stimulus (i.e., the reason), the sender, the message, the medium, the receiver, and the feedback.
- Environmental factors, the relationship between the sender and the receiver, the context of the communication, and the individual's attitudes, beliefs, knowledge, and perception all influence communication.

- Nonverbal communication cues involve all five senses. Ninety percent of communication is nonverbal. Verbal and nonverbal communication need to be congruent for the communication to be effective.
- Interpersonal communication (i.e., communication between two or more people) can be collegial, social, or therapeutic.

CHAPTER SUMMARY—cont'd

- The three purposes of therapeutic communication are to facilitate patient self-expression for the promotion of healthy growth, to understand the significance of the patient's problems, and to assist with the identification and resolution of the problems.
- Empathy is an important quality of therapeutic communication. It is necessary to the success of the nurse–patient relationship and to the patient's progress toward treatment goals.
- Some responding techniques that enhance therapeutic communication are silence, active listening, support, reassurance, the giving of information, restating, reflecting, clarifying, and role-playing.

- Self-disclosure by the nurse is an effective technique when it is used for the right reasons, such as for the benefit of the patient.
- Resistance, transference, countertransference, and boundary violations are obstacles to therapeutic communication.
- Certain therapeutic responding techniques correspond with the specific steps of the nursing process and the phases of the nurse–patient relationship.
- Issues that relate to the nurse's skill and self-awareness levels, the patient's length of stay in treatment, the patient's physical and emotional impairments, the patient's age, and language and cultural differences are all challenges to effective communication.

REVIEW QUESTIONS

1. A patient with paranoid schizophrenia tells the nurse, "I'm here on a top secret mission for the President. Don't tell anyone I am here." Which response by the nurse would be most therapeutic?
    1. "Let's talk about something other than your mission for the President."
    2. "Your admission papers do not list you as an employee of the President."
    3. "You have lost touch with reality, which is a symptom of your illness."
    4. "It sounds like you have some concerns about your privacy. You are safe here."
2. A nurse assesses a newly admitted patient. Which of the following examples demonstrates the offering of the self?
    1. "I've had some very stressful experiences in my life, too. Hospitalization isn't so bad, really."
    2. "Tell me why you felt you had to be hospitalized for the treatment of your depression."
    3. "I know you will feel better after we get your medication adjusted."
    4. "I'd like to spend some time helping you to get comfortable talking with me."
3. A military wife tearfully tells a nurse about her husband's death in a helicopter crash 6 months earlier. The patient cries on a daily basis. She says, "I think I'm losing it. I'll never be the same." What is the nurse's best response?
    1. "You will eventually get back to normal. Just start doing the things that used to be fun for you."
    2. "When you find yourself starting to cry or feel sad, distract yourself by getting busy with an activity."

3. "Your husband died for our country. You should be proud of him rather than absorbed in grief."
    4. "Crying and the feelings that you describe are normal after such a loss. It may take you a long time to grieve his death."
4. A psychiatric nurse who works in a day treatment program for patients with serious and persistent mental illness helps a group of patients to plan a Halloween party. One patient says, "Halloween is a celebration of demons and evil." Select the nurse's most therapeutic response.
    1. "Perhaps you could stay home from the center on the day of the party."
    2. "Maybe it would be better if we provided you with alternative activities on the day of the party."
    3. "Don't be silly, your participation doesn't mean you believe in demons."
    4. "The party is part of the programming here at the center. You are expected to participate."
5. A child's parent enters the nurse's station yelling, "What is wrong with you people? My daughter cut herself and you allowed it to happen. I thought my child would be safe here." Select the assertive response for the nurse.
    1. "I can't help you right now. Your child is assigned to another nurse today."
    2. "I can't hear you if you're yelling. Let's sit down and talk about it."
    3. "Why are you always screaming when you come for visits?"
    4. "I am sorry this incident happened. We were short staffed today."

REFERENCES

Arkowitz H et al: *Motivational interviewing in the treatment of psychological problems*, New York, 2008, The Guilford Press.
Arnold E, Boggs K: *Interpersonal relationships: professional communication skills for nurses*, ed 5, St. Louis, 2007, Saunders.

Aronson Fontes L: *Interviewing clients across cultures: a practitioner's guide*, New York, 2008, The Guilford Press.
Balzer Riley J: *Communication in nursing*, ed 6, St. Louis, 2007, Mosby Elsevier.
Berlo D: *The process of communication*, New York, 1960, Holt, Rinehart and Winston.

Carpenito LJ: Nurses, always there for you, *Nurs Forum* 35:3-4, 2000.

Deering C: To speak or not to speak: self-disclosure with patients, *Am J Nurs* 99:34-36, 1999.

Dellasega C: Bullying among nurses, *Am J Nurs* 109:52-58, 2009.

Fortinash KM, Holoday Worret PA: *Psychiatric nursing care plans*, ed 5, St. Louis, 2007, Mosby.

Gelkopf M et al: The effect of humorous movies on inpatients with chronic schizophrenia, *J Nerv Ment Dis* 194:880-883, 2006.

Fox L et al: *Professional assault crisis training*, San Clemente, Calif, 2010, Pro-ACT, Inc.

Higueras A et al: Effects of a humor-centered activity on disruptive behavior in patients in a general hospital psychiatric ward, *Int J Clin Health Psychol* 6:53-64, 2006.

Health Literacy Institute: *About health literacy and plain language* (website): www.healthliteracyinstitute.net/about.html. Accessed April 20, 2010.

The Joint Commission: *Sentinel Event Alert* (website): www.jointcommission.org/SentinelEvents/SentinelEventAlerts/sea_40.htm. Accessed April 23, 2010.

Kemp P et al: Work-based learning with staff in an acute care environment: a project review and evaluation, *Mental Health Practice* 12:31-35, 2009.

Leininger M: Founder's focus: transcultural nursing is discovery of self and the world of others, *J Transcult Nurs* 11:312-313, 2000.

Luft J, Ingham H: *The Johari window: a graphic model for interpersonal relations*, Los Angeles, 1955, University of California Western Training Laboratory.

Milton C: Boundaries: ethical implications for what it means to be therapeutic in the nurse-person relationship, *Nurs Sci Quarterly* 21:18-21, 2008.

Morse J et al: Beyond empathy: expanding expressions of caring, *J Adv Nurs* 53:75-90, 2006.

National Center for Cultural Competence at Georgetown University Center for Child and Human Development: Home page (website): http://nccc.georgetown.edu/index.html. Accessed April 27, 2010.

Peplau HE: *Interpersonal relations in nursing*, New York, 1952, Putnam.

Peplau HE: *Interpersonal relations in nursing: a conceptual frame of reference for psychodynamic nursing*, New York, 1991, Springer.

Shattell M et al: 'Take my hand, help me out': mental health service recipients' experience of the therapeutic relationship, *Int J Mental Health Nurs* 16:274-284, 2007.

Shives LR: *Basic concepts of psychiatric mental health nursing*, ed 7, Philadelphia, 2007, Lippincott.

Walker K, Alligood M: Empathy from a nursing perspective: moving beyond borrowed theory, *Arch Psychiatr Nurs* 15:140-147, 2001.

Wheeler K: *Psychotherapy for the advanced practice psychiatric nurse*, St. Louis, 2008, Mosby.

Adaptation to Stress

Pamela E. Marcus

"Adopting the right attitude can convert a negative stress into a positive one."

Hans Selye

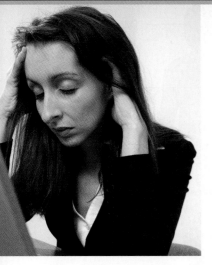

⊝volve WEBSITE

http://evolve.elsevier.com/Fortinash/

OBJECTIVES

- Define the two types of stress.
- Describe the functions of the brain, the nervous system, and the hormonal system when an individual is confronted by a stressor.
- Discuss the General Adaptation Syndrome.
- Explain the role that an individual's locus of control has in the adaptation to stress.

- Identify three interventions that promote positive adaptation to stress.
- Describe the use of "Stop, Divert, and Reframe" when negative thinking is potentially sabotaging problem solving in response to a stressor.
- Discuss the use of Mindfulness-Based Stress Reduction as a problem-solving modality.

KEY TERMS

alarm stage of the GAS
compartmentalization
distress
eustress
exhaustion stage of the GAS

fight-or-flight response
General Adaptation
   Syndrome (GAS)
limbic-hypothalamic-
   pituitary-adrenal axis

locus of control
Mindfulness-Based Stress
   Reduction
resistance stage of the
   GAS

Social Readjustment
   Rating Scale
stress
stressor

All living creatures experience stress. While in nursing school, the student confronts new learning material as well as the need to synthesize this information and use it in a variety of settings, including in the clinical area providing patient care, in the simulation laboratory, and during test taking. The student is constantly challenged in school and often feels stressed, and this stress can become further complicated by other important personal issues.

WHAT IS STRESS?

There are a number of definitions for stress. Chandler (2010) defines stress as the interaction between the individual and the environment that causes strain and challenges the person's ability to cope. The stimulus that is causing the stress is called the stressor. Stressors can be internal or external to the

individual. An example of an internal stressor is when peak physical performance is demanded of a person who has not eaten properly and has only slept 4 hours per night for several nights in a row. The body cannot sustain the stress of inadequate nutrition and the lack of sleep. The individual becomes irritable, is unable to sustain a fully awake state, and falls into a light sleeping state while studying. An example of an external stimulus is when that same individual goes to school the next morning without having prepared for class. The professor calls on that student to be part of the student team to demonstrate the study material in the simulation laboratory. The student does not know the information and demonstrates physical signs of stress, such as dry mouth, sweaty palms, and rapid heart rate.

There are two types of stress defined in the research. *Distress* is stress that is damaging to the individual. An example of distress is when a person has an argument with his or her spouse before leaving for work. On the way to work, the individual thinks about what could have been said instead and experiences physical sensations, such as an upset stomach or headache as a result of the stress of arguing with someone significant in his or her life. This stressor can become chronic if the relationship becomes further strained and the conflict is not resolved. Distress can take a toll on an individual's body as well as on his or her emotional state.

Eustress occurs as a result of a positive event. Examples of this may be the anticipation of the birth of a baby, buying a new house, or planning a wedding. Although these events may have positive outcomes, there are physical and emotional responses to the eustress that are similar to those caused by distress as a result of the psychologic and physical adjustments that occur in the mind and body with both types of stress.

Physical Responses to Stress

Stress signals the body that something is off course or not quite right. The body reacts in an effort to protect itself and to establish equilibrium. In 1932, Walter Cannon described the fight-or-flight response. There are several systems involved in the physical response to stress, including the neurologic, cardiovascular, and hormonal systems. The brain (specifically the medulla oblongata) is responsible for the heart rate, the blood pressure rate, and the respiration rate. When a stressor is detected, the autonomic nervous system tells the medulla oblongata to increase the blood flow to certain organs (e.g., the muscles) to allow the individual to prepare for fight or flight. The brain receives an increase in oxygenated blood to increase awareness and the ability to think and respond to the stressor. The blood in the brain has an increase in glucose, epinephrine, and nor-epinephrine to assist the individual with reacting to the stressor. The reticular formation supports the coordination of the sensory and motor tract of the individual's brain. This provides the individual with the ability to fight or flee (Baier, 2009). The limbic-hypothalamic-pituitary-adrenal axis is initiated when the person's brain perceives a stressor. The limbic area of the brain communicates with the hypothalamus that the stress is occurring, and the hypothalamus secretes corticotropin-releasing factor, which alerts the pituitary gland regarding the need for action against the stressor. The pituitary gland secretes adrenocorticotropic hormone, which stimulates the adrenal cortex to release cortisol. Cortisol is involved in helping the entire body to react to the stress by mobilizing the energy reserves so that the body can rapidly respond (Fontaine, 2009; Alters and Schiff, 2006) (Figure 5-1).

Recent research involves understanding the role that the neurotransmitter gamma-aminobutyric acid (GABA) has on the limbic-hypothalamic-pituitary-adrenal axis. It is thought that GABA may assist the limbic-hypothalamic-pituitary-adrenal axis with decreasing the intensity of the neurologic and hormonal reactions to prevent chronic stress-related illnesses (Cullinan et al, 2008). Research is also exploring the

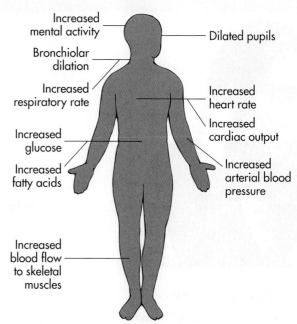

FIGURE 5-1. The fight-or-flight response. (From Potter PA, Perry AG, editors: *Fundamentals of nursing,* ed 7, St. Louis, 2009, Mosby Elsevier, p. 486, Figure 31-1.)

relationship between the serotonin and GABA pathways in the brain; this study is identifying the role that anxiolytics can play in reducing the effect that stress has on both neurotransmitter pathways (Vinkers et al, 2010). These research projects will involve the use of medications to initiate the GABA and serotonin systems to reduce the physical responses of chronic stress (see Chapters 6 and 25).

Hans Selye and the General Adaptation Syndrome

Hans Selye described the General Adaptation Syndrome (GAS) as a three-stage physical and psychologic reaction to stress. The first stage is called the *alarm stage.* The alarm reaction involves the physical reaction described as the fight-or-flight response. During this stage, the body's brain, cardiovascular system, and hormonal system become activated so that the person is able to react to the stressor (Figure 5-2). The physical changes can last between 1 minute and several hours. The second stage is called the *resistance stage.* The body stabilizes and returns to normal homeostasis. The neurotransmitters, cardiovascular system, and hormonal system return to the normal level of functioning during the resistance stage (see Figure 5-2). If the individual's body does not adapt and the stressor continues to be prominent, then the third stage, called the *exhaustion stage,* occurs. The physiologic and psychologic responses to the stressor continue in the alarm-stage format. The body becomes exhausted and is unable to sustain the necessary changes that are activated during the alarm stage. The exhaustion stage can manifest itself in the form of illnesses such as infections, headaches, hypertension, asthma attacks, chronic fatigue syndrome, depression, anxiety disorders, and many other chronic conditions. If the exhaustion stage continues for a long period of

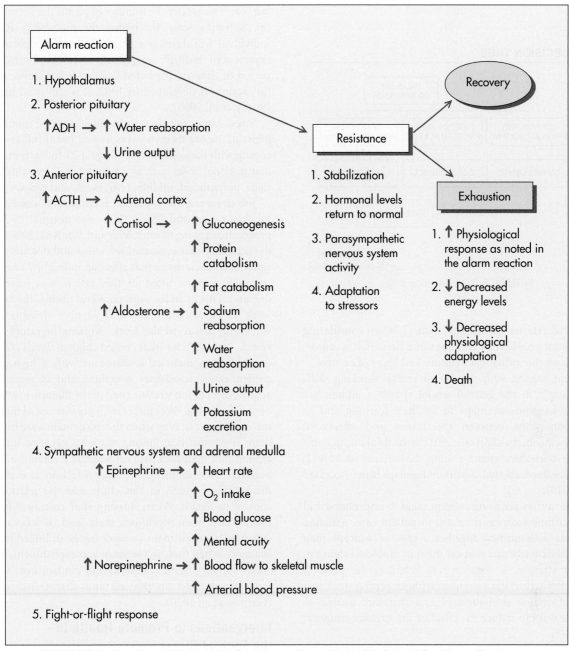

FIGURE 5-2. The General Adaptation Syndrome. (From Potter PA, Perry AG, editors: *Fundamentals of nursing*, ed 7, St. Louis, 2009, Mosby Elsevier, p. 487, Figure 31-2.)

time, it can result in the individual's death (Zuck and Frey, 2006; Baier, 2009).

Personal Control and Stress

Stress is part of an individual's everyday life. Some people cope with stress in a healthier adaptive manner than others. What causes two people to react differently to the same stressor? Each person has his or her own method of problem solving. Some individuals have learned how to make stress a challenge, whereas others perceive the stressor as devastating and too big to solve. How individuals perceive the issues around them will determine how they will respond to untoward events.

Rotter (1975) described the locus of control in his paper about generalized expectancies. His hypothesis was based on how different people perform a task with regard to their own sense of goal attainment. The locus of control can be measured along a continuum between internal and external control. An individual's locus of control includes his or her thoughts, beliefs, behaviors, aptitudes, culture, and value system. Individuals who demonstrate an internal locus of control view their capability to have personal success or failure as having to do with their own efforts and their ability to complete a task. An individual with an external locus of control views task completion as having to do with circumstances beyond his or her control, such as luck and the

DECISION TREE

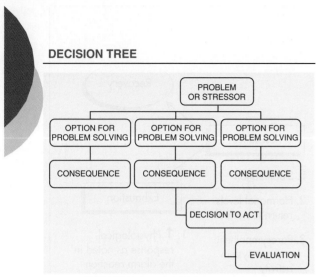

FIGURE 5-3. A decision tree.

influence of external forces (e.g., nature). When considering how different people cope with the same stressor, it is important to assess the individual's culture and locus of control.

Problem solving with the use of critical-thinking skills is now taught in the general school system. Children are taught to use concept maps to facilitate learning and to make connections between the causes and effects of events (www.somers.k12.ny.us, 2010; www.thinkbuzan.com\US\articles\view\how-create-a-mind-map. Accessed May 1, 2010; www.bookladymel.com\thinkingmaps.htm. Accessed May 1, 2010).

Student nurses are using concept maps to understand and evaluate complex concepts related to patient care. Assisting individuals with putting together a type of concept map called a *decision tree* can support them in problem solving to address a stressor. A decision tree enhances the person's ability to think through a problem without getting stuck in a pattern of feeling overwhelmed and therefore unable to determine ways to reduce the effect of the stressful situation (Figure 5-3).

The decision tree pictured here provides individuals with opportunities to problem solve by breaking down a problem or a stressor into smaller increments. Defining a problem clearly and determining three options for solving it can help a person to think about more than one way to work on the problem or stressor. Determining the possible consequences of each option further broadens the ability to problem solve. Individuals who are rigid or constricted in their ability to determine more than one option for problem solving tend to experience more stress.

Life Events That Trigger Stress

In 1967, researchers Holmes and Rahe developed the Social Readjustment Rating Scale (Table 5-1). This rating scale outlines 43 stressors that are each assigned a point value. The individual adds up the number of points on the basis of the life events that he or she has experienced within the

last year. The greater the number of points the person receives on the rating scale, the higher the probability is that the individual will develop a physical illness. People who have experienced multiple major life stressors during a short period of time are predicted to develop an illness. Although this scale was developed in 1967, it is still used in research (Scully et al, 2000).

Stress can occur as an individual ages and matures. Each phase of life has its own stressors and healthful strategies for coping with these issues. See Chapter 21 to learn more about maturational crises such as adolescence, career choices, marriage, parenthood, midlife, retirement, and old age.

Job stress is a life event that is commonly cited as a cause for frustration and illness. It is not unusual to hear that people dread going to work. Way and MacNeil (2006) searched the literature that evaluated job stress and described organizational characteristics that affect an individual's health. One common stressor listed in this article was increased job demand. This includes work pace and timing, the amount of work to be accomplished, and whether there is an overwhelming nature to the work. Nursing literature was surveyed, and articles that noted higher levels of worker dissatisfaction included institutions with a high nurse-to-patient ratio, mandatory overtime, and increased patient acuity. Another job stressor cited in the literature is the degree of social support. Workplaces with positive social interactions involve less stress, even when the job demands are high. When there is competition among workers, negative interactions among staff members, and no assistance when the workload becomes overwhelming, job dissatisfaction is evident. The third stressor noted in this study was the relation of job control to health. When nursing staff members had more control over their workload, their level of job satisfaction increased. Commitment to work has been linked to job satisfaction. When there is a sense of accomplishment, increased social support, team cohesion, and control over workflow, injuries sustained on the job and absenteeism decreased (Garrosa et al, 2010).

Interventions to Promote Health in the Face of Stress

Understanding the causal factors of stress gives the nurse the opportunity to assess a patient to determine if there are areas in that patient's life that demonstrate an unhealthy coping pattern. Identifying the type of stress and the pattern of the stressor can lead to successful interventions. The American Institute of Stress (www.stress.org) has identified 50 behaviors that are common signs and symptoms of stress, including the following: frequent headaches; cold and sweaty hands and feet; dry mouth; frequent colds and infections; chest pain; frequent urination; increased anger, frustration, and depression; increased or decreased appetite, including weight gain or loss; sleep disturbances; social isolation; fatigue; and an increase in smoking, alcohol, or drug use. These are examples of some of the symptoms that the nurse may encounter in individuals who are experiencing an increase in stress.

TABLE 5-1	SOCIAL READJUSTMENT RATING SCALE	
RANK	LIFE EVENT	MEAN VALUE
1	Death of spouse	100
2	Divorce	73
3	Marital separation	65
4	Jail term	63
5	Death of close family member	63
6	Personal injury or illness	53
7	Marriage	50
8	Fired at work	47
9	Marital reconciliation	45
10	Retirement	45
11	Change in health of family member	44
12	Pregnancy	40
13	Sex difficulties	39
14	Gain of new family member	39
15	Business readjustment	39
16	Change in financial state	38
17	Death of close friend	37
18	Change to different line of work	36
19	Change in number of arguments with spouse	35
20	Mortgage over $10,000	31
21	Foreclosure of mortgage or loan	30
22	Chance in responsibilities at work	29
23	Son or daughter leaving home	29
24	Trouble with in-laws	29
25	Outstanding personal achievement	28
26	Wife begin or stop work	26
27	Begin or end school	26
28	Change in living conditions	25
29	Revision of personal habits	24
30	Trouble with boss	23
31	Change in work hours or conditions	20
32	Change in residence	20
33	Change in schools	20
34	Change in recreation	19
35	Change in church activities	19
36	Change in social activities	18
37	Mortgage or loan less than $10,000	17
38	Change in sleeping habits	16
39	Change in number of family get-togethers	15
40	Change in eating habits	15
41	Vacation	13
42	Christmas	12
43	Minor violations of the law	11

One area to consider when planning an intervention is the use of health-promoting defense mechanisms. Humor is an example of such a defense mechanism, because it allows the individual to reframe the stressor by poking fun at the situation. While telling others about the stressor in a humorous manner, sometimes the person can plan a different way to problem solve that can reduce the effect of the stress. Another healthy defense mechanism is compartmentalization. The person who uses compartmentalization learns to leave the stressor in a designated space. An example of this mechanism is to plan 10 to 15 minutes to read a novel before going home after a stressful workday. After reading for a few minutes, the stress of work is left at work, and the individual can proceed home without thinking about the workday (Miller and McGowen, 2010). Another example of compartmentalization is when there is a conflict at work; one could to use a decision tree (see Figure 5-3) to plan an alternative approach to the conflict and then think about another aspect of work until it is time to implement the new option for solving the problem. See Chapter 10 for more information about defense mechanisms.

Exercise, a healthy diet, and sufficient sleep are ongoing recipes for health. This is especially important when there is an increase in stress in a person's life. There is a tendency for people to skip exercise when stressed, particularly when there is an increase in fatigue. Individuals tend to eat more haphazardly when they are confronted with stress or to increase their intake of fat, chocolate, or sugar as a coping strategy. Disrupted sleep can lead to an increase in physical stress, because the body does not have the sufficient amount of restorative rest. Making time for exercise, healthful eating, and rest is emphasized in all of the literature as a method to reduce the effects of stress on the body and to promote health (www.stress.org/topic-effects.htm. Accessed August 13, 2010).

People need people to prevent isolation to promote their ability to deal with stress. In a study, Floyd and colleagues (2007) found that individuals who had significant relationships that involved an expression of affection had a reduction in the fight-or-flight response when stressed. Women who regularly received hugs from their romantic partners had a decrease in resting heart rate and a healthy functioning limbic-hypothalamic-pituitary-adrenal axis. Conversely, individuals who experienced conflict within their families showed a higher level of stress and an increased possibility of developing an illness.

A well-researched therapeutic modality called *cognitive behavioral therapy* is used in a variety of inpatient and outpatient mental health settings to assist individuals with recognizing when their automatic thought patterns increase their anxiety and whether these thoughts contain erroneous core beliefs of negative self-worth (Beck, 1976; see Chapter 26). If an individual is attempting to solve a problem created by a stressor and encounters a negative core belief, some of the principles of cognitive behavioral therapy may be indicated to decrease the stressor. A way of thinking about such an intervention that is based on the principles of cognitive behavioral therapy and appropriate for reducing the effect of a stressor is called Stop, Divert, and Reframe, which is described as follows:

Stop, Divert, and Reframe

You are a student nurse who is preparing to take a test. During the preparation, you begin to tell yourself, "I do not

BOX 5-1	STOP, DIVERT, AND REFRAME METHOD

Stop: Interrupt the negative train of thought. This is best accomplished by telling yourself, using your name, that this type of thinking is going to sabotage the test.

For example: "Kristin, stop this train of thought so that you can successfully pass the test!"

Divert: Think about something that will rapidly reduce the stress. An example may be a favorite prayer or quote; something beautiful like an animal, a picture, or a tree; or the lyrics of a favorite inspirational song.

Reframe: Use this step to reinforce what you *can* do to reduce the stressor. What type of test-taking skills can assist you during the test? Find the key word in each question to determine what the professor is asking. Think through the concept that is being tested. Tell yourself that you can work this way and complete the test to obtain a good grade.

understand the concepts, I can't understand how this applies to patient care, and I do not understand the recent lecture the professor gave." Your anxiety begins to climb. You are having trouble sleeping, and you are irritable with your family on the morning of the test. As the test is being passed out, you begin to feel your heart rate increase, and your palms become sweaty. As you begin to take the test, you tell yourself, "I don't understand this stuff. How am I going to pass this course? I need to pass it to become a nurse!" You recognize the need to interrupt this pattern of negative self-talk that is increasing the stress of taking the test and that may sabotage your grade. You decide to use the method of Stop, Divert, and Reframe (Box 5-1).

By using a cognitive method to address the stressor, there is a possibility of a positive outcome and a reduction of the negative physical effects of stress.

Research has shown that mindfulness meditation can reduce the effects of stress on the individual and also reduces negative emotions. Lane and colleagues (2007) trained healthy adults in the use of meditation for stress reduction. The authors found that the research subjects showed improvement with regard to mood and their perception of the stressor. The more often the individual was able to meditate, the stronger the positive outcome became. In another study, Oman and colleagues (2008) found that the use of mindfulness meditation reduced stress and increased forgiveness among college undergraduates (see Chapter 27).

Mindfulness-Based Stress Reduction (Kabat-Zinn, 1994) and Transcendental Meditation (www.stress.org\topic-red uction.htm. Accessed August 13, 2010) (http:\\www.umassm ed.edu\csrn\srp\index.asp\. Accessed April 4, 2010) based on the traditional practices of Asian religions. It is helpful to teach individuals a generic method of relaxation by concentrating on the rhythm of breathing. Paying attention to each breath one takes in during inhalation and releases during expiration provides a focus for the meditation. A sound, word, or brief phrase can also enhance the individual's ability to concentrate. There are commercial products to assist with meditation. Nurses in the Victoria Province in Australia developed a CD entitled *A Guide to Relaxation* that has three choices for relaxation exercises. One track consists of guided progressive muscle relaxation, the second track involves the use of visualization to enhance relaxation, and the third track is a relaxation exercise for children. This CD is available through the Integrated Primary Mental Health Service website at www.ipmhs.org.au, and it does not have any copyright restrictions (Ahrens, 2008).

Living a balanced life assists with stress reduction. The integration of arts, music, reading, spirituality, and recreation is important. If one focuses on only one aspect of his or her life, such as work, there is a greater opportunity for stress to build (see Chapters 26 & 27).

CHAPTER SUMMARY

- Two types of stress have been identified: distress and eustress. The physical and emotional responses are similar for both types of stresses.
- The fight-or-flight response involves the neurologic, hormonal, and cardiovascular systems. The limbic-hypothalamic-pituitary-adrenal axis makes use of hormones to assist the body with quickly mobilizing to respond to the stressor.
- Hans Selye defined the GAS as a three-stage physical and psychologic reaction to stress. By understanding this theoretic framework, nursing interventions can be formulated to protect the body from the exhaustion stage of the GAS.
- The locus of control is the individual's perception of his or her ability to problem solve. An individual with an

internal locus of control believes that he or she has the ability to problem solve with the use of his or her own efforts. Individuals with an external locus of control rely on external factors, such as luck and circumstances beyond their control, to problem solve.
- The nurse can identify several different interventions to assist a person who is experiencing stress. These include the use of humor, compartmentalization, regular exercise, eating a healthy diet, and obtaining sufficient sleep. Cognitive interventions to reduce the impact of stress include an offshoot of cognitive behavioral therapy called Stop, Divert, and Reframe as well as the use of meditation.

REVIEW QUESTIONS

1. A woman who is anticipating her wedding ceremony in a week comes to the urgent care clinic with a headache that has been ongoing for 3 days' duration as well as a pounding feeling in her chest. She is concerned that she may be having a stroke or a cerebral vascular accident. All of her medical tests are negative. The woman wonders what is happening to her, because she feels that she is unable to function. What is the best response?
   1. " You are having difficulty coping with your upcoming wedding."
   2. "You are experiencing distress as a result of your upcoming wedding."
   3. "You are experiencing eustress as a result of your upcoming wedding."
   4. "You are being warned by your body that you may have hypertension."

2. Which intervention has been shown in the research to reduce the increase in the activity of the limbic-hypothalamic-pituitary-adrenal axis that accompanies the reaction to a stressor?
   1. Talking on the phone to a friend
   2. Hugging a significant person in your life
   3. Confronting the person who created the stressor
   4. Assigning blame to the causal factor of the stressor

3. When assessing an individual who has had several infections in a short period of time, it is important to ask which of the following questions?
   1. Does the person have an autoimmune disease?
   2. Does the person have a genetic history for a depressed immune system?
   3. Does the person come in contact with multiple children?
   4. Has the person had a recent increase in stressful events in his or her life?

4. An individual says, "I am able to think through problems, and I like to piece together the causes and effects of the issues." Which of the following is this person demonstrating?
   1. Internal locus of control
   2. External power while problem solving
   3. External locus of control
   4. Eustress when problem solving

5. The identified categories of job stress include which of the following?
   1. Job satisfaction, staffing patterns and work conflict
   2. Work hardiness, repetitious task completion, and staffing patterns
   3. Job demand, negative social interactions, and lack of control
   4. Job demand, staffing patterns, and repetitious task completion

REFERENCES

Ahrens J: Relaxation to combat stress, *Aust Nurs J* 16(4):44-45, 2008.

Alters S, Schiff W: *Essential concepts for healthy living*, ed 4, Sudbury, Mass, 2006, Jones and Bartlett Publishers.

Baier M: Stress and coping. In Potter PA, Perry AG, editors: *Fundamentals of nursing*, ed 7, St. Louis, 2009, Mosby Elsevier.

Beck AT: *Cognitive therapy and the emotional disorders*, New York, 1976, International Universities Press.

Chandler B: Stress. In Long JL, editor: *Gale encyclopedia of nursing and allied health*, vol 4, ed 2, Detroit, Thomson Gale 2010.

Cullinan WE et al: Functional role of local GABAergic influences on the HPA axis, *Brain Struct Funct* 213(1-2):63-72, 2008.

Fontaine KL: *Mental health nursing*, ed 6, Upper Saddle River, NJ, 2009, Pearson Prentice Hall, p. 106.

Floyd K et al: Human affection exchange: XIV. Relational affection predicts resting heart rate and free cortisol secretion during acute stress, *Behav Med* 32(4):151-157, 2007.

Garrosa E et al: The relationship between job stressors, hardy personality, coping resources and burnout in a sample of nurses: a correlational study at two time points, *Int J Nurs Stud* 47(2):205-215, 2010.

Holmes TH, Rahe RH: The social readjustment rating scale, *J Psychosom Res* 11:213-218, 1967.

Kabat-Zinn J: *Catastrophe living: using the wisdom of your body and mind to face stress, pain, and illness*, New York, 1994, Guilford Press.

Lane JD et al: Brief meditation training can improve perceived stress and negative mood, *Altern Ther Health Med* 13(1): 38-45, 2007.

Miller MN, McGowen R: Strategies to avoid burnout in professional practice: some practical suggestions, *Psychiatric Times* 27(2):1-5, 2010.

Oman D et al: Meditation lowers stress and supports forgiveness among college students: a randomized controlled trial, *J Am Coll Health* 56(5):569-579, 2008.

Rotter JB: Some problems and misconceptions related to the construct of internal versus external control of reinforcement, *J Consult Clin Psychol* 43:56-67, 1975.

Scully JA et al: Life event checklists: revisiting the social readjustment rating scale after 30 years, *Educ Psychol Meas* 60(6):864-877, 2000.

Vinkers CH et al: 5-HT1A receptor blockade reverses GABA(A) receptor alpha3 subunit-mediated anxiolytic effects on stress-induced hyperthermia, *Psychopharmacology (Berl)* 211(2):123-130, 2010.

Way M, MacNeil M: Organizational characteristics and their effect on health, *Nurs Econ* 24(2):67-76, 2006.

Zuck M, Frey R: General adaptation syndrome. In Longe JL, editor: *Gale encyclopedia of medicine*, vol 3, ed 3, Detroit: Thomson Gale, 2006.

Online Resources

The American Institute of Stress: www.stress.org
American Psychological Association: www.apa.org

Center for Mindfulness at the University of Massachusetts Medical School: www.umassmed.edu/cfm/srp/index.aspx
Integrated Primary Mental Health Service (Australia): www.ipmhs.org.au. Accessed August 15, 2010.
MedicineNet.com: www.medicinenet.com/stress/article.htm
Thinking Maps (concept maps for school-aged children): www.bookladymel.com/thinkingmaps.htm

ThinkBuzan.com (Web site about the creation of concept maps): www.thinkbuzan.com/us/articles/view/how-to-create-a-mind-map
Transcendental Meditation: www.tm.org. Accessed April 20, 2010.

Neurobiology in Mental Health and Mental Disorder

Candice A. Francis

"Man's mind, once stretched by a new idea, never regains its original dimensions."

Oliver Wendell Holmes

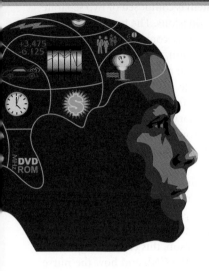

ⓔvolve WEBSITE

http://evolve.elsevier.com/Fortinash/

OBJECTIVES

- Identify the basic anatomic structures of the central nervous system.
- Describe the physiologic functions of the central nervous system.
- Describe the normal functioning of neurons.
- Discuss the role of common neurotransmitters in the functioning of the central nervous system.
- Describe the electrochemical mechanism of the central nervous system.

- Identify criteria for patient care related to neuroimaging testing.
- Identify emerging technologies with a significant impact on the future of psychiatric nursing.
- State uses for current neurobiologic research findings when planning care for patients with a psychiatric disorder.
- Identify potential areas for further nursing research related to neurobiology.

KEY TERMS

action potential	cerebellum	limbic system	peripheral nervous system
adrenergic	cerebrum	neuroendocrinology	pyramidal tract
amygdala	cholinergic	neuroimaging	stem cells
aphasia	chronobiology	neuroinformatics	sulci
autonomic nervous system	circadian rhythm	neuron	synapse
basal nuclei	cortex	neuroplasticity	Wernicke's area
Broca's area	diencephalon	neuroscience	
central nervous system	hypothalamus	neurotransmitter	

An explosion of information occurred during the last decade of the twentieth century regarding the subject of the human brain and the central nervous system, and this explosion continues today. The 10-year period between 1990 and 1999 was designated the "Decade of the Brain" in a joint research initiative by the Library of Congress, The National Institutes of Mental Health, and the National Institutes of Health. More was learned about the brain and the neurosciences than during all of the combined time that preceded that decade. A floodgate of research in the neurosciences opened and remains open today. It has revealed that the human brain—which weighs approximately 3 pounds and has approximately 100 billion neurons—is the most sophisticated computer ever created.

This continually evolving neuroscientific research provides new strategies for addressing mental disorders, which benefits clinicians who provide care, as well as patients and families who seek answers to their problems. The majority of the population now recognizes mental disorders as brain-based illnesses.

Because of a lack of information and education about the topic, some still misunderstand mental disorders and stigmatize those who have the disorders. However, new research into brain biology and the publicizing of information has helped to reshape perceptions of mental illness.

To understand treatment approaches to psychiatric illness, the psychiatric mental health nurse requires a firm foundation in the fundamentals of neurobiology, physiology, and genetics, and how these affect the treatment of psychiatric disorders. This chapter reviews the fundamentals of neurobiology and related topics and examines concepts and clinical approaches to the treatment of mental illness in relation to our growing knowledge of neuroscience.

NEUROBIOLOGY AND HUMAN BEHAVIOR

The biologic model of psychiatric illness has become increasingly more sophisticated as a result of the creation and availability of new tools. Science has advanced far beyond merely making educated guesses about how the brain works; it has developed scientific models that facilitate the diagnosis of brain-based disorders and the development of new and effective treatments and interventions (Bear et al, 2007).

The best psychiatric mental health care begins with the understanding that the symptoms associated with psychiatric disorders are usually manifested behaviorally. Patients with psychiatric disorders frequently behave in ways society considers different, strange, or abnormal. Their disorders are expressed through responses such as hearing voices that no one else hears, having paranoid thoughts that everyone is out to hurt them, or wearing a winter coat on a hot summer day. These abnormal perceptions, thoughts, and behaviors usually have a neurobiologic basis.

Knowledge of normal brain structure and function helps mental health care providers to offer an optimal level of treatment to people with brain-based illnesses. With an understanding of the structural or neurochemical defects that affect patients with psychiatric disorders, psychiatric nurses are able to effectively assess patients' responses, plan interventions, and provide optimal treatment.

NEUROANATOMY

The most rudimentary of human perceptions, thoughts, feelings, impulses, and actions begin in the central nervous system. The brain acts as the primary mediator organ that controls and determines how people interact with the world. All human responses are the result of the complex interaction between underlying neuroanatomy and neurophysiology as well as the genetic, environmental, and developmental factors that influence those systems.

The Brain

The brain is one of the most important structures in the human body. Although it weighs only approximately 3 pounds, the brain contains approximately 100 billion cells, and it is the most complex and vital of human organs (Figure 6-1). The human nervous system is composed of two separate but interconnected anatomic divisions. The first division, the central nervous system (CNS), is composed of the spinal cord and brain. The second division, the peripheral nervous system (PNS), contains peripheral nerves, 12 pairs of cranial nerves that originate just outside of the brainstem, and 31 pairs of spinal nerves that arise from the spinal cord. These peripheral nerves transmit sensory (incoming) information toward the CNS and motor (outgoing) information away from the CNS to muscles and glands that are controlled by the CNS.

Although the PNS and certain interactions with the autonomic nervous system are of critical importance to human functioning, the understanding of psychiatric disorders depends on the in-depth understanding of the structure and function of the CNS. For that reason, this chapter focuses on the anatomy and physiology of the CNS and how the nurse will use that knowledge to provide care to individuals who have psychiatric and neurologic disorders.

Brain Cells

Brain cells belong to one of two large categories: neurons and neuroglia. About 10% of the cells that make up the CNS are neurons. Neurons are highly specialized to generate and conduct electrical signals, and they are the cells that we most commonly think about when we consider the nervous system. Neuroglia are the other neural cells that provide the mechanical and physiologic support for neurons and that produce an important insulating material called *myelin*. White matter found in the brain and spinal cord is composed of the axons of neurons that are insulated by myelin and the glial cells that produce it. White matter makes up the core of major brain structures such as the cerebrum and the cerebellum. The gray matter or cortex typically covers the surface of these organs and lacks myelin. The gray matter found in the cortex is the functional area of the brain where neurons communicate with each other by way of synapses and where neurotransmitters are concentrated.

Of the billions of cells that make up the human brain, only about 10% are neurons. The neurons are directly responsible for impulse conduction that allows the brain to initiate signals and process information. Each neuron has thousands if not hundreds of thousands of connections to other neurons. These connections, which are called *synapses*, allow various areas of the brain to communicate with each other, to interpret sensory information, and to initiate stimuli that travel along neural pathways and that activate several areas of the brain.

This constant brain nerve cell (neuronal) activity accounts for the complex perceptions and behaviors that make us human. The vast numbers of synaptic interconnections make the brain far more complex and sophisticated than any computer.

There are several types of neurons in the brain. Nuclei and other major organelles are typically in a region of the cell known as the *cell body* or *cyton*. Two kinds of processes originate from the cell body region. Dendrites carry electrical

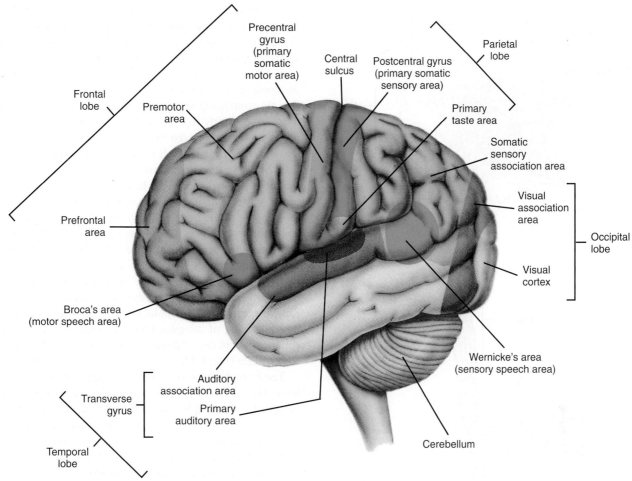

FIGURE 6-1. Functional areas of the cerebral cortex. (From Thibodeau GA, Patton KT: *Anatomy & physiology,* ed 7, St. Louis, 2009, Mosby.)

impulses toward the cell body, whereas axons carry impulses away from the cell body. Some axons are more than a meter in length. Axons end at the telodendron, where small presynaptic axon terminals or synaptic knobs are located. Figure 6-2 illustrates one common type of neuron, called a *motor neuron,* which stimulates glands and muscle cells.

Cerebrum

The cerebrum is the largest part of the brain, and it is divided into two halves called *cerebral hemispheres.* The cerebral hemispheres contain important functional areas such as the cerebral cortex, the basal nuclei, and the limbic system.

The cerebral hemispheres account for more than 70% of the neurons in the CNS, and they are responsible for functions such as hearing, vision, language, cognitive functions, control of muscles, and sensory interpretation. The left hemisphere is dominant in almost 95% of people and mainly controls the motor and sensory functions on the right side of the body. The right hemisphere controls functions on the left side of the body, and vice versa. This observation dates back to the time of Hippocrates.

Effective coordinated human activity requires a complex interrelationship and communication within and between the two hemispheres. A large bundle of white matter called the *corpus callosum* connects the two hemispheres. Sensorimotor information constantly flows between the two hemispheres via nerve pathways in the corpus callosum. The corpus callosum has to be intact for full, smooth, and coordinated communication between the hemispheres.

The outermost surface of the cerebral cortex contains ridges that are separated by grooves and indentations. Shallow grooves are called *sulci,* and the deeper grooves that extend deep into the brain are called *fissures.* The raised areas are called *gyri.* The sulci and gyri dramatically increase the overall surface area of the cerebrum. The cerebral cortex is typically composed of only six layers of cells, but it covers an area that, if spread out, is equal almost 2.5 square feet. By contrast, the cortex of a chimpanzee would cover only a single sheet of paper, whereas a rat's cortex occupies an area roughly equal to the size of a postage stamp (Gribbin, 2002). Most discussions of cerebral function focus on the outer gray layer, which is the cerebral cortex. Reductions in the thickness of the surface area of the cortex are associated with some age-related disorders (Dickerson et al, 2009).

Anatomically, the cerebrum is divided by the major fissures into four distinct functional regions called *lobes.* These

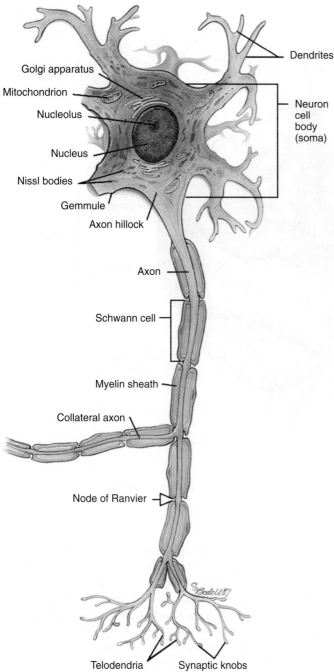

Golgi apparatus

Mitochondrion

Nucleolus

Nucleus

Nissl bodies

Gemmule

Axon hillock

Dendrites

Neuron
cell
body
(soma)

Axon

Schwann cell

Myelin sheath

Collateral axon

Node of Ranvier

Telodendria   Synaptic knobs

FIGURE 6-2. Structural features of neurons: dendrites, cell body, and axon. (From Lewis SM et al: *Medical-surgical nursing: assessment and management of clinical problems,* ed 7, St. Louis, 2007, Mosby.)

are the *frontal, temporal, occipital,* and *parietal* lobes. Although these lobes often work together, each has distinct functions. The normal functions of each lobe, along with typical symptoms of disturbances in each cerebral cortical region of the brain, are described in Table 6-1. Many symptoms that are exhibited by patients with neurologic and mental disorders are the result of disturbances in the normal functioning of one or more these cerebral lobes.

The frontal lobe is the largest lobe in the human brain. Much of what makes human behavior unique is a result of the functioning of the frontal lobe. The frontal lobe contains several important structures. The primary motor cortex lies in front of the large central sulcus, and it is also called the *precentral gyrus.* As the primary cortex, it is responsible for directly controlling the voluntary motor activity of specific muscles. Neurons that originate from the primary motor cortex are directly traced to peripheral nerves that innervate the muscles of the body. It is near the medulla of the brain that the nerve tracts cross over or decussate to the opposite side of the spinal cord. This helps to explain why the right motor cortex actually controls voluntary motor activity on the left side of the body and why the left motor cortex controls motor activity on the right side of the body. As the nerve tracts leave the brain, they form a bulge that is shaped like a pyramid and that is sometimes called the *pyramidal tract.* Extrapyramidal symptoms (EPS) in relation to some psychotropic medications are described in Chapters 13 and 25. Knowledge of this neurobiology will facilitate the nurse's understanding of complex pharmacologic interactions and enhance patient care. Patients suffer when nurses lack knowledge of EPS (Box 6-1).

The frontal lobe also contains two other important structures. The premotor cortex is responsible for the coordinated movement of multiple muscles, and the somatic association cortex integrates motor commands. Researchers have identified a number of brain regions as association regions. In fact, some estimate that 70% to 75% of all cortical regions are association regions that integrate functions in the primary region. The primary regions are generally involved in analysis, initiation, interpretation, and integrative activities. In the case of the frontal lobe, the somatic association cortex is the area of the brain that is responsible for coordinating learned motor skills. Cognition, memory, and analytic functions are largely functions of a third region of the frontal lobe known as the *prefrontal cortex.* Damage to this area of the frontal lobe may cause changes in personality.

Other functions of the prefrontal cortex, which are sometimes called *executive functions,* include reasoning, planning, prioritizing, sequencing behavior, insight, flexibility, and judgment. Normal frontal cortical functions help suppress and moderate more primitive impulses and actions. The frontal cortex also allows a person to appropriately process incoming sensory stimuli, reason, focus on tasks, and respond to social cues. Difficulty with performing these activities often manifests as symptoms of psychiatric disorders. Two key functions—working memory and behavioral inhibition—have increasingly become targets of research as scientists explore the neurobiology of psychiatric disorders (Dubin, 2002). Another important area that is usually localized only in the left frontal lobe is Broca's area, the speech area. Accidents or strokes that damage Broca's area may result in the inability to speak (i.e., motor aphasia).

The temporal lobe is responsible for some functions of language, memory, and emotion. Wernicke's area is a specialized area of the temporal lobe and is responsible for

TABLE 6-1	NORMAL FUNCTIONS AND SYMPTOMS OF DYSFUNCTION OF THE CEREBRUM		
LOBE	**LOCATION**	**NORMAL FUNCTION**	**SYMPTOMS OF ALTERATIONS IN BRAIN FUNCTIONING**
Frontal	Anterior (front area) of brain	Programming and execution of motor functions Higher thought processes such as planning, ability to abstract, trial-and-error learning, and decision making Intellectual insight and judgment Expression of emotion	Changes in affect, such as flattening Alteration in language production Alteration in motor functioning Impulsive behavior Impaired decision making Concrete thinking
Parietal	Posterior to the central sulcus	Sensory perception: taking in information from the environment, organizing it, and communicating this information to the rest of the brain Association areas that allow for such things as accurately following directions on a map, reading a clock, building a birdhouse, or dressing oneself	Altered sensory perceptions, such as decreased consciousness of pain sensation Difficulty with time concepts, such as an inability to keep appointment times Alteration in personal hygiene Alteration in ability to calculate numbers Inability to adequately perform the common motor actions of writing Mixing up of the right and left Poor attention span
Temporal	Lies beneath the skull on both sides; commonly called the *temples*	Primarily responsible for hearing and receiving information via the ears	Auditory hallucinations Increased sexual focus Decreased motivation Alterations in memory Altered emotional responses Sensory aphasia
Occipital	Most posterior of the brain lobes; the back of the head	Primarily responsible for seeing and receiving information via the eyes	Visual hallucinations

organizing words so that they will be recognized and express the correct emotional content. Effects of long-term alcohol abuse can damage this area and are described in Chapter 15. Written words, verbal speech, and visual recognition that is critical to communication are all functions of the temporal lobe. Language is one example where two distinct regions—Broca's area in the frontal lobe and Wernicke's area in the temporal lobe—work together to facilitate normal communication. Aphasia, which is a communication disorder, sometimes has several origins within the brain, most notably in Wernicke's area of the temporal lobe and Broca's of the frontal lobe. The auditory association area of the temporal lobe is involved with memories, especially those that are connected to visual and auditory cues.

Communication disorders may involve several regions of the frontal and temporal cortices. Effective communication is vital to appropriate social interaction. The hippocampus is located deep within the temporal lobe. It has direct connections with the diencephalon, and it plays a major role in the encoding, consolidation, and retrieval of memories. Patients with Alzheimer's disease have damage to the hippocampus, which results in difficulties with short-term memory and learning ability.

The primary visual cortex is located in the occipital lobe. Color recognition, the ability to visually recognize and name objects, and the ability to track moving objects are functions

of the occipital lobe. The occipital lobe is sensitive to hypoxia, and trauma to this region of the brain sometimes results in blindness, even if the optic nerves and eyes remain intact. Lesions of the occipital lobe can cause visual hallucinations and other abnormalities of visual functioning, such as alexia (i.e., the inability to read).

The parietal lobe of the brain functions as the primary sensory processing center. The postcentral sensory gyrus area of the parietal lobe, which is also known as the *somesthetic cortex,* interprets sensory information. Posterior to the somesthetic cortex is the somesthetic association area. Again, as an association area, it is responsible for organizing, integrating, and analyzing sensory information that the primary sensory cortex in the postcentral gyrus will interpret more specifically.

Basal Nuclei. The basal nuclei, which are also known as *basal ganglia,* are concentrations of cell bodies that are closely involved with motor functions and association. Basal nuclei are gray matter located within the white matter of the cerebrum and the midbrain. They have countless connections to both the superficial cortex above and the deep midbrain structures below. Among the most well-known basal nuclei are the caudate lobe, the putamen, the globus pallidus, and the substantia nigra. These basal nuclei mediate movements such as walking while it is happening, and they also modulate and correct muscle functioning that allows movements to

---

BOX 6-1 EXTRAPYRAMIDAL SYMPTOMS: ADVERSE EFFECTS FROM ANTIPSYCHOTIC MEDICATIONS

- *Acute dystonia.* This condition is marked by prolonged and often painful muscle contractions that primarily occur in the eye (oculogyral crisis), the tongue (glossospasm), the neck (torticollis), and the back (retrocollis). The nurse assesses a patient who complains of a stiff neck, backache, or other muscle aches and pains after receiving antipsychotic medication to either rule out or treat this extrapyramidal symptom. Treatment includes antiparkinson medication.
- *Akathisia.* This condition is possibly a result of the blockade effect of these drugs on the neurotransmitter dopamine. Signs include motor restlessness, a subjective sense of anxiety, and an inability to lie down or sit still.
- *Pseudoparkinsonian symptoms.* This condition is marked by decreased motor movements, muscle rigidity, drooling,

mask-like facies (i.e., a blunted or flat facial expression), and a shuffling gait (walk). Treatment includes antiparkinson medication.
- *Tardive dyskinesia.* This is a significant adverse effect of antipsychotic drug therapy. Usually an irreversible and late-onset complication, it is characterized by the presence of abnormal, stereotyped, rhythmic movements of the limbs and torso; tongue protrusion; and chewing movements. It will affect any muscle in the body, including the diaphragm, and it usually occurs after the abrupt termination of the drug, a reduction in dosage, or after long-term, high-dose therapy. Nurses can minimize incidence with careful dose management, drug holidays, and the administration of antiparkinson drugs.

---

occur in a coordinated manner. The basal nuclei aid in the learning and programming of motor behavior so that it becomes automatic. Complex motor activities such as walking, eating, and driving become so natural that a person does not have to think consciously to perform them. This helps to explain why some people with dementia retain some of these complex behaviors long after severe memory or language loss has occurred.

Conditions such as Huntington's disease and Parkinson's disease are associated with basal nuclear dysfunction and the inability of these structures to effectively communicate with the motor cortex (Montoya et al, 2006). Some medications that are used to treat psychiatric disorders alter basal nuclear function (Box 6-1). For example, chlorpromazine (Thorazine) and haloperidol (Haldol) and other older neuroleptic antipsychotic medications sometimes cause hypertonicity, or dystonia, a condition that is marked by excessive muscle tone.

Limbic System. Instincts, primitive drives, sexual arousal, fear, aggression, and other primitive emotions are part of the mechanisms that help us to survive. These functions are localized in structures deep within the brain called the limbic system or the *limbic lobe.* It is often called a *system* because researchers believe its functions are a result of the interrelated and closely coordinated actions of its various brain structures (Table 6-2 and Figure 6-3).

The amygdala is part of the limbic system and is instrumental in emotional functioning and in the regulation of affective responses to events. The amygdala modulates common emotional states such as feelings of anger, aggression, love, and comfort in social settings. The limbic system's function of emotional regulation is linked with the olfactory pathways that connect with the amygdala. Some suggest that this explains why certain smells evoke strong emotional responses and memories in some individuals. The limbic system holds increasing interest for researchers who are trying to identify the biologic etiology of bipolar disorder. Some researchers hypothesize that the rapid misfiring of neurons in the amygdala plays an important role in the

TABLE 6-2	STRUCTURES OF THE LIMBIC SYSTEM
STRUCTURE	**FUNCTION**
Amygdala	Modulates emotional states
	Regulates affective responses to events
Thalamus	Relays all sensory information except smell
	Filters incoming information regarding emotions, mood, and memory to prevent the cortex from becoming overloaded
Hypothalamus	Regulates basic human functions such as sleep–rest patterns, body temperature, and the physical drives of hunger and sex
Hippocampus	Controls learning and the recall of an event with its associated memory

development of the typical symptoms of bipolar disorder. Researchers are also studying the amygdala in an attempt to better understand abnormal fear reactions, such as panic and violent rage behaviors (Carlson, 2009).

DIENCEPHALON

The thalamus, the hypothalamus, and the epithalamus are parts of the brain that are collectively referred to as the *diencephalon.* Functionally, these are also part of the limbic system.

The thalamus is a structure that acts primarily as a gateway for directing sensory information to the cerebral cortex. All sensory information except smell comes from the PNS to the cerebral cortex of the CNS via the thalamus. This critical structure helps to filter incoming sensory information and to direct it to specific regions of the cortex, where it can be

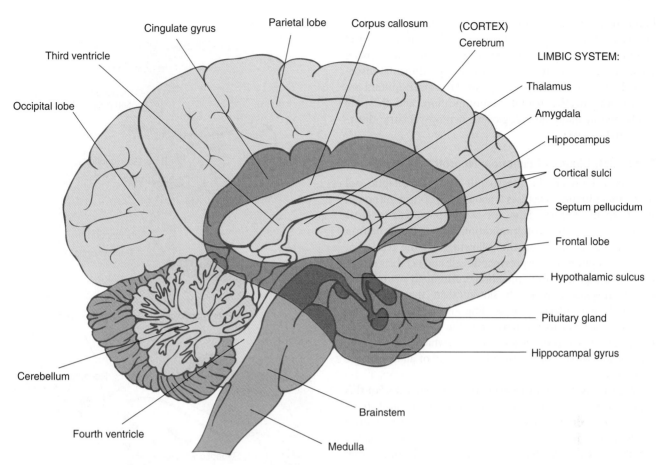

FIGURE 6-3. The limbic system.

interpreted and evaluated more fully. This includes sensory information that influences emotions, mood, and memory.

The hypothalamus is another functional part of the limbic system that rests deep within the brain and helps to regulate some of the most basic human functions, including sleep-rest patterns, body temperature, thirst, and the physical drives of hunger and sex. Research indicates that some symptomatic behaviors—such as appetite and sleep problems in the depressed patient, the seasonal mood changes of seasonal affective disorder, and temperature regulation problems in patients with schizophrenia (e.g., wearing winter coats in the summer)—are the result of hypothalamic dysregulation.

Cerebellum

The cerebellum, like the cerebrum, is bilobed, and it has a core of white matter that is covered with gray matter. Functionally, the cerebellum is most frequently associated with activities such as motor coordination and balance. However, because it communicates with the cerebrum, it also is identified as having a role in cognition, and it is a potential player in such complex disorders as schizophrenia and autism (Bullock et al, 2008).

Brainstem

The brainstem consists of two major components: the pons and the medulla. Although most often these two regions are

thought of as relay centers that control such critical life functions as respiration and heart rate, there is reason to believe that they may also play a role in some psychiatric disorders such as obsessive-compulsive disorder and eating disorders (Patel et al, 2008).

Neurophysiology
Nerve Cell Electrical Function: Action Potential

All neurons are capable of detecting, processing, generating, and conducting electrical signals known as *action potentials*. Neurons have special properties that allow for rapid changes in the concentrations of electrically charged ions such as sodium, potassium, and chloride. The differences in the distribution of electrically charged ions on the two sides of the membrane create an electrical potential, which is the ability to conduct an electrical current. An action potential occurs as a result of the rapid movement of ions across the cell membrane, thus temporarily shifting the electrical charge on each side of the nerve cell membrane.

Many types of events initiate action potentials given sufficient stimulus strength. Of particular interest to nurses is when this phenomenon involves the transmission of chemical substances called *neurotransmitters*. When an action potential reaches the synaptic terminal, it causes a change in the permeability of the membrane, thereby allowing chemical neurotransmitter substances stored in the synaptic knobs to be released into the gap (i.e., the synaptic cleft) between adjacent neurons. Figure 6-4 illustrates a typical synaptic structure. Specific neurotransmitters have been identified and directly associated with several mental disorders. Table 6-3 illustrates this point. Neurotransmitters are critical for effective neural communication, and they are implicated in many neurologic and neuropsychiatric disorders (Stahl, 2008).

Nerve Cell Chemical Function: Neurotransmitters

The space between the presynaptic and postsynaptic cell membranes in most synapses is about 20 to 30 nm. Although this is small, it is too large for action potentials to cross directly. As a result, communication between one neuron and another depends on the following: (1) the release of neurotransmitters by the presynaptic cell; and (2) their reception on the postsynaptic membrane. Although neurotransmitter movement is much slower than that of action potentials, it is effective for sending and regulating signals from one neuron to the next. It is the specificity of neurotransmitter receptor sites on the postsynaptic membrane that forms the basis of the chemical control of all neurologic functions.

Neurotransmitters are categorized in several ways. For this chapter, they are classified according to their chemical structure. In addition, they are also identified as either excitatory or inhibitory in nature when they reach the postsynaptic membrane. Considerable available research identifies brain regions with the highest concentrations of various transmitter substances and associates various brain functions and malfunctions with specific neurotransmitters. Although more than 100 substances are identified as neurotransmitters or probable neurotransmitters, Table 6-3 summarizes the most widely recognized neurotransmitter substances of the CNS (Box 6-2).

Many synthetic and naturally occurring toxins, street drugs, anesthetics, and medications that are used to treat psychiatric disorders function at the level of the synapse, where cell sites have specific receptors. Similarly, an increasing number of neurologic dysfunctions are attributed to abnormalities that are associated with neurochemical transmitter substances.

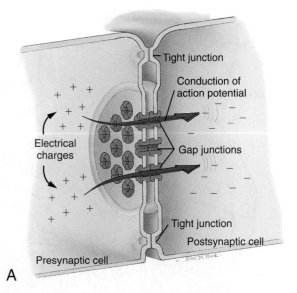

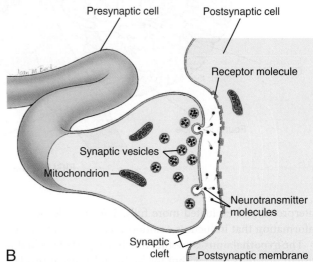

FIGURE 6-4. Electrical and chemical synapses. **A,** Electrical synapses involve gap junctions that allow action potentials to move from cell to cell directly by allowing electrical current to flow between cells. **B,** Chemical synapses involve transmitter chemicals (neurotransmitters) that signal postsynaptic cells, possibly inducing an action potential. (From Thibodeau GA, Patton KT: *Anatomy & physiology,* ed 7, St. Louis, 2009, Mosby.)

TABLE 6-3	RELATIONSHIP OF NEUROTRANSMITTER DYSFUNCTION TO MENTAL DISORDERS	
NEUROTRANSMITTER	**DYSFUNCTION**	**MENTAL DISORDER**
Dopamine	Increase	Schizophrenia
Serotonin	Decrease	Depression
Norepinephrine	Decrease	Depression
γ-Aminobutyric acid	Decrease	Anxiety disorders
Acetylcholine	Decrease	Alzheimer's disease

After an action potential reaches the synaptic knob, the neurotransmitter leaves the area via the natural diffusion of a substance from an area of high concentration to one of low concentration. A neurotransmitter is attracted to the postsynaptic membrane at receptor sites that are specific for the particular neurotransmitter. It is typically deactivated by enzymatic degradation and reassimilated within the presynaptic cell. This process is repeated over and over.

Specific Neurotransmitters. Specific neurotransmitters are located in different regions and areas of the brain to allow for the highly differentiated regional functions of the brain. The intricate interaction of nerve cells and the distribution of various neurotransmitters in different areas of the brain form the basis for all complex activities of the CNS.

Acetylcholine (ACh) was the first substance that was discovered to be a neurotransmitter. It is almost everywhere in the brain, but particularly high concentrations occur in the basal nuclei and the motor cortex of the brain. Neurons that make use of ACh as a neurotransmitter are often called *cholinergic*. There are two types of acetylcholine receptors: muscarinic and nicotinic. Many drugs, such the older neuroleptic antipsychotics, interact with ACh and its receptor sites to produce anticholinergic side effects, which occur when muscarinic acetylcholine receptors are blocked. Side effects include dry mouth, blurred vision, constipation, and urinary retention. These side effects are troubling to patients, and they are a common reason why patients stop using their medications and fail to comply with their treatment regimens. In severe cases, muscarinic receptor blockade produces confusion and delirium, especially among older patients.

Nicotinic receptors respond positively to nicotine and are common in neuromuscular synapses as well as in some CNS and PNS regions. Nicotine, which is found in tobacco, binds with the nicotinic receptor sites. It is able to mimic the effects of ACh released in some centers of the brain that are associated with pleasure, thus making nicotine highly addictive. Exposure to excessive levels of nicotine will sometimes cause paralysis, and, because of this, it is an effective insecticide. The nicotine found in cigarettes is a common cause of poisoning in children.

Glutamate (glutamic acid) is an amino acid that is an excitatory neurotransmitter in the brain. The brain's principal inhibitory neurotransmitter, γ-aminobutyric acid (GABA), is chemically derived from glutamate. Nerve cells that are stimulated by inhibitory neurotransmitters such as GABA will be turned off, which slows or stops actions completely in the postsynaptic neurons. Glutamate and GABA are the subject of extensive research in disorders such as Alzheimer's disease and schizophrenia (Schinder, 2009).

Dopamine is a neurotransmitter that is well localized in several brain regions, including the substantia nigra, the midbrain, and the hypothalamus. Dopamine-containing cells in the midbrain project into the limbic cortex. Researchers think that these areas are the parts of the brain that malfunction in patients with schizophrenia. Dopamine antagonists are prescribed for the treatment of some psychoses.

Norepinephrine or noradrenaline is concentrated in a small area of the brain known as the *locus coeruleus.* Many studies now indicate that patients with mood disorders, particularly major depression, have a deficiency of norepinephrine. Sympathetic nerves that innervate smooth muscles in the blood vessels have a heavy concentration of norepinephrine, which helps to explain norepinephrine's role in the elevation of blood pressure during the fight-or-flight response. When it is released directly into the bloodstream, norepinephrine acts as a hormone that enhances the effect of locally released norepinephrine at neuromuscular junctions. Both norepinephrine and its chemical relative epinephrine are synthesized from the amino acid tyrosine. Foods that are high in tyrosine and tyramine are avoided by patients who are taking certain psychotropic medications; see Chapter 25 for an explanation of this important nursing alert and teaching opportunity. Norepinephrine, epinephrine, dopamine, serotonin, and histamine belong to the class of neurotransmitters known as *monoamines.* Norepinephrine-producing neurons are sometimes referred to as *adrenergic*, whereas neurons that produce acetylcholine-like substances are identified as *cholinergic.*

Serotonin has a pattern of action that is similar to that of norepinephrine and that is made from tryptophan, which is another amino acid. Serotonin production occurs in the brainstem, and it is also widely dispersed throughout the cerebral cortex and the spinal cord. Serotonin helps to regulate a constant internal environment in relation to the maintenance of a normal body temperature, normal eating and sleep–rest patterns, and normal moods. All of these depend on adequate levels of serotonin. Clinically significant problems occur when patients have low levels of serotonin, and many behavioral symptoms related to depression occur when available serotonin is low or depleted.

Researchers suspect that two gases—carbon monoxide and nitric oxide—function as neurotransmitter-like substances. Carbon monoxide and nitric oxide are both poisonous and unstable gases that are byproducts of automobile emissions and other forms of combustion. Nitric oxide is not stored in synaptic vesicles; in fact, it actually works in the opposite

---

BOX 6-2	**CRITERIA FOR A SUBSTANCE TO BE LABELED A NEUROTRANSMITTER**

- The chemical is synthesized in the neuron.
- The chemical is present in the presynaptic terminal and released in amounts that are sufficient to exert a specific effect on a receptor neuron.
- When applied exogenously (i.e., via a drug) in a reasonable concentration, the drug mimics the action of the endogenously released neurotransmitter.
- A specific mechanism exists for removing the chemical from its site of action (i.e., the synaptic cleft).

TABLE 6-4	COMMON CNS NEUROTRANSMITTERS		
MOLECULAR CLASS	NAME OF NEUROTRANSMITTER	ACTIVITY	DISTRIBUTION
Biogenic amine (catecholamine)	Acetylcholine	Excitatory	Motor neurons, pons, and forebrain
Amino acids	Aspartate	Excitatory	CNS
	Glutamate	Excitatory	Primary exciter in the CNS
	γ-Aminobutyric acid	Inhibitory	Primary inhibitor in the CNS
	Glycine	Inhibitory	Spinal cord
Monoamines	Dopamine	Excitatory	Basal nuclei and limbic system
	Serotonin	Excitatory	Brainstem, pons, and medulla
	Norepinephrine	Excitatory	Pons and medulla
Neuropeptides	Many	Excitatory	CNS and PNS
Gases	Nitrous oxide	Uncertain	Brain and blood vessels
	Carbon monoxide		

direction and feeds back toward the presynaptic neurons, and it has no known specific receptor sites. However, it functions as a chemical messenger in the brain and in the peripheral blood vessels. It is involved in blood vessel contraction in the clitoris and penis during sexual arousal. Research suggests that nitric oxide plays a role in the brain's memory function, and it is possibly part of the complex illness of major depression (Zhou et al, 2007). Research indicates that carbon monoxide acts in similar ways.

Other larger neuropeptide molecules such as cholecystokinin and endorphins, which have functions that are still being researched, occur at multiple sites in the brain. Researchers think that these molecules play a role in the complex functioning of the brain.

Clinical Significance of Neurotransmitters. Extensive research is earmarked for the development of new drugs that operate at the synaptic level within the brain. Any chemical that mimics, competes, destroys, or prevents a neurotransmitter from binding to specific receptor sites on the postsynaptic membrane alters the effectiveness of communication between neurons. Researchers have made countless advances in the treatment of psychiatric disorders; this is the result of an increased understanding of neurotransmitters as well as an understanding of the way that neurotransmitters are synthesized and deactivated. A brief discussion of some of the more common brain-related illnesses linked to neurotransmitter dysfunctions follows. Table 6-4 summarizes specific disorders and the related neurotransmitters.

Depression. Serotonin and its close chemical relatives, dopamine and norepinephrine, are the neurotransmitters that are most widely involved in various forms of depression. The two major classes of antidepressants—tricyclic antidepressants and selective serotonin reuptake inhibitors agents—differ primarily with regard to their effects on either norepinephrine or serotonin levels. This explains why certain drugs that specifically target serotonin (e.g., fluoxetine, paroxetine) may not be effective for some patients but will work well for others (see the Case Study presented later in the chapter). The selective serotonin reuptake inhibitor class of antidepressants inhibits the reuptake of serotonin by the presynaptic secreting cells. This reduces the availability of

serotonin for subsequent release. Other antidepressants function as monoamine oxidase inhibitors. Monoamine oxidase is an enzyme that typically deactivates serotonin and dopamine. Deactivating this enzyme leaves the system unable to turn off the effects of these transmitter substances on postsynaptic neurons. Conversely, an enzyme or drug that acts opposite of monoamine oxidase or that is a monoamine oxidase *inhibitor* reduces the transmission of signals between neurons. Catechol-O-methyltransferase, which is an enzyme that is normally responsible for deactivating norepinephrine, is sometimes present in excess in certain synapses. Too much of this enzyme prevents adrenergic neurons from effectively communicating with one another. Antidepressants that inhibit or reduce catechol-O-methyltransferase levels restore neuronal communication ability. Because norepinephrine is also important for regulating activities such as heart rate and blood pressure, antidepressants that operate on the norepinephrine system may have adverse side effects that interfere with these functions (see Chapter 12).

Anxiety. A number of conditions related to anxiety, such as panic disorders and extreme phobias, are triggered by an overproduction of some excitatory neurotransmitters, which causes a hyperexcitability of the postsynaptic membrane. GABA, which is one of the key inhibitory neurotransmitters in the CNS, normally counteracts the effect of these transmitters. Many antianxiety medications (e.g., diazepam [Valium], alprazolam [Xanax]) act by stimulating GABA synthesis, which then modulates the effect of excitatory neurotransmitters. This produces a calming effect in patients who are experiencing anxiety (see Chapter 10).

Schizophrenia. A complex disorder such as schizophrenia most likely has multiple contributing factors, including genetic predisposition, prenatal development, and the environment. The direct cause of the symptoms manifested in patients with schizophrenia is a disruption of normal neurotransmitter activity, particularly dopamine. One plausible explanation for schizophrenia is the dopaminergic theory, which hypothesizes that the dopamine levels in people with schizophrenia are elevated. Some maintain that at least six other neurotransmitters—glutamate, serotonin, norepinephrine, ACh, GABA, and cholecystokinin—are also involved in schizophrenia. The most commonly prescribed antipsychotic drugs suppress dopamine and similar transmitter substances. Current treatment continues to focus primarily on the dopaminergic theory (see Chapter 13).

Parkinsonism. Most researchers agree that the immediate cause of parkinsonism is a deficiency of dopamine, particularly in the basal nuclei that are involved in motor coordination. Characteristically, patients with Parkinson's disease display tremors, a shuffling gait, a progressive lack of motor control, a loss of facial motor control, slurred speech, and facial expressions that are flat or mask-like. Public figures such as the late Pope John Paul II, boxer Muhammad Ali, and actor Michael J. Fox display these symptoms, thus raising public awareness of the condition. The causes of dopamine deficiency in patients with Parkinson's disease appear to be both genetic and environmental. Currently, parkinsonism is treated with levodopa, which is a dopamine precursor that is capable of crossing the blood–brain barrier of the brain. According to the theory, brain cells that contain the appropriate enzymes will convert levodopa into dopamine.

Alzheimer's Disease. Alzheimer's disease is among the leading causes of disability and death among older adults in the United States, and the number of affected persons increases each year as the population ages. ACh is the neurotransmitter that is primarily involved in this condition. Decreased levels of ACh produce many of the behavioral manifestations of the disease, such as memory loss and disorientation. Donepezil (Aricept) and other similar drugs inhibit the cholinesterase enzyme that breaks down ACh. This increases the amount of available ACh, thereby delaying the onset of symptoms (Trinh et al, 2003) (see Chapter 16).

Both Parkinson's disease and Alzheimer's diseases are examples of recognized organic brain disorders. They are included in this discussion because of their relationship to specific transmitter substances and because the devastating effects of these degenerative conditions are clearly linked to the mood disorders and dementia that occur in patients and that are encountered by psychiatric mental health nurses. The following case study describes the neurodegenerative disorder multiple sclerosis, which frequently involves symptoms that are associated with mental disorders.

CASE STUDY

AD, a 43-year-old woman, was diagnosed with multiple sclerosis 5 years ago. She was taking gabapentin (Neurontin) and paroxetine (Paxil). Muscle pains and migraine headaches made it difficult for her to sleep. She also complained of feeling depressed and hopeless as a result of the recent exacerbation of the debilitating symptoms of her condition. AD reported a 10 pound weight loss that occurred during the previous 2 months.

Critical Thinking
1 What questions will the nurse ask at this time?
2 What changes will the nurse suggest to improve AD's insomnia?

INTERRELATED BODY SYSTEMS

Although psychiatric disorders are primarily brain based, it is important to examine other biologic etiologies. The brain operates in delicate balance with other body systems, and the mind–body connection is undeniable. Research demonstrates that the CNS both affects and is affected by the immune system, the endocrine system, the body's natural biologic rhythms, as well as other systems. The following are some examples of interactions among body systems and how the disruption of these systems sometimes results in mental, emotional, and behavioral dysfunction and disorder.

Psychoneuroimmunology

Psychoneuroimmunology is the study of the relationship between the neurologic, endocrine, and immune systems and the behaviors associated with these systems. Cytokines are chemical messengers that are exchanged among immune cells. Their function is to signal the brain to produce changes of activity in the endocrine system as well as the immune system. Research studies focus on the relationship of cytokines and the pathophysiology of medical diseases such as cancer, allergies, and autoimmune diseases. More recent studies have focused on psychiatric disorders such as major depression, schizophrenia, and Alzheimer's disease (Potvin et al, 2008).

Brain receptor sites for neuropeptides produced by the immune system are associated with changes in emotions and behaviors. Stress causes the discharge of corticotropin-releasing factors that suppress the immune system. Studies indicate that negative emotions, anxiety, and psychiatric disorders such as schizophrenia and mood disorders are sometimes associated with decreased functioning of the immune system. Posttraumatic stress disorder is associated with long-term immunosuppression (Miura et al, 2008).

Neuroendocrinology

Neuroendocrinology is the study of the relationship between the nervous system and the endocrine system. Because of its close physical association with the pituitary, hypothalamic activity influences hormonal regulatory events attributed to the pituitary as well (i.e., the hypothalamic-pituitary-adrenal HPA axis). A number of hormones, including epinephrine, actually function as neurotransmitter-like substances. This affects chemical communication among many cells, even the ones that are distant from the source of the hormone. Several hormonally based disorders result in medical conditions that produce psychiatric symptoms. The neuroendocrinologic relationship between stress and brain function continues to intrigue researchers (Chrousos, 2009).

Research studies correlate hypothyroidism with depressive symptoms and Addison's disease with depression and fatigue. Other endocrine disorders are linked to autoimmune conditions such as Graves' disease, which causes excessive thyroid secretion. This sometimes follows an acute infection, which suggests an immunologic origin for Graves' disease. People with Graves' disease commonly report symptoms of emotional stress, nervousness, fatigue, weight loss, heat intolerance, and gastrointestinal symptoms. In addition, schizophrenia and other psychiatric disorders occur more frequently during the reproductive period of life, when sex hormones are most active. This suggests that there may be an endocrine-related origin of these disorders in some individuals.

Chronobiology

Chronobiology is the study of the biologic rhythms of the body, which are commonly referred to as the *circadian rhythms*. These rhythms manifest as changes or interruptions in metabolic rate, the sleep-wake cycles, blood pressure, hormone levels, and body temperature. Researchers have shown that the brain controls these rhythms through their interactions with various endocrine organs. Many psychiatric and medical disorders occur more frequently or are exacerbated when sleep patterns and biologic rhythms are disrupted (i.e., there is a strong correlation).

Many hypothesize that dreams result from the activation of electrical activity in brain regions that recall recent memories and that reinforce long-term memories. One theory maintains that mental disorders are the result of brain circuits that are not activating competently because of abnormal brain wave patterns. When incompetent brain circuits are activated while the individual is awake, patients often report hallucinations and illusions. Psychoactive drugs modify brain waves in psychotic patients, which temporarily restores more normal brain circuits. Antidepressants increase brain waves and suppress or reduce rapid eye movement sleep. Electroconvulsive therapy suppresses abnormal brain waves, thereby allowing for more typical brain wave patterns. Additional information about sleep disorders can be found in Chapter 19.

Sundowning or *sundown syndrome* is the exacerbation of psychotic or depressive symptoms during the afternoon or evening that results in disorientation and confusion. Some studies associate sundowning with a disturbance of circadian rhythms. Psychiatric and medical conditions such as Alzheimer's disease also disrupt the patient's circadian rhythms. Decreased exposure to light during the winter months has also been shown to produce depressive symptoms among patients with seasonal affective disorder. The role of the hormone melatonin is being investigated for its role in chronobiologic disorders (Srinivasan et al, 2006). Patients benefit when psychiatric mental health nurses are aware of chronobiologic disruptions that produce symptoms of mental illnesses and intervene with effective treatment methods.

Genetics

Genes are the hereditary units in chromosomes that determine specific characteristics in an organism. Much information evolved in the 1990s during the focused scientific research period called the Decade of the Brain, and probably none was more important than the Human Genome Project. This project began during the 1990s, and it resulted in the identification of all of the genes contained on the 23 pairs of human chromosomes. The knowledge of the precise locations of the genes responsible for every human biologic characteristic as well as their biochemical structure, has opened up endless possibilities for research into the genetic causes of nearly every human disease or condition, including psychiatric disorders. However, recognizing that genes only determine the potential to develop any normal or abnormal condition significantly complicates the problem of identifying genetic causes of specific psychiatric disorders. Excellent evidence attributes disorders such as Huntington's disease and Parkinson's disease to specific genes. Both diseases have been linked to genes found on chromosome number 4, but evidence for the genetic causes of some other specific neurologic disorders is not so clear.

Familial tendencies appear with some disorders, and researchers are attempting to specify schizophrenia genes. According to the most current literature, there are as many as 150 genes on nearly a dozen different chromosomes that contribute to the causes of schizophrenia, thereby making the situation more complex. Research indicates that schizophrenia results from the interaction of multiple genes rather than from a single gene (Hashimoto et al, 2006).

In theory, defective genes code for the incorrect synthesis of neurotransmitters or their deactivating enzymes, or other factors interfere with the proper transmission of vital chemical agents. The genetic origins of several other psychiatric disorders (e.g., attention-deficit/hyperactivity disorder, antisocial personality disorder, violent behaviors) are being explored (Siebner et al, 2009; Craddock et al, 2005).

Research has also identified genes that are linked to bipolar disorder and substance dependence (Schindler et al, 2001). This helps to explain why certain psychiatric disorders recur in families and why the first degree-relatives of individuals with psychiatric disorders have an increased risk for developing the same or similar disorders.

Although few researchers believe that any one single gene causes a psychiatric illness, genetics clearly plays a significant role in influencing mental health and disorder. The interaction of genes is highly complex, and the link of genes to behavior remains controversial. It appears that many genes influence psychiatric illness and the dysfunctional behaviors that are symptomatic of those illnesses (Petronis et al, 2003). There is increased evidence that environmental and developmental conditions in utero contribute to the expression of these genes that subsequently manifests as abnormal behavior.

Stem Cell Technology

Stem cell technology is perhaps the most controversial and promising technique that will lead to treatments and cures for neurobiologic disease and injury. Stem cells are cells that have the complete genome intact and that have not yet differentiated or developed into a specific cell type. Research continues on both embryonic and adult stem cells.

A fertilized egg is totipotent, which means that it has the total potential to develop into an entire human being.

As some genes are turned on and others are turned off, embryonic cells become specialized. *Adult stem cells* have begun to develop to a certain degree. For example, some adult stem cells have already developed into epithelia rather than connective tissue, or muscle tissue, or nervous tissue cells. Although there are adult stem cells in a variety of tissues (including bone marrow, some connective tissues, and even brain tissue), the ability to successfully culture them and use them for therapeutic purposes is somewhat limited.

Stem cell technology is promising for many reasons. A primary reason is that undifferentiated stem cells from embryos have the potential to develop into any type of cell, and researchers are able to deliberately control gene expression. Specialized stem cells can be developed into organs for transplants and have fewer complications from tissue rejection.

Despite research gains in this field, it continues to be controversial because of differing opinions about the use of embryonic tissue to harvest the cells for use. Regardless of the source of the stem cells (i.e., adult or embryonic), several technical challenges remain, but the potential for the therapeutic application of this research seems unlimited at this time. Active research continues regarding numerous neurobiologic conditions, including brain and spinal cord injuries; neurogenetic disorders that affect brain development; and degenerative conditions such as amyotrophic lateral sclerosis, Parkinson's disease, and Alzheimer's disease. Recent studies have looked at the role of stem cell therapy in the repair of damaged adult brain tissue (van Velthoven et al, 2009). The implications of stem cell research for the future of psychiatric nursing are promising, as is the potential of stem cell therapy itself.

Neuroplasticity

The brain is a dynamic and constantly changing environment, and researchers are continually discovering more about its complexities. Neuroplasticity, or the ability of the brain to change its structure and function, is providing insights into the role of certain brain areas in the development of illness and mood disorders (Carlson et al, 2006). The increased understanding and application of the concepts of the neuroplastic nature of brain tissue are leading to new approaches to the treatment of disorders. Until now, many believed that the capacity of the brain to repair itself after injury or to replace degenerative cells was minimal, particularly in adults; however, current research reveals that brain cell regeneration is possible in several conditions.

These implications for patients, families, and nurses are many. For example, patients who in the past may not be expected to recover from major traumatic injuries or damage to the brain as the result of a traumatic accident or cerebrovascular accident are now being treated more hopefully. Research and actual findings regarding the brain's neuroplasticity affected changes in treatment plans.

NEUROTECHNOLOGY: PSYCHOBIOLOGIC TOOLS

Neuroimaging

Before modern neuroimaging techniques were available, clinicians had few noninvasive tools for examining the human brain, with the exception of radiography, but much about the brain remained a mystery. The development of imaging techniques since the early 1980s has dramatically changed the understanding of brain structure and function. Brain anatomy and physiology have now been mapped in exquisite detail, which has provided valuable information via the use of a variety of techniques. Useful neuroimaging techniques available today include ultrasonography, computed tomography (CT) scanning, magnetic resonance imaging (MRI), functional magnetic resonance imaging (fMRI), positron emission tomography (PET), and single photon emission computed tomography (SPECT) (Figure 6-5). Unlike older radiography technology that involved the use of film, these techniques make use of computers to generate images. Table 6-5 identifies common nursing considerations for patients who are undergoing neuroimaging tests.

Ultrasonography

Ultrasonography, which is also known as *echoencephalography,* involves the use of high-frequency sound waves to form images of brain spaces and masses. Because ultrasonography does not involve harmful radiation, many prefer this technique for the examination of developing brains. It has been widely used to create images of developing fetuses as well as of various organs within the body, including the brain.

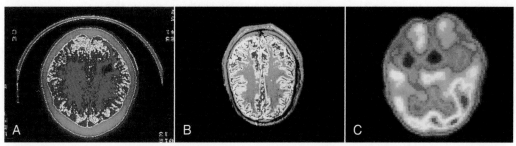

FIGURE 6-5. Neuroimaging techniques. **A,** Computed tomography scanning. **B,** Magnetic resonance imaging. **C,** Positron emission tomography. (From Thibodeau GA, Patton KT: *Anatomy & physiology,* ed 7, St. Louis, 2009, Mosby.)

TABLE 6-5   NURSING CONSIDERATIONS WITH NEUROIMAGING PROCEDURES

TEST	GENERAL CONSIDERATIONS	COMMON NURSING CARE	COMMON CONTRAINDICATIONS
Anatomic Imaging			
Computed tomography scanning	Three-dimensional view of brain structures Differentiates fine-density structures, unlike normal radiography film Examination time: 15–30 min Clear-liquid diet before test	Explain the purpose of the test and all procedures. Reassure the patient that the test is safe and that radiation exposure is not a concern. Assess the patient's anxiety level and monitor for symptoms of claustrophobia. Reassure the patient that hearing monotonous noise is common. Instruct the patient to lie still to ensure good imaging. If contrast iodine is used, monitor the patient for gastrointestinal upset, flushing, and perceptions of excess warmth.	Allergy to iodine (although not all computed tomography scanning requires iodine) Inability to lie completely still Claustrophobia
Magnetic resonance imaging	Three-dimensional view of brain structures Separates view of white matter tissue from gray matter tissue Examination time: 15–60 min	Explain the purpose of the test and all procedures. Reassure the patient that the test uses magnets rather than radiation and that radiation exposure is not a concern. Assess the patient's anxiety level and monitor for symptoms of claustrophobia. Instruct the patient to lie still to ensure good imaging. Instruct the patient that a clear plastic helmet with an antenna will be put over his or her head. Reassure the patient that hearing monotonous noise is common.	Inability to lie completely still Claustrophobia Pacemakers Metallic implants, plates, or screws Life-support equipment needed for patient Infusion pumps Generally not used when the patient is pregnant
Functional Imaging			
Positron emission tomography	Two-dimensional view of brain structures Measures physiologic and chemical functioning (e.g., the glucose uptake of cells in the brain) and provides information about anatomic structures Isotopes with short half-lives used	Explain the purpose of the test and all procedures. Inform the patient that isotopes are radioactive and discuss the patient's concerns. Assess the patient's anxiety level and monitor for symptoms of claustrophobia. Explain that there will be time interval of about 45 min between the injection of the isotope and the scanning procedure. Explain that the patient may be blindfolded and have earplugs placed to decrease environmental stimuli during testing. Instruct the patient to lie still to ensure good imaging. Make sure that the patient does not fall asleep during the procedure, because this will affect the test results.	Inability to lie completely still Claustrophobia Severe anxiety level Recent use of sedating or tranquilizing medication, because these medications alter cellular glucose use patterns Breast-feeding Requires expensive cyclotron
Single photon emission computed tomography	Two-dimensional view of brain structures Measures physiologic and chemical functioning (e.g., the glucose uptake of cells in the brain) and provides information about anatomic structures Isotopes with long half-lives used No onsite cyclotron required	As for positron emission tomography above	Breast-feeding Inability to lie completely still Claustrophobia

Computed Tomography Scanning

After the development of sonography, a neuroimaging technique based on radiography was developed in 1972. Scientists conducted research to develop this technology at EMI, a branch of Capitol Records, with money from the sale of Beatles records partly funding the research.

This technique, which was once called *computerized axial tomography,* is now more commonly is referred to as *CT scanning.* It provides three-dimensional views of the brain by imaging serial thin sections of brain matter. These multiple sections help to differentiate fine differences or changes occurring throughout the organs being visualized. Anatomic abnormalities in the brain as revealed by CT scans are not specific to any type of psychiatric disorder, and CT scanning does not serve as a specific test for such disorders. However, these tests do provide suggestive evidence of brain-based problems. For example, patients with diagnoses of schizophrenia, bipolar disorder, certain other mood disorders, alcoholism, multi-infarct dementia, and Alzheimer's disease have demonstrated nonspecific brain abnormalities on CT scans. The CT scan is often used because it is available and cost effective. Disadvantages of CT scanning include a lack of screening sensitivity, the underestimation of brain atrophy, and the inability to image in the sagittal and coronal views.

Magnetic Resonance Imaging

MRI has become an excellent substitute for actual invasive exploratory brain surgery. It is also advantageous because it makes use of radio waves rather than harmful radiation and because it provides three-dimensional images that are sharper than those obtained with CT scanning. MRI is unaffected by bone, and, unlike CT, it is capable of revealing views of brain structures that are close to the skull. It is also able to differentiate between white matter tissue and gray matter tissue. Of significance to psychiatric diagnosticians is that MRI shows neuroanatomic changes in patients with schizophrenia that include increased ventricle size, temporal lobe reductions, hippocampal reductions, and cortical atrophy (as evidenced in Figure 13-1).

MRI is not appropriate for all patients, and contraindications are noted in Box 6-3. In addition, patients with claustrophobia are often unable to complete this type of study, because the MRI machine is enclosed, and patients are required to remain motionless. Because of the confining environment and the excessive noise of the equipment, nurses focus on patient teaching before the test and closely monitor the patient's anxiety levels during testing. Newer open-structured MRI equipment has made MRI testing easier for patients.

Functional MRI. fMRI is a modification of the basic MRI that detects brain activity by measuring oxygen consumption and metabolic differences in various parts of the brain. fMRI reveals that patients with Alzheimer's disease often have lower glucose metabolism in the cortical regions of the brain (Alexander et al, 2002). In addition, it is an effective tool for identifying specific functional areas of the brain that are associated with certain behaviors. The science of neuroinformatics, which makes use of techniques such as fMRI, has become the equivalent of the Human Genome Project of the 21st century by helping with the mapping of the human brain.

> **BOX 6-3 PATIENT GROUP CONTRAINDICATIONS FOR MAGNETIC RESONANCE IMAGING**
>
> - Individuals with pacemakers
> - Individuals with metallic objects such as screws, prostheses, and orthopedic devices
> - Patients on life-support systems

Positron Emission Tomography and Single Photon Emission Computed Tomography

A PET scan is a neuroimaging technique that produces a three-dimensional image of the structures and functions of the brain. It is based on technology that is similar to that of a CT scan, and remains at the forefront in neuroimaging procedures. PET scans consist of introducing a radioactive substance into the blood supply of the brain in order to trace compounds, most commonly glucose. Glucose metabolism is related to the functional activity in specific areas of the brain, which is useful for identifying anomalies. PET scans can also detect oxygen use, blood flow, and neurotransmitter-receptor interactions in the brain. When positron-emitting radionuclei interact with electron molecules, an image is produced that is converted into photons and detected as color variations that are indicated on a computer screen. The machine and the procedure require a support team of physicists, chemists, and computer experts, which greatly increases its expense of operation. (See Figures 6-5 and 13-1 for examples of PET scans.)

PET and the related technology of SPECT are also called *radionuclide scanning techniques,* because both involve the introduction of radioactive substances into the blood supply. Because the brain has such extensive blood supply, SPECT is particularly useful for visualizing vascular structures in the brain and for diagnosing conditions such as cerebrovascular accidents or anomalies.

These techniques are particularly useful for demonstrating variable levels of brain activity and associated blood flow within the brain. SPECT scans have detected abnormalities in the frontal cortex, the occipital and temporal lobes, and the parahippocampal gyrus in patients with panic disorders (Zipursky et al, 2007).

PSYCHIATRIC NURSING AND NEUROBIOLOGY

Knowledge of the neurobiologic basis of psychiatric disorders is essential for effective psychiatric mental health nursing practice. Nurses include biologic principles in all aspects of nursing care, from assessment to evaluation, to ensure comprehensive and quality nursing care. New information about the neurosciences will continually be made available, and, because of this, the role and function of the psychiatric mental health nurse will continue to evolve. Staying current with dynamic developments in this field helps to ensure that the professional psychiatric mental health nurse is offering patients best-practice–level of care.

Increasingly, a strong background in neurobiology is part of the standards of practice for psychiatric mental health nursing (American Nurses Association, 2006). The nurse's synthesis of the findings of the nursing assessment (practically applied in most chapters) coupled with an understanding of psychobiologic theory and practice results in effective nursing care that assists psychiatric patients to achieve or regain wellness.

PATIENT AND FAMILY TEACHING GUIDELINES

Biologic Basis of Psychiatric Disorders

- Determine a mutually acceptable time and location for the teaching session.
- Select an environment that is favorable for learning.
- Identify the patient's readiness for learning.
- Identify the patient's motivation for learning.
- Identify the patient's knowledge about the topic and accuracy of that knowledge.
- Identify with the patient the specific content that is requested and required.
- Define a measurable outcome with the patient to determine that learning has occurred.
- Define the evaluation method used to determine the effectiveness of teaching.
- Use multiple teaching-learning approaches, such as visual and auditory, based on the patient's needs.
- Monitor the patient's anxiety level during the teaching session, as increased anxiety will decrease information processing.
- Identify alternative resources available to the patient to increase learning potential.
- Identify the process that the patient will follow to access support persons if the patient requires more reinforcement.

Much of the stigma attached to psychiatric illness was due to a lack of understanding of the biologic basis of these disorders. Therefore, effective patient, family, and public teaching is an important function of the role of the psychiatric mental health nurse as researchers discover new information regarding the structures and functioning of the CNS. The Patient and Family Teaching Guidelines box displays the highlights of effective patient teaching regarding the biologic basis of psychiatric disorders. Psychiatric mental health nurses continue to play an important role by directly assisting patients with brain-based disorders and by teaching and informing patients, families, and the general public about advances in neurobiology.

New research findings continue to change the way that people with psychiatric disorders are cared for and treated. The Research for Evidence-Based Practice box highlights the importance of critical thinking as psychiatric mental health nurses approach and plan modifications of care on the basis of new research findings.

RESEARCH FOR EVIDENCE-BASED PRACTICE

Gross-Isseroff R et al: The suicide brain: a review of postmortem receptor transporter binding studies, *Neuroscience and Biobehavior Review* 22:653, 1998.

Some research has reported that the brains of individuals who commit suicide are different from the brains of individuals who have died of natural causes. Postmortem examination of the receptor/transport binding sites of the brain tissue of suicide victims and of individuals who have died of natural causes show that the brains of suicide victims have unique, specific neurochemical characteristics that make "suicide brains" different from the brains of individuals who have died of natural causes. Scientists are using such studies to formulate a hypothesis of molecular markers that will possibly help define and identify individuals at risk for suicidal behavior. Researchers are developing tests to measure identified markers. When these markers are specifically identified and prove to be reliable in their ability to predict suicidal behavior, the test will likely become a routine aspect of mental health evaluation.

▮ CHAPTER SUMMARY

- Current research findings involving the brain and its functions are continually advancing.
- The brain is the most complex and one of the most important organs in the human body because of its multiple functions.
- Psychiatric disorders are brain-based illnesses with anatomic or physiologic components.
- It is imperative for nurses to understand the anatomy and physiology of the brain and other body systems that interact with the nervous system.
- One key to understanding treatment strategies for psychiatric disorders is to recognize the role that

neurotransmitter substances play in neural communication.
- Nurses become familiar with psychobiologic approaches to the treatment of psychiatric disorders by recognizing the importance of the brain's neuroplasticity.
- Modern brain neuroimaging techniques help to explain the brain's structure and function and their relationship with psychiatric illnesses.
- Emerging fields in neuroscience (e.g., genetics, stem cell research) continue to develop advanced technologies that lead to improved medical and nursing care for patients with neurobiologic disorders.

REVIEW QUESTIONS

1. Which statement made by a family member of a person with schizophrenia demonstrates effective learning about the disease?
   1. "The disease was probably caused by problems with several genes. These genes cause changes in how certain brain chemicals work."
   2. "The disease could be cured if our politicians and laws allowed for more stem cell research. Adult stem cells hold so much promise."
   3. "The disease probably resulted from the mother's smoking during pregnancy. Nicotine is actually a neurotransmitter."
   4. "If our family had more money, we could afford the promising psychoneuroimmunologic treatments available in other countries."
2. Which assessment finding best indicates the release of norepinephrine?
   1. The pulse rate changes from 70 bpm to 62 bpm.
   2. The pupil size changes from 8 mm to 3 mm.
   3. The patient begins complaining of intestinal cramping.
   4. The blood pressure changes from 126/70 mm Hg to 158/84 mm Hg.
3. The following patients are scheduled to undergo MRI. For which patients should additional assessment information be gathered before the diagnostic procedure? You may select more than one answer.
   1. A patient with a history of wounds caused by exploding shrapnel during military service
   2. A patient with a concurrent diagnosis of bleeding peptic ulcers for the past 3 years
   3. A patient with current complaints of extreme sensitivity to loud noises
   4. A patient with reports of allergies to iodine, eggs, and shellfish
   5. A patient with a 3-year history of Parkinson's disease
4. An adult has panic attacks. Which neurotransmitter is most likely to be implicated in this problem?
   1. Norepinephrine
   2. ACh
   3. Serotonin
   4. GABA
5. A nurse plans the care for an adult with a tumor in the brain's frontal lobe. Initial interventions should focus on the patient's anticipated problems with which of the following?
   1. Motor function and judgment
   2. Sensory and calculation abilities
   3. The interpretation of visual stimuli
   4. Hearing and hygiene

REFERENCES

Alexander GE et al: Longitudinal PET evaluation of cerebral metabolic decline in dementia: a potential outcome measure in Alzheimer's disease treatment studies, *Am J Psychiatry* 159: 238-245, 2002.

American Nurses Association: *Scope and standards of psychiatric mental health practice*, Washington, DC, 2006, American Nurses Publishing.

Bear MF et al: *Neuroscience: exploring the brain*, ed 3, Baltimore, 2007, Lippincott Williams & Wilkins.

Bullock M et al: Altered expression of genes involved in GABAergic transmission and neuromodulation of granule cell activity in the cerebellum of schizophrenic patients, *Am J Psychiatry* 165:1594-1603, 2008.

Carlson NR: *Physiology of behavior*, ed 10, Boston, 2009, Allyn & Bacon.

Carlson PJ et al: Neural circuitry and neuroplasticity in mood disorders: insights for novel therapeutic targets, *Neurotherapeutics* 3:22-41, 2006.

Chrousos GP: Stress and disorders of the stress system, *Nat Rev Endocrinol* 5:374-381, 2009.

Craddock N et al: The genetics of schizophrenia and bipolar disorder: dissecting psychosis, *J Med Genet* 42:193-204, 2005.

Dickerson B et al: Differential effects of aging and Alzheimer's disease on medial temporal lobe cortical thickness and surface area, *Neurobiol Aging* 30:432-440, 2009.

Dubin MW: *How the brain works*, Williston, Vt, 2002, Blackwell Science.

Gribbin J: *How the brain works: a beginner's guide to the mind and consciousness*, New York, 2002, Dorling Kindersley.

Gur R: Functional imaging is fulfilling some promises, *Am J Psychiatry* 159:693-694, 2002.

Hashimoto R et al: Susceptibility genes for schizophrenia, *Psychiatry Clin Neurosci* 60:S4-S10, 2006.

Miura H et al: A link between stress and depression: shifts in the balance between the kynurenine and serotonin pathways of tryptophan metabolism and the etiology and pathophysiology of depression, *Stress* 11:198-209, 2008.

Montoya A et al: Brain mapping and cognitive dysfunction in Huntington's disease, *J Psychiatry Neurosci* 31:21-29, 2006.

Patel AS et al: Central pontine myelinolysis as a complication of refeeding syndrome in a patient with anorexia nervosa, *J Neuropsychiatry Clin Neurosci* 20:371-373, 2008.

Petronis A et al: Monozygotic twins exhibit numerous epigenetic differences: clues to twin discordance? *Schizophrenia Bull* 29:169-178, 2003.

Potvin S et al: Inflammatory cytokine alteration in schizophrenia: a systematic quantitative review, *Biol Psychiatry* 63:801-808, 2008.

Schinder AF, Morgenstern NA: Adult neurogenesis is altered by GABAergic imbalance in models of Alzheimer's disease, *Cell Stem Cell* 5:573-574, 2009.

Schindler KM et al: Candidate genes for schizophrenia: further evaluation of KCNN3, *Prim Psychiatry* 8:51-53, 2001.

Siebner HR et al: From the genome to the phenome and back: linking genes with human brain function and structure using genetically informed neuroimaging, *Neuroscience* 164:1-6, 2009.

Srinivasan V et al: Melatonin in Alzheimer's disease and other neurodegenerative disorders, *Behav Brain Funct* 2: 15, 2006.

Stahl SM: *Essential psychopharmacology: neuroscientific basis and practical applications*, ed 3, New York, 2008, Cambridge University Press.

Trinh N et al: Efficacy of cholinesterase inhibitors in the treatment of neuropsychiatric symptoms and functional impairment in Alzheimer disease: a meta-analysis, *JAMA* 289:210-216, 2003.

van Velthoven CT et al: Regeneration of the ischemic brain by engineered stem cells: fueling endogenous repair processes, *Brain Res Rev* 61:1-13, 2009.

Zhou Q et al: Neuronal nitric oxide synthase contributes to chronic stress-induced depression by suppressing hippocampal neurogenesis, *J Neurochem* 103:1843-1854, 2007.

Zipursky RB et al: PET and SPECT imaging in psychiatric disorders, *Can J Psychiatry* 52:146-157, 2007.

Online Resources

American Academy of Sleep Medicine: www.aasmnet.org
American Society of Neuroimaging: www.asnweb.org
Center for Sleep & Circadian Biology: www.northwestern.edu/cscb
Encyclopedia of Psychology: Psychobiology: www.psychology.org/links/publications/psychobiology
International Society of Developmental Psychobiology: www.isdp.org
National Institute of Mental Health: The Human Brain Project: www.apps.nimh.nih.gov/index.shtml
National Sleep Foundation: www.sleepfoundation.org
Society for Light Treatment and Biological Rhythms: www.sltbr.org

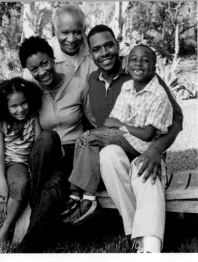

Human Development Across the Life Span

Linda Hollinger-Smith

"What lies behind us and what lies before us are tiny matters compared to what lies within us."

Ralph Waldo Emerson

⊖volve WEBSITE

http://evolve.elsevier.com/Fortinash/

OBJECTIVES

- Describe the importance of human development from a life span perspective.
- Discuss the key elements of developmental theories and the forces that affect human development.
- Describe how developmental theories have expanded to encompass a life span perspective.
- Discuss how biologic, psychologic, and social factors influence life span transitions across the process of aging.

- Describe distinctions between normal and abnormal physical and psychosocial processes of aging.
- Discuss the meaning of health and wellness for older adults.
- Describe how new research into successful aging is demonstrating that such concepts as learning and creativity continue to be important for adults as they age.

KEY TERMS

activity theory	disengagement theory	locus of control	rites of passage
adaptation	functional ability	moral development	self-actualization
ageism	gerontology	nature versus nurture	successful aging
cognitive theory	interpersonal theory	psychosexual theory	
continuity theory	life stages	psychosocial theory	

Across the human life span, a person's growth and development travels a pathway of transition and transformation that is marked by key milestones. Mental health problems influenced by human developmental factors may occur at distinct points along this path. Understanding stages of human development is important for psychiatric mental health nurses for assessing and applying psychosocial interventions that are appropriate for particular phases of the life span.

The process of aging, which is described as a sequence of physical and psychosocial changes, begins at the moment of birth. Developmental theorists make distinctions about these aging changes in accordance with life stages, eras, or periods. Early theorists who studied human development primarily focused on children and adolescents because they believed

that cognition, intellect, personality, and social abilities are all acquired at early ages.

More recently, researchers have debated that human development extends well beyond adolescence into adulthood and even into old age. Many external social and environmental factors are modifiable through psychosocial interventions and thus may impact human development across the life span. In addition, with many people living longer as a result of advances in the health sciences and technology, enhancing quality of life across those extended years is important to optimal physical and mental health. Having a clear understanding of these factors and applying this knowledge to practice is essential for psychiatric mental health nurses.

DEVELOPMENTAL THEORIES

How individuals adapt and respond within dynamic environments is core to developmental theories. Human development is a result of heredity and environment, which interact in ways that are still puzzling to researchers. Development is affected by the following: (1) a predetermined plan that is genetically built into the individual; (2) one's previous developmental history; and (3) an accommodation to one's environmental circumstances (Sroufe et al, 1992).

Few debate how much nature versus nurture influences human development today. Researchers are studying connections between genetics and human development to better understand how genetic and environmental factors interact with regard to influencing behavior development. They are also studying how interactions between human behavior and the environment influence future behavior.

CHILD AND ADOLESCENT DEVELOPMENT

Psychosexual Theory

Sigmund Freud (1856-1939) developed psychosexual theory, which views children's development as a biologically driven series of conflicts and internal needs. According to his theory, infants are primarily focused on meeting their own internal needs. Through parental interactions, infants experience conflict between internal selfish desires and parental controls that require them to learn to reduce tensions from these conflicting situations in socially acceptable ways.

Freud (1923) described a child's development as a series of psychosexual stages. The confrontation of two forces—the id (representing primitive drives for pleasure) and the superego (representing morals and principles)—characterizes each stage. During the early years of life, one's sense of reality, which Freud referred to as the *ego*, begins to develop, and it serves as mediator between the id and superego. The individual learns from past conflicts and begins to use defensive processes (i.e., ego defense mechanisms) to maintain balance in life. Freud believed that who you are and everything that you become are determined during the first few years of life. At each stage of development, the individual increases the ability to tolerate clashes between the id and the superego because of previous childhood experiences. Freud supposed that libido or sexual energy influences a person's ability to deal successfully with life's conflicts and challenges.

Freud identified five stages of development: oral, anal, phallic, latency, and genital. The following outlines some of the developmental issues that he believed occur at each stage:

- *Oral stage (birth to about 1 year of age).* Because the mouth is the source of nurturing and pleasure, primary activities of infants focus on receiving and taking. Later in life, overeating or smoking is an oral fixation.
- *Anal stage (2 to 3 years of age).* Children begin to contend with rules and regulations for the first time with toilet training. As adults, anal fixation appears as being overly tidy or miserly.
- *Phallic stage (4 to 5 years of age).* Some boys experience the Oedipus conflict, which consists of sexual longings for their mothers and perceptions of their fathers as rival figures. This stage for girls is referred to as the Electra conflict.
- *Latency stage (7 to 12 years of age).* This stage represents a period of no particular developmental trials.
- *Genital stage (around 13 years of age).* The final developmental stage reflects sexual feelings for the opposite sex. Freud stated that these feelings bring up anxieties as the child recalls feelings for parents that occurred during the phallic stage.

Critics of Freud's theory point to some fundamental weaknesses in the initial development and testing of the theory's basic premises on the basis of Freud's adult patients' recall of childhood memories, dreams, and free associations rather than from studies of children.

Regardless of criticisms of Freud's work, one of his most important contributions remains his theory of how past trauma may result in mental and physical health problems later in life. On the basis of this much earlier theory, research into posttraumatic stress disorder began in earnest with Vietnam War veterans, and it continues to evolve with the growing frequency of terrorism threats worldwide (Shalev, 2009). Researchers do not fully understand the impact of both manmade and natural disasters on children, although these possibly have a significant influence on their development.

Psychosocial Theory

Erik Erikson (1902-1994), who was a student of Freud, disagreed with his mentor regarding the factors that drive human development and behavior. In contrast with Freud's focus on biologic instincts, Erikson saw social interaction as the driving source that influences human development. Erikson also believed that human development extends across the entire life span. Combining the effects of the social environment on biologic maturation, Erikson formulated the psychosocial theory of human development, which he considered "the eight stages of man" (Erikson, 1963).

Building on previous stages and influenced by past experiences, each of the eight stages represents a particular psychosocial crisis that the ego needs to resolve, either successfully or unsuccessfully, before moving to the next stage. The source of the crisis is internal (biologic) or external (social). A pair of specific traits—one positive and one negative—represents each stage. Resolution of these crises is typically not an all-or-nothing situation. In some cases, future experiences cause the individual to mistrust the social environment. Overall, an individual's psychosocial development is successful if he or she is comfortable trusting the social environment in most situations, and thus one trait dominates the other.

The following provides a brief overview of Erikson's first five stages, which deal with child and adolescent development. Erikson's final three stages are discussed later in the chapter and deal with adult developmental theory.

- **Trust versus mistrust.** To successfully resolve the psychosocial crises of mistrust experienced during the first stage, the infant develops the belief or trust that the social environment will meet basic physiologic or psychologic needs through care that satisfies the most basic oral and sensory needs, such as feeding and cuddling.
- **Autonomy versus doubt.** When toddlers realize that they are able to trust their social environment, they begin to see their behaviors as their own and to develop a sense of independence and self-confidence with the encouragement of their parents. Alternatively, if parents overprotect or overly disapprove of expressions of independence, feelings of self-doubt or shame may develop.
- **Initiative versus guilt.** During early childhood and preschool, children are exposed to a larger social world and need to learn to take responsibility for demonstrating more socially acceptable behaviors and expressing initiative. If parents are inconsistent or strict disciplinarians, children may develop feelings of guilt regarding their behaviors.
- **Competence versus inferiority.** During the school years (6 to 12 years of age), children's social environment continues to expand as they make new friends and develop new relationships. Children gain new knowledge, learn new skills, and grow more competent. If they lack successes in learning or productivity, children may develop a sense of inferiority.
- **Identity versus role confusion.** As they enter the adolescent years (13 to 18 years of age), children begin to develop their social identities. Adolescents consider how they appear to their peers, and they begin to think about what sort of careers or jobs they will have in the future as their senses of identity are emerging. Adolescents who experience difficulties fitting in with their peers and who suffer from low self-esteem may suffer from role confusion.

As compared with Freud's view of the ego, Erikson's theory places more importance on the ego for the resolving of conflict situations independent of the id and the superego (Erikson, 1982). Erikson's focus on personality development was broader and included the impact of social, cultural, and environmental factors rather than just the effects of sexuality. Erikson's model stands as one of the most important contributions to human development theory across the life span.

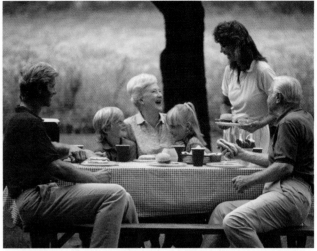

FIGURE 7-1. Healthy intergenerational involvement benefits the entire family. ©2007 Jupiterimages Corp.

Interpersonal Theory

The **interpersonal theory** of human development created by Harry Stack Sullivan (1892-1949) emphasizes interpersonal behaviors and relationships as the central factors that influence child and adolescent development across six eras, from infancy to late adolescence. There are two dimensions to interpersonal behaviors: (1) the need to satisfy social attachments; and (2) the longing to meet biologic and psychologic needs (Figure 7-1).

Interpersonal behaviors also invite social reactions that either complement or discredit behaviors (Sullivan, 1953). For example, children learn that behaviors that result in praise from their parents are preferable to behaviors that result in discipline, which increases the child's anxieties. Parents' overreactions to negative behaviors, such as an extreme reaction or the punishment of an occasional "accident" during toilet training, will produce intense anxieties in the child, thus interfering with the child's ability to separate the mood and the reactions of parents from the biologic act of excretion.

Sullivan described some of the developmental issues that are faced during each era:

- **Infancy era.** The first 2 years of life represents a phase of dependency on parents to meet all biologic and survival needs. Parents empathetically communicate their moods so that the child feels comforted when the parents communicate tenderness, and the child feels anxiety when parents communicate frustration. Sullivan identified the development of the infant's "good me" when gratification needs are met and parents react positively and the opposite "bad me" when needs are not met, parents react negatively, and anxiety increases.

Continued

- **Childhood era**. The childhood era (2 to 6 years of age) extends from the beginning of language development to the beginning social relationships with peers. Children's coping mechanisms (i.e., "good me" and "bad me") continue to develop from learned interpersonal interactions with parents, teachers, and other caregivers.
- **Juvenile era**. From the ages of 6 to 10 years, children begin to develop friendships with peers, which represents a widening of social circles. At this stage, children learn to develop elements of their conscience and personalities that will help them to succeed in society. Along with group membership, they learn various ways to exclude individuals from the "in group" to the "out group" by forming stereotypes about these individuals, usually on the basis of culture. The self-system is also developing and internalizing personality patterns that develop during the juvenile era, are refined over the subsequent years, and remain throughout life.
- **Preadolescent era**. From the ages of 10 to 13 years, friendships with same-sex friends deepen because of the need for alliances in meeting mutual needs. Social groups continue to evolve their self-identity and to become goal-focused. Preadolescents learn the importance of reciprocity (the exchange of favors or privileges) and equality in interpersonal relationships.
- **Adolescent era**. The adolescent era (13 to 17 years of age) begins at puberty with individuals experiencing sexual attraction and feelings of lust for the first time. Low self-esteem, insecurity, anxiety, and loneliness will develop if adolescents are constantly criticized or disciplined by parents for sexual thoughts or behaviors.
- **Late adolescent era**. During this era (17 to 19 years of age), adolescents develop the ability to be comfortable with intimate relationships while meeting the socially acceptable expectations of society. Adolescents who have not learned to develop intimate relationships sometimes move back to the juvenile era and remain with an egocentric personality throughout life, unable to develop satisfying interpersonal relationships.

Cognitive Theory

Jean Piaget (1896-1980), a Swiss philosopher and psychologist, dedicated his life's work to observing and interacting with children to determine how their thinking processes differed from those of adults. His study of cognitive learning influenced generations of educators who applied his constructivist learning concepts to elementary level education by focusing on the child's abilities to continuously create and test

new knowledge (Gallagher and Reid, 1981). As a result, Piaget's work continues to be directly applicable to current theories of moral development. Cognitive theory explains how thought processes are structured, how they develop, and their influence on behavior. The structuring of thought processes occurs through the development of schema (i.e., mental images or cognitive structures). When the child encounters new information that is recognized and understood within existing schema, the assimilation of that new information occurs. If the child is not able to link the new information to existing schema, the child has to learn to develop new mental images or patterns through the process of accommodation. As long as the child is able to assimilate new knowledge or accommodate it adequately, then he or she is able to achieve equilibrium or mental balance. When schemas are inadequate to facilitate learning, disequilibrium occurs.

Piaget viewed the development of thought processes as progressing over four stages (Piaget, 1970). During each stage, the development of cognitive images or structures influences the child's actions and behaviors. The child must successfully achieve the goals of each stage before moving onto the next.

- **Sensorimotor period**. From birth to 2 years of age, infants learn about the environment through the senses in a trial-and-error fashion that Piaget called *instrumentality*. Gradually, infants begin to recognize the difference between the self and others in the environment, which is the process of decentering. Theorists originally believed that object permanence, which is the ability to recognize that an object or person is in a given area or continues to exist even outside of the field of vision, begins to develop as early as 6 months of age.
- **Preoperational period**. From 2 to 7 years of age, children's use of verbal and mental symbols to represent persons, objects, and actions develops. Children also begin to exhibit pretend play, to experience difficulty with distinguishing reality from fantasy, and to focus solely on the present. Thought processes are egocentric in nature in that children consider only their own viewpoints, and aspects of their self-esteem begin to show. Children's emotional states are constantly changing, and they are able to focus on only one emotion at a time. Later during this period, the unconditional acceptance of authority begins to develop.
- **Concrete operations period**. From 7 to 11 years of age, children's thought processes are only concrete in character, which fosters their ability to sort objects and to place them in some order. Children recognize thoughts about the past and the present but not thoughts about the future. Children are also able to understand

TABLE 7-1	APPLICATION OF COGNITIVE DEVELOPMENT THEORY TO EDUCATIONAL ACTIVITIES

Preoperational period. From 2 to 7 years of age, the use of verbal and mental symbols to represent persons, objects, and actions develops.

EDUCATIONAL APPLICATION	EXAMPLE ACTIVITIES
Provide physical practice with facts and fundamental skills that serve as building blocks for future development.	• Use cutout letters or block letters to build words. • Use drawings or illustrations to teach words that describe what children are seeing, doing, touching, or tasting.
Provide opportunities to manipulate physical objects that change shape but that retain mass to help students understand the concept of conservation and to ready them for the understanding of two-way logic that is needed during the next stage.	• Use physical materials such as clay and foam. • Encourage students to talk about what they are experiencing when manipulating objects.

Concrete operations period. From 7 to 11 years of age, thought processes are concrete in character, thereby fostering the child's ability to sort objects and to place them in some order.

EDUCATIONAL APPLICATION	EXAMPLE ACTIVITIES
Provide concrete models or props as visual aides, particularly with conceptual studies.	• Show visual timelines for history lessons. • Use three-dimensional models or experiments to explain scientific concepts.
Use familiar examples to explain more complex ideas to help students assimilate new information.	• Compare student's own lives to the lives of characters in a story. • Use story problems when teaching mathematics concepts.

Formal operations period. From 11 to 16 years of age, systematic ways to think about and solve problems develop.

EDUCATIONAL APPLICATION	EXAMPLE ACTIVITIES
Provide opportunities to explore hypothetical problems.	• Target student discussions about topics that may have multiple potential solutions, such as social issues. • Ask students to justify their positions on such issues.
Teach broad concepts (rather than just facts) with the use of ideas that are relevant to the student.	• When teaching about historical issues, relate how these issues may have current implications. • Use current song lyrics or poetry to reflect on current issues.

conservation, which is the principle that an object is able to change shape but retain the same volume. They are able to acknowledge the viewpoints of others and to appreciate feelings such as friendship, truthfulness, and integrity.

• **Formal operations period.** During this final period (11 to 16 years of age), individuals develop systematic ways to think about and solve problems. Individuals are able to think in abstract (i.e., explaining metaphors) or hypothetical terms (i.e., "what if" statements). Thinking in terms of the future and solving or debating problems in a logical manner are also characteristic of this period.

Cognitive development represents humans' constant attempts to adapt to and make sense of their environment. Piaget's stages of cognitive development are associated with particular age spans, but they typically vary among individuals. Educators have also applied Piaget's theory to learning activities for specific elementary school grades. Table 7-1 provides some examples of these applications according to the preoperational, concrete operations, and formal operations stages. When applying Piaget's theory to education, it is the important role of teachers to provide students with opportunities for personal growth and discovery through problem solving rather than focusing on norms.

Attachment Theory

John Bowlby (1908-1990) recognized the importance of maternal bonding in child development, and this is a consistent phenomenon across all cultures. From initial animal studies, Bowlby saw bonding as a type of "protective" response by the youngster in a dangerous situation (Bowlby, 1988). Ainsworth (1989) expanded the concept of attachment to include all caregivers or "primary attachment figures" and found that infants from all cultures of the world showed the same types of distress (although to different degrees) when attachment is disrupted. Positive interactions with caregivers build secure attachments, whereas negative interactions result in insecure attachments. Bowlby viewed attachment as the core of all human development and the foundation of building relationships. Responses of the caregiver to the infant's distress over time result in what Bowlby called "internal working models of self and parent." These formed models influence the development of social interactions.

According to attachment theory, children who experienced secure attachments develop into resilient, happy, and capable individuals, whereas those who faced insecure attachments tended to become antisocial, helpless, passive, or needing attention. Critics point out that this places undue emphasis on the "nurture assumption," which is the idea that how parents raise their children shapes the children's characters. To address these issues, Bowlby further recognized that other figures influence a child's development as his or her social circle expands. For example, a child who experiences helpless or passive behaviors is positively affected by a caring elementary schoolteacher who encourages, supports, and nurtures the child toward a more positive developmental process. Alternatively, a child who is greatly affected by the loss of a parent faces a more negative developmental pathway. Bowlby explained these experiences as a process of adaptation.

Current attachment theory researchers have looked toward linking attachment theory and psychoanalysis together through the cognitive science of *mentalization*, which is the theory of mind. Mentalization is the ability of humans to estimate—with some accuracy—the thoughts, emotions, and intentions behind subtle behaviors such as facial expressions (Thompson, 2008). A study of the connections between the theory of mind and these types of behaviors may lead to new attachment theory frameworks.

Behavioral Theories

Behavioral or learning theories focus on the basic relationship between a stimulus and a response so that researchers can accurately predict responses. For psychologists who were concerned with developing behavioral theories, it was also a way to break with the biologists and psychiatrists who believed that instincts drive all human behavior and that patterns of behavior are determined at early ages. It is interesting to note that early behavioral scientists were also American, which was in contrast with the domination of European scientists who were involved in the previously described development theories.

Classical and Operant Conditioning

The early influences on behavioral theory are credited to the scientific works of John B. Watson (1878-1958) and B.F. Skinner (1904-1990). With the use of research techniques designed by Ivan Pavlov, Watson showed that humans learn new behaviors through *classical conditioning*. He demonstrated that a conditioned stimulus paired with an unconditioned stimulus elicits a conditioned response or a behavior change. When the researcher removed the unconditioned stimulus, the conditioned stimulus continued to result in the same conditioned response.

Skinner expanded on Watson's work, believing that learning occurred through the association of a behavior with a particular consequence. Skinner referred to this process as *operant conditioning*. He identified three basic consequences or responses to learning situations: *reinforcement*, *extinction*, and *punishment*. *Reinforcement* is a positive response, which then increases a particular behavior; or it is a negative response, *extinction*, which removes or eliminates the behavior. *Punishment* or an unpleasant response reduces the frequency of the behavior.

Social Learning Theory

Social learning theory is a general theory that is used to explain human behavior. The term *social learning theory* first appeared in a 1941 publication by Miller and Dollard entitled *Social Learning and Imitation*. They outlined the concepts that formed the foundation of several versions of social learning theory. From their early work, behaviorists were able to empirically test and validate their hypotheses.

One of the pioneers of social learning theory, Julian Rotter (1916-), moved away from the view that biologic motives determine human behavior. Instead, he selected the *empiric law of effect* as the motivating factor that drives human behavior. Basically, individuals are motivated to search for positive stimulants or reinforcers and to avoid negative stimulants. He went further to say an individual's personality is essentially linked to his or her environment. His approach to clinical psychology included the study of not just one's life history, personality, and experiences but also of one's awareness of and response to the environment. In contrast with other child development theorists, Rotter also believed that personality continues to evolve with new life experiences or new learning opportunities, although, as one ages, stimulants have to be more intense to affect the same degree of personality change.

Rotter's social learning theory (1982) has the following four main components:

- **Behavior potential** is the degree of probability that individuals will engage in specific behaviors in particular situations. For each specific behavior, there is a corresponding behavior potential. Rotter believed that people seek behaviors with the greatest potential.
- **Expectancy** is the likelihood that a behavior will lead to a certain outcome, and it is based on past experiences. Because people are more likely to seek positive outcomes or reinforcers, they will select behaviors with the highest expectancy of achieving positive outcomes.
- **Reinforcement value** is the desirability of behavior outcomes, so those outcomes that one rates the highest have the greatest reinforcement value. Reinforcement value is subjective and influenced by past experiences. For most children, parental punishment is a negative outcome with low reinforcement value. However, for some children who suffer from neglect, parental punishment has a high reinforcement value, because it is more desirable than abandonment.

> • **Psychologic situation** represents how different individuals have different explanations of the same circumstances. Individuals' behaviors are the result of their subjective analyses of the environment.

Rotter's work on social learning theory formed the basis for the concept of locus of control (Rotter, 1992). The locus of control is an aspect of personality that addresses an individual's belief about who is in control—the self or some outside force. Some have mistakenly attempted to categorize people with internal locus of control personalities or external locus of control personalities. Rotter explained that, under specific situations, "internals" sometimes function more like "externals," or vice versa, on the basis of previous experiences, which again reinforces the interaction of the individual and the environment.

Albert Bandura's (1986) addition to social learning theory emphasized the importance of observation and modeling the actions, emotions, and attitudes of others. By copying the behaviors of others, individuals encode information that forms the basis for new behaviors. For example, children often imitate other children or adults. By role-playing and dressing up as the mother and father, children are programming their own future behaviors. Cognitive, environmental, and behavioral factors interact during observational learning processes and have four basic parts:

- Paying *attention* to the modeled behavior
- *Retention* or storing images of the behavior
- *Reproduction* of the behavior
- *Motivation* through reinforcement of the reproduced behavior

Individuals are more likely to act out behaviors if they perceive that outcomes will be valuable or result in positive reinforcement. Thus, if someone recognizes and rewards the behavior, this will further strengthen the new behavior.

Bandura expanded his social learning theory to include the concept of self-regulation as a way for persons to examine their experiences, to consider their own thinking processes, and to adjust their thinking as a result. Self-efficacy is a form of self-regulation that affects one's behaviors and that is a central focus of Bandura's research. Basically, individuals develop perceptions about their own effectiveness, and this guides their behavior. Self-efficacy determines what individuals attempt to achieve and the amount of effort that they give to achieve their goals.

Social learning theory has greatly contributed to many fields, including education, health care, and behavior therapy. Most recently, researchers have applied social learning theory to the study of how children internalize the morals and values of society. Self-control therapy is based on self-regulation concepts, and is used to change habitual behaviors such as smoking and overeating. For example, keeping track of one's smoking behaviors with the use of a behavioral diary helps to identify cues associated with the habit. Taking steps to then remove or avoid some of the cues is a way to alter the environment.

Moral Development

Moral development focuses on moral judgment or reasoning processes and involves making decisions about right or wrong actions in a particular situation. Piaget examined the concept of moral development and determined that there were two stages (Piaget, 1970). Before the ages of 10 or 11 years, children considered moral dilemmas differently from older children. These two different views are based on how children view rules. For younger children, rules are absolute and come from an authority figure. Older children learn that rules are changeable in certain situations. According to Piaget, younger children base moral judgment on consequences, whereas older children base judgment on motives. For example, if a child has to select which situation represents the greater wrong—the child who steals food every day to feed his poor family or the child who steals money once to buy a toy—the younger child will say that the child who steals food daily is doing the greater wrong on the basis of the consequences or amount of harm. By contrast, the older child judges wrongness according to the motives present in the situation.

Lawrence Kohlberg built on Piaget's work in the area of moral development and focused his research on the moral issues faced by children and adolescents (Kohlberg, 1973). In accordance with Piaget's schema, Kohlberg identified three stages of moral development that are each categorized into two levels. The three stages describe how children learn to discriminate right from wrong while developing an increased appreciation for morality as a lifelong task.

> The <u>first level</u>, preconventional morality (4 to 10 years of age), consists of the following two stages:
> • **Punishment and obedience orientation** is present when children realize that there are physical consequences in the form of punishment for bad behaviors. During this stage, children reason that authority figures lay down the rules of what is moral and believe that they have to obey these decisions without question or punishment results.
> • **Instrumental relativist orientation** is present when children focus on satisfying their own instrumental needs and occasionally the needs of others. Moral judgment is based on the question, "What do I get out of this decision?"
>   The <u>second level</u>, the conventional level (10 years of age through adolescence), seeks conformity and loyalty as key behaviors and also consists of two stages:
> • **Interpersonal concordance** deals with the give-and-take nature of helping or good behaviors. Children receive approval from others for doing good works. Intent and

Continued

character traits (e.g., "she means well," "he is a loving father") are also taken into account and grow in importance as children attempt to assist others.

- **Law-and-order orientation** is a stage of doing good and making moral decisions out of respect for authority or as a result of the duty to maintain the social order.

The third level, the postconventional or principled level (from early adulthood onward), seeks to define moral judgment and values in terms of the universal good. It consists of two stages:

- The **social-contract legalist orientation** focuses on the legal point of view but is also open to considering what is moral and good for society.
- The **universal ethical-principle orientation** deals with abstract and ethical moral value, rather than concrete moral rules. These include universal principles such as equality, justice, and beneficence.

Carol Gilligan, an associate of Kohlberg, considered his premises as sometimes being sexually biased. Because Kohlberg's sample consisted of all men, Gilligan thought that the stages represented masculine values that were focused on moral rules and responsibilities. She saw female moral values as being based in interpersonal relationships and reality situations rather than in abstract concepts. Gilligan (1982) raised another possibility to explain gender differences in the formation of moral values. She suggested that moral development progresses along more than one pathway: one focused on ethics, justice, and other abstract concepts, and the other focused on interpersonal relationships. At some point, each gender tends toward making one of these paths more dominant.

Theories of moral development have gained more focus in that moral education has grown to be an important topic in both the fields of psychology and education. Reports of increased violent juvenile crimes, teen pregnancy, and suicide have resulted in many declaring that there is a moral crisis in the United States. Although morality may not be at the root of all of these social issues, there is a growing trend to link these problems to the presence of absence of teaching of moral and social values in school systems. The impact of schools on the moral development of youth continues to be a subject of debate and controversy.

ADULT DEVELOPMENT

Since the time of the Chinese philosopher Confucius (511-479 BC), many have viewed development on a continuum, with childhood and adolescence on one end and adulthood and old age at the other. There is a lack of adult development research as compared with studies of infancy, childhood, and adolescence. Judith Stevens-Long (1992) attributed this fact

to social, psychologic, and economic issues. Much of the emphasis on child development was in the fields of education, biology, and psychology. When education became a requirement for all children, teachers wanted to develop and test optimal teaching methodologies. Biologists and psychologists studied child development to understand human evolution.

Another reason for the lack of focus on adult development is the unsupported belief that human development plateaus at adulthood. For many years, the assumption was that adulthood was a period when external events (e.g., marriage, jobs, raising children) influenced human development rather than the internal processes that occurred during childhood. Research in adult development began evolving during the mid 1970s to include a more complex view of adulthood as a continuous and active process of growth and development. In earlier times, researchers perceived adulthood as the period of the basic maintenance of the family. Little effort or time was available for creativity, self-expression, and new learning opportunities.

As human development theorists expanded in their attempts to explain concepts of personality, cognition, motivation, emotions, and intellect, it soon became apparent that values, cognitive abilities, mental and physical health, and many other factors continue to change throughout adulthood. Many life experiences occur only during adulthood (e.g., marriage, raising children, starting or ending a career) that will significantly affect growth and development during those years. Arnold Van Gennep was one of the pioneers of adult development theory. In his book *The Rites of Passage* (1909), he described rites of passage as significant and meaningful rituals that mark and celebrate the milestones and transitions of life.

Life Stage Theories

Several researchers have proposed life stage theories over the past several years. These theories divide the life span into a series of sequential transitions with a series of age-appropriate developmental tasks to complete during each stage. These tasks may focus on cognitive abilities, learning, or self-concept development over the adult life span.

Carl Jung's life stage theory (1971) was based on psychoanalytic theory, which states that as one goes through life, one develops inner exploratory abilities that add meaning to life. The degree to which one is able to open up to new and unfamiliar experiences affects transitions to future life stages. He also postulated that personality differences between males and females become less distinct as people age. The final life stage deals with maintaining a balance between wisdom and senility during old age. The older person who is successful in life does not attempt to compete with youth but rather is able to deal with the changes of aging.

Jung considered adult development on a continuum across the life cycle. He found that adults between the ages of 20 and 35 years continue to develop their individuality and other personality patterns while they are establishing their families. Jung was one of the first to describe the midlife transition, which is a period of the growing awareness of the masculine and feminine aspects of personality that are present in each individual.

Erikson was the most well-known of the life stage theorists, and he identified eight stages of psychologic development. Each stage of development involves maintaining a balance between the *syntonic* (state of stability) and the *dystonic* (state of disorder) (Erikson et al, 1986). A person has to adjust to move forward to the next level. The first five stages focused on children and adolescents, as described previously in this chapter. The remaining three stages followed adulthood from young adulthood to old age:

- **Intimacy versus isolation.** During young adulthood, individuals develop the ability to have loving relationships, and they begin to establish long-term commitments in their relationships. Some individuals retain a sense of self-absorption and find it difficult to make and keep intimate relationships; therefore, they tend to isolate themselves.
- **Generativity versus stagnation.** During middle adulthood, individuals seek opportunities to guide the development of the next generation. As the children of adults grow more independent, their aging parents become more dependent. Those in middle adulthood then face new roles, responsibilities, and challenges. Generativity also includes the ability to evaluate and appreciate past life experiences, embrace the future, assume new relationships and responsibilities, and develop creativity. For adults who cannot achieve such outcomes and who view their lives at this point as boring or unfulfilling, their existence feels stagnant or empty.
- **Ego integrity versus despair** During late life, older adults develop a sense of acceptance of how they lived their lives and the importance of the relationships that they acquired throughout their lives. This stage is sometimes the climax of the previous seven stages. The individual with ego integrity is prepared to defend the dignity of his or her own lifestyle and life choices. Individuals who have not successfully accomplished development tasks of earlier stages will lack ego integrity and thus feel despair about a lack of life fulfillment and death. When describing the final stage of life, Erickson stated that "the process of bringing into balance feelings of integrity and despair involves a review of and a coming to terms with the life one has lived thus far" (Erikson et al, 1986, p. 54).

Theorists focused on successful aging have developed a psychologic model that encompasses life span development called *selective optimization with compensation* (Baltes et al,

1992). Individuals who age successfully are those who select and modify activities to enrich their lives despite energy declines. With the growth of the old-old population (i.e., those 85 years old and older), theorists are applying selective optimization with compensation as a model to understand transitions from healthy aging that is more commonly seen in older adults up to about the age of 80 years (termed *the third age*) to a nonreversible declining aging that seems to begin around the age of 85 years (termed *the fourth age*) (Hyer and Intrieri, 2006). Accordingly, physical and psychologic resources shift to managing the losses that are experienced later in life. For example, an older adult was a professional landscaper for most of his life. Now that he is older and less mobile, he becomes selective by caring for a small garden (optimization) and by setting it up in raised containers for ease of reach (compensation).

Human Motivation and Development Theory

Many view Maslow's motivation and development theory (1962) as a valuable framework for understanding human needs and values from a holistic point of reference. Maslow's theoretic construct is a hierarchy of needs that is diagrammed in the form of a pyramid (see Figure 1-1). Maslow identifies five levels of needs, with the most basic representing the base of the pyramid. From the most basic (1) to the highest (5) level, these needs include the following:

1. Biologic and physiologic needs
2. Safety and security needs
3. Affiliation or sense of belonging needs
4. Self-esteem needs
5. Self-actualization needs

Ebersole and Hess (1999) conceptualized Maslow's hierarchy of needs and applied his theory to the identification of the special needs of older adults at each level. Table 7-2 identifies some of these specific needs as well as potential strategies for the meeting of those needs.

Contemporary Theorists

During adulthood, development focuses on the ability to interact with transitional aspects of life experiences and the environment. Recognition and acceptance of the finiteness of time and the inevitability of death are essential to adult development.

Daniel Levinson, a psychosocial theorist, examined life stages from early through late adulthood (1986), with a broad view based in Erikson's work. In contrast with Erikson, Levinson focused less on changes within the person and more on the connection between the self and the interpersonal world. His psychosocial theory of adult development addressed the assessment of one's self within the world, the functioning of the individual self, and the relationship between the self and the environment (Newton and Levinson, 1979). Psychosocial theory focuses on one's connection to the self and the environment, living life's experiences, and the creative potential of human variability.

Levinson proposed a universal life cycle that consists of specific eras that are sequenced from birth to old age. The *era*

TABLE 7-2   SPECIAL NEEDS OF OLDER ADULTS ACCORDING TO MASLOW'S HIERARCHY OF NEEDS

MASLOW'S HIERARCHY OF NEEDS	NEEDS OF OLDER ADULTS	STRATEGIES TO MEET THOSE NEEDS
Self-actualization	Finding meaning in life and death	Identify the value and contributions of the individual.
	Transcendence throughout the aging process	Encourage a continuity of participation in decision-making processes.
	Creativity and mastery	Reflect about the past in relation to the present and the future.
Self-esteem	Responsible roles	Maintain aspects of roles that are important to the individual.
	Social supports	Facilitate socialization.
	Locus of control	Promote the maintenance of the physical appearance.
	Cognitive awareness	Facilitate decision making.
Belonging	Relationships	Identify the impact of loss on the individual.
	Intimacy	Support the needs for intimacy and sexuality.
	Affiliations	Facilitate changes in lifestyle.
Safety and security	Sensory awareness	Obtain the necessary equipment or supplies for home independence.
	Environmental safety	Assist with obtaining legal or financial help.
	Legal and economic issues	Educate the older person and the family about home safety.
Biologic integrity	Biologic needs	Provide for physical comfort.
	Comfort needs	Provide for nutritional needs.

From Ebersole P, Hess P: *Toward healthy aging: human needs and nursing responses*, ed 5, St. Louis, 1998, Mosby.

refers to a basic unit of the life cycle, and it lasts approximately 20 years. A person experiences stable periods of 6 to 7 years followed by transitional periods of 4 to 5 years. Each period consists of specific tasks for a person to encounter and achieve. From a clinical viewpoint, therapists found this framework to be useful for identifying transitional periods that were often times of internal conflict and thus motivation for seeking treatment (Myers, 1998). The following summarizes key events that occur during Levinson's stages and transitions:

- **Preadulthood** lasts up to about the age of 17 years, and the early adult transition occurs from the ages of 17 to 22 years, during which time individuals begin to modify their relationships with family and friends.
- The **early adulthood** stage, between the ages of 17 and 45 years, is characterized by periods of vitality, contradiction, and stress. Individuals are faced with major life tasks, including achieving goals, raising families, and establishing their positions in society.
- The **midlife transition** occurs between the ages of 40 and 45 years. Individuals face the realization that the failure to accomplish all of life's goals leads first to disappointment and then to the reformulation of earlier goals.
- **Middle adulthood** lasts from the ages of 40 to 65 years. During these years, adults have the greatest potential to have a positive impact on society.

- The **late adult transition** occurs between 60 and 65 years of age, and individuals experience some anxiety regarding their physical decline.
- The **late adulthood** era occurs after 65 years of age, and individuals learn to accept the realities of the past, present, and future.

The Harvard Study of Adult Development, which is the longest and most thorough study of aging ever attempted, has followed the life course of two very different groups of men from 1939 to the present: the Harvard cohort, which consists of 268 Harvard graduates from the classes of 1939 through 1944, and the inner-city cohort, which consists of 456 men who grew up in the inner-city neighborhoods of Boston. Every 2 years, both groups are surveyed about their physical and mental health, their relationships, their careers, and their adjustment to aging.

The current director of the study, George Vaillant, is studying adult adaptation related to ego defense mechanisms. He identified behaviors that promote adaptation as well as those that promote maladaptation (Vaillant, 2002). In addition to the two groups of men in the Harvard Study, Vaillant added a third group that consists of 90 middle-class, intellectually gifted women who were born in or near 1910.

Vaillant identified six factors of middle adulthood that promote longevity:
- Experiencing a warm and caring marriage
- Having effective adaptive or coping strategies
- Not smoking heavily
- Not abusing alcohol

BOX 7-1   VAILLANT'S HIERARCHY OF ADAPTIVE MECHANISMS

Level I: Psychotic Mechanisms (Common With Psychosis, Dreams, and Childhood)
Denial (of external reality)
Distortion
Delusional projection

Level II: Immature Mechanisms (Common With Severe Depression, Personality Disorders, and Adolescence)
Fantasy (schizoid withdrawal, denial through fantasy)
Projection
Hypochondriasis
Passive-aggressive behavior
Masochism or turning against the self
Acting out (compulsive delinquency, perversion)

Level III: Neurotic Mechanisms (Common in Everyone)
Intellectualization (isolation, obsessive behavior, undoing, rationalization)
Repression
Reaction formation
Displacement (conversion, phobias, wit)
Dissociation (neurotic denial)

Level IV: Mature Mechanisms (Common in Healthy Adults)
Altruism
Suppression
Anticipation
Humor

From Vaillant GE: *Adaptation to life,* Boston, 1977, Little Brown.

- Getting adequate exercise
- Being at a recommended weight

Vaillant's study built on the intrapsychic styles of adaptation that were first described by Freud. The ego mechanisms of defense are the major channels toward managing instinct and affect. Ego defense mechanisms are either adaptive or pathologic in nature. Vaillant (1977) developed a theoretic hierarchy of ego defenses, and he grouped them according to their relative maturity and pathology (Box 7-1). Because ego defense mechanisms are dynamic and mature throughout the life cycle, individuals who successfully adapt are able to select from a range of defense mechanisms to deal with problems. In healthy adults, these successful mechanisms include altruism, suppression, anticipation, and humor.

The adaptation theory as described by Vaillant (1977) is more of a conceptual model that categorizes the changes that are brought about by aging. Vaillant identified a series of shifts and tradeoffs that occur during the aging process. The ability of the individual to let go of parts of the past while pursuing quality of life is critical to successful adaptation. For example, the older person often experiences sensory losses, especially in the areas of vision and hearing, and he or she adapts to such losses by facilitating the quality of the remaining sensory perceptions. The use of large-print books, direct lighting, or hearing aids enhances the older person's remaining sight and hearing. Encouraging the use of other sensory perceptual systems such as touch or taste is another way for the older individual to gather information from the environment (see the Research for Evidence-Based Practice box #1).

RESEARCH FOR EVIDENCE-BASED PRACTICE #1

Kotter-Gruhn D et al: Self-perceptions of aging predict mortality and change with approaching death: 16-year longitudinal results from the Berlin Aging Study, *Psychol Aging* 24:654-667, 2009.

In this research study, more than 400 older adults between the ages of 70 and 100 years were followed as part of the 16-year Berlin Aging Study to examine how satisfaction with aging is an indicator of positive well-being and possibly predicts death. Researchers found that feeling older and being dissatisfied with how one is aging are related to an increased mortality risk over time. Persons who were satisfied with their aging or who felt "younger than their years" generally had longer survival. Self-perception of aging predicted mortality even after controlling for known mortality predictors such as illness, old age, gender, and socioeconomic status.

Midlife Transitions

Many young adults anxiously anticipate a midlife transition as they enter middle adulthood. As previously discussed, Levinson noted that, for many, this transition is a period of struggle or crisis (Myers, 1998). Levinson believed that up to 80% of individuals experience such a period of crisis. Researchers have examined the possibility of a possible midlife crisis and whether it is universal throughout cultures and genders.

Physical changes and new responsibilities of taking care of children, grandchildren, and older parents typically characterize middle age. In addition, middle-aged adults sometimes assume new work responsibilities and subsequently feel the need to reappraise their life situations and to make changes while they still have the time. The term *midlife crisis* describes a point in time when individuals experience a life crisis as their own mortality becomes real (Shek, 1996). These realizations often result in negative outcomes such as perceptions that health is deteriorating, bad feelings about marital relations or work, the inability to enjoy leisure time, and stress from caring for aging parents. The focus shifts from "How long have I lived?" to "How many years do I have left?"

Daniel Shek examined the concept of midlife crisis among adults of Chinese descent. He found that some participants were unhappy with work and personal achievements, but most did not indicate that their dissatisfaction was at a crisis level. Other studies (McCrae, 1984) also support the view that the midlife crisis is not a universal phenomenon and that it does not cluster around any particular age group.

Role of Stress in Adult Development

The negative effects of stress on aging are well documented. A growing body of research confirms that stress plays a part in hastening cognitive and memory decline, particularly among older adults who are already experiencing mild cognitive decline (Peavy et al, 2009). The effects of stress on adult development are complex.

Some researchers are examining the possibility that stress actually has a positive effect on adult development. In many cases, individuals who experience a stressful life event find that they have learned from the experience in the long run as a result of gaining new coping skills, increasing their self-knowledge, or enhancing their social networks. Some believe that these stressful experiences made them better people. Further research is necessary in this area, because it is difficult to generalize these findings across all adult populations.

Gender Differences in Adult Development

As research in adult development evolved, particularly in the areas of adult personality and adult learning concepts, gender differences became apparent. Some studies focused on a trait approach to adult personality, which suggests that personality is constant or stable over time. These studies also highlight gender differences in their approaches to adult development.

Personality is continuous for the most part, but there are some gender- and age-related differences. The most stable aspects of personality include coping styles, life satisfaction factors, and goal-directed behaviors. Bernice Neugarten (1979) noted the following changes that occur with aging:

- From the ages of 40 to 60 years, there is a shift from feeling in control over one's environment to perceiving the environment as more threatening, which is referred to as a change from *active* to *passive mastery.*
- Older adults become more introspective and self-reflective as they age.
- There are shifts in sex-role expressiveness between men and women. Men take on a more nurturing role, and women become more accepting of their aggressive tendencies.
- Older adults tend to become more introverted.

Positive Psychology and Aging

Erikson (1974) described what is necessary to sustain a person's opportunity and ability to grow and mature. He noted that vital individual strengths come from the stages of life. These strengths include faith, willpower, purposefulness, competence, fidelity, love, care, and wisdom. Slowly, the typical model of the elderly is changing as a result of increased longevity. Growth and maturity are now considered dynamic processes, many of which are under the control of individuals, which leads to new opportunities and rewards in later life.

Positive psychology, which is the scientific study of the traits and virtues that enable people and communities to thrive, was built on the pioneering work of Erikson and other theorists including Maslow and Vaillant (Seligman and Steen, 2005). Some of these traits include the following:

- Creativity
- Persistence
- Kindness
- Fairness
- Forgiveness
- Gratitude

Positive psychologists believe that the factors that affect positive emotions or character traits are not simply the opposite (or lack) of those that affect negative emotions or traits. In other words, the factors that make people happier may not necessarily be contrary to those that result in stress. Positive aging is a relatively new area of study that is building on the science of positive psychology. Researchers are just beginning to examine the application of positive interventions to nurture the strengths of older adults.

ADULT DEVELOPMENT IN LATER LIFE

Advances in the health care sciences have ensured that a larger proportion of people will be living longer with a better quality of life. More than ever, as we enter the 21st century, aging has become an evolutionary process. Aging is a complex process that involves biologic, psychologic, social, and environmental factors. How a person adapts to aging is very individualized, and no single theory adequately explains the effects of aging from a developmental perspective. Newer theories of aging are attempting to integrate biologic and behavioral changes to view aging as a series of life events.

It is important that psychiatric nurses understand normal and abnormal aging changes and their impact on such factors as activities of daily living (ADLs), mental processes, social supports, sexuality, and role development. For older adults, their physical and mental health represents the summation of health care beliefs and practices across the years. The psychiatric mental health nurse needs to consider the older person's perceptions of health and wellness as key information during the assessment and the management of care.

Changing attitudes and images of aging have important implications for the psychiatric mental health nurse. Jung stated that we would not grow to be 70 or 80 years old if this longevity had no meaning for the species. Two decades ago, that concept was poetically stated as follows: "The afternoon of human life must also have a significance of its own and cannot be merely a pitiful appendage to life's morning" (Campbell, 1979). This is even more significant in the new millennium. Scientists are beginning to pay attention to those words and to focus on successful aging processes as a reality rather than an ideal.

Overview of the Older Adult Population

It is projected that the population aged 65 years old and older will increase from 35 million in 2010 to 55 million in 2020, which is a 36% increase in one decade. By 2030, there will be approximately 72.1 million older adults; that is nearly double the number present in 2008, with the most significant growth rates among the oldest-old cohort of those 85 years old and older (Administration on Aging, 2009).

To that end, it is imperative for all health care professionals to understand basic gerontology. Gerontology is the study of the aging process across multiple disciplines and settings. Gerontologists who receive specialized training and education in the field of aging are in many disciplines, including nursing, medicine, psychiatry, social services, pharmacology, biology, and the humanities. The term *geriatrics* broadly refers to the health care and human services that are provided to older adults (Eliopoulos, 2001).

Demographics

Since the beginning of the 20th century, the average growth rate of the population 65 years old and older has greatly surpassed the overall population rate according to the U.S. Census Bureau (2008). From 1900 to 2000, the older population increased more than 11 times, from 3 million to 35 million. By comparison, the total population tripled during that same period. By 2050, projections show a marked increase in the older population to more than 88.5 million persons. With the aging of the baby boomers, one in five individuals will be more than 65 years old in 2030. Older adult minority groups, including African Americans, Asians and Pacific Islanders, Native Americans, and Hispanics, will see substantial population growth into the middle of the 21st century.

The most rapidly growing group of the older population is the group of those 85 years old and older, who are called the *oldest old*. Currently, 1.3% of the U.S. population is in this age group. By 2050, this group will grow to 19 million, or almost one fourth of the entire older population (U.S. Census Bureau, 2008). Table 7-3 presents a profile of the aging U.S. population that demonstrates several important characteristics of this growing group now and in the future.

Health Status

Overall, older adults report that their health is good to excellent (Rowe and Kahn, 1998). Socioeconomic status and the availability of social support have direct effects on reports of health. Minority groups and those with low incomes consistently report poorer health, even when the results are controlled for age. Because both males and females are living longer, a greater proportion of couples are surviving into old age. Older adults of today are more educated, with a greater portion having completed some college. More than 22% of persons age 65 years old or older completed at least one year of college; this was true of only 12.5% of individuals in 1970. Older adults also maintain better health care practices than some younger-age groups. The most recent data from the Agency for Healthcare Research and Quality (2003) reported that older persons had better dietary habits and smoked and consumed alcohol to a lesser extent than those who were younger than 65 years old. Only in the area of physical exercise did older adults report less activity than younger age groups.

Although a majority of older adults across all settings suffer from at least one chronic condition, illness in itself does not appear to influence individual perception of health status if functional abilities are not impaired. Functional ability is

TABLE 7-3	PROFILE OF THE OLDER U.S. POPULATION: 2010 AND 2050 COMPARISONS	
ETHNIC GROUP	**OLDER POPULATION IN 2010 (%)**	**OLDER POPULATION IN 2050 (%)**
Caucasian	80.2	58.5
African American	8.3	11.2
Hispanic	7.1	19.8
Asian and Pacific Islander	3.4	8.6
Other races	1.0	1.9

OTHER FACTS

Florida has the highest proportion of persons 65 years old and older (17%), followed by Pennsylvania and West Virginia (>15% each).

Older women outnumber older men in the United States, and this is similar in most countries worldwide. In the United States, women account for 58% of the population 65 years old and older and for 68% of the population 85 years old and older.

Older women are more than twice as likely as older men to live alone (39% and 19%, respectively).

The living arrangements of older adults differ by race and Hispanic origin. Older black, Asian, and Hispanic women are more likely than non-Hispanic white women to live with relatives other than a spouse.

In 2006, 9% of people 65 years old and older lived below the poverty threshold (this decreased significantly from 35% in 1959).

Poverty rates differ with age, gender, and race among older adults, with older women (12%) more likely than older men (7%) to be living in poverty. Those who are more than 75 years old are more likely to live in poverty than those between the ages of 65 and 74 years (10% and 9%, respectively). Minority older adults are also more likely to be living in poverty (23% for older African Americans and 19% for older Hispanics as compared with 7% of non-Hispanic whites).

Modified from U.S. Bureau of the Census: *Population estimates* (website): www.census.gov/popest/estimates.html. Accessed October 26, 2010; and Federal Interagency Forum on Aging Related Statistics: *Older Americans 2008, key indicators of well-being*, Washington, DC, 2008, U.S. Government Printing Office.

categorized as ADLs and instrumental ADLs (IADLs). Nurses include physical and psychosocial functions in a functional assessment. There is a discussion of the assessment of the functional abilities of older adults later in this chapter.

A Life Span Perspective of Aging

Gerontologists in a variety of scientific fields have attempted to explain the developmental processes of aging from biologic and behavioral perspectives. A variety of theories on aging exist because scientists do not agree on a single definition of aging. The literature has described chronologic, biologic, psychologic, and social definitions of aging extensively, but there is no adequate description of the process of aging. Therefore, scientists and philosophers have developed theories to explain the meaning, causes, and factors related to the aging process.

Biologic Theories of Aging

Biologic theories of aging are classified into various categories on the basis of causative factors. Most biologic theories view the process of aging as either a normal, gradual wearing down of all systems or an abnormal series of cellular damages or mutations that eventually lead to the body's inability to make repairs (Schneider and Rowe, 1990).

One method of classifying biologic theories of aging relates to categorizing predisposing factors as intrinsic or extrinsic to the organism. Intrinsic or genetic theories focus on the process of aging as internal to the organism. Researchers estimate that genetic factors account for about 30% of variance in life expectancy, with lifestyle and environmental influences having more profound effects on aging than was previously thought (Lao et al, 2005). Certain genetic diseases, including several types of cancers and high-cholesterol syndromes that lead to heart disease, have a negative impact on life expectancy (Rowe and Kahn, 1998).

Extrinsic or nongenetic theories propose that aging occurs as a result of environmental factors that act on the organism, such as radiation, ozone, drugs, and toxic substances, which, researchers have theorized, damage cellular structures, thereby leading to aging and death. Researchers have not agreed about any single biologic theory to explain the aging process. A combination of genetic and environmental factors best explains why individuals age differently. Four biologic theories of aging that have been most examined by researchers follow.

Genetic Theory. The genetic theory of aging represents a group of basic aging theories, all of which focus on an internal genetic code driving the aging process. Genetic theory basically states that the life span is determined primarily by genes that we inherit from our parents and other ancestors. The basis of the theory is that genes are categorized as juvenescent or senescent. Juvenescent genes promote and maintain growth and vigor through the adult years, whereas senescent genes become active during middle adulthood and later years and initiate a process of decline and deterioration. However, this theory lacks empiric evidence to support that there is an "aging" gene.

Another popular genetic theory is the biologic clock theory (Schneider and Rowe, 1990), which suggests the existence of a programmed internal genetic clock that regulates an organism's development and subsequent decline. This internal clock runs down over a predetermined length of time. Supporters of this theory point to certain normal physiologic changes in humans that happen with time, such as hair graying and menopause.

Although the biologic clock theory gives dramatic evidence for boundaries of the human life span, there are limitations to this theory. One limitation is the inability to generalize in vitro studies to in vivo studies. Second, the theory does not

explain what factor triggers the end of cellular replication and the beginning of cellular degeneration. Finally, the theory does not explain extreme cases of longevity.

Researchers have a suggested a final genetic theory, known as *error theory*, to explain the development of harmful genes that interfere with biologic processes such as protein synthesis (Hayflick, 1985). Damage to biologic synthesis results in the development of damaged cells that interfere with normal biologic functions. The proliferation of cancerous cells is an example of a process in which normal cells become unusual through some error process.

Immunologic Theory. Most biologists agree that changes in the immunologic system after puberty influence the process of aging. Antibody production declines, and autoimmune responses change in response to the decline. The result is that the body's ability to differentiate normal tissue from abnormal or foreign substances fails. This response occurs sometimes in cases of tissue rejection after organ transplantation.

Immune function significantly declines with aging. By the age of 85 years, an individual's immune system functions at 5% to 10% of the system's level at puberty. Rheumatoid arthritis and mature-onset diabetes are two diseases that are commonly experienced during older age that are caused by alterations to the immune system. Although no one knows exactly how or why the immune system exhibits a functional decline with aging, the appearance of autoantibodies in the serum of older persons is common. Autoantibodies are antibodies that are particular to an individual's own normal serum or tissue. Researchers hypothesize that their appearance signals declines in immune system function (Navratil et al, 2004).

Cross-Linkage Theory. Collagen tissue, which is an important component of connective tissue that maintains the structure of cells, tissues, and organs, changes with aging. Collagen provides the elasticity that is necessary in many types of tissue, such as cardiac and muscle. With age, the combination of chemical changes and external stimuli causes the formation of molecular bonds in collagen—known as *cross-links*—that tend to stabilize the collagen fibers, thereby resulting in rigid and fragile tissue. Scientists do not understand the mechanism that triggers the formation of cross-links, but they believe that the most active period of cross-link development is between 30 and 50 years of age.

Cross-links also form in elastin in connective tissue. Elastin is similar to collagen in that it maintains tissue flexibility and permeability. The effects of cross-linking in elastin fibers are most pronounced in the changes that occur in facial skin with aging. Skin becomes brittle, dry, and saggy, and it appears translucent. The formation of cross-links is probably not the only cause of aging, but collagen alterations at the cellular level affect the structural and functional changes that are associated with aging.

Cross-linkage theory has recently been at the forefront of new antiaging research and product development. Researchers are testing various substances in terms of their abilities to inhibit cross-linking and thereby slow aging processes.

Resveratrol—a compound found in the skins of red fruits and in grapes, seeds, some berries, peanuts, red wine, and several herbs—is currently under much study regarding its antiaging potential (Valenzano et al, 2006).

Free Radical Theory. Biologists theorize that some environmental stimuli (e.g., radiation, ozone, certain chemicals) interfere with cellular activity, thereby resulting in the production of free radicals; these are compounds that the body produces in cells as a result of environmental stimuli. They sometimes interact with various cellular structures and cause damage to normal cellular function. Free radicals are also formed during the normal process of cellular oxygenation when the cell removes waste products. Although the cell is capable of neutralizing and removing such byproducts, researchers theorize that, over time, the cell loses its capacity to eliminate waste and repair itself. Researchers are continuing to study the potential effectiveness of antioxidants such as vitamins A, C, and E for the protection of cellular structures.

Sociologic Theories of Aging

Sociologists have observed that an individual's role, relationships, and social experiences change as he or she ages. Sociologic theories of aging attempt to explain the social aspects of the aging process. Sociologists developed three of the earliest theories during the 1960s. These three theories—*disengagement, continuity,* and *activity*—all take a different approach to the social aspects of aging. Common to the three theories is the focus on action and adaptation by the individual (i.e., the aging person needs to change or adjust to new situations). Relocation to a nursing home is often traumatic for the older person who is not able to adjust to the highly structured institutional routines. Social theories that focus more on the interaction between the aging individual and the environment have evolved.

Disengagement Theory. The disengagement theory was the first sociologic aging theory developed by social gerontologists. In 1961, Cumming and Henry published the results of their exploratory study of 275 healthy, financially stable persons between the ages of 50 to 95 years who lived in Kansas City. They theorized that a process of mutual withdrawal naturally occurs between the aging individual and society that is inevitable and universal in its occurrence. The retirement process is an example of this disengagement. Society clearly identifies the age of 65 years as the time for retirement. Identifying a retirement marker or target is also a mechanism for society to open the opportunity for a young person to enter the workforce. According to Cumming and Henry (1961), if the older person is prepared for retirement, he or she will then have an easier time "disengaging" from society.

The disengagement theory has been the most controversial of the social aging theories. Most of the criticism focuses on its presumed universality and on the fact that it does not allow for biologic, personality, or cultural differences. In addition, it presumes that the individual will see disengagement as an obligation to society. How ready and accepting

older persons are to change roles determines their ability to adjust and, subsequently, their life satisfaction.

Havighurst and colleagues (1968) reexamined the original data that were used to formulate the disengagement theory and arrived at different conclusions in support of disengagement. For example, they found that individual personality traits and past experiences influence how an individual in society adapts to aging. A person who is withdrawn early in life will probably continue to withdraw and adapt if his or her social ties also support withdrawal behaviors. Society today is less insistent that older adults completely disengage. For example, some industries are hiring retired persons on a part-time or per-diem basis or using them as expert consultants. It is a combination of one's personal preferences and the needs of society rather than personal preference or societal needs alone that determine the degree and pattern of disengagement.

Continuity Theory. Theorists developed the continuity theory out of Havighurst and colleagues' reformulation of the disengagement theory. The basis of the continuity theory is the idea that people adapt best when they are allowed to be who they are. With aging, people become "more like themselves" in that they attempt to maintain the continuity of habits, beliefs, norms, values, and other aspects of the personality. If a person is having difficulties adjusting to changes such as retirement or relocation, the continuity theory says that it is not the process of aging interfering with adaptation but rather personality factors or the individual's social environment influencing adaptation. The continuity theory allows for individual differences in the aging process and theorizes that each individual's personality contains a self-maintaining component, which means that the individual's longstanding behavior patterns affect coping and adjustment to new situations across the life span (Atchley, 1989).

Activity Theory. Those who support the activity theory believe that maintaining an active lifestyle and social roles offsets the negative effects of aging (Figure 7-2). Activity theorists postulate that by retaining a high level of participation in his or her social environment, the older individual will report a higher level of overall life satisfaction and a more positive self-concept. Four propositions were initially identified during the conceptualization of the activity theory (Lemon et al, 1972):

- The greater the loss in social roles (both formal and informal), the less the activity participation.
- The more activity maintained, the greater the social role support for the older person.
- Maintaining the stability of social roles supports a person's positive self-concept.
- The more positive a person's self-concept, the greater the degree of life satisfaction experienced.

Many do not accept this activity theory because of the lack of empiric evidence to support these postulates. The importance, type, and availability of a particular activity as

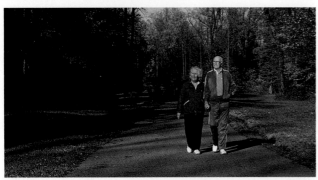

FIGURE 7-2. Continuing interest and activity in a favorite hobby helps to preserve cognitive and physical function. From Sorrentino SA: *Mosby's textbook for nursing assistants,* ed 4, St. Louis, 1996, Mosby.

perceived by the older person is an essential consideration that affects self-concept and life satisfaction. It is possible that the activity theory only applies to older persons who are able to participate in meaningful activities and social interactions.

Newer Theories and Emerging Models of Aging

In the field of theory, aging theories are in their infancy. This is especially true of psychologic theories, most of which theorists developed after World War II. Newer theories of aging include behavioral genetics, gerotranscendence, and gerodynamics theories. Emerging models of aging focus on successful aging and explore the complexities of health and aging from the perspective of older adults.

Behavioral genetics theory examines the relevant impact of genetic and environmental factors on biologic and behavioral differences among individuals across the life span (DeFries et al, 2000). Gerotranscendence theory looks at aging from three levels: cosmic, the self, and social relations. The theory implies that aging brings on changes such as (1) changes in time perception; (2) the acceptance of the mysteries of life and death; (3) altruistic behavior; and (4) an increased need for solitude and reflection (Wadensten and Hagglund, 2006). Gerodynamics theory is based on several physics theories, including general systems theory and chaos theory. Gerodynamics postulates that individuals pass through a series of transformations or life events and are thereby changed in some way (Schroots, 1995). Individuals respond differently to these events, which either weaken or strengthen the individual. Those who age successfully have the ability to cope with traumatic events and to maintain healthy lifestyles. Currently, these theories require additional testing to support their concepts.

Models of healthy aging are beginning to come from explorations of reports made by older adults of their perceptions regarding the attributes of successful aging. Later in this chapter, what researchers are learning about healthy aging is discussed in terms of how this knowledge will restructure views about developmental aging. New models of healthy aging go beyond what is typically considered the dimensions

of health (i.e., physical, functional, psychologic, and social) and attempt to understand how older adults interpret their health and well-being (see the Research for Evidence-Based Practice box #2).

Process of Aging

The process of aging incorporates physiologic and psychosocial changes within the individual. As described in several of the biologic and psychosocial theories of aging, external or environmental factors affect aging in many ways. The physiologic changes that come with aging are universal. Because the changes that characterize normal physiologic aging reflect pathologic changes, health care providers often confuse normal and abnormal aging processes. Although aging is ultimately irreversible, people are still able to significantly delay disease and disability, even into very old age (Rowe and Kahn, 1998).

Psychosocial changes during aging in the areas of cognition, personality, social interactions, sexuality, and roles are even less distinct. Personality and socioenvironmental factors play a huge role in determining psychosocial aging changes. Particular aspects of such processes as cognition and memory decline with aging, whereas other aspects remain the same or are even enhanced with advanced age.

Physiologic Aging

The physiologic aging changes that are considered part of normal aging affect all body systems, but not necessarily at the same rates. It is important to have an understanding of the common physiologic aging changes, because some of these changes indicate the development of pathologic conditions. Many of these changes begin as early as the fourth and fifth decades of life. There are also individual differences in the rates of aging of some biologic systems as a result of factors such as heredity, environment, lifestyle, and nutrition (Kane et al, 2003). In keeping with the focus of this textbook, the following section discusses the physiologic changes of the nervous system.

Nervous System. Unlike cells of other body systems, the cells of the nervous system reproduce more slowly. There is a loss of nerve cells with normal aging, but the degree of loss differs, depending on the structure of the nervous system. The aging pigment, lipofuscin, is deposited in nerve cells, and neurofibrillary plaques and tangles form in the aging brain. These plaques and tangles sometimes indicate Alzheimer's disease, but they are also apparent in normal aging brains in the absence of dementia (see Chapter 15).

The number of some neurotransmitters present in the brain also decreases with normal aging. A decrease in acetylcholine and epinephrine sometimes causes changes in cognitive functioning (e.g., memory storage). Because of the redundancy of nerve cells, it is impossible to generalize that all older persons have diminished memory or cognitive abilities. Decreases in another neurotransmitter, serotonin, is also part of normal aging. Serotonin is important for the regulation of activities such as sleeping, drinking, and breathing. Serotonin also affects temperature regulation, heart rate, and affect. Reductions in the amount of serotonin result in the older person's inability to respond to physical and psychologic stressors in an appropriate manner (see Chapters 6, 11, and 24).

❖ CLINICAL ALERT #1

Because many drugs are excreted through the kidneys, it is important to test creatinine clearance, which is an indicator of the proportion of the body's muscle mass. Reduced creatinine clearance indicates a decrease in muscle mass, so dosages of medication that the kidneys absorb will sometimes need to be reduced for older clients who lose muscle mass.

❖ CLINICAL ALERT #2

It is important for psychiatric mental health nurses to recognize that many mental health problems develop or are identified at certain ages. For instance, schizophrenia is most often diagnosed during late adolescence or early adulthood, but it is uncommon after the age of 50 years. Certain forms of dementia are also more commonly identified at particular ages. For example, symptoms of Pick's disease are often evident by middle age, but symptoms of Alzheimer's disease are typically observed by the age of 75 years.

Functional Assessment. In view of all of the physiologic changes that older adults experience throughout the life span, most individuals are able to cope with the minor aches and pains that are attributed to normal aging. Coping mechanisms usually fail when the older person is unable to function and to carry out ADLs independently. Most situations that bring the older person to the primary care practitioner involve an inability to carry out specific functional tasks.

BOX 7-2   ADL AND IADL FUNCTIONAL ASSESSMENT CATEGORIES

ADL Categories
Bathing
Dressing
Hair care
Mouth care
Nutrition/assist with feeding
Ambulation/mobility
Mental status
Elimination

IADL Categories
Shopping
Meal preparation
Transportation
Use of telephone
Medication usage
Housekeeping
Laundry
Financial management

Therefore, it is important to assess the older person's functional status and its effect on the person's daily life.

Functional assessment usually consists of evaluating two areas. The first area, ADLs, includes categories of personal care such as bathing, grooming, toileting, and transferring. The second area, IADLs, addresses activities that are important for the individual to be able to function in the community. IADLs include shopping, preparing meals, and getting around. Box 7-2 shows the major categories of ADL and IADL assessment.

Activities of Daily Living (ADL). ADLs focus on the physical skills that are necessary to function from day to day. Nearly 31% of adults aged 65 years old or older reported some degree of activity limitations caused by physical, mental, or emotional problems (Centers for Disease Control and Prevention, 2004). Older African Americans and Hispanics tended to have more difficulties with ADLs (Federal Interagency Forum on Aging Related Statistics, 2008). Older adults reported having the greatest amount of difficulty bathing, walking, and transferring between a bed and a chair.

Instrumental Activities of Daily Living (IADL). The ability of the individual to function in the community is an important aspect of the functional assessment. Approximately 17.5% of older adults report difficulty with at least one IADL. Performing heavy housework was a problem for more than 31% of older adults, followed by problems with shopping (17%), doing light housework (12%), and managing money (11%) (National Centers for Health Statistics, 2002).

There are both subjective and objective components of IADLs. Assessing the ability of the older person to perform the daily skills needed to function in the community is important. In addition, the nurse needs to assess the meaning of the activity to the individual. For example, taking care of shopping needs is not as important to some individuals as housekeeping or meal preparation. An older individual who fears going out into the community because of safety issues will essentially become isolated. Another older person may have difficulty chewing and swallowing, so meal preparation may seem like a difficult task.

Both aspects of the functional assessment—ADLs and IADLs—are relevant indicators for identifying outcomes of both physical and mental illness. Often changes in ADLs and IADLs are the indication of a new illness. Individuals respond differently to physical aging changes, so the ability to function independently is more predictive of outcomes of aging than physical aging changes alone.

Psychosocial Aging

Psychosocial aging changes typically focus on an individual's responses to particular events across the life span. Past coping mechanisms are not always effective for adjusting to stressful events in later life. Because the life events of old age differ from those of younger ages, adaptation is sometimes more difficult for older adults. Miller (1990) distinguished the life events of older adults as follows:

- They are viewed as losses rather than gains.
- They are most likely to occur close together with less time to adjust to each event.
- They are more intense and demand greater energy than is available for the coping process.
- They are longer lasting and often become chronic problems.
- They are inevitable and bring a feeling of powerlessness.

Preparing for some life events will facilitate adjustment during old age. For instance, some employers offer preretirement counseling for older employees. Psychosocial aging changes are reflected in several areas, including cognition, memory, personality, social support, sexuality, and role status. From a developmental perspective, the meaningfulness of life events is important for determining patterns of psychosocial aging in these particular areas. A great deal of research is necessary before researchers are able to draw any conclusions regarding normal versus abnormal psychosocial aging. The following section explores the current state of knowledge of psychosocial aging from a developmental perspective.

Cognition and Memory. Probably no other area of aging research has been studied to such an extent as cognition, especially in the areas of intelligence and memory. Cognitive behaviors are divided into several interrelated processes that include intelligence, memory, attention, reaction time, and problem solving. These divisions are random, and researchers base them on how they typically study cognitive behaviors.

Several factors contribute to the variability in cognitive functioning observed among older adults. These factors include health status, genetic profile, socioeconomic status, education, and lifestyle behaviors (Herzog and Wallace, 1997). In turn, cognitive losses often result in functional impairment and physical disabilities, which cause a spiraling decline for the older person. Evidence of the development of cognitive function into old age is becoming clearer with

studies that follow older subjects over time. It is apparent that cognitive functioning shows as much variability during aging as physiologic indicators do (MacDonald et al, 2003).

Intelligence and Aging. Studies of intelligence during the 1940s reported that older adults experienced declines in all aspects of intelligence, including knowledge acquisition, calculating, vocabulary, and abstract thought. The problem with these early studies was that researchers used the cross-sectional method to collect the data and compared younger age groups with older adult groups. The younger age groups consistently had higher intelligence scores on the various tests, thus prompting researchers to conclude that intelligence declines with aging (Woodruff, 1983). Subsequent studies that followed the same older subjects over a period of time found that intelligence showed little or no decline among healthy aging persons. Declines that did occur were in the oldest age group (Schaie and Willis, 1991).

Horn and Cattell (1967) theorized that age-related differences in intelligence are possibly due to distinctions between two types of intelligence that seem to develop from birth. Crystallized intelligence develops from knowledge gained through the accumulation of experience and education. Crystallized intelligence declines slightly, remains the same, or even increases with aging, depending on one's life experiences. Alternatively, neurophysiologic processes across the life span affect fluid intelligence. Declines in the nervous system with aging that affect one's attention span or reaction time reflect a loss of fluid intelligence. Instruments that measure intelligence with the use of performance standards show declines in intelligence with aging (Birren and Schaie, 1985), and even some gerontologists have questioned these conclusions. Some older adults have demonstrated an increased time needed to complete intelligence performance tests because they are more cautious and take additional time to make correct choices.

Memory Processes and Aging. Much aging research is devoted to the study of memory processes during aging. It is unfortunate that society equates aging with memory loss. Older persons are often portrayed on television or in movies as forgetful. A common joke is, "There are three telltale signs you are getting old. The first is loss of memory, and the other two . . . I forget." There is much that we still do not know about the process of memory perception, storage, and retrieval.

Most of the early theories of memory focused on the three components of memory: (1) perception or encoding; (2) storage; and (3) retrieval. Memory was categorized as short or long term or as primary, secondary, or tertiary. These categorizations were based on the length of storage time and the process of retrieval.

Other memory theories focused on the encoding processes, which involved different types of information in various ways. For example, information that the brain processes in a more complex manner (e.g., algebraic equations) is stored in a deeper area of memory and will last longer. Information that the brain easily recognizes requires less attention. For example, tasks such as starting a car are almost automatic. Researchers believe that the automatic processing of information does not change with aging (Friedman, 2000). Offering cues to older adults will help them to recall information that is stored in deeper areas of memory.

Theorists developed the contextual theory of memory from the information-processing model. This theory expands the information-processing model by including individual factors that sometimes affect memory, such as learning behaviors, past experiences, personality, degree of motivation, physical health, and socioeconomic status (Perlmutter et al, 1987).

Certain types of memory decline as a part of normal aging. Explicit memory, which is the ability to recall a specific name or place, tends to decline with aging (Rowe and Kahn, 1998). Working memory, which is the type of memory that is needed to perform daily activities, does not show an aging decline. Because older adults often take longer to process information (which is also normal with aging) and have some specific recall problems, they often fear that this is an indicator of Alzheimer's disease. It is important to explain to them that this is not the case and to encourage older adults to seek ways to improve cognitive functioning through training and practice.

Self-perception of memory changes and self-efficacy also influence memory performance (Ryan and See, 1993). The term *metamemory* refers to one's self-perceptions of memory changes and their effect on memory processes (Hertzog et al, 1990). For example, an older person falsely believes that memory loss is part of aging and perceives that forgetfulness indicates the start of memory decline. In reality, forgetting information is also the result of a lack of attention to detail in a particular situation. Further study is necessary to determine whether an individual is able to mentally control or influence the development of memory across the life span.

Other Cognitive Functions. The term *attention span* refers to one's ability to concentrate throughout the performance of some task. With aging, the ability to maintain the attention span through the completion of complex tasks diminishes, because complex tasks require dividing one's attention among several tasks at the same time. Some misinterpret these normal aging changes that involve the attention span as dementia. Two other segments of attention also show some decrements with aging. Vigilance, which is the ability to sustain attention over longer periods of time, and selective attention, which is the ability to discriminate and focus on relevant information, are less acute among older adults.

Increased reaction time that results in decreased speed of performance on intelligence tests is one of the most obvious changes that occurs with normal aging, but researchers still do not fully understand why this happens. Anxiety caused by unfamiliarity with performance or the fear of failure may affect the reaction time of older adults.

Problem-solving ability is a higher cognitive function. The complexity of the problem, past experiences, the amount of information that is irrelevant to the situation, and the individual's level of education are factors that influence problem solving. There is little knowledge regarding normal changes

in higher cognitive functioning during aging. Most older persons are able to live and function effectively in the community.

Personality. Personality traits develop over the life span, and they are influenced by internal and external environmental factors. An individual's ability to cope with stress and to adapt to change molds an individual's personality. How individuals perceive themselves (i.e., the self-concept) reflects their personality. In general, most personality traits remain stable during the aging process. Personality influences how an individual interacts and reacts within the social environment (see Chapter 14).

Personality theorists have attempted to identify specific traits that predict successful aging. Individuals who are described as introverted are more self-centered and internalize behaviors and responses. Extroverted personalities focus more on the outside world and are described as outgoing. Certain personality traits assist individuals with adapting to aging better than others. The individual's ability to adapt to change determines successful aging more than a particular category of personality traits.

Some traits intensify with aging, such as cautiousness, which is often an effective safety mechanism for older adults. For example, the older person tends to drive a car with more caution, to drive only during daylight hours, or to avoid high speeds. In unfamiliar situations or when several choices are available, older adults tend to act more cautiously. They also tend to prefer familiar tasks, places, and situations. The locus of control is another aspect of personality that remains stable over time (Reid et al, 1977). Individuals with an internal locus of control perceive that they actively control their own destiny. Alternatively, individuals with an external locus of control believe that they have no control over their destinies and that their behaviors have no effect on any outcomes. Another phenomenon, the secondary locus of control, describes individuals with an external locus of control who learn to adapt to their beliefs; this has also been called *learned helplessness.* These individuals learn dependency and prefer that others make decisions for them.

Social Support and Interactions. In an extensive review of the literature, Broadhead and colleagues (1983) presented Kahn and Antonucci's comprehensive definition of social support as interpersonal transactions that include one or more of the following behaviors: (1) expressing positive affect between individuals; (2) affirming or approving of another person's behaviors; and (3) providing direct aid or assistance to another. Different individuals within one's social network provide different types of support.

Hyde (1988) suggested that the quality rather than the quantity of social relationships is significantly related to life satisfaction among older adults. The quality of social support is a key area for interventions in the training of health care providers. Social support is part of a communication process in which the facilitation of communication skills improves the quality of support (Albrecht and Adelman, 1984).

Social networks are generally the web of social ties that surround a person and include several characteristics that are

TABLE 7-4	SOCIAL RELATIONSHIP ASSESSMENT	
COMPONENTS	**CHARACTERISTICS**	**SAMPLE QUESTIONS**
Social network	Marital partner/confidant	Are you married? Is there any one special person who you feel very close and intimate with?
Structure and composition	Number and kinship Proximity Frequency and type of contact	How many children or close family members do you have? How many live within an hour's drive? How many do you have phone or letter contact with at least once per month?
Type and amount of social support and function	Emotional Tangible aid Guidance	How frequently did someone try to make you feel better about your illness during the past month? How frequently did someone help you get your medication during the past month? How frequently did someone suggest that you call the doctor during the past month?
Perceived adequacy of social support	General Specific	During the past year, did you need more help with daily tasks than you received? How helpful was it for your children to try to make you feel better about your illness?

From Oxman T, Berkman L: Assessment of social relationships in elderly patients, *Int J Psychiatry Med* 20:65-84, 1990.

important in the study of the health and well-being of older adults. These include the following:

- The size of the social network
- The frequency of social contacts
- The quality of the interactions
- The degree of intimacy or closeness among members
- The strength of the relationships
- The geographic location of the members
- The reciprocity of assistance

Social networks and social supports are different concepts; the social network is the web or structure of the group, and the social support is the emotional or tangible assistance that is obtained from the social network. Not all social ties are supportive, and not all social supports come from the closest social network, such as a son or daughter living near older parents. Oxman and Berkman (1990) proposed a three-component model of social relationships that included the quantitative and qualitative nature of social relationships. Because many have associated social relationships with subsequent physical and mental illness in older adults, an assessment tool that addresses the multidimensional aspects of social relationships is important. Table 7-4 presents examples of some relevant assessment questions (Oxman and Berkman, 1990).

Sexuality and Intimacy. Physical aging changes related to the reproductive system occur in men and women. Several factors influence psychologic aspects of sexuality and intimacy in older adults, including past experiences, attitudes toward intimacy, societal views about sexuality in older adults, and functional status.

Many older adults feel a newfound freedom with regard to their sexual behaviors because they no longer need to focus on concerns regarding pregnancy. The unavailability of an acceptable partner, stereotypes that suggest that older adults are asexual, and fears of an inability to initiate or maintain sexual performance frustrate some of these feelings. Older women probably experience the greatest effects, because many become widowed or suffer from the effects of long-standing values about sexual taboos. Only in recent years have older persons, especially those more than 80 years old, been the subjects of studies of sexuality (see the Research for Evidence-Based Practice box #3).

RESEARCH FOR EVIDENCE-BASED PRACTICE #3

Lindau ST et al: A study of sexuality and health among older adults in the United States, *N Engl J Med* 357:762-774, 2007.

In this large national survey of more than 3000 older adults, the researchers examined the little known relationships among sexual behaviors, sexual function, age, and health status in this population. The prevalence of sexual activity declined with increasing age, but it was still prevalent into the later years: 73% of individuals were sexually active between the ages of 65 and 74 years, and 26% were sexually active from the ages of 75 to 85 years. Nearly half of those who were sexually active reported at least one bothersome sexual problem, with many of them discussing these problems with their physicians. The most common reason for sexual inactivity was the partner's poor physical health rather than a lack of interest or other reasons. Overall, the majority of older adults are engaged in intimate relationships and feel that sexuality is an important part of their lives.

Role Transitions. Older persons also experience role changes along with other changes that occur with aging. Some of these role variations are more obvious than others, and individuals adapt to role changes in different ways. How important the role is influences how well the older person is able to cope with a role transition. From a developmental perspective, roles include various tasks that a person has to perform in life, and each role involves different life tasks. Some tasks are new to the person if the role is a completely new one, whereas other tasks are similar to those that have been performed early in life (e.g., role reversals).

Retirement. Retirement involves a major role transition for many individuals. Because individuals live longer and retire earlier, the retirement period may last for 30 to 40 years. Only recently have researchers begun to explore gender differences with regard to adaptation to retirement. Life events that surround retirement affect adaptation more than the retirement process itself (Reitzes and Mutran, 2004). Particular life events often force retirement. For example, a middle-aged woman takes an early retirement because she needs to care for her older mother with Alzheimer's disease at home. This individual's adjustment to retirement is negative because of a conflict between the woman's role in the workforce and her caregiver role.

Loss of a Spouse. A major role transition occurs after the loss of one's spouse, when adaptation requires the survivor to perform tasks that the partner previously performed. Couples who have shared responsibilities across the life span have less difficulty with the role changes. Personality traits seem to influence adjustment to widowhood. For example, a widow who let her husband take care of finances finds herself overwhelmed by the new responsibility, or the husband who lost his wife and who never learned how to cook or clean and is also overwhelmed. If the surviving spouse adapts to change, he or she will rapidly adjust and learn these tasks. Widows or widowers sometimes finds themselves at the center of attention of family members who want to assist them as well as members of the opposite gender who are looking for companionship.

Grandparent Role. The role of the grandparent is another transition. The grandparent who adjusts successfully provides grandchildren with a viewpoint that often differs from the parents but that is equally positive. Many grandparents take on the role of full- or part-time surrogate parents. According to the U.S. Census (2008), grandparents raising grandchildren is a growing issue nationwide, with 2.4 million families being maintained by grandparents caring for one or more grandchildren. Studies report that such caregiving may cause higher levels of physical burden than parenting one's own children (Bachman and Lindsay, 2005). As a result, grandparents often face greater stress and subsequent health problems believed to be related to the increased focus on their grandchildren's health and welfare rather than on their own.

Role Reversal. When physical or mental deterioration is present, this often reverses the roles of the parent and the child. Most often the oldest female child, on reaching middle age, provides care for the incapacitated older parent. This is an especially difficult transition for the female middle-aged child who has just completed raising her own children and who was planning her own retirement in a few years. If the caregiver is a middle-aged man, it is often an awkward

situation, because his wife has to adapt to a role for which she sometimes has no emotional connection (i.e., caring for the older parent-in-law). Supporting the caregiver is as important as supporting the care receiver under these circumstances. Table 7-5 summarizes some normal aging changes that are discussed in this section as well as some areas for functional assessment.

Mental Assessment. Gerontologists are attempting to develop adequate standardized tests that are designed specifically for older adults to assess their mental status and cognitive functioning. Designing reliable instruments for older adults continues to be a challenge because of the interrelationships among several factors, including health status, physical and mental aging changes, socioenvironmental variables, and life events. Thus, the context of what many consider normal development for an older individual is the focus of any mental status assessment.

Several mental status assessment instruments are available to evaluate mental and cognitive functions. Most instruments examine mental status in view of the individual's ability to function in daily living activities. However, the mental status assessment is not sufficient to provide a diagnosis of a disorder. Other sources of information (e.g., health history, physical examination, diagnostic and laboratory tests, psychosocial factors) are necessary for diagnosis.

The mental status assessment of older adults includes the following areas: appearance, mood, communication, thought processes, perceptual and motor abilities, attention, memory, consciousness, and orientation. Appearance, behaviors, and responses of the older client are areas for attention by the health care provider who is performing the assessment. For instance, the older person states that he or she has no suicidal ideations, but his or her appearance indicates self-neglect, and behaviors include withdrawing from social networks and accumulating drugs. It is important to identify such inconsistencies.

Several screening instruments are available for the health care provider to use for a quick assessment of mental status. Each instrument addresses different areas of the mental status examination. Often these brief instruments provide an initial baseline of cognitive functioning for use in further in-depth assessment and screening for diagnosis and subsequent interventions.

The Mini-Mental State Examination (MMSE) is one of the most commonly used instruments for screening for cognitive disorders among older adults (Folstein et al, 1975). It assesses several dimensions of cognitive function, including orientation, memory, attention, and speech. Criticisms of the MMSE focus on its inability to discriminate between persons with mild dementia and those who do not have dementia as well as its bias against persons with little education. The MMSE is a copywritten instrument that is designed for trained professional use. More information about obtaining the MMSE for clinical use may be found at www.minimental.com.

An alternative to the MMSE is the short and simple-to-use Blessed Orientation-Memory-Concentration Test (BOMC) (Katzman and Rowe, 1992). The short version of the BOMC

TABLE 7-5   FUNCTIONAL ASSESSMENT OF COMMON PSYCHOSOCIAL AGING CHANGES

AREA	NORMAL AGING CHANGES	AREAS FOR FUNCTIONAL ASSESSMENT
Cognition and memory	Normal crystallized intelligence ↓ Fluid intelligence (slight, gradual) ↑ Reaction time ↓ Divided attention ↓ Vigilance ↓ Selected attention ↑ Information-processing time ↑ Cautiousness	Degree of external stimulation Environmental distractions Assess barriers to learning (e.g., sensory impairments, relevancy or level of information, learning environment) Assess factors that influence the memory process (e.g., education level, learning style, past experiences, physical and mental health, motivation)
Personality	Stability of most personality traits ↑ Cautiousness ↑ Rigidity (slight)	Adaptive coping strategies Decision-making processes Adjustment to change (e.g., retirement, change in housing, loss)
Social support and interactions	Perceived social support affected by several factors (e.g., personality, health status, past experiences, coping style) Changes in social network (e.g., size, intimacy, geographic location, reciprocity of assistance) Changes in sources of social support with aging	Attitudes and perceptions regarding social support Past experience with social support Social network Types of social support needed Sources of social support
Sexuality and intimacy	Sexual behaviors and interests maintained across life span in the absence of physical and mental disorders ↓ Sexual activity in males ↓ Intensity of sexual responses Lack of partner is the greatest factor that affects sexual activity	Attitudes toward expressions of sexuality and intimacy Means to maintain sexual behaviors and interests Availability of privacy in environment Risk factors that block sexual behaviors
Role transitions	Retirement Widowhood Grandparenting	Importance of past roles and tasks Responses to retirement Effects of retirement on spouse Impact of loss of spouse Ability to take on new tasks in activities of daily living and instrumental activities of daily living Social support and network Relationships with children and grandchildren Parenting role

is six items in length, and the psychometric properties of the tool are well documented (Katzman et al, 1983). Three items test orientation, two items test recall, and one item tests the ability to concentrate. Unlike the MMSE, which requires some degree of motor dexterity, the BOMC requires only verbal responses and thus may be used in telephone interviews as well as for in-person screenings. Components of the BOMC short version are presented in Box 7-3.

Human Development During the Twenty-First Century

On January 1, 2011, the first baby boomer turned 65 years old. Society's entire perception of aging will continue to evolve for the following 20 to 30 years as the older adult population experiences unprecedented growth during that time frame. Images of aging and attitudes toward older persons are gradually changing for the better. As the aging population grows more ethnically and racially diverse, a reexamination of cultural values regarding aging is necessary. In fact, the entire body of knowledge on human development will probably need revising, because research in aging has begun to refocus its efforts to understand successful aging. In particular, scientists are examining health, learning, and creativity as areas to promote quality of life among older adults.

Images of Aging

Images of aging and the attitudes of society toward older adults have been changing over the past several years. Unfortunately, society has usually focused on the negative aspects of aging. The term *ageism* has been used to describe the stereotypic views of older adults (Butler, 1987). The myth of the "burden of the elderly" has been gradually rejected with the growing body of scientific evidence that disproves the notion that to be old is to be sick (Rowe and Kahn, 1998).

In 1995, the American Association of Retired Persons published a study titled *Images of Aging in America* (Speas and

BOX 7-3   THE BLESSED ORIENTATION-MEMORY-CONCENTRATION TEST, SHORT VERSION

QUESTION	MAXIMUM ERROR	SCORE MULTIPLIER	WEIGHT
1. What year is it now?	1	___ × 4	=
2. What month is it now?	1	___ × 3	=
Repeat this phrase: "John Brown, 42 West Street, Chicago"			
3. About what time is it (within one hour)?	1	___ × 3	=
4. Count backward from 20 to 1.	2	___ × 2	=
5. Say the months in reverse order.	2	___ × 2	=
6. Repeat the phrase just given.	5	___ × 2	=
		Total error score = ___ /28	

Scoring:
- Allow up to three trials for learning the phrase ("John Brown..."). If the subject has not learned the phrase after three trials, code this as a "9," and proceed with test.
- Items 4 and 5: If no errors, score "0"; if one error, score "1"; if two or more errors, score "2."
- Item 6: Score of "1" for each incorrect response. An answer of either "Market" or "Market Street" is acceptable.
- Maximum weighted error score = 28; cutoff score >16.

Obenshain, 1995). The purpose of this report was to examine knowledge, perceptions, and attitudes about aging. One's personal experience with older adults was the strongest predictor of perceptions and attitudes toward aging. Most Americans had misconceptions about older adults that reflected a lack of knowledge about aging. On a positive note, many subjects showed a lack of stereotypes and myths about aging. These findings have important implications for health care professionals who work with older adults.

In 2004, researchers repeated this study and obtained noticeably similar results. Many people continued to have false impressions about aging and older adults. Less knowledge about the aging process was related to greater anxiety about getting older. In addition, adults with fewer economic resources and significant health issues expressed the greatest anxiety about getting older. Similar to the 1990s study, the later study found little evidence of intergenerational conflict (Abramson and Silverstein, 2006).

Cultural Impact

Cultural beliefs also influence one's attitudes toward older adults. Culture affects the responses of older adults to health, illness, and treatment. Some cultures subscribe to health care practices or home remedies that are in direct opposition to modern health care practices. The health care professional needs to examine his or her own feelings toward differing cultural beliefs and health care practices of older clients. The incorporation of some home remedies into the older client's care plan sometimes increases compliance, but only if these remedies do not conflict with treatment.

Various cultures hold different views regarding aging. Since ancient times, the contributions of older adults to society have affected the status of older adults within a particular cultural group. For example, Eastern cultures value the wisdom of elders and hold the older population in high respect. By contrast, some primitive cultures have considered older adults a burden because they are unable to hunt and provide for the tribe. Such cultures have sometimes sent older adults away from the tribe.

In the current Western culture, there is greater support for views of successful aging. Focusing on age presents issues that relate to functional, economic, and political aspects of aging that future older persons will experience. The situation of today's older population is possibly the most optimistic in terms of the availability of social and economic resources, but future generations of older persons face difficult resource issues (Conrad, 1992). Costs may outweigh contributions by future older persons in society, and cultural values toward older adults may change.

Refocusing on Healthy Aging

Perceptions of health and wellness develop across the life span and affect an individual's attitudes and behaviors related to health care practices. For older adults, physical and mental health represent the result of health care beliefs and practices across the years. During the period from 2004 to 2006, 74% of older adults rated their health as good to excellent, which were similar to results obtained a decade earlier. As older adults age, the percentage who report good to excellent health declines, regardless of gender or race. Regardless of age group or gender, Caucasians overall report good to excellent health as compared with other ethnic groups (Federal Interagency Forum on Aging Related Statistics, 2008).

The MacArthur Foundation Study (Rowe and Kahn, 1998) has brought together 10 years of scientific knowledge and expertise related to aging. The study identified three components that were necessary for successful aging:

1. The avoidance of disease and risk factors
2. The maintenance of high cognitive and physical abilities
3. The engagement with life through productive relationships and behaviors

The early identification of risk factors and disease-prevention/health-promotion behaviors has a significant impact on the development and progress of several chronic diseases. For example, exercise is beneficial for helping older adults to prevent heart disease, hypertension, and diabetes. A regular moderate program of aerobic and strength training for older adults is both safe and effective for the improvement of function.

Challenging the mind as well as the body is important for the maintenance of mental capabilities. Not all cognitive processes decline with aging, and most of these changes occur very late in life. Older persons who maintain a high level of self-efficacy, which is a measure of one's self-esteem, appear to manage well both mentally and physically.

Maintaining social relationships and continuing some sort of meaningful activities contribute positively to aging. Social networks often shrink for older adults who outlive their peers and relatives. Older persons find support in caring relationships with friends or family members. Grandparents find joy in having their grandchildren visit for extended periods, which also offers a break to the children's parents. In terms of productive activities, many older retirees remark that they are much busier after retirement, with new projects and volunteer work. With the aging of the baby boomers, the focus on successful aging is more of a reality than an ideal.

Refocusing on Learning and Aging

A large body of literature has focused on adult learning theory. In contrast with children, adults prefer self-directed learning and incorporate past experiences into new opportunities. Adults also prefer to learn about things that apply to their daily lives. Older adults continue to learn well into their 70s or 80s. Physical limitations affect the speed of learning, so teaching methods need to be adapted for older learners. Older adults also need to have a choice regarding how they best learn certain material (i.e., auditory, visual, or tactile).

When teaching older adults, nurses need to link their lessons to experiences or activities that older adults are familiar with or have enjoyed, especially social activities. For example, encourage older adults who enjoyed the years they spent raising their own children to join a foster grandparent program or a senior volunteer program where they develop new relationships and learn about new resources. Intergenerational programs are also growing in popularity. Elementary and high schools are joining with senior communities to share learning experiences. For example, retired persons teach young people about skills such as woodcrafting, and young people give teach the older persons about computers and the Internet.

Refocusing on Creativity and Aging

In his book, *The Creative Age: Awakening Human Potential in the Second Half of Life* (2000), Gene D. Cohen provided evidence that the human potential for creativity continues well into old age. He found that, although information processing slows down as one ages, older persons are able to go on to learn new information by modifying how they process this information; they will slowly digest bits of data or thoughtfully ask questions to clarify key points. Studies of the computer training of individuals 65 years old or older reported that practicing increased both the speed and accuracy of their computing.

In another example, older persons tend to have difficulty bringing up certain words. By contrast, persons in their 80s who keep on challenging themselves by reading, writing, or doing crossword and word game puzzles have continued to grow their vocabularies. Research has even demonstrated links between creative activities and the consequential positive feelings with the increased production of protective immune cells. Creativity is also possibly linked to delaying the onset of Alzheimer's disease. Continually challenging oneself mentally is a way to build up reserves of neurologic structures and connections.

CHAPTER SUMMARY

- Whatever the directions and results of future studies of aging and human development, it is clear that human development does not occur in isolation. The constant influence of biologic, psychosocial, and environmental factors creates a dynamic system in which human development occurs across the life span.
- Human development also begins at a much earlier age than previously believed, and it continues into much later years than researchers ever anticipated.
- It is important for the psychiatric mental health nurse to consider development as a continuous process. Although there are common markers of human development at particular ages, there is a great degree of human variation.
- External factors such as culture and traditions also have a significant influence on human development, so the nurse needs be aware of these factors and to take them into account when caring for clients.
- Understanding that many aspects of human development continue to grow and change well into old age provides the nurse with additional opportunities to promote and stimulate successful aging.

REVIEW QUESTIONS

1. To assess whether a 4-year-old child is in Erikson's initiative-versus-guilt developmental stage, the nurse asks the parent which of the following?
   1. "Can your child put on socks without help?"
   2. "What activities does your child participate in with other children?"
   3. "Does your child get upset when you leave the room?"
   4. "Does your child do chores to help you out at home, such as picking up toys?"

2. A 10-year-old child has this nursing diagnosis: *Delayed growth and development related to insufficient opportunities to interact with other children as evidenced by inability to engage in group play.* Select the best outcome for this child's plan of care. Within 2 months, the child will:
   1. Voluntarily join a team sport.
   2. Find useful ways to engage in solitary play.
   3. Attend three sessions with a certified child psychologist.
   4. Have an improved sense of self and peers.

3. A nurse cares for a 77-year-old retired physician who is hospitalized with pneumonia. Which form of address would be the most appropriate to use with this client?
   1. The client's first name
   2. "Mr." or "Ms.," followed by the client's surname
   3. "Dr.," followed by the client's surname
   4. An endearing term, such as "Honey" or "Sweetie"

4. Which neurotransmitter changes are expected during the normal aging process? You may select more than one answer.
   1. Decreased serotonin
   2. Increased glutamate
   3. Decreased acetylcholine
   4. Decreased epinephrine
   5. Decreased lipofuscin

5. A nurse offers an educational presentation in a senior citizens center. Which activities might the nurse suggest to promote healthy, successful aging? You may select more than one answer.
   1. A water aerobics class
   2. Woodworking
   3. Watching television
   4. Crossword puzzles
   5. Drinking four to six glasses of wine daily

REFERENCES

Abramson A, Silverstein M; American Association of Retired Persons: *Images of aging in American 2004* (website): www.assets.aarp.org/rgcenter/general/images_aging.pdf. Accessed October 27, 2010.

Abramson A, Silverstein M: *Key Predictors of Knowledge and Anxiety About Aging,* Washington DC, 2006, Gerontological Society of America.

Administration on Aging: *A profile of older Americans: 2009.* Washington, DC, 2009, U.S. Department of Health and Human Services.

Agency for Healthcare Research and Quality: *Medical expenditure panel survey,* Rockville, Md, 2003, Agency for Healthcare Research and Quality.

Ainsworth M: Attachments beyond infancy, *Am Psychol* 44:709, 1989.

Albrecht T, Adelman M: Social support and life stress: new directions for communication research, *Hum Commun Res* 11:3, 1984.

Atchley R: A continuity theory of normal aging, *Gerontologist* 29:183, 1989.

Bachman HJ, Lindsay P: Custodial grandmothers' physical, mental, and economic well-being: comparisons of primary caregivers from low-income neighborhoods, *Family Relations* 54:475, 2005.

Baltes P et al: Life-span developmental psychology, *Annu Rev Psychol* 23:65, 1992.

Bandura A: *Social foundations of thought and action: a social cognitive theory,* Englewood Cliffs, NJ, 1986, Prentice-Hall.

Birren J, Schaie K: *Handbook of the psychology of aging,* ed 2, New York, 1985, Van Nostrand Reinhold.

Bowlby J: *A secure base: clinical applications of attachment theory,* London, 1988, Routledge.

Broadhead W et al: The epidemiologic evidence for a relationship between social support and health, *Am J Epidemiol* 117:521, 1983.

Butler R: Ageism. In Maddox G, editor: *The encyclopedia of aging,* New York, 1987, Springer.

Campbell J: *The portable Jung,* New York, 1979, Penguin Books.

Centers for Disease Control and Prevention: *Basic actions difficulty and complex activity limitation among adults 18 years of age and over, by selected characteristics: United States, selected years 1997–2007* (website): http://www.cdc.gov/nchs/data/hus/hus09.pdf#055. Accessed December 12, 2010.

Cohen G: *The creative age: awakening human potential in the second half of life,* New York, 2000, Avon Books.

Conrad C: Old age in the modern and postmodern western world. In Cole T et al, editors: *Handbook of the humanities and aging,* New York, 1992, Springer.

Cumming E, Henry W: *Growing old: the process of disengagement,* New York, 1961, Basic Books.

DeFries J et al: *Behavioral genetics,* New York, 2000, Worth.

Ebersole P, Hess P: *Toward healthy aging: human needs and nursing responses,* ed 5, St. Louis, 1999, Mosby.

Eliopoulos C: *Gerontological nursing,* ed 5, Philadelphia, 2001, JB Lippincott.

Erikson EH: *Eight stages of man in childhood and society,* New York, 1963, WW Norton.

Erikson EH: *Childhood and society*, ed 2, New York, 1974, WW Norton.

Erikson EH: *The life cycle completed*, New York, 1982, WW Norton.

Erikson EH et al: *Vital involvement in old age: the experience of old age in our time*, New York, 1986, WW Norton.

Federal Interagency Forum on Aging Related Statistics: *Older Americans 2008: key indicators of well-being* (website): www.agingstats.gov. Accessed October 27, 2010.

Folstein M et al: "Mini-mental state": a practical method of grading the cognitive state of patients for the clinician, *J Psychiatr Res* 12:189, 1975.

Friedman D: Event-related brain potential investigations of memory and aging, *Biol Psychol* 54:175, 2000.

Freud S: *The ego and the id*, New York, 1923, WW Norton.

Gallagher J, Reid D: *The learning theory of Piaget and Inhelder*, Monterey, Calif, 1981, Brooks/Cole.

Gilligan C: *In a different voice*, Cambridge, Mass, 1982, Harvard University Press.

Havighurst R et al: Disengagement and patterns of aging. In Neugarten B, editor: *Middle age and aging*, Chicago, 1968, University of Chicago Press.

Hayflick L: Theories of biological aging. In Andres R et al, editors: *Principles of geriatric medicine*, New York, 1985, McGraw-Hill.

Hertzog C et al: Relationships between metamemory, memory predictions, and memory task performance in adults, *Psychol Aging* 5:215, 1990.

Herzog A, Wallace R: Measures of cognitive functioning in the AHEAD study, *J Gerontol* 52:37, 1997.

Horn J, Cattell R: Age differences in fluid and crystallized intelligence, *Acta Psychol* 26:107, 1967.

Hyde R: Facilitative communication skills training: social support for elderly people, *Gerontologist* 28:418, 1988.

Hyer L, Intrieri R: *Geropsychological interventions in long-term care*, New York, 2006, Springer.

Jung C: The stages of life. In Campbell J, editor: *The portable Jung*, New York, 1971, Viking Press.

Kane R et al: *Essentials of clinical geriatrics*, New York, 2003, McGraw-Hill.

Katzman R et al: Validation of a short orientation-memory-concentration test of cognitive impairment, *Am J Psychiatry* 140:734, 1983.

Katzman R, Rowe J: *Principles of geriatric neurology*, Philadelphia, 1992, FA Davis.

Kohlberg L: Stages and aging in moral development: some speculations, *Gerontologist* 13:497, 1973.

Lao J et al: Genetic contribution to aging: deleterious and helpful genes define life expectancy, *Ann N Y Acad Sci* 1057:50, 2005.

Lemon B et al: An exploration of the activity theory of aging: activity types and life satisfaction among inmovers to a retirement community, *J Gerontol* 27:511, 1972.

Levinson DJ et al: *The seasons of a man's life*, New York, 1986, Ballantine Books.

MacDonald S et al: Performance variability is related to change in cognition: evidence from the Victoria Longitudinal Study, *Psychol Aging* 18:510, 2003.

Maslow A: *Toward a psychology of being*, New York, 1962, Van Nostrand.

McCrae RR, Costa PT: *Emerging lives, enduring dispositions: personality in adulthood*, Boston, 1984, Little, Brown and Co.

Miller C: *Nursing care of older adults: theory and practice*, Glenview, Ill, 1990, Scott Foresman.

Miller N, Dollard J: *Social learning and imitation*, New Haven, Conn, 1941, Yale University Press.

Myers D: Adulthood's ages and stages, *Psychology* 5:196, 1998.

National Centers for Health Statistics: *Limitation of activity: difficulty performing instrumental activities of daily living*, 2002 (website): www.cdc.gov/nchs, accessed February 7, 2011.

Navratil JS et al: Apoptosis and immune responses to self, *Rheum Dis Clin North Am* 30:193, 2004.

Neugarten BL: Time, age, and the life cycle, *Am J Psychiatry* 136:887, 1979.

Newton PM, Levinson DJ: Crisis in adult development. In Lazare A, editor: *Outpatient psychiatry: diagnosis and treatment*, Baltimore, 1979, Williams & Wilkins.

Oxman T, Berkman L: Assessment of social relationships in elderly patients, *Int J Psychiatr Med* 20:65, 1990.

Peavy GM et al: Effects of chronic stress on memory decline in cognitively normal and mildly impaired older adults, *Am J Psychiatry* 166:1384, 2009.

Perlmutter M et al: Aging and memory, *Annu Rev Gerontol Geriatr* 7:57, 1987.

Piaget J: *The science of education and the psychology of the child*, New York, 1970, Grossman.

Reid D et al: Locus of desired control and positive self-concept of the elderly, *J Gerontol* 32:441, 1977.

Reitzes DC, Mutran EJ: The transition to retirement: stages and factors that influence retirement adjustment, *Int J Aging Hum Dev* 59:63, 2004.

Rotter J: *The development and application of social learning theory*, New York, 1982, Praegor.

Rotter JB et al. *Incomplete sentences blank*, ed 2, New York, 1992, Psychological Corporation.

Rowe J, Kahn R: *Successful aging: the MacArthur Foundation Study*, New York, 1998, Pantheon Books.

Ryan E, See S: Age-based beliefs about memory changes for self and others across adulthood, *J Gerontol* 48:199, 1993.

Schaie K, Willis S: *Adult development and aging*, Boston, 1991, Little Brown.

Schneider E, Rowe J: *Handbook of the biology of aging*, ed 3, San Diego, 1990, Academic Press.

Schroots J: Gerodynamics: toward a branching theory of aging, *Can J Aging* 14:74, 1995.

Seligman ME, Steen TA: Positive psychology progress—empirical validation of interventions, *Am Psychol* 60:5, 2005.

Shalev A: Posttraumatic stress disorder and stress-related disorders, *Psychiatr Clin North Am* 32:687, 2009.

Shek D: Mid-life crisis in Chinese men and women, *J Psychol* 130:109, 1996.

Speas K, Obenshain B; American Association of Retired Persons: *Images of aging in America: final report*, Chapel Hill, NC, 1995, FGI Integrated Marketing.

Sroufe LA et al: *Child development: its nature and course*, ed 2, New York, 1992, McGraw Hill.

Stevens-Long J: *Adult life: developmental processes*, ed 4, Palo Alto, Calif, 1992, Mayfield.

Sullivan H: *The interpersonal theory of psychiatry*, New York, 1953, WW Norton.

Thompson RA: Early attachment and later developments. In Cassidy J, Shaver PR, editors: *Handbook of attachment: theory, research and clinical applications*, New York and London, 2008, Guilford Press.

U.S. Census Bureau: *Census of population: population projections by race and Hispanic origins for persons 65 and older: 2000 to 2050*

(2008), Washington, DC, 2008, US Department of Commerce, Economics and Statistics Administration.

Vaillant G: *Adaptation to life*, Boston, 1977, Little Brown.

Vaillant G: *Aging well: surprising guideposts to a happier life from the landmark Harvard study of adult development*, New York, 2002, Little Brown.

Valenzano DR et al: Resveratrol prolongs lifespan and retards the onset of age-related markers in a short-lived vertebrate, *Curr Biol* 16:296, 2006.

Van Gennep A: *The rites of passage*, Chicago, 1909, University of Chicago Press.

Wadensten B, Hagglund D: Older people's experience of participating in a reminiscence group with a gerotranscendental perspective: reminiscence group with a gerotranscendental perspective in practice, *Int J Older People Nursing* 1:159, 2006.

Woodruff D: A review of aging and cognitive processes, *Res Aging* 5:139, 1983.

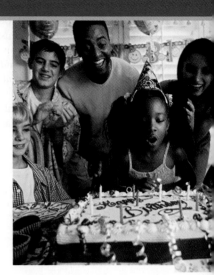

Culture, Ethnicity, and Spirituality

Ruth N. Grendell

"Cultural values give an individual a sense of direction as well as meaning to life."

Josepha Campinha-Bacote

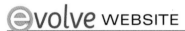

WEBSITE

http://evolve.elsevier.com/Fortinash/

OBJECTIVES

- Differentiate the concepts of culture, race, and ethnicity.
- Discuss characteristics that are common to all cultures.
- Discuss the need for a nurse's self-evaluation to provide competent cultural care to persons from other sociocultural backgrounds.
- Analyze selected socialization issues—acculturation, assimilation, ethnocentrism, and xenophobia—as they relate to cultural heritage, mental health beliefs, and practices.
- Perform a cultural assessment with the use of the Heritage Assessment Tool.

- Formulate potential nursing diagnoses related to a patient's cultural or ethnic orientation.
- Discuss adaptive methods for planning and implementing therapeutic nursing interventions that consider a patient's cultural or ethnic orientation.
- Conduct a self-assessment of your spiritual beliefs.
- Develop a spiritual assessment to use when pastoral care is not available.
- Describe a therapeutic plan of care for a person who is in spiritual distress.

KEY TERMS

acculturation	cultural heritage	ethnocentrism	racism
ageism	culture	faith	religion
assimilation	culture of poverty	health literacy	sexism
cultural awareness	culture shock	heritage consistency	spirituality
cultural competence	ethnicity	heterosexism	xenophobia

THE MANY FACES OF CULTURE

The term *culture* is usually associated with minority and ethnic groups. It is the defining boundary that makes one culture different from another. However, *culture* is a multifaceted term that can refer to many groups such as gender, age, socioeconomic status, membership in social or sport groups or in organizational environments, employment status, mental or physical disability, political affiliation, and education level. Culture consists of the values, beliefs, and behaviors of the members of a social group, and it must be

viewed as more than the sum of its parts; however, those parts are interrelated and interdependent (Catalano, 2009; Giger and Davidhizar, 2007).

Culture, then, is an integral part of all lived experiences. An individual can belong to more than one cultural group at any given time. Therefore, a stereotypic view is not a valid perspective, because each person brings uniqueness to every interaction. Until individuals view the world through the lenses of persons of another culture, they cannot understand how prejudgments and fears affect their perceptions and interactions. The following discussion addresses many of these diverse cultural issues as they relate to holistic and culturally competent nursing interventions and health care.

Cultural Heritage

The integrated pattern of human behavior of members of a racial, religious, or social group that is passed on to future generations results in the development of a **cultural heritage**. The cultural background is a core component of **ethnicity**, which is a race or group of people who have common traits and customs. An example of an ethnicity is the more than 200 Native American groups. These groups share many common cultural values, but they have different life patterns. The groups have their individual languages, traditions, values, and symbols. Each group belongs to the Native American culture, but each subculture perceives itself as distinct. Ethnic pride sometimes leads to conflict among subcultures (Spector, 2008). **Heritage consistency** is how closely a person's lifestyle matches or reflects the typical lifestyle of one's own culture. Common themes and roles that all cultures address include the family, marriage, parenting roles, education, health, work, and methods of education. A major component of heritage consistency is a cultural, ethnic, or national religion or a belief in a divine or superhuman power or powers. **Religion** consists of a system of beliefs, practices, and ethical values (Spector, 2008). Many cultures view physical and mental illnesses as spiritual problems or as punishment for behaviors that oppose the religious codes and morals of the cultural group. Some cultures believe that traditional healers, rituals, talismans, and folk medicines and practices will restore health.

Individuals also express their cultural heritage through language; works of art, music, and dance; ethnic clothing; customs and traditions; holiday celebrations; diet; and expressions of spirituality. Culture includes behavioral responses and decisions regarding significant life experiences such as birth, right-of-passage ceremonies, illness, pain, death, and mourning. Culture is a learned process or socialization that begins at birth and continues throughout the person's life span. Individuals rarely consider the influence of culture unless they purposely study their own culturally determined behavior (Clark, 2008). In other words, cultural values are powerful forces that affect all aspects of a person's life, both consciously and unconsciously.

An illustration of strong cultural heritage is Mardi Gras, which is an important celebration for residents of New Orleans, Louisiana. Despite the tragedies caused by Hurricane Katrina in August 2005, the people of New Orleans decided that they had to demonstrate their spirit of survival and to celebrate this special event. Displaced residents returned to share in the celebration. Many of those who remained struggle with posttraumatic stress disorder, the exacerbation of mental and physical illnesses, unemployment, and loss of housing; they are waiting for assistance with cleaning up the debris. Although many worry that coming hurricane seasons may bring more disaster, the Mardi Gras celebration is a treasured tradition, and the population of New Orleans believes that it is important for instilling hope for the future.

CHANGING TRENDS

Since the mid-1960s, there has been a massive migration of immigrants and refugees from many countries into the United States, Canada, Britain, and several European nations; these individuals are seeking political and religious freedom and economic opportunities. The melting pot theory—a common belief that **acculturation**, which is the acceptance of the values and traditions of the host country that takes place as immigrants adjust to their new environment—is no longer true. Acculturation is sometimes referred to as *assimilation*, which is the gradual process of developing a new cultural identity. The process is complete when the individual becomes fully merged into the dominant cultural group.

Examples of cultural assimilation include developing the ability to speak fluently in the host country's language, assuming a new name, and moving to a nonethnic neighborhood. Marital assimilation occurs through the intermarriage of members of different cultures, thus forming a new subculture. Structural assimilation occurs primarily through social interactions and the development of friendships between different cultural groups; this includes engaging in personal and social activities in impersonal settings such as church, school, and the workplace (Spector, 2008).

Many immigrants experience **culture shock**—a sudden or violent disturbance of emotions that involves a sense of anxiety, fear, and distrust—when confronted with different standards of living, opposing worldviews, and societal expectations. They have difficulty abandoning their cultural traditions to take on a strange new way of life. They prefer to live in their own communities for social support and to maintain their cultural heritage. Children and young adults usually adapt to their new surroundings more quickly, although they are subject to the traditions of the older family members. It takes approximately three generations or longer for members of a minority group to integrate into the dominant culture environment (Catalano, 2009).

The transition from a society with one dominant culture to a multicultural society has resulted in many challenges with regard to meeting the needs of all of the people. The particular disparities for minority and ethnic groups from other cultures are access to the host nation's health care services and the receiving of culturally competent health care. The U.S. Office for Minority Health issued national standards in 2000 for appropriate cultural and linguistic services. Another major barrier for minority and ethnic groups is their lack of **health literacy**, which is the ability to understand basic health information and the services available to assist them with the making of appropriate health decisions. The Office for Minority Health has assisted health organizations with implementing interpretation and translation services, health and illness prevention education materials, and diagnostic screening information, and it has provided technical assistance to support the organizations with developing policies and educating health care providers (Graham, 2008).

Several nursing education programs have integrated narrative pedagogy (i.e., a way of teaching) into the curriculum as a framework for designing innovative strategies for patient-centered care. Storytelling—whether through oral or written words, media presentations, or the fine arts—has proven to be a very effective method for providing opportunities for a personal relationship between the reader/observer and the characters in the story. Individuals can "see" the world from another's point of view and reflect on the influence of their own personal beliefs and values. The act of reflecting on the meaning of the story's content and how to apply it is an essential ongoing part of the process (Giger and Davidhizar, 2007; Halloran, 2009; Haviland et al, 2009).

Stories such as *The Spirit Catches You and You Fall Down* by Anne Fadiman (1997) is required reading in many colleges and universities across the United States to introduce students and faculty to concepts related to cultural awareness. It is a fascinating true account of conflicts and misunderstandings between cultures. The story describes how a Hmong refugee family from Laos interacted with the culture of the Western (allopathic) health care system during the treatment of Lia, a young child who had been diagnosed with epilepsy. Lia's parents believed that she was ill because she lost one of her three souls and that soul had been replaced by a spirit. They described her seizures as "the spirit catches you and you fall down." Their beliefs and the beliefs of the Western health care providers clashed during every interaction, which led to disastrous results and, eventually, to Lia's death. Many other stories have been used for these same purposes, including *Three Cups of Tea* by Greg Mortensen and David Relin (2009), which is a story about life in Pakistan, and *When I was Puerto Rican* by Esmeralda Santiago (2006), which describes an escape from the effects of poverty. Other examples of narratives to consider include living with a chronic illness or a life-threatening disease, surviving an abusive relationship, and adjusting to life transitions.

Subcultures

There are subcultures within each major culture. Subcultures develop when members of the group develop new values that they honor more than the values of their dominant culture (Catalano, 2009). Although these groups accept many of the traditional values of the main culture, they modify or abandon some values because of influences within or outside of the different subculture groups. Sometimes individuals actually belong to several subcultures related to age, gender, occupation, socioeconomic status, geographic location, family style, alternative lifestyle, and ethnicity. Teenagers, young adults, and older adults are representatives of subcultures. Some individuals also belong to several subsets within a subculture. For example, some students in a high school belong to clubs (e.g., sports, music, drama), use a special language (e.g., slang), wear a particular clothing style, develop specific habits and lifestyles, or have friendships and values that differ from those of the other subset groups. These

TABLE 8-1	CURRENT U.S. GENERATION SUBCULTURES	
GENERATION	**BIRTH YEARS**
G.I., World War I, or Greatest Generation	1900–1924
Silent Generation (includes Korean War veterans)	1925–1945
Baby Boomers	1946–1964
Baby Busters	1958–1968
Generation X	1965–1981
Generation Y	1984–2004
Generation Z (the Millennials)	2005–2025

differences sometimes lead to intrapersonal and interpersonal conflicts.

Many studies have been published regarding generation gaps among the age groups within a culture, particularly in the Western world. Each generation has its separate group awareness, a particular lifestyle, and a belief system and worldview that define its social norms. Each generation has a particular impact on society and its own mental and physical health problems. Table 8-1 outlines the current generations in the United States. Consider how the social and physical environments, the advances in science and technology, and the specific mental and physical health care needs have influenced each generation. Members of the G.I. Generation are currently the old and frail elderly, and 95% of the members of the Silent Generation have entered retirement. The eldest members of the Baby Boomer Generation are entering senior age status.

A subculture that is important to include in this discussion is the culture of poverty. The term *poverty* refers to not being able to obtain what is necessary to adequately live in a particular cultural context (Cutheral et al, 2010; Rogalsky, 2009) (Figure 8-1).

The concept of a culture of poverty was developed during the 1950s on the basis of the belief that the poor remain poor because their lives and behaviors were determined by shared expectations and negative attitudes—hopelessness, dependency, powerlessness, and being convinced that their fate was to remain poor—that were transmitted from one generation to the next. However, although this perspective is still popular today, it does not fully explain many of the factors that are involved or contribute to strategies that could assist with eliminating the many barriers that maintain the poverty culture. Concerted efforts to inform educators, the public, and officials and to procure funds for programs to meet the needs of children, parents, and others living in poverty have demonstrated effectiveness in some urban areas (Rogalsky, 2009).

Poverty has become a global social and economic burden because of the increased numbers of people entering and remaining in poverty during the past several decades. The characteristics, special needs, and issues related to living in poverty are diverse and complex. The affected groups include

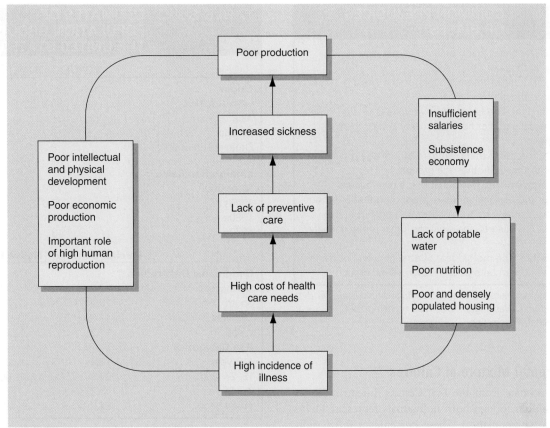

FIGURE 8-1. The cycle of poverty. (From Spector RE: *Cultural diversity in health and illness,* ed 6, Upper Saddle River, NJ, 2004, Pearson.)

several subsets of individuals with mental illnesses, teenage runaways, families, the poor elderly, individuals who are addicted to drugs or alcohol, and those who suffer from posttraumatic stress disorders, such as war veterans, refugees, and legal or illegal immigrants.

A subset in the culture of poverty is the *working poor,* which is made up of people who receive the minimum wage and exist on housing and food allowances through public assistance or pensions. The working poor group also includes people who receive survivor benefits, persons with mental or physical disabilities, children of incarcerated parents, and single-parent families and large families with children younger than 18 years of age (U.S. Department of Health and Human Services, 2006).

An estimated 1.7 million American youth are homeless as an alternative to living in dangerous home situations, or they may be runaways from foster care or homeless due to gender issues. An 18-month study of youth between the ages of 16 and 21 years revealed that many of these youth distrust adults. They seek remote or abandoned buildings as living places. They often shy away from health care and social services that could be of help to them; however, their lifestyles are detrimental to their biopsychosocial health. They frequently form new "families" among themselves for protection, and they create their own languages, symbols, and rules; many belong to Wicca, which is an ancient Celtic pagan religion that is

mixed with aspects of the New Age philosophy. Their primary survival methods include drug dealing for money or to supply their own needs, panhandling, and prostitution (O'Sullivan-Oliveira and Burke, 2009).

All of these individuals experience discrimination and live under the stigma that is associated with poverty. Many live for the moment and cannot plan for the future. Access to health care is minimal, and it is most often received for emergency circumstances. These people are frequently unable to see the importance of prescribed therapy, or they are unable to self-manage the treatment requirements.

Cultural Diversity

Different characteristics of cultures are either primary characteristics or secondary characteristics. Examples of primary characteristics are nationality, race, color, gender, age, and religious beliefs. Secondary characteristics are socioeconomic status, occupation, education, gender issues, geographic place of residence, length of time absent from the country of origin, and sexual orientation. The secondary characteristics sometimes have a more powerful effect on an individual's cultural identity, although these characteristics are sometimes more difficult to identify than the primary characteristics. Nurses avoid generalization or stereotyping on the basis of minimal information about the individual or the culture (Box 8-1).

BOX 8-1	COMMON PREJUDICES OR BIASES

- **Racism.** The belief that members of one race are superior to those of other races.
- **Sexism.** The belief that members of one sex are superior to those of the other sex.
- **Heterosexism.** The belief that everyone is or should be heterosexual and that heterosexuality is best, normal, and superior.
- **Ageism.** The belief that members of one age group are superior to those of other age groups.
- **Ethnocentrism.** The belief that one's own cultural, ethnic, or professional group is superior to that of others. One judges others by his or her own yardstick and is unable or unwilling to see what the other group is really about.
- **Xenophobia.** The morbid fear of strangers and of those who are not members of one's own ethnic group.

From the American Nurses Association: *Multicultural issues in the nursing workforce,* Washington, DC, 1993 (updated 2006), American Nurses Association.

Environmental Mixture of Cultures

A current estimate from the U.S. Census Bureau indicates that 33.5 million foreign-born individuals represent 11.7% of the nation's population. These percentages are rapidly changing because of the increase in the number of immigrants each year (Table 8-2). The foreign-born category includes naturalized citizens, lawful permanent residents (immigrants), temporary migrants (foreign students), refugees (humanitarian migrants), and people who are living in the United States illegally. Persons born in the United States and its islands such as Puerto Rico or persons born abroad to American parents are considered to be "native born." Many immigrants obtain U.S. citizenship after the 5-year residency requirement; however, fewer foreign-born persons under the age of 25 years have graduated from high school. They usually marry at an early age and have larger families than the comparative native-born group. Approximately 16.6% live below the poverty level as compared with 11.5% of native-born individuals. Many of the children of immigrant parents who are younger than 18 years old were born in the United States (U.S. Census Bureau, 2003).

The U.S. population reached the 300 million mark in 2006. Most of this growth is the result of natural causes (i.e., more births than deaths). However, 42% of the current population increase is a result of the arrival of immigrants. Many of the immigrants are young and in their prime childbearing years (Kim, 2006). Approximately 18% (47 million) of the nation's population speaks a language other than English in the home (U.S. Census Bureau, 2003). Consider the contributions and challenges that these facts bring.

Western Health Care System as Culture

At the beginning of this chapter, the Western (allopathic) health care system was referred to as a culture. Consider how

TABLE 8-2	ESTIMATES OF POPULATION GROUPS IN THE UNITED STATES: 2003

	POPULATION (%)*	
Origin		
Latin America	53.3	
Asia	25	
Europe	13.7	
Other world regions	8	
Immigration Rates		
Since 2000	13.6	
1990s	36.6	
1980s	24	
1970s	13	
	Foreign Born (%)	**Native Born (%)**
Geographic Distribution		
Northeast	22.2	18.5
South	29.2	36.5
Midwest	11.3	24.1
West†	37.3	21
Age Categories		
<18 years	8.9	27.8
18–24 years	80.1	60
25–44 years	45.1	21
45–64 years	24.7	23.5

From the U.S. Census Bureau: *Current population survey, 2003 annual social and economic supplement.* In Larsen LJ: *The foreign-born population in the United States 2003,* Current Population Reports, P20-551, Washington, DC, 2004, U.S. Census Bureau.
*33.5 million foreign-born individuals (11.7% of the total U.S. population).
†52.7% of immigrants from Central America reside in the West.

the defining characteristics apply. Health care providers in this system are socialized into their various specialty areas through education, internalized beliefs and values, traditions, clothing, habits, standards, and language, all of which are transmitted to them by the previous generation. Scientific evidence is the primary acceptable method for establishing truth and gaining new knowledge. Members believe that the Western system of health care delivery is superior to any other method. They are privileged to know specific items of information related to health and illness, and they perceive themselves as the experts when it comes to stating what health care should be (Phillippe, 2009).

The beliefs of the Western health care system consist of standard definitions of health and illness, the necessity for routine physical examinations and diagnostic procedures, compliance with prescribed treatment regimens, and the advantages of technology. The known causes of disease are bacteria, viruses, chemical carcinogens, environmental pollutants, and lifestyles, among other factors. For centuries, allopathic medicine followed a philosophy of dualism (i.e., the separation of the body from the mind and spirit), and therefore treatment was directed primarily toward physiologic issues. Health care providers viewed pain as a cultural phenomenon, and responses to pain varied according to the person's cultural background. Health care providers stereotyped individuals from different cultures according to their emotional and behavioral pain responses. We are currently aware that pain is simply what the person says it is and that it exists when the affected person says it does (McCaffrey and Pasero, 2004; McGinnis, 2009). Pain, along with its physiologic and emotional effects, is currently considered as the fifth vital sign to be included in the routine patient assessment.

The public's increased interest in and use of alternative therapies challenges the Western health care culture. Immigrants from all of the other cultures present in the United States have introduced their own traditional methods, and many patients, fearing criticism, do not share with their health care providers information about any of these methods that they may be employing. Until recently, many health care providers have not inquired about the patient's self-care practices, or they were unaware of the many types of alternative therapy that patients use. Within the past several years, health care providers have become more aware of alternative therapies, and they have included some in the plan of care as complementary measures. Some of these include biofeedback and meditation. Most of the alternative and complementary therapies from China and other Eastern countries are now widely accepted.

Cultural Awareness

Cultural awareness is the initial step toward effective interaction among individuals from different cultures. This awareness develops through an understanding and valuing of all aspects of another person's culture. It also involves an awareness of one's own culture, including the overt and covert prejudices and biases that it may harbor toward other cultures (Smith-Miller et al, 2010; Erickson and al-Timimi, 2001).

Various self-assessment tools are available. These tools encourage listening to comments from individuals from a different culture and reflecting on how your culture affects these individuals. Such comments also help you to recognize behaviors that may offend people from other cultures. Examples of items on an assessment tool include reflecting on one's personal prejudices and biases, one's ability to think in and speak a second language, the degree of knowledge that one has about the history and traditions of different cultures, one's personal interest in understanding more about other cultures, and whether one has had any meaningful interactions with people of other cultures (Giger and Davidhizar, 2007).

The self-assessment tool in Box 8-2 allows for the calculation of points from the responses that indicate a high, average, or low degree of cultural awareness. Several resources and classes are available to help individuals to develop cultural awareness. Not all self-assessment tools are accurate. However, these tools help people to gain insight and understanding of the important factors in the development of cultural awareness. It is important to realize that cultural values are neither right nor wrong. Many groups established certain values for survival purposes, but, in another culture's view, these values may be harmful (Catalano, 2009). This is especially true when dealing with health care issues.

Culturally Competent Health Care

Cultural competence requires respect for diversity and an understanding of the attitudes, beliefs, behaviors, practices, and communication patterns of multiple cultures and their languages (Medrano et al, 2005). Culturally competent health care requires the development of interpersonal skills, communication skills, and awareness and sensitivity to the uniqueness of individuals. It is also an ongoing process, because each new encounter presents the opportunity to gain additional knowledge and skills. Establishing trust is an important aspect of the development of an effective relationship between the patient and the care provider. Nurses need to use a gradual approach to complete an accurate assessment that includes initially asking general questions to ease the patient's anxiety and to demonstrate interest in the patient as an individual before that patient will reveal personal information.

Transcultural Communication

Effective communication is necessary for culturally competent care. Clear and effective communication is important in any exchange between individuals, and it is especially important when there are cultural and language differences. Learning to listen is fundamental to the communication process, which is extremely complex and involves multiple verbal and nonverbal components. The nurse and other health care providers need to be aware of the meaning of gestures, body positions, facial expressions, eye movements, and the tone of voice during all communication with individuals from various cultures (Catalano, 2009). Sometimes health care professionals speak authoritatively and use too many medical terms, which is a practice that does not contribute to a patient's health literacy.

Some groups, including Native Americans, use a soft tone of voice. Members of Arab groups sometimes use dramatic emotional communication styles that seem hostile. Other groups, such as Asian and Pacific Islanders, nod their heads and smile to show respect, but health care providers from other cultures often interpret these behaviors as understanding and agreement when in fact they represent neither.

High-Context and Low-Context Cultures. One set of factors that dramatically influences communication and understanding between people of different cultures is the values of each culture regarding the decision-making process. A model that is taken from anthropology, sociology, and psychology defines behaviors and communication styles of cultural societies as low context (individualistic) or high context (collectivistic). The model suggests that an individualistic or low-context society is one in which people care for themselves and their immediate families. Low-context societies emphasize thinking and values that are centered on

BOX 8-2   SELF-ASSESSMENT OF CULTURAL AWARENESS

I understand that the term *culture* implies an integrated pattern of human thoughts, communication methods, actions, customs, beliefs, values, and institutions of a racial, ethnic, religious, or social group. I also understand that the term *competence* implies a capacity to function effectively. Therefore, within this perspective, I will use this self-assessment tool to determine my ability to provide culturally competent care to individuals who belong to various cultural groups.

Responses: A = strongly agree, B = agree, C = disagree, D = I don't know

_____ 1 I acknowledge cultural differences and similarities that exist, and I refuse to label one culture superior or inferior to another.

_____ 2 I understand that the therapeutic relationship is based on respect for the patient and adherence to acceptable social and cultural communication patterns.

_____ 3 I understand the features of a culture to take into consideration when planning and implementing culturally competent care.

_____ 4 I am aware that I have subconscious biases and prejudices that affect my ability to adequately assess the needs of individuals from other cultures.

_____ 5 I always try to determine the norms for nonverbal communication within a culture and family that affect my interactions with people from that culture or family.

_____ 6 I use various resources to determine the diseases and disorders that are endemic (common) to a culture.

_____ 7 I respect the uniqueness of individuals from different cultures and avoid stereotyping.

_____ 8 I look for educational information that reflects different cultures.

When interacting with individuals and families who have limited English proficiency, I always keep the following in mind:

_____ 9 A person's limitation for communicating in English is not a reflection of intelligence.

_____10 I am willing to work with the individual, the family, and others to find effective methods of communication.

_____11 During an interview, I ask about the individual's beliefs and practices.

_____12 I inquire about the individual's and his or her culture's customs and beliefs related to major life events.

_____13 I provide written instructions and alternative illustrations as often as possible to accompany any verbal communication, and I make sure that the patient understands the content.

_____14 I am comfortable working with an interpreter, and I take time to clarify the content that the interpreter presents to the patient.

_____15 I am aware of the resources that are available to me at my institution and on the Internet that will assist me with developing educational materials for patients from different cultures.

_____16 I inquire about family colloquialisms (i.e., dialects and expressions) that affect communication.

_____17 I am able to intervene when I observe others being insensitive toward patients from different cultures.

_____18 I avoid imposing my values on people from different cultures.

_____19 I accept and am considerate of the fact that male and female roles vary significantly among different cultural and ethnic groups and that the patient may be reluctant to discuss certain matters or to receive care provided by me.

_____20 I accept that religion and other beliefs influence how individuals and families respond to illness, disease, and death.

_____21 I stay informed of the major health concerns and issues for ethnically and racially diverse patient populations that reside in my local area.

_____22 I have taken professional development and training courses to enhance my knowledge and skills in the provision of service and support to culturally, ethnically, racially, and linguistically diverse groups.

_____23 I am actively involved in developing educational materials that account for average literacy and that are culturally appropriate for individuals and families who receive care at my facility.

Modified from Giger J, Davidhizar R: *Transcultural nursing*, ed 4, St. Louis, 2007, Mosby.

the individual: autonomy, individual initiative, the right to privacy, emotional independence, and universalism (i.e., arriving at rules of conduct that are applied to everyone). Although there are wide variations among persons in any culture, these qualities are generally characteristic of persons who function in a democratic environment in which most members of the society have a legal voice and advocate for themselves. These cultures emphasize individual thinking and an analytic style of approaching a situation without considering the context or social situation in which the individual is acting. In general, this kind of thinking is typically American, and it is also found in other Western cultures.

Successful communication in this type of culture includes being assertive (including making direct eye contact), advocating for oneself, thinking through problems independently, and arguing for a point of view. It is typical for Americans to use this style of interaction as a standard. However, the rest of the world does not always function with these understandings.

By contrast, a high-context society is one in which people are included in strong groups throughout their lifetimes. These individuals stress a "we" consciousness, a collective identity, group solidarity, sharing, group decision making, collective duties and obligations, emotional dependence, and particularism (i.e., arriving at rules of conduct that are applied to persons depending on their particular role in society) (Ito, 2005; Autgis and Raneer, 2004; Giger and Davidhizar, 2007).

Several high-context cultural cues are present and noticeable to the observer. For example, those from a high-context culture tend to use communication that is more global and that is based on standards that are external to the person, such as social position. Successful communication in this culture depends on the physical context and the cultural information that has been internalized by the communicators. More of the message comes from nonverbal symbolization and cultural roles in the society.

Many Asian and some South American, French, Hispanic, African-American, and Native American cultures share high-context culture characteristics. This cultural environment supports the development of persons who base their decisions on group input. Sometimes people from these cultures do not want to argue in public; they use indirect language to communicate, and they are also hesitant to make direct eye contact. Roles of women and men in some cultures determine their appropriate interaction with professional persons or those outside of the family (Harris, 2003).

The globalization effects created by social, political, educational, and economic interchanges have resulted in an increased acceptance of the values held by Westernized low-context cultures by some of the high-context societies. Remember, however, that wide individual variations exist within any culture, and knowing that a patient is from a particular culture is just a starting point.

Guidelines for Communicating with Non–English-Speaking Patients. Consider the following when interacting with patients (Box 8-3):

Personal Space. Personal space or territory is an important consideration when interacting with individuals from various cultures. The space may be perceived as being violated when the distance between two individuals is too close or too far. In some cultures (e.g., Jewish, Arab, Turkish, Middle Eastern), people are comfortable with standing close together when speaking to each other. These individuals may interpret an American health care provider as being cold and distant (Catalano, 2009).

Touch. Touch also has different cultural meanings, which range from implying a person's power or authority, anger, or sexual arousal to expressing empathy and friendliness. Some consider touching inappropriate, and it is sometimes a cause of miscommunication. In some Arab cultures, men and women do not display affection or touch each other when they are in public. Some Native American cultures interpret eye contact as stealing the soul from the body. Mexican-American and other South American groups believe that eye contact invokes the *mal de ojo*, which translates to "the evil eye." In some cultures, individuals embrace and kiss each other on both cheeks when greeting and again when departing. It is important to know the appropriate methods for greeting people, when touching such as a handshake is acceptable, or whether physical contact is forbidden. Some people

---

BOX 8-3 GUIDELINES FOR COMMUNICATING WITH NON–ENGLISH-SPEAKING CLIENTS

- Use interpreters rather than translators. Translators just restate the words from one language in another. An interpreter decodes the words and provides the meaning behind the intended message.
- Use dialect-specific interpreters whenever possible.
- Use interpreters who have been trained in the health care field.
- Give the interpreter time alone with the patient.
- Provide time for translation and interpretation to occur.
- Be aware that interpreters affect the reporting of symptoms, insert their own ideas, or omit information.
- Avoid the use of relatives as interpreters; these individuals sometimes distort information, and they may not be objective.
- Avoid using children as interpreters, especially when dealing with sensitive topics.
- Use same-age and same-gender interpreters whenever possible.
- Maintain eye contact with both the patient and the interpreter to elicit feedback and to read nonverbal cues. (Note: Some cultures interpret constant eye contact as disrespectful or aggressive.)
- Remember that patients usually understand more than they can express; thus, they need time to think in their own language. They are alert to the health care provider's body language, and they sometimes forget some or all of their English during times of stress.
- Speak slowly without exaggerating mouthing, allow time for translation, use the active rather than the passive tense, wait for feedback, and restate the message. Do not rush, and do not speak loudly. Use a reference book with common phrases, such as *Roget's International Thesaurus* or *Taber's Cyclopedic Medical Dictionary*.
- Use as many words as possible in the patient's language, and use nonverbal communication when you and the patient are unable to understand each other's languages.
- If an interpreter is unavailable, the use of a translator is acceptable. Be aware that translation sometimes leaves out parts of the message, distorts the message, and involves the sending of information that is not provided by the speaker. In addition, sometimes the patient will not fully understand the messages.

Modified from: Catalano J: *Nursing now! Today's issues, tomorrow's trends,* ed 2, Philadelphia, 2009, FA Davis; and Giger JN, Davidhizar RE: *Transcultural nursing: assessment & intervention,* ed 2, St. Louis, 2007, Mosby.
Note: Social class differences between the interpreter and the patient sometimes results in the interpreter not reporting information to the health care provider that the interpreter perceives as superstitious or unimportant.

perceive physical contact as inappropriate when a person from a different culture or gender performs a physical examination, takes a pulse, provides personal care, or performs a procedure. It is necessary to explain what is happening and its purpose before performing the physical contact. Some cultures, including some African and Arab groups, require that a hospitalized female patient have a female companion present and be treated only by female health care providers (Catalano, 2009; personal experience).

Time Orientation. Time orientation is also a factor in communication with patients. In some cultures, time is of little importance, and people from these cultures pay little attention to the exact time of an appointment; living in the present is the norm. In Western cultures, people are more future oriented and prefer designing plans, making schedules, and organizing activities. Differences in time orientation interfere with adherence to medication schedules and to the treatment regimen, and this may result in the patient's failure to meet the intended outcomes of long-term health care plans. Some health care providers are frustrated by this discrepancy and avoid talking with such patients. When a breakdown in communication occurs, the patient sometimes feels isolated, distrusts the provider, withdraws or becomes angry, and eventually abandons the health care system.

Biologic Characteristics. The assessment also considers biologic characteristics related to susceptibility to certain diseases, variability of skin and body structures, the metabolism of medications, enzyme deficiencies, and high-risk behaviors such as smoking and substance addiction (Catalano, 2009). The assessment of a person's spiritual beliefs is discussed later in this chapter.

Translation Services. Guidelines for obtaining translation services are important. Communicating an important and often complex health care matter is difficult without the use of the patient's specific language. Nurses often use translation services, so a good interview question before accepting a position in a particular health care facility is whether professional translation services are available. It is important to acquire accurate translation with the use of an educated, credentialed, or certified translator, if possible. Using a family member or an additional hospital staff member is often convenient, but it is not recommended, because the patient may wish to avoid embarrassing the translator or revealing information that is culturally inappropriate.

Many factors affect the accuracy of the translation, so the translator needs to take care to avoid bias. It is a good idea to use standard communication techniques when asking questions through an interpreter, beginning with general information and asking sensitive questions after establishing communication. Some communication patterns in low-context cultures use fewer words and more nonverbal communication. Therefore, it may seem as though the translator is not asking the questions that have been posed by the interviewer. It is important to consider the communication context and the preferences of the patient and the translator. The care team needs to incorporate a plan of adequate translator involvement for the sufficient ongoing assessment of the patient's status. Important cultural considerations also include dietary needs. In addition, reading materials—especially patient education materials—need to be in the patient's language.

SPIRITUALITY

It is often difficult to separate religious and spiritual values from ethnic and cultural beliefs. People often use the terms *religion* and *spirituality* synonymously. However, the nature of spirituality is broad, and it involves the search for answers to questions such as the following:

- Why are we here?
- What am I supposed to be doing with my life?
- How am I to make meaning out of my suffering?
- What really happens to the soul after death?
- Why did this happen to me?
- Why is God punishing me?

Advances in technology, global disasters, wars, threats of nuclear destruction, and the genome mapping project have created additional questions that are often disturbing to the integrity of the self and the meaning of life. Spirituality is (1) an integrative energy that produces inner harmony or wholeness; (2) a sense of coherence; (3) the driving force that permeates all aspects that give meaning to life; and (4) a sense of transcendence over reality that involves living fully in the moment and feeling strengthened through a sense of inner knowledge (Catalano, 2009). Spirituality provides a set of self-determined values that are the basis for living. Hope is a central concept of spirituality, and the faith factor helps to provide coping skills. Religion is a personal set or institutionalized system of shared religious attitudes, beliefs, and practices (Koenig and Cohen, 2006; Koenig, 2004). Faith is the belief and trust in God or a supreme being. It is also the ability to draw on spiritual resources without having physical and empiric proof. It is an internal certainty that comes from one's own experience with the divine. Although faith is only a part of spirituality, it is an essential component. It is through one's experience of faith that a deep individual spirituality assists one with the challenges and celebrations of life. The goals of faith are as follows:

- To provide an image of the divine
- To provide an image of humanity
- To provide an understanding of the relationship between the divine and humanity
- To help with the examination of thoughts of divine punishment, reward, or neutrality
- To help with giving belief and meaning to life
- To help with finding a sense of duty, vocation, calling, or moral obligation
- To help with examining one's experience of the divine and the sacred
- To help with coping with situations and conflict that involve spiritual understanding
- To provide a format for spiritual rituals and practices

- To provide a faith community
- To provide authority and guidance for one's system of belief, meaning, and ritual

Religion usually includes a set of beliefs that help with explaining the meaning of life, suffering, health, and illness. A religious perspective of spirituality views the soul as a means of relating to a supreme being and to others. Some call the supreme being *the divine creator of the universe, God,* or *the divine mystery,* or they may use other similar names. Religious practices nurture the soul. Religion determines the important rituals that are meaningful during transitions in life, the types of foods to eat, the times for fasting, and the services to attend. Examples of rituals that surround the birth process include the baptism of the infant at a specific time, circumcision, postpartum practices for the new mother, and a specific burial site for the placenta. Certain traditional rites of passage into adulthood are honored as well as the rituals that surround death.

Some express spirituality by participating in an organized religious community and by adhering to a set of rules of behavior. Traditional spiritual healing practices include the use of prayer, meditation, fasting, belonging to religious support groups, reading scriptures and religious literature, and listening to inspiring music. One study revealed that 63% of the individuals who responded indicated that they wanted their spiritual needs considered in the plan of care (Myerstein, 2004).

A secular perspective of spirituality is made up of a set of positive values such as love, honesty, truth, and optimism that the person chooses as a standard or purpose to live by. The person renews spirituality through loving relationships; through experiencing the beauty of nature, art, music, poetry, and literature; and through other activities that assist with the fulfilling of life goals. The soul does not need to be a religious concept; rather, it is an image of the person that extends beyond the physical self such (i.e., an energy field or aura) that is characterized by a color and movement. The soul is often considered as a life force; it is referred to as *chi* in the Chinese culture, as *ki* in the Japanese culture, and as *prana* in Indian faith systems. Reiki, shiatsu, and therapeutic touch are practices that renew or balance the energy force. Some believe that the use of herbs, aromatherapy, and other techniques provides a balance between all living things, the earth, and the universe (Catalano, 2009).

Some major spiritual considerations include the fear of death and loss, both of oneself and of others. Spirituality allows one to cope with these feelings by providing a sense of hope and meaning to experiences that would otherwise be crippling. A spiritual understanding that one's connection with creation is more than merely a physical existence helps to ease the fear and pain of loss. Feeling connected to the divine eases feelings of abandonment, grief, and alienation, and it promotes self-acceptance. Spirituality is often a key component in the healing process, and it is an integral part of the patient's treatment plan.

Significant spiritual questions tend to remain constant, regardless of the health care need. Issues such as loss, fear, death, abandonment, and feelings of alienation are sometimes present in patients who have both physical and psychiatric illnesses. Responses to these feelings range from finding new meaning and strength to acceptance, grief, and a sense of hopelessness. An objective in a spiritual intervention is to first acknowledge and validate these feelings and then to help the patient to consider ways to rewrite his or her life story in a way that includes these experiences. One's spirituality can be a significant help during these times.

A spiritual crisis may occur when religious or spiritual beliefs conflict with a necessary procedure or a treatment protocol, such as agreeing to a therapeutic abortion, permitting a blood transfusion, or making end-of-life decisions. Situational spiritual distress is sometimes related to the death or illness of a significant other; to beliefs that the family, peers, or health care providers oppose; or to other separations (e.g., divorce). Spiritual distress also occurs when a person is separated from his or her spiritual or cultural support systems and when personal beliefs and values are challenged. In some cases, spiritual beliefs and practices are harmful to a person's mental and physical health (Myerstein, 2004; Ackley and Ladwig, 2007).

Spiritual Support

Before caregivers provide effective spiritual interventions, it is critical to identify people who are at significant spiritual risk. *Spiritual distress* is a nursing diagnosis that is defined as a disruption in the value and belief system that pervades the person's state of being and that transcends the physical and psychosocial self (Ackley and Ladwig, 2007). Individuals at spiritual risk are those who have a high spiritual need coupled with low spiritual resources to meet that need. These individuals have more risk for poor outcomes, and they are the primary focus for outcome-based spiritual care (Koenig and Cohen, 2006; Koenig, 2004).

The traditional definitions of mental health and illness differ among cultures and individuals. However, many cultural beliefs do not separate illnesses of the body from illnesses of the mind. Ancient beliefs attributed illnesses of the body or mind to the work of evil spirits outside of the body (e.g., witchcraft, voodoo curses) or to evil spirits that entered the body or mind. Some societies believed that evil was caused by someone within the community who was different. It was believed that, if that person was punished or removed from the community, then a cure could be found. Special healers used their skills to remove the power of the spirits. Healing methods included the use of purgatives, bloodletting, the application of leeches, and herbal mixtures, among others. Sometimes groups have said special prayers and incantations and made sacrifices on the ill person's behalf. Modern societies consider these practices to be primitive. However, some people consider these traditions sacred and continue to use them. Today, some religious faiths promote praying to saints, lighting candles, making pilgrimages to shrines, and anointing with oil. Faith healers and practitioners of therapeutic touch often perform the "laying on of hands" as a healing practice.

Culturally competent care includes providing spiritual support and pastoral counseling to patients in the psychiatric setting. The provision of these services and assurance of access for all patients is a standard set forth by credentialing organizations. In general, one of the pastoral services offered by institutions or within communities is to contact appropriate representatives of the patient's faith tradition. Having these services available is often of great comfort to the mentally ill. Certified pastoral counselors are skilled at communicating with mentally ill persons. The nurse's role is to find out if patients wish to make use of these persons by visitation, prayer, or other faith tradition. Part of the typical psychiatric intake assessment includes determining whether there are any spiritual or religious concerns. Usually the nurse will contact a representative of the patient's faith tradition to meet with the patient or the health care team to discuss the patient's preferences and concerns and to make plans to meet the individual's needs.

Visits from a religious practitioner often comfort patients with depression or who are in crisis. Frequently, representatives of faith traditions such as elders, rabbis, priests, ministers, imams, and other spiritual leaders come to psychiatric units to visit people from their communities. Occasionally, individuals with serious mental disorders experience delusions that are spiritual or religious in nature. As is explained in Chapters 12 and 13, challenging or debating the truth of a person's delusions is not therapeutic, and spiritual delusions are no exception. The nurse does not agree with the patient's delusions but rather avoids arguing or debating the specifics of a delusion and focuses on decreasing the person's anxiety or agitation.

Nurses need to be consciously aware of their own personal beliefs or lack of beliefs about spirituality and religion and not impose them on patients. Nurses remain neutral and unbiased. For example, advising the patient that a particular spiritual practice will cure a mental illness is inappropriate, even if the nurse believes this to be true. Engaging in spiritual or religious practice with individuals on a psychiatric unit is also inappropriate. The nurse elicits information about what is causing the person distress without discussing specific spiritual or religious content. Certified pastoral counselors are skilled with regard to counseling patients and consulting with staff about these problems, and they assist the health care team in ways that address the particular concerns of individual patients. Many times, an individual will make a decision that is difficult for the health care provider to accept. In some settings, the certified pastoral counselor will meet with the staff to assist them with understanding and accepting what they believe to be controversial decisions made by the patients and their families (Catalano, 2009).

Intervention Tools

There are a variety of spiritual interventions for use that range from formal to informal rituals and practices. For example, formal Christian rituals include sacraments such as baptism, communion, and anointing. Additional formal practices include worship and memorial services as well as formal confession and absolution. On many of these occasions, a chaplain involves members of a local faith community, either in a leadership role or a support role. Often the agency chaplain is in contact with local worship communities to provide appropriate information for formal prayer services at a local church or synagogue when requested by a patient.

Informal rituals and practices include pastoral counseling; the use of individual or group prayer at the hospital; the reading of scripture; and the distribution of devotional books, cards, and other related materials. The use of rosaries or prayer beads, the playing of music, and the use of icons or pictures often allow patients to express the more experiential, noncognitive side of their spirituality. Some individuals use visual imagery, such as in the telling of sacred stories from various traditions. Access to audiotapes and videotapes of the patient's own religious community worship services or activities can be especially helpful.

Religious practices are often beneficial for patients, but, for those who do not have a formal religion, other spiritual interventions are useful. Group therapies that encourage patients to extend themselves and to find meaning in life are helpful. In addition, several other creative forms of expression such as art, music, and dance therapy often address patients' spiritual needs.

Spiritual Assessment

Assessing an individual's spiritual needs and determining interventions that will be helpful and appropriate for addressing those needs are essential components of the chaplain's role in a health care system. Discovering the patient's perception of his or her spirituality requires the ability of the chaplain to acknowledge his or her own biases and a willingness to put them aside during the interaction.

A pastor or chaplain usually addresses spirituality. If there is no pastoral care department in the facility and if the patient has no specific faith community, then these spiritual issues may not be addressed. Even when the patient has a faith community, he or she may be reluctant to examine areas of spirituality that deal with mental illness. Therefore, nursing interventions that address spirituality are important. The core factors that underlie spiritual assessment are belief and meaning. An individual views life in terms of what he or she perceives to be important and to give meaning to life. Some areas that the interviewer will consider are as follows:

- What beliefs does the person have that give meaning and purpose to life?
- What are the important symbols that reflect these beliefs?
- How does the person's life story reflect or demonstrate these underlying themes?
- Do any areas of the person's life story come into conflict with these underlying foundational beliefs?

- Do any current situations or problems come into direct conflict with these beliefs?
- Is the person able to consciously communicate these beliefs?
- In what ways are these beliefs an unconscious part of the person's worldview?

The assessment tool is brief, patient centered, and focused on specific information. Religious experts or facility ethics committee will approve the content before use.. The question to pose to the patient is, "How do you wish us to address these issues in your health care?" (LaRocca-Pitts, 2008)

Vocation and Obligation

Out of one's perception of belief and meaning comes a sense of how to live life. The following axis is closely linked to the one that was presented earlier, and demonstrates that people usually do what they consider to be important. If a task, action, or thought has no meaning, then the person is much less likely to perform that action or to follow through on thoughts about that task. When life circumstances place the person in a position in which actions come into conflict with core beliefs and meaning systems, crisis and significant stress may result. The following questions are included in this axis:

- What sense of duty, vocation, calling, or moral obligation does this person have?
- How actively has this patient been able to express these in the past?
- What impact does the patient's current situation or illness have on these perceptions?

Experience

The interviewer examines both hopeful and worrisome questions that surround the emotional experiences of a person of faith. Questions to examine in this axis include the following:

- What experience of the divine or sacred has this person had?
- What emotions or moods are associated with these contacts?
- How does the patient's current situation relate to these experiences?

Courage and Growth

This axis examines how the person adapts to situations that confront and conflict with the patient's core beliefs and meanings. Questions in this axis examine how a patient may deal with extremely stressful and challenging issues and include the following:

- How spiritually adaptable is the patient?
- How has the patient coped in the past with situations that were in conflict with his or her current spiritual understanding?
- Must new experiences fit into existing belief systems, or can the person's beliefs adapt with new experiences?
- How concrete is the person's spirituality?
- How adaptable is the person currently?

Ritual and Practice

- What are the spiritual rituals and practices of this individual?
- Are they formal or informal?
- Does the individual experience them on a regular basis?
- How do they support the individual?
- How do the patient's current circumstances affect these rituals?

Community

- *Family of origin.* How did the patient's family of origin share spiritual experiences?
- *Current family structure.* How does the patient's current family share spiritual experiences? How does the patient view participation in a faith community?
- *Faith community of origin.* How formal was the patient's faith community of origin? How informal? How active or inactive was the patient?
- *Current faith community.* How formal is the patient's current faith community? How informal? How active or inactive is the patient?

Authority and Guidance

- What is the source of this patient's system of belief, meaning, and ritual?
- When faced with problems, tragedy, or doubt, where does the patient look for guidance?
- Does the patient look for answers from internal or external sources?
- Is this source fixed, or is it flexible? (Fitchett, 2002)

Stages of Faith

A key concept for understanding spiritual development is that a person's faith tends to become internalized as one develops. During development, one's sense of faith, meaning, moral values, and judgment moves from an external locus of control to an internal locus of control. When determining how best to assist a patient with using his or her spirituality to address mental illness, it is essential to determine the patient's stage of spiritual development. This is important for determining what interventions, if any, are appropriate. Several significant models of both faith development and moral and spiritual development will help to inform a chaplain regarding the patient's spiritual needs.

The first model is James Fowler's (1981) stages of religious development theory (Box 8-4). In this theory, Fowler states that an individual passes through various stages in a linear fashion on the basis of age. This theory is much like many of the other individual development theories.

Stages of Moral Development

A second important model that helps with the assessment of a patient's spirituality and how illness or the current situation has challenged the patient's spirituality is Kohlberg's six stages of moral development theory. Kohlberg theorized that individuals move in a linear fashion with age through key areas

BOX 8-4	FOWLER'S STAGES OF RELIGIOUS DEVELOPMENT

Stage 1: Intuitive-Projective Faith
A developmental stage that begins during early childhood
Intuitive images of good and evil
Fantasy and reality are the same

Stage 2: Mythical-Lyrical Faith
A developmental stage that can begin during middle to late childhood
More logical and involves concrete thought
Literal interpretation of religious stories
God is like a parent figure

Stage 3: Synthetic-Conventional Faith
A developmental stage that can begin during early adolescence
More abstract thought
Conformity to the religious beliefs of others

Stage 4: Individuating-Reflexive Faith
A developmental stage that can begin during late adolescence or early adulthood
Individuals begin to take full responsibility for their religious beliefs
In-depth exploration of one's values and religious beliefs

Stage 5: Conjunctive Faith
A developmental stage that can begin during middle adulthood
Individuals become more open to paradox and opposing viewpoints
Stems from an awareness of one's finiteness and limitations

Stage 6: Universalizing Faith
A developmental stage that can begin during late adulthood
Individuals transcend belief systems to achieve a sense of oneness with all beings
Conflicting events are no longer viewed as paradoxes

of faith and spiritual reasoning. The theory indicates that individuals all move through one or more of the following stages:

Preconventional	I	Avoids breaking rules to avoid punishment
	II	Bases moral action on satisfying needs
Conventional	I	Pleases others and does what is expected
	II	Maintains order and follows the law
Postconventional	I	Determines moral actions on the basis of individual rights and community standards
	II	Believes in universal ethical principles that can guide actions

On the basis of the work of Kohlberg and Fowler, the following model looks at four areas of spirituality, each of which has implications for effective pastoral interventions.

Impartial Spirituality

- They believe that individuals are amoral.
- They tend to do things that are in their own interest (i.e., "What's in it for me?").
- They are generally individuals who are not involved in faith communities.
- Some have a casual cultural acquaintance with a formal faith community.
- They represent a significant minority of the population.

Institutional Spirituality

- These individuals are regular church attendees.
- They follow institutional rules.
- They do things because they are told to do them.
- They follow a good person/bad person concept.
- They probably make up the largest percentage of the population.

Individual Spirituality

- These individuals are seekers who have left a formal religious community.
- They often challenge the beliefs of formal religious communities.
- They seek new answers or personal answers to questions, problems, or crises.
- They appear on the surface to be in the impartial stage of faith.
- They represent a smaller minority of the population.

Integrated Spirituality

- These individuals have internalized their faith.
- These people obey rules because they fully accept them and feel that they are just and right.
- They may or may not belong to formal faith communities.
- They are seen as teachers or mystics.
- They make up a very small percentage of the population.

An accurate assessment of the patient's stage of faith is important, because it helps determine the type of interventions that a nurse will use. As always, these models also have their limitations, and individuals tend to move along a continuum of spirituality and faith rather than being locked into a particular stage. In some instances, a crisis is the initiator of a person's movement in either direction along the continuum. An individual in the first stage might likely be operating out of a "bargaining" position when dealing with a spiritual crisis that questions a core meaning held by the individual. An intervention that helped that individual to become connected with a faith group or perhaps a return to a youthful experience of faith provides some additional spiritual tools that were not otherwise available to the person. It is probably less effective to attempt to use interventions that encourage and support challenges to existing spiritual norms for a person in either the first or second stage; however, it is an effective intervention to use when dealing with an individual in the third stage. For individuals who are in the fourth stage, who are often older adults, the best possible pastoral intervention is in learning from them and accepting their unique spiritual legacy.

Selected Cases of Clinical Spiritual Interventions

Pain

Kathleen, a patient with depression and anxiety, also had a serious case of pancreatitis, which required an inpatient stay of several days. A few weeks after her discharge, she returned to talk. As she talked, she confessed that the experience had made a significant impact on her faith and her spiritual viewpoint. When faced with agonizing pain for the first time in her life, this middle-aged woman confided that the physical agony she felt connected her emotionally for the first time with the concept of "torment and damnation." Although her existing spiritual beliefs helped her to cope with the symptoms of her illnesses, the experience of excruciating pain caused her to question some of the fundamental spiritual principles that had guided her up to that point. Especially challenged during this illness were her understanding of the relationship between the divine and humanity and her concept of ultimate punishment and reward.

Spiritual Torment

Steven, a devout Mormon in his mid-50s, was in spiritual torment. His permanent developmental delay coupled with his bipolar illness had prevented him from marrying. His own understanding of his religious principles, whether or not they were completely accurate according to that faith tradition, led him to believe that he would never "be able to enter heaven." He usually made this statement as part of a tearful, tormented lament. His own strong faith was "punishing" him. An appropriate intervention in this case was to listen to and acknowledge Steven's pain and to help connect him with responsible members of his faith community with whom he could discuss his concerns.

Punishment

Mary, a woman in her mid-50s, was a devout Catholic. She believed that her lifelong bouts of major depression were an appropriate "punishment" for the sexual abuse that she had experienced as a child. She clung to the belief that she was responsible for the abuse and that the attention she received and the enjoyment she felt at the time only confirmed her worthlessness and her lack of capacity to be loved as an adult. In this case, because Mary deeply believed in her denominational faith system, religious authority figures held much more authority for her than either physicians or other health care team members. Mary was introduced to an empathetic priest who was also a trained psychotherapist. The interventions all centered on Mary's own belief system and included helping Mary to see herself as a survivor of abuse rather than as the responsible party. A sacramental ritual particular to her denomination was also included to eliminate Mary's deeply held "need" to be punished.

Voices

Fred, a patient with schizophrenia and a member of a charismatic Protestant group, stated that he had the "gift of wisdom." Fred's schizophrenic symptoms included auditory hallucinations. After further discussion, Fred revealed that, during worship services, it was quite common for him and others to rise and to "speak in tongues." He also revealed that the voices he heard were negative and that they frequently told him to harm himself. In Fred's case, the hospital chaplain provided the interventions. Without challenging the faith experience that Fred described having during worship services, the chaplain was able to help Fred to see a difference between the negative voices that told him to harm himself and any prophetic experience that Fred had within the understanding of his own religious concepts. From this distinction, Fred's reluctance to maintain his antipsychotic medication regimen diminished. This improved medication maintenance gave Fred a better quality of life and fewer hospitalizations.

Guilt

Terry, a woman in her mid-40s with bipolar disorder, felt guilty because of how she behaved during previous manic phases of her illness. These actions included both risky sexual behaviors and irresponsibility with her finances. Terry came from a mainstream liturgical Protestant tradition with a culture that emphasized both personal responsibility and spiritual consequences for one's own actions. Terry believed that she was "condemned" and that there was nothing she could do to change that. During ongoing discussions, the nurse educated Terry about her illness and instructed her regarding how to manage her symptoms more effectively by correctly using and monitoring her medications. Terry was eventually able to view her illness in the same way that she viewed a chronic physical illness such as diabetes, and this decreased her feelings of guilt. To help maintain her medication compliance, Terry also began to incorporate part of her faith tradition in her ongoing care by using the daily prayer rituals of her faith to help her to take her medication.

Hyperreligiosity

Hank, a religiously preoccupied individual with schizoaffective disorder, often lectured others when anyone engaged him in conversation. Any attempt to relate to Hank using the more traditional religious language of his own faith background caused him to begin a long, rambling, confused, and pressured ranting about his "special connection" to God "as a prophet." To engage Hank in spiritual discussions for either assessment or intervention purposes, it was necessary to use language that he did not identify as religious. By engaging Hank in discussions about meaningful areas of spirituality in ordinary language rather than spiritual language, the staff avoided the words that usually triggered

Hank's tangential responses. He then had more meaningful conversations with staff.

SELECTED TRADITIONAL AND CULTURAL MENTAL HEALTH BELIEFS

In some cultures, there is no distinction between physical and mental illness. Symptoms are somaticized by complaints of fatigue, dizziness, weight loss, nausea, headache, chest pain, or insomnia. Some African Americans consider stress as a source of physical problems. Latinos often view the person with mental illness as a victim of circumstances with no responsibility for the illness, such as a blow on the head, a sudden fright, anxiety, or witchcraft. People from some cultures believe alcohol or drug addiction is the result of a moral weakness. Puerto Ricans perceive evil spirits to be the cause of mental illness. Mental illness is a cause of shame for Chinese and Japanese families. In some cultures, people seek help only when psychosomatic symptoms appear.

An overview of the mental health beliefs and practices of different selected cultures follows. This information is not intended to stereotype any group but rather merely to describe the known traditional means that some members or families of a given group use to cope with a mental health problem.

Native American Communities

The traditional beliefs of Native American communities equate health with living in total harmony with nature and possessing the ability to survive under exceedingly difficult circumstances. Evil spirits and witchcraft are sometimes felt to be the causes of illness. The medicine man or woman may chew on the root of jimson weed, which induces a trancelike state and a vision to identify the specific evil cause of the person's illness. In some tribes, the healer builds a sand painting or sprinkles pollen around the sick person and then sits in meditation regarding the possible causes of the illness. The government hospitals on Navajo reservations include a hogan for the medicine man to use when treating patients.

Remedies include purification ceremonies, immersion in water, and the use of sweat lodges, herbal medicines, and special rituals. Singers chant to ease the spirit of the sick person. Purification or cleansing contributes to spiritual renewal and to preparation for meditation (Spector, 2008).

Mental illness includes "ghost sickness," which is a preoccupation with death and with a deceased person that is thought to be the result of witchcraft. Alcohol addiction, suicide, and domestic violence are major mental health problems in this community.

Asian and Pacific Islander Communities

The Asian and Pacific Islander populations are a diverse mixture of people from many cultures who speak multiple languages. In addition, several dialects are often spoken within cultures, thus further limiting communication among the groups. The nations of origin include China, Japan, Hawaii, the Philippines, Vietnam, Asian India, Korea, Samoa,

Guam, and the remaining Asian and Pacific islands. Health is believed to be a state of spiritual and physical well-being that involves harmony with nature and a balance of the forces of yin (i.e., the inner body, viscera, or the front of the body) and yang (i.e., the outer surface or back part of the body). Yin restores life strength, and yang protects the body from outside forces. The person lives in peaceful interaction between the mind and body when the forces are in balance. The universe is indivisible, and each person has a function within it. Health care practices are based on the ancient philosophies of Buddha, Confucius, and Tao; most of these individuals make use of versions of Chinese medicine such as acupuncture, acupressure, massage, moxibustion (the application of heat), cupping, bleeding with the use of leeches, herbal remedies, and consultation with traditional healers (see Chapter 27).

Mental illness creates stigma and shame for the family, and the family often cares for the patient in private. Individuals often seek health care much later during the course of the disease, when they have developed a feeling of hopelessness. Mental illnesses are often identified in somatic terms. Such illnesses include the anger syndrome, which is caused by the suppression of anger, anxiety, paranoia symptoms, compulsive neuroses, depression, and fear that body or its functions will be offensive to others (Spector, 2008).

Black American (African-American) Communities

Members of the black American communities in the United States have their origins in Africa and a cultural heritage that is a mixture of Caribbean, Native American, and northern European cultures. In 2006, there were 40.2 million African Americans in the United States (13.4% of the total population), and approximately one third were reported to be living in poverty (U.S. Census Bureau, 2008).

In this culture, health means that the person is in harmony with nature. The body, mind, and spirit are viewed as one entity. Illness is the result of demons or spirits or of actions made of the person's own accord. The family often has a matriarchal structure, and there are strong, large, extended family networks. There is a continuation of tradition and a strong religious connection within the community. Prayer and the laying on of hands are common methods for treating illness. Many black Americans tend to use traditional medicines and healers to treat physical and mental illnesses when they are knowledgeable in this area and have access to such resources. Diagnostic techniques include the use of biblical phrases and material from folk medicine books, observation, and entering the spirit of the patient. Some black Americans stay away from health clinics because they do not trust the health care system, feel discriminated against, or lack funds.

Individuals who follow the Muslim faith believe that foods affect thoughts and behaviors; therefore, they eat kosher foods to protect themselves from illnesses. Fasting is a part of traditional Muslim celebrations such as Ramadan.

Voodoo is a traditional practice of both white (harmless) magic and black (dangerous) magic. Slaves from the West Indies brought voodoo to the United States during the late

1700s and the early 1800s. Some individuals have integrated the rituals and practices into Christian rituals used by some black communities today. Black people may attribute their illness to a "fix" or a "hex" put on them by a person who is angry with them. Bad voodoo is greatly feared. A voodoo priest or an elderly woman healer sometimes uses herbal remedies to treat mental illnesses.

Hispanic Communities

Members of Hispanic communities include Mexico, Puerto Rico, Cuba, Central and South America, and Spain among their countries of origin. These individuals comprise the fastest-growing group in the United States. The term *Chicano* is used as a universal identifier of all Americans of Mexican descent. These individuals believe that the natural world is not separated from the supernatural world. The traditional definition of health is related to evil spirits or forces that cause mental illness. Folk healers or *curanderos* are well known within their communities for their holistic services, which have roots in Aztec, Spanish, spiritualistic, homeopathic, and scientific elements. The *curandero* may be born with the gift of healing, learn by apprenticeship (especially the use of herbs), or receive a calling to be a healer. The *santeria* or *santero*, which is the folk healer of the Puerto Rican culture, uses storytelling to help people to cope with their daily difficulties.

Religious rituals are common healing practices. The types of practices include making promises, visiting shrines, and offering candles, medals, flowers and prayers to saints. Altars, shrines, and pictures of saints are placed in many homes.

Mental illnesses are thought to be hereditary; others are believed to occur because of a hex, worry, fright, or injury. Emotional illnesses are believed to be the result of jealousy or rage. Drug addiction is a vice or a moral illness, and others will judge the person on the basis of his or her immoral behaviors (Spector, 2008).

Arab-American Communities

There are many mistaken conceptions about the diverse population of immigrants who are considered Arab Americans. There are approximately 2 to 3 million people who have come from more than 19 countries with different social structures, languages, beliefs, values, and traditions. Their differences are also classified according to the three time periods of immigration that represent distinct demographic characteristics. The first wave of people, who immigrated between the 1800s and World War I, were mainly from Syria and Lebanon; they were merchants and farmers who blended well into the general population, and many were Christian. The second wave began in 1948. Several of these immigrants were well-educated individuals or students seeking higher education; some were refugees from Palestine, and more were Muslims. The third wave came after 1967, and these individuals came to the United States primarily to escape an unstable political situation. This group has been more negatively received in the United States. Instead of assimilating to U.S. norms, they have created their own schools and communities, they worship in their own mosques, and they wear traditional garments to signify their ethnic identity. They have a cautious and apprehensive worldview with regard to Western society.

Commonalities associated with these diverse groups include the family as the central core of life in which all decisions are made, including those that address mental health issues and other illnesses. Individuality is not valued, and family honor is very important. Religion and its traditions are part of everyday life. It is imperative that health care providers become knowledgeable about these diverse populations and their needs and preferences to provide culturally appropriate quality care (Erickson and al-Timimi, 2001).

Communities of European Origin

Members of this community have origins throughout Europe; in 2003, they made up 15% of the foreign-born population of the United States (www.census.gov). The 2000 census counted 211,460,626 people who indicated their heritage as European; this was 75.1% of the total U.S. population at that time. Those who noted themselves as having two races (if Caucasian was one) constituted 77.1% of this population. In general, this population expresses a low-context cultural heritage and speaks a variety of languages. They typically value individual strengths and independence, and they do not emphasize community identification as much as some of the other groups. Traditional religious practice is common, and many nationalities are represented in this group. Careful assessment, as in all the other groups, is key to understanding the individual. Individuals in this population often seek traditional medical care; many use alternative health care before seeking allopathic treatment. This culture is beginning to have a clearer understanding of mental illness, but many individuals in this population still view mental illness as a moral failing.

The Jewish population is a subculture of the European population, although Jews have emigrated from countries all over the world. There is an emphasis on community and multigenerational continuity. Most Jews celebrate the important religious holidays. Their religious beliefs range from completely secular to the orthodox traditions. Some of the aging survivors of the Holocaust experience survivor guilt and present symptoms of chronic posttraumatic stress disorder. Some survivors with dementia can still recall their experiences, which affects their behaviors and requires sensitivity to their particular needs (Sable, 2009). In biblical times, the Jews perceived mental illness as demon possession; visions were proof of contact with the divine. Currently, some still view mental illness as punishment for disobedience, creating a social stigma; however, today there is more acceptance of therapeutic measures. The most common mental symptoms among this group include paranoia and neuroses. The patterns of illness are related to religious and cultural experiences. Certain holidays, such as days of mourning, are triggers for dysfunctional mental symptoms, including suicidal thoughts.

Healing practices include prayer, reading Psalms and religious texts, participating in religious rituals, and activities that provide a distance and the opportunity to reflect and find new options (Myerstein, 2004).

THE ROLE OF THE NURSE

Nursing traditionally maintains a holistic view when caring for patients and their families. The profession has incorporated cultural and spiritual content within the academic context and in all levels of actual patient care, including all phases of the nursing process and discharge planning. Psychiatry also now recognizes the necessity of the inclusion of cultural and spiritual content. The *Diagnostic and Statistical Manual of Mental Disorders* (DSM-IV-TR) includes several problems that may cause noncompliance with treatment. Among those are the patient's personal cultural or religious beliefs, values, and judgments with regard to the advantages and disadvantages of accepting a treatment regimen (American Psychiatric Association, 2000). In the first report on mental health by the U.S. surgeon general, multiple entries appear that emphasize the influence of culture and spirituality in the area of mental wellness and illness (U.S. Department of Health and Human Services, 1999). The report covers many aspects of mental health and illness that the American Psychiatric Association will address during upcoming decades.

Definitions of mental health and illness as well as the entire concepts of mental health and illness are different within different societal structures. The DSM-IV-TR (American Psychiatric Association, 2000) provides information about syndromes that occur in particular cultures (i.e., culture-bound syndromes) (Table 8-3). The DSM-V, which will be released in 2013, will have diagnostic changes in several areas.

The purpose of cultural competence is to ensure that the nurse gives patients of all cultures every opportunity to receive information about treatment in ways that they understand, with consideration given to their education, acculturation, and language (Box 8-5). The Research for Evidence-Based Practice box describes how learning about the traditions and beliefs of a culture will lead to culturally responsive care. However, it is essential to address the individual's specific needs while working within the framework of his or her culture.

As mentioned previously, it is necessary to use a gradual approach for obtaining information from individuals from another culture. Because most patients with mental health problems do not react well to pencil-and-paper questionnaires, it is helpful to be knowledgeable of the scope and nature of these questions to gather information effectively. In some mental care institutions, patients respond to a crisis questionnaire and a recovery questionnaire. The questions ask what the patient believes the crisis event is and how the health care providers can assist with the meeting of a positive recovery outcome.

The nurse and other health care providers are important advocates for helping patients and families to understand various treatment methods in multilingual and ethnically diverse environments. This is particularly important in the area of mental health given the complex terminology and multiple behaviors and symptoms that require accurate interpretation by a culturally aware staff. Interpreters need to be able to attach accurate meaning and purpose to a patient's

---

BOX 8-5   L-E-A-R-N MODEL FOR CROSS-CULTURAL HEALTH CARE

Listen to the patient and the family's concepts of the illness, their reactions to the Western health care system approaches, and their desires for therapy.

Explain your assessment with the use of drawings, videotapes, and test results.

Acknowledge differences and similarities between a person from a different culture and the health care system perspective; emphasize the similarities.

Recommend the diagnostic and therapeutic approaches, and listen to the patient and the family's responses.

Negotiate all areas of care to accommodate the patient and the family's cultural beliefs and practices.

Modified from Her C, Culhane-Pera K: Culturally responsive care for Hmong patients, *Postgrad Med* 116:39-46, 2004.

RESEARCH FOR EVIDENCE-BASED PRACTICE #1

Garrett PW et al: Cultural competency from a patient's perspective: a qualitative study, *Ethn Health* 13(5):479-496, 2008.

Seven language-specific focus groups with 59 hospitalized patients and their caregivers participated in a study to determine their perspective of cultural competency care in their overall hospital experience. Critical factors that were identified included communication in a language that they could not understand; feelings of powerlessness as a result of staff attitudes; inattention to cultural mores and beliefs; and expressions of racism in some instances. These individuals valued positive engagement; communication; information; compassionate, kind, and respectful treatment; and negotiation for the involvement of their family in their care. Some of the specific things that were mentioned included the following:

"They didn't respect my modesty and preference for a female care provider."

"I didn't know what was happening. No one explained things to me."

"I was frustrated because I wanted to express my feelings, but I could not."

"They took away my teeth, and I couldn't chew the food."

"The nurse was so kind. She spent time with me. She even gave me a hug."

"My family was allowed to stay and help care for me."

"My family and I were included in the discharge instructions."

TABLE 8-3	**CULTURE-BOUND SYNDROMES**		
CULTURE	**IDIOM**	**BEHAVIOR**	**POTENTIAL RELATIONSHIP WITH DSM-IV-TR AXIS CLASSIFICATION**
Malaysia Polynesia Puerto Rico Navajo Indian	*Amok* *Cafard* or *cathard* *Mal de pelea* *lich' aa*	Brooding, episodes of intrusive thoughts, violent outbursts, aggressive behavior followed by exhaustion, amnesia	Occurs at onset or exacerbation of a chronic psychotic process or during a brief psychotic episode
Latino (especially women from the Caribbean and Latin Mediterranean populations)	*Atique de nervios*	Uncontrollable screaming, crying, trembling May exhibit aggressive behavior Fainting and seizures sometimes occur Suicidal intent Behaviors frequently occur after a stressful event related to the person's family	Anxiety, mood, dissociation, or somatoform disorders Distinguished from panic attack classification by no expressions of fear or apprehension
Latino	*Bilis, colerea, muina*	Perceived cause is inner core imbalance (of hot/cold or material/spiritual) caused by the suppression of anger or rage Symptoms: headache, nervous tension, trembling, screaming, gastric upset, possible loss of consciousness Chronic fatigue after acute episode	
West Africa, Haiti	*Boufee delirante*	Sudden outburst of agitation, aggressive behavior, confusion, jerky movements May have hallucinations (visual and auditory) and paranoid behavior	Resembles brief psychotic disorder episode
West Africa	*Brain fog, brain tiredness*	Difficulty concentrating or remembering, feeling that brain is "fatigued" Other somatic symptoms include pain, pressure in the head and neck, blurred vision, heat or burning Often expressed by high school or university students	Resembles symptoms of anxiety, depressive, and somatoform disorders
Far East, India, Sri Lanka, China	Folk terms *dhat* (or *jiryan*) *sukrapraena* *shen-k uei*	Severe anxiety associated with weakness, exhaustion, and discharge of semen or white discoloration of urine	
Southern United States and Caribbean groups	Falling out Blacking out	Sudden collapse (usually preceded by dizziness or "swimming in the head") Temporary loss of vision Feels paralyzed	Compared to conversion disorder or dissociation disorder
Several Native American tribes	Ghost sickness	Preoccupation with death or a deceased individuals Fear of danger Anxiety, hallucinations, confusion, anorexia, fainting, dizziness	
Korean folk syndrome	*Hwa-byung (wool-hwa-byung)* English term: anger syndrome	Caused by the suppression of anger Insomnia, panic, fear of impending death, palpitations, dyspnea, chest pressure, indigestion, generalized aches and pain	
Malaysia China Assam Thailand	*Koro* (and other local terms) *Shuk yang, shook yong* *Jinjinia bemar* *Rok-joo*	Sudden severe anxiety that the penis in the male or the vulva and nipples in the female will recede into the body and possibly cause death	Symptoms meet criteria for a DSM-IV-TR mood or anxiety disorder Diagnosis included in *Chinese Classification of Mental Disorders*

Continued

TABLE 8-3   CULTURE-BOUND SYNDROMES—cont'd

CULTURE	IDIOM	BEHAVIOR	POTENTIAL RELATIONSHIP WITH DSM-IV-TR AXIS CLASSIFICATION
Malaysia, Indonesia Siberian groups Thailand Ainu, Sakhalin, Japan,	*Latah* *Amurakh, irkunii, ikota, olan, myriachit, menkeiti*	Syndrome seen in many parts of the world More prevalent among middle-aged females in Malaysia	Dissociation disorder
Philippines	*Bah tschi, bah-tsi, baah-ji* *Imu* *Mali-mali, silok*	Dissociation or trancelike behavior Echolalia (parrot-like repetitions) and echopraxia (imitation of actions of others)	
Latino (United States and Latin America)	*Locura*	Severe form of psychosis Possibly caused by inherited vulnerability to many of life's difficulties Poor social skills Auditory and visual hallucinations, unpredictable behavior Some exhibit violent behavior	
Mediterranean cultures and other parts of the world	*Mal de ojo* (evil eye)	Children are especially vulnerable; also seen among women Sleep disturbances, crying, diarrhea, vomiting, fever in a child or infant	
Latino (United States and Latin America) Greeks in North America	*Nervios* *Nevra*	Broad term to describe vulnerability to stressful life experiences Headache ("brain aches"), irritability, gastrointestinal disturbances, sleep disturbances, dizziness *(mareos)*	
Arctic and subarctic Eskimo communities	*Pibloktoq* (term may vary by region)	Sudden dissociation event; convulsive seizures and sometimes coma follows Before the episode, the person is withdrawn and irritable or exhibits bizarre behavior	
Chinese	Qigong psychotic reaction	Acute dissociation episode, paranoia Can occur after the practice of qigong, which is a health-enhancing exercise Vulnerability increases with overinvolvement with exercise	Included in the *Chinese Classification of Mental Disorders*
Southern United States among African-American, European-American, and Caribbean societies Latino societies	*Rootwork* *Mal puesto* *Brujeria*	Anxiety, gastrointestinal disturbances, fear of being poisoned or killed ("voodoo death") Attributed to hexes, spells, roots; a "root doctor" (a traditional healer) is able to remedy this situation	
Portuguese Cape Verde Islanders and immigrants to the United States	*Sangue dormido* (i.e., "sleeping blood")	Pain, numbness, tremors, convulsions, paralysis, blindness, heart attack, infection, miscarriage	
China	*Shenjing shairuo* (neurasthenia)	Fatigue, headache, pain, difficulty concentrating, sleep disturbances	Symptoms meet criteria for a mood or anxiety disorder Diagnosis included in the *Chinese Classification of Mental Disorders*
Taiwan China	*Shen-k'uei* *Shenkui*	Severe anxiety and panic symptoms, numerous somatic complaints, and sexual dysfunction Often considered life threatening	

TABLE 8-3	CULTURE-BOUND SYNDROMES—cont'd		
CULTURE	IDIOM	BEHAVIOR	POTENTIAL RELATIONSHIP WITH DSM-IV-TR AXIS CLASSIFICATION
Korea	Shin-byung	Anxiety with numerous somatic complaints Sometimes develops into dissociation Thought to be caused by possession by ancestral spirits	
African and European Americans from the Southern United States	Spell	Trance state with the ability to "communicate" with the deceased or spirits Folk tradition does not consider these episodes as medical problems; often misinterpreted in clinical settings	
Latino (Mexico, Central America, South America); similar syndromes and beliefs are found throughout the world	Susto ("soul loss"); also referred to as espanto, pasmo, tripa ida, perdida del alm, chibih	Presumed cause is a frightening event Multiple somatic symptoms occur shortly after the fright or a long time later Considered life threatening, ritual healings are used	Related to posttraumatic stress disorder and somatoform disorder
Japan	Taijin kyofusho	Phobia that own body parts and functions are offensive to others	Resembles social phobia Syndrome is in the official Japanese diagnostic system for mental disorders
Ethiopia, Somalia, Egypt, Sudan, Iran and other North African and Middle Eastern societies	Zar	Possession by a spirit Episodes of dissociation, bizarre behavior, and sudden verbal outbursts Withdrawal from social group and has a "relationship" with the spirit Not considered as an illness by the community	

Data from the American Psychological Association: *Diagnostic and statistical manual of mental disorders,* ed 4, text revision, Washington, DC, 2000, American Psychological Association; and the U.S. Department of Health and Human Services and the Substance Abuse and Mental Health Services Administration: www.mentalhealth.samhsa.gov.

language so that the patient will clearly understand nursing implications for effective treatment. Cultural diversity helps nurses and professionals in other health care disciplines to recognize that people are more alike than different and that everyone deserves the best possible physical and psychologic treatment, regardless of language, culture, or ethnicity.

Several theories are proposed for incorporating cultural content while making use of the nursing process. Madeleine Leininger's *Culture Care Diversity and Universality: A Theory of Nursing* (1991) is the only nursing theory text that specifically addresses the patient's holistic cultural needs. Leininger noted that there are common or similar patterns, values, and meanings related to health and illness that are manifested by many cultures and that the differences are based on the worldview and the spiritual, social, and environmental context of a particular culture. Her sunrise enabler model is a tool that examines the influences of the multiple factors that are involved in the designing of efficient cultural care. Watson's theory of human caring and Neuman's systems model are other nursing models that are used frequently when designing and implementing culturally congruent health care plans (Fawcett, 2005).

THE NURSING PROCESS

The principal nursing tool in mental health is the therapeutic use of self. Often in the nurse–patient relationship, sensitive cultural issues manifest themselves and affect patient care. Therefore, understanding the significance of culture and its influence on patients' mental and physical health is important for nurses in all settings of health care delivery. This understanding will affect every step of the nursing process as well as the patient's interpretation of life events.

ASSESSMENT

The assessment process is the foundation for all other steps of the nursing process. During assessment, the nurse formulates a perspective of the patient's needs and problems. The nurse's personal biases, assumptions, cultural meanings, and nursing experience all influence the process.

The use of the Heritage Assessment Tool (Box 8-6) when assessing patients is an entry point for gathering culture-specific data. In some instances, a more comprehensive assessment is necessary. Some assessment tools include

BOX 8-6   HERITAGE ASSESSMENT TOOL

1 Where was your mother born?
2 Where was your father born?
3 Where were your grandparents born?
  a Your mother's mother?
  b Your mother's father?
  c Your father's mother?
  d Your father's father?
4 How many brothers and sisters do you have?
5 What setting did you grow up in?
  a Urban
  b Rural
  c Suburban
6 What country did your parents grow up in?
  a Father
  b Mother
7 How old were you when you came to the United States?
8 How old were your parents when they came to the United States?
  a Mother
  b Father
9 When you were growing up, who lived with you? *(ask this way)*
  a Nuclear family
  b Extended family
  c Single-parent family
  d Other
10 Have you maintained contact with any of the following:
  a Aunts, uncles, and cousins? (1) Yes (2) No
  b Brothers and sisters? (1) Yes (2) No
  c Parents? (1) Yes (2) No
  d Your own children? (1) Yes (2) No
11 Did most of your aunts, uncles, and cousins live near your home when you were growing up?
  a Yes
  b No
12 Approximately how often did you visit your family members who lived outside of your home when you were young?
  a Daily
  b Weekly
  c Monthly
  d Once a year or less
  e Never
13 Was your original family name changed?
  a Yes
  b No
14 Do you have a religious preference?
  a Yes (if yes, please specify)
  b No (1 point for yes, 0 for no)
15 Is your spouse the same religion as you?
  a Yes
  b No
16 Is your spouse from the same ethnic background as you?
  a Yes
  b No
17 What kind of school did you go to?
  a Public (0)
  b Private
  c Parochial

18 As an adult, do you live in a neighborhood where the neighbors have the same religion or ethnic background as you do?
  a Religion (1) Yes (2) No
  b Ethnicity (1) Yes (2) No
19 Do you belong to a religious institution?
  a Yes
  b No
20 Would you describe yourself as an active member?
  a Yes
  b No
21 How often do you attend your religious institution?
  a More than once a week
  b Weekly
  c Monthly (0)
  d Special holidays only (0)
  e Never
22 Do you practice your religion in your home?
  a Yes (please specify, 1 point for each example)
  b Praying
  c Bible reading
  d Diet
  e Celebrating religious holidays
  f No
23 Do you prepare foods related to your ethnic background?
  a Yes
  b No
24 Do you participate in ethnic activities?
  a Yes (please specify, 1 point for each example)
  b Singing
  c Holiday celebrations
  d Dancing
  e Festivals
  f Costumes
  g Other
  h No
25 Are your friends from the same religious background as you?
  a Yes
  b No
26 Are your friends from the same ethnic background as you?
  a Yes
  b No
27 What is your native language (i.e., the language that your parents may have spoken other than English)?
28 Do you speak this language?
  a Prefer
  b Occasionally (0)
  c Rarely (0)
29 Do you read this language?
  a Yes
  b No

The greater the number of "yes" answers, the more likely the patient is to strongly identify with a traditional heritage. (The one "no" answer that indicates heritage identity is "Was your name changed?") This assessment may be scored by giving 1 point for each "yes" from question 10 (except where noted as 0) and 2 points for "no" if the person's family name was not Americanized. Again, a high score (usually >15 points) indicates identification with a traditional background.

From Spector RE: *Cultural diversity in health and illness,* ed 6, Upper Saddle River, NJ, 2008, Prentice Hall.

additional information that is related to the interpretation of time; attitudes related to personal space or territory; the format for names, social greetings, and departures; family roles; expected and taboo behaviors; nutrition and deficiencies; pregnancy and childbearing practices; rituals related to illness and death; and the use of folklore practices (Catalano, 2009).

NURSING DIAGNOSIS

The nurse needs to be as specific as possible when conducting an assessment to determine the patient's needs and problems and to identify specific nursing diagnoses. Nursing diagnoses are the same for patients from diverse cultural backgrounds, with a few exceptions. Actual culture-related nursing diagnoses include those that are related to communication barriers, sociocultural conflicts, language barriers, and differences in health and illness beliefs and practices.

The process of making a nursing diagnosis is important because these diagnostic categories often help other staff members to frame a patient's health concerns and potential outcomes. Accurate nursing diagnoses reflect the patient's unique cultural perspective. If the assessment is inaccurate, the nursing diagnosis will be incorrect; a nurse who views patient behavior through an ethnocentric lens may interpret the patient's behavior as dysfunctional when in fact it is acceptable in the patient's own culture. Box 8-7 describes common mistakes that nurses make as a result of culture-related misunderstandings when they are making nursing diagnoses.

❖ CLINICAL ALERT

Mrs. Williams is a 50-year-old woman whose husband died about 14 months earlier as a result of a myocardial infarction. She came to the family practice clinic because she began to have chest pain, and she wondered if she also had cardiac problems. While obtaining a history from Mrs. Williams, the practitioner noticed that Mrs. Williams was still dressed in black and added the diagnosis of "delayed bereavement" to her history. The practitioner failed to assess Mrs. Williams in terms of her cultural expression of grief. Mrs. Williams is Hispanic, and it is customary for people of many Hispanic cultures to wear black for a year or longer; it would be socially unacceptable for Mrs. Williams to do otherwise. Nurses need to avoid the making of assumptions about others' behaviors.

OUTCOME IDENTIFICATION

The nurse's understanding of cultural issues is crucial to ensure that the outcomes involve patient participation; this also ensures that the outcomes fit the patients' needs and wishes. Often patients fail to achieve desired outcomes because those outcomes are inconsistent with their cultural worldviews. Many patients will agree with the nurse, whom they see as the expert. In reality, however, these patients do

---

BOX 8-7 COMMONLY MISAPPLIED NURSING DIAGNOSES

Common North American Nursing Diagnosis Association nursing diagnoses that are frequently misapplied as a result of a lack of understanding of cultural issues include the following:

- **Defensive coping and noncompliance.** Patients from minority cultures that have experienced discrimination, bias, and stereotyping are often resistant to appropriate nursing interventions, especially in the area of teaching and discharge planning. Suspicion and mistrust cause the nurse to misunderstand a patient's behaviors and to then mislabel them.
- **Ineffective role performance and impaired parenting.** The use of these diagnoses requires an understanding of the patient's culture-specific roles and parenting activities. They are often different from those of the nurse and the majority culture.
- **Impaired social interaction and impaired verbal communication.** Misunderstanding occurs when the nurse fails to take into account culture-specific interaction patterns. Silence, infrequent eye contact, shame, fear, and language barriers all affect a patient's ability to interact. The gender of the nurse and the gender of the patient also influence communication, because many cultures have specific gender-role behavioral codes.
- **Disturbed thought processes.** Thought patterns and processes that appear to be distorted are sometimes related to culture-specific expressions of anxiety and fear. Careful assessment will enable the nurse to accurately diagnose anxiety or fear in many patients rather than assume that underlying thought processes are altered.

---

not plan or are unable to follow through with the educational and discharge planning because, from their perspective, the plans make no sense to them and are not relevant to their problems. This leads to further misdiagnoses and especially to the diagnosis of noncompliance. This happens most often when a patient wants to use a traditional healing method or another culture-specific approach and sees the allopathic-oriented nursing intervention as conflicting with his or her traditional ways of achieving health.

PLANNING

A nurse is more likely to include a patient's beliefs in the mental health care plan when the nurse considers the meaning of the patient's behavior and communication in the context of that patient's culture and traditions. When establishing goals of care and planning nursing interventions, the nurse considers each patient's particular situation and challenges. Ideally, the family and the patient's community are partners in developing and implementing the patient's treatment plan.

IMPLEMENTATION

Holistic and culturally sensitive care plans that fit with the patient's culture and needs evolve over time. The care plan is a living document, and the nurse adjusts the plan as goals are met and as other goals are identified. For example, if the patient is using culturally specific medications, the nurse determines their type and how they react with conventional medications. In addition, it is important to maintain effective verbal and nonverbal communication between the patient and the caregivers and to obtain an interpreter, if necessary. Promoting the patient's understanding of the allopathic system and the rationale for the care often increases compliance.

Patients who are members of cultural communities often mistrust the system in general and the nurse in particular, especially if the nurse comes from a different cultural background. Trust issues are important in mental health nursing care, and, because of the nurse's professional role, responsibility for the therapeutic relationship rests primarily on the nurse. For example, researchers have noted that race is a powerful issue in treatment. In particular, it affects how medication is administered, the level and frequency of interventions, and the outcome of intervention. Symptom presentation and the prevalence of certain disorders also differ across cultural groups.

Faison and Mintzer (2005) reported that the elderly population is growing in size and in racial and ethnic diversity worldwide. Growing public health concerns include depression and suicide among the elderly, and different cultural communities have not always understood access to mental health service. There is a great need for care providers and the public to understand mental health issues in the diverse aging population and to develop strategies to meet the needs of this population. Cohen and colleagues (2005) noted that blacks born in the United States and those from African Caribbean islands (both English and French speaking) were more likely to seek services and be treated. A majority of participants in the treatment group in this study were diagnosed with depression; they were younger, they experienced impaired abilities related to daily functions, and they had a family history of mental illness and minimal social or religious supports. The use of social support systems during the intervention process is crucial for effectively caring for these older patients (Kim, 2002). Involving family members and other members of the patient's cultural group in the assessment, planning, and intervention processes facilitates nursing care and ensures more effective patient outcomes.

EVALUATION

The nurse evaluates whether the patient has been able to maintain his or her cultural beliefs with regard to mental health and illness. To do this, the nurse evaluates mental health care from a multicultural nursing perspective to determine whether the patient outcomes have been achieved. The nurse respects the patient's needs and beliefs and remains open to communication. The discharge plan needs to be realistic and culturally congruent. If the patient does not feel invested in the treatment choices, he or she is less likely to be effective after discharge. Thus, the evaluation of nursing interventions is based on culturally sensitive and realistic patient outcomes. The Case Study on page 163 demonstrates the use of assessment and intervention tools.

▌ CHAPTER SUMMARY

- Cultural awareness is the initial step toward effective interaction among individuals from different cultures, and it involves an awareness of one's own culture, including its prejudices and biases toward other cultures.
- Cultural competence requires a respect for diversity and the understanding of the attitudes, beliefs, behaviors, practices, and communication patterns of multiple cultures and their languages.
- Culture is a set of values, beliefs, and behaviors that influence the way that members of a group express themselves; it is also the integrated pattern of human behavior of members of a racial, religious, or social group that is transmitted to succeeding generations as a cultural heritage.
- The communication aspects of language, space, and time orientation have various practices among different cultures.
- Secondary characteristics of cultural diversity (i.e., socioeconomic status, occupation, education, gender issues, geographic place of residence, length of time absent from the country of origin, sexual orientation) have a powerful effect on an individual's cultural identity, although these characteristics are not as easy to identify as the primary characteristics.
- Heritage consistency is the concept that describes how much a person identifies with his or her cultural background.
- The nurse and other health care providers need to be aware of the meaning of gestures, body positions, facial expressions, eye movements, and tone of voice during all communications with individuals from various cultures.
- Religious beliefs are a part of the cultural heritage, and they have a strong influence on lifestyle, ethics, health care, and life decisions.
- Religion is a personal set or institutionalized system of religious attitudes, beliefs, and practices.
- Spirituality is composed of the following: (1) an integrative energy that can produce inner harmony or wholeness; (2) a sense of coherence; (3) a driving force that permeates all aspects that give meaning to life; and (4) a sense of transcendence over reality.
- Faith is the belief and trust in God or a supreme being and the ability to draw on spiritual resources without having

This case illustrates the use of the assessment and intervention tools referred to in this chapter. It also reflects some of the significant aspects of spiritual care as they apply to both patients and nurses, and it demonstrates the value of spiritual care as perceived by a patient and a physician.

Holistic Assessment

The patient is a 66-year-old woman who has been hospitalized for an extensive period (approximately 6 weeks). Her initial problems were major depression, anxiety, and a degenerative spinal condition that required several surgeries. The spinal condition is treatable, but the process will leave her with some permanent restrictions in movement and some possible residual pain. The patient currently has significant chronic leg and lower back spasms, and she states that medication gives her little relief. Both the pain and the restrictions that resulted from the surgery have exacerbated her depression and anxiety.

The patient has been divorced for almost 40 years. Immediately after her divorce, she and her four children moved 1500 miles away from her family and friends so that she could seek employment in a manufacturing environment. Although two of her children live close by, only one child is in regular contact with the patient. The patient has a Lutheran background, but she has no local connection to a congregation, and she has not attended church regularly since leaving her hometown. Both the patient and her physician are extremely interested in her having regular visits for spiritual care, and both have stated that the visits provide the patient with significant help and support.

The Patient's Beliefs and Meanings

Being independent, strong, and self-sufficient are important goals in life, which are to be valued and pursued.

The Patient's Vocations and Obligations

The patient's goal was to support, raise, and care for herself and her children without being dependent on others. She still seeks to care for her adult daughter: she asks the spiritual caregiver to meet with her daughter to talk about performing a marriage ceremony.

The Patient's Experiences and Emotions

The patient has had a life of struggle, which has been balanced with the rewards of accomplishing her goal of being independent and her pride in being self-sufficient.

The Patient's Courage and Growth

The patient is now struggling to find some meaning in her pain and suffering.

The Patient's Ritual and Practice

The patient has a strong and dependent need to have the poem "Footprints," Psalm 23, and the Lord's Prayer read to her; she requests few other institutional rituals.

The Patient's Community

The patient's community is small and consists mainly of her children, their spouses, and several grandchildren, most of who live some distance from the patient.

The Patient's Source of Authority and Guidance

The patient's source of authority and guidance is largely external and comes from her early Midwestern social norms and experiences with institutional religion. She grants pastors a great deal of power, authority, and control; the patient also believes that common religious articles such as the Bible and prayer cards have an almost magical authority and power.

The Patient's Stage of Faith Development

The patient is basically in stage 1, which is the impartial stage of faith. She is now possibly seeking to move into the early phase of stage 2, which is the institutional religion stage.

Level of Spiritual Risk

This patient is at significant spiritual risk. She has an extremely high need for spiritual care, and she has limited to nonexistent resources with which to meet this need. When making a triage assessment of how to assign scarce pastoral care resources, this patient's particular situation calls for a significant amount of qualified pastoral care.

Spiritual Care Plan

With the use of the assessment tools that have been previously described, the spiritual pastoral care plan was to see the patient often—daily, if possible. During these visits, the spiritual intervention tools of prayer, presence, and short scripture readings were used to help bolster the patient's sense of God's care for her and to support her in the healing process. Another intervention strategy was to help the patient to explore her stated desire to be connected to a local Lutheran church and to help identify ways in which to do this. In addition, the spiritual caregiver helped the patient explore, to the extent of her desire and capability, what meaning there is for her in this illness and in her future physical limitations. The intent of this goal was to help the patient to find possible new meanings in her life as a result of this illness.

The benefit to the patient of pursuing these spiritual care plan goals was the provision of help, support, and comfort. This spiritual support helped to ease her sense of torment and pain, thereby resulting in a reduced experience of suffering. The benefit to the hospital of pursuing these spiritual care plan goals was greater patient satisfaction. As the patient experienced significant relief during the periods after her spiritual care, her requests for nursing interventions decreased. The patient was also more satisfied with her overall care, and she was less anxious about her prognosis. The patient's physician reported that she was quite satisfied with the hospital's ability to address the patient's spiritual needs and that by doing so the hospital helped the patient to experience less pain and discomfort.

Critical Thinking

1 Assess and prioritize the patient's psychiatric, physical, and spiritual areas of concern to ensure that all areas are addressed.
2 Describe the benefits of collaborating with the hospital chaplain when addressing the patient's spiritual needs as part of a holistic assessment.
3 Given your knowledge of the stages of faith and the patient's spiritual and religious background, which stage of faith best fits this patient? What is the rationale for your choice?
4 How can your assessment of this patient's family history of struggle, pride, and pain be used to guide you in your spiritual assessment? Consider the stages of the spiritual dimension as a guide.

CHAPTER SUMMARY—cont'd

physical and empiric proof. It is an internal certainty that comes from one's own experience with the divine.

- Health is three dimensional in that it encompasses the body, mind, and spirit.
- Belief and meaning make up the central core principles that underlie an individual's spiritual dimension, and culture and life experiences influence this dimension as well.
- Spirituality is an essential human dimension that helps to connect people to each other, the community, and the world. Patients express their spirituality in a variety of ways.

- There is a growing belief that a quality spiritual assessment is significantly beneficial for reducing a patient's feelings of powerlessness and despair.
- For some individuals, a chaplain represents the ultimate authority for one's spiritual health, just as the nurse or physician is often the authority regarding one's physical or mental health.
- Research on spirituality and healing has grown, but a greater focus on mental health and spirituality is needed.

REVIEW QUESTIONS

1. A family immigrates to the United States from Honduras. Which members of the family are most likely to experience culture shock? You may select more than one answer.
   1. Father
   2. Mother
   3. Teenage daughter
   4. 8-year-old son
   5. 3-year-old son
2. A nurse assesses an adult patient with a foot ulcer that will not heal. The patient is of Cuban heritage, has been in the United States for 2 years, and is fluent in English. Which question should the nurse include in the assessment?
   1. "Do you believe evil spirits caused your problem?"
   2. "What are your main cultural values and beliefs?"
   3. "Have you used any folk medicine treatments on your foot?"
   4. "How have you been treating your foot sore at home?"
3. An adult patient who has been recently diagnosed with cancer states, "I've lived my life according to the Bible. I don't understand why God has forsaken me." Which nursing diagnosis applies?
   1. Spiritual dysfunction
   2. Disturbed thought processes
   3. Hopelessness
   4. Spiritual distress

4. A nurse provides discharge instructions to a patient of Vietnamese heritage who immigrated to the United States 1 year ago. Which strategy would be important for ensuring the patient's understanding of the instructions?
   1. Use a professional interpreter.
   2. Handwrite the instructions.
   3. Show the patient a video.
   4. Contact a bilingual translator.
5. A Native American adult is hospitalized. The emergency department assessment indicates auditory and visual hallucinations. The patient states, "My dead father told me to kill myself to save me from the bad spirits." What would be an appropriate nursing intervention for the nursing care plan?
   1. Consult the family, with the patient's consent, for a spiritual healer from the patient's tribe.
   2. Initiate a consultation between the hospital chaplain and the patient.
   3. Assign only Native American staff members to provide this patient's care.
   4. Provide the patient with frequent periods alone for meditation and prayer.

REFERENCES

Ackley BJ, Ladwig GB: *Nursing diagnosis handbook: an evidence-based guide to planning care*, ed 5, St. Louis, 2007, Mosby.

American Psychiatric Association: *Diagnostic and statistical manual of mental disorders*, ed 4, text revision, Washington, DC, American Psychiatric Association, 2000.

Autgis T, Raneer A: Personalization of conflict across cultures: a comparison among the U.S., New Zealand and Australia, *J Intercultural Commun Res* 33:109-119, 2004.

Catalano JT: *Nursing now! Today's issues, tomorrow's trends*, ed 2, Philadelphia, 2009, FA Davis.

Clark MJ: *Community health nursing: advocacy for population health*, ed 5, Upper Saddle River, NJ, 2008, Pearson Prentice Hall.

Cohen C et al: Comparison of users and non-users of mental health serves among depressed older urban African Americans, *Am J Geriatr Psychiatry* 13:545-553, 2005.

Cutheral K et al: Examining the culture of poverty: promising practices, *Preventing School Failure* 54(2):104-110, 2010.

Erickson C, al-Timimi N: Providing mental health services to Arab Americans: recommendations and considerations, *Cultur Divers Ethnic Minor Psychol* 7(4):308-327, 2001.

Fadiman A: *The spirit catches you and you fall down*, New York, 1997, Farrar, Straus & Giroux.

Faison W, Mintzer M: The growing ethnically diverse aging population: is our field advancing with it? *Am J Geriatric Psychiatry* 13:541-544, 2005.

Fawcett J: Leininger's theory of culture care diversity and universality. In *Analysis and evaluation of contemporary nursing knowledge*, Philadelphia, 2005, FA Davis.

Fitchett G: *Assessing spiritual needs: a guide for caregivers*, Minneapolis, 2002, Augsburg Fortress.

Fowler JW: *Stages of faith*, San Francisco, 1981, Harper.

Giger JN, Davidhizar RE: *Transcultural nursing: assessment & intervention*, ed 2, St. Louis, 2007, Mosby.

Graham G: *The role of Office of Minority Health (OMH) in eliminating health disparities*, presentation to Congress, 2008.

Halloran L: Teaching transcultural nursing through literature, *J Nurs Educ* 48(9):523-528, 2009.

Harris J: Learning to listen across cultural divides, *Listening Professional* 2:4, 20-21, 2003.

Haviland VS et al: Making the journey toward cultural competence with poetry, *Multicultural Perspectives* 11(1):19-26, 2009.

Ito K: A history of manga in the context of Japanese culture and society, *J Pop Cult* 38:456-475, 2005.

Kim G: U.S. Population is nudging toward the 300 million mark, *San Diego Union Tribune*, p A-3, Jan 30, 2006.

Kim M et al: Primary health care for Korean immigrants: sustaining a culturally sensitive model, *Public Health Nurs* 19:191-200, 2002.

Koenig H: Religion, spirituality and medicine: research findings and implications for clinical practice, *South Med J* 97:1194-1205, 2004.

Koenig H, Cohen HJ: Spirituality across the lifespan, *South Med J* 99(10):1157-1158, 2006.

LaRocca-Pitts MA: FACT: Taking a spiritual history in a clinical setting, *Journal of Healthcare and Chaplaincy* 15(1):1-12, 2008.

Leininger MM: *Culture care diversity and universality: a theory of nursing*, New York, 1991, National League for Nursing Press.

McCaffery M, Pasero C: *Pain: clinical manual*, ed 2, St. Louis, 2004, Mosby.

McGinnis D: *Exit wounds: a survival guide to pain management for returning veterans and their families*, Washington, DC, 2009, American Pain Foundation and Waterford Life Science.

Medrano M et al: Self-assessment of cultural and linguistic competence in an ambulatory health system, *J Health Care Manage* 50:371-385, 2005.

Mortensen G, Relin DO: *Three cups of tea*, New York, 2009, Penguin Publishers.

Myerstein I: Psychopathology and psychotherapy: a clinician's view, *J Relig Health* 43:329-341, 2004.

O'Sullivan-Oliveira J, Burke P: Lost in the shuffle: culture of homeless adolescents, *Pediatr Nurs* 35(3):154-161, 2009.

Phillippe MY: Valuing corporate culture, *Profiles in Diversity Journal* 11(4):72, 2009.

Author. Putting a face on poverty, *Canada & World Backgrounder* 70:8-12, 2005.

Rogalsky J: "Mythbusters": dispelling the culture of poverty: management in the urban classroom, *Journal of Geography* 108(4/5):198-209, 2009.

Sable J: Caring for older Jews, *Nursing and Residential Care* 11(12):621-623, 2009.

Santiago, C: *When I was Puerto Rican*, Cambridge, MA, 2006, De Capo Press.

Smith-Miller C et al: "Leaving the comfort of the familiar": fostering workplace cultural awareness through short-term global experiences, *Nurs Forum* 45(1):18-28, 2010.

Spector R: *Cultural diversity in health and illness*, ed 6, Upper Saddle River, NJ, 2008, Prentice Hall Health.

U.S. Census Bureau: 2003; www.census.gov/prod/2004/pubs/p20-s51/pdf.

U.S. Census Bureau; 2008: http://www.census.gov/mso/www/pres_lib/blackpop_files/outline/index.html.

U.S. Department of Health and Human Services: *Mental health: a report of the Surgeon General*, Rockville, MD, 1999.

U.S. Department of Health and Human Services: The 2006 HHS poverty guidelines (website): http://aspe.hhs.gov/poverty/06poverty.shtml. Accessed October 31, 2010.

Online Resources

National Consumer Supporter Technical Assistance Center: Cultural Competency Initiative Toolkit: www.ncstac.org/content/culturalcompetency/index.htm

Transcultural Nursing: www.madeleine-leininger.com

CHAPTER

9

Legal and Ethical Aspects in Clinical Practice

Robert L. Erb, Jr.

"The law is reason, free from passion."

Aristotle

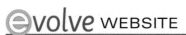 WEBSITE

http://evolve.elsevier.com/Fortinash/

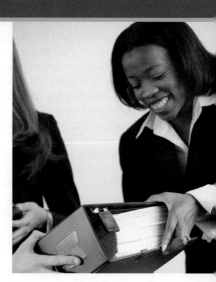

OBJECTIVES

- Review key events in the history of mental illness and its legal treatment.
- Describe and discuss the various forms of admission to mental health facilities.
- Explain the difference between confidentiality and privileged communication.
- Discuss the impact of federal legislation on patient privacy.
- Identify situations in which the duty to warn is applicable.

- List the rights of mental health patients, and identify how these rights apply in practice.
- Distinguish between the concepts of competency to stand trial and the insanity defense.
- Apply the elements of malpractice to a current practice situation.
- Describe the purpose and implementation of psychiatric advance directives.

KEY TERMS

breach of duty
clear and convincing
    evidence
commitment

competency to stand trial
duty to warn
expert witness
forensic psychiatric nurses

least restrictive alternative
legal duty
mandatory outpatient
    treatment

privileged communication
psychiatric advance
    directives

HISTORIC REVIEW

According to Sales and Shuman (1994), law and mental health have been linked for many years. Even in ancient Rome, the law was concerned about the legal status of the mentally disabled. Should the individual have a guardian? Could the individual enter into a contract? According to Roman law, the person with a mental disability could not form a marriage contract; if the law made a person a ward (i.e., a dependent), then the person did not have any legal rights (Brakel et al, 1985).

During the Middle Ages, people believed that mentally ill individuals were possessed by demons. The king could hold

custody of the property of these patients, and then any profits were applied to the maintenance of the individuals and their households. When a person was thought to be incompetent as a result of mental illness, a jury of 12 men decided whether or not to commit the individual to the care of a friend, who received an allowance for taking care of the individual (Brakel et al, 1985).

In the American colonies of the 17th century, the lack of facilities meant that families had to care for people with mental illnesses. If a person had no family or friends, then that individual wandered from town to town, in some instances in the company of transient groups. There was no distinguishing between a homeless person and a person with a mental illness; therefore, all were treated as itinerant poor people. As early as 1676, the state of Massachusetts passed a law to manage people who had mental illnesses and were dangerous. The individual could be detained, but generally there were no procedures for the commitment of a person with a mental illness at this time (Brakel et al, 1985).

It was not until 1752 that Pennsylvania Hospital in Philadelphia opened to treat people with mental illnesses (Laben and MacLean, 1989). In Williamsburg, Virginia, in 1773, the state opened a facility specifically for the treatment of people with mental illnesses. The next state institution built was in Lexington, Kentucky, in 1824 (Brakel et al, 1985).

In 1841, American educator Dorothea Dix began her crusade to place individuals with mental illnesses in specially built hospitals rather than in poorhouses and jails. During the following years, Dix traveled throughout the United States working for the moral and humane treatment of people with mental illnesses (Harshey-Meade, 2006).

During the late 19th and early 20th centuries, various states passed laws addressing civil commitment procedures for people with mental illnesses. From 1900 to 1955, the population in mental institutions grew from 150,000 to 819,000 inpatients in state and county mental hospitals (LaFond, 1994). The passage of the Community Mental Health Centers Act of 1963 authorized funds to build community treatment centers. Shortly thereafter, civil rights lawyers began to challenge the treatment of people with mental illnesses. During the Vietnam War era, a distrust of government appeared. Activism began with concern about the treatment of people with mental illnesses and their rights. Society gave more consideration to individual rights, and the longstanding practice of hospitalizing individuals for many years—in some instances without much treatment—was especially questioned (LaFond, 1994).

Large numbers of individuals were released into the community, which raised concerns that there were not appropriate facilities and services to adequately care for them. Because of the increasing number of people with mental illnesses in the community and the appointment of more conservative judges who were reluctant to become involved in the administration of hospitals, recommendations for expanding mental health commitment laws began. In California, state legislation passed an act (i.e., the Lanterman-Petris-Short Act of 1969) that allowed psychiatrists and other designated professionals to hold individuals for an evaluation period of 72 hours. The individuals had to be a danger to themselves, a danger to others, or "gravely disabled" (i.e., unable to provide or use food, clothing, or shelter for themselves) on the basis of a mental disorder.

In an extensive review of the literature, Lamb and Weinberger (1998) described a variety of factors that limit adequate access to mental health services: the closure of long-term treatment facilities (state hospitals), a lack of developed treatment resources in the community, a lack of understanding by police officers and the general population, and the creation of strict civil commitment standards. As a result, a large number of mentally ill individuals are now in jails and prisons; surveys estimate that up to 15% of inmates have severe mental illness (Lamb and Weinberger, 1998).

The impact of managed behavioral health organizations on hospitals, clinics, and patients themselves is a growing concern with ethical and legal consequences. In an effort to control the rising costs associated with psychiatric treatment, many insurance plans carve out the management of mental health benefits to managed behavioral health organizations. Authorization for access to treatment and the ongoing use of mental health benefits is often a complicated maze for patients and clinicians alike. Insurance mental health benefits (if they are offered at all) have historically had many more restrictions on their use or are paid at significantly lower rates than health benefits for other chronic medical illnesses such as diabetes and heart disease. This is largely a result of the stigma that is still associated with mental illness.

Nurses and physicians need to consider their legal and ethical responsibilities when managed care organizations pressure to limit or deny patient access to treatment or payment for services. Pressure to prematurely discharge patients from inpatient facilities is increasing (Simon, 1998). The advocacy role of nurses to help patients to obtain, maintain, and fully make use of mental health benefits is critical. Although managed care organizations will deny authorization or stop paying for mental health services, the potential liability for denying services remains with the physician, the nurse, and the hospital (Simon, 2001).

COMMITMENT

Commitment is a term that refers to the various ways that an individual enters mental health treatment. States have varying terms and mechanisms associated with commitment, but, in general, there are three common types: (1) voluntary commitment; (2) emergency commitment; and (3) longer-term judicial or civil commitment.

An important concept related to the location and nature of mental health treatment is the concept of the least restrictive alternative; this involves providing mental health treatment in the least restrictive environment with the use of the least restrictive treatment. During the mid-1960s, an elderly woman who was hospitalized at St. Elizabeth's Hospital in Washington, DC, filed a writ of habeas corpus so that she could be released into the community. At that time, there were few alternatives to hospitals for treatment. The court ruled that there needed to be alternatives to inpatient facilities, including halfway houses, nursing homes, and day treatment programs (*Lake v. Cameron*, 1966).

Developing a treatment plan involves the consideration of all alternatives, including such options as inpatient treatment, partial hospitalization, intensive outpatient treatment, home health services, and foster and respite care. An individual who resides in a community that has developed many care options is the least likely to be hospitalized. The cost of health care services is also an important factor. The nurse needs to select the least restrictive, most clinically appropriate, and most cost-effective intervention to assist the patient.

Voluntary Commitment

Nurses are the most familiar with patients who access treatment voluntarily by consenting to be admitted and treated. Nurses treat voluntarily admitted patients whose clinical conditions vary widely with regard to their psychiatric severity. However, voluntary patients who are seeking a discharge from the hospital but who are an immediate danger to themselves or others may be placed on an emergency commitment status pending further evaluation and treatment.

Emergency Commitment

Severe mental illness sometimes affects a patient's cognitive functions so that he or she refuses treatment for a variety of reasons. Some individuals with psychosis, paranoia, delusions, or hallucinations reject psychiatric treatment for fear of being harmed or on the basis of some strange rationale that only they understand. Persons who suffer from severe mood disturbances and who are depressed and suicidal sometimes refuse to enter treatment because of a sense of hopelessness and a wish to die. When the effects of the patient's mental illness result in an immediate risk of self-harm or harm to others, an emergency commitment is appropriate. In some states, if the effect of the mental illness is such that the patient is unable to provide food, clothing, or shelter for himself or herself (i.e., "gravely disabled"), an emergency commitment is also appropriate (see Chapter 30).

Emergency commitment differs from a judicial or indefinite commitment. Emergency commitment is for a shorter period and generally has more restrictive criteria for admission. Usually a state requires that a mental health official such as a physician, psychologist, social worker, or advanced practice nurse see the individual; some states require a licensed physician. After the individual is brought to the inpatient unit, a second mental health professional, usually a psychiatrist, has to make an examination. This procedure protects the rights of the individuals. Usually within a short period (5 days or less, excluding weekends and holidays) a probable cause hearing has to take place to continue the person's hospitalization.

Taking away an individual's freedom through a commitment procedure is a serious matter. The U.S. Supreme Court has established the standard of clear and convincing evidence as the standard of proof that must be met for commitment. The criminal standard of "beyond a reasonable doubt" is not used.

Civil or Judicial Commitment

A judicial or civil commitment is for a longer amount of time than an emergency commitment. The legal basis for the extended detention of an individual for treatment lies in the *parens patriae* power of the state to protect and care for individuals with disabilities and the police power of the state to protect the community from persons who are a threat. For a judicial commitment, the individual has to be given time to prepare a defense that states why hospitalization is not necessary. The patient has the right to have his or her attorney cross-examine the mental health

professionals regarding the necessity for continued inpatient treatment.

Although many states usually use judicial or civil commitment for longer-term inpatient or residential treatment, at least 35 states have passed legislation for mandatory outpatient treatment (Cullen-Drill and Schilling, 2008). In California, AB 1421 Court-Ordered Outpatient Treatment went into effect on January 1, 2003, but it was applicable only in those counties that adopted a resolution to authorize its application. The purpose of mandating outpatient mental health treatment is to break the cyclic pattern of patients who, when discharged from an inpatient treatment facility, discontinue their medications, deteriorate, exhibit dangerous behavior, and subsequently require readmission to the acute psychiatric care setting. Nurses need to acknowledge their advocate role and yet balance patients' need for progressive mental health treatment. This includes activating patients' participation in outpatient treatment programs that effectively address the recurring nature of chronic mental illness.

PSYCHIATRIC ADVANCE DIRECTIVES

Virtually all states have developed statutes to govern the use of advanced directives that focus on anticipatory planning regarding general medical and psychiatric care (Appelbaum, 2004). Some states have special provisions and have made psychiatric models that allow a competent person to describe warning signs of declining mental health and consent to or refuse a treatment method. These models also allow a competent person to agree to commitment in a psychiatric care facility for a determined period of time and to appoint a surrogate (substitute) decision maker (Backlar et al, 2001).

In accordance with the principle of medical advance directives for health care, psychiatric advance directives are legal documents that are used when a patient is unable to participate in the decision-making process (O'Connell and Stein, 2005). The implementation of psychiatric advance directives reduces the average hospital length of stay, affects the burden on the mental health legal system, and significantly decreases involuntary commitments (Sherman, 1998; Backlar and McFarland, per PubMed, 1996).

CONFIDENTIALITY

The Health Insurance Portability and Accountability Act (HIPAA) of 1996 now regulates the protection and privacy of health information. This law guarantees the security and privacy of health information and outlines standards for enforcement. The final HIPAA Privacy Rule went into effect on April 14, 2003, for all health care providers (i.e., individuals or organizations that send bills or that are paid for health care). The Privacy Rule defines protected health information as any individually identifiable health information that an organization keeps, files, uses, or shares in an oral, electronic, or written form (Sharp HealthCare medication guidelines, 2002). Both civil and criminal penalties of fines and prison sentences were established under HIPAA for the knowing violation of patient privacy. Hoffman (2010) reviewed the new legal duty to disclose security breaches established by the 2009 HITECH Act regarding mental health records, including those related to psychotherapy and drug and alcohol treatment; these types of information have special additional privacy protection under the regulation (see Legal Case Report: Clinical Case Implications).

Nursing Implications

Nurses need to be knowledgeable about federal and state privacy regulations and understand their relevance to information management in the nurse's practice area. The American Nurses Association code of ethics (American Nurses Association, 1982) also defines the importance of keeping a patient's information confidential. At the time of admission to a mental health facility, admission staff often request that patients sign a release-of-information document. The release of information usually includes the following:

- The information that will be released
- The persons or parties that the information will be shared with, such as other health care providers and insurance providers
- The purpose of the release of the information
- The period of time during which the information will be released

The release of confidential patient information even for the best-intended purposes is risky. Even when presented with a subpoena for the release of protected health information, consulting with an attorney from the nurse's place of employment before such as release is advisable.

The confidentiality of the patient's information and the necessity of having a signed release from the patient before releasing information—even to family members who are closely involved with the patient's daily care—present challenges for the nurse. For instance, a paranoid patient who refuses to sign a release of information for his parents who are the caregivers will result in the nurse having to tell the parents when they telephone, "I'm sorry, but I'm not able to give you any information at this time." However, it is possible to also say, "However, if you have information that you think it would be important for me to know, I can listen to you." In this way, the family is able to communicate important medical or behavioral history to the treatment facility without the nurse releasing any information about the patient without that patient's permission.

PRIVILEGED COMMUNICATION

Privileged communication is different from confidentiality. It is enacted by statute to designated professionals such as clergy, attorneys, psychologists, or physicians. Several states are now including nurses and other health care professionals under these conditions; this reflects a major change in direction. The provisions of these statutes allow certain information given to professionals by patients to remain secret during any litigation. The privilege belongs to the patient, and only the patient can assert or waive this privilege. These statutes

---

LEGAL CASE REPORT: CLINICAL CASE IMPLICATIONS

Sexually Violent Predator: Commitment Standard • Kansas v. Hendricks (1997)

In a controversial 5-to-4 decision, the U.S. Supreme Court upheld a statute enacted by the state of Kansas. Leroy Hendricks had been convicted of sexual offenses against children. He had a 40-year history of sexual involvement with children, and he had been convicted on several occasions. Before his release, the state of Kansas petitioned to have Hendricks civilly committed under the state's Sexually Violent Predator Act. When he was stressed or pressured, he was unable to control his impulses. A jury in a lower state court found him to be a sexually violent predator, and the court civilly committed him. The court defined his pedophilia as a mental abnormality, but, on appeal to the Kansas State Supreme Court, the commitment was overturned. Hendricks' mental abnormality did not meet the commitment standard, which was based on mental illness. On appeal to the U.S. Supreme Court, the justices remarked that over the years, states have used many specialized terms to define mental health concepts. These definitions did not precisely fit with the terminology used by the medical community. The Court also said that the person must be unable to control his or her behavior and can be held until he or she no longer poses a danger to others. During the jury trial, Hendricks admitted that he could not control his behavior. The admission of a lack of control, along with a predictor of future dangerous behavior, satisfactorily distinguishes Hendricks from other dangerous persons who are more appropriately managed exclusively through criminal proceedings. Hendricks' diagnosis as a pedophile, which is considered a "mental disability" under the Act, is a clear qualification for due process. Because no effective treatment was offered at this stage, treatment was "nonexistent." The Court stipulated that it had never held that the constitution prevents states from detaining those for whom no treatment is available, yet still pose a danger to others. Treatment is not required for those who are dangerously mentally ill. There are built-in safeguards to ensure against an indefinite duration. The commitment is reviewed annually, and if the person no longer demonstrates dangerous behavior in the future, he or she can be released.

The dissenting opinion focused on several issues; the act was meant to segregate violent sexual offenders and to be a meaningful attempt to provide treatment. This had not been accomplished. "At the time of Hendricks' commitment, the state had not provided funds for treatment, it had not entered into treatment contracts, and it had few, if any, qualified staff. Offenders were not committed until sentences were near completion, there were no less restrictive alternatives, and any treatment available was not offered until the sentence had been completed.

Since this ruling, some states have moved toward enacting laws that would place sexual offenders who have completed their sentences in mental health facilities. This action places a responsibility on mental health professionals to develop programs of intervention that will lead to reducing the symptoms of these sexual offenders.

exclude the mandatory reporting of child, elder, impaired adult, and (in some instances) domestic violence; some communicable diseases that affect public safety; and information that will prevent a felony (e.g., murder) from occurring (see Legal Case Report: Clinical Case Implications).

LEGAL CASE REPORT: CLINICAL CASE IMPLICATIONS

Privileged Communication • Jaffee v. Redmond *(1996)*

In a U.S. Supreme Court decision, the justices ruled that a social worker—according to Illinois law and the Federal Rule of Evidence 501—did have privileged communication and that her patient could use privilege in keeping communications between them confidential. The patient, Mary Lu Redmond, was a police officer who had in the process of her duties shot and killed Ricky Allen. In a wrongful death lawsuit filed by Allen's estate after his death, the social worker and Redmond declined to answer questions about what took place during their therapeutic sessions. The judge directed the jury that the notes about the sessions must be negative in relation to the defendant. The jury sent back a verdict of $545,000 against the defendant, Redmond, on state and federal claims. Although the therapist was not an advanced practice nurse, if a state has a nurse-therapist–patient privilege, it seems likely that federal courts, on the basis of this decision, would recognize the privilege. Nurses need to be aware of the privileged communication statutes in the state in which they are practicing.

DUTY TO WARN AND PROTECTION: TARASOFF

During the mid-1970s, a landmark case changed the manner in which mental health professionals dealt with warning their patients' intended victims. That case, *Tarasoff v. Regents of the University of California* (1976), was about a young University of California student from India, Prosenjit Poddar. He had a relationship with Tatiana Tarasoff, and he had misinterpreted a New Year's Eve kiss as a serious romantic gesture. After several months had passed, Tarasoff told Poddar that she wished to date other men and that she did not view their relationship as serious. Poddar subsequently became depressed and sought mental health counseling. He communicated to his therapist that he would harm Tarasoff, who at that time was in South America. One day, he ran out of the therapist's office, and he was detained by campus police and then released. After Tarasoff's return, Poddar went to her home and fatally wounded her with a knife. The family of the victim brought suit against the University of California, and, after the case reached the Supreme Court of California, the justices ruled "protective privilege ends where the public peril begins." (*Tarasoff v. Regents of the University of California*, 1976). This ruling, called *duty to warn*, established the responsibility of a treating mental health professional to notify an intended and identifiable victim. Other states have

enacted similar statutes since *Tarasoff v. Regents of the University of California* to ensure that mental health professionals warn potential identifiable victims.

Nursing Implications

Nurses need to be aware of any case law related to duty to warn/Tarasoff policies within their jurisdictions. Nurses—especially advanced practice nurses—should know when to refer a patient for commitment and when to warn their patient's potential intended victims. Many mental health treatment facilities have duty-to-warn/Tarasoff policies and procedures in place that will guide nurses and other clinicians in the notification and documentation processes.

RIGHTS OF CLIENTS

Up until the last quarter of the 20th century, few gave any attention to the rights of individuals in mental health facilities; mental health laws that protect patient rights are therefore relatively new. These days, when individuals enter a mental health facility, they usually retain their civil rights, unless such rights are clearly restricted via the use of due process to certify that an individual lacks the capacity or competence to have them. These individuals retain the right to vote, to manage financial matters, to enter into contractual relationships, and to assert the constitutional right to seek the advice of an attorney. Other basic rights usually include the rights to send and to receive unopened mail, to wear one's own clothes, to receive visitors, to keep and use personal possessions, and to have access to a telephone.

Patients also have a right to be informed about potential risks, benefits, and reasonable alternatives before giving consent for any specific therapy, surgery, or treatment, including medication. Nurses need to disclose serious side effects that will be uncomfortable or irreversible to the patient. Patients are able to give informed consent unless there has been a judicial ruling to the contrary. In documented emergency or endangering situations, however, nurses are able to administer medications and treatment without the patient's consent.

Many states require that all patients receive a written summary of their rights in their own language on admission to an inpatient facility. In California, a list of patient rights (including the name and telephone number of the Office of Patient Advocacy) is required to be publicly posted in every mental health treatment facility. For non–English-speaking patients, it is important that the patient rights are in the patient's own language or presented via a qualified interpreting service. Treatment facilities are expected to know the dominant languages of the patients that they serve and to make provisions to have patient rights available in those languages.

Nursing Implications

The education of patients regarding their rights is an ongoing advocacy process and a major focus for nurses. Patients' diminished mental status and cognitive function at the time of admission when patient rights are reviewed often means that nurses have to use a variety of educational methods and repeat the material as a part of the treatment plan.

SECLUSION AND RESTRAINTS

Since the Middle Ages, mental health facilities have used seclusion and restraints (S/R) to control the behavior of persons with mental disorders. In October 1998, the *Hartford Courant* published a five-part investigative series of articles entitled "Deadly Restraints." It included a national survey that documented 142 deaths over the most recent decade that were directly related to the use of S/R. Congressional hearings followed, and federal reforms were proposed and implemented shortly thereafter (see the Research for Evidence-Based Practice box).

RESEARCH FOR EVIDENCE-BASED PRACTICE #1

Johnson ME: Being restrained: a study of power and powerlessness, *Issues Ment Health Nurs* 19:191-206, 1998.

Researchers conducted a phenomenologic study with 10 adult participants (5 men and 5 women) relating to their experiences of being restrained. Interviews were transcribed in their entirety. All participants had been controlled with leather restraints on a psychiatric unit. Generally, the attitude of psychiatric nurses had been that assisting patients with external limits helped them to feel safe and protected. Usually the restraint resulted from the patient's failure to conform to unit rules or from a feeling on the part of the staff that the behavior of these patients was escalating and out of control. Results of the study indicated that the participants felt coerced, vulnerable, helpless, and dehumanized. Johnson commented that, "We need to use restraints as a last resort." This study supports the need to use least restrictive interventions to help patients regain control, such as talking to patients, presenting anxiety-reducing strategies, or offering medications before using physical restraint, whenever possible.

As of August 2, 1999, the Health Care Financing Administration—now called the U.S. Centers for Medicare & Medicaid Services (CMS)—introduced new standards for the use of S/R for all Medicare and Medicaid participating hospitals. CMS declared that "the patient's right to be free of restraints is paramount" (Pennsylvania Department of Public Welfare, 2000). The new rules stated that health care professionals were to use S/R only when less restrictive alternatives to ensure patient safety had failed, such as talking to the patient. Coercion, discipline, punishment, and staff convenience were unacceptable reasons for placing a person in S/R. However, the most notable change was the implementation of the "1-hour rule," which requires a face-to-face evaluation by a licensed independent practitioner (LIP) within 1 hour of the initiation of restraints that were being used for

behavioral management. The face-to-face assessment is required even if the patient has been released from restraints before the arrival of the LIP. The definition of the LIP varies by state. In addition to physicians, psychologists and advanced practice nurses are sometimes able to order restraints, depending on the individual's license.

The second major reform came from the Joint Commission on Accreditation of Healthcare Organizations, now known as The Joint Commission (TJC). TJC issued new Restraint and Seclusion Standards for Behavioral Health that were made effective January 1, 2001 (Restraint and Seclusion Standards, 2000). The new TJC standards concurred with the CMS's "1-hour rule"; in addition, these standards required that the patient's family and legal representatives be notified when restraints are used, and the LIP is required to engage the clinical staff when reviewing alternative interventions. The staff is also now required to perform continuous in-person observation of any patient in restraints for the duration of the restraint procedure. Patients who are in seclusion are only to be monitored in person for the first hour. After that, the staff is able to use audio and video equipment.

The third set of reforms was in the Children's Health Act of 2000, which included national standards restricting the use of S/R in psychiatric facilities and in nonmedical community children's programs that were previously not covered by CMS and TJC standards.

The health care community has dramatically reduced the use of S/R, partly as a result of the new standards but also because of a new commitment on the part of mental health professionals to focus on restraint reduction as the best psychiatric nursing practice. From 1997 to 2000, Pennsylvania successfully reduced the incidence of S/R in its nine state hospitals by 74%, with no increase in staff injuries and without any additional funds. The state hospitals implemented key concepts, including identifying the use of S/R as a treatment failure, restriction of the use of S/R to emergency situations only, having adequate numbers of staff, and providing staff training in crisis prevention and nonviolent intervention.

Nursing Implications

In inpatient settings, nurses play a primary role in maintaining or changing unit culture with regard to the use of S/R. The leadership role of nurses in staff training, treatment planning, and performance improvement activities related to decreasing S/R is critical. "Never underestimate the difference one person can make" (Sharp HealthCare medication guidelines, 2002).

RIGHT TO TREATMENT

In the 1980s, a movement began in Alabama for the right to treatment for people with mental illnesses. With financial limitations within the mental health system, employees at Bryce Hospital were laid off because of a budget shortfall. As a result of this situation, a class action suit on behalf of the employees and patients was filed, alleging that with fewer employees the patients could not receive the proper treatment. The case was settled by consent decree in 1986. Many jurisdictions continue to follow some of the standards and guidelines specified, including the right to privacy and dignity, the right to the least restrictive treatment, and individual treatment plans. These plans included a statement of problems and intermediate and long-range treatment goals, with a timetable for attainment and rationales for the specified treatments.

The U.S. Supreme Court ruled that health care professionals cannot keep an individual in a mental hospital without treatment if he or she is not dangerous and is capable of defining and carrying out a plan of self-care in the community. Consider the following: Mr. Donaldson had been hospitalized in Florida for more than 14 years and wanted to be released. Because of his religion, he declined to take medication or to undergo other treatments. He was denied the privilege of going out on the grounds. He had a friend who was willing to assist him after discharge from the hospital. The ruling was limited, but it did set the standard that the state cannot detain individuals who are not dangerous without providing some mode of treatment (O'Connor v. Donaldson, 1975).

In the later decision *Youngberg v. Romeo* (1982), the U.S. Supreme Court ruled that a young man with profound retardation was entitled to "minimally adequate training" to provide him with safe conditions. The court stated that a qualified professional's judgment about this matter is "presumptively valid." There was great concern at the time that the right-to-treatment movement was over, but that is not entirely true: courts have upheld the concept of providing adequate treatment (*Woe v. Cuomo,* 1986). Therefore, the new generation of mental health nurses has a professional obligation to help patients seek out and engage treatment for mental illness at the least restrictive level. This will provide the greatly needed protective care regarding health care discrimination for this underserved population (Mental Health Equitable Treatment Act of 2001).

RIGHT TO REFUSE TREATMENT

During the late 1970s and the early 1980s, two well-known cases were litigated in the states of Massachusetts and New Jersey that were based on the right to refuse psychotropic medication. In the New Jersey case, Mr. Rennie was diagnosed with a psychotic disorder (schizophrenia) at one point and manic depression (bipolar disorder) at another time. There was no agreement about the appropriate medication to be administered. He was given the antipsychotics fluphenazine (Prolixin) and chlorpromazine (Thorazine) at different times. He suffered from documented side effects such as akathisia (a restlessness manifested by the inability to lie down or sit still) and wormlike movements of the tongue (a symptom that was indicative of tardive dyskinesia, which is a very serious side effect). He refused to take his medication. Rennie filed suit to prevent the involuntary administration of medications. After the courts heard the suit on four different occasions, they decided that voluntary and involuntary patients had the right to refuse medication.

During emergency situations, if there is potential danger, patients can be forcibly medicated. In the case of an involuntary patient, as long as nurses follow due process guidelines as established and the administration complies with accepted professional judgment, medication can be given (*Rennie v. Klein,* 1979, 1982). The administrative procedure includes the physician communicating with the patient about his or her mental health condition and outlining the plan of care with the patient when possible. If the patient refuses treatment, the medical director of the facility reviews the treatment recommendations and is authorized to call in an outside psychiatrist for consultation.

Rogers v. Okin was originally filed in 1975 (Rogers, 1979, 1980) as a class-action suit to stop a state hospital from certain seclusion practices and forcibly medicating patients. In this case, the courts reached a different conclusion. Instead of deferring to administrative procedures that rely on professional judgment, the right to refuse treatment is upheld if the patient is involuntary and competent. If the person is ruled incompetent, the judge uses the substituted judgment standard to determine the administration of medication (Muramatsu et al, 2010). The judge looks at whether the patient, if competent, would have chosen medication administration. With this decision, the court ruled that only a judicial authority—and not the decision of the physician or the guardian—was vital.

Nursing Implications

Nurses practicing in mental health facilities need to be aware of the state and case laws and policies and procedures for that jurisdiction regarding the administration of medication to voluntary and involuntary competent patients. Frequent nursing assessment for side effects and the careful documentation of patients' complaints related to side effects are essential for the adjustment or discontinuance of medication. Nurses need to carefully analyze and question the reason for the refusal of medication: is it because of the patient's denial of the illness or of the symptomatology of the condition, or is it because of side effects or displeasure with the treatment staff? Patient and family medication education by nurses, physicians, and pharmacists and a reassuring therapeutic relationship will greatly assist with medication adherence and minimize refusal (Sharp HealthCare medication guidelines, 2002) (see Chapter 25).

ELECTROCONVULSIVE THERAPY

The administration of electroconvulsive therapy (ECT) is still controversial, in part as a result of its portrayal in movies as a traumatic procedure. However, in many instances, it is an effective treatment for life-threatening depression. The patient needs to give informed consent for the procedure, which includes being knowledgeable about the risks and benefits. A potential side effect is memory loss that is usually temporary but that is sometimes irreversible.

The question of who can give informed consent is an issue. Previously, the American Psychiatric Association (1978) advised that, if an incompetent patient could not give informed consent, then a relative of the patient is sufficient. Later, if there is a question regarding competence, legal consultation or court guidance takes place. California recognizes that both voluntary and involuntary patients are sometimes capable or incapable of giving informed consent. A court hearing is held for incapable patients to determine whether the ECT treatment will be administered.

In the state of Washington, a patient has the right to refuse ECT unless there is clear and convincing evidence that it is necessary. The state must have compelling evidence that ECT is necessary and would be effective and that other forms of treatment have not been beneficial or are not available (www.ncbi.nim.nih.gov/pubmed/17032966. 1993). Some states, such as Tennessee, have regulations related to the administration of ECT to minors (Tennessee Code Annotated §33-3-105). Other states limit the number of treatments that a health care provider is able to give to an individual within a certain time frame. California limits the duration of the validity of the patient's informed consent to 30 days, during which a maximum of 15 treatments may be administered. In addition, an oversight ECT committee consisting of three ECT-qualified psychiatrists have to review each series of ECT treatments to determine the appropriateness and efficacy of that treatment (California Health & Safety Code, Title 9). Health care facilities have to report data on a quarterly basis to the state Department of Health. Data include the number of ECT treatments administered by age group and any serious medical complications (see Chapter 26 for more information about ECT, including nursing implications; see also Legal Case Report: Clinical Case Implications).

RESEARCH

The federal government has established guidelines that apply to research on human subjects. The major objective is to provide informed consent to the person who has agreed to participate in research projects. Some of the guidelines include a clear statement of the following:

- Purpose of the research
- Risks and possible discomforts to the subject
- Possible benefits to the individual or to others
- Alternative treatment procedures
- Confidentiality of records
- Sources for further information
- Availability of compensation if injury occurs

It is most important to note that the research is voluntary and that it clearly reflects autonomy on the participants' part (45Code of Federal Regulations [CFR] §46.116; Box 9-1).

Alzheimer's disease and other dementias will increase in number as the population ages. Because there are no animal models of this degenerative process, human experimentation is necessary. The National Institutes of Health has discovered that patients in the early stages of dementia are able to select health care proxies (substitutes) despite some "minimal

LEGAL CASE REPORT: CLINICAL CASE IMPLICATIONS

Involuntary Commitment • In the Interest of RAJ (1996)

In a recent case, a son petitioned for the involuntary commitment of his 62-year-old father, RAJ. The court found probable cause at a preliminary hearing to commit RAJ for no more than 14 days to the state hospital. At the hospital, he was diagnosed with bipolar disorder and alcohol abuse. At a later hearing, it was not concluded that he had a chemical dependency, but a judgment was issued that he was mentally ill, had impairment, and could be hospitalized for up to an additional 90 days. Because he was refusing to take medication, the court ordered that this intervention was the least restrictive option and that RAJ could be involuntarily medicated with haloperidol (Haldol) and carbamazepine (Tegretol) or with risperidone (Risperdal) and carbamazepine for 90 days. RAJ then appealed the decision related to the forced medication order. He contended that he had agreed to take the risperidone but not the other medication. The hospital argued that, if just one medication was refused, that would indicate that the patient had "effectively refused treatment that was necessary." The court noted that it must find by clear and convincing evidence that the treatment was necessary, that the patient refused it, that medication was the least restrictive alternative, and that the benefits outweighed the risks. The following items were also taken into consideration:

- The danger that the patient represented to himself or others
- The patient's current condition
- The patient's treatment history
- The results of previous medication trials
- The efficacy of current or past treatment modalities for this patient
- The patient's prognosis
- The effect of the patient's mental condition on his capacity to consent

The court ruled that the refusal to take one medication instead of the two prescribed amounted to the refusal of treatment in accordance with the forced medication statute. The medication haloperidol could be given in injectable form if RAJ refused the oral risperidone. The benefits outweighed the risks, and medication was the least restrictive form of treatment.

memory problems and word-finding difficulties"; in the early stages, they continue to "possess the capacity to make independent decisions" (www.alz.org/diagnostic_criteria/2010). As a safeguard to this process, a biochemist assesses all patients in these studies. In this manner, as the disease progresses and the research participants are no longer capable of giving informed consent, patients will have a health care proxy to speak for them (see Chapter 16)

Nursing Implications

Nurses need to be aware of research guidelines in their particular area of practice, especially when they are involved with

BOX 9-1	EXPERIMENTAL SUBJECT'S BILL OF RIGHTS

1 A statement that the procedure or treatment involves research, an explanation of the purposes of the research, the expected length of the subject's participation, an estimate of the subject's expected recovery time after the experiment, and identification of any procedures that are experimental.

2 An explanation of the procedures the subject will follow and any drug or device to be used, including the purposes of such procedures, drugs, or devices. If researchers are giving a placebo to a portion of the subjects involved in a medical experiment, all subjects need to be informed of this fact; however, they need not be informed as to whether they will actually receive a placebo.

3 A description of any reasonably foreseeable or expected risks or discomforts to the subjects.

4 A description of any benefits to the subject or to others that may reasonably be expected from the research.

5 A disclosure of appropriate alternative procedures or courses of treatment, if any, that will possibly be advantageous to the subject and their relative risks and benefits.

6 A statement describing how the researchers will maintain the confidentiality of records that identify the subject. For research subject to the U.S. Food and Drug Administration (FDA) regulations, this statement also has to specify that the FDA has the right to inspect the records of subjects participating in studies involving a drug or device subject to FDA regulation.

7 For research involving more than minimal risk, an explanation as to whether any compensation or medical treatments are available if injury occurs. This includes a description of the compensation and where a subject can obtain further information.

8 A statement that participation is voluntary, refusal to participate will involve no penalty or loss of benefits to the subject, and the subject has the right to end participation at any time without penalty or loss of benefits.

9 The name, institutional membership, if any, and address of the person or persons actually performing and primarily responsible for conducting the experiment.

10 The name of the sponsor or funding source, if any, or manufacturer if the experiment involves a drug or device, and the organization, if any, under whose general authority the experiment is being conducted.

11 The name, address, and telephone number of an impartial third party not associated with the experiment for the subject to address complaints about the experiment.

12 An offer to answer any questions concerning the experiment or procedures involved, a person to contact for answers to relevant questions about the research and the research subject's rights, and the person to contact in the event of a research-related injury.

From California Health and Safety Code Section 24172.

research projects to fulfill educational or clinical requirements. Many health care facilities are encouraging staff nurses to participate in research, and a thorough awareness of guidelines, including legal and regulatory implications, is imperative (Kotzalidis et al, 2008).

THE AMERICANS WITH DISABILITIES ACT

The Americans with Disabilities Act (42 United States Code [USC] §12101) is a substantial breakthrough in discrimination against people with mental illnesses; however, there are specific exclusions. The definition includes mental barriers that limit the ability of the individual in one or more major activities. Enforcement of the statute depends on the person's limitations. Courts have ruled that, if a person's mental condition is stabilized, then there is no disability (*Mackie v. Runyon*, 1992). However, such people are protected if the fact that they once had a mental disability (e.g., depression) is used against them in the employment situation. Some exclusions include persons who use controlled substances for unlawful purposes and individuals who take prescribed drugs without the supervision of a health care professional. In addition, people who are a direct threat to others are excluded. However, it is important to recognize that this must be based on the actual behavior of the individual and not on the mental disability itself.

An employer cannot ask a person about his or her history of mental health treatment as part of an application process for employment. The employer can only evaluate the individual regarding his or her ability to perform the job functions. Questions about the prior use of health care insurance coverage are also not permissible.

ADVOCACY

The term *advocacy* refers to speaking in favor of or arguing for a cause. As a result of the mental health movement that began during the 1970s, states developed advocacy programs for patients. Many states initiated internal grievance procedures to allow patients to express their views about their treatment. Under the Protection and Advocacy for Mentally Ill Individuals Act of 1986, all states were required to designate an agency that is responsible for maintaining the rights of people with mental illnesses. The names vary from state to state. For example, in Tennessee, Tennessee Protection and Advocacy, Inc., is the organization that is responsible for the implementation of this Act. There has been some controversy about this movement; some mental health professionals say that advocacy sets up adversarial relationships. Advocates need to have some understanding of the nature of mental illness and how the mental health system works.

Nursing Implications

With the increasing prevalence of managed care, patient advocacy has become a major part of the nurse's responsibility, especially in the case of nurse psychotherapists and psychiatric case managers who are seeking appropriate care for their patients from third-party payers. Simon (1998) has written that psychiatrists have to advocate with managed care organizations for the care that psychiatrists consider necessary. This strategy incorporates nurses calling managed care companies to obtain authorization for patient care. Nurses need to be well informed about the patient's right to appeal the denial of services that a mental health provider believes are medically necessary. Nurses need to help patients strongly pursue appeals, particularly in cases in which the patient is living in the community and the mental health provider believes that there is a potential for danger to the patient himself or herself or to others. Documentation that the patient has been clearly informed about these rights is also advisable. In addition to the responsibility to pursue appeals, the nurse is often responsible for providing adequate data so that a utilization reviewer is able to make an informed decision.

It is critical that nurses have a keen understanding of each patient's rights and that the nurse report to the health care provider and administration when those rights are violated. Nurses have a long history of being in the best position to serve as outspoken advocates for the patient; to continue in this role, they need to be aware of the changing laws and guidelines relative to mental health treatment (Rossetti et al, 2005).

FORENSIC EVALUATIONS

Individuals who have mental health problems and who are charged with or convicted of crimes fall within the category of forensic mental health services. During the 1960s and the 1970s, there were many exposés in professional journals and newspapers regarding the treatment of these individuals. In many instances, persons were sent to institutions for evaluation and remained there for years without the resolution of criminal charges. Procedural due process for many was nonexistent. Many forensic units were isolated and provided inadequate treatment. These conditions began to change in 1972 with the landmark decision *Jackson v. Indiana*. Mr. Jackson was mentally challenged and hearing and speech impaired. He was found incompetent to stand trial. Because of his disabilities, he probably would never become competent to stand trial. At that time, Indiana required hospitalization in a mental hospital until return to competency. Jackson was not going to become competent, so hospitalization would literally sentence him to a form of detention for life. His criminal charge was a robbery of a total of $9.

The U.S. Supreme Court ruled that an individual could be hospitalized only for a reasonable length of time (although this was not defined) and that the 3.5 years that Jackson had been detained was too long. If the state wanted to hospitalize him longer, he had to be civilly committed, which meant that he had to meet commitment standards, or else he had to be released. Recent technology advancements have arrived in the form of telepsychiatry and videoconferencing, which bring both effectiveness as well as legal issues that require nurses to

be both knowledgeable and well versed in the forensic domain (Antonacci et al, 2008).

Competency to Stand Trial

Competency to stand trial is a narrow concept. Criteria include the following:
- Does the individual charged with the crime understand the criminal charges?
- Is there an understanding of the legal process and the consequences of the charges?
- Can the individual advise an attorney and defend the charges?

Essentially, it is the person's awareness of the legal process that the mental health professional has to evaluate (see the Research for Evidence-Based Practice box).

RESEARCH FOR EVIDENCE-BASED PRACTICE #2

Appelbaum KL, Fisher WH: Judges' assumptions about the appropriateness of civil and forensic commitment, *Psychiatr Serv* 48:710-712, 1997.

Researchers completed a survey of Massachusetts district court judges related to forensic evaluations; 58 of 160 responded. The judges were asked the following: when civil commitment was available and the charge was a minor offense, why were individuals committed for a 20-day forensic evaluation for competency to stand trial? An overwhelming majority (93.1%) admitted concerns about the treatment of individuals in civil commitment in a mental health facility. Some of the reasons for this strategy included that the defendant did not meet commitment standards and that, on some occasions, psychiatric hospitals deny admission to offenders who meet commitment criteria unless the court orders the admission. A forensic commitment does not allow for early discharge; the defendant must remain for 20 days and must appear in court before discharge. This study confirms suspicions that judges order pretrial evaluations to fill perceived gaps in the civil system."

If the judge, prosecuting attorney, or defense attorney believes that competency is an issue, a request by the attorney results in a court-ordered evaluation to ask for an evaluation of the person's competency to stand trial. Many states recognize not only psychiatrists as competent evaluators of this issue but also psychologists, social workers, and advanced practice psychiatric nurses who have been educated and trained in this evaluation process. Many of these individuals now perform these evaluations on an outpatient basis, which results in a return to the courts and a more timely resolution of the charges (Laben and McLean, 1989).

Criminal Responsibility (Insanity Defense)

Competency to stand trial relates to the present mental condition of the defendants and their current ability to make a defense in court. The insanity defense relates to the state of mind at the time of the offense. This concept comes from the legal doctrine of *mens rea.* For a person to be found guilty, the individual must be able to form intent. If, because of mental illness, intent cannot be formed and the person is possibly responding to hallucinatory voices, there is no guilt involved (Melamed, 2010).

The first well-known case came from England, where the M'Naghten rule was declared. The set of circumstances involved Daniel M'Naghten, who shot and mistakenly murdered the secretary to the prime minister instead of his intended victim, Sir Robert Peel. M'Naghten intended to kill Peel because he had an irrational belief that Peel was plotting against him. He was found not guilty by reason of insanity, which caused great anxiety in England. Subsequently, a panel of 15 judges met and defined what has become known as the *M'Naghten rule.* An accused will not be held responsible if, at the time of the commission of the act, he or she was laboring under such a defect of reason, from disease of the mind, as to not know the nature and quality of the act he was doing, or if he did know it, that he did not know he was doing what was wrong" (Pridmore, 2004).

Much criticism of this doctrine emerged during the 1960s and the 1970s, and some states subsequently adopted a modern interpretation of the insanity defense, which states that a person is not responsible for criminal conduct if at the time of such conduct, as a result of mental disease or defect, the person lacks substantial capacity either to appreciate the criminality (i.e., wrongfulness) of the conduct or to conform his or her conduct to the requirements of the law (*Graham v. State of Tennessee,* 1977).

After a person is found not guilty by reason of insanity, he or she is usually hospitalized and sent to a psychiatric unit for evaluation of commitability. Many states have stricter release standards for individuals who are found not guilty by reason of insanity, because, although they have been found not guilty, they have committed a criminal act.

Guilty but Mentally Ill

Several states have adopted a new plea of guilty but mentally ill. The individual is found guilty, but, because of the plea that mental illness caused the person to commit the crime, the person is sent to prison and treated for the mental illness. Many thought that fewer people would adopt an insanity defense with the guilty but mentally ill plea. However, this has not always proved to be the case. In Michigan, the number of individuals pleading guilty but mentally ill has increased; while in Georgia, the number of individuals pleading guilty but mentally ill has decreased.

Nursing Responsibilities in the Criminal Justice System

In several states, advanced practice nurses can testify regarding the issue of competency to stand trial. Nurses should not take this lightly, and they should seek special education before testifying about this issue. In most states, psychologists with doctoral degrees and psychiatrists testify for the insanity defense. Many states have highly specialized psychiatric units staffed with forensic psychiatric nurses trained in clinical-legal observation and the treatment of victims and violent offenders (Kent-Wilkinson, 2010).

MALPRACTICE

Because of the irreversible side effects of some medications given to individuals with mental health problems and the trend of short-term hospitalizations, nurses working in psychiatric settings need to be aware of situations that will potentially lead to a malpractice lawsuit. Negligence, which is the primary basis for malpractice lawsuits, is a civil dispute between two or more citizens or between an individual and a health care facility. A person alleges that a professional ignored or committed an act that a reasonably prudent professional would not have done. The action of the professional causes injury that results in measurable damages.

Elements of a Malpractice Suit Based on Negligence

To bring a suit, the plaintiff must establish that a nurse had a legal duty or relationship to that person to provide a certain standard of care. The second aspect to establish in that relationship is a breach of duty. The care is then measured by the reasonably prudent nurse standard: what would another nurse working in a mental health facility have done in the same situation? The clarification of the community standard and the nursing care standard in practice at a given facility may be presented via the use of fact witnesses, who bring to the court given facts without opinion regarding the case. Usually expert witnesses testify regarding adherence to or departure from the standard of care and provide opinions about the impact of these on the issues of the case. Some jurisdictions look to a reasonably prudent nurse standard; however, the standards of care of the American Nurses Association and the American Psychiatric Nurses Association in relationship to psychiatric nursing practice can also be applied in a lawsuit (Statement on Psychiatric Mental Health Nursing Practice, 1994). A poor outcome does not necessarily mean that an act of negligence has occurred. The next element that a court explores is whether the injury (i.e., damages) was predictable on the basis of the nurse's actions and the set of circumstances that followed. The court explores whether the nurse was the causal link in the injury that occurred. This is defined by establishing the connection between the nurse's acts of negligence and the alleged damages with the use of two tests that are accepted throughout the United States: (1) the "but for" test, which questions whether the alleged damages would not have occurred but for the act of negligence; and (2) the substantial factor test, which investigates whether the negligence was a substantial factor in causing the alleged damages. For example, did the nurse give the wrong medication, or did the nurse not know about drug interactions with certain medications that led to the injury? The last element that a court has to determine is whether there is a proven injury because of the nurse's behavior. The most damaging and reckless behavior that a nurse could be associated with would involve gross negligence, which is defined as acting with willful and conscious disregard for the rights and safety of others.

Documentation

The state or the mental health facility in which the nurse is practicing often regulates the information that needs to be documented in a mental health record. Although many mental health professionals view comprehensive charting as a challenge, reflected clinical information is not just a record of the care of the patient; it is also a legal document that is valuable in any litigation that takes place.

Adequate and legible documentation is the best means of defense against a lawsuit and the best way to validate that the nurse and other health care professionals adhered to their scope of practice and to a safe standard of care. It is important to be specific and to document symptoms by writing in quotes what the patient expresses to you, such as "I am hearing voices that say I am a bad person." Recording the actual words of the patient is more definitive than simply noting, "The patient is hallucinating," especially if the words are destructive to the patient or others. Nurses need to chart

in a timely and legible manner. Recording at the time that something happens is more adequate than block charting, which is usually briefer and not as definitive (*Nurse's Legal Handbook*, 2004). A patient's record is a sequential document; thus, it does not save space for late entries. Nurses need to label late entries as such and initial them (see Legal Case Report: Clinical Case Implications)

In a mental health record, it is especially important to document when the person has achieved the goals outlined in the treatment plan. If the individual has an exacerbation of the illness, the treatment plan needs to reflect the change. Informed consent regarding the giving of psychiatric medications is an important aspect of the chart, especially medications such as some neuroleptics, which cause irreversible side effects or provide chemical restraint.

Records are an excellent source for communicating with other mental health professionals on the staff as well as with other agencies. Records are also used to validate reimbursement for care that the agency gave the patient. Because managed care is becoming more common, nurses need to carefully record a clear outline of all of the patient's

---

LEGAL CASE REPORT: CLINICAL CASE IMPLICATIONS

Nurse's Responsibility • Hatley v. Kassen *(1992)*

Pennie Johnson had been mentally ill for 10 years. She had been an outpatient in a forensic unit, because long-term inpatient treatment was considered nontherapeutic. Because of her long-term history, a difficult patient file had been established to assist treating physicians. In February 1988, a state trooper picked Johnson up on a toll road, at which time she threatened suicide. She was taken to a county hospital. During the nursing assessment, Johnson stated that she was feeling increasingly depressed and that she had ingested medication that exceeded the prescribed dosage. She continued to take this medication in front of the hospital staff, at which time it was removed from her.

She was examined by Dr. Kalra, who decided to discharge her, because he thought her condition had not changed. Johnson asked both the nurse who assessed her and the nursing supervisor, Ms. Kassen, RN, to return her medication. She announced that if they did not return the medication, she would throw herself in front of a car. Kassen told Johnson that, if she would return home in a taxicab paid for by the hospital, Kassen would return the medication. Johnson declined the offer. A security officer was instructed to escort Johnson out of the hospital. There was disputed testimony as to whether the physician knew about Johnson's threats. Thirty minutes after leaving the hospital, Johnson stepped in front of a truck and was killed.

Johnson's parents brought an action for damages against Kassen. In the lower court decision, a summary judgment (which is granted when no genuine issue of material fact is presented) was awarded to the physician and the hospital, and a directed verdict was entered in favor of Kassen (this is a decision that is directed to the jury by the judge because the opposing party has not sufficiently presented its case) (Weiner and Wettstein, 1993). The Court of Appeals of Texas reversed

the decision and sent the case back to the lower court for further litigation, stating that the doctor and the nurse were not entitled to official immunity because they were employed at a government hospital.

The court, in its decision, did note the testimony of three expert witnesses regarding Kassen's nursing care. Two nurse experts testified that Kassen's actions were substandard when she knew that Johnson had communicated suicidal intentions with a specific plan. A psychiatric expert in the field of suicidology testified that Kassen should have sought the advice of the physician or supervisor before releasing Johnson after the suicide threats.

One judge wrote a dissenting opinion. This justice believed that Johnson had threatened for 10 years to commit suicide and had never done so; therefore, it was not foreseeable that Johnson would follow through with her threat, and thus it was not negligence on Kassen's part. The judge held that threats of suicide could not enslave the intended victim to either submission or damages—especially threats that have been "empty" for years.

This case was sent for retrial, so the final results are unknown. However, elements of the case are useful for analytic purposes. The nurses and the doctor had a duty to a patient who was brought to the emergency department. Several experts testified that, when a patient has a suicide plan, some form of hospitalization should be instituted or, at minimum, a supervisor should be notified or another discussion held with the physician. On the basis of this testimony, it might be concluded that the nurse's actions fell below the standard of care. Because the nurse permitted the patient to leave the hospital, she could be targeted as a causal agent in the resulting death, and damages could be awarded for the incident (Weiner and Wettstein, 1993).

symptoms to document the necessity for continued care or for an increased or decreased level of care (e.g., controlled structured environment, increased observation, medication stabilization, and continued hospitalization). For example, if routine hospitalization is for 5 days but the patient continues daily to verbalize suicidal thoughts, recording this information is critical for extended permission to continue the hospitalization.

Do not use improper abbreviations that the agency does not authorize. Nurses need to obtain records from other facilities or other treating professionals to provide an accurate long-term picture of how the patient was treated on previous occasions.

Nurses need to document in writing all patient education, aftercare plans, participation in a treatment team, and referral to other agencies for care. The accurate recording of vital signs is essential, especially when patients are taking psychotropic medications. Nurses will need to define and communicate their observations about the efficacy of prescribed medication in the chart and to the physician. Clearly document all notifications and order clarifications. Nurses also need to complete any nursing assessments that the organization requires. Careful documenting also means spelling words correctly and making sure that sentences are grammatically correct. If a nurse makes an error in documentation, he or she needs to place a single line through the words without making them illegible and then initial the error (see Legal Case Report: Clinical Case Implications).

Sexual Misconduct

From studies that have been conducted with social workers, psychiatrists, and psychologists, researchers have estimated that up to 14% of these professionals have had a sexual relationship with a patient (Somer and Nachmanil, 2005). There has not been a study of nurses; however, cases for the removal of a nursing license for such activity are on record (*Heinecke v. Department of Commerce*, 1991). All mental health professions consider such behavior unethical, and, in many states, this behavior is criminal, especially if it is within a few months of the therapeutic relationship. Some states have mandatory reporting laws for a second therapist who learns about such behavior.

Many of the cases are settled out of court (*Hall v. Schulte*, 1992). When information about the relationship is presented to a jury, members tend to be sympathetic to the patient, except when a patient appears to have encouraged the relationship. Because the patient comes to a therapist with a problem, the issue of the transference phenomenon becomes pronounced, thus resulting in a true lack of consent with regard to becoming involved with the therapist.

Suicide and Homicide

Malpractice suits and wrongful death actions for homicidal patients' injury to a third party and death from suicide have become more common. Some states have ruled that individuals working in government agencies have sovereign immunity and are protected from liability in malpractice situations

(*Poss v. Department of Human Resources*, 1992; *Smith v. King*, 1993). When conducting nursing assessments that include a suicidal component, use extreme caution. For example, when an individual threatens intent of suicide with a defined plan and demonstrates lethality and access to the means to commit suicide, nurses must communicate this information, in a timely manner, to a mental health provider. Then health care providers must follow the appropriate steps to provide patient safety, including involuntary commitment, to escape liability. If there is a question, the nurse should seek legal consultation. However, "clinicians are not liable for errors of clinical judgment; they are liable only for departures from the relevant standard of care, given the clinical situation." (Weiner and Wettstein, 1993, p. 119).

Because of the previously described decision regarding *Tarasoff v. Regents of the University of California*, it is important to communicate with the mental health treatment team when a patient threatens to harm someone. Many states require that health care providers notify a potential victim or police of this occurrence. Some states have limited the warning to include only identifiable victims (*Leonard v. Iowa*, 1992; Rudegair and Appelbaum, 1992). Failure to comply with the required notification will lead to exposure and major liability.

ETHICAL ISSUES

Ethical issues are connected to legal implications for nursing care. Ethics is that body of knowledge that explores the moral problems surrounding specific issues. In nursing practice, look at the rules, principles, and ethical guidelines that the nursing profession has developed to guide conduct. Laws reflect the moral character of a society and are developed (it is hoped) with an ethical basis; therefore, consider ethical principles when evaluating a dilemma or a problematic situation. Many ethical problems occur in the arena of mental health law when statutes conflict with a nurse's personal beliefs.

Autonomy

The term *autonomy* refers to having respect for an individual's decisions or self-determination regarding health care issues. This point is especially important with problems such as the right to die and, in mental health, treatment with the use of the least restrictive alternative. When involuntary commitment is necessary, it is difficult for mental health providers to have to follow the law rather than to do what the patient currently desires. The caregiver will want to allow the patient to make decisions, but, if the individual is demonstrating intent by threatening suicide with an active plan, proceeding against the wishes of the person is necessary for safety and compliance with the law. This kind of decision in ethical terms is called a *paternalistic decision* or *parentalism* (Purtilo, 1993). This often causes a great deal of anxiety for the new health care professional.

In addition, it is sometimes difficult for families when the member who is mentally ill and refusing treatment has to be

Matt Morgan was playing a card game with his parents and his sister when he left the room, returned with a gun, and shot and killed his parents. His sister was injured but survived. Matt had problems during his senior year of high school, and, after graduation, he had difficulty retaining employment. He was verbally abusive to his parents, and they had become afraid of him. In January 1990, police removed him from his home as he was attempting to fight with his father.

After a period of wandering, Matt eventually presented to the emergency department at a hospital in Philadelphia. He was diagnosed with schizophreniform disorder and transferred to a mental health facility. He had delusions that the government was affecting his body and the airwaves so that he was unable to watch television or listen to tapes or radio, and he had delusions of persecution, ideas of reference, and thought broadcasting. He was given thiothixene (Navane), and he was admitted to a respite unit.

During the 12-week stay at the respite unit, Matt continued to receive thiothixene and intensive therapy. He had paranoia concerning his family, but this decreased, and he was able to admit that the medication helped him to manage his symptoms. He acknowledged that his conflicts with his family, especially his relationship with his father, could be attributed to his mental illness. The treating physician thought that it was in Matt's best interest to return to his home and to be followed at the Fairfield Family Counseling Center (FFCC). His parents came to get him at the end of June 1990, and he was first seen in the FFCC on July 16, 1990.

A psychotherapist initially saw Matt, and then Matt was referred to Dr. Brown, a contract psychiatrist for medication evaluation, on July 19, 1990. Dr. Brown reported that Matt had been in some sort of mental health facility in Philadelphia and that he was out of medication. Dr. Brown noted that "Matt came to the mental health clinic for his medication, continued care, and help in completing a Social Security Disability form." Dr. Brown concluded that Matt had some form of atypical psychosis and that he did not appear to have a thought disorder or schizophrenia. Dr. Brown also noted that he thought Matt might be malingering in an attempt to obtain disability. Dr. Brown wrote that it was more prudent to defer diagnosis, continue taking the medication, obtain Matt's records from Philadelphia, and schedule another appointment in a month. When Matt returned for his appointment, the records from the mental health unit in Philadelphia were available, but the court reported that it was clear from Dr. Brown's testimony that he never read them or attempted to contact the treating physician.

Dr. Brown reduced the dosage of thiothixene and wrote again about the possibility of malingering. Dr. Brown saw Matt on October 11, 1990, for the last time; he prescribed a tapering and discontinuation of the thiothixene. He stated that Matt would continue in psychotherapy. Matt was referred to a vocational counselor to assist him with finding employment. Between October 1990 and January 1991, Matt remained in psychotherapy and vocational counseling. However, his mother reported that Matt's condition was deteriorating. He was pacing and showed a quiet demeanor, withdrawal, and irritability. She said that Matt had given a deposit toward the purchase of a gun and asked that he be placed back on medication. The vocational counselor thought that the mother was overprotective. When Matt failed to keep his appointment with the psychotherapist in January 1991, it was decided that the only person who should see him was the vocational counselor.

Matt's condition continued to worsen, his parents became afraid of him, and he once again developed symptoms of paranoia. During May 1991, Matt's mother continued to report Matt's deterioration. An appointment was scheduled with Dr. Brown, but Matt did not keep it. Matt's employer remarked that Matt did not have the strength to push a lawnmower, was on the verge of fainting, and he did not appear to be in complete touch with reality. On June 14, 1991, Matt's mother wrote a letter to FFCC seeking help for her son. She explained her concerns about his potential violence. The vocational counselor and a licensed social worker conducted an assessment. FFCC had an unwritten policy that no involuntary commitment would be initiated without family involvement; however, when the family attempted such a course of action, the probate court informed them that it would need the vocational counselor's approval.

On July 20, 1991, Matt's parents sent a letter to a psychologist employed at FFCC who reviewed the record, talked with the vocational counselor and social worker, and determined that Matt could not be given medication against his will and could not be hospitalized. Another social worker commented on July 25, 1991, that Matt was losing weight and deteriorating. That evening, Matt shot his family.

In an action for negligence brought by the parents' estate, expert witnesses for the plaintiffs, (the Morgan estates) testified that Dr. Brown's treatment of Matt was negligent for failure to read the prior treatment reports, for failure to diagnose, for discontinuing needed medication, and for failure to closely monitor Matt after discontinuation of the medication. The fact that a vocational therapist was making commitment decisions was of particular concern. One expert testified that it was foreseeable that, without medication, this created a potential for violent behavior. The expert stipulated that "The only reason Matt killed his parents was because he was taken off medication and didn't receive proper care."

The expert witnesses testified that, when Matt refused medication due to his deteriorating condition, the action at that point should have included strong involvement by his family, making Matt's participation in vocational therapy contingent upon ongoing treatment, and telling Matt that he faced involuntary hospitalization unless he began taking his medication.

The court in its ruling stipulated that the relationship between a psychotherapist and a patient in an outpatient setting is considered a special relationship; therefore, it is the duty of the psychotherapist to protect against the patient's violent tendencies. The court went on to say that "the outpatient environment provides sufficient, effective measures of control to justify imposing the duty to protect on the psychotherapist. The duty to protect is also in the public's best interests as it protects the public from patients with violent tendencies, in accordance with Ohio law."

The trial court had dismissed this action, and the court of appeals affirmed in part and reversed in part. The Supreme Court held that the psychotherapist had a duty to protect against the patient's potentially violent behavior. The case was returned to the trial court to settle the issues of whether the defendants were negligent and whether a summary judgment in the defendant's favor was warranted.

What nurses need to learn from this case is that any treating therapist needs to be aware of the duty to hospitalize and protect families and the public when appropriate. Consultation by nurse clinicians with mental health professionals who have legal authority to commit is essential.

involuntarily hospitalized. Educating the family about the illness, being supportive, and allowing all of the family members to express their frustration, anxieties, and any anger will be helpful for the family.

Olsen (1998) has raised an interesting question about autonomy and privacy in relation to the video monitoring of psychiatric patients who are placed in seclusion. One loses autonomy when secluded or restrained, and compounding this situation with video monitoring is threatening to a patient. To justify the use of such strategies, Olsen has recommended that health care providers keep a record that acknowledges that a monitor is being used and the therapeutic reason for such use. The patient needs to be informed of the monitoring, perhaps with the placement of a sign in the seclusion room. Olsen contends that only staff with clinical responsibility for the care of the patient should have access to the monitor, that only clinically competent staff should monitor patients, and that the nurse should perform personal visualization and assessment of the patient. Ethical experts stipulate that "ethical treatment is determined by weighing the benefits of a safer environment with the risk of harm that could result from a loss of privacy."

Beneficence

Individuals who work in the health care field have a special duty and responsibility to act in a manner that is going to benefit rather than harm patients. The term *beneficence* refers to bringing about good (Purtilo, 1993). The goal in mental health treatment is to assist individuals with returning to a mentally healthy way of life.

The moral rule of *primum non nocere* ("first do no harm") is vital in clinical interventions with persons who have mental illnesses. Situations in which this issue will possibly occur include giving neuroleptic medications when certain side effects are irreversible. Another instance is the consideration of giving ECT to a patient who has failed to respond to antidepressive medication and who continues to be suicidal. It is known that memory loss is sometimes a side effect of ECT. Do the beneficial aspects of the treatment outweigh its possible side effects? This dilemma causes anxiety for the patient, the family, and the mental health professional during the decision-making process.

Certainly, when a mental health professional considers a sexual relationship with a patient, preventing harm is the major consideration. According to the literature, the professional who becomes involved with a patient uses denial and rationalizes that the patient desires the relationship, that the therapeutic relationship has ended, or that it took place outside of the therapeutic time (Russell, 1993). Russell writes

that it is important for students to become aware of their own sexual feelings for and possible attraction to a patient and that this is an important part of the mental health curriculum, especially for students who later hope to specialize in this area.

Distributive Justice

According to Purtilo (1993), the term *distributive justice* refers to the "comparative treatment of individuals in the allotment of benefits and burdens." "The principle of justice holds that a person should be treated according to what is fair, given what is due or owed" (Chally and Loriz, 1998, p. 17). During times of health care cost constraints, who is going to get treatment and the cost of the treatment are frequent topics of debate. In managed care, mental health care is not always treated equally with physical health; the mental health needs of patients are often compromised. Many nurses who work in a mental health setting find that, to access mental health care, it is necessary to become an active advocate for the patient with the primary care provider. When there is an annual cap (i.e., a limit) on the amount of money that a managed care organization is allowing for each individual in a health care plan, resistance to treating a person with a serious and persistent mental illness will occur, especially when this person needs a variety of services over a long period of time.

A major question is the treatment site for individuals with medical and mental health problems. It is not uncommon for a mental health unit to not want to admit a person with serious physical health problems, and a medical unit may not want to admit someone with severe mental health problems who also has a physical problem. These issues are going to become more widespread as the nation moves more toward managed care to control health care costs. How is the United States going to divide the health care dollar, and where will individuals with mental illnesses fit into the picture (Lazarus, 1994)?

An editorial in the *American Journal of Psychiatry* reported that "under managed care, the actual dollar amounts spent on all mental illness treatment have decreased" (Leslie and Rosenheck, 1999, p. 1250). There is growing concern that, because people with the diagnosis of major depression have high rates of health care use, the managed care organizations will "dump" them or fail to provide adequate care, thus resulting in a longer duration of illness.

Mental health parity (equality) bills have been introduced and passed in some states. In addition, some states have passed their own statutes that give patients a bill of rights in relation to reimbursement for mental health care.

CHAPTER SUMMARY

- Balancing the rights of the mentally ill with those of the community has been and continues to be a struggle.
- Alternatives to inpatient mental health treatment need to consider the least restrictive environment and make use of the least restrictive treatment.
- There are three types of commitments for a patient with a mental illness: an emergency commitment, a voluntary commitment, and an involuntary indefinite commitment.
- Patients need to be informed about treatment, including its risks and alternatives, on admission.
- The civil or judicial commitment of a patient is legally based in *parens patriae,* which is the power of the state to protect and care for disabled individuals, and the police power of the state to protect the community from persons who are a threat.
- Half of the states in the United States have enacted preventive or mandatory outpatient treatment in which patients can be returned to the hospital if they discontinue treatment or medication, deteriorate, or exhibit dangerous behavior after discharge.
- Patients with mental illnesses retain their civil rights when they enter a mental hospital or another inpatient treatment center. Patients need to receive a summary of their rights when they are admitted.

- Restrain patients only to prevent physical injury to the patients themselves or to others. Only a psychiatrist or a licensed physician is able to order nonemergency seclusion or restraint.
- Patients who are ruled competent and who are voluntarily or involuntarily committed have a right to refuse treatment and medication.
- The U.S. Supreme Court ruled that individuals charged with or convicted of a crime could only be hospitalized for a reasonable length of time. To be committed longer requires a person to be civilly committed or released.
- Competency to stand trial is based on a person's current awareness of the legal process as evaluated by a mental health professional.
- The insanity defense comes from the concept that, for a person to be found guilty, the person must be able to form intent and relate to his or her state of mind at the time of the offense.
- Several states have adopted a new plea: guilty but mentally ill. Because the plea states that mental illness caused the commission of the crime, the person is sent to prison and treated for mental illness.
- Nurses working in psychiatric settings need to be aware of situations that will possibly lead to malpractice lawsuits.

REVIEW QUESTIONS

1. An individual is found not guilty by reason of insanity after planting explosive devices in a local church. What would be the nurse's expectations regarding this person?
   1. The individual will be treated for mental illness in a prison or another forensic setting.
   2. The individual will be unable to provide useful assistance to the defense attorney.
   3. The individual will have a new trial after psychiatric stability has been attained.
   4. The individual will have been unable to act with intent at the time of the offense because of mental illness.
2. An adult patient assaulted another patient in an acute psychiatric unit and was unable to be managed through less restrictive means. The patient was restrained at 13:45. By what time must the patient have a face-to-face assessment by the physician?
   1. 14:45
   2. 15:45
   3. 17:45
   4. 13:45 on the following day
3. Which individual with a mental illness may require emergency or involuntary hospitalization for mental illness?
   1. The individual who sees visions of angels dancing on the television screen.
   2. The individual who throws a lamp at the owner of a local department store.

   3. The individual who resumes using cocaine after 1 year of being clean.
   4. The individual who stops taking prescribed antipsychotic medications.
4. A nurse at a local mental health clinic prepares to give a patient with schizophrenia a regularly scheduled monthly antipsychotic medication injection. Just before the nurse gives the injection, the patient says, "Wait! I've changed my mind. I don't want to take that medicine anymore." Which initial action by the nurse would be legally and ethically appropriate?
   1. Saying, "You have a right not to take it, but let's talk about how that could affect your illness."
   2. Reminding the patient that this medication has been used for months with no adverse effects
   3. Assessing the patient for evidence of dangerousness to self or others
   4. Calling for assistance to restrain the patient and proceeding with the scheduled injection
5. A nurse's neighbor asks, "Why aren't people with mental illnesses kept in state institutions anymore?" Select the nurse's accurate response or responses. You may select more than one answer.
   1. "Better drugs for mental illness now make it possible for many people to live in their communities."

REVIEW QUESTIONS—cont'd

2. "There are less restrictive settings available now to care for individuals with mental illness."
3. "Our nation has fewer people with mental illness; therefore, fewer hospital beds are needed."
4. "Psychiatric institutions are no longer popular as a consequence of negative stories in the press."
5. "Funding for the treatment of mental illness has shifted to community rather than institutional settings."
6. Benjamin Franklin invented the lightning rod, a device that saved lives and property in early American history. He refused to patent the invention, because he wanted it widely shared for the well-being of humankind. Franklin's action can best be correlated with which ethical principle in health care?
1. Autonomy
2. Beneficence
3. Distributive justice
4. Parity

REFERENCES

American Nurses Association: *Code for nurses*, Kansas City, Mo, 1982, American Nurses Association.

American Psychiatric Association: *Electroconvulsive therapy: task force report 14*, Washington, DC, 1978, The Association.

Americans With Disabilities Act (42 United States Code [USC] §12101).

Antonacci DJ et al: Empirical evidence on the use and effectiveness of telepsychiatry via videoconferencing: implications for forensic and correctional psychiatry, *Behav Sci Law* 26:253-269 2008.

Appelbaum P: Law & psychiatry: psychiatric advance directives and the treatment of committed patients, *Psychiatr Serv* 55:751-763, 2004.

Backlar P et al: Consumer, provider, and informal caregiver opinions on psychiatric advanced directives, *Adm Policy Ment Health* 28:427, 2001.

Backlar P, McFarland H: A survey on use of advanced directives for mental health treatment in Oregon, *Psychiatr Serv* 47:1387, 1996.

Brakel SJ et al: *The mentally disabled and the law*, ed 3, Chicago, 1985, American Bar Foundation.

California Health & Safety Code 24172, Experimental subject's bill of rights, California Welfare & Institutions Code, Title 9 (45 Code of Federal Regulations [CFR] §46.116).

Cullen-Drill M, Schilling K: The case for mandatory outpatient treatment, *J Psychosoc Nurs Ment Health Serv* 46:33, 2008.

Chally PS, Loriz L: Ethics in the trenches: decision making in practice, *Am J Nurs* 98:17, 1998

General requirements for informed consent, Department of Health and Human Services, National Institutes of Health, Office for Protection of Research Risks 45 C.F.R. § 46.116, 1991.

Graham v. State of Tennessee, 541 SW2d 531 (Tenn 1977).

Hall v. Schulte, 836kP2d 989 (Ariz Or of App 1992).

Harshey-Meade G: Dorothea Dix: she was a nurse, advocate and lobbyist, *Ohio Nurses Rev* 81:6, 2006.

Health Insurance Portability and Accountability Act of 1996.

Heinecke v. Department of Commerce, 810 P2d 459 (Utah App 1991).

Hoffman S: Breach notification and the law, *J Clin Ethics* 21(1):42-43, 2010.

Jackson v. Indiana, 406 US 715 (1972).

Johnson ME: Being restrained: a study of power and powerlessness, *Issues Ment Health Nurs* 19:191-206, 1998.

Kent-Wilkinson AE: Forensic psychiatric/mental health nursing: responsive to social need, *Issues Ment Health Nurs* 31:425, 2010.

Kotzalidis G et al: Ethical questions in human clinical psychopharmacology: should the focus be on placebo administration? *J Psychopharmacol* 22:590-597, 2008.

Laben JK, McLean CP: *Legal issues and guidelines for nurses who care for mentally ill*, Owings Mills, Md, 1989, National Health Publishing.

LaFond JQ: Law and the delivery of involuntary mental health services, *Am J Orthopsychiatry* 64:409, 1994.

Lake v. Cameron, 364 F2d 657 (DC Cir 1966 en banc).

Lamb HR, Weinberger LE: Persons with severe mental illness in jails and prisons: a review, *Psychiatr Serv* 49:483, 1998.

Lanterman-Petris-Short Act of 1969.

Lazarus A: Disputes over payment for hospitalization under mental health "carve out" programs, *Hosp Community Psychiatry* 45:115, 1994.

Leonard v. Iowa, 491 NW2d 508 (Iowa Sup Ct 1992).

Leslie DL, Rosenheck R: Shifting care to outpatient mental health care: use and cost under private insurance, *Am J Psychiatry* 156:1250, 1999.

Mackie v. Runyon, 804 F Supp 1508 (1992).

Melamed Y: Mentally ill persons who commit crimes: punishment or treatment? *J Am Acad Psychiatry Law* 38:100, 2010.

Mental Health Equitable Treatment Act of 2001.

Muramatsu RS et al: Alternative formulations, delivery methods, and administration options for psychotropic medications in elderly patients with behavioral and psychological symptoms of dementia, *Am J Geriatr Pharmacother* 8:98, 2010.

Nurse's legal handbook, 5th ed, Springhouse, Pa, 2004, Springhouse.

O'Connell M, Stein C: Psychiatric advance directives: perspectives of community stakeholders, *Adm Policy Ment Health* 32:241, 2005.

O'Connor v. Donaldson, 422 U5 563 (1975).

Olsen DP: Ethical consideration of video monitoring psychiatric patients in seclusion and restraint, *Arch Psychiatr Nurs* 12:90, 1998.

Pennsylvania Department of Public Welfare, Office of Mental Health and Substance Abuse Services: *Leading the way toward a seclusion and restraint-free environment—Pennsylvania's seclusion and restraint reduction initiative,* Harrisburg, Pa, 2000, Office of Mental Health and Substance Abuse Services.

Poss v. Department of Human Resources, 426 SE2d 635 (Go Or App 1992).

Pridmore S: M'Naghten rules, *Aust N Z J Psychiatry* 37:478, 2004.

Purtilo R: *Ethical dimensions in the health professions,* ed 2, Philadelphia, 1993, WB Saunders.

Rennie v. Klein, 416 F Supp 1294 (1979); 653 F2d 836 (3rd Cir 1981); 454 US 1978 (1982).

Restraint and seclusion standards for behavioral health (effective January 1, 2001). Joint Commission for the Accreditation of Healthcare Organizations (websites). www.jointcom mission.org/2009, www.2.ed.gov/policyseclusion/seclusion-state-summaryhtml-July, 2009. Accessed November 2000.

Rogers v. Okin, right to refuse treatment for a mental illness, 478 F Supp. 1342 (Mass, 1979); F .2d 1 (1st Cir, 1980).

Rossetti J et al: Advocating for the rights of the mentally ill: a global issue, *Int J Psychiatr Nurs Res* 11:1211, 2005.

Rudegair TS, Appelbaum PS: On the duty to protect: an evolutionary perspective, *Bull Am Acad Psychiatry Law* 20:419, 1992.

Russell J: *Out of bounds sexual exploitation in counseling and therapy,* London, 1993, Sage.

Sales BD, Shuman DW: Mental health law and mental health care: introduction, *Am J Orthopsychiatry* 64:172, 1994.

Sharp HealthCare medication guidelines, San Diego, Calif, 2002.

Sherman PS: Computer-assisted creation of psychiatric advanced directives, *Community Ment Health J* 34:351, 1998.

Simon RI: Psychiatrists' duties in discharging sicker and potentially violent inpatients in the managed care era, *Psychiatr Serv* 49:62, 1998.

Simon RI: *Psychiatry and law for clinicians,* ed 3, Washington, DC, 2001, American Psychiatric Publishing.

Smith v. King, 615 So2s 69 (Ala Sup Ct 1993).

Somer E, Nachmanil I: Constructions of therapist-client sex: a comparative analysis of retrospective victim report, *Sexual Abuse: A Journal of Research and Treatment* 17: 47-62, 2005.

Statement on psychiatric mental health nursing practice and standards of psychiatric mental health clinical nursing practice, Washington, DC, 1994, American Nurses Publishing. American Psychiatric Nurses Association.

Tarasoff v. Regents of the University of California, 529 P2d 553 (Cal 1974) and 551 P2d 334 (Cal 1976).

Tenn Code Ann §33-6-201, 33-10-103, 33-3-105.

Weiner BA, Wettsein RM: *Legal issues in mental health care,* New York, 1993, Plenum Press.

Woe v. Cuomo, 638 F Supp 1506 (ED NY 1986).

Wyatt v. Stickney, 344 F Supp 373 (1972).

Youngberg v. Romeo, 461 US 308 (1982).

10

Anxiety and Anxiety Disorders

Pamela E. Marcus

"Anxiety does not empty tomorrow of its sorrows, but only empties today of its strength."

Charles Spurgeon

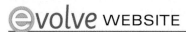 WEBSITE

http://evolve.elsevier.com/Fortinash/

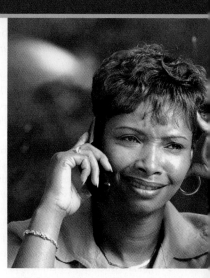

OBJECTIVES

- Discuss the four stages of anxiety and their manifestations.
- Describe the various defense mechanisms that an individual uses when feeling anxious.
- Identify the defining characteristics of anxiety in the North American Nursing Diagnosis Association classification.
- Describe the coping mechanisms of trauma victims that assist the nurse with evaluating the risk for posttraumatic stress disorder.

- Apply the nursing process to provide comprehensive nursing care to patients with anxiety disorders.
- Relate the biologic model to target symptoms and therapeutic agents for psychopharmacologic intervention for patients with anxiety and related disorders.
- Design a teaching plan for family members of patients with obsessive-compulsive disorder.
- Discuss the usefulness of clinical rating scales for evaluating the treatment outcomes of patients with anxiety disorders.

KEY TERMS

agoraphobia	compulsions	obsessions	phobias
anxiety	defense mechanisms	panic anxiety	repression
anxiolytic	dissociation	panic attacks	stress

Anxiety is an integral part of the universal human experience. For most people, it is a vague, subjective feeling of uneasiness with no identifiable object that results from an external threat to one's integrity. The function of anxiety is to warn the individual of impending threat, conflict, or danger. Anxiety is also a state of tension, dread, or impending doom that results from external influences that threaten to overwhelm the individual. When a person receives a signal of approaching danger, he or she is motivated to act, whether it means fleeing the threatening situation or controlling dangerous impulses. Some people freeze or do not act.

A helpful way to conceptualize the physiologic and behavioral changes that occur during stress is by understanding the General Adaptation Syndrome identified by Hans Selye, who was a pioneer in stress research (see Chapter 5).

Defense mechanisms are the primary methods that the ego (i.e., the self) uses to control or manage anxiety (Table 10-1). Defense mechanisms protect us from threats to the physical, mental, and social aspects of ourselves. We all use defense mechanisms unconsciously in various stages of life. For example, a person with a history of being abused as a child unconsciously uses the defense mechanism of repression to control the anxiety related to the trauma. Repressing the painful event enables the individual to engage in normal activities, such as school, sports, making friends, and even marriage and parenthood. If the pain of the trauma eventually becomes too difficult to repress, the person unconsciously uses dysfunctional methods to manage anxiety, which disrupts the person's life. Psychotherapy helps these individuals to confront the traumatic event and the effects of the trauma.

TABLE 10-1	DEFENSE MECHANISMS	
DEFENSE MECHANISM	**DEFINITION**	**EXAMPLE**
High Adaptive Level		
Humor	Using humor assists the person with the management of everyday stressors	The comedian talks about his substance abuse and current recovery with humorous stories that the audience can identify with
Sublimation	Channeling maladaptive thoughts and feelings such as aggression into socially acceptable behaviors	A young man experienced being bullied as a child and becomes a policeman; he channeled his feelings of anger and the inability to deal directly with the bully into observing law and order and protecting others
Suppression	Avoiding thinking about problem areas intentionally (unlike repression, which is unintentionally put into play)	The student nurse focuses all his energy on his school assignments to avoid several problems that are happening at home
Mental Inhibitions: Compromise Formation Level		
Displacement	Transferring a feeling or response toward one person onto another less threatening person or object	A mother was angry with her teenage daughter for doing poorly in school and disobeying, so she goes to the gym and plays a rigorous game of racquetball
Dissociation	An alteration in an awake state during which the person feels detached from his or her surroundings	The patient describes feeling detached from his body and looking down at his body from the corner of the room
Repression	Unintentionally pushing back disturbing thoughts, desires, or experiences from the conscious mind (more intense than suppression, which is intentional)	When describing a childhood that included sexual abuse, the patient is unable to recall a lot of her early experiences and appears to be detached from them
Minor Image-Distorting Level		
Devaluation	Attributing negative qualities to the self or others	The patient finds fault in every aspect of the hospitalization experience
Disavowal Level		
Denial	Unconsciously refusing to acknowledge some painful reality or subjective experience that others identify	The patient consumes a six-pack of beer every day; he does not identify a problem with alcohol consumption
Projection	Attributing strong conflicting feelings or faults to another person	The patient is angry at the nurse for setting limits but accuses the nurse of being angry with him
Major Image-Distorting Level		
Splitting of the self-image or of the image of others	Inability to integrate positive and negative aspects of the self or others or to integrate own strengths and weaknesses; viewing self, others, and situations as being either all good or all bad	The patient cannot identify anything about the self or others that is positive and only identifies the negative characteristics; views things only in black and white and cannot see shades of gray

From the American Psychiatric Association: *Diagnostic and statistical manual of mental disorders*, ed 4, text revision, Washington, DC, 2000, American Psychiatric Association.

The person's level of functioning increases as he or she learns to manage anxiety in a healthier way.

An example of a commonly used defense mechanism called *identification* is seen in a teenager who dresses and grooms like the most popular girls in school. She is unconsciously using the defense mechanism to identify with the peers she admires to diffuse her own identity with theirs and thus be accepted as one of the group. Being different carries the threat of rejection, and this creates overwhelming anxiety in most teens. Eventually, many young people grow into confident adults who find their own identities. All defense mechanisms reduce anxiety, and most people unconsciously use a variety of them occasionally to get through a difficult time or to meet the challenges of a developmental milestone. Individuals who use defense mechanisms rigidly or consistently will not grow and develop emotionally as healthy, responsible beings. This is often noted in individuals who are diagnosed with personality disorders. For example, a person with an antisocial personality disorder often relies on the defense mechanism of projection to control anxiety

TABLE 10-2	**RESPONSES TO ANXIETY**		
ANXIETY LEVEL	**PHYSIOLOGIC**	**COGNITIVE/PERCEPTUAL**	**EMOTIONAL/BEHAVIORAL**
Mild	Vital signs normal; minimal muscle tension; pupils normal and constricted	Perceptual field is broad; awareness of multiple environmental and internal stimuli; thoughts are often random but controlled	Feelings of relative comfort and safety; relaxed and calm appearance and voice; performance automatic; habitual behaviors occur
Moderate	Vital signs normal or slightly elevated; tension experienced; patient is uncomfortable or experiences pleasure (labeled as *tense* or *excited*)	Alert; perception narrowed and focused; optimum state for problem solving and learning; attentive	Feelings of readiness and challenge; energized; engages in competitive activity and learns new skills; voice and facial expression interested or concerned
Severe	Fight-or-flight response; autonomic nervous system excessively stimulated (vital signs increased, diaphoresis increased, urinary urgency and frequency increased, diarrhea present, dry mouth occurs, appetite decreased, pupils dilated); muscles rigid and tense; senses affected; hearing decreased; pain sensation decreased	Perceptual field greatly narrowed; problem solving difficult; selective attention (focuses on one detail); selective inattention (blocks out threatening stimuli); distortion of time (things seem faster or slower than they actually are); dissociative tendencies; detachment; vigilambulism (automatic behavior)	Feels threatened and startles with new stimuli; feels on "overload"; activity increases or decreases (may pace, run away, wring hands, moan, shake, stutter, become very disorganized or withdrawn, freeze in position, or be unable to move); appears and feels depressed; demonstrates denial; complains of aches or pains; is agitated or irritable; need for space increases; eyes move around room or gaze is fixed; some patients close eyes to shut out the environment
Panic	Above symptoms increase until sympathetic nervous system release occurs; person becomes pale; blood pressure decreases; hypotension occurs; muscle coordination poor; pain and hearing sensations minimal	Perception totally scattered or closed; unable to take in stimuli; problem solving and logical thinking highly improbable; perception or unreality about self, environment, or event; dissociation often occurs	Feels helpless, with a total loss of control; patient is angry or terrified; becomes combative or totally withdrawn, cries, or runs away; completely disorganized; behavior is usually extremely active or inactive

From Green E et al: Practice guideline for management of anxiety. In Green E, Katz J, editors: *Clinical practice guidelines for the adult patient*, St. Louis, 1995, Mosby.

by projecting his own inadequacies onto another person or situation. In one sense, projection effectively reduces anxiety; however, by constantly using projection, the individual fails to confront and deal with his vulnerabilities and thus ceases to grow (see Chapter 14).

Psychoanalytic theory says that, at an unconscious level, the consequence of ignoring anxiety signals is the threat of "being destroyed" or of no longer existing. Anxiety responses exist on a continuum (Table 10-2), and individuals are more or less successful at using various defense mechanisms to control their own anxiety experiences. Those who are less successful at using these mechanisms or who rely primarily on less adaptive defense mechanisms sometimes develop the symptoms of anxiety disorders because they have not successfully managed anxiety. Treatment for anxiety disorders, therefore, includes functional methods to reduce anxiety, which are discussed later in this chapter (see Chapters 5, 11, and 14).

HISTORIC AND THEORETIC PERSPECTIVES

In *Interpersonal Relations in Nursing*, Hildegard Peplau (1952), a pioneer of psychiatric mental health nursing,

identified the stages of anxiety on a continuum. Her work illustrates the view of anxiety and tension developed by Harry Stack Sullivan, a prominent American-born psychiatrist and an expert in developmental theory. Nurses further began to explore these stages while providing care with the use of clinical practice guidelines. Figure 10-1 describes the anxiety continuum as mild, moderate, severe, and panic. Optimally functioning people generally operate in the mild range of anxiety. The mild stage facilitates learning, creativity, and personal growth. Nursing students and other learners often experience mild anxiety as they strive to excel in their work. Occasional movement to the moderate stage is an adaptive mechanism to cope with pleasant or unpleasant situations. For example, a nursing student who is giving an important oral presentation or who is anticipating a difficult test experiences moderate anxiety. When the student manages the stressor, he or she will then move back along the continuum to mild anxiety. Moderate and severe anxiety are either acute or chronic. With severe anxiety, the person focuses energy primarily on reducing the pain and discomfort of anxiety rather than on coping with the environment. Consequently, this impairs the individual's level of functioning, and the

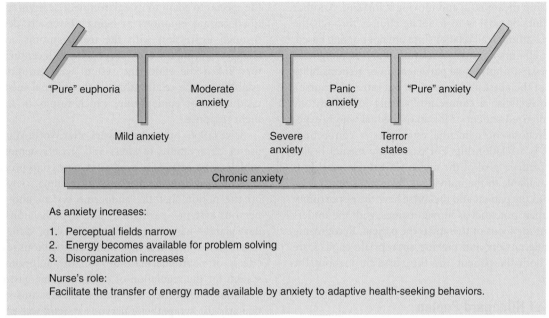

FIGURE 10-1. Hildegard Peplau's construction of the anxiety continuum. (From Peplau H: *Interpersonal relations in nursing: a conceptual frame of reference for psychodynamic nursing,* New York, 1991, Springer.)

person often requires help to reverse the situation. With panic-level anxiety, the individual is disorganized, with increased motor activity, a distorted visual-perceptual field, a loss of rational thought, and a decreased ability to relate to others. Table 10-2 fully explains the responses to the different stages of anxiety.

In addition to varying degrees of anxiety, there are also different types. Signal anxiety is the type of anxiety that is experienced when a person identifies a precipitant. It is important to note that, although signal anxiety is learned, it results from situations that have been successfully repressed or coped with by making use of another defense mechanism. Consequently, the precipitant is successfully excluded from one's consciousness. Signal anxiety is the predominant etiologic factor in phobic disorders. A cue in the environment causes anxiety, which becomes severe in nature and results in a panic attack. The individual is unaware of the cue initially; the original experience involving the cue is repressed. For example, Hannah is shopping at a grocery store, and she becomes severely anxious when passing an individual who smells of alcohol. Hannah had an uncle who drank alcohol heavily and was abusive when intoxicated. When she passed this person who had similar characteristics to those of her uncle, it reminded her of the fear that she experienced when her uncle visited her family after drinking.

Trait anxiety is a function of personality structure. As a part of developmental processes or events, some individuals have more traumatic experiences or have less success coping with these events, thereby resulting in unresolved conflict or confusion. These individuals have an anxiety diathesis or a predisposition to anxiety when stressed. They have a higher probability of worrying than someone who does not have trait anxiety as part of his or her personality structure. Situations that recreate or represent the original conflict or experience evoke a more severe anxiety response in persons with a higher level of trait anxiety. For example, a woman worries excessively about her own children being injured or catching colds because her mother was chronically ill for much of her childhood. As a result, she limits their activity and is anxious and overprotective. These anxious behaviors can be passed on to her children and continue to affect future generations.

State anxiety develops in situations that have been identified as conflictual or stressful and in which the individual experiences limited control. This is often perceived as anxiety that has occurred before. The "butterflies in the stomach" feeling that some students experience before an important examination is an example of mild state anxiety. A person who was bitten by a dog in the past and who experiences an increased heart rate when seeing a large dog walking down the street is displaying a more moderate form of state anxiety. A woman with a strong family history of cancer who delays making an appointment with her primary health care provider after noticing a lump in her breast demonstrates severe and maladaptive state anxiety. Free-floating anxiety is a pervasive sense of dread or doom that is unattached to any idea or event. This type of anxiety often results in a panic state if stressors exceed the person's ability to cope.

Anxiety in the Context of Psychiatric Mental Health Nursing

Many people use the term *anxiety* in a variety of contexts. However, it is important to be precise when using it. Inherent in all nurse–patient relationships is the nurse's goal of making the relationship meaningful and moving it forward. Another important nursing goal is to facilitate choices through the relationship. Although all relationships are not nursing based, the basis for all nursing care is a relationship. A nursing relationship does not imply equal participation or responsibility on the part of the nurse and the patient but rather the nurse's intention to establish a connection. Caring for an unconscious anesthetized patient or for an individual who is experiencing psychosis or dementia establishes a connection; therefore, it is a relationship. For psychiatric mental health nurses, the primary goal of the nurse–patient relationship is to become available to the individual. By establishing a relationship, both the patient and the nurse have the opportunity to develop their potential as human beings, with the understanding that the focus of therapy is the patient. Recognizing and managing anxiety and making appropriate choices are critical for both the patient and the nurse throughout the relationship.

Influence of Hildegard Peplau

During the 1950s, Peplau described the nurse as a person who relates *to* the patient rather than *with* the patient. She presented the phases of the nurse–patient relationship in a social learning model. Hildegard Peplau is considered the matriarch of psychiatric mental health nursing.

According to Peplau, it is critical that nurses recognize the choices or potentials that exist in the emerging relationship between the patient and the nurse. In *Interpersonal Relations in Nursing*, Peplau (1952) addressed the term *unexplained discomfort,* which includes the needs, frustrations, and conflicts that occur within the relationship. She considers them experiences that influence behavior by providing energy for the relationship. According to Peplau, nurses need to examine anxiety as it occurs in nurses and patients and in the communication that occurs in the interpersonal relationship.

Peplau also presented a method for the nurse to examine the relationship between the nurse and the patient called *process recording.* Process recording helps the nurse to develop self-awareness about the way that he or she relates to the patient and emphasizes the value of the nurse–patient relationship (see Chapter 4). The defining purpose of process recording is to provide a practical vehicle for the nurse to reflect on the content of the interaction in a safe, effective manner. The nurse reviews his or her responses to the patient to develop a growing awareness of his or her responses. This is a critical factor in helping patients achieve their goals and function optimally. Peplau's anxiety continuum is a theory that is helpful to use during the treatment of patients with anxiety disorders.

ETIOLOGY

Biologic Model

The roots of the biologic model for anxiety disorders date back to the 19th-century writings of Charles Darwin. Darwin postulated that emotional expression and anatomic structures both changed during the course of evolution to enable the species to adapt to its environment. Darwin further identified certain emotions as being universally demonstrated through expression with the use of motor and postural changes. During the early part of the 20th century, investigators linked the endocrine system with emotions, first by establishing the relationship of the adrenal medulla in the production of epinephrine, which results in the fight-or-flight response.

Selye (1956) built on this work after World War II with the use of observations of stress and anxiety demonstrated by soldiers who served in combat. A new conceptualization of stress replaced the former "psychic trauma." Selye expanded on the notion that the endocrine system and the central nervous system—particularly the hypothalamus and pituitary gland—have a reciprocal relationship. At the same time, researchers conducted important investigations regarding the effects of neuropharmacology on the autonomic nervous system for the regulation of cardiovascular, gastrointestinal, and motor responses. The autonomic nervous system, particularly the sympathetic nervous system, was responsive to environmental stimuli, including emotional states. A comprehensive discussion of Selye's theory appears in Chapter 5.

As the ability to understand the physiologic state by observing the living brain with imaging techniques such as positron emission tomography and functional magnetic resonance imaging has developed, the role of stress and brain functioning has become more apparent. The amygdala and the hippocampus are particularly important to understand as they relate to the fear response. Researchers are currently studying the amygdala and the hippocampus with regard to changes in size and function when an individual is experiencing symptoms seen with anxiety disorders, such as posttraumatic stress disorder (PTSD), social phobia, and generalized anxiety disorder (GAD). The amygdala is involved in the fight-or-flight response, and some have hypothesized that different anxiety disorders affect different parts of the amygdala. One current hypothesis that is being evaluated is the possibility that there may be a reduction in the size of the amygdala and the hippocampus in adults with generalized social phobia (Irle et al, 2010). The medial prefrontal cortex organizes the response to a traumatic episode, and the hippocampus has the spatial and contextual memory of the trauma. Chronic stress possibly causes changes in the amygdala, the hippocampus, and the prefrontal cortex (Irle et al, 2010).

Genetic considerations are important when assessing individuals with anxiety disorders. When performing functional magnetic resonance imaging, researchers found that some of the research subjects had one or two copies of a short variant of the human serotonin transporter gene as opposed to the long variant of this same gene. The transporter gene helps to code protein in the neuronal area that recycles secreted serotonin from the synapse. Lau and colleagues (2009) compared gene variants in healthy adults and teens as well as in teens with anxiety disorders. They found that adults with one long gene and one short gene tended to be more anxious than those with two copies of the long gene. According to the research, the adults who have one version of the short gene have a higher reaction in the amygdala than individuals with two long versions of the serotonin transporter gene. Adolescents who have one copy of the short version of the serotonin transporter gene show less amygdala reaction than adolescents who have two copies of the long version of the gene. This demonstrates the need for further research on the cellular level to understand the role the serotonin transporter genes and their effect on the amygdala when predicting the differences between adolescent and adult reactions to stress.

Research is being performed to evaluate whether there are deficits in the brain circuits that contribute to fear extinction that are not effective in individuals with anxiety disorders (Likhtik et al, 2008). Fear extinction is the individual's ability to note an environmental cue that may increase anxiety and then use a cognitive response to decrease the fear. Individuals with normal brain circuits that contribute to fear extinction can respond to stimuli with the use of a problem-solving approach rather than a fight-or-flight or freeze response. This is an important concept to consider when planning the care of an individual with anxiety disorders (e.g., phobias).

By studying and understanding brain functioning and genetics, researchers are making advances in the use of pharmaceutical agents and psychotherapeutic approaches to assist patients with anxiety-related disorders (see Chapter 25).

Psychodynamic Model

In psychoanalytic terms, anxiety is a warning to the ego that it is in danger from either an internal or external threat. Anxiety is involved in the development of personality and personality functioning and in the development and treatment of neuroses and psychoses. Freud's work is the basis for anxiety neurosis existing as a separate classification.

Three types of anxiety are identified in psychoanalytic theory: reality anxiety, moral anxiety, and neurotic anxiety. Reality anxiety is a painful emotional experience that results from the perception of danger in the external world, such as the fear of the possibility of a terrorist attack. Fear is the response to external danger, and, consequently, anxiety parallels fear. Moral anxiety is the ego's experience of guilt or shame. An example of moral anxiety is experiencing guilt for expressing anger at a family member. Neurotic anxiety is the perception of a threat according to one's instincts. According to Freud's theory of "signal anxiety," anxiety is a signal of the impending emergence of threatening unconscious mental content. Neurotic symptoms develop in an attempt to defend against anxiety, including somatic symptoms, obsessions, compulsions, and phobias (these are described more fully in this chapter and in Chapter 11).

Behavioral Model

Clinicians who believed that the psychoanalytic model and methods were lacking designed behavioral models in psychiatry and psychology. They identified experimental psychology as a resource for ideas from which to develop new treatments.

In behavioral models that are based on learning theory, the etiology of anxiety symptoms is a generalization from an earlier traumatic experience to a benign setting or object. An example is an awkward child whose parents ridiculed him while he was bowling. As a result, he associates embarrassment and shame with sports events in indoor facilities and develops panic attacks during basketball games. The same kinds of cognitive operations that link embarrassment with sporting events link the cognition of the expectation of embarrassment with the idea of a sporting event, and the individual begins to experience panic attacks while reading the sports page. Consequently, in this model, anxiety occurs when an individual encounters a signal that predicts a painful or feared event.

Early behavioral therapists directed their efforts toward the anxiety disorders. In 1958, a physician named Joseph Wolpe (1915-1997) who was working with soldiers who were experiencing symptoms of PTSD reported success with the use of systematic desensitization applied to simple phobias (Wolpe, 1973). Systematic desensitization is a method that comes from the learning theory. The therapist exposes a deeply relaxed patient to a graded hierarchy of phobic stimuli. Others have redefined this method further into in vivo desensitization, whereby the therapist exposes the individual progressively to more anxiety-provoking situations. These live exposure treatments take a variety of forms, including graded practice, participant modeling, and prolonged or brief duration. In 1981, behaviorists demonstrated that 60% to 79% of patients with agoraphobia experienced clinically significant improvement with the use of the methods of systematic desensitization.

Table 10-3 demonstrates the clinical manifestations of anxiety, which take into account the biologic, cognitive, behavioral, and affective patterns of behavior. This table is a good tool to help nurses recognize the manifestations that anxiety has on body systems as well as on thought patterns and behavior.

Epidemiology and Age of Onset

A National Institute of Mental Health study called *The Numbers Count: Mental Disorders in America* (2010) describes the statistics of behavioral disorders in America. This report states that 40 million adults aged 18 years old and older have an anxiety disorder. These disorders are often co-occurring with other emotional illness, such as affective disorders, substance abuse, and other anxiety disorders. Anxiety disorders often occur when the patient is about 21 years old. The statistics demonstrate that approximately 6 million adults have experienced a panic disorder. Agoraphobia with panic attacks occurs among one in three people who have panic disorders. Approximately 2.2 million adults have obsessive-compulsive disorder (OCD). OCD begins during childhood and adolescence, with a median age of onset of 19 years. PTSD occurs after an incident that is violent or that the individual perceives as life threatening, such as war, a violent personal attack, an accident, or a natural disaster. Approximately 7.7 million adults have developed PTSD.

TABLE 10-3	CLINICAL MANIFESTATIONS OF ANXIETY: SYMPTOMS AND RESPONSES	
MANIFESTATION	**SYMPTOM/RESPONSE**
Physiologic	
Cardiovascular system	Palpitations, racing heart, increased blood pressure, fainting, decreased blood pressure
Respiratory system	Rapid and shallow breathing, pressure in the chest, shortness of breath, gasping, lump in the throat
Gastrointestinal system	Loss of appetite or increased appetite, abdominal discomfort or feeling of fullness, nausea, heartburn, diarrhea
Neuromuscular system	Hyperreflexia, insomnia, tremors, pacing, clumsiness, restlessness, flushing, sweating, muscle tension
Genitourinary system	Decreased libido, increased frequency or urgency of urination
Cognitive	Decreased attention, inability to concentrate, forgetfulness, impaired judgment, thought blocking, fear of injury or death
Behavioral	Rapid speech, muscle tension, fine hand tremors, restlessness, pacing, hyperventilation
Affective	Irritability, impatience, nervousness, fear, uneasiness

Studies are ongoing to understand the effect of psychologic trauma on war veterans, such as those who have participated in the Vietnam War, the Gulf War, and wars in Iraq and Afghanistan. There are approximately 6.8 million adults with GAD. The median onset of GAD is the age of 31 years, although symptoms can begin anytime during an individual's life. Social phobia symptoms develop during childhood and adolescence, usually beginning when the patient is about 13 years old. Approximately 15 million adults have social phobia (National Institute of Mental Health, 2010).

Almost all patients who present with agoraphobia in clinical samples have a current diagnosis or history of panic disorder. Agoraphobia occurs when an individual experiences an overwhelming fear of places where there is no means of escape, if needed. An example of agoraphobia is when a person is unable to fly in an airplane as a result of a fear that the plane may crash and the person may not be able to escape and therefore will die. Agoraphobia is more common among women than men. Approximately 1.8 million adults have agoraphobia without panic disorder (National Institute of Mental Health, 2010).

Simple phobia is common in the general population, with approximately 19.2 million adults being affected. Specific phobias begin during childhood and start at approximately the age of 7 years. The prevalence of simple phobia is higher among women than men (National Institute of Mental Health, 2010).

Cultural Variance

Most research that supports the development of the *Diagnostic and Statistical Manual*, ed 4, text revision (DSM-IV-TR) classification occurred in the United States; consequently, symptoms that define disorders are representative of U.S. culture. However, take care to establish cultural norms when evaluating patients for anxiety and related disorders. For example, some cultures restrict women's participation in public activities; thus, agoraphobia is less commonly diagnosed. Fears of magic and spirits are present in many cultures and are pathologic only when they are deemed excessive in the context of that culture. Many cultures have rituals to mark important events in people's lives. The observation of these rituals is not indicative of OCD unless it exceeds norms for that culture, is exhibited at times or places that are inappropriate for that culture, or interferes with social functioning.

It seems that, with the exception of OCD and social phobia, anxiety and related disorders exhibit a higher prevalence among women than men. This observation possibly represents a cultural variation. Overall, women are more likely than men to present for treatment or to come in contact with health care providers (American Psychiatric Association, 2000).

Comorbidity (Co-occurrence)

It is important for the nurse to understand the co-occurrence of anxiety disorders with other Axis I disorders to provide comprehensive treatment. There is a high comorbid rate of anxiety and depression. Often patients with these disorders are at an increased risk for suicidal ideation as compared with patients who have neither disorder. There is a substantial co-occurrence between substance abuse disorders and anxiety disorders as the individual attempts to medicate his or her symptoms of anxiety with medications or alcohol (American Psychiatric Association, 2000).

OCD exists with other anxiety disorders as well as with substance abuse, major depression, and eating disorders. There is a possibility for an individual who has OCD to develop a hypochondriac focus on body feelings and functions. An individual with OCD may also develop Tourette's syndrome; this may be more common among children who have symptoms of OCD. Children with OCD also have a higher incidence of the development of disruptive learning disorders (American Psychiatric Association, 2000). Acute and posttraumatic stress disorders have an increased risk for major depression, other anxiety disorders, somatization disorder, and substance abuse disorders. Because of the nature of the disorder and its presentation after a significant event, it is difficult to determine whether the co-occurring condition developed before the stress disorder or as a consequence of it.

CLINICAL DESCRIPTION

Panic

Freud first named panic attacks as occurring when "the connection between anxiety and threatened danger is entirely lost from view … spontaneous attacks … represented by intensely developed symptoms … tremor, vertigo, palpitations of the heart" (Freud, 1963). Freud also noted the co-occurrence of the anxiety disorders and depression.

World Wars I and II contributed to the development of the knowledge base of the anxiety disorders, as did the work of the noted cardiologist Paul Dudley White. He and his colleagues collected data from a number of patients with symptoms such as cardiac palpitations, tremors, or vertigo, who did not have organic heart disease. They named the clinical syndrome *neurocirculatory asthenia*. In the same institution, neuropsychiatrists identified a similar symptom complex and named it *anxiety neurosis*. Both the cardiologists and the neuropsychiatrists were describing what we today call *panic disorder*.

Panic anxiety involves anxiety symptoms that occur during panic attacks. Panic anxiety is differentiated from generalized anxiety by the sudden onset of distressing physical symptoms in combination with thoughts of dread, impending doom, and death and the fear of being trapped.

Panic Attack

It is important to note that panic attacks are not listed in the DSM-IV-TR classification as psychiatric illnesses. Rather, panic attacks are symptoms that potentially meet some of the defining characteristics of many of the disorders described in this chapter. Panic attacks are sudden, spontaneous episodes that are accompanied by symptoms such as a racing heart, palpitations, dizziness, dyspnea, and a feeling that death is imminent.

Panic attacks occur with a variety of anxiety disorders, including panic disorder, social phobia, simple phobia, and PTSD. Panic attacks occur in specific, cued situations (e.g., with simple phobias, such as seeing a snake), or they may be unexpected (i.e., uncued, with nothing in the environment to cue the individual) (American Psychiatric Association, 2000). The DSM-IV-TR Criteria box lists the symptoms of a panic attack.

Panic Disorder

An individual is diagnosed with panic disorder if the following two criteria are met: (1) recent and unexpected panic attacks are present; and (2) at least one of the attacks has been followed for 1 or more months by (a) persistent concern about having additional attacks; (b) worry about the

---

DSM-IV-TR CRITERIA

Panic Attack

A distinct period of intense fear or discomfort in which four or more of the following symptoms develop abruptly and reach a peak within 10 minutes:

1 Palpitations, pounding heart, or accelerated heart rate
2 Sweating
3 Trembling or shaking
4 Sensations of shortness of breath or smothering
5 Feelings of choking
6 Chest pain or discomfort
7 Nausea or abdominal distress
8 Feeling dizzy, unsteady, lightheaded, or faint
9 Derealization (feelings of unreality) or depersonalization (being detached from oneself)
10 Fear of losing control or going crazy
11 Fear of dying
12 Paresthesias (numbness or tingling sensations)
13 Chills or hot flushes

From the American Psychiatric Association: *Diagnostic and statistical manual of mental disorders,* ed 4, text revision, Washington, DC, 2000, American Psychiatric Association.

---

implications of the attack or its consequences (e.g., losing control, having a heart attack, "going crazy"); or (c) a significant change in behavior related to the attacks.

For patients with panic disorder without agoraphobia, the individual is free from agoraphobic symptoms, the panic attacks are not related to the direct effects of a substance (e.g., illicit drugs, medication), and the attacks are not the result of a physiologic condition (e.g., hyperthyroidism). An individual with panic disorder with agoraphobia must meet the criteria for panic disorder in addition to experiencing debilitating agoraphobic symptoms. These agoraphobic symptoms involve feeling anxiety about being in areas from which it is difficult to escape or where no assistance is available, such as in a crowd, on a bridge, or in a subway train. The individual with agoraphobia avoids these situations or stays home if the agoraphobia involves a fear of being outside of the house alone (See assessment section later in chapter).

Phobias

The prominent feature of phobic disorders or phobias is that the patient experiences panic attacks in response to particular situations or has learned to avoid the situations that cause panic attacks.

Agoraphobia

To meet the first DSM-IV-TR criterion for panic disorder with agoraphobia, the person must experience recurrent, unexpected panic attacks, with at least one attack followed by one of the following for a month: (1) persistent concern about having additional attacks; (2) worry about the implications of the panic attacks; or (3) a significant change in behavior as a result of the attacks.

The second criterion is that the individual experiences agoraphobia. Agoraphobia is when the individual experiences fear when perceiving that he or she is unable to escape from a situation that is restricting, like a moving automobile, or from an embarrassing situation when help is not available if there in an unexpected panic attack. Agoraphobia can occur with or without the presence of a panic disorder. Agoraphobic fears typically involve the following: being outside of the home alone; being in a crowd or standing in line; being on a bridge; and traveling in a bus, train, or car.

The third criterion is that the person avoids agoraphobic situations or has anxiety about having a panic attack. This person will not go to an area or event where he or she has experienced an agoraphobic reaction without being with a trusted friend or companion.

The fourth criterion states that panic attacks are not caused by the direct effects of a substance, a medication, or a medical condition (American Psychiatric Association, 2000).

Specific Phobias

The DSM-IV-TR criteria define a specific phobia as an overwhelming fear that is in excess of that experienced by others that is cued by the presence of a specific objects or situations, such as animals, insects, heights, flying, or seeing blood. When the person is exposed to the stimulus, he or she will have a cued panic attack. Children express their phobias by crying, throwing tantrums, freezing, or clinging. Adults with a simple phobias recognize that their fears are more than what others experience. These individuals either avoid phobic situations or endure them with distress (American Psychiatric Association, 2000).

Social Phobia

Social phobia or social anxiety disorder occurs when the individual experiences an overwhelming fear of being in a social situation or having to interact with many people at once. An individual with social phobia has great concern that people are criticizing him or her, and he or she worries about acting in a manner that will be humiliating or embarrassing. Children with this condition demonstrate extreme anxiety when interacting with peers or others whom they do not know that well. For example, the child tells his mother that he will not go to camp because the other campers will think that he is stupid. Children express their fear by crying or exhibiting tantrum-like behavior. Adults who have social phobia acknowledge that their fear is excessive or unreasonable. Individuals with social phobia avoid social or performance situations or endure them with intense anxiety and distress (American Psychiatric Association, 2000).

Individuals with social phobia are unable to work well in a group. If an individual is in the psychiatric hospital for a co-occurring disorder such as substance abuse, the use of the group format may cause this person a great deal of anxiety and therefore may not be therapeutic for this patient. The care of this individual would include working on problem areas with individual attention and medications such as the

selective serotonin reuptake inhibitor antidepressant paroxetine (Paxil) (Case Study #1) (American Psychiatric Association, 2009).

Posttraumatic Stress Disorder

PTSD was first defined as a diagnostic category in DSM-III. Before that time, the pattern of response after a traumatic event was most common among soldiers, and the syndrome was called *shell shock* or *combat fatigue*.

The term *PTSD* is used to describe an individual's reaction to traumatic events such as war, sexual abuse, physical

---

CASE STUDY #1

Jacob is a 19-year-old freshman at a local college. His friends brought him to the emergency department from a fraternity party one Saturday night with acute alcohol intoxication. He is referred to the college health service.

During Jacob's initial evaluation, the nurse asks him about his patterns of drinking. He reports that he began drinking at the age of 14 years when one of his friends suggested having a beer or two before attending a school dance. He reported that, ever since he started school, he has been unable to participate in the easy conversation or social chitchat that is common among his peers. He did not report the same experience with family members. He was afraid that he would not have anything to contribute to conversations with his schoolmates. He began to worry about his appearance and his tendency to "trip over his own feet."

When Jacob reached high school, he found that this uneasiness was beginning to isolate him from others in his age group. At home, his parents usually began dinner parties with a glass of wine or a cocktail, so when his friend suggested a beer before the dance, Jacob eagerly accepted. To his surprise, he found that, when he arrived at the dance, he was relaxed and able to interact. He was even able to ask two girls to dance.

He continued to drink before arriving at parties, dances, football games, and just about any other social activity or class that involved active participation. He was worried that he was an alcoholic. The nurse practitioner at the health service talked with Jacob at length about social phobia and prescribed the antidepressant paroxetine (Paxil). Jacob also began attending a group that was focused on behavioral strategies to cope with anxiety disorders, including social phobia. (see Chapter 26).

Critical Thinking

1 What cues does Jacob offer that will lead to the most appropriate nursing diagnoses for him?
2 What two beliefs did Jacob form that led to his experience at the fraternity party?
3 According to information presented in this chapter and in Chapter 15, what would be the prognosis for Jacob?
4 What is an alternative pharmacologic choice for Jacob (see Chapter 25)?
5 How would you describe the advantages of group therapy to Jacob?

abuse, disasters, accidents, and the grieving process. Cases of PTSD are expected to rise as a result of disasters such as the events of September 11, 2001; Hurricanes Katrina and Rita; earthquakes such as the one that occurred in Haiti; the massive oil spill in the Gulf of Mexico; and the wars in Iraq and Afghanistan. These disasters will have an impact on the health care system for years to come. Controversy still exists with regard to refining the level of intensity required of an event or an experience to meet the definition of trauma and the separation of PTSD symptoms from other co-occurring disorders, including substance abuse, depression, and anxiety.

To demonstrate the symptoms of PTSD, the individual must have experienced or witnessed a traumatic event that involved a feeling of being threatened with death or severe injury. The person's response to the trauma includes intense fear, helplessness, or horror. If there is a child exposed to an event that causes psychologic trauma, that child will demonstrate his or her response by behaving in an agitated or disorganized manner.

One defining behavior that is seen when an individual has PTSD is that the person reexperiences the traumatic event. This takes place by having recurrent and intrusive disturbing recollections of the trauma, including thoughts, images, or perceptions about the incident. The person sometimes experiences recurrent dreams of the incident, acts or feels as though the event was recurring in the present, and feels the experience of psychologic distress when internal or external cues resemble the trauma. This includes physiologic reactions after exposure to internal or external cues that resemble the incident. An example of this would be the following: Amy was raped when she was 15 years old by a neighbor. While watching a popular television program about crime, she began to have body sensations as though she were being raped again. She began to have dreams about the rape that happened years ago and was unable to function at home or at school as a result of not being able to concentrate because she was experiencing recurring thoughts of the rape.

The person with PTSD avoids stimuli associated with the trauma and experiences a numbing of general responsiveness if reminded of the incident via certain cues. Numbing and avoidance are evidenced by at least three of the following:

- Efforts to avoid thoughts, feelings, or conversations about the trauma
- Efforts to avoid persons or places that evoke memories of the trauma
- Inability to remember an important aspect of the trauma (i.e., **repression**)
- Diminished interest or participation in significant activities
- A feeling of estrangement or detachment from others
- Restricted range of affect
- A sense of impending doom (i.e., no expectation of a career or a normal life span)

A person who has PTSD experiences increased arousal after the incident. This increased arousal is demonstrated by the following symptoms: sleep disturbances, irritability or angry outbursts, difficulty concentrating, hypervigilance, and an exaggerated startle response (American Psychiatric Association, 2000).

Acute Stress Disorder

Acute stress disorder differs from PTSD in three ways: (1) the individual experiences at least three symptoms indicating dissociation; (2) the time frame of the development and duration of symptoms is shorter; and (3) the dissociative symptoms prevent the individual from adaptively coping with the trauma. The person demonstrates the following symptoms of dissociation: a subjective sense of numbing or detachment, a reduced awareness of his or her surroundings (being in a daze), derealization (unreal feeling), depersonalization (feeling alienated), and dissociative amnesia. The symptoms of dissociation occur during the traumatic experience or develop immediately afterward. The person is unable to function in his or her usual social or occupational role. For example, the individual who has experienced the trauma is unable to perform some necessary task, such as obtaining necessary medical or legal assistance or mobilizing personal resources to cope with the incident.

Generalized Anxiety Disorder

GAD occurs when a person experiences excessive anxiety and worry that impedes the person's ability to function at home, at work or school, and in the community. This anxiety involves concerns about many aspects of the person's life. The individual experiences difficulty when trying to control the worry. The person describes feeling restless or on edge, being easily fatigued, and having difficulties with concentration, irritability, muscle tension, and sleep disturbances. Box 10-1 offers a self-test for GAD.

Obsessive-Compulsive Disorder

OCD involves symptoms that cause the person to experience the presence of either obsessions, compulsions, or both. DSM-IV-TR defines obsessions as recurrent and persistent thoughts that are intrusive to the individual and that cause a marked increase in anxiety. The individual attempts to suppress or ignore these thoughts and impulses or to neutralize them with some other thought or action. People with OCD recognize that the obsessive thoughts are part of their own thoughts as opposed to coming from somewhere else as occurs with thought insertion, which may be present with schizophrenia (see Chapter 13).

Compulsions are repetitive behaviors that the person feels driven to perform in response to an obsession. Some examples include repeated hand washing and checking many times to ensure that appliances are unplugged before leaving the house (see Case Study #2). The behaviors or thoughts are an attempt to prevent or reduce the distress invoked by the obsession or to prevent some dreaded threatening situation from occurring (e.g., a fire in the example of checking appliances). However, these behaviors or thoughts are not a realistic way to prevent a dreaded situation and are often excessive as well as anxiety producing.

BOX 10-1   GENERALIZED ANXIETY DISORDER SELF-TEST

The following questions will help you to determine if you are experiencing symptoms of GAD. Simply answer yes or no, and then take this questionnaire to your health care professional to see if further evaluation and treatment are necessary.

YES/NO	ARE YOU TROUBLED BY THE FOLLOWING?
Y N	Excessive worry that has occurred more days than not for at least 6 months
Y N	Unreasonable worry about a number of different situations, such as work, school, or health
Y N	Your inability to "shut off" your worry

	ARE YOU BOTHERED BY AT LEAST THREE OF THE FOLLOWING:
Y N	Restlessness or feeling keyed up or on edge
Y N	Being easily tired
Y N	Concentration problems
Y N	Irritability
Y N	Muscle tension
Y N	Trouble falling asleep, trouble staying asleep, or restless or unsatisfying sleep
Y N	Anxiety that interferes with your daily life

Having more than one illness at the same time makes it difficult to diagnose and treat the different conditions. Conditions that sometimes complicate anxiety disorders include depression and substance abuse, among others. The following information will help your health care professional to evaluate you for GAD.

YES/NO	IN THE LAST YEAR, HAVE YOU EXPERIENCED THE FOLLOWING?
Y N	Changes in sleeping or eating habits
Y N	Feeling sad or depressed more days than not
Y N	A disinterest in life more days than not
Y N	A feeling of worthlessness or guilt more days than not
Y N	An inability to fulfill responsibilities at work, school, or home because of alcohol or drug use
Y N	Being arrested because of alcohol or drugs
Y N	The need to continue using alcohol or drugs even though doing so is causing problems for you or your loved ones

Modified from the Anxiety Disorders Association of America, www.adaa.org/living-with-anxiety/ask-and-learn/screenings/screening-generalized-anxiety-disorder-gad. Accessed October 26, 2010.

CASE STUDY #2

Jason is a 31-year-old accountant who has been disabled from his job with a national firm for 8 months. He reports that he has been hospitalized for the treatment of depression, which he has experienced since college. Despite his depression, he graduated with honors, was certified as a public accountant, and finished graduate school.

Jason first was treated for OCD 2 years after graduate school, when he began experiencing trouble with his supervisor. A number of the firm's clients had complained that Jason was unable either to give them completed tax forms or to file for the necessary extensions in a timely manner.

Treatment with paroxetine relieved Jason from his counting and checking behaviors, but he presently spends his time preoccupied with thoughts about killing himself. He is unable to decide on a method of suicide that will not endanger his family's entitlement to his accidental death insurance policies. However, he has plans to have a fatal automobile accident. After relating this lethal suicidal plan to his nurse psychotherapist, Jason is admitted to an inpatient facility to prevent a suicidal gesture and to stabilize the medication regimen.

Critical Thinking

1 What type of treatment plan is indicated for Jason, with safety being a priority?
2 What three collaborative treatment approaches are important for Jason's long-term therapy?
3 Which methods can be used to measure the outcomes that Jason achieves as a result of his treatment?

Individuals with obsessions or compulsions experience marked distress, because these thoughts are time consuming, and they significantly interfere with the person's normal routine or occupational functioning. School nurses need to be aware of this disorder in children. OCD is often undetected in children as a result of shame, so the symptoms are often hidden. It is only when the child is unable to play, socialize, and concentrate in school that OCD may be discovered and treated (Helbing and Ficca, 2009) (see Patient and Family Teaching Guidelines box).

PROGNOSIS

The prognosis for anxiety disorders is related to factors that are specific to the disorder, the patient, and the clinician. Patients who are treated for panic disorder with or without

PATIENT AND FAMILY TEACHING GUIDELINES

Obsessive-Compulsive Disorder

Teach the Patient's Family

- Obsessive-compulsive disorder is a chronic anxiety disorder that responds to different treatment strategies.
- The patient experiences recurrent thoughts that interrupt his or her day-to-day functioning. To decrease the overwhelming anxiety felt as a result of the thought pattern, the patient manifests compulsions or behavior patterns. Some of the thoughts involve counting, checking (i.e., to see if the stove is off or the door is locked), and concern about germs.
- Thoughts, impulses, and images are involuntary and worsen with stress.
- Books and Internet resources can be helpful (e.g., *Loving Someone with OCD* by KJ Landsman (2005) or the website of the International OCD Foundation [www.ocfoundation.org]).

Teach the Patient

- It is important to apply behavioral and cognitive strategies to manage the anxiety and reduce the symptoms of the disorder by doing so when the thought patterns are more intense and the compulsions are most disruptive.
- Obtain psychotherapy that is oriented toward problem solving (e.g., cognitive behavioral therapy) to reduce the symptoms of OCD.
- Medication management is an effective treatment modality that usually involves treatment with a drug in the antidepressant category.
- Different classes of drugs have different side-effect profiles; recognizing and reporting side effects are important for managing the patient's drug therapy.
- Achieving symptom control through pharmacotherapy may take up to 6 weeks.
- Obtaining information via self-help books or websites can be helpful.

---

agoraphobia generally demonstrate some symptoms during the course of their lives after their initial episodes. Follow-up studies indicate that, 6 to 10 years after treatment, 30% of patients are well, 40% to 50% are improved but still symptomatic, and 20% to 30% are the same or slightly worse (American Psychiatric Association, 2000).

Specific phobias that persist into adulthood are generally chronic. The course of social phobia is often continuous, with onset or reemergence after stressful or humiliating experiences. The prognosis for OCD is similar to that for other anxiety disorders, with increasing and decreasing symptoms related to stressors. However, 15% of patients demonstrate a chronically deteriorating course with the progressive compromise of social and occupational functioning.

The prognosis for acute stress disorders and PTSD is related to the individual's exposure to the stressful event, the patient's premorbid functioning (i.e., their functioning just

before onset of illness), and their ability to recognize and make use of support systems. People with acute stress disorder either recover within 4 weeks or are diagnosed with PTSD. Approximately half of those who are diagnosed with PTSD recover in 3 months, whereas the other half continues to experience symptoms that persist for more than a year after the trauma. It is more likely that the individual will have a good recovery if there are few competing stressors at the time that the symptoms develop, if the patient seeks early treatment and follows it, and if the affected person has above-average intelligence (American Psychiatric Association, 2000).

DISCHARGE CRITERIA

The patient will do the following:

- Identify situations and events that trigger anxiety and select ways to prevent or manage them.
- Describe anxiety symptoms and levels of anxiety.
- Discuss the connection between anxiety-provoking situations or events and anxiety symptoms.
- Explain relief behaviors openly.
- Identify adaptive and positive techniques and strategies that relieve anxiety.
- Demonstrate behaviors that represent reduced anxiety symptoms.
- Use learned anxiety-reducing strategies.
- Demonstrate the ability to problem solve, concentrate, and make decisions.
- Verbalize feeling relaxed.
- Sleep through the night.
- Use appropriate supports from the nursing and medical communities, family, and friends.
- Acknowledge the inevitability of the occurrence of anxiety.
- Discuss the ability to tolerate manageable levels of anxiety.
- Seek help from appropriate sources when anxiety is not manageable, including websites such as www.adaa.org (i.e., the website of Anxiety Disorders of America)
- List the medication that are used to control the symptoms as well as the appropriate dosage and scheduled times.
- Continue postdischarge anxiety management, including medication and therapy.

THE NURSING PROCESS
ASSESSMENT

Assessing patients for the presence of anxiety disorders is conducted in a variety of settings. New treatment modalities have improved the quality of life and the level of participation in activities for people with anxiety disorders. Nurses no longer expect to encounter patients with psychiatric disorders only in traditional psychiatric settings. It is important for all nurses to identify dysfunctional manifestations of anxiety so that treatment can be implemented promptly (see Chapter 3).

Nurses primarily see individuals with panic disorders in ambulatory settings. Nurses are among the first health care providers to come in contact with patients who are experiencing their first symptoms of panic disorder, either in a clinic, a physician's office, or, more typically, in a hospital emergency department. The sudden onset of physical symptoms and the pervasive feelings of impending doom are frightening, and the patient often responds by seeking reassurance from a caregiver. It is these physical symptoms that bring patients to the emergency department with the concern that they are experiencing a heart attack and impending death.

The patient with agoraphobia sometimes comes to the attention of a nurse when the nurse is preparing a patient for diagnostic testing that includes a computed tomography scan or magnetic resonance imaging. The patient who is agoraphobic may become visibly anxious at the prospect of entering a confined space when the nurse describes the procedure and the equipment.

Most often patients with anxiety symptoms do not present with anxiety as their primary reason for seeking treatment. Anxiety by definition is a vague and nonspecific feeling of discomfort. Nurses who use an assessment tool that addresses each identified human response pattern will obtain cues from the patient who is experiencing anxiety that indicate further assessment.

NURSING DIAGNOSIS

To determine which nursing diagnoses will most effectively guide the treatment of patients with anxiety and related disorders, the nurse relies on information obtained during the assessment process. The nurse identifies defining characteristics of the target diagnoses from the patient. The nurse and the patient jointly identify etiologic factors or risk factors.

Etiologic factors influence the selection of the intervention. It is impossible to anticipate each potential diagnosis for all of the disorders that are discussed in this chapter. Diagnoses are prioritized according to patient's needs. Typical diagnoses for patients with anxiety disorders include the following:

- Risk for suicide
- Anxiety
- Death anxiety
- Stress overload
- Self-mutilation
- Hopelessness
- Powerlessness
- Social isolation
- Disturbed sensory perception
- Disturbed thought processes
- Insomnia
- Impaired memory
- Deficient knowledge
- Fear
- Fatigue
- Chronic low self-esteem
- Disturbed body image
- Risk-prone health behavior

- Ineffective role performance
- Ineffective coping
- Defensive coping
- Ineffective denial
- Impaired social interaction
- Compromised family coping
- Interrupted family processes
- Spiritual distress
- Decisional conflict
- Noncompliance
- Posttrauma syndrome
- Risk for posttrauma syndrome

OUTCOME IDENTIFICATION

Outcome criteria differ according to the characteristics of each patient's nursing diagnoses and associated DSM-IV-TR diagnoses. Determining outcomes before implementing the plan will guide both nursing interventions and evaluation. Nursing diagnoses are associated with outcomes (i.e., goals) to serve as a guide for outcome development. In practice, nurses generally determine outcomes by the patient's presentation of clinical manifestations.

Generalized Anxiety Disorder

The patient will do the following:
- Demonstrate a significant decrease in the physiologic, cognitive, behavioral, and emotional symptoms of anxiety.
- Demonstrate effective coping skills.
- Exhibit an enhanced ability to make decisions and problem solve.
- Demonstrate the ability to function adaptively in mild anxiety states.
- Discuss the medication regimen and take the medications as prescribed.
- Identify when to call the therapist for more visits when a crisis occurs.
- Demonstrate the use of mindfulness meditation when experiencing symptoms of heightened anxiety (see Box 10-2)

BOX 10-2   MINDFULNESS MEDITATION

- The individual learns meditation to reduce stress by concentrating on her or his body.
- The individual pays attention to the act of breathing to enhance concentration.
- The individual observes the act of breathing, attending to the inhaling and exhaling of each breath.
- Meditation discourages intrusive thoughts; the patient agrees to deal with the subject of the intrusive thought at a later time.
- The individual benefits by feeling in control of his or her body. There is a reduction of pain and anxiety, and the individual feels hopeful.

From Ott MJ: Mindfulness meditation: a path of transformation and healing, *J Psychosoc Nurs Ment Health Serv* 42(7):22-29, 2004.

Obsessive-Compulsive Disorder

The patient will do the following:

- Participate actively in learned strategies to manage anxiety and to decrease obsessive-compulsive behaviors, such as using mindfulness meditation (see Box 10-2).
- Describe an increasing sense of control over intrusive thoughts and ritualistic behaviors.
- Demonstrate the ability to cope effectively when thoughts or rituals are interrupted.
- Spend less time involved in anxiety-binding activities and instead use the time gained to complete activities of daily living and to participate in social or recreational activities.
- Successfully manage times of increased stress by integrating knowledge that thoughts, impulses, and images are involuntary, thereby reducing the sense of responsibility and consequent anxiety. The use of conscious thought extinction techniques taught in cognitive behavioral therapy can assist the patient with decreasing the attention paid to the repeated thought patterns that increase anxiety (see Chapter 26).
- Discuss the medication regimen and take the medications as prescribed.
- Identify when to call the therapist for more visits when a crisis occurs.

Posttraumatic Stress Disorder

The patient will do the following:

- Demonstrate concern for personal safety by beginning to verbalize worries.
- Participate actively in a support group, individual therapy, or both.
- Identify and involve a significant support system.
- Assume a decision-making role for his or her own health care needs.
- Acquire and practice strategies for coping with anxiety symptoms, such as breathing techniques; progressive relaxation exercises; thought, image, and memory substitution; and assertive behaviors (see Chapters 26 and 27).
- Discuss the medication regimen and take the medications as prescribed.
- Identify when to utilize an as-needed medication to decrease the heightened anxiety response to a cue in the environment.
- Contact the therapist for immediate help when a crisis occurs.
- Identify the need to call the therapist for more visits when symptoms increase.

PLANNING

Treatment planning for the patient with anxiety disorders in the current health care environment is complex and varied. Patients with severe OCD were formerly hospitalized for structured behavioral programs.

Today, both clinicians and administrators in inpatient facilities are struggling to balance effective treatment with the high costs that are associated with these specialty units.

Inpatient hospitalization is increasingly only available for short periods of time for patients who are at risk to themselves or others. Rather than assuming their traditional roles of providing direct care to patients in inpatient facilities, nurses are becoming case managers. As case managers, nurses provide information about treatment alternatives to patients and their families.

IMPLEMENTATION

The role of a nurse in the implementation of a care plan for patients with anxiety and related disorders depends on the setting. The following interventions are useful for patients with anxiety symptoms, regardless of diagnosis or treatment setting.

Nursing Interventions

1. Maintain safety for the patient and the environment. A patient's anxiety can escalate to a panic state, which can frighten and harm the patient and others. The nurse's first priority is to protect the patient and the environment.
2. Assess your own level of anxiety, and make a conscious effort to remain calm. Anxiety is readily transferable from one person to another.
3. Recognize the patient's use of relief behaviors (e.g., pacing, wringing of hands) as indicators of anxiety. Early interventions help to manage anxiety before symptoms escalate to more serious levels.
4. Inform the patient of the importance of limiting caffeine, nicotine, and other central nervous-system stimulants. Limiting these substances prevents or minimizes the physical symptoms of anxiety (e.g., rapid heart rate, jitteriness).
5. Teach the patient to distinguish between anxiety that is connected to identifiable objects or sources (e.g., illness, prognosis, hospitalization, known stressors) and anxiety for which there is no immediately identifiable object or source. Knowledge of anxiety and its related components increases the patient's control over the disorder.
6. Instruct the patient in the following anxiety-reducing strategies. These help to lessen anxiety in a variety of ways, and they distract the patient from focusing on the anxiety (see Chapters 26 and 27):
   a. Progressive relaxation techniques
   b. Mindfulness meditation (Box 10-2)
   c. Slow deep-breathing exercises
   d. Focusing on a single object in the room
   e. Listening to soothing music or relaxation tapes
   f. Visual imagery or nature-related DVDs
   g. Exercise
7. Help the patient to build on the coping methods that the patient used to manage anxiety in the past. Coping methods that were previously successful will generally be effective in subsequent situations.
8. Help the patient to identify support persons who will help the patient to perform personal tasks and activities

that current circumstances (e.g., a partial hospitalization program, a short-stay hospitalization) make difficult. A strong support system will help the patient to avoid anxiety-provoking situations and activities.

9. Assist the patient with gaining control of overwhelming feelings and impulses through brief and direct verbal interactions. Individual interactions that are executed at appropriate intervals will reduce or manage the patient's anxious feelings and impulses.

10. Help the patient to structure the environment so that it is less noisy. A less stimulating environment creates a calming and stress-free atmosphere that reduces anxiety.

11. Assess the presence and degree of depression and suicidal ideation in all patients with anxiety and related disorders. A thorough assessment results in early intervention that will possibly prevent self-harm.

12. Administer anxiolytic (antianxiety) medication as a least restrictive measure. Medication is often the first appropriate method for reducing debilitating anxiety.

13. Help the patient to understand the importance of the medication regimen and to take it as prescribed. Medication is an effective addition to other psychosocial therapeutic interventions, when necessary.

Additional Treatment Modalities
Biologic Interventions

Pharmacologic Interventions. Pharmacologic interventions alone or in combination with cognitive behavioral interventions are among the most successful treatments for anxiety and related disorders. Since the early 1960s, benzodiazepines have been used widely for the treatment of anxiety disorders. They are relatively safe and effective for short-term use to control the debilitating symptoms of anxiety. However, longer-term treatment with these drugs raises issues of tolerance, abuse, and dependence.

Selective serotonin reuptake inhibitors, which are antidepressants that are now widely used for the treatment of anxiety disorders, are particularly effective for the treatment of OCD and panic disorders. Fluoxetine and fluvoxamine are for OCD; paroxetine is for GAD, OCD, panic disorder, PTSD, and social phobia. Sertraline is for OCD, panic disorder, and PTSD; venlafaxine is for GAD. Benzodiazepines are useful for the initial treatment of anxiety disorders. As a result of the side effects of tolerance and dependence, this group of medications is best used for the short term (Ravindran and Ravindran, 2009). Pharmacologic treatment for PTSD is largely symptomatic. The American Psychiatric Association clinical practice guideline for the treatment of individuals with acute stress disorder and PTSD suggests that sertraline (Zoloft) and paroxetine (Paxil) are the first-line treatment for symptoms of PTSD. Individuals with PTSD have shown improvement in global functioning and a reduction of symptoms (e.g., reexperiencing the trauma) with the use of certain tricyclics, such as imipramine (Tofranil) (Benedek et al, 2009; American Psychiatric Association, 2004) (see Chapter 25). (see Medication Key Facts box)

⬤ MEDICATION KEY FACTS BOX
Anxiety Disorders

Pharmacologic treatment includes benzodiazepines (e.g., alprazolam [Xanax], clonazepam [Klonopin], diazepam [Valium], lorazepam [Ativan]) and nonbenzodiazepines (e.g., buspirone [Buspar]). Other medications include antidepressants and pregabalin (Lyrica).

Benzodiazepine
- This drug may cause physical and psychologic dependence.
- Alcohol and other central nervous system depressants may potentiate the action of this drug, especially in elderly patients.
- Blood dyscrasias (e.g., fever, sore throat, bruising, rash, jaundice) are rare.
- *Herbal considerations:* Kava kava and St. John's wort may potentiate the action of this drug.
- *Dietary considerations:* Grapefruit juice may increase blood concentration and the risk of toxicity.

Nonbenzodiazepine (Buspirone)
- Monoamine oxidase inhibitors may increase blood pressure; *do not use these drugs together.*
- This drug has a lower potential for abuse, addiction, or tolerance.

Psychotherapy

Psychotherapeutic intervention takes place in group or individual settings. One advantage of group therapy is the opportunity for the patient to learn from the successes and failures of others with similar symptoms. Behavioral and cognitive behavioral therapies have been widely effective for the treatment of a variety of anxiety disorders (see Chapter 26) (Benedek et al, 2009).

Behavioral Therapy. Behavioral treatments, including systematic desensitization, are among the most effective treatments for panic disorder with agoraphobia. First, the therapist and the patient define the phobic stimulus. Together, they define a hierarchy for the phobic stimulus. The patient and the therapist then expose the patient to events on the hierarchy that increase the patient's degree of anxiety. As the patient and therapist move through the hierarchy, the patient progressively masters increasing levels of anxiety until he or she encounters the phobic stimulus (see Chapter 26).

Cognitive Behavioral Therapy. Cognitive behavioral therapy is widely used for the treatment of anxiety disorders. The success of this approach centers on the patient's understanding that the symptoms are a learned response to thoughts or feelings about behaviors that occur in daily life. The patient and therapist identify the target symptoms and then examine the circumstances associated with the symptoms. Together, they plan strategies to change either the cognitions or the behaviors. Cognitive behavioral therapy is short-term and demands active participation on the part of both the patient and the therapist (see Chapter 26) (Roy-Byrne et al, 2010).

Psychologic First Aid. Psychologic first aid is currently recommended as an initial response if a person or a group of individuals encounters a traumatic event or loss. This involves protecting individuals who have experienced or witnessed the trauma from any further injury or harm by reducing their psychologic arousal. Support for individuals who are demonstrating distress is obtained by keeping families together so that there is support among family members. Information about stress reduction and common side effects of trauma must be given to individuals who have been involved with the trauma to help them to return to their pre-event psychologic state. It is important to provide information about where they can receive further assistance for their psychologic needs. The research suggests that brief cognitive behavioral therapy may be the intervention of choice to prevent further trauma-related maladaptive responses. Research into the use of critical incident stress debriefing has been inconclusive with regard to the prevention of individuals from developing acute stress disorder or PTSD after a traumatic incident (Benedek et al, 2009).

Additional treatment modalities and collaborative interventions include consultation with occupational therapists, vocational rehabilitation counselors, and psychologists, depending on the particular treatment needs of the patient. A summary of additional treatment modalities appears in the Additional Treatment Modalities box and in Chapter 26.

EVALUATION

A number of valid and time-tested tools are available that yield reliable information about anxiety disorders. Although

---

ADDITIONAL TREATMENT MODALITIES
Anxiety Disorders

- Biologic
  - Pharmacologic
    Benzodiazepines
    Selective serotonin reuptake inhibitors
    Tricyclic antidepressants
    Monoamine oxidase inhibitors
- Psychotherapy
  - Behavioral therapy
  - Cognitive behavioral therapy
  - Psychologic first aid

---

these tools are not specifically for nurses, clinical rating scales offer a method for tracking changes in symptoms over time with a numeric value. These changes are correlated with discrete interventions (e.g., instituting a behavioral program or a change in medication). Three rating scales that are commonly used with patients who exhibit anxiety disorders are the Yale-Brown Obsessive-Compulsive Scale, the Beck Anxiety Inventory, and the Hamilton Anxiety Scale.

Ideally, the nurse evaluates patient progress toward the identified outcomes during every interaction with the patient. If the patient does not make satisfactory progress, the nurse modifies either the expected outcomes or the interventions. The nurse examines all factors that relate to the outcomes, including what occurred during the previous phases of the nursing process, the role of the nurse in setting patient and clinician expectations, the clarity of communicating patient goals with the patient, and other intervening events that have occurred since the outcomes were set.

◎ CONCEPT MAP CASE STUDY 10-1

Wendy, a 47-year-old woman, presented to the employee health department of a teaching hospital after walking there from her office. She was complaining of chest pain and shortness of breath. The staff instituted the standard cardiac workup for patients with new-onset chest pain. Wendy's medical history included psoriasis. Her vital signs were remarkable for a pulse of 116 bpm, but her electrocardiogram and laboratory work were within normal limits.

Wendy mentioned to the staff that her son had died 3 months ago. She was referred to a research team that was conducting a study on panic disorder, and she saw a clinical specialist in psychiatric mental health nursing. Wendy participated in the research protocol after giving informed consent. During the course of the interview, she revealed that her deceased son, who was her only child, had been an alcoholic whose death was a suicide. She was presently considering separating from her husband of 27 years who was involved in a long-term extramarital affair. Her screening was positive for limited-symptom panic attacks that were increasing in frequency. She agreed to an extended evaluation after her initial interview.

During the evaluation, Wendy and the nurse explored Wendy's symptoms of anxiety and depression, the exacerbation of her psoriasis, and her chronic headaches, which had become worse since her son's death. After moving back from the West Coast, Wendy had obtained her first job in 24 years. In addition to concern about financial matters and her son's alcoholism, she now worried frequently about her performance at work. She revealed that her husband's extramarital affair had been occurring for several years, and she related his behavior to their sexual difficulties. The nurse recommended a medication trial. Wendy refused medication because of her fears of addiction and loss of control. See Figure 10-2.

DSM-IV-TR Diagnoses
Axis I Generalized anxiety disorder (with limited-symptom panic attacks)
      Bereavement
      Partner relational problem
Axis II Deferred
Axis III Psoriasis
      Headaches
Axis IV Problems with primary support system
Axis V GAF = 60 (current); GAF = 75 (past year)

Nursing Diagnosis *Anxiety related to changes in role functioning, recent loss of son (complicated grieving), threat to socioeconomic status, and stressors exceeding ability to cope as evidenced by uncertainty, intermittent sympathetic nervous system stimulation, restlessness, and exacerbation of medical condition (psoriasis)*

NOC Anxiety self-control; Symptom control; Psychosocial adjustment: life change; Neurologic status: autonomic, coping
NIC Anxiety reduction; Anticipatory guidance; Teaching: individual; Counseling; Coping enhancement

Nursing Diagnosis *Complicated grieving related to ineffective coping response to son's death as evidenced by anxiety on returning home; disturbed sleep pattern; expression of guilt, sadness, and crying; difficulty with concentration*

NOC Grief resolution; Psychosocial adjustment: life change; Role performance; Sleep; Coping; Family coping
NIC Grief work facilitation, Guilt work facilitation, Emotional support, Family support, Family integrity promotion, Coping enhancement

Nursing Diagnosis *Decisional conflict related to uncertainty surrounding personal values and beliefs as evidenced by delayed decision making and physical signs of distress when faced with decisions, specifically regarding her relationship with her husband*

NOC Information processing, Decision making, Personal autonomy, Family social climate, Family functioning, Family coping
NIC Self-awareness enhancement, Values clarification, Decision-making support, Mutual goal setting, Support system enhancement

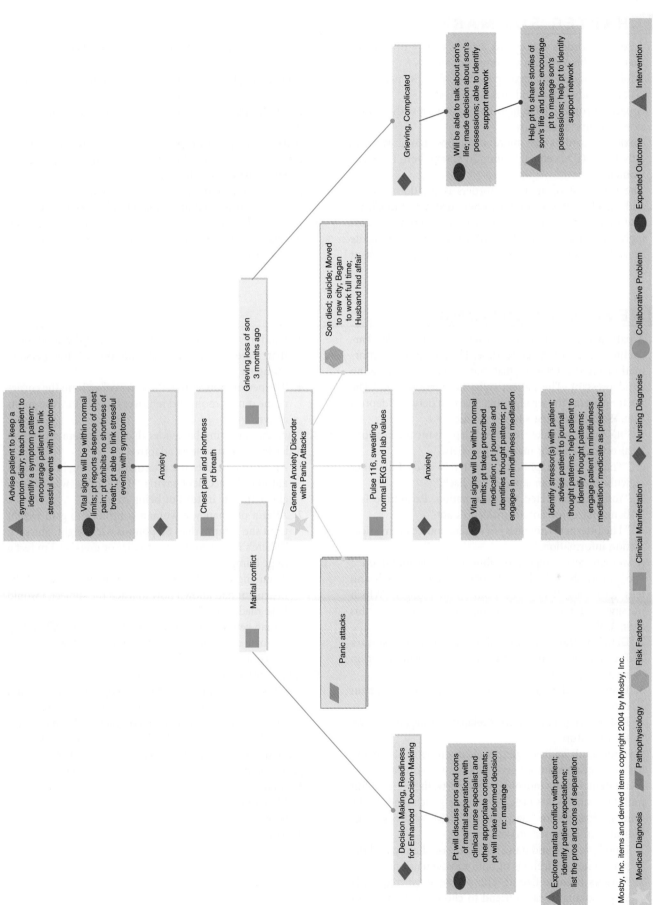

FIGURE 10-2. Concept map: anxiety with panic symptoms.

Mosby, Inc. items and derived items copyright 2004 by Mosby, Inc.

Medical Diagnosis   Pathophysiology   Risk Factors   Clinical Manifestation   Nursing Diagnosis   Collaborative Problem   Expected Outcome   Intervention

CHAPTER SUMMARY

- Anxiety disorders encompass a wide variety of illnesses that share the common symptoms of anxiety.
- Etiologic models for anxiety include biologic, psychosocial, psychodynamic, and social theories.
- Anxiety disorders have high co-occurrence with depression and substance abuse.
- Anxiety disorders are more common among women, although OCD is equally common among both men and women.
- The treatment of anxiety disorders is multidisciplinary and usually involves more than one treatment modality.
- The inpatient treatment of anxiety disorders is increasingly rare and is generally confined to managing acute exacerbations if the person becomes a danger to self or others or if the symptoms are so severe that they greatly reduce self-care functions.
- The nursing role in the treatment of patients with anxiety symptoms varies. Nurses in all treatment settings will assist the patient and family with education about the disorders and their treatment.
- Nursing care plans for patients with symptoms of anxiety reflect the understanding that managing anxiety effectively is part of daily living.
- Nurses actively participate in behavioral interventions that have been structured to decrease phobic responses.
- Rating scales are an effective means for nurses to measure the success of strategies that have been implemented to reduce anxiety.

REVIEW QUESTIONS

1. A patient with GAD receives a new prescription for Paroxetine (Paxil) 10 mg at bedtime. The patient finds information on the Internet that states that the drug is an antidepressant. The patient calls the nurse saying, "The doctor gave me the wrong drug. I have anxiety, not depression." Select the nurse's best response.
   1. "It's not a mistake. Some antidepressant medications also work well for managing anxiety."
   2. "Thank you for phoning about this error. I'll confer with the physician and call you back."
   3. "You misinterpreted the information. Paroxetine is a benzodiazepine not an antidepressant."
   4. "The Internet is not always a reliable source for medication information."

2. A woman gets a report of abnormal cells found on a Pap smear. She calls her attorney to prepare a will and tells her family, "I won't be around much longer." Which nursing diagnosis and etiology best apply to this situation?
   1. Deficient knowledge related to reasons for Pap smears
   2. Fear related to misinterpretation and misinformation regarding Pap tests
   3. Disturbed thought processes related to malignant cancer
   4. Risk-prone health behavior related to a negative vision for the future

3. A young adult invites eight people to dinner. This person has never given a dinner party and wants to prepare every menu item. On the morning of the party, the young adult multitasks and makes progress preparing each food. As the time approaches for the guests to arrive, which change indicates an increased anxiety level?
   1. Blood pressure and pulse rates increase slightly, and the person notices feelings of mild muscle tension.
   2. Muscles become flaccid. The person must frequently stop cooking to call a friend to check the accuracy of a recipe.
   3. Fond memories of family reunions and the good foods that were served drift in and out of the person's thoughts.
   4. The person notices that there are cobwebs in the corner of the dining room and removes them before the guests arrive.

4. Place the following behaviors that result from anxiety in order from most to least adaptive.
   1. An adult describes the aftermath of being in a serious automobile accident saying, "I felt like I was floating above the car instead of being in it."
   2. After a pregnancy, a woman continues to gain weight until she is more than 80 pounds overweight. She says, "There's no reason for me to diet or exercise. I'm just a huge blimp."
   3. A nursing student fails a major exam and states, "If the instructor had known how to teach the subject, I would have made an A."
   4. A man gets a chocolate stain on his necktie while eating a cookie and chuckles, "Oh well, I guess that's the way the cookie crumbles."

5. After 3 weeks of hemoptysis (coughing blood), a person finally seeks treatment. A chest radiograph is taken, and the person waits for the results. When the physician explains the report, the person complains, "I can't understand what you're saying. You're talking so fast. All I hear is a loud clicking on my watch." The patient is wet with perspiration. Which level of anxiety is evident?
   1. Mild
   2. Moderate
   3. Severe
   4. Panic

REFERENCES

American Psychiatric Association: *Diagnostic and statistical manual of mental disorders*, ed 4, text revision, Washington, DC, American Psychiatric Association, 2000.

American Psychiatric Association: *Clinical practice guidelines: acute stress disorder and post traumatic stress disorder*, Washington, DC, American Psychiatric Association, 2004.

American Psychiatric Association: *Clinical practice guidelines: panic disorder*, ed 2, Washington, DC, American Psychiatric Association, 2009.

Benedek DM et al: *Guideline watch (March 2009): practice guideline for the treatment of patients with acute stress disorder and posttraumatic stress disorder*, Washington, DC, 2009, American Psychiatric Association.

Freud S: Introductory lectures on psychoanalysis. In Freud S, editor: *The standard edition of the complete psychological works*, London, 1963 (originally published in 1917), Hogarth Press.

Helbing MC, Ficca M: Obsessive-compulsive disorder in school-age children, *J School Nursing* 25(1):15-27, 2009.

Irle E et al: Reduced amygdalar and hippocampal size in adults with generalized social phobia, *J Psychiatry Neurosci* 35(2):126-132, 2010.

Landsman KJ et al: *Loving someone with OCD: help for you and your family*, Oakland, Calif, 2005, New Harbinger.

Likhtik E et al: Amygdala intercalated neurons are required for expression of fear extinction, *Nature* 454(7204):642-645, 2008.

National Institutes of Mental Health: The numbers count: mental disorders in America (website): www.nimh.nih.gov/health/publications/the-numbers-count-mental-disorders-in-america/index.shtml. Accessed October 19, 2010.

Peplau H: *Interpersonal relations in nursing*, New York, 1952, Putnam.

Ravindran AV, Ravindran L: Depression and comorbid anxiety: an overview of pharmacological options, *Psychiatric Times* 26(6):53-58, 2009.

Roy-Byrne P et al: Delivery of evidence-based treatment for multiple anxiety disorders in primary care: a randomized controlled trial, *JAMA* 303(19):1921-1928, 2010.

Selye H: *The stress of life*, New York, 1956, McGraw-Hill.

Wolpe J: The practice of behavior therapy, ed 2, New York, 1973, Pergamon Press.

Online Resources

Anxiety Disorders Association of America: www.adaa.org
International OCD Foundation: www.ocfoundation.org
Mental Health America: www.nmha.org
National Center for Post-Traumatic Stress Disorder: www.ncptsd.va.gov
National Alliance on Mental Illness: www.nami.org
National Institute of Mental Health: www.nimh.nih.gov
Posttraumatic Stress Disorder Alliance: www.ptsdalliance.org

11

Somatoform, Factitious, and Dissociative Disorders

Pamela E. Marcus

"After great pain, a formal feeling comes. The nerves sit ceremonious, like tombs."

Emily Dickinson

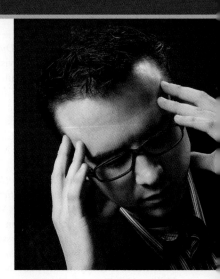

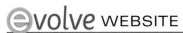 WEBSITE

http://evolve.elsevier.com/Fortinash/

OBJECTIVES

- Name four physical symptoms that are reported by patients with somatization disorder.
- Discuss two treatment strategies that reduce the symptoms of somatization disorder.
- Apply the nursing process for managing patients with somatization disorder.
- List two symptoms of pain disorder and interventions that are useful for the reduction of symptoms.
- Describe a major symptom of conversion disorder and an effective nursing response to this symptom.
- Identify two symptoms of hypochondriasis and two appropriate nursing interventions.

- Describe the symptoms of body dysmorphic disorder.
- Formulate three nursing assessment questions to ask an individual with suspected body dysmorphic disorder.
- Describe the symptoms of factitious disorder.
- Identify two nursing interventions that are helpful for the reduction of symptoms of factitious disorder.
- Relate the biologic patterns to target symptoms and therapeutic agents for psychopharmacologic interventions for somatization disorder and body dysmorphic disorder.

KEY TERMS

body dysmorphic disorder
conversion disorder
countertransference

dissociation
factitious disorder
hypochondriasis

la belle indifference
pain disorder
somatization disorder

HISTORIC AND THEORETIC PERSPECTIVES

Somatoform disorders include a group of disorders that convert anxiety into physical symptoms for which there is no identifiable physical diagnosis. Theorists believe that the physical symptoms are linked to psychobiologic factors that are not intentional or under the conscious control of the patient. *Soma* is the Greek word for body, and somatization is the expression of psychologic stress through physical symptoms. The etiology of somatoform disorders and other

disorders that express anxiety through physical symptoms can be traced to the work of Briquet, for whom somatization disorder was originally named (i.e., Briquet syndrome). In 1859, a French physician Paul Briquet (1796-1881), wrote about somatization in his book *Treatise on Hysteria*. For more than 10 years, he followed 430 patients who had a diagnosis of hysteria with a focus on bodily concerns and sensations. Briquet disputed the belief that hysteria originated in the female reproductive system via what was termed a "wandering uterus." His hypothesis was that hysteria was caused by an impact on the nervous system as a result of life stressors, such as marital conflict, child abuse, and family losses.

The results of Briquet's study found that 14% of his patients demonstrated symptoms after a psychologic trauma, such as a rape, witnessing a fire, or witnessing a sibling jumping from a high window. He described other stressors that were related to conflict in the individual or the family, such as unplanned pregnancy, conflict in the marriage, or issues related to in-laws' input into their adult children's marital dynamics.

Briquet's research subjects were 87 individuals who were younger than 12 years old who had been abused or neglected. He described these children as being held constantly in fear. Briquet also studied nuns, household servants, and prostitutes. The results of his research demonstrated that hysteria was rarely found in nuns. There were 197 prostitutes in his research population. Of these prostitutes, 104 had hysteria. An additional 29 prostitutes had intense nervous reactions that were similar to mild forms of hysteria (Briquet, 1859).

ETIOLOGY

Somatoform disorders reflect complex interactions between the mind and the body, with serious impairment in the person's social and occupational functioning. Psychoanalytic theory suggests that psychogenic complaints of pain, disease, or loss of functioning are generally related to repressed aggression or sexuality. For example, with conversion disorder, the individual may be expressing a forbidden thought or wish by converting it into physical symptoms that are more appropriate and acceptable and that also elicit sympathy, care, and attention from others. Some theorists see hypochondriasis as an acceptable way to express anger or hostility that results from past losses or disappointments. The physical symptoms supply the person with the help and concern needed to make up for his or her troubled past. Others see hypochondriasis as a defense against guilt or a low self-concept. In this case, the physical symptoms may be viewed as a well-deserved punishment. With pain disorder, the pain may be the person's way of gaining the love and care of others or a reprimand for actual or perceived wrongful acts. With body dysmorphic disorder (BDD), some theorists believe that the person gives a special meaning to the body or body part that is related to an event that occurred early during his or her psychosexual development. The body part is the symbol of the earlier event that is repressed. Examples of BDD may be seen in people who undergo extensive and painful cosmetic surgeries that seem distorting and disfiguring to others.

Biologic Theory

In biologic terms, changes in the structure and function of the brain caused by prolonged stress or trauma can result in somatoform disorders by altering the individual's perceptions and interpretations of bodily functions. It is puzzling why some persons develop an anxiety disorder and others develop a somatoform disorder, although many patients experience both. There is speculation that there may be a disruption in the physical sensation signals that are part of the cortical system. Somatoform disorders may be caused in part by a misinterpreted cortical perception of distress. Neurotransmitters such as serotonin and norepinephrine are closely involved with depression and anxiety, but they are also known to modulate pain. Individuals who experience severe pain generally have abnormal levels of neurotransmitters, particularly serotonin (Marcangelo and Wise, 2007).

Behavioral Theory

Behaviorists believe that some individuals learn to use somatic symptoms to communicate helplessness and to manipulate others. Attention from others tends to exacerbate somatic symptoms in these individuals. Nurses and doctors in the United States are trained to respond to patients who report pain. Pain is considered the fifth vital sign in this country, and it must be addressed during admission and throughout the patient's hospital stay. In a study to determine if there is a correlation between alexithymia and somatization, an objective tool called the Toronto Alexithymia Scale was used. The concept *alexithymia* is defined as the inability of an individual to describe his or her feelings in words. An individual who has alexithymia tends to express feelings with somatic concerns. An example of this is a woman who is angry with her boss. Instead of being able to discuss her angry feelings with her friend, she reports stomach pain and frequently calls in sick to work. The study that examined the association between alexithymia and somatization showed results from the Toronto Alexithymia Scale that demonstrated that individuals who scored high in areas relating to "difficulties identifying feelings" also showed a strong relationship between alexithymia and somatization (Mattila et al, 2008).

Cognitive Theory

Cognitive theorists believe that patients with somatic symptoms misinterpret the meaning of body functions and sensations and become overly alarmed by them. Cognitive theorists advocate cognitive therapy to help patients to reinterpret the meaning of body sensations; this is discussed later in this chapter and in Chapter 26.

EPIDEMIOLOGY

The epidemiologic data of this group of disorders differ with regard to incidence and prevalence (Box 11-1). With these disorders, it is interesting to note that some believe that an increase in diagnoses may be caused by a greater awareness of the disorder, whereas others think the increase is the result of overdiagnosis of the disorder in highly suggestible individuals. The committee that is evaluating diagnostic categories for the fifth edition of the *Diagnostic and Statistical Manual of Mental Disorders* (DSM) is discussing the best way to define the somatic disorders, including somatization disorder, hypochondriasis, and pain disorder. Most of

---

BOX 11-1   **EPIDEMIOLOGY OF SOMATOFORM, FACTITIOUS, AND DISSOCIATIVE DISORDERS**

Somatoform Disorders
Somatization Disorder
Widely variable lifetime prevalence, from 0.2% to 2% among women and less than 0.2% among men
Occurs in all cultures; most prevalent in South America, where 60% to 80% of the population may have somatic symptoms without a known organic cause

Conversion Disorder
Widely varied prevalence; reported cases from 11 per 100,000 to 500 per 100,000 in the general population
Reported in up to 3% of outpatient referrals to mental health clinics
Conversion symptoms identified in 1% to 14% of general medicosurgical patients

Pain Disorder
Prevalence unknown
Association with both psychologic issues and general medical condition seems fairly common
Association with only psychologic factors appears much less common

Hypochondriasis
Seen in 1% to 5% of the general population
Seen in 2% to 7% of primary care outpatients

Body Dysmorphic Disorder
Prevalence unknown
Seen in 5% to 40% of patients in mental health settings with concurrent anxiety or depressive disorders
Seen in 6% to 15% of patients in cosmetic surgery and dermatology settings

Factitious Disorder
Limited information about prevalence because this disorder generally involves deception, which is difficult to recognize
More common among females than males; Munchausen is the most chronic and severe form, in which a person feigns illness or injures the self to gain sympathy; more common among males
Higher prevalence in specialized treatment settings

Dissociative Disorders
Dissociative Amnesia
Recent increase in reported cases involving previously forgotten early childhood memories

Dissociative Fugue
Seen in 0.2% of the general population
Prevalence may increase during times of extraordinarily stressful events

Dissociative Identity Disorder
Recent increase in reported cases

Depersonalization Disorder
Lifetime prevalence in community and clinical settings unknown
Half of all adults may experience a single brief episode during their lifetimes, usually as a result of stress

Data the from American Psychiatric Association: *Diagnostic and statistical manual of mental disorders,* ed 4, text revision, Washington, DC, 2000, American Psychiatric Association.

---

the discussion revolves around clarifying the definition for clinicians, for medicolegal purposes, and with a consideration for cultural reactions to stress (Marcangelo and Wise, 2007; www.dsm5.org, 2010).

CLINICAL DESCRIPTION

Somatoform Disorders
Somatization Disorder

Somatization disorder was formerly called *hysteria* and *Briquet syndrome* (Briquet, 1859). Briquet developed a checklist of somatic concerns that are commonly voiced by the population as a whole. If a patient had reported concerns in 13 out of 35 items, the individual was considered to have Briquet syndrome. The checklist was shortened for DSM-IV-TR, and is discussed in the following narrative. The characteristic pattern of patients who present with somatization disorder is one of frequently seeking and obtaining medical treatment for multiple and clinically significant somatic complaints. To meet the DSM-IV-TR criteria, the symptoms

must begin before the patient is 30 years old and not be adequately explained by any general medical disorder or the direct effects of a substance. For example, patients with multiple sclerosis, systemic lupus erythematosus, or other chronic debilitating diseases that have an onset during early adulthood frequently present with multisystem complaints; however, they do not have somatization disorder because they have general medical conditions that better explain their symptom complexes.

The distribution of symptoms with somatization disorder requires that symptoms have a distinct pattern that differs from general medical conditions if the following three criteria are met: (1) there is involvement of multiple organ systems (e.g., gastrointestinal, reproductive, neurologic); (2) the symptoms exhibit an early onset and a chronic course without the development of physical signs or structural abnormalities; and (3) the clinical laboratory abnormalities that are commonly associated with general medical conditions are absent. The specific diagnostic criteria are listed in the DSM-IV-TR Criteria box. Nurses in a general hospital or clinical practice setting are more likely to encounter patients with somatization disorder than those who are working in inpatient psychiatric units.

Pain Disorder

The predominant focus of the clinical presentation in **pain disorder** is pain in one or more anatomic sites. The severity of the pain calls for clinical attention and causes clinically significant impairment in one or more areas of functioning. Psychologic factors have an important role in the onset, severity, exacerbation, or maintenance of the pain. This experience of pain is not the result of a mood, anxiety, or psychotic disorder, and it does not meet the criteria for dyspareunia (i.e., painful coitus or intercourse). This disorder is a pain disorder that is associated with psychologic factors. If a general medical condition plays a major role in the maintenance of the syndrome, the disorder is pain disorder associated with both psychologic factors and a general medical condition. Both types of disorders can be either acute (if the duration is less than 6 months) or chronic (if the pain extends beyond 6 months) (American Psychiatric Association, 2000).

Conversion Disorder

Patients who present with conversion symptoms exhibit one or more symptoms that affect voluntary motor or sensory function. These symptoms appear to be related to a neurologic or general medical condition; however, they are not caused by a general medical condition, the direct effects of a substance, or a culturally sanctioned behavior or experience. The symptom is not intentionally produced, and it is not limited to pain or sexual dysfunction. The conversion symptoms cause clinically significant distress or impairment in social, occupational, or other important areas of functioning. Common symptoms are blindness, paralysis, deafness, seizures, anesthesia, or abnormal motor movements (American Psychiatric Association, 2000) (see Case Study #1).

The critical defining characteristics of **conversion disorder** are as follows: (1) psychologic factors are identified as being related to the onset or exacerbation of the symptom; (2) specific and identifiable conflicts or stressors precede the development of the conversion symptoms; and (3) the person demonstrates an obvious lack of concern about the seriousness of the symptoms, which is inconsistent with the problem. This lack of concern is called *la belle indifference* or "beautiful indifference," which is a hallmark symptom of conversion disorder.

Hypochondriasis

"Don't be such a hypochondriac!" is a common theme in American culture and perhaps in other cultures as well. Parents say it to children who complain about having stomachaches before school on the day of an important test. Sometimes even nursing students say it to each other as they worry about potential signs and symptoms while learning and acquiring knowledge related to medical, surgical, or psychiatric mental health nursing. However, such instances

---

DSM-IV-TR CRITERIA
Somatization Disorder

A A history of many physical complaints beginning before age 30 that occur over several years and result in treatment being sought or significant impairment in social, occupational, or other important areas of functioning.

B Each of the following criteria must have been met, with individual symptoms occurring at any time during the course of the disturbance:

1 Four pain symptoms: a history of pain related to at least four different sites or functions (e.g., head, abdomen, back, joints, extremities, chest, rectum, during menstruation, during sexual intercourse, or during urination).

2 Two gastrointestinal symptoms: a history of at least two gastrointestinal symptoms other than pain (e.g., nausea, bloating, vomiting other than during pregnancy, diarrhea, or intolerance of several different foods).

3 One sexual symptom: a history of at least one sexual or reproductive symptom other than pain (e.g., sexual indifference, erectile or ejaculatory dysfunction, irregular menses, excessive menstrual bleeding, vomiting throughout pregnancy).

4 One pseudoneurologic symptom: a history of at least one symptom or deficit suggesting a neurologic condition not limited to pain (conversion symptoms such as impaired coordination or balance, paralysis, or localized weakness; difficulty swallowing or lump in throat; aphonia (loss of voice); urinary retention; hallucinations; loss of touch or pain sensation; double vision; blindness; deafness; seizures; dissociative symptoms such as amnesia; or loss of consciousness other than fainting).

C Either 1 or 2:

1 After appropriate investigation, each of the symptoms in criterion B cannot be fully explained by a known general medical condition or the direct effects of a substance (e.g., a drug of abuse or a medication).

2 When there is a related general medical condition, the physical complaints or resulting social or occupational impairment is in excess of what would be expected from the history, physical examination, or laboratory findings.

D The symptoms are not intentionally produced (as in factitious disorder or malingering).

From American Psychiatric Association: *Diagnostic and statistical manual of mental disorders,* ed 4, text revision, Washington DC, 2000, American Psychiatric Association.

---

probably do not reflect true **hypochondriasis** as defined in the DSM-IV-TR.

Six major criteria are associated with this diagnosis. First, the individual focuses on fears of having or the idea of having a serious medical disorder on the basis of his or her misinterpretation of bodily symptoms. Second, this misinterpretation of symptoms persists despite appropriate medical

Carlos is a 34-year-old patient on a neurologic unit in a Department of Veterans Affairs medical center. He has been treated by the psychiatric service in this facility for a number of years, and he was diagnosed with schizophrenia primarily on the basis of his prominent and constant visual and auditory hallucinations involving his former drill sergeant. In the past, he has taken the antipsychotic medication haloperidol (Haldol).

Carlos was born in Puerto Rico, and he joined the Marines in San Juan when he turned 18. He was unable to complete basic training because he experienced a psychotic episode during which he assaulted his drill sergeant. Carlos was admitted to the neurology department when one morning he told his family that he was unable to walk. Carlos had no recent falls or other injuries. Providers did not find any abnormalities on his physical examination or on a computerized tomography scan. During a mental status examination, Carlos reported that he no longer heard any voices. The nursing assessment also revealed Carlos' lack of concern about this inability to walk. The psychiatric mental health nurse specialist learned from Carlos' family that, about a month before his admission, Carlos' appeal for a service-related disability was turned down. His family was depending on that financial supplement to help them obtain better housing, which is a goal that they had voiced on many occasions.

Critical Thinking

1 What are two symptoms that indicate that Carlos is experiencing a conversion disorder?
2 How does the recent behavior of Carlos' family play a role in his current symptomatology?
3 Which of Carlos' symptoms might be labeled *la belle indifference*?
4 How does Carlos' assaultive behavior during his psychotic episode influence his perceived paralysis?
5 What are two behavioral outcomes that would indicate Carlos' ability to better cope with his disorder?

evaluation and reassurance. Third, the individual's preoccupation with symptoms is not as intense or distorted as it would be with a delusional disorder nor is it as restricted as it would be with BDD. The fourth criterion states that the preoccupation causes clinically significant distress or impairment in social, occupational, or other major areas of functioning. To meet the fifth criterion, the duration of the disturbance must be at least 6 months. The sixth criterion is that the hypochondriasis is not caused by another anxiety disorder, somatoform disorder, or major depressive episode (American Psychiatric Association, 2000; Brier and Halverson, 2009)

Body Dysmorphic Disorder

Body dysmorphic disorder occurs when a patient is preoccupied with a self-perceived defect in appearance. If the individual has a slight physical anomaly, the person's concern is markedly focused on this deficit. This preoccupation causes clinically significant distress or impairment in social or occupational functioning, and it is not the result of another mental disorder.

BDD usually begins during adolescence, but it sometimes may begin during childhood. Diagnosis may take years because patients hide their symptoms, and the onset can be gradual or abrupt (American Psychiatric Association, 2000). Depending on how the patient experiences the severity of the symptoms or the extent to which the patient focuses on the perceived deficit, behavior patterns sometimes cause difficulties at school or at work. Examples of symptoms include excessive grooming, checking in the mirror, skin picking, and multiple cosmetic surgeries to "fix" the deficit. Often the patient reports poor grades as a result of this preoccupation with his or her body's imperfections. An example of a patient with BDD is an individual who is preoccupied with his or her hair and uses a mirror to check on the status of how the hair appears multiple times a day. With this disorder, patients stop participating in sports, they have numerous school absences, and, if the symptoms are severe, students may even quit school. When they are experiencing severe symptoms, patients often become hesitant to even leave the house. Some become violent and angry when they are frustrated about the perceived deficit. For example, a person who is preoccupied with a perceived problem with his hair, breaks the bathroom mirror by throwing a brush against it in a fit of anger (see Case Study #2).

During the last several years, there has been a focus on famous people in the news. This coverage includes actors and actresses, athletic heroes, and newscasters. Part of this attention has been on the style and appearance of these individuals. Some people have compared their appearance with that of these popular icons and become obsessed with the deficits that they perceive in their own appearances. It is important when assessing an individual who is suspected of having BDD to determine if there is an influence of this nature (Haas et al, 2008; Knoesen et al, 2009).

There is a high risk of completed suicide among patients with BDD. In their study population of 185 subjects followed for 4 years, Phillips and Menard (2006) found out that two individuals completed suicide during this study period (see Research for Evidence-Based Practice box).

When assessing the individual with BDD, it is important to ask if the patient has any worries about his or her body appearance. This includes hair, facial features, hips, fingers, and any other body area that the patient identifies as concerning. Ask directly about the concern and how the person perceives the deficit. Determine the amount of time that the patient spends thinking about the imagined defect and looking in the mirror or engaged in grooming. What actions does the person take to hide or get rid of the deficit (e.g., makeup, surgery, baggy clothes)? How has the concern about the deficit affected the person's ability to function at school, at work, socially, and within his or her family? Understanding the patient's subjective experience will assist the nurse with planning care that considers the individual's needs (Phillips and Menard, 2006; Feusner et al, 2005).

Factitious Disorder

Individuals with factitious disorder intentionally produce physical or psychologic signs and symptoms to assume the sick role. The individual performs this behavior for economic gain, to avoid school or legal responsibilities, or to improve his or her physical well-being. Although the patient has created the signs and symptoms of the physical disorder, there is often an unconscious aspect to the patient's behavior and thought pattern; this is an important aspect of this disorder. Individuals who have factitious disorder may also have a personality disorder. Their relationships are often disturbed, they may have few attachments, and they may have some delusions of grandiosity as well as some thought distortions. Some individuals distort the infliction of pain as an indication of caring (Epstein and Stern, 2007). Men and women can both have symptoms of factitious disorder. Peebles and colleagues (2005) described six cases of this disorder among girls between the ages of 9 and 15 years. Two of these girls were avoiding attendance at school; the other four had unresolved psychologic conflicts. This illness is often unreported. Some adults demonstrate factitious disorder in prison and in the military. Some individuals develop factitious disorder after an actual physical illness. Some patients also have symptoms of depression, hypochondriasis, anxiety, borderline personality disorder, conduct disorder, and antisocial disorder. The adult patients are often knowledgeable regarding medical terminology, and many work in the health care

system. Providers often make the diagnosis of factitious disorder on the basis of inexplicable laboratory results (Krahn et al, 2003).

Health care providers are often reluctant to make this diagnosis. These patients frequently undergo expensive procedures that can endanger their lives. Countertransference, in which the nurse's responses to a patient are associated with a significant person in the nurse's life, may cause staff members to be abrupt and inappropriately confront the patient; this damages the therapeutic relationship and does not provide the patient with appropriate care. There is still no clear evidence that indicates the best method of intervention for these patients. Confrontation can be ineffective as a means of intervention unless this intervention is performed in an empathic and nonthreatening style. One intervention that is necessary for treatment is a supportive empathetic relationship that helps the patient to change the maladaptive behaviors. The use of the multidisciplinary team approach with one practitioner being responsible for the care of the patient provides consistent comprehensive care and has the greatest success with regard to decreasing the symptoms of factitious disease. This team consists of medical practitioners as well as psychiatric practitioners. Note that malingering differs from factitious disorder in that individuals who malinger have external incentives (e.g., relief from work) and no intrapsychologic need to maintain the sick role.

Dissociative Disorders
Dissociative Amnesia

People with dissociative amnesia have one or more episodes of inability to recall important personal information that is usually of a traumatic or stressful nature, and the loss of memory is too extensive for ordinary forgetting to explain (i.e., dissociation). The disturbance does not occur exclusively during the course of dissociative identity disorder, and it does not result from the effects of a substance (e.g., blackouts during ethyl alcohol intoxication) or a general medical condition (e.g., amnesia after head trauma) (American Psychiatric Association, 2000).

Further study of this disorder is ongoing. The committee that is reviewing diagnostic categories for the fifth edition of the DSM is considering a clarification of this diagnosis in that edition, which is due to be published in 2013 (www.dsm5.org).

Dissociative Fugue

Dissociative fugue is a sudden and unexpected travel away from home or one's customary place of work with an inability to recall one's past or where one has been. The individual demonstrates confusion about personal identity or assumes a new identity, which is sometimes partial (i.e., "filling in the blanks"). As with dissociative amnesia, the disturbance does not occur in the context of a dissociative identity disorder, and it is not caused by the effects of a substance or a general medical condition (American Psychiatric Association, 2000).

Dissociative Identity Disorder

No other disorder in current psychiatric classification has aroused as much controversy as dissociative identity disorder. The DSM-IV-TR criteria for dissociative identity disorder are straightforward. The first criterion is that the individual must demonstrate two or more distinct identities or personality states, each with its own relatively enduring pattern of perceiving, relating to, and thinking about the environment and the self. Second, at least two of these personality states recurrently take control of the person's behavior. The individual is unable to recall important personal information to a degree that is too extensive for ordinary forgetting to explain. These behavior patterns and thoughts do not result from the effects of a substance or a general medical condition. In children, the symptoms are not the result of imaginary playmates or other fantasy play (American Psychiatric Association, 2000).

Depersonalization Disorder

Essential features of depersonalization disorder are persistent or recurrent episodes of feelings of detachment or estrangement from one's self. Sensations of being outside of one's body or mental processes or of being an observer of one's body often occur. Various types of sensory anesthesia, lack of affective response, and a sense of lacking control of one's actions or speech are often present. The individual has intact reality testing and awareness of the situation. Depersonalization is a common experience, and the diagnosis is made only if symptoms are severe enough to cause marked distress or impaired functioning. A separate diagnosis is not made if the experience occurs exclusively during the course of another mental disorder (e.g., schizophrenia, panic disorder, acute stress disorder, another dissociative disorder) or if it is caused by the physiologic effects of substance use or a general medical condition (American Psychiatric Association, 2000).

PROGNOSIS

With the exception of conversion disorder, the somatoform disorders are chronic and fluctuating conditions that rarely remit fully. The prognosis for persons with somatization disorder is related to factors that are specific to the disorder, the patient, and the clinician. One follow-up study of BDD indicated that, after 1 year, full remission was 0.09% and partial remission was 0.21% (Phillips et al, 2006).

In that study, 84.2% of the subjects were receiving mental health treatment. The authors concluded that the probability of relapse was 0.15% among patients whose symptoms were partially or fully remitted (Phillips et al, 2006). Conversion disorders usually remit within 2 weeks; however, there is recurrence in 20% to 25% of cases. A single recurrence of symptoms is predictive of future episodes. Factors that have been identified with a good prognosis are identifiable stressors at the time that symptoms develop, early treatment, and above-average intelligence. The dissociative disorders have varying prognoses that range from a rapid and complete recovery (i.e., for fugue) to both episodic and continuous chronic courses (i.e., for dissociative identity disorder). Dissociative identity disorder frequently reemerges during periods of stress or during a relapse of substance abuse (American Psychiatric Association, 2000).

DISCHARGE CRITERIA

The patient will do the following:
- Identify situations and events that trigger somatic concerns or dissociative states and select adaptive ways to prevent or manage these situations.
- Describe somatic symptoms and thoughts or stressors that may have increased his or her level of anxiety.
- Discuss the connection between anxiety-provoking situations or events and somatic symptoms or dissociation.
- Explain relief behaviors openly.

- Identify adaptive positive techniques and strategies that relieve anxiety and decrease the focus on somatic concerns.
- Demonstrate behaviors that represent reduced somatic focus or dissociation states.
- Use learned stress-reducing strategies, such as mindfulness meditation.
- Demonstrate the ability to solve problems, concentrate, and make decisions.
- Sleep through the night.
- Use appropriate supports from the nursing and medical community, family, and friends.
- Determine the difference between somatic concerns and illness states, with an understanding of laboratory and other objective tests that are used to provide confirmation of pathology.
- Discuss the ability to tolerate manageable levels of stress and emotionality.
- List the medications that are used to control his or her symptoms as well as the appropriate dosage and scheduled times for each.

THE NURSING PROCESS

ASSESSMENT

It is important for the nurse to thoroughly assess each patient without considering the possibility that the patient is feigning the physical symptoms. Obtaining a collaborative history with the assistance of family members and other treating practitioners will help staff to provide the patient with comprehensive care. Understanding the possible anxiety precipitants of the somatic concerns will help the patient to reduce his or her focus on the physical sensations.

NURSING DIAGNOSIS

To determine which nursing diagnoses will most effectively guide the treatment of patients with somatoform disorders, factitious disorders, and dissociative disorders, the nurse relies on information that is obtained during the assessment process. The nurse identifies defining characteristics of the target diagnoses from the patient, and together the nurse and patient jointly identify etiologic factors. Etiologic factors influence the selection of the appropriate interventions. Nursing diagnoses are prioritized according to patients' needs. Typical diagnoses for patients with somatoform disorders, factitious disorders, and dissociative disorders include the following:
- Risk for suicide
- Risk for self-directed violence
- Risk for other-directed violence
- Self-mutilation
- Risk for self-mutilation
- Anxiety
- Death anxiety
- Hopelessness

- Powerlessness
- Insomnia
- Chronic pain
- Fatigue
- Fear
- Health-seeking behaviors
- Disturbed body image
- Chronic low self-esteem
- Ineffective coping
- Defensive coping
- Social isolation
- Risk for loneliness
- Risk-prone health behavior
- Ineffective role performance
- Noncompliance
- Impaired social interaction
- Ineffective denial
- Impaired memory
- Disturbed sensory perception
- Disturbed thought processes
- Deficient knowledge
- Imbalanced nutrition: less than body requirements
- Imbalanced nutrition: more than body requirements
- Activity intolerance
- Impaired physical mobility
- Spiritual distress
- Sexual dysfunction
- Interrupted family processes
- Compromised family coping
- Decisional conflict
- Relocation stress syndrome

OUTCOME IDENTIFICATION

Outcome criteria differ according to the characteristics of each patient's nursing diagnoses and collaborative DSM-IV-TR diagnoses. Determining the intended outcomes before implementing the plan will guide both nursing interventions and evaluations. Nursing diagnoses are associated with outcomes (i.e., goals) and serve as guides for outcome development. In practice, nurses generally determine outcomes in accordance with the patient's presentation of clinical manifestations.

General Outcome Expectations

The patient will do the following:
- Contact the nursing staff members if he or she is experiencing thoughts or desires that are suicidal or harmful toward others.
- Identify situations and events that trigger somatic concerns or dissociative episodes and select ways to prevent or manage them.
- Describe somatic symptoms that occur with an increase in the level of anxiety.
- Discuss the connection between anxiety-provoking situations or events and somatic symptoms or dissociative states.

- Explain relief behaviors and thoughts openly.
- Identify adaptive and positive techniques and strategies that relieve anxiety and decrease somatic focus or the dissociative episodes.
- Demonstrate behaviors that represent reduced somatic symptoms or that provide him or her with a means of reassociation when experiencing a dissociative state.
- Use learned anxiety-reducing strategies such as mindfulness meditation (see Box 10-3).
- Demonstrate the ability to solve problems, concentrate, and make decisions.
- Verbalize the feeling of being relaxed and less concerned about somatic sensations or disorders.
- Sleep through the night for 6 to 8 hours.
- Use appropriate supports from the nursing and medical community, family, and friends.
- Learn to manage anxiety at tolerable levels without dissociating or focusing on somatic sensations.
- Seek help from appropriate sources when there is an awareness of new somatic concerns.
- List the medications that are used to control the symptoms as well as their appropriate dosages and scheduled times.
- Continue postdischarge symptom management, including medication and other therapies.

Somatization Disorder

The patient will do the following:
- Construct an exercise program that includes anxiety-reducing techniques.
- Address two positive somatic responses (e.g., massage therapy, the satisfied feeling after a successful exercise session).
- Keep a journal to document somatic preoccupation and stressors, including intrusive thoughts and concerns.
- Help the therapist to coordinate the information from the primary care provider and any other involved specialists.
- Take medications as prescribed and be able to identify the rationales for the medications.
- Contact the therapist for more frequent visits if somatization increases.

Dissociative Identity Disorder

The patient will do the following:
- Alert the therapist or use a hotline such as or 1-800-273-TALK when feeling suicidal.
- Respond to his or her name when addressed by a member of the treatment team.
- Refer to himself or herself in the first-person pronoun form (e.g., "*I* think...").
- Identify periods of increasing anxiety.
- Inform others about dissatisfaction in a nonthreatening manner.
- Use assertive-response behaviors to meet his or her needs (see Chapters 4 and 26).
- Keep a written journal to identify stressors and when the dissociation occurs.

- Take medications as prescribed.
- Identify when to use an as-needed medication to decrease a heightened anxiety response to a cue in the environment.
- Contact the therapist if symptoms increase.

PLANNING

Treatment planning for patients with somatic, factitious, and dissociative disorders in the current health care environment is complex and varied. Patients with severe BDD often require hospitalization to prevent a suicidal occurrence. In the past, treatment for dissociative identity disorder occurred in special units with prolonged hospitalization. Currently, the individual with dissociative identity disorder is treated in an outpatient setting and often with the use of several different modalities, including individual psychotherapy, group therapy, family therapy, and art therapy. Children and adolescents who have trauma-related dissociative symptoms experience a decrease in these symptoms when they participate in therapeutic modalities of play therapy and gestalt techniques (Weber, 2009).

Today, both clinicians and administrators who manage inpatient facilities are struggling to balance effective treatment with the high costs associated with these specialty units. Increasingly, inpatient hospitalization is available only for short periods of time for patients who are at imminent risk to themselves or others. Rather than assuming their traditional roles of providing direct care to patients in inpatient facilities, nurses are increasingly involved as case managers. In this role, nurses provide patients and families with information about treatment alternatives, and they also provide comprehensive discharge planning.

IMPLEMENTATION

The role of a nurse in the implementation of a care plan for patients with somatization disorders depends on the setting. The following interventions are useful for patients with somatic symptoms, regardless of the diagnosis or treatment setting.

NURSING INTERVENTIONS

1. *Identify the degree of suicidal ideation and depression in patients with all types of anxiety and associated disorders.* A thorough evaluation of patients with anxiety disorders and associated disorders will help to prevent suicide and other destructive behaviors early during the intervention process.
2. *Monitor your own level of anxiety, and make a conscious effort to remain calm.* Anxiety is readily transferable from one person to another. Individuals with somatoform illnesses have a risk of an increase in symptoms during times of increased anxiety.
3. *Recognize that the patient's use of relief behaviors focuses on somatic sensations as indicators of anxiety.* Early inter-

ventions help to manage anxiety before symptoms escalate to more serious levels.

4. *Educate the patient about the importance of limiting caffeine, nicotine, and other central nervous system stimulants.* Limiting these substances prevents or minimizes physical symptoms of anxiety (e.g., rapid heart rate, jitteriness) that may cue other somatic concerns.

5. *Teach the patient to distinguish between somatic sensations that are connected to identifiable objects or sources (e.g., symptoms of a cold, pain from a fall) and somatic concerns for which there is no immediate identifiable object or source but that are a reaction to an increase in anxiety.* Knowledge of anxiety and its related components increases the patient's control over the disorder.

6. *Instruct the patient to perform the following strategies to reduce anxiety and to distract his or her focus on somatic concerns* (see Chapter 26):
   a. Progressive relaxation techniques
   b. Mindfulness meditation
   c. Slow deep-breathing exercises
   d. Focusing on a single object in the room
   e. Soothing music
   f. Visual imagery (guided imagery)

7. *Help the patient to build on coping methods that have helped with the management of his or her anxiety in the past.* Coping methods that were previously successful will generally be effective in subsequent situations.

8. *Encourage the patient to contact support people who will increase socialization and provide emotional support as the patient attends work or school, even when patient is feeling poorly.* A strong support system helps the patient to avoid anxiety-provoking situations or activities.

9. *Help the patient to gain control of overwhelming feelings and impulses through brief and direct verbal interactions.* Individual interactions at appropriate intervals help to reduce or manage a patient's anxious feelings or impulses.

10. *Help the patient to understand the importance of the medication regimen and the need to take the medications as prescribed.* Medication is an effective adjunct to other psychosocial therapeutic interventions, when necessary.

✎ MEDICATION KEY FACTS

Somatoform, Factitious, and Dissociative Disorders

Pharmacologic interventions are symptom oriented. Medications include the following:
- Anxiolytics for associated anxiety
- Antidepressants for associated depression and for intense focus on somatic concerns
- Antipsychotics for any underlying psychosis

Additional Treatment Modalities
Biologic Interventions

Pharmacologic Interventions. Pharmacologic interventions alone or in combination with cognitive behavioral interventions are among the most successful treatments for somatoform disorders. Selective serotonin reuptake inhibitors, which are antidepressants that are now widely used to treat somatoform disorders, have been particularly effective for the treatment of BDD. The pharmacologic treatment of dissociative identify disorder is largely symptomatic. Varying combinations of antidepressants, antipsychotics, and, to a lesser extent, benzodiazepines are used. Researchers are currently studying the best medication regimen for individuals with somatoform disorders. It has been shown that patients who have chronic somatoform disorders have demonstrated a reduction in their symptoms with the use of a combination of somatization-focused cognitive behavioral therapy and antidepressants and specifically with the use of a selective serotonin reuptake inhibitor or venlafaxine (Marcangelo and Wise, 2007). For more specific information about dosages and their side-effect profiles, see Chapter 25.

Psychotherapy

Psychotherapeutic intervention takes place in group or individual settings. One advantage of group therapy is the opportunity for the patient to learn from the successes and failures of others with similar symptoms. Behavioral and cognitive behavioral therapies have widely been effective for the treatment of a variety of anxiety disorders (see Chapter 26).

Cognitive Behavioral Therapy. Many therapists use cognitive behavioral therapy to treat patients with somatoform disorders and dissociative disorders. The success of this approach involves the patient's ability to understand that physical symptoms are a response to thoughts or feelings about behaviors that occur in daily life. The patient and the therapist identify target symptoms and then examine the circumstances associated with the symptoms. Together they plan strategies to change either the cognitions (thoughts) or the behaviors. Cognitive behavioral therapy is a short-term treatment that demands active participation on the part of both the patient and the therapist (see Chapter 26).

EVALUATION

Ideally the nurse and the patient together evaluate the patient's progress toward the identified outcomes during every interaction. If the patient does not make satisfactory progress, the nurse modifies either the expected outcomes or the interventions. The nurse examines all factors that relate to the outcomes, including what occurred during the previous phases of the nursing process, the role of the nurse in setting patient and clinician expectations, the clarity of communicating patient goals with the patient, and other intervening events that have occurred since the outcomes were set. It is important for the nurse to remember that the somatoform disorders and the dissociative disorders are chronic and enduring. It takes patience and support for the patient to determine the pattern of his or her behavior and to incorporate methods to initiate change.

◎ CONCEPT MAP CASE STUDY 11-1

Emma is a 40-year-old woman who has seen four primary practitioners in the past 2 weeks. A nurse is currently evaluating her for chronic constipation and intolerance of several different foods. At her gynecologic appointment last week, she had concerns about having excessive menstrual bleeding and cramps. Emma went to the chiropractor during the early part of this week with vague back pain. She reports several concerns about her ability to walk; sometimes she has weakness in her knees, and overall she feels tired and weak. She has been having arguments with her boyfriend, and she has been concerned that he will end the relationship because of her significant complaints about her body. Emma has been having some stress at work. She has been calling in sick frequently, and her employer is requesting a note from her practitioner each time that she calls in. Emma is afraid that her supervisor will reprimand her for absenteeism.

The nurse practitioner performed a thorough physical examination, which was negative. Emma's recent laboratory values were within normal limits. The nurse practitioner obtained Emma's past medical records with Emma's permission and noticed a pattern of multiple physician visits with similar complaints assessed during the past 2 weeks. The nurse practitioner made the diagnosis of somatization disorder.

DSM-IV-TR Diagnoses

Axis I   Somatization disorder

Axis II   Deferred

Axis III   History of gastroesophageal reflux disease, chronic constipation, and intolerance of several different foods
Headaches and back pain
Sexual dysfunction (inability to lubricate), excessive menstrual bleeding, and cramps
Weakness in the knees that results in concerns about ambulating
Reports of feeling tired and weak

Axis IV   Problems with primary support system
Occupational concerns

Axis V   Global Assessment of Functioning (GAF) = 60 (current); GAF = 75 (past year)

Nursing Diagnosis *Disturbed sensory perception related to subjective experience of feelings of pain, weakness, and gastrointestinal and genitourinary symptoms as evidenced by chronic constipation, intolerance of several different foods, excessive menstrual bleeding and cramps, and vague back pain*

NOC Stress level, Distorted thought self-control, Cognitive orientation, Neurological status: spinal sensory/motor function
NIC Anxiety reduction, Cognitive restructuring, Neurologic monitoring, Surveillance: safety, Self-esteem enhancement, Environmental management

Nursing Diagnosis *Impaired social interaction related to multiple somatic concerns that restrict the patient's ability to socialize as evidenced by the patient's boyfriend voicing frustration with the patient's somatic concerns; the patient's girlfriends have also stopped asking the patient to join them on outings because of her frequent somatic concerns*

NOC Stress level, Fear level, Social involvement, Self-esteem, Social interaction skills, Role performance
NIC Anxiety reduction, Coping enhancement, Socialization enhancement, Self-esteem enhancement, Support system enhancement

Nursing Diagnosis *Health-seeking behaviors related to multiple somatic concerns as evidenced by going to four practitioners during a 2-week period to report many health concerns*

NOC Health beliefs; Knowledge: health promotion; Participation in health care decisions; Personal health status; Personal well-being
NIC Health education; Self-modification assistance; Coping enhancement; Teaching: individual; Decision-making support; Mutual goal setting

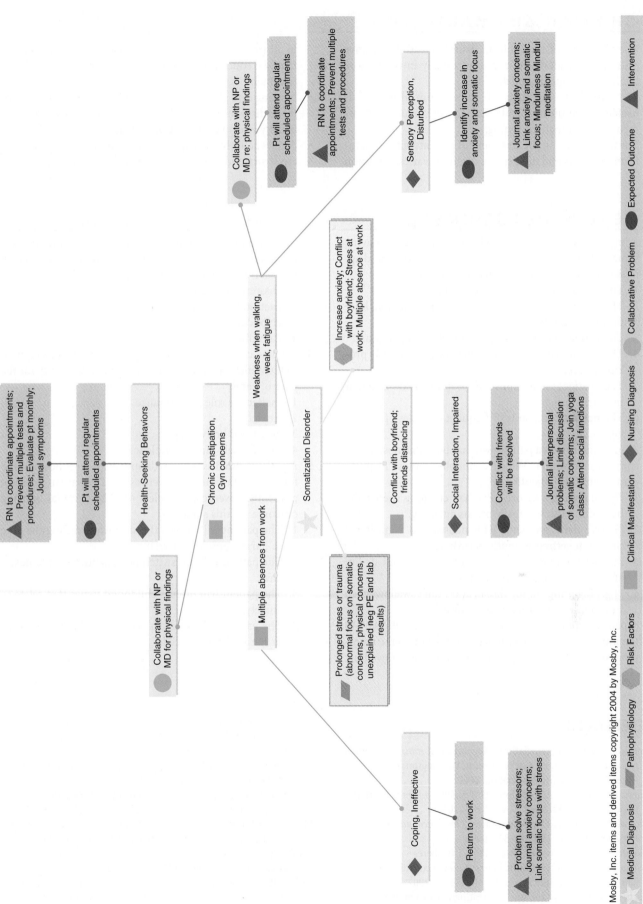

FIGURE 11-1.   Concept map: Somatization Disorder.

CHAPTER SUMMARY

- The treatment of somatoform disorders and dissociative disorders is multidisciplinary and usually involves more than one treatment modality.
- The inpatient treatment of somatoform disorders is usually the result of suicidal risk and the failure of treatment in an outpatient setting.
- The nursing role in the treatment of patients with somatoform disorders and dissociative disorders varies. Common to all treatment settings is the nurse's role in patient and family education about the disorders and their treatment.
- Nursing care plans for patients with symptoms of somatoform disorders reflect the understanding that managing anxiety effectively is part of daily living.
- Nurses actively participate in behavioral interventions that are structured to decrease the somatic responses.

REVIEW QUESTIONS

1. A nurse assesses a patient who is suspected of having somatization disorder. Which findings support the diagnosis? You may select more than one answer.
   1. The patient is currently 46 years old.
   2. The patient reports headaches, burning urination, knee problems, and hemorrhoids.
   3. The patient has been diagnosed with Graves' disease.
   4. The patient names six physicians that are currently providing care.
   5. The patient complains of skimpy and irregular menstruation.
   6. The patient complains of frequent episodes of double vision.
2. A nurse interviews a patient who has been diagnosed with conversion disorder. Which comment is most likely to come from this patient?
   1. "Since getting a divorce, I've had crushing chest pain, but I don't think it really means anything."
   2. "I have daily problems with nausea and vomiting. I think I'm getting seriously dehydrated."
   3. "Sexual intercourse is so painful that I avoid it. I'm afraid that's going to destroy my marriage."
   4. "I get big lumps in my throat, and I can't swallow when I eat. I'm afraid I might have cancer."
3. A patient reports fears of having breast cancer and says to the nurse, "I've missed so much work having three mammograms in the past 6 months. No problems showed up, but I'm sure that's because the radiologic technicians were not qualified to correctly perform mammograms." Which disorder would the nurse suspect?
   1. Dissociative fugue
   2. Factitious disorder
   3. Hypochondriasis
   4. Pain disorder
4. A nurse counsels a patient who has been diagnosed with BDD. Which nursing diagnosis would be a priority for the plan of care?
   1. Ineffective role performance
   2. Anxiety
   3. Disturbed body image
   4. Risk for self-directed violence
5. A patient with dissociative identity disorder is hospitalized for the fourth time after overdosing. The patient does not remember overdosing. Select the best initial nursing outcome for this situation.
   1. The patient will inform the staff when feeling the urge to harm himself or herself.
   2. The patient will not switch personalities for the next 7 days.
   3. The patient will discuss childhood issues that relate to anxiety.
   4. The patient will assume a decision-making role for his or her health care needs.

REFERENCES

American Psychiatric Association: *Diagnostic and statistical manual of mental disorders*, ed 4, text revision, Washington, DC, American Psychiatric Association, 2000.

American Psychiatric Association: *DSM-5 development* (website): www.dsm5.org. Accessed November 3, 2010.

Brier M, Halverson L: Hypochondriasis, *The clinical advisor: for nurse practitioners* 12(7):81-83, 2009.

Briquet P: *Traits de l'hysterie*, Paris, 1859, J Baillière.

Epstein LA, Stern TA: Factitious illness: a 3-step consultation-liaison approach, *Curr Psychiatry* 6(4):54-58, 2007.

Feusner J et al: Beyond the mirror: treating body dysmorphic disorder, *Curr Psychiatry* 4(10):1-10, 2005.

Haas CF et al: Motivating factors for seeking cosmetic surgery: a synthesis of the literature, *Plast Surg Nurs* 28(4):177-182, 2008.

Knoesen N et al: To be Superman: the male looks obsession, *Aust Fam Physician* 38(3):131-134, 2009.

Krahn LE et al: Patients who strive to be ill: factitious disorder with physical symptoms, *Am J Psychiatry* 160:1163-1169, 2003.

Marcangelo MJ, Wise T: Resistant somatoform symptoms: try CBT and antidepressants, *Curr Psychiatry* 6(2):101-115, 2007.

Mattila AK et al: Alexithymia and somatization in general population, *Psychosom Med* 70(6):716-722, 2008.

Peebles R et al: Factitious disorder and malingering in adolescent girls: case series and literature review, *Clin Pediatr* 44:237-244, 2005.

Phillips KA et al: A 12-month follow-up study of the course of body dysmorphic disorder, *Am J Psychiatry* 163:907-913, 2006.

Phillips KA, Menard W: Suicidality in body dysmorphic disorder: a prospective study, *Am J Psychiatry* 163:1280-1283, 2006.

Weber S: Treatment of trauma- and abuse-related dissociative symptom disorders in children and adolescents, *J Child Adolesc Psychiatr Nurs* 22(1):2-7, 2009.

Online Resources

American Psychiatric Association, DSM-5 Development: www.dsm5.org

Body Dysmorphic Disorder Information, Awareness, and Support: www.bddcentral.com

Mental Health America: www.nmha.org

National Alliance on Mental Illness: www.nami.org

National Institute of Mental Health: www.nimh.nih.gov

VHA/DoD clinical practice guidelines for the management of medically unexplained symptoms: chronic pain and fatigue (brief summary): www.guideline.gov/summary. aspx?doc_id=3415.

12

Mood Disorders: Depression, Bipolar, and Adjustment Disorders

Bonnie M. Hagerty and Kathleen L. Patusky

"When you are mad, mad like this, you don't know it. Reality is what you see. When what you see shifts, departing from anyone else's reality, it's still reality to you."

Marya Hornbacher (Madness: A Bipolar Life)

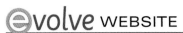 WEBSITE

http://evolve.elsevier.com/Fortinash/

OBJECTIVES

- Describe theories that address the etiology of mood disorders, including biologic and psychosocial theories.
- Discuss the etiology and characteristics of adjustment disorders.
- Compare and contrast the *Diagnostic and Statistical Manual of Mental Disorders* (ed 4, text revision) classifications of depressive, bipolar, and adjustment disorders.

- Discuss the epidemiology and course of depressive, bipolar, and adjustment disorders.
- Apply the nursing process to patients with mood and adjustment disorders.
- Describe independent and collaborative interventions that nurses and other mental health care providers use with patients who have mood and adjustment disorders.

KEY TERMS

adjustment disorders	flight of ideas	neuroplasticity	seasonal affective disorder
affect	hypomania	neurotransmission	selective gene expression
anhedonia	kindling	nihilism	temperament
atypical depression	learned helplessness	postpartum mood disorder	unipolar depression
bipolar disorder	melancholic depression	psychomotor agitation	
dysthymia	mood	psychomotor retardation	
euthymia	mood disorders	schemata	

MOOD DISORDERS

Mood disorders are a group of psychiatric illnesses in which the predominant symptom is the dysregulation of mood or emotion. Mood disorders occur throughout the lifespan, and often cause personal suffering, difficulty with relationships, impaired functioning, and high costs to society and health care systems. These illnesses are also sometimes fatal, with a high risk of suicide. Major depressive disorder often called *depression*, and bipolar disorder formally known as *manic-depressive illness*, are two severe mood disorders that pose significant public health problems that require attention and often long-term treatment. Depression is the world's leading cause of disease burden or years lost to disability. Bipolar disorder, is the seventh cause of disease burden for men and the eighth for women (World Health Organization, 2008).

Mood disorders are characterized by shifts in mood which is a subjective feeling state. Although mood dysregulation is a major sign of these illnesses, other symptoms are also prominent, including changes in physiology, cognition, and behavior. Depression is also linked to illnesses such as cardiovascular disease, stroke, cancer, and acquired immunodeficiency disorder (AIDS), and it can influence morbidity and mortality. As a result of these serious consequences, health care researchers are investigating the etiologies, clinical courses, outcomes, and treatment modalities for mood disorders. Mental health care providers are becoming more aware of the importance of assessing and intervening with patients who are experiencing these major illnesses.

Depression and elation can be normal responses to life events; however, mood disorders involve dysfunctional mood expression that includes incapacitating depression, irritability, and intense elation. For example, a person who has suffered a loss will feel grief and sadness and sometimes even experience physical symptoms and problems with thinking. Adjustment disorder can occur as a time-limited response to an environmental stressor. Success or exciting life events generate mood elevation, elation, and euphoria. Most people experience mood swings associated with loss or success, but these feelings are usually time-limited and not extreme. The mood changes that occur with mood disorders, though, are more pronounced, and they are characterized by their *pattern* over time, which includes frequency of occurrence, duration, and intensity. Additional symptom clusters that occur with mood disturbance include changes in sleep, appetite, thinking, activity, self-worth, and suicidal thinking. These illnesses affect the total person and not just that person's mood.

Mood disorders can be characterized as **unipolar** or **bipolar**. The term *unipolar mood disorder* refers to patients who usually have only depressive episodes or, rarely, only manic episodes. Bipolar disorders occur when people experience periods of depression that alternate with periods of elevated mood, impulsivity, and hyperactivity, which is known as *mania*. Mental health professionals currently recognize that there are various forms of unipolar and bipolar disorders that include a broad spectrum of mood disorders with varied features and clinical characteristics. Mood disorders have commanded more public attention as a result of their pervasiveness and the recognition of their serious and damaging consequences. New treatments, including the use of medications such as fluoxetine (Prozac) and electroconvulsive therapy, have created social controversy.

Despite mood disorders being recognized as serious illnesses, stigma still exists. People are embarrassed to acknowledge that they have mental illnesses, and the public often views someone with a mental illness as being "weak" or "crazy." Famous people with high media profiles such as Robin Williams, Billy Joel, Brooke Shields, and Buzz Aldrin have publicly acknowledged their struggles with mood disorders. Historians have identified many prominent people who experienced serious mood disorders, including Abraham Lincoln, Winston Churchill, Vincent van Gogh, Ernest Hemingway, Sylvia Plath, and Herman Melville.

ETIOLOGY

There are multiple explanations for the genesis of mood disorders. Major theories of etiology include biologic and psychosocial factors that contribute to the development of depression and mania. Each theoretic perspective helps to explain some aspect of mood disorders, but none fully accounts for their development.

Biologic Theories

Biologic research has been a major focus for understanding the cause of depression and bipolar disorder. Although some of this research has shown possible links between physiology, genetics, and mood disorders, none has established direct cause-and-effect relationships. Important biologic theories include those related to altered neurotransmission, neuroendocrine dysregulation, and genetics.

Neurotransmission

The ways in which neurotransmitters work in the brain have been examined for decades. Researchers initially became interested in neurotransmission after investigating the action of antidepressant drugs. In 1954, scientists discovered that patients who had been treated with reserpine for hypertension developed depression. Several years later, they found that isoniazid had an antidepressant effect on persons being treated for tuberculosis. Imipramine was then introduced as an antidepressant in 1958, and research began into its mechanisms of action in the brain. Results from this line of research became the basis for discovering the important role of neurotransmitters in psychiatric disorders. Brain neurotransmitter functioning affects mood regulation and controls a wide range of behaviors and functions, including appetite, arousal, sleep, cognition, and movement.

Early investigation of neurotransmitter systems implicated norepinephrine and serotonin, their metabolites, and their receptors as somehow being altered during episodes of depression and mania. Neurotransmitter availability and receptor change theories have described less-than-normal neurotransmission activity during depression and more-than-normal activity during mania.

Neurotransmitter theories of mood disorders are simplistic and incomplete. More recent investigations have focused on changes in receptors; ion channel processes that involve sodium, potassium, and calcium; and neurotropic growth factors (e.g., brain-derived neurotropic factor) that nourish neurons. Deficits of or alterations in neurotrophins cause brain cells to atrophy or to fail to regenerate under stressful conditions (Duman, 2009).

These complex physiologic mechanisms are consistent with theories that propose the development of long-term changes in the brain that occur with mood disorders. Post (1992) described an important phenomenon called kindling in which stress initially alters neurotransmission mechanisms, and results in a first episode of depression or mania. This initial episode creates an electrophysiologic sensitivity to future stress, thereby requiring less stress to trigger another depressive or manic state. In essence, kindling creates new hardwiring of the brain or long-lasting alterations of neuronal functioning that influence many changes in cellular processes, brain structures, cell dendrites, and cellular metabolism.

This process is based on **neuroplasticity**, which is the ability of neurons to regenerate or restructure (Pittenger and Duman, 2008). The kindling model is consistent with the cyclic and progressive nature of mood disorders and suggests the importance of health care providers treating patients early for their mood episodes and maintaining these patients on medication for extended periods to avoid brain physiologic alterations and deterioration over time.

New brain imaging techniques provide additional support for brain disturbances during depression and mania. Positron emission tomography (PET scans) enables researchers to examine the brain physiology of depressed persons as compared with normal control subjects and to focus on the metabolism of glucose and oxygen. This allows for the comparison of brain functioning in individuals during their depressive episode and after their recovery. Figure 12-1 depicts the differences that are apparent with the use of positron emission tomography scanning of depressed, recovered, and normal control brains. Figure 12-2 indicates alterations in blood flow in the brains of depressed persons. Positron emission tomography scanning has shown that the prefrontal cerebral cortex and the limbic system (including the amygdala) appear to have physiologic and anatomic changes in the brains of persons who are experiencing depression (Duman, 2009). Researchers also use magnetic resonance imaging and single photon emission computed tomography to produce images of the functioning of the brain.

The complexity of the biologic, structural, and physiologic changes that occur with mood disorders continues to pose challenges for investigators. Neurotransmission is a complex activity that includes multiple processes, such as neurotransmitter synthesis and release, receptor site function and change, interactions among the various neurotransmitters and hormones, and the action of these transmitters and hormones on genes.

Neuroendocrine Dysregulation

Mood disorders have been linked to dysregulation of the limbic hypothalamic–pituitary–adrenal (HPA) axis. The hypothalamus, the pituitary, the adrenal glands, and the hippocampus make up the HPA axis, which controls physiologic responses to stress. The hypothalamus regulates endocrine functions and the autonomic nervous system. It is also related to the fight-or-flight response, eating, sleep, and sex. The hypothalamus manufactures serotonin, which is a major neurotransmitter that is implicated in mood disorders. In response to stress, the hypothalamus releases corticotropin-releasing hormone, which stimulates the anterior pituitary to secrete adrenocorticotropic hormone. Adrenocorticotropic hormone, in turn, triggers the release of cortisol from the adrenal cortex into the blood. Serum cortisol is elevated during stress, and it stimulates the autonomic nervous system, thereby increasing levels of epinephrine and norepinephrine. Through an elaborate feedback mechanism, levels of cortisol signal the hypothalamus via the hippocampus to increase or decrease corticotropin-releasing hormone production.

Researchers do not yet fully understand the specific physiologic mechanisms through which stress signals this process to begin.

The HPA axis is often hyperactive in patients with depression. Patients with moderate to severe depression may exhibit elevated serum cortisol levels. Over time, high levels of cortisol can damage the hippocampus. There is evidence that associates decreased hippocampal volume with stress and recurrent and chronic depression (Frodl et al, 2008). Serious consequences include cognitive impairment and particularly memory difficulties.

The functioning of the HPA axis is related to the 24-hour cycle of circadian rhythms that control physiologic processes. Patients with mood disorders have disrupted or irregular cyclic patterns. Blood cortisol is normally low during the night and peaks during the day, although constantly higher levels are often apparent in depression. Disrupted sleep–wake cycles are associated with mood disorders. Patients with mania have a decreased need for sleep, whereas many patients with depression experience hypersomnia (excessive sleep). During depression, patients experience decreased rapid eye movement latency and decreased shallow and slow delta wave sleep, thus fragmenting the sleep–wake cycle. Even seasonal patterns appear to have some relationship with mood disorders, with episodes of depression often occurring during periods of decreased light. Thus, many alterations are evident in the normal body rhythms.

Genetic Transmission

Mood disorders tend to occur in certain families, and many believe that genetics are responsible for their manifestation (Kendler et al, 2006). Studies of families, twins, adoption, and molecular genetics provide data regarding the heritability of mood disorders.

In family studies, researchers select families who exhibit mood disorders and then examine the risks that relatives have for developing these disorders. This risk is then compared with the general population. Results of these studies consistently demonstrate that first-degree relatives of persons with bipolar disorder and unipolar depression have a greater risk for the development of a mood disorder. This risk is particularly high for relatives of persons with bipolar disorder, which possibly indicates that genetics plays a greater role in bipolar disorder than in unipolar depression (Nomura et al, 2002).

Twin studies have been based on the assumption that monozygotic twins share the same genes and that dizygotic twins have about 50% of their genes in common. Results of twin research provide additional evidence for the genetic transmission of mood disorders. If one monozygotic twin suffers from bipolar disorder, there is a strong chance that the other twin will have a disorder as well. In some studies, up to 100% of the other twins developed a mood disorder (usually bipolar illness). Although there are high rates of concordance for dizygotic twins, the rates tend to be less than those for monozygotic twins. For unipolar disorders, the concordance rates continue to be higher for monozygotic twins, and both

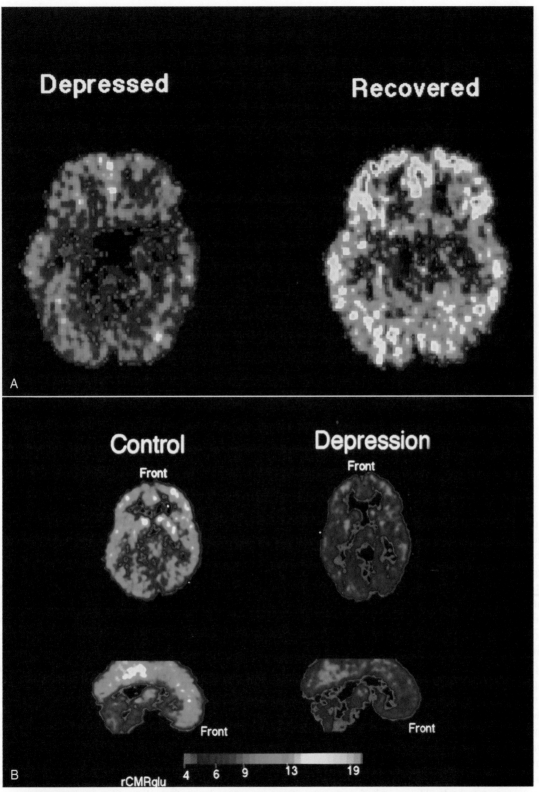

FIGURE 12-1. A, Positron emission tomography scans of the brain of the same individual during depression *(left)* and after recovery as a result of treatment with medication *(right)*. Several brain areas, particularly the prefrontal cortex *(top)*, show diminished activity *(darker colors)* during depression. **B,** Positron emission tomography scans of a normal subject *(left)* and a depressed subject *(right)* reveal reduced brain activity *(darker colors)* during depression, especially in the prefrontal cortex. A form of radioactively tagged glucose was used as a tracer to visualize levels of brain activity. *Courtesy of Mark George, MD, National Institute of Mental Health Biological Psychiatry Branch, U.S. Department of Health and Human Services, Washington, DC.*

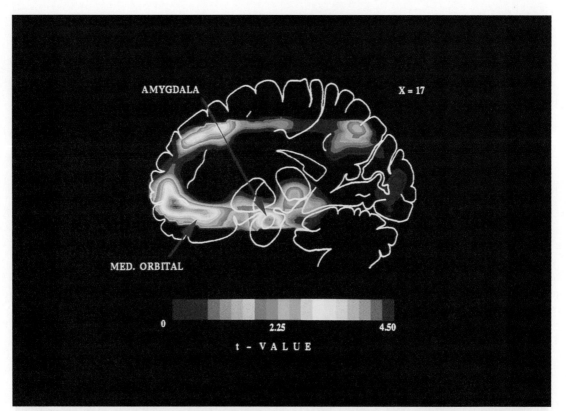

FIGURE 12-2. Positron emission tomography scans indicate increased blood flow in the amygdala and prefrontal cortex of individuals with major depression of the familial pure depressive disease subtype. This scan is a composite of images from 13 individuals. Courtesy of Wayne C. Drevets, MD, Department of Psychiatry, Washington University School of Medicine, St. Louis.

twin types have a higher concordance than individuals in the general population (Kendler, 2001).

With the use of adoption studies, researchers examine the contributions of both the environment and genetic transmission. In general, adoption studies also demonstrate that genetic factors play some role in mood disorders. Most studies focus specifically on bipolar disorder, and reveal that the biologic parents of adult adoptees who are diagnosed with bipolar disorder have a much higher incidence of the disorder than parents of adoptees with no mood disorders.

Although all of the preceding information indicates that genetics is partially responsible for the development of mood disorders, research continues to probe for specific genes or genetic mechanisms. A genetic predisposition will involve at least several genes with different variants. In addition, it is unclear how genes and the environment interact to affect behavior (Keltikangas-Jarvinen and Salo, 2009). This interaction between genes and the environment further complicates genetic research. The search for the specific genetic basis of mood disorders continues, with special emphasis on genetic location and genetic processes. Many researchers agree that genetic expression, the genetic transmission of mood disorders, and how these interact with the environment hold the key to future major advances in understanding, diagnosing, and treating depression and bipolar disorders.

Psychosocial Factors
Evolutionary Psychology and Biology

The basic idea in *evolutionary psychology* is that natural selection designed the human mind to solve problems of adaptation. All human minds develop reasoning and regulatory mechanisms that organize the interpretation of experiences, account for recurrent concepts and motivations, and provide universal meaning structures that help us to understand the behavior of others. *Evolutionary biology* is a related field that examines the selective advantages of human traits and biology. Both areas explore how human beings have adapted and are still adapting to changes in the environment. They also try to identify defenses that seem like diseases but that are actually evolved protective mechanisms. When exploring mood disorders, the focus is on proximate explanations such as brain chemistry, past experiences, and personality. From an evolutionary perspective, the focus is on the *purpose* of a mood disorder and why it persists in the present.

On the surface, depression and its main symptoms (i.e., lack of energy, fearfulness, loss of interest, sleep and eating disorders) do not seem to promote survival; however, depression possibly serves as a cry for help. Sometimes it forces the loser of a social conflict to accept defeat, thereby stopping the winner's oppressive behavior. Depression also possibly forces a partner to have greater involvement. Depression may serve a social rumination function, and the symptoms permit the individual to focus on and analyze social problems. Depression may have a social motivation function in that the severity of symptoms may influence reluctant social partners to provide help or withdraw demands. Nesse (2009) also suggested that depression prevents wasted effort by allowing the individual to disengage from unreachable goals.

Psychodynamic Theory

The basic premise of psychoanalytic theory is that unconscious processes result in the expression of symptoms, including depression and mania. Freud (1957) distinguished between depression and normal grief, citing both as responses to real or symbolic loss. According to Freud, loss generates intense hostile feelings toward the lost object. The person then turns these feelings inward onto the self, thereby creating guilt and loss of self-esteem. Thus, depression is linked with loss and aggression.

Psychodynamically, mania is a defense against depression. The patient denies feelings of anger, low self-esteem, and worthlessness and reverses his or her affect so that there is a triumphant feeling of self-confidence. Mania represents a conquered superego with little inclination to control id impulses; however, over time, this distorted view of reality waivers, and the patient demonstrates outward hostility toward others, often focusing on the weaknesses of others that are similar to the internal weaknesses that they are avoiding.

Few data support the psychodynamic theories of depression and mania, but there is some evidence that patients with depression have experienced more early childhood loss and trauma than persons without depression (Brown and Harris, 1978). Clinicians also note that anger is often associated with depression, although the relationship between anger and depression remains obscure. Many people who experience early childhood loss and anger never experience depression, whereas many who do not experience a visible or acknowledged loss do experience depression. Psychoanalytic theory is only one of many explanations that attempt to explain the intrapsychic dynamics of depression and mania. The relevance of this theoretic perspective is in its references to the early childhood environment in which loss, disruption, or chaos triggers stress that, in turn, triggers the physiologic mechanisms described previously.

Cognitive Theory

Errors of logical thinking may be one causative factor of depression. This perspective assumes that underlying cognitive structures, some of which are not fully conscious, influence mood. These cognitive structures are shaped by early life experiences, and they are predisposed to the negative processing of information. In a diatheses–stress model, when individuals who are predisposed to depression with negative schemata encounter stress, the negative processing is activated, thereby resulting in depressive thinking (Beck, 1967).

Beck (1967) differentiated among levels of cognition that influence depression: automatic thoughts, schemata or assumptions, and cognitive distortions. Automatic thoughts are thoughts that a person responds to but usually does not recognize as a basis for behavior and thinking. They form the person's perception of a situation, and it is this perception—rather than the objective facts about the situation—that results in emotional and behavioral responses. If the perceptions are distorted, inferences and responses will be maladaptive. For example, a businessman was offered a substantial job promotion that required frequent travel. He was afraid to fly and did not take the job because of his fear. His basic automatic thought was that planes crash and that he had a good chance of dying in a plane crash. He was unable to look at data that demonstrate that flying is the safest form of transportation. He compromised his career because of this thinking. Schemata are internal representations of the self and the world. They facilitate information processing, because the mind uses them to understand, code, and recall information. Beck (1967) proposed a triad of thinking (schemata) that gives rise to the development of depression:

1. Negative, self-deprecating views of the self
2. Pessimistic views of the world, which result in life experiences being interpreted in a negative way
3. The belief that negativity will continue into the future, which promotes a negative view of future events

These mind-sets result in the misinterpretation of events and situations so that the patient sees the self as worthless, and the world and the future as hopeless. This faulty cognitive processing leads to assumptions and continued errors of logic that result in depressive symptoms and an ongoing negative view of life. This is exemplified when people state that they know that they will never make it through college. Cognitive distortions link schemata and automatic thoughts. Faulty information processing includes cognitive distortions, such as *all-or-nothing thinking* (i.e., seeing only two opposite categories or options), *discounting the positive* (i.e., not believing that positive experiences matter) and *magnification* (i.e., placing a distorted emphasis on a single event or error). The following example illustrates each of these types of distortion. A young woman was engaged to be married, but her fiancé called off the wedding, telling her that he did not think he loved her enough to get married. She was convinced that, if he would not marry her, no one ever would (all-or-nothing thinking). When the woman's friends tried to tell her that she was wonderful, lovely, and talented, she insisted that her achievements did not count (discounting the positive). She believed that, when she did not want to go out with her fiancé one evening several weeks earlier, the incident ruined their relationship (magnification).

Learned Helplessness/Hopelessness Theory

Cognitive theory presumes that depression results from altered cognition. One such altered cognition involves learned helplessness, which is demonstrated by the development of helplessness, apathy, powerlessness, and depression. According to the original theory as proposed by Seligman (1975), uncontrollable stressful events that a person experiences result in a lack of motivation to act in response to the environment.

Learned helplessness theory was modified to specify that, in the face of current events and past experiences, individuals have the expectation (cognition) that external events are uncontrollable (Abramson et al, 1978). This in turn results in helplessness, passivity, and sadness, which lead to other symptoms of depression, such as decreased appetite and low self-esteem.

The hopelessness theory of depression is a further revision of learned helplessness. In this theory, hopelessness is a sufficient cause of depression. The individual's inferred negative outcomes and negativity about the self are key elements of depression. Helplessness is only a part of hopelessness. With the occurrence of an unpleasant event, persons who are at risk for depression and who have negative expectations attribute instability, globalization, and excessive importance to those events. For example, a patient perceives that she is not able to recover from divorce (instability), that her entire life is ruined (globalization), and that her former marriage is the only focus of her life (importance). A lack of social support during times of negative life events often leads to increased helplessness, hopelessness, and depression.

Life Events and Stress Theory

Researchers have been interested in the quantity and nature of life events and in the size and perceived support from the patient's social network as they relate to depression. In their early research, Brown and Harris (1978) reported that stressful social factors (e.g., the lack of an intimate, confiding relationship with a significant other; having three or more children at home; being unemployed; the loss of one's mother before the age of 11 years) contributed significantly to vulnerability for depression.

Holmes and Rahe (1967) indicated that all life events, even pleasant ones, are capable of causing various degrees of stress. Thus, even a vacation or a promotion may generate high levels of stress. The person's perception or appraisal of an event is as important as the change in daily life caused by the event. Factors such as social support and the person's perception of that support as wanted or unwanted and as sufficient or insufficient also influence the effect of an event. Ravindran and colleagues (2002) associated depressive illness with increased stress perception, reduced perception of positive events, reliance on coping styles that make use of emotion rather than rational thought, and quality of life.

Early life stress, including child abuse and loss, influences the development of depression, most likely by disrupting the functioning of the HPA axis. The chronic hypersecretion of corticotropin-releasing factor and cortisol, and the autonomic nervous system activation that occurs during neurologically vulnerable times of development, sensitize physiologic stress responses and even generate brain changes (Gillespie and Nemeroff, 2005). Thus, individuals who experience early life stress become vulnerable with regard to how their stress response influences the onset and course of depression. Life events most likely influence the development and recurrence of depression through the psychologic and

ultimately the biologic experiences of stress (Heim et al, 2008).

Researchers have examined the occurrence of stressful life events and depression with regard to gender differences. Stressful life events triggered episodes of depression in women that were mediated by genetic risk factors. Although women reported more interpersonal stressors, men reported more legal and work-related stressful life events. At the same time, most life events influenced the risk for depression in men and women in similar ways. Researchers concluded that the greater prevalence of depression among women as compared with men was not the result of differences in the rate of reported stressful life events or of a greater sensitivity of women to the harmful influences of stressful life events (Kendler et al, 2001). Marital status has been a risk factor for a higher severity of depressive symptoms among women as compared with men. Greater role demands and more chronic family stress among women as well as higher education and the presence of children in the household may explain the difference (Barnow et al, 2002). There are less data regarding the relationship between stressful life events and bipolar disorder, although studies have suggested a role for disrupted social routines or circadian rhythms. Malkoff-Schwartz and colleagues (2000) studied the influence of social rhythm disruption as a stressful life event on patients with mania, depression, cycling episodes, and recurrent unipolar depression. The researchers found that stressful life events, especially social rhythm disruption, influenced the onset of manic episodes. The authors suggested that interventions to minimize stress and social rhythm disruption in patients with a history of mania will help to prevent the onset of manic episodes.

Adjustment Disorders

Life stressors sometimes can lead to adjustment disorders, which are different from major depression. The main distinction between an adjustment disorder and major depression is that a specific psychosocial stressor can be identified for the adjustment disorder. Adjustment disorders or adjustment reactions can occur in response to any type of stressor, including but not limited to loss, personal tragedy, change in lifestyle, maturational crisis, or even success or gain. In acute cases, the adjustment disorder occurs within 3 months of a stressor. In chronic cases, symptoms last more than 6 months after the occurrence of the stressor. During this time, individuals have difficulty functioning in their roles or interpersonal relationships, and they demonstrate great distress. Symptoms usually decrease after the stressor is removed. In some cases, symptoms disappear outside of the setting that is linked with the stressor, especially when the stressor is specific to a location (e.g., the work setting).

An adjustment disorder can occur in anyone, regardless of age, gender, or socioeconomic status, when a single stressor or multiple stressors overwhelm a person's coping skills. There is often no preexisting mental disorder, and the symptoms of adjustment disorder are time limited. The stress response is highly individualized, and what one person experiences as highly stressful is sometimes perceived as an irritant or a challenge to another person.

EPIDEMIOLOGY

Mood disorders, particularly depression, are common. According to the National Institute of Mental Health (2010), about 9.5% of the U.S. population or 20.9 million people 18 years old or older in any given year have a mood disorder. About 6.7% of the population 18 years old or older or 14.8 million people suffer from major depression, whereas about 2.6% or 5.6 million adults over the age of 18 years are affected by bipolar disorder. Chronic depression or dysthymic disorder occurs in about 3.3 million adults or 1.5% of adults older than the age of 18 years. Data from the National Comorbidity Survey Replication suggest that the lifetime prevalence of developing major depressive disorder is 16.2%, with twice as many women as men developing the disorder (Kessler et al, 2005). Women have a lifetime prevalence of 21.3% for major depression and 8.0% for dysthymia, whereas men have a lifetime prevalence of only 12.7% for major depression and 4.8% for dysthymia. These gender differences begin to occur around the age of 13 years. Researchers have proposed a number of theories to account for gender differences in the rates of depression, including hormonal or biologic differences, social roles, and cognitive processing. However, no one has adequately explained these gender differences for depression, and additional research is necessary to determine why women are at higher risk.

The first episode of a mood disorder seems to be occurring at younger ages (Beesdo et al, 2009). The average age for the onset of bipolar illness is the late teens to the early twenties, and children now being diagnosed (Merikangas and Pato, 2009). Although the most frequent age of onset for depression is between 25 and 44 years, people in younger age groups have an ever-increasing risk of developing depression. Data indicate that, when the onset of depression is at an early age (i.e., teens or early 20s) or at the age of 55 years or more, it is usually more prolonged and chronic (Greden, 2001). Persons who present with depression that is diagnosed during their 20s or 30s often report not having had depression during their early years. Rates of depression do not significantly increase during menopause. The risk of developing depression and mania increases if there is a positive family history of mood disorders (Perlis et al, 2006).

Sociocultural factors are sometimes related to the onset of depression and mania. Depression seems to occur less frequently among African Americans than among either white or Hispanic groups in the United States. It also appears that depression is more frequent in lower socioeconomic groups, whereas bipolar disorders are more frequent in higher socioeconomic groups. Although depression and mania occur throughout the world, ethnicity and culture influence the expression of symptoms. For example, people from Asian countries describe more somatic symptoms of depression, whereas people from Western cultures tend to describe more mood and cognitive changes. There are differences in the use of therapies for depression on the basis of ethnicity and race; Mexican Americans and African Americans have the lowest rates of care for depression (Gonzalez et al, 2010).

In an increasingly stressful society that is characterized by mobility, family disruptions, and economic stressors, women and younger persons are manifesting depression more than they have in previous generations. Persons with depression often seek help from their primary care providers for physical symptoms such as fatigue, insomnia, headache, and loss of appetite. Primary care providers do not always correctly diagnose depression or treat it appropriately (Solberg et al, 2005). (Epidemiology data for mood disorders are summarized in box 12-1).

The adjustment disorders have received little attention, despite their frequent occurrence. These disorders occur in 5% to 21% of adults in outpatient psychiatric settings, 7.1% of adults in psychiatric inpatient settings, and 13.7% of medical inpatients (Jones et al, 2002). Reliable data are not available for children or adolescents, although adjustment disorders are common in these age groups.

Nurses need to anticipate the frequent diagnosis of adjustment disorders among children and adolescents. Children and adolescents are going through the developmental processes of acquiring coping skills. The occurrences of stressors—particularly those that appear suddenly, involve loss, or disrupt a sense of family security—can overwhelm their coping skills. Stressors include a death in the family and the disruption of the family because of a natural disaster, a divorce, or the diagnosis of a physical illness. The potential for suicidal ideation and behavior, especially among adolescents, necessitates immediate treatment. A comparison of nonsuicidal adolescents with suicidal-adjustment–disordered adolescents revealed that the suicidal patients were more

---

BOX 12-1 **EPIDEMIOLOGY OF MOOD AND ADJUSTMENT DISORDERS**

- 16.2% of the general population will develop a mood disorder.
- 21.3% of women and 12.7% of men will develop major depression.
- The median age of onset for bipolar illness is 25 years.
- The median age of onset for depression is 32 years.
- Depression is diagnosed more frequently among whites and Hispanics than among African Americans.
- Depression is diagnosed more frequently among members of lower socioeconomic groups.
- Bipolar disorders are diagnosed more frequently among members of higher socioeconomic groups.
  - The highest suicide rates in the United States are among white men who are more than 85 years old.
  - Four times as many men as women die as a result of suicide, but women attempt suicide two to three times as often as men do.
- Adjustment disorders occur in 5% to 21% of adults in psychiatric outpatient settings.

likely to have received previous psychiatric treatment, to demonstrate poor psychologic functioning, to report the recent suicide of a significant other, to report dysphoric mood, or to display psychomotor restlessness (Pelkonen et al, 2005).

Children and Adolescents

Depression and bipolar disorder can begin during early childhood and adolescence. As compared with knowledge about adults, less is known about the diagnosis and treatment of mood disorders in this younger age group. Mood disorders that present during childhood or adolescence are significant: (1) they generate extraordinary pain and distress for young individuals who are not prepared to understand or deal with the resulting emotions and behaviors; (2) they initiate major difficulties during a period of time that is essential to psychosocial development; (3) they produce tremendous stress and concern for the entire family unit; (4) they affect the educational experience, because teachers can become frustrated and angry and not understand the basis for the symptoms, which may result in them treating the child differently; and (5) they influence biologic processes and brain functioning to create changes that will have lifelong effects.

Labeling a child with a mental illness generates social and health care debate. This is influenced by the lack of clarity of diagnostic criteria and symptom expression as well as a lack of agreement about appropriate treatment. Symptoms of mood disorders in children and adolescents often appear different from those seen in adults. Depressed youth often exhibit declining academic performance, with school grades dropping for no apparent reason. Other indicators include behavioral problems, aggression, difficulty with peer relationships, withdrawal, and moodiness. Those symptoms may override depression and sadness as key features. Boys often exhibit acting out and the external expression of symptoms, whereas girls tend to exhibit more internalization of the illness in ways such as withdrawal, sadness, and self-deprecation (Bailey et al, 2007).

Childhood depression may occur as early as infancy. Research into the emergence of mood disorders in children has placed greater emphasis on the understanding of inborn and early environmental issues rather than genetics. Temperament is one inborn factor that affects behavior. In one study of young children, the temperamental trait of behavioral disinhibition was associated with higher rates of mood disorders (Hirshfeld-Becker et al, 2002).

The diagnosis of early-onset bipolar disorder (EOBD) has gained acceptance. Bipolar disorder was once thought to emerge around early adulthood, but the diagnosis has been made as early as the age of 5 years. The symptom profile of EOBD overlaps with that of other childhood psychiatric disorders, some of which may be comorbid. It may be difficult to distinguish between EOBD and attention-deficit/hyperactivity disorder. Both of these conditions are manifested by hyperactivity, impulsivity, irritability, and inattention. One differentiating characteristic seems to be that EOBD symptoms show a cyclic pattern that is not evident with other disorders, including attention-deficit/hyperactivity disorder.

Older Adults

Just as the picture of mood disorders has changed for children and adolescents, new information has emerged regarding mood disorders among older adults. Estimates of late-life depression have ranged from 3% to 57%. The recognition of late-life depression has increased with the understanding that depressed older adults are less likely to report depressed mood; however, they tend to describe somatic symptoms, including apathy, fatigue, difficulty sleeping, and loss of interest in usual activities. Confounding this are the losses that older adults may be experiencing, such as of a spouse or friends. This requires the health provider to sort through the patient's symptoms to determine if these symptoms represent depression or if they are consistent with the patient's life experiences and general health. Symptoms such as feeling guilty, low self-worth, suicidal thinking, and irritability may indicate depression. A personal or family history of depression may be a helpful determinant. Older adults respond well to treatment, especially when pharmacotherapy and psychotherapy are combined.

Nurses need to consider social differences in the treatment plans for older adults with depression. Often these patients have no available support system. Getting a family's help is sometimes difficult, and this may add to the older adults' stress level, depending on the relationship. Some family members view depressive symptoms as a part of normal aging, so they require instruction regarding the nature, treatment, and positive prognosis of depression. Furthermore, the values and attitudes of the older adult will influence treatment participation. Generational differences in the acceptance of psychiatric treatment can lead the older adult to refuse care. When asked if they are depressed, some older adults deny it. However, asking about somatic and activity changes (e.g., "What activities do you enjoy these days?" "Are you participating in the same activities that you did a few months ago?") will provide a clearer picture of depressive symptoms.

Apart from the direct effects of depression in older adults, findings demonstrate that the association of depression with cognitive disorders is of particular concern. It is possible depression is an early sign of dementia or a risk factor for dementia, or it may be depression initiates physiologic effects that result in damage to the hippocampus, which later manifests as dementia. The criteria for diagnosing depression in older adults include requiring three (instead of five) depressive symptoms from the DSM-IV list; the expansion of the symptom list to include irritability and social isolation or withdrawal; assessing for decreased positive affect rather than loss of interest; and no longer requiring that symptoms occur nearly every day but rather determining that they represent a change from previous behavior.

Ultimately, depression is of particular concern with older adults because the symptoms often result in life-threatening situations within a rather short time. For example, vegetative symptoms in which the patient sleeps, slows down, and regresses lead to dehydration and electrolyte imbalance, and they compromise any existing medical conditions. Higher mortality among older adults with depression is the result of suicide, comorbid medical conditions, and the impairment of physical functioning. Late-onset depression has been associated with mortality for both men and women.

Mood disorders at either end of the life span are responsive to treatment. However, less is known about how best to use available treatments. Medications are prescribed, but exact standards for type, dosing, and knowledge about side effects are not uniform.

CLINICAL DESCRIPTION

Mood disorders are defined by a pattern of episodes over time and by a pattern of symptoms in each episode, including onset, severity, frequency, and duration. Although mood is the predominant symptom of these disorders, there are changes in cognition, physiologic functioning, and behavior.

Mood disorders are classified in the DSM-IV-TR as depressive disorders (unipolar), bipolar disorders, or other mood disorders. A mood disorder diagnosis is currently based on clinical symptoms; however, future classifications and descriptions will likely encompass biologic markers and further define subtypes of mood disorders with different characteristics. The following sections describe the signs and symptoms of mood disorders.

Types of Mood Disorders
Depressive Disorders

Persons who are diagnosed with a depressive disorder (unipolar depression) have experienced only episodes of depression with no manic or hypomanic episodes. This is also referred to as *unipolar depression*. The DSM-IV-TR Criteria box lists criteria for a major depressive episode. The clinical symptoms of depressive disorders are listed in the Clinical Symptoms box later in this chapter.

Major Depressive Episode, Single or Recurrent. A specific episode of major depression is indicative of a first episode or of a recurrent episode of major depression. Symptoms occur as a result of the disorder and not from the effects of a substance, a medical condition, or the loss of a loved one within the previous 2 months.

Emotional Symptoms. Two primary symptoms of major depression are depressed mood and anhedonia, which is a loss of interest and the capacity to experience pleasure. For patients to be diagnosed with major depression, one of these symptoms must be present most of the day, nearly every day, for at least 2 weeks. Patients describe their mood as depressed, sad, empty, or numb. They report difficulty experiencing pleasure or satisfaction from their usual activities, including eating, sex, or going out with friends. Although patients describe feelings of sadness or frequent crying, some persons with depression are unable to describe their feelings and report disinterest, disconnection, or an inability to feel emotion. Anxiety, irritability, or anger is also sometimes present. Patients also report feelings of loneliness, helplessness, or hopelessness. Affect is the emotional state observed by others, whereas mood is the patient's report of his or her own emotional state. The affect of a person with depression is flat and constricted, with minimal expression; however, that person can appear rather normal as he or she attempts to disguise inner struggles.

Cognitive Symptoms. The criteria for major depression that involves cognition include a diminished ability to think, concentrate, or make decisions; recurrent thoughts of death; and an excessive focus on self-worthlessness and guilt. Concentrating on a task, reading a newspaper, or following a conversation can be overwhelming. Patients are sometimes unable to make decisions about routine concerns, such as what clothing to put on in the morning or what to buy at the grocery store. They have problems at their jobs, including problems with memory and executive functions that originate in the frontal lobe of the brain, which results in an inability to organize, initiate, and complete their work. Recurrent thoughts of death are often evident, including thoughts of suicide, death from natural causes, or existential thoughts about dying. At times, these thoughts occupy a large portion of the patient's waking hours. Negative thinking may be apparent, with feelings of worthlessness and excessive guilt. Patients think about past deeds and focus on their negative view of themselves and the world. Patients with severe depression sometimes become delusional, with fixed beliefs that cannot be changed by logic; these delusions focus on persecution, punishment, nihilism (i.e., a belief in nonexistence or nothingness), or somatic concerns.

Behavioral Symptoms. Behavioral symptoms that are the criteria for major depression are significant weight loss or gain, changes in appetite, insomnia or hypersomnia, psychomotor agitation or psychomotor retardation, and fatigue. Weight gain or loss is significant when it represents a 5% change in body weight within 1 month. Sometimes the weight change is not apparent, but the patient may report a major change in appetite. Sleep disturbances are common, and patients report not being able to sleep (insomnia) or sleeping too much (hypersomnia). Psychomotor agitation is evident when the patient appears to be restless, paces, fidgets, or is irritable. With psychomotor retardation, the patient appears slowed down in movement and in speech. The entire body is slowed, which results in symptoms such as constipation and difficulty digesting food. Persons with diverse depression may appear listless and disheveled. They sometimes do not carefully attend to their dress, appearance, or hygiene, and they may exhibit stooped posture and make little eye contact. Many patients report feelings of fatigue and loss of energy, and they may cite an inability to accomplish tasks and an increased need for naps. They often appear very tired. Fatigue causes many patients to visit a family physician or a nurse practitioner, believing that the fatigue is indicative of a physical problem. Thus, depression is often initially diagnosed during a visit with the primary care provider.

Social Symptoms. For major depression to be diagnosed, the symptoms must cause personal distress and significant

DSM-IV-TR CRITERIA

Major Depressive Episode

A Five (or more) of the following symptoms have been present during the same 2-week period and represent a change from previous functioning; at least one of the symptoms is either (1) depressed mood or (2) loss of interest or pleasure.

NOTE: Do not include symptoms that are clearly due to a general medical condition or mood-incongruent delusions or hallucinations.

1 Depressed mood most of the day, nearly every day, as indicated by either subjective report (e.g., feels sad or empty) or observation made by others (e.g., appears tearful). Note: In children and adolescents, it can be irritable mood.

2 Markedly diminished interest or pleasure in all, or almost all, activities most of the day, nearly every day (as indicated by either subjective account or observation made by others).

3 Significant weight loss when not dieting or weight gain (e.g., a change of more than 5% of body weight in month) or decrease or increase in appetite nearly every day. Note: In children, consider failure to make expected weight gains.

4 Insomnia or hypersomnia nearly every day.

5 Psychomotor agitation or retardation nearly every day (observable by others, not merely subjective feelings of restlessness or being slowed down).

6 Fatigue or loss of energy nearly every day.

7 Feelings of worthlessness or excessive or inappropriate guilt (which may be delusional) nearly every day (not merely self-reproach or guilt about being sick).

8 Diminished ability to think or concentrate, or indecisiveness, nearly every day (either by subjective account or as observed by others).

9 Recurrent thoughts of death (not just fear of dying), recurrent suicidal ideation without a specific plan, or a suicide attempt or a specific plan for committing suicide.

B The symptoms do not meet criteria for a mixed episode.

C The symptoms cause clinically significant distress or impairment in social, occupational, or other important areas of functioning.

D The symptoms are not due to the direct physiologic effects of a substance (e.g., a drug of abuse, a medication) or a general medical condition (e.g., hypothyroidism).

E The symptoms are not better accounted for by bereavement (i.e., after the loss of a loved one, the symptoms persist for longer than 2 months or are characterized by marked functional impairment, morbid preoccupation with self-worthlessness, suicidal ideation, psychotic symptoms, or psychomotor retardation).

From the American Psychiatric Association: *Diagnostic and statistical manual of mental disorders*, ed 4, text revision, Washington, DC, 2000, American Psychiatric Association.

CLINICAL SYMPTOMS

Symptom Comparison

Major Depression

Emotional
Anhedonia
Depressed mood and sadness
Irritability

Cognitive
Diminished ability to think, concentrate, or make decisions
Recurrent thoughts of death
Excessive focus on self-worthlessness and guilt

Behavioral
Significant weight loss or gain or a change in appetite
Insomnia or hypersomnia
Psychomotor agitation or retardation
Fatigue
Sleep disturbances

Social
Withdrawal from family and social interactions
Problems at work as a result of the inability to organize, initiate, or complete work
Financial problems

Dysthymic Disorder

Emotional
Depressed mood
Anhedonia
Irritability or angry mood

Cognitive
Feelings of low self-esteem and inadequacy
Feelings of guilt and brooding about the past
Difficulty with concentration, memory, and decision making
Attitudes of pessimism, despair, and hopelessness

Behavioral
Chronic fatigue

Social
Social withdrawal

The rapid discontinuation of some antidepressants results in withdrawal symptoms. *Tricyclic antidepressant discontinuation syndrome* sometimes results in gastrointestinal symptoms (nausea, vomiting, abdominal cramps, diarrhea), general distress (headaches, lethargy, sweating), sleep disturbances (insomnia, excessive dreaming, nightmares), affective symptoms (anxiety, agitation, low mood, mania, hypomania), movement disorders, or cardiac arrhythmias. Selective serotonin reuptake inhibitor (SSRI) discontinuation syndrome sometimes manifests as gastrointestinal symptoms (nausea, distress), general distress (flu-like symptoms, lethargy, sweating), sleep disturbances, affective symptoms (anxiety, irritability, crying spells, agitation, confusion), problems with balance (dizziness, lightheadedness, vertigo, ataxia), or sensory abnormalities (paresthesias, numbness, tremor). SSRI discontinuation syndrome is especially likely with the shorter-lasting selective serotonin reuptake inhibitors, and it is most problematic with fluvoxamine (Luvox), nefazodone (Serzone), paroxetine (Paxil), and venlafaxine (Effexor). The nurse needs to instruct patients to avoid missing doses of antidepressants, to reassure patients that withdrawal symptoms are usually mild and short lived, and to anticipate that most antidepressants will need to be tapered off gradually.

impairment in social and occupational functioning. Some patients withdraw from family and social interactions. Although some people are able to function at work with relatively little obvious impairment, this often comes at great personal and family expense as their energy for social interaction is exhausted.

When the person is unable to work, financial problems often jeopardize the family. Family members begin to feel confused, angry, guilty, abandoned, and sad. During an episode, the patient's erratic behavior, mood, and cognition may alienate loved ones who become frustrated with not knowing how to help. Marital distress may continue even after the acute episode subsides.

These descriptions of cognitive, behavioral, and social symptoms depict individuals with moderate to severe depression. Depression can be insidious, and sometimes people who are experiencing these symptoms can conceal the extent to which they interfere with their functioning. It is possible for someone to work, maintain a home, go to school, or care for children and still be experiencing depression. Eventually the symptoms can become overwhelming, and the individual's level of functioning will begin to decline.

Dysthymic Disorder. Dysthymia differs from major depression in that it is a chronic, rather than episodic, low-level depression. To receive this diagnosis, the patient must have had a depressed mood and at least three of the following symptoms for most of the day, nearly every day, for at least 2 years (1 year for children and adolescents): poor appetite or overeating, insomnia or hypersomnia, low energy, low self-esteem, poor concentration or difficulty making decisions, and feelings of hopelessness. There cannot have been a manic

or hypomanic episode. The patient may have experienced an episode of major depression before the onset of dysthymia, provided that there were at least 6 months with no signs or symptoms of depression. After 2 years of dysthymia, some patients are diagnosed with major depression superimposed on dysthymia if symptoms increase in severity. The dysthymic disorder is not a result of the effects of a substance or a medical condition. Psychotic features are usually not present with this disorder.

Emotional Symptoms. The predominant symptom that must be present for the diagnosis of dysthymia is depressed mood. Patients report feeling chronically "down," "gloomy," or "sad." Many are unable to remember a time when they felt good or their usual self. Another symptom that is indicative of dysthymia is a generalized loss of interest or pleasure in activities; however, unlike with major depression, anhedonia is not a primary emotional symptom. Another symptom is irritability or angry mood. Some patients find themselves feeling impatient with family members or coworkers and having angry outbursts. Many feel bad about their irritable state but are unable to control it.

Cognitive Symptoms. Cognitive symptoms of dysthymia include low self-esteem and inadequacy; guilt and brooding about the past; difficulty with concentration, memory, and decision making; and negative thinking evidenced by pessimism, despair, and hopelessness. Patients with dysthymia often have little regard for themselves and are overwhelmed by a sense of inadequacy and a lack of self-confidence. They reflect on past actions and attribute personal guilt to their circumstances. Negativity is pervasive in what they do and say; life seems hopeless, and situations are full of pessimism and despair. Patients often report poor memory and decreased concentration on tasks, and they have problems making decisions. However, the impairment is usually not as severe as the impaired cognition that occurs with major depression.

Behavioral Symptoms. Patients with dysthymia commonly complain of chronic fatigue. They are exhausted by usual activities, and they often believe that they have a physical illness or chronic fatigue syndrome. Patients make repeated visits to their health care providers in the hope of determining the cause of their fatigue. Along with the fatigue, patients display decreased activity and productivity. Everything becomes a chore, and it often becomes difficult to complete tasks in the usual amount of time.

Social Symptoms. Social withdrawal is common with dysthymia. Patients are tired, irritable, and depressed, and they no longer experience satisfaction from outings or activities with family and friends. Patients' mood states and negativity prevent people from wanting to be with them, thereby increasing their isolation from others.

Depressive Disorders not Otherwise Specified. There are types of depression that do not meet the criteria for the depressive disorders presented thus far or that will be disorders in their own right. Some of these include premenstrual dysphoric disorder, minor depressive disorder, recurrent brief depressive disorder, and the postpsychotic depression of schizophrenia. The term *dysphoria* refers to a depressed and sad mood. The reader is referred to the DSM-IV-TR classification for more extensive descriptions of these diagnoses.

Bipolar Disorders

A bipolar disorder occurs when the patient experiences both episodes of depression and episodes of mania or hypomania over time. Bipolar disorders are characterized by a pattern of manic, hypomanic, and depressed episodes. These depressed and manic episodes are not the result of the effects of a substance (e.g., antidepressant medication), electroconvulsive therapy, or light therapy. Patients may be diagnosed with a bipolar I or a bipolar II disorder. The primary characteristics of bipolar I disorder include the occurrence of one or more manic episodes or mixed episodes as described below; depressed episodes may have occurred in the past. The primary feature of bipolar II disorder is a clinical course of major depressive episodes accompanied by at least one hypomanic episode. The public often refers to bipolar disorders as *manic depression*. A bipolar disorder encompasses the range (spectrum) of possible disturbances in mood. Bipolar disorder is being viewed increasingly as a spectrum disorder rather than several separate illnesses. The clinical symptoms of bipolar disorders are listed in the Clinical Symptoms box.

Manic Episode. Manic episodes occur when there is an abnormally and persistently elevated, expansive, or irritable mood for at least 1 week. At least three of the following symptoms must also be present: inflated self-esteem, decreased need for sleep, more-than-usual talkativeness, racing thoughts, distractibility, increase in goal-directed activity, and excessive involvement in pleasurable activities (see the DSM-IV-TR Criteria box). Mixed episodes occur when both manic and major depressive criteria are met nearly every day for 1 week (see the DSM-IV-TR Criteria box).

Emotional Symptoms. To be diagnosed as having a manic episode, the patient must exhibit an abnormally and persistently elevated, expansive, or irritable mood for at least 1 week. The patient appears euphoric, with periods that are punctuated by irritability and anger. Some patients report minimal euphoria and instead consider irritability to be their primary mood. Emotional lability, with which mood and affect fluctuate between euphoria and anger, is common.

Cognitive Symptoms. Inflated self-esteem and grandiosity are common symptoms of mania. Patients report that they are confident and capable and that they can do things better than others can. As the mania becomes more intense, patients describe themselves in glowing terms, and they may believe that they are capable of amazing feats and achievements. Delusions of grandeur are sometimes evident during severe episodes of mania, because patients believe that they possess extraordinary gifts and talents, are famous, or that they personally know someone famous. These delusions of inflated self-worth and ability represent mood-congruent psychotic features of mania. Cognitively, patients with mania also experience thought-flow disturbances with racing thoughts and flight of ideas. Flight of ideas is a type of thought disorder in which somewhat connected thoughts occur quickly, which

---

CLINICAL SYMPTOMS

Bipolar Disorders

Manic Episode
Emotional
Excessively and persistently elevated, expansive, or irritable mood

Cognitive
Thoughts of inflated self-esteem and grandiosity
Thought-flow disturbance with racing thoughts and flight of ideas

Behavioral
Increased talkativeness
Decreased need for sleep
Increased goal-directed behavior or agitation
Excessive involvement in activities thought to be pleasurable, risky, or even dangerous

Social
Increased sociability and sexuality
Intrusive, interruptive, and disruptive during conversations or activities
Fluctuations between euphoria and anger

Perceptual
Distractibility
Hallucinations

Cyclothymic Disorder
Behavioral
Periods of hypomania
Periods of depressed mood and anhedonia
Irritability or angry mood
Chronic fatigue

Cognitive
Feelings of low self-esteem and inadequacy
Feelings of guilt and brooding about the past
Difficulty with concentration, memory, and decision making
Attitudes of pessimism, despair, and hopelessness

Social
Social withdrawal

---

results in little elaboration and the rapid changing of subjects. It becomes difficult to block out incoming stimuli, and the patient becomes distractible, responding to irrelevant stimuli. Patients with mania often deny the seriousness of their status, and they lack judgment regarding personal, social, and occupational needs and activities.

Behavioral Symptoms. Increased talkativeness, increased goal-directed behavior or agitation, and excessive involvement in pleasurable activities are notable symptoms of mania. As the mania progresses, patients become more talkative, and their speech is pressured (delivered with urgency). The rate of speech often increases and becomes rapid. There is a decreased need for sleep, and patients do not feel tired. Some patients exhibit extremes in appearance and start wearing

---

DSM-IV-TR CRITERIA

Manic, Mixed, and Hypomanic Episodes

Manic Episode

A A distinct period of excessively and persistently elevated, expansive, or irritable mood, lasting at least 1 week (or any duration if hospitalization is necessary).

B During the period of mood disturbance, three (or more) of the following symptoms have persisted (four if the mood is only irritable) and have been present to a significant degree:
1 Inflated self-esteem or grandiosity
2 Decreased need for sleep (e.g., feels rested after only 3 hours of sleep)
3 More talkative than usual or pressure to keep talking
4 Flight of ideas or subjective experience that thoughts are racing
5 Distractibility (i.e., attention too easily drawn to unimportant or irrelevant external stimuli)
6 Increase in goal-directed activity (either socially, at work or school, or sexually) or psychomotor agitation
7 Excessive involvement in pleasurable activities that have a high potential for painful consequences (e.g., engaging in unrestrained buying sprees, sexual indiscretions, or foolish business investments)

C The symptoms do not meet criteria for a mixed episode.

D The mood disturbance is sufficiently severe to cause marked impairment in occupational functioning or in usual social activities or relationships with others, or to necessitate hospitalization to prevent harm to self or others, or there are psychotic features.

E The symptoms are not due to the direct physiologic effects of a substance (e.g., a drug of abuse, a medication, or other treatment) or a general medical condition (e.g., hyperthyroidism).

Note: Manic-like episodes that are clearly caused by somatic antidepressant treatment (e.g., medication, electroconvulsive therapy, light therapy) should not count toward a diagnosis of bipolar I disorder.

Mixed Episode

A The criteria are met both for a manic episode and for a major depressive episode (except for duration) nearly every day during at least a 1-week period.

B The mood disturbance is sufficiently severe to cause marked impairment in occupational functioning or in usual social activities or relationships with others, or to necessitate hospitalization to prevent harm to self or others, or there are psychotic features.

C The symptoms are not due to the direct physiologic effects of a substance (e.g., a drug of abuse, a

medication, or other treatment) or a general medical condition (e.g., hyperthyroidism).

Note: Manic-like episodes that are clearly caused by somatic antidepressant treatment (e.g., medication, electroconvulsive therapy, light therapy) should not count toward a diagnosis of bipolar I disorder.

Hypomanic Episode

A A distinct period of excessively and persistently elevated, expansive, or irritable mood, lasting throughout at least 4 days, that is clearly different from the usual nondepressed mood.

B During the period of mood disturbance, three (or more) of the following symptoms have persisted (four if the mood is only irritable) and have been present to a significant degree:
1 Inflated self-esteem or grandiosity
2 Decreased need for sleep (e.g., feels rested after only 3 hours of sleep)
3 More talkative than usual or pressure to keep talking
4 Flight of ideas or subjective experience that thoughts are racing
5 Distractibility (i.e., attention too easily drawn to unimportant or irrelevant external stimuli)
6 Increase in goal-directed activity (either socially, at work or school, or sexually) or psychomotor agitation
7 Excessive involvement in pleasurable activities that have a high potential for painful consequences (e.g., engaging in unrestrained buying sprees, sexual indiscretions, or foolish business investments)

C The episode is associated with an unequivocal change in functioning that is uncharacteristic of the person when not symptomatic.

D The disturbance in mood and the change in functioning are observable by others.

E The episode is not severe enough to cause marked impairment in social or occupational functioning or to necessitate hospitalization, and there are no psychotic features.

F The symptoms are not due to the direct physiologic effects of a substance (e.g., a drug of abuse, a medication, or other treatment) or a general medical condition (e.g., hyperthyroidism).

Note: Hypomanic-like episodes that are clearly caused by somatic antidepressant treatment (e.g., medication, electroconvulsive therapy, light therapy) should not count toward a diagnosis of bipolar II disorder.

From the American Psychiatric Association: *Diagnostic and statistical manual of mental disorders*, ed 4, text revision, Washington, DC, 2000, American Psychiatric Association.

---

bright colors, unusual dress, and heavy makeup. Patients begin and engage in more activities, taking on additional tasks and initiating new projects. Productivity appears to increase, but, as the mania becomes more intense, actual productivity decreases as patients become more distractible, disorganized, and agitated. They begin to physically move faster,

pacing, fidgeting, and rarely letting their bodies remain still. It becomes more difficult for the patient to eat and drink because of excessive movement and activity. As insight and judgment become more impaired, patients become involved in activities that they perceive as pleasurable but that carry a high risk for harm or negative consequences. Patients often report engaging in extramarital affairs, promiscuity, spending sprees, gambling, wild driving, risk taking, and unwise business deals. These behaviors often have serious health, financial, legal, and interpersonal consequences.

Social Symptoms. At first, mania seems to promote sociability, and patients become more outgoing and active; however, before long, insight and judgment fail, and these same patients become intrusive; they interrupt others' conversations and activities, change from a euphoric to an angry mood, and disrupt social interactions. Patients with mania find it difficult to set both physical and emotional boundaries, and they interfere in the physical space and personal issues of others. The funny, witty patient may become angry and isolated as the mood escalates and intensifies.

Perceptual Symptoms. One symptom of mania is distractibility, in which attention is easily and frequently drawn to irrelevant external stimuli. Patients appear to be unable to screen out secondary stimuli (e.g., noises, other voices, and visual attractions) that are not necessary or relevant to the task at hand. Distractibility interferes with attention, concentration, and memory. Perceptual disturbances also may occur in the form of hallucinations. Manic hallucinations occur in any sensory mode, but they are usually auditory, with themes that pertain to grandiosity, power, and, occasionally, paranoia. These symptoms indicate manic psychosis.

Hypomanic Episode. Manic and hypomanic episodes share symptom criteria, and they differ primarily with regard to their severity and duration. Hypomanic episodes are not severe enough to cause significant impairment in social and occupational functioning or to require hospitalization. However, for diagnosis, it must be evident that the mood and behavioral disturbances of hypomania represent a definite change in the person's usual functioning that lasts for at least 4 days. During a hypomanic phase, patients appear extremely happy and agreeable, at ease with social conversation, and humorous. Although the moments of elevated mood seem desirable, they represent dysfunctional affective states during which the patient is not fully in control of his or her moods and accompanying behavior. Many patients often report that they like the experience of hypomania. They perceive that, during these episodes, they are productive, creative, and functioning at a higher level. However, this is a dangerous time, because hypomania can escalate to mania. As judgment declines, patients sometimes fail to recognize the consequences of their actions. Some patients report going off of their medications to experience hypomanic episodes during which they feel productive and creative. The criteria for hypomanic episodes are presented in the DSM-IV-TR Criteria box.

Cyclothymic Disorder. Cyclothymic disorder is a chronic mood disturbance of at least 2 years' duration (1 year for children and adolescents), with many periods of hypomanic symptoms, depressed mood, and anhedonia. Patients with cyclothymic disorder have not been without the symptoms for more than 2 months over a period of 2 or more years; however, these symptoms are less severe or intense than those seen with major depressive or manic episodes.

Additional Types of Mood Disorders

The DSM-IV-TR also provides diagnostic criteria for mood disorders that result from general medical conditions and from substance use. In these instances, the depressed or elevated mood and the accompanying symptoms are the result of some general medical condition or the ingestion of or withdrawal from medications or other substances. Box 12-2 lists examples of the types of medical conditions and substances that are commonly associated with the development of mood disorders. See the Clinical Symptoms box.

CLINICAL SYMPTOMS
Additional Mood Disorders

Melancholic Depression
Emotional
Anhedonia
Increased depression in the morning

Cognitive
Excessive feelings of guilt

Behavioral
Waking at least 2 hours before normal and being unable to fall back to sleep
Psychomotor retardation or agitation
Significant weight loss

Atypical Depression
Emotional
Mood reactivity
Ability to react to positive stimuli

Cognitive
Sensitivity to interpersonal rejection

Behavioral
Significant weight gain or increase in appetite
Hypersomnia
Leaden paralysis

Seasonal Affective Disorder
Emotional
Depression between October/November and March/April

Postpartum Depression
Behavioral
Difficulty caring for child

Medical Conditions and Mood Disorders

When mood disorders and medical conditions are concurrent, the presentation, treatment, and prognosis of both are often complicated and compromised. Comorbidity (co-occurrence) is identified in several ways:

- A medical patient develops a mood disorder as a stress response to a serious medical condition.
- A medical patient develops a mood disorder as a physiologic response to either medical pathology or medications.
- A psychiatric patient with a persistent mood disorder develops common medical disorders.

BOX 12-2	SELECTED MEDICAL CONDITIONS AND SUBSTANCES ASSOCIATED WITH MOOD DISORDERS

Medical Conditions
Hypothyroidism/hyperthyroidism
Mononucleosis
Diabetes mellitus
Cushing's disease
Pernicious anemia
Pancreatitis
Hepatitis
Human immunodeficiency virus
Multiple sclerosis

Substances
Digitalis
Thiazide diuretics
Reserpine
Propranolol
Anabolic steroids
Oral contraceptives
Disulfiram
Sulfonamides
Alcohol and other substances of dependence
Marijuana

- A psychiatric patient with a persistent mood disorder has an exacerbation of symptoms as a result of medical pathology or treatment.
- Health care providers identify previously unrecognized relationships between mood and medical disorders.

Medical conditions are often stressful and frightening, and some result in a depressive reaction to the situation or major depression. A variety of medical disorders are associated with depression.

The pathophysiology of a medical condition or a response to the medications given for a medical condition sometimes results in a mood disorder. Research has implicated disorders of nearly every body system with co-occurring mood disorders. Cardiovascular disorders have been linked with major depression. Major depression and depressive symptomatology are common in patients with coronary artery disease, and they significantly increase risk and complicate recovery from a range of cardiac events (Shin et al, 2010). Depression after myocardial infarction increases mortality, especially during the first 18 months after the myocardial infarction. Neurologic disorders are closely linked with depression, and depression after stroke is particularly common. Estimates suggest that up to 80% of poststroke patients have depression (Carota, 2005). The early treatment of poststroke depression has a significant influence on the rehabilitation and recovery of function related to activities of daily living among stroke patients. Depression is a significant symptom of Parkinson's disease. Clinical manifestations include apathy, psychomotor retardation, memory impairment, pessimism, irrationality,

and suicidal ideation without suicidal behavior. When depression occurs among patients with Parkinson's disease, Alzheimer's disease, or epilepsy, the consequences can include increased mortality, suicide, and need for institutionalization (Evans et al, 2005).

Endocrine disorders are also involved in the emergence of psychiatric disorders. There seems to be a relationship between type 2 diabetes mellitus and bipolar I disorder that is separate and apart from the effects of age, race, gender, medication, and body mass (Regenold et al, 2002).

Additional disorders that result in mood disturbances are also the focus of much research, including cancer, thyroid disease, and human immunodeficiency virus. Alternatively, a number of medical conditions mimic psychiatric illness. The problem lies in determining the root cause of symptoms and whether they are the result of medical, pharmacologic, psychiatric, or psychologic pathology. During the process of treatment, nurses must take care to ensure that medication administration does not further complicate illnesses. Many medical drugs are associated with the emergence of mood disorders. At the same time, many side effects of psychotropic drugs are initially assessed as being medical in nature (e.g., cardiac or blood pressure changes seen with certain antidepressant drugs). Ultimately, the assessment of medical patients must include the psychiatric component.

Psychiatric patients are at least as likely as individuals without psychiatric disorders to develop medical problems that range from the common cold to serious medical disorders. This is particularly problematic because psychiatric patients have not always received timely or adequate medical care. Consequently, psychiatric patients tend to present at more advanced stages of illness, with more complicated psychosocial factors influencing care. Patients with a preexisting psychiatric disorder will present for treatment at any hospital inpatient unit or outpatient clinic. Unless the treatment plan considers the psychiatric disorder along with the medical illness, problems often occur with medication compatibility, accurate interpretation of patient behavior by staff, patient cooperation with and involvement in care, and patient ability to follow treatment instructions after hospitalization. For example, bipolar disorder increases the risk for human immunodeficiency virus, thereby increasing the morbidity of illnesses related to human immunodeficiency virus.

Among psychiatric patients, the pathophysiology of or the treatment received for a medical disorder can promote the return of psychiatric symptoms or the emergence of a new disorder. For example, when patients are admitted to the hospital, a complete history of previous medications is not always available. If the patient does not continue to take psychotropic medications, the symptoms of a preexisting mood disorder will return, or the patient will experience a withdrawal response as a result of not taking the medications.

Comorbidity

Current research is expanding our awareness of medical and psychiatric comorbidity, with new knowledge and questions available every day. There is a high co-occurrence of mood

---

❖ **CLINICAL ALERT #2**

Be alert to suicidal ideation and intent among patients with depression and patients with mania who are cycling into depression or whose insight and judgment are impaired. A particularly high-risk time is 1 to 6 weeks after the initiation of antidepressant therapy, before therapeutic levels are reached.

---

disorders with other major mental illnesses (Rush et al, 2005), especially substance abuse and dependence. Psychiatric patients are living longer than they did during previous generations. Consequently, clinics are seeing an increase in the number of patients with comorbid medical and psychiatric disorders who are also showing signs of dementia. Epidemiologic data indicate that from 30% to 50% of patients with Alzheimer's disease have significant depressive symptoms. As a result, researchers are trying to develop criteria that will define the course of depression in patients with Alzheimer's disease. Others are making an effort to identify criteria for vascular depression, which is a subtype that occurs with acute and chronic cerebrovascular pathology. Thus, two new diagnostic categories will become available that are separate from existing depressive disorders. Ultimately, nurses need to be aware of the comorbidity of mood and medical disorders in all treatment settings.

Additional Symptom Features of Mood Disorders

The DSM-IV-TR recognizes that there are features of mood disorders that indicate various subtypes of unipolar and bipolar disorders. Persons who are experiencing an episode of major depression, whether it is part of a unipolar or bipolar pattern, sometimes demonstrate melancholic, atypical, or seasonal features. Postpartum onset represents another type of mood disorder.

Features of melancholic depression include anhedonia and a lack of reactivity to any pleasurable stimulus; a distinct quality of mood in which the patient perceives the depression as different from the feeling after the death of a loved one; depression that is worse in the morning (diurnal variation); sleep disturbance of early morning awakening at least 2 hours before the usual time; marked psychomotor retardation or agitation; significant weight loss or loss of appetite; and excessive guilt.

Features of atypical depression include mood reactivity; the loss of the ability to react to positive stimuli; significant weight gain or increase in appetite; hypersomnia; leaden paralysis or a heavy feeling in the arms and legs; and a longstanding pattern of being sensitive to interpersonal rejection. Of particular concern is that atypical depression may be associated with suicide attempts more often than other types of depression (Sanchez-Gistau et al, 2009).

A seasonal pattern occurs when there is a regular temporal relationship between the onset and remission of an episode of major depression (unipolar or bipolar) at a particular time of the year. This pattern must be evident for 2 consecutive years with no intervening nonseasonal episodes. Seasonal episodes of altered mood must outnumber any nonseasonal episodes over a lifetime. This pattern is commonly called *seasonal affective disorder* (SAD). Patients with SAD often develop depression during October or November and find it diminishing in March or April, although some demonstrate an unusual pattern in which their depression occurs during the summer months. Atypical features are also associated with SAD. A seasonal pattern also occurs with bipolar disorder, particularly bipolar II disorder, in which increased light triggers manic or hypomanic episodes.

Some women will experience a postpartum mood disorder that includes depression or mania after the birth of a child. This is the most common childbirth complication, with about 15% to 20% of new mothers exhibiting this disorder (Beck, 2008). This usually occurs within 3 months of the birth. Postpartum depression consists of the symptoms of depression or mania described earlier in this chapter. With the severe form of this disorder, new mothers become psychotic, hearing voices and experiencing delusions. Some new mothers who are clinically depressed have a great deal of difficulty providing childcare; in fact, the child is sometimes at risk for neglect or harm. Many women describe transient mood changes after delivery that are less severe and that end within a few weeks.

A summary of the clinical symptoms of these additional types of mood disorders is provided in the Clinical Symptoms box on page 232.

ADJUSTMENT DISORDERS

Adjustment disorders occur in response to major life stressors, and manifest with a variety of symptoms, most of which are similar to other psychiatric disorders, particularly mood disorders. Sadness or mood disturbances, withdrawal, and preoccupation with the stressors lead the clinician to conclude that the person is experiencing major depression. However, adjustment disorders are generally of a briefer duration. The nervousness and distress of adjustment disorders sometimes mimics a generalized anxiety disorder, but the criteria symptoms for generalized anxiety disorder are not met for the required time frame. Although acute stress disorder and posttraumatic stress disorder are also responses to a stressor, the nature of the stressor with these disorders is much more severe and perceived as life threatening.

The diagnostic criteria for adjustment disorders are listed in the DSM-IV-TR Criteria box. These disorders occur when the level of distress exceeds usual expectations or when social, occupational, or school functioning is impaired. For example, a conflict with a coworker results in prolonged sleep disturbance and depressed mood or a pattern of calling in sick to work. Adjustment disorder is often diagnosed if a stressor is identified and the patient's symptoms are not severe enough to meet criteria for a more severe disorder.

The diagnostic category of adjustment disorders has been controversial for many reasons. Its criteria are seen as overlapping with those of depressive and anxiety disorders, so many have questioned the category's validity. Reactions to stress are highly individualized, both in perception and in expression, so specific symptoms are difficult to identify. The absence of biologic markers, the close link with environmental factors, and the lack of clear measurable criteria are problematic. Some have questioned how adjustment disorders differ from normal adaptive reactions, with a concern that current diagnostic and treatment practices overmedicalize a process that is not truly pathologic.

DSM-IV-TR CRITERIA

Adjustment Disorders

A The development of emotional or behavioral symptoms in response to an identifiable stressor(s) occurring within 3 months of the onset of the stressor(s).

B These symptoms or behaviors are clinically significant as evidenced by either of the following:
  1 Marked distress that is in excess of what would be expected from exposure to the stressor
  2 Significant impairment in social or occupational (academic) functioning

C The stress-related disturbance does not meet criteria for another specific Axis I disorder and is not merely an exacerbation of a preexisting Axis I or Axis II disorder.

D The symptoms do not represent bereavement.

E Once the stressor (or its consequences) has terminated, the symptoms do not persist for more than an additional 6 months.

  Specify if:

Acute: if the disturbance lasts less than 6 months

Chronic: if the disturbance lasts for 6 months or longer

  Adjustment disorders are coded based on the subtype, which is selected according to the predominant symptoms. The specific stressor(s) can be specified on Axis IV.

With depressed mood

With disturbance of conduct

With anxiety

With mixed disturbance of emotions and conduct

With mixed anxiety and depressed mood

Unspecified

From the American Psychiatric Association: *Diagnostic and statistical manual of mental disorders,* ed 4, text revision, Washington, DC, 2000, American Psychiatric Association.

PROGNOSIS FOR MOOD DISORDERS

Mood disorders are usually lifetime illnesses. The bipolar disorders historically have been perceived as recurrent, with cycles of mania and depression interspersed with periods of euthymia or normal mood. The pattern of cycles varies from person to person, with episodes of depression, mania, and euthymia varying widely in duration. Some individuals experience rapid shifts in mood, which is known as *rapid cycling*. It is often more difficult to treat individuals who exhibit this pattern. The bipolar disorders have a high rate of recurrence and relapse. Factors that contribute to relapse

include the number of and recovery from previous episodes, a family history of bipolar disorder, functional incapacity associated with episodes, past psychotic episodes, and past suicide attempts (Consensus Development Panel, 1985). Many recurrences are controllable with proper treatment and monitoring.

There is evidence of differences between the depression period of bipolar disorder and the depression of major depressive disorder, including family history of bipolar disorder, earlier age of onset, more depressive episodes, and individual symptom differences. Symptom differences include more sadness, insomnia, cognitive difficulties, and somatic complaints with bipolar disorder (Perlis et al, 2006). The depression cycle of bipolar disorder may be very difficult to treat.

Major depression is a serious and recurrent disorder for the majority of persons with the illness (Greden, 2001). A large percentage of patients with an episode of major depression experience a subsequent episode, and recurrent episodes tend to be increasingly intense, with shorter time periods between episodes. Data suggest that nearly two thirds of people who experience major depression will suffer at least one recurrence within 10 years. Negative long-term effects impair self-care, productivity, social functioning, occupational functioning, and physical health (Greden, 2001). The long-term outcomes of major depressive disorder tend to be less than positive: each succeeding episode sets up the brain for future negative changes (Yiend, 2009). A major study, the STAR*D, was a multisite project that tracked patients who had been treated for depression and that examined those patients who became symptom free and those who were resistant to the original medication. The research attempted to determine successes and how to intervene with those who retained at least some residual symptoms (National Institute of Mental Health, 2006). However, education, lifetime monitoring, adherence to treatment, and maintenance treatment for many persons with mood disorders can promote health and reduce the risk of recurrence. Patients need to be aware of the recurrent nature of their disorders and educated about the importance of recognizing symptoms and seeking help early when these symptoms begin. Unfortunately, many persons do not recognize the onset of their recurrences (Hagerty et al, 1997), and less than a third of the people who experience depression seek help, which puts them at risk for future and more severe depression.

Dysthymia often continues for years before individuals seek assistance for their symptoms. Many people are unaware that the chronic, low-level depression that is draining their energy is a form of depression that is treatable. Unfortunately, many people with dysthymia go on to develop major depression.

With proper treatment, the prognosis for maintaining individual functioning with a mood disorder is favorable. Inevitably, failure to seek help, lack of education about the disorder, lack of proper diagnosis and appropriate treatment, not following a treatment plan, and resistance of the symptoms to usual interventions mean that some persons will become so impaired that their daily functioning will diminish for long periods.

Discharge Criteria

Most patients with mood disorders are seen in primary care settings rather than specialty clinics. Patients go to their primary care provider with symptoms such as fatigue, insomnia, or weight loss. They are often not properly diagnosed in the primary care setting, and inappropriate intervention may occur. When depressed patients do receive care through mental health services, most are not hospitalized but instead receive outpatient treatment. Because of insurance constraints and the availability of services, both inpatient and outpatient settings have become increasingly limited with regard to the amount of time available to patients for treatment. Inpatient stays are often for only several days unless symptoms are severe, and outpatient visits are usually limited by insurance. Consequently, the goals of treatment are quite different for hospital treatment as compared with outpatient treatment, and realistic outcomes within the available time frame sometimes differ from ideal expectations. When patients are discharged from the hospital, the expectation is for outpatient treatment to begin so that progress will continue. Patients require attention to ensure that they at least meet the following realistic criteria for each setting before discharge.

Hospital Discharge Criteria
Realistic

The patient will do the following:
- Verbalize plans for the future, including an absence of imminent suicidal intent or behavior.
- Verbalize plans for seeking help (a contract) if suicidal thoughts become intensified or if thoughts progress to plans.
- Demonstrate the ability to manage basic self-care needs, such as personal hygiene, or verbalize strategies for acquiring assistance.
- Identify psychosocial or physical stressors that have negative influences on mood and thinking.
- State positive and helpful strategies to cope with threats, concerns, and stressors.
- Identify signs and symptoms of the mood disorder, including prodromal (early) signs that indicate the need to seek help.
- Describe how to contact appropriate sources for validation or intervention when necessary.
- Verbalize knowledge about medication treatment and necessary self-care strategies.

Ideal

The patient will do the following:
- Describe his or her mood state and demonstrate the ability to identify changes from euthymic mood.
- Verbalize realistic perceptions of himself or herself and his or her abilities that are positive and hopeful.

- Verbalize realistic expectations for himself or herself and for others.
- Use learned techniques and strategies to prevent or minimize symptoms.
- Engage family members or significant others as sources of support.
- Structure his or her life to include appropriate activities that promote social support, that minimize stress, and that facilitate healthy living (e.g., diet, exercise).

Outpatient Discharge Criteria
Realistic

The patient will do the following:
- Verbalize plans for the future, including an absence of imminent suicidal intent or behavior.
- Verbalize plans for seeking help (a contract) if suicidal thoughts become intensified or if thoughts progress to plans.
- Demonstrate an ability to manage basic self-care needs, such as personal hygiene, or verbalize strategies for acquiring assistance.
- Describe his or her mood state and demonstrate the ability to identify changes from euthymic mood.
- Identify psychosocial or physical stressors that have negative influences on mood and thinking.
- State positive and helpful strategies for coping with threats, concerns, and stressors.
- Identify signs and symptoms of the mood disorder, including prodromal (early) signs that indicate the need to seek help.
- Describe how to contact appropriate sources for validation or intervention when necessary.
- Use learned techniques and strategies to prevent or minimize symptoms.
- Verbalize knowledge about medication treatment and necessary self-care strategies.

Ideal

The patient will do the following:
- Verbalize realistic perceptions of himself or herself and his or her abilities that are positive and hopeful.
- Verbalize realistic expectations for himself or herself and for others.
- Engage family members or significant others as sources of support.
- Structure his or her life to include appropriate activities that promote social support, that minimize stress, and that facilitate healthy living (e.g., diet, exercise).

THE NURSING PROCESS
ASSESSMENT

Mood is the key variant in mood disorders, and it may be prolonged over a course of time, whereas affect may be highly changeable. The term *temperament* refers to observable differences in the strength and duration of a patient's

BOX 12-3   MENTAL STATUS CRITERIA

- **Mood:** The internal manifestation of a subjective feeling state
- **Affect:** The external expression or manifestation of a feeling state
- **Temperament:** Observable differences in the intensity and duration of arousal and emotionality
- **Emotion:** The experience of a feeling state
- **Emotional reactivity:** The tendency to respond to internal or external events with emotion
- **Emotional regulation:** The ability to control or modify the occurrence and intensity of feelings
- **Range of affect:** The span of emotional expression experienced and displayed by an individual

tendency to respond to circumstances and the degree of emotionalism expressed. Many consider this to be a product of a person's biologic constitution. The term is generally applied when speaking about infants or children, but temperament patterns influence a variety of phenomena that extend into adulthood, including impulse control and attachment. Emotion is the patient's experience of a feeling state, and patients are often able to identify previous experiences that are highly intense and variable. Emotional or affective reactivity is the degree to which a patient tends to respond to external and internal changes with feeling states; this is evident in how the patient responds to questions. Emotional regulation is the patient's ability to control or modify the occurrence and intensity of feeling states. The range of affect is the span of emotional expression that the patient shows. Limitations of range are described as *restricted, blunted,* or *flat* (Box 12-3).

The prevalence and incidence of mood disorders demand that nurses be alert for symptoms of depression and mania. Most persons who are experiencing a mood disorder (particularly depression) never seek psychiatric care; more often, they will visit family practitioners, clinics, or emergency departments and report symptoms of fatigue, lack of activity, or vague physical complaints. Many do not realize that they are experiencing a mood disorder. They may be treated for a medical problem such as an acute cardiac event, cancer, or stroke but have an underlying mood disorder that increases their risk for morbidity and mortality.

Patients with mood disorders pose a challenge because their primary symptom is one of depression or emotional elation. Their affective dysregulation often evokes emotional responses in nurses who find themselves feeling depressed, anxious, or angry while caring for these individuals. The negativity of depression or the expansive euphoria, hyperactivity, and grandiosity of mania may also promote fatigue, irritability, and negativity in the nurse. Therefore, when caring for patients with mood disorders, nurses must maintain awareness of their own personal reactions to the patient and the ways in which these reactions affect the nurse–patient relationship and subsequent care.

Patients who are experiencing mood disorders are in emotional pain and are suffering. In fact, high psychologic pain during an episode of depression may be associated with higher suicide risk (Olie et al, 2010). These patients are unable to change their emotional state at will. However, many have heard people close to them—including health professionals—make comments such as, "Pull yourself together" or "Get a hold of yourself." These patients require validation that their emotional state is not their fault and that they are experiencing psychiatric disorders. In other words, they need acceptance and respect.

It is important that nurses appear confident, straightforward, and hopeful. Reassuring comments such as "I know you'll feel better soon" are not helpful, because they provide false reassurance. It is appropriate to express hope with comments such as, "I've known many patients with depression, and they have felt better within several weeks after starting their medications."

Severity of depression determines communication with a depressed person. Patients with severe depression are frequently physically and cognitively slowed down and have problems with attention, concentration, and decision making. Simple and clear communication is most helpful in this situation. The nurse needs to be more directive if the person is having a difficult time making decisions and functioning (e.g., "It's time for lunch. I'll go with you" rather than "Would you like to go to lunch?"). As patients' conditions improve, they cognitively process more complex information, concentrate better, and make decisions more easily.

Communication with patients who are experiencing mania is often challenging as well. Their hyperactivity, their expansive or irritable mood, and their inability to filter stimuli are barriers to effective communication. Nurses need to be simple, clear, direct, and firm. Patients need to know that the nurse cares about them and that he or she is concerned about their behavior. It is not appropriate to have patients examine their feelings in depth when they are experiencing acute episodes of mania. Interactions need to be brief and direct to minimize unnecessary stimuli. It is also important to not threaten or challenge a patient during a manic episode; in some situations, the patient will escalate and respond with anger or rage.

Information from the patient who is experiencing a mood disorder is sometimes minimal or inaccurate because of the patient's cognitive impairment, altered mood, or behavioral disturbances. A family member or significant other is an important source of information when the patient is not reliable. Interviews need to be short and more direct if the patient is having behavioral or cognitive difficulty.

The assessment of patients with depression or mania includes information about their presenting problem and mental status, their past psychiatric history, their social and developmental history, their family history, and their physical health history. Assessment instruments assist with the specificity of data collection. Several instruments are used to assess depression, including the Beck Depression Inventory-II and the Carroll Rating Scale for Depression.

One scale that is used to assess mania is the patient's self-report with the use of the Altman Self-Rating Mania Scale. Nurses can ask patients to assess their own levels of depression or mania by having the patients rate these items on a 10-point scale (e.g., "If 0 represents feeling fine and 10 represents the worst depression that you have ever experienced, how would you rate your current depression?"). This allows for daily comparisons of mood with the use of specific empiric data.

Physiologic Disturbances

Body physiology changes during episodes of depression and mania. During moderate or severe depression, body processes frequently slow down. The patient with depression reports and exhibits neurovegetative signs of depression, which include psychomotor retardation, fatigue, constipation, anorexia (loss of appetite), weight loss, decreased libido (sex drive), and sleep disturbances. These symptoms relate to changes in body processes that cause disruption and the slowing of normal physiology. Some patients also describe vague physical symptoms such as headache, backache, gastrointestinal pain, and nausea. Sleep disturbance is a common problem. Patients describe initial insomnia (i.e., the inability to fall asleep after going to bed), middle insomnia (i.e., waking up in the middle of the night and being unable to return to sleep easily), and terminal or late insomnia (i.e., waking up in the early hours of the morning and being unable to return to sleep). Hypersomnia occurs when the patient sleeps excessively but never feels rested. Patients with depression have a decreased or increased appetite with corresponding changes in weight. Patients often describe food as being tasteless. Sometimes patients with depression exhibit hyperactivity rather than psychomotor retardation. In this type of *agitated depression*, patients are restless, moving, and pacing and may be irritable.

The patient who is experiencing mania also has difficulty sleeping. Not feeling the need for sleep, the patient sleeps only a few hours a night or not at all but may still feel rested. Hyperactive behavior and the inability to attend to tasks often prevent the patient from eating properly, which results in dehydration and inadequate nutrition. As the patient becomes increasingly stimulated, metabolic activity increases, and vital signs become elevated. Without proper intervention, patients with mania are at physical risk for dehydration, malnutrition, hypertension, fever, and even cardiac arrest, which may lead to death.

NURSING DIAGNOSIS

The nurse uses objective and subjective data obtained during the assessment of patients with mood disorders and adjustment disorders to arrive at relevant nursing diagnoses. Data from all sources—including the patient, significant others, and other professionals—are organized into a pattern of relationships that reflects the patient's major areas of health care needs (see the previous Case Study Mood the Nursing Assessment Questions box). Box 12-4 lists nursing diagnoses that

---

CASE STUDY #1

Maureen, who is 30 years old, arrives at the primary care clinic for her annual physical. She complains of frequent headaches and muscle aches, extreme fatigue, difficulty falling asleep and never feeling well rested, and a loss of 20 pounds during the past month without dieting. She has stopped attending the reading group and dance classes that she used to enjoy, stating she has no energy for them. Her mother suffers from bouts of depression and thinks that this may be Maureen's problem, but Maureen says she does not feel particularly depressed. Her affect is blunted, and she admits to feeling sad at times with no reason.

You are assessing Maureen before the nurse practitioner enters the examination room.

Critical Thinking

1 What are important questions for the nurse to ask Maureen at this time?
2 What laboratory tests will be appropriate?
3 What risk factor suggests that Maureen may be prone to depression?
4 What specific signs and symptoms suggest that Maureen may be depressed?
5 Why is it important for Maureen to get help immediately for her depression?

---

are relevant to patients who are experiencing mood or adjustment disorders. Nurses will prioritize diagnoses in accordance with patient needs and problems.

OUTCOME IDENTIFICATION

Outcome criteria for patients with mood disorders include short- and long-term patient behaviors and responses that indicate improved functioning. Patient safety and health are of utmost importance. These criteria are based on nursing diagnoses, and they are achieved through the implementation of planned nursing care. Outcomes are established for phases of treatment, including the acute phase of the illness, the continuation of treatment to prevent relapse, and long-term maintenance. Outcome criteria provide the nurse with direction for evaluating patient responses to treatment and the ongoing maintenance of health. Outcomes for patients with adjustment disorder will be related to the nature of the stressor and to strategies for managing it as well as to current symptomatology (e.g., sleeping problems) that require focused interventions.

Outcome Criteria

The patient will do the following:
- Remain safe and free from harm.
- Verbalize suicidal ideations and commit to a contract to not harm himself or herself or others.
- Verbalize the absence of suicidal or homicidal intent or plans.
- Express the desire to live and to not harm others.

BOX 12-4	NANDA NURSING DIAGNOSES FOR DEPRESSION AND MANIA

Depression
Risk for suicide
Ineffective health maintenance
Hopelessness
Powerlessness
Self-care deficit: bathing/hygiene; dressing/grooming; feeding
Impaired social interaction
Ineffective coping
Ineffective activity planning
Adult failure to thrive
Anxiety
Constipation
Death anxiety
Deficient diversional activity
Disturbed energy field
Impaired environmental interpretation syndrome
Fatigue
Risk for complicated grieving
Insomnia
Deficient knowledge
Risk for loneliness
Noncompliance
Imbalanced nutrition: less than body requirements
Imbalanced nutrition: more than body requirements
Risk for impaired parenting

Disturbed sleep pattern
Self-neglect

Mania
Risk for self-directed violence
Risk for other-directed violence
Disturbed thought processes
Ineffective health maintenance
Impaired social interaction
Noncompliance
Risk-prone health behavior
Caregiver role strain
Impaired verbal communication
Compromised family coping
Defensive coping
Ineffective coping
Ineffective denial
Disturbed energy field
Impaired environmental interpretation syndrome
Interrupted family processes
Risk for deficient fluid volume
Disturbed sleep pattern
Deficient knowledge
Risk for loneliness

From North American Nursing Diagnosis Association International: *NANDA nursing diagnoses: definitions and classification 2007-2008*, Philadelphia, 2007, North American Nursing Diagnosis Association International.

CASE STUDY #2

Robert, who is 32 years old, has been brought to the emergency department by his mother, who visited Robert after not hearing from him for several weeks. Robert is in the midst of a contentious divorce, and he complains of not being able to fall asleep and then not feeling like getting out of bed the next day. He alternates between irritability and feelings of guilt, and he cries easily about not being a "good enough" father to his two children, who are currently in his wife's custody. He reports being hypersensitive to the reactions of others. He states that his children would be better off if he were dead because then they would at least have his life insurance money. He has gained 25 pounds in 2 months, and he attributes this to no longer attending daily workouts at the gym.

Critical Thinking
1 What information suggests that Robert may be experiencing atypical depression?
2 What additional information would be helpful for the nurse to know about Robert to develop nursing diagnoses and goals?
3 What are the care priorities for Robert at this point?
4 Which nursing diagnoses would be relevant for this patient?
5 What long- and short-term outcomes, on the basis of the nursing diagnoses, might be established with Robert?

- Make plans for himself or herself for the future and verbalize feelings of hopefulness.
- Engage in self-care activities in accordance with ability, health status, and developmental stage.
- Develop a plan to manage inadequate sleep.
- Develop a plan to achieve and maintain adequate nutrition.
- Establish a pattern of rest and activity that enables the fulfillment of role and self-care demands.
- Make decisions on the basis of the examination of options and problem solving.
- Report the absence of hallucinations and delusions.
- Initiate satisfying social interactions with and assistance from significant others or peers.
- Demonstrate participation in milieu, group, and community activities.
- Report increased communication and problem solving among family members regarding issues related to the disorder.
- Describe alternative coping strategies for responses to stressors in addition to his or her perceived strengths and limitations.
- Report increased feelings of self-worth and confidence.
- Engage in activities and behaviors that promote confidence, belonging, and acceptance.
- Describe information about the disorder, including the course of illness, personal symptom patterns, and available ongoing resources.

NURSING ASSESSMENT QUESTIONS

Mood Disorders

1   How do you describe your mood? *To assess the patient's insight into his or her own feeling state*

2   Have you noticed a change in your behavior within the past month? *To determine the patient's awareness of behavioral changes*

3   Have people told you they notice changes in your behavior, such as irritability or hyperactivity? *To determine the patient's sensitivity to others' observations of his or her behavioral changes*

4   What activities have you found enjoyable during the past month? Did you enjoy them as much as you previously did? Can you imagine an event or situation that would give you pleasure? Have you been able to enjoy food or sex during the past month? *To determine the patient's current quality of life*

5   When did you first begin to feel depressed or elated? Did others comment that your mood seemed more depressed (or higher) than usual? Have you ever felt this way before? When? What was it like? *To establish the patient's behavioral patterns*

6   How has your sleep been? Are you able to fall asleep at night? To stay asleep? Do you find yourself waking up early and being unable to return to sleep? Are you sleeping more than usual in a 24-hour period? How much? Are you sleeping less than usual? How much? *To determine the patient's sleep patterns*

7   How has your appetite been during the past month? How much weight have you lost or gained during the past month? *To determine the patient's nutritional and metabolic status*

8   How has your energy level been? Do you feel tired every day? Do you ever feel as though your limbs are heavy? Do you have more energy than usual? *To assess the patient's fatigability*

9   How has your concentration been? Are you able to attend to things such as reading the newspaper? Can you

concentrate on projects or activities long enough to finish them? What has your decision making been like? Have you had racing thoughts? *To evaluate the patient's cognitive abilities*

10 How have you felt about yourself lately? Have you felt guilty more than usual about things that you have done? *To determine the patient's level of self-worth and self-esteem*

11 Have you felt particularly slowed down? Have others told you that you seem to move or speak more slowly than usual? *To determine presence of sensorimotor retardation in the patient*

12 Have you felt particularly "speeded up" to the point at which you noticed it or someone told you this? *To evaluate for the presence of mania or hypomania in the patient*

13 Have you had thoughts of death or suicide? How often? What specifically have you thought about doing to harm yourself? What prevented you from committing suicide? Have you had thoughts of harming or killing someone else? How often? What specifically have you thought about doing to harm someone else? *To determine the presence of suicidal or homicidal intent or plans in the patient*

14 What have you been doing lately to manage your feelings? Has it helped? *To assess the patient for effective coping mechanisms or strategies*

15 How has your mood affected your job? Your family? Your social life? Your interpersonal relationships? *To assess the pervasiveness of the patient's present mood state*

16 Have you received treatment from a mental health professional in the past? What kind of treatment? Did it help? *To determine the presence and effectiveness of any past treatment of the patient*

- Identify medications, including their actions, dosages, side effects, therapeutic effects, and self-care issues.
- In conjunction with a mental health provider, practice self-management of the illness, including monitoring and identifying prodromal (early) symptoms of recurrence and initiating strategies to deal with recurrent symptoms.
- Follow prescribed professional and self-care treatment strategies.

PLANNING

Nurses provide care to patients with mood disorders in every setting (e.g., the community, medical-surgical units, psychiatric inpatient units, pediatric clinics). Nursing care addresses not only the acute episodes of the disorder but the patient's ongoing risk for recurrent episodes. Interventions during the

acute depressive or manic episodes are effective, but too often the patient is left with little understanding of the clinical course of the illness and of the importance of long-term management and self-care strategies. Nurses need to plan interventions for each patient on the basis of that patient's particular behaviors, needs, and concerns. When planning patient care, the nurse purposefully involves and includes the patient, the patient's significant others, and additional health care providers. With the use of prioritized nursing diagnoses derived from assessment data, interventions are selected and planned to facilitate the achievement of desired patient outcomes.

IMPLEMENTATION

The plan of action for patients with mood disorders varies depending on whether the patient's mood is depressed or manic. In the short term, nursing and collaborative interventions are available that are effective for reducing the acuity of the episode and for promoting more optimal functioning. With short-term hospitalizations, nurses in the hospital setting may not have the opportunity to observe the patient's recovery from the acute episode. Nurses document and communicate projected treatment responses to other nurses, mental health professionals, and significant others who will care for the patient in the community. Nurses who work with patients in the community are able to see treatment responses and outcome achievement over time. Initial treatment responses help to dictate continued care and to assist with the prevention of recurrences over time. Interventions for patients with adjustment disorders will consider the nature of the stressor as well as the patient's immediate symptoms that need to be addressed.

Although mood disorders are primarily disturbances in mood regulation, they affect the whole person: physically, cognitively, socially, and spiritually. Short-term interventions in the hospital or community address priority issues such as preventing self-harm; promoting physical health (e.g., adequate nutrition, bathing, grooming, sleep); monitoring the effects of medications; and assisting with altered thought flow and impaired communication. Other concerns to address include promoting social interaction; improving self-esteem; understanding the mood disorder and its treatment; the need to follow the treatment plan; and the plan for discharge and the continuation of services. One goal is to help patients to improve their quality of life. Because episodes of depression and mania affect the entire family, involving the patient's significant others provides an opportunity for them to understand the disorder and to support patients during their recovery.

Nursing interventions for patients with mood disorders cover a wide range of biopsychosocial areas, with consideration of the effects of depression and mania on the physiologic, cognitive, psychologic, behavioral, and social domains. Intervention for patients who are experiencing depression and mania requires that nurses maintain self-awareness and boundaries regarding their own reactions to patients, because patient depression, irritability, anger, negativity, euphoria, and hyperactivity can readily influence nursing responses. It is potentially difficult and exhausting to interact with patients who provoke personal feelings and reactions during highly emotional encounters. Nurses initiate and maintain a therapeutic connection with patients by being consistent, caring, concerned, empathetic, and genuine. Patients with mood disorders often have a difficult time developing a therapeutic alliance, and they can avoid making an interpersonal connection with others. A knowledgeable, nondemanding, and matter-of-fact approach is reassuring to patients and promotes their confidence in the nurse.

Nursing Interventions

1. Conduct a suicide assessment as necessary *to ensure the patient's safety and to prevent harm to the patient or others*. Patients with mania (not just those with depression) also need to be assessed for suicidal thinking. As patients cycle out of mania into depression, suicidal risk increases.

2. Maintain a safe, harm-free environment through close and frequent observations *to minimize the patient's risk of self-harm or violence*. This intervention requires that the nurse conduct an assessment of the patient's environment to determine if there are items or physical space issues that could facilitate self-harm. Patients with depression or mania may require close observation to ensure safety.

3. Establish rapport and demonstrate respect for the patient *to facilitate the patient's willingness to communicate his or her thoughts and feelings*. Creating a connection with patients helps them to communicate with the nurse.

4. Assist the patient with verbalizing feelings *to promote a healthy and expressive form of communication*. During an acute episode (particularly mania), the nurse's goal is to focus on acute symptoms such as cognitive impairment, diminished self-care, and hyperactivity. It is more appropriate to encourage a substantial discussion of feelings when the patient is able to focus, concentrate, and reflect.

5. Identify the patient's social support system, and encourage the patient to use it *to minimize isolation and loneliness and to provide assistance with monitoring the illness and its treatment*. Support from loved ones conveys caring and concern and helps to promote functioning.

6. Praise the patient for attempts at alternate activities and interactions with others *to encourage socialization and to promote self-esteem*. Positive feedback reinforces behavior that helps the patient to make more adaptive changes.

7. Gently refuse to be part of secrecy agreements with the patient; instead, encourage the patient to share important and relevant information with staff *to promote the patient's participation in care and his or her responsibility for his or her own actions*. Sometimes patients may confide thought of self-harm or other intentions or experiences that should be known by others for the prevention of harm and the provision of therapeutic care.

8. Monitor and implement strategies to ensure adequate fluid intake and output, food intake, and weight *to ensure adequate nutrition and hydration and adequate weight for body size and metabolic needs*. Patients with depression or mania may not eat or drink, thereby putting their physical health at risk.

9. Promote self-care activities (e.g., bathing, dressing, feeding, grooming) *to establish the patient's level of functioning and to increase his or her self-esteem*. During acute depression, patients may not have the energy or motivation to care for themselves. Patients who are manic may be so hyperactive that they may not be able to slow down long enough to manage these activities.

10. Assist the patient with establishing daily goals and expectations *to promote structure and direction and to minimize cognitive difficulties*. For patients who are experiencing cognitive difficulties such as disorientation, memory

impairment, or flight of ideas, clear direction and structure enable them to function better with more cognitive clarity.

11. Plan self-care activities around those times when the patient has more energy or less manic behavior *to enable the patients to focus on the task.* To conduct self-care activities, patients need to attend to the task and to complete a series of sequential actions to achieve a goal.

12. Reduce choices of clothing, activities, and tasks and then increase choices as the patient improves cognitively *to make decision making easier and to minimize stress.* Choice requires planning, focus, and judgment, all of which might be impaired in a patient with depression or mania.

13. Assess the patient's cognitive and perceptual processes *to ascertain the existence of hallucinations or delusions that are troubling or harmful to the patient.* Patients with depression or mania can become psychotic with delusional thinking or hallucinations. These experiences can be potentially harmful when patients respond to these altered thinking and perceptual experiences.

14. Assist the patient with the identification of negative, self-defeating thoughts and with modifying them into more realistic thoughts *to promote more accurate and positive thoughts about the self and others.* Patients with depression focus on the negative, whereas patients with mania are often grandiose. Both types of thinking require modification to promote healthy functioning and coping.

15. Encourage the patient to attend therapeutic groups and activities that provide feedback about thinking *to reframe thinking with the support of others.* Depressed patients may not be motivated or energized to attend activities, and they may require encouragement to do so. Groups and activities can be helpful for patients with mania when they are able to focus and remain still, thereby not disrupting the group. Group support and input from other patients can help to clarify or raise issues that involve thinking and perspective.

16. Provide simple, clear directives and communication in a low-stimulus environment *to assist with the patient's focus, attention, and concentration with minimal distractions.* Clear communication is helpful for patients with cognitive difficulties.

17. Teach the patient and his or her significant others about the patient's disorder and its treatment when the patient is able to learn *to increase knowledge, to promote adherence to treatment, and to minimize guilt regarding the disorder.* Mood disorders are recurrent illnesses that require ongoing monitoring, intervention, and self-care. Patients who understand the biologic nature of their illnesses may be more motivated to adhere to treatment.

18. Gradually increase levels of activity and exercise for patients with depression *to minimize fatigue and to increase activity tolerance.* As patients with depression improve, exercise and activity promote biologic changes that can help to minimize depression and generate energy.

19. Identify sources of external stress and assist the patient with coping with them in a more effective manner *to minimize stressors and to promote adaptive coping mechanisms.* As patients with depression and mania improve, identifying coping strategies that help them to deal with external stressors can prevent or minimize future episodes.

20. Establish limits with patients with mania in a firm, consistent, and caring way *to provide acceptable boundaries for behavior.* During mania, patients have difficulty setting boundaries or creating structure. Failure to respect boundaries can have damaging consequences.

21. Teach the patient and significant others how to self-manage the illness at home, including identifying prodromal (early) symptoms, seeking help, and implementing appropriate strategies *to prevent or minimize recurrent episodes.* Self-management helps to prevent or minimize future episodes, and it empowers the patient.

22. Direct the patient's energy into constructive activities when he or she is manic *to allow for the release of energy in a focused and acceptable way.* Helping patients to channel their activity can help to promote functioning in a positive way.

23. Establish a low-stimulus environment for patients with mania *to reduce sensory input.* An environment with many stimuli (e.g., noise, music, many people) can promote the escalation of the manic symptoms.

Additional Treatment Modalities
Psychopharmacology

Although there is no "cure" for mood disorders, since the 1950s, there have been major advances in the use of medications to treat the associated symptoms. Investigation of the neurobiology of depression and mania has provided directions for the development of these new medications. In addition to a focus on the effects of antidepressants on neurotransmitters, research suggests that these medications produce changes in gene expression and neuroplasticity (Yamada et al, 2005). Because there are multiple types of medications that seem to work with various individuals and with different types of depression and mania, selecting the drug and the dosage that is effective for any individual is often a difficult process. Nurses need to explain to patients that some individuals do not respond to the first or even the second medication prescribed but that most people do find a medication that works well for them.

✎ MEDICATION KEY FACTS
Adjustment Disorders

Pharmacologic interventions for adjustment disorders focus on treating symptoms that may cause clinically significant functional impairment. Medications that are prescribed include antianxiety drugs, antidepressants, and, occasionally, antipsychotics.

There are various types of antidepressant medications used to treat persons with episodes of major depression and some persons with dysthymia. These include tricyclics, heterocyclics, monoamine oxidase inhibitors (MAOIs), selective serotonin reuptake inhibitors (SSRIs), and joint serotonin and norepinephrine reuptake inhibitors. These medications have powerful effects not only on mood but also on the entire syndrome of depression symptoms, including the neurovegetative symptoms. As with all medications, these can cause side effects that create discomfort and even danger. Taken in large quantities, many drugs, including the tricyclics and the MAOIs, are toxic or even lethal. In addition, these medications usually have a lag period of 1 to 6 weeks for the initiation of therapeutic effects, during which time the side effects are often the most pronounced. As the medication begins to exert its therapeutic effect, many of the side effects usually diminish. The nurse needs to be aware that a time for higher suicide risk occurs within several weeks after the patient has started an antidepressant. In the light of data regarding the recurrent nature of depression and how it impairs functioning over time, many patients are now taking these medications for years or for an entire lifetime. Debate continues about the safety, benefits, and problems associated with taking antidepressants during pregnancy.

There is some evidence that herbal substances may have an effect on depression. St. John's wort and omega-3 fatty acids have some effect on mild to moderate depressive symptoms (Clement et al, 2006). It is important that nurses know all of the medications that their patients are taking, including herbal, alternative, and complementary remedies, because these can influence the effects and safety of antidepressant medications.

Mood stabilizers are effective for the treatment of mania in patients with bipolar disorders. The most widely used mood stabilizer for bipolar disorder is lithium. Lithium acts as a salt within the body, and its blood levels are closely linked to the patient's hydration and sodium intake. Side effects of lithium include neuromuscular and central nervous system effects (tremor, forgetfulness, slowed cognition), gastrointestinal effects (nausea, diarrhea), weight gain, hypothyroidism, and renal effects (polyuria). Nurses monitor lithium blood levels to ensure an adequate but not toxic level. Usually blood levels of 0.6 mEq/L to 1 mEq/L are appropriate for maintenance therapy; for the treatment of acute mania, levels of up to 1.5 mEq/L are necessary. The therapeutic-range blood level for lithium is narrow; toxicity can occur quickly, and it is evidenced by tremors, vomiting, oversedation, ataxia, and, finally, seizures. Lithium blood levels of more than 1.5 mEq/L are toxic. Lithium is excreted through the kidneys, so nurses need to use caution with patients with renal disease and to warn patients to use diuretics only with extreme caution and under close supervision, because diuretics elevate lithium blood levels quickly. Changes in hydration through perspiration, vomiting, and restricted fluid intake promote elevated lithium levels and toxicity.

Anticonvulsants are now being prescribed for mood stabilization. These medications, which include carbamazepine, valproate, gabapentin, and lamotrigine, are used when the patient is unable or unwilling to take lithium or when other medications have been ineffective. In many settings, anticonvulsants are the drugs of choice for mood stabilization. Lamotrigine is especially promising, because research indicates that it is useful as a mood stabilizer, particularly with patients who are experiencing bipolar depression that has been difficult to treat.

Other medications that have been prescribed for patients during episodes of depression or mania include benzodiazepines on a time-limited basis for associated anxiety symptoms; sedative-hypnotics or trazodone for sleep regulation; and antipsychotics for relief from hallucinations, delusions, and extremely agitated behavior. Although antidepressants and mood stabilizers assist with minimizing and regulating symptoms related to anxiety and sleep, their therapeutic effects take longer to occur than the other medications mentioned here.

Although physicians or advanced practice nurses prescribe medications, the nursing care related to the administration of psychopharmacologic agents is extensive. The nurse needs to understand the mechanisms of action, dosages (therapeutic), side effects, and self-care considerations of each medication. This enables the nurse to explain the medications to patients and to observe for intended and unintended effects. By teaching patients more about their medications, the nurse promotes and encourages adherence to the treatment plan and helps with the minimization of negative effects. Patients are able to discuss their concerns and to make informed decisions about their treatments.

Many of these medications require special considerations that patients need to understand to ensure efficacy and safety. Because many patients discontinue their antidepressants and mood stabilizers too early or do not take them as prescribed, nurses need to emphasize the importance of staying on the medication to prevent relapse, recurrence, and the continuation of changes in the brain. Nurses teach patients specific self-care activities associated with their medications, such as the required dietary restrictions for MAOIs, precautions regarding hydration and salt intake for lithium, and the management of the anticholinergic effects of the tricyclics. With permission from patients, it is helpful for significant others to understand the medications. This allows them to help monitor therapeutic and side effects, and it may help the patient to better adhere to the medication regimen.

Other Types of Interventions

Electroconvulsive Therapy. Electroconvulsive therapy (ECT) involves the use of electrically induced seizures to treat severe depression or, less frequently, intense mania that is not controlled with lithium or antipsychotics. Although scientists introduced ECT during the 1930s, its use decreased after the discovery of antidepressants and lithium. Procedures have been developed for ECT that make it a safe and effective treatment for many individuals who have not achieved a treatment response with medication or other types of treatment.

MEDICATION KEY FACTS

Depressive Disorders

Cyclic Antidepressants
Selective Serotonin Reuptake Inhibitors (SSRIs)
Citalopram (Celexa), fluoxetine (Prozac), paroxetine (Paxil), sertraline (Zoloft), venlafaxine (Effexor), fluvoxamine (Luvox), and escitalopram (Lexapro)
- First-line antidepressant therapy
- May cause fatal reactions with MAOIs by causing serotonin syndrome, hypertensive crisis, rigidity, and neuroleptic malignant syndrome
- A life-threatening condition called *serotonin syndrome* can occur when medicines that are used to treat migraine headaches (5-hydroxytryptamine receptor agonists [triptans]) and medicines that are used to treat depression (SSRIs and serotonin–norepinephrine reuptake inhibitors (SNRIs), which are medicines from different classes) are used together.
- Episodes of self-harm and potential suicidal behavior are reportedly higher among patients who are younger than 18 years old.
- Use with caffeine increases agitation; use with alcohol increases sedation. Effectiveness is decreased with cigarette smoking.
- These drugs should not be taken with lithium.
- *Herbal considerations*: St. John's wort and SAM-e may cause serotonin syndrome. Use with coffee or tea results in precipitation. Use with ascorbic acid (e.g., grapefruit juice) may alter the elimination of the drug and its plasma concentration.

Atypical New-Generation Antidepressants
- May cause fatal reaction with MAOIs by causing neuroleptic malignant syndrome, serotonin syndrome, and autonomic instability
- Elderly patients are more sensitive to the drugs' anticholinergic, cardiovascular, and sedative effects.
- *Herbal considerations*: St. John's wort and SAM-e may increase the patient's risk for serotonin syndrome.

Specific Atypical New Generation Antidepressants
Selective Serotonin–Norepinephrine Reuptake Inhibitors
Venlafaxine (Effexor) and duloxetine (Cymbalta)
- Indicated for social anxiety disorder and general anxiety disorder
- Venlafaxine is not approved for indications in children and adolescents because of the lack of efficacy and concerns about increased hostility and suicidal ideation.

Norepinephrine Dopamine Reuptake Inhibitors
Bupropion (Wellbutrin)
- Second-line agent in cases of depression that is resistant to SSRI or SNRIs
- Wellbutrin-SR and Zyban indicated for smoking cessation
- Lowers seizure threshold; should not be used for patients with seizure disorders or eating disorders because of increased seizure incidence in this group
- *Herbal considerations*: Ephedra may cause hypertensive crisis

Serotonin-2 Antagonist/Reuptake Inhibitors
Trazodone (Desyrel) and nefazodone (Serzone)
- May increase risk for hypertensive crisis when taken with MAOIs
- Trazodone may be used to treat insomnia; it may be associated with priapism, and it may contribute to dysrhythmia in patients with preexisting cardiac disease.

Noradrenergic/Specific Serotonergic Antidepressant
Mirtazapine (Remeron)
- Poses a higher risk of seizures than tricyclic antidepressants (mirtazapine)
- Use with MAOIs may increase the risk of hyperpyretic crisis, hypertensive episodes, and severe seizures
- Episodes of self-harm and potential suicidal behaviors reported among patients who are younger than 18 years old and taking this drug

Nonselective Cyclic Agents
Tricyclic Antidepressants (TCAs)
Amitriptyline (Elavil), clomipramine (Anafranil), imipramine (Tofranil), desipramine (Norpramin), doxepin (Sinequan), nortriptyline (Aventyl), protriptyline (Vivactil), amoxapine (Asendin), and trimipramine (Surmontil)
- Overdose, as with suicidality, can cause life-threatening toxicity; prescribed amounts at any one time should be limited.
- Use with MAOIs may increase the risk of neuroleptic malignant syndrome, seizures, hypertensive crisis, and hyperpyrexia.
- Use with oral anticoagulants can result in bleeding. Use with clonidine can cause severe hypertension.
- *Herbal considerations*: St. John's wort and SAM-e may increase the patient's risk for serotonin syndrome.

Monoamine Oxidase Inhibitor Agents
Phenelzine (Nardil), tranylcypromine (Parnate), isocarboxazid (Marplan), moclobemide (Manerix), and selegiline transdermal patch (Emsam)
- Prescribed as third-line agents after SSRIs and tricyclic antidepressants have been tried
- Signs of toxicity include increased headaches and palpitations.
- MAOIs should not be used within 14 days of taking SSRIs.
- Avoid anticholinergics, anesthetics, amphetamines, appetite suppressants, nasal decongestants, antihypertensives, central nervous system depressants (including alcohol), sympathomimetics, and cyclic and newer antidepressants, because these may increase hyperpyretic crises, seizures, hypertensive episodes, or serotonin syndrome. Some over-the-counter cough and cold medications contain sympathomimetics; it is prudent to consult the pharmacist when purchasing over-the-counter medicines when taking MAOIs.
- Oral selegiline (Eldepryl) has been helpful with refractory depression.

MEDICATION KEY FACTS—cont'd

- *Herbal considerations*: Parsley and St. John's wort pose some risk for serotonin syndrome.
- *Dietary considerations*: Avoid caffeine, chocolate, and all tyramine-containing foods (e.g., aged cheese) within several hours of ingestion of MAOIs, because the combination may cause sudden and severe hypertension or hypertensive crisis.

New Agent: Selegiline Transdermal System (Emsam)
- A patch version of a monoamine oxidase inhibitor for adults with major depression

- *Dietary considerations*: No tyramine dietary modifications are needed at a dosage of 6 mg per 24 hours, because monoamine oxidase activity in the digestive system is not affected at this level. Higher doses increase the patient's risk for hypertensive crisis, and tyramine-containing foods and beverages should be restricted.

Note: Definitions and descriptions of the adverse reactions to medications appear in Chapter 25.

MEDICATION KEY FACTS

Bipolar Disorders

Mood Stabilizers
- Pharmacologic treatment for acute mania in bipolar disorder includes lithium, carbamazepine, divalproex, and lamotrigine.
- Second-generation (atypical) antipsychotics are approved for the treatment of acute bipolar mania, and olanzapine is indicated for the treatment of acute bipolar depression (see Chapters 13 and 25).
- Antidepressants are typically used only in combination with other medications because of their risk for switching the patient into mania or accelerating the rate of mood cycling.
- Antidepressants (citalopram, fluoxetine, paroxetine, bupropion, venlafaxine) are also indicated for the treatment of acute bipolar depression. Clonazepam (a benzodiazepine) is used as treatment or adjunct therapy for acute mania (see Chapters 10 and 25).

Lithium Salts
Lithium carbonate (Lithotabs, Eskalith, Lithobid)
- These require therapeutic drug monitoring to prevent toxicity. The therapeutic serum level is 0.6 mEq/L to 1.2 mEq/L; the toxic serum level is greater than 1.5 mEq/L.
- A lithium serum concentration of 1.5 mEq/L to 2.0 mEq/L may produce vomiting, diarrhea, drowsiness, confusion, lack of coordination, coarse hand tremor, muscle twitching, and T-wave depression on electrocardiogram.
- Acute toxicity may be characterized by seizures, oliguria, circulatory failure, coma, and death.
- Lithium may not work or its side effects may be intolerable in more than half of patients with bipolar disorder. Anticonvulsants may be needed.
- *Herbal considerations*: Dandelion, goldenrod, juniper, and parsley increase lithium's effects and toxicity.
- *Dietary considerations*: Monitor the patient's sodium intake, because significant changes will alter lithium excretion. Black and green tea, coffee, cola nut, guarana, plantains, and yerba maté may all decrease lithium levels.

Anticonvulsants
Divided into three classes (first, second, and third generation) and indicated for manic symptoms

First-Generation Anticonvulsants
Klonopin (Clonazepam)

Second-Generation Anticonvulsants
Carbamazepine (Tegretol), valproic acid (Depakene), and divalproex sodium (Depakote)
- Require a therapeutic serum level of 50 µg/mL to 100 µg/mL; a toxic serum level is greater than 100 µg/mL.
- Toxic reactions include blood dyscrasias.
- Do not use with MAOIs, because this may cause fatal reactions (i.e., seizures and hypertensive crisis).
- *Herbal considerations*: Gingko and quinine increase anticonvulsant action.
- *Dietary considerations*: Grapefruit and grapefruit juice may increase the absorption and blood concentration of carbamazepine.

Third-Generation Anticonvulsants
Gabapentin (Neurontin), topiramate (Topamax), lamotrigine (Lamictal), and oxcarbazepine (Trileptal)
- Gabapentin (Neurontin) has been found to be ineffective for the treatment of bipolar disorders.
- The abrupt withdrawal of these drugs may increase seizure frequency.
- Use caution with lamotrigine, especially in children, as a result of the possibility of a potentially life-threatening rash (Stevens-Johnson syndrome); a slow titration of the dosage is warranted. Patients should be instructed to go to the emergency department immediately if such a rash develops.
- *Herbal considerations*: Ginkgo increases these drugs' anticonvulsant effects, and ginseng and santonica decrease their effects.

❖ CLINICAL ALERT #3

Serotonin syndrome is an idiosyncratic medication reaction with a fairly rapid onset that occurs with the excessive accumulation of serotonin (5HT1A). In depressed patients, serotonin syndrome results from high doses or the concurrent use of such medications as serotonin reuptake inhibitors (including tricyclic antidepressants), serotonin precursors (e.g., l-tryptophan), serotonin agonists (e.g., buspirone), MAOIs, or other medications that influence serotonin levels (e.g., cold or allergy preparations, cocaine, lithium, ginseng, St. John's wort). Risk factors include genetic predisposition (MAO activity), acquired disorders (liver, pulmonary, or cardiovascular disease), and iatrogenic situations (medications). At least three of the following symptoms contribute to the diagnosis: mental status changes, agitation, myoclonus, hyperreflexia, fever, diaphoresis, ataxia, and diarrhea. Symptoms also include abdominal pain, elevated blood pressure, tachycardia, irritability, hostility, increased motor activity, and mood change. Severe reactions manifest as high fever, cardiovascular shock, and death. Early identification is important. The nurse will obtain a full history of all medications that the patient is taking (including those available over the counter); instruct the patient and family to report immediately any subtle changes that involve confusion, unusual behavior, or agitation; and monitor the patient's vital signs carefully. If a nurse suspects serotonin syndrome, he or she will discontinue the patient's medications and notify the physician.

❖ CLINICAL ALERT #4

Patients need to avoid foods that contain tyramine while taking MAOI antidepressants to prevent hypertensive crisis. These foods include avocados; yogurt; aged cheese; smoked or pickled fish, meat, or poultry; processed meats; yeast; overripe fruit; chicken or beef liver pate; red wine; beer; liqueurs; and fava beans. Foods to use in moderation include caffeine beverages, cottage and cream cheese, soy sauce, chocolate, and sour cream. Medications to avoid include over-the-counter cough and cold medicines, appetite suppressants, muscle relaxants, allergy remedies, hay fever remedies, narcotics, analgesics, and several prescription medications. The nurse needs to ask the patient to contact the physician or nurse before taking any over-the-counter medications. Tell the patient to avoid common cold remedies and diet medications.

PATIENT AND FAMILY TEACHING GUIDELINES
Serotonin Selective Reuptake Inhibitors

Teach the Patient the Following:
- The purpose of SSRIs is to treat depression. These medications alter brain nerve cells, thus increasing the availability of serotonin. A deficiency of serotonin in the brain is possibly related to the onset of depression.
- It is important to take the medication as prescribed; changing the dosage or missing a dose will prevent it from helping the depression. Do not stop the medication suddenly; work with a health care provider to taper the dosage.
- Common side effects of SSRIs include nausea, increased anxiety, and insomnia. These side effects often diminish when the medication begins to exert its therapeutic effect.
- Do not take these medications with grapefruit juice to avoid changing the amount of medication in the bloodstream.
- The medication usually does not immediately improve symptoms of depression. It usually takes 1 to 6 weeks before you will feel the effects of the medication. At first, you will still feel depressed, but you will have more energy and look less depressed. These medications often work from the outside inward.
- The medication needs to be taken as prescribed, even after you feel better. It needs time to have positive effects on the brain that will minimize the chances for future episodes of depression.

Researchers do not know how ECT alleviates depression and mania, but they believe that it is related to the alteration of neurotransmission. A more complete discussion of ECT is presented in Chapter 26.

Transcranial Magnetic Stimulation. Transcranial magnetic stimulation is a noninvasive procedure in which an electromagnet is placed on the scalp. Electrical current is generated by rapid pulsing in the magnetic field, which causes the cortical neurons to depolarize. Although the specific mechanisms involved in its antidepressant effect remain unclear, this intervention increases monoamine concentrations in the brain when it is used repetitively. Research has been encouraging with respect to its effects with unipolar depression (Fitzgerald et al, 2009).

Vagal Nerve Stimulation. Vagal nerve stimulation is induced with a *vagal nerve stimulator device* that is implanted in the left chest wall under the collarbone to electrically stimulate the vagus nerve. This treatment has been helpful, particularly for patients with treatment-resistant depression (George, 2010).

Deep Brain Stimulation. With this treatment, an electrode is inserted deep into the brain, and an electrical current stimulates the brain. The application of this treatment to patients with mood disorders is recent; current research examines its use for patients with treatment-resistant depression (George et al, 2006).

Phototherapy. Phototherapy is one type of treatment that has effectively lessened symptoms of SAD. Researchers believe

PATIENT AND FAMILY TEACHING GUIDELINES
Lithium

Teach the Patient the Following:

- Lithium is a mood stabilizer for individuals with mania and depression.
- Lithium alters brain neurotransmission. It is not clear how lithium specifically stabilizes mood.
- Before starting lithium, health care providers will perform laboratory tests to ensure the adequate functioning of the heart, the kidneys, the thyroid gland, and the electrolytes.
- It is important to take lithium daily as prescribed to maintain a steady blood level of the medication. Do not skip doses or take extra doses to make up for missed doses.
- Lithium sometimes takes a week or more to begin working and to develop a steady blood level. Your health care provider will have you get your blood drawn to check your lithium blood levels. Blood for the lithium level must be drawn about 12 hours after the last dose of lithium (e.g., if you take your dose at 8 PM, your blood level must be drawn at 8 AM).
- Common side effects of lithium include increased urine output, increased thirst, fine tremors, muscle weakness, nausea, weight gain, and diarrhea.
- Lithium levels can increase rapidly, which leads to toxicity. Signs of toxicity include nausea and vomiting, marked tremors, muscle weakness, muscle twitching, lack of coordination, sluggishness, drowsiness, confusion, seizures, and coma. Toxicity can occur as blood levels rise above 1.5 mEq/L.
- It is important to maintain a stable blood level of lithium. Do not change the amount of sodium (salt) in your diet, because decreasing salt will increase the amount of lithium in the blood.
- Avoid caffeine, because it interferes with lithium's effectiveness. Drink at least 2 quarts of water each day.
- Any activity or situation that affects your fluid and salt intake or output will change the level of lithium in your blood. Episodes of fever, hot weather, exercise, sunbathing, and vomiting are examples of situations in which you lose salt and fluid, thereby increasing your lithium level. It is important to contact your health care provider if you believe that your lithium level changed or if you experience any side effects or early toxic signs.
- Other drugs can affect your lithium level. Certain medications (e.g., diuretics, ibuprofen, verapamil) can raise lithium levels. Be sure to check with your health care provider before taking any new prescribed or over-the-counter medications.
- Lithium causes birth defects if it is taken during the first trimester of pregnancy. Tell your health care provider if you intend to become pregnant or are pregnant.

that exposure to morning light causes a circadian rhythm shift (i.e., a phase advance) that regulates the normal relationships between sleep and circadian rhythms and that ultimately affects mood regulation (Golden et al, 2005).

Patients are referred for phototherapy after a careful and complete psychiatric history that documents the occurrence of SAD. Phototherapy that consists of a minimum of 2500 lux is usually administered when the patient wakes in the morning. Patients sit or lie in front of the light box for 30 minutes to several hours, depending on the strength of the light source. An antidepressant effect usually occurs within 2 to 4 days and is complete after 2 weeks. Maintenance therapy consists of sitting in front of the lights for about 30 minutes each day. Side effects are rare, although some patients do report irritability, headaches, or insomnia. Phototherapy is not effective for everyone with a diagnosis of SAD; some fail to respond, and others experience only a partial response. Because phototherapy requires a large amount of time each day, alternative methods to acquire the additional light are being used, including the use of light visors and lights that shine onto the bed during the early morning before awakening.

Family Intervention

Mood disorders affect the entire family, not just the patient who is experiencing the depression or mania. Most often the family or significant others become known to the nurse during the patient's acute episode of depression or mania.

Conflicts and communication problems that existed in the family network before the onset of the episode intensify, and usual role functioning is disrupted. There are often negative effects of a depressed parent on children and adolescents (Marshall and Harper-Jaques, 2008).

Nurses in both the hospital and the community interact with the patient's family, who often appreciate the opportunity to vent feelings of confusion, anger, concern, or frustration. Teaching family members about the patient's disorder, especially the biologic nature of the disorder, allows them to rethink the situation and to minimize blaming the patient. Many are relieved to hear that their loved one's behavior can be explained and is manageable. They also find it helpful to know that the patient's behavior is not intended as a personal offense to other family members but rather is part of the symptomatology of depression or mania. Nurses run family education groups in the hospital and in the community and invite family and patients to learn more about these disorders and their impact.

Nurses also work together with other mental health professionals, including advanced practice nurses, to assess the need for family therapy. Nurses observe patient–family interactions, listen to concerns, and identify potential problem areas. Nurses also make referrals for marital therapy or family therapy.

Interventions that include preparing the family for a patient's discharge from the hospital facilitate the patient's return to functioning in the community. Even after symptoms stop, the patient who has experienced affective episodes may continue to have difficulty with his or her interpersonal and occupational functioning.

Group Intervention

Group intervention provides multiple benefits to patients with mood disorders, including socialization, education about their disorders, the discussion of more useful coping mechanisms, the opportunity to vent feelings, the establishment of personal goals, and the realization that others have similar problems. These benefits help to reduce isolation and hopelessness. Nurses assess patients' ability to participate in groups on the basis of their behavior, mental status, psychologic readiness in view of the nature of the particular group, and physiologic status. For example, patients with mania who are hyperactive and extremely agitated are not able to focus on the group discussion, and they become overstimulated and disruptive in the group. Some patients with severe depression with psychomotor retardation and cognitive impairment have a difficult time and become overwhelmed by a formal group. Certain types of groups (e.g., a unit community meeting, an activity group) are less structured and less imposing to patients than formal group therapy.

In addition to assessing patients' readiness for groups, nurses encourage their attendance at appropriate functions. Some patients need to be directed with statements such as, "It's time for group now. I'll walk there with you." Others require only encouragement or reminders.

Nurses who are qualified conduct groups along with other nurses or therapists. Nurses initiate and lead groups such as social skills training and educational groups. Patients often need to discuss their experiences and reactions after the completion of a group. Nurses listen, allow patients to ventilate feelings, and reinforce the new insights or perceptions that patients experience.

Psychotherapeutic Intervention

Although the effectiveness of antidepressant and mood-stabilizing medications is undisputed, psychotherapeutic interventions are also important for the treatment of mood disorders. Psychopharmacologic agents pose a number of problems for many patients. These medications often have major side effects that create discomfort, interfere with usual functioning, and promote noncompliance. Alternative treatment is necessary for the 20% to 30% of persons with mood disorders who do not respond to medications. In addition, although mood disorders represent alterations in neurobiologic functioning, numerous psychologic, social, and interpersonal issues that require psychotherapeutic intervention are associated with episodes of depression and mania.

Types of psychotherapy that are used to treat mood disorders and associated psychosocial issues include cognitive therapy, behavioral therapy, interpersonal relationship therapy, and psychodynamic therapy. Although each of these differs with respect to its underlying theoretic framework, goals, and approach, there are some commonalities.

Therapeutic success is related to several factors: the nature of the relationship between the therapist and the patient; the provision of understanding, support, help, and hope; the establishment of a framework for understanding and interpreting patients' problems; and the provision of an opportunity to explore and try out new coping strategies.

Cognitive Therapy. Cognitive therapy as outlined by Beck (1967) addresses systematic errors in the patient's thinking that maintain negative cognitive processing. The goal of the therapy is to identify underlying cognitive schemata and specific cognitive distortions. Nurses ask patients to identify their automatic thoughts, silent assumptions, and random inferences so that they are able to examine negative thoughts and assumptions logically. This helps the patient to compare these thoughts with realistic attributes and subsequently validate or refute them.

Cognitive therapy has been effective for the treatment of outpatients with mild to moderate unipolar depression. The use of cognitive therapy increases the rate of symptom improvement in patients with depression.

Behavioral Therapy. Behavioral therapy, which is often used as outpatient therapy in conjunction with cognitive therapy for mild to moderately depressed patients, is an effective treatment for depression and compares favorably with medication and cognitive therapy. There is less information about its usefulness for persons who are experiencing mania.

The behavioral approach is based on learning theory. Troublesome behaviors that occur in depression and mania represent behaviors that are acquired as a result of aversive (negative) environmental events. Positive environmental responses to the maladaptive behaviors or the avoidance of negative consequences reinforce these. The behavioral therapist works with patients to determine specific behaviors to identify and modify the factors that evoke and reinforce these behaviors. With the use of role modeling, role-playing, and situational analysis, nurses assist patients with learning and practicing different adaptive behaviors that bring positive environmental reinforcement. The therapy is not concerned with understanding underlying issues or pathopsychology; rather, it is concerned only with those behaviors that are changeable. Behavioral therapy has several advantages (e.g., shorter treatment duration than other types of therapy, focus on specific behaviors to modify), and it is applicable to various types of patients.

Interpersonal Therapy. The therapist who uses interpersonal therapy views depression as developing as a result of pathologic early interpersonal relationship patterns that continue to be repeated in adulthood. The emphasis is on social functioning and interpersonal relationships, with particular emphasis on the milieu or the environment. Life events including change, loss, and relationship conflict trigger earlier relationship patterns, and the patient experiences a sense of failure, decreased importance, and loss. The goal of the therapy is to understand the social context of current problems on the basis of earlier relationships and to provide symptomatic relief by solving or managing current interpersonal problems. The patient and the therapist select one or two current interpersonal problems and examine new communication and interpersonal strategies for managing relationships more effectively.

Interpersonal therapy is often effective for patients with mild to moderate depression, although there is no indication that it is more effective than other types of psychotherapy.

Psychodynamic Therapy. Psychodynamic therapy is based on Freud's psychoanalytic model. In this model, depression is a result of the early childhood loss of a love object and ambivalence about that object; the projection of anger onto the ego, thereby resulting in the blockage of the libido (sex drive); and unresolved intrapsychic conflict during the oral or anal stage of psychosexual development. These damage self-esteem, and the person repeats the primary loss pattern throughout life. Through the relationship with the therapist, the patient uncovers repressed past experiences, experiences a catharsis or a release of feelings, confronts defenses, interprets current behavior, and works through early loss and cravings for love.

Scientists have not fully researched the effect of psychodynamic psychotherapy on depression or mania. Many have modified the techniques used in this type of therapy over time, and there have been problems with standardizing the approach for research purposes. For some patients, psychodynamic psychotherapy assists with the development of insights that promote behavioral change. However, many patients—including those with severe depression—are unable or unmotivated to participate in this type of therapy; for some, problems such as self-care deficits, psychomotor retardation, and fatigue take priority.

Self-Management Intervention

In the current health care environment, which involves fewer financial resources and difficulty with access to health care, patients have had to be more involved in self-managing their chronic illnesses. Self-management approaches for chronic illnesses such as asthma and cardiac disease have reduced health care costs and improved longer-term health outcomes. There is little documentation of specific interventions to teach and help patients and their families to better manage their mood disorders on an ongoing, daily basis. Related research has shown that depression management and relapse prevention strategies, including extra visits with a depression specialist and follow-up telephone calls, result in greater adherence to antidepressant medication regimens and fewer depressive symptoms (Katon et al, 2001).

Nurses have a major role in educating patients with mood disorders about their illnesses and in helping these patients develop strategies for ongoing management of the disorders and the subsequent impact on their lives. Nurses are able to teach patients self-management strategies such as identifying early symptoms of recurrence (see the Research for Evidence-Based Practice box), problem solving regarding potential options for intervention, and building a collection of self-management strategies for times of increased stress and potential recurrence.

RESEARCH FOR EVIDENCE-BASED PRACTICE

Hagerty BM et al: Prodromal symptoms of recurrent major depressive episodes: a qualitative analysis, *Am J Orthopsychiatry* 67:308-314, 1997.

Hagerty and colleagues conducted a qualitative study to determine patients' experiences with the onset of symptoms with recurrent depression. Participants in four focus groups with 16 persons had at least three well-documented episodes of major depression. With the use of the phenomenologic analysis of transcribed audiotapes and videotapes, the researchers identified themes in the focus group content. The distinct phases that participants experienced as they were entering a recurrent episode of depression were termed "Something's not right," "Something's really wrong," "the Crash," and "Connection." Sometimes these phases occurred over a short period of time, such as a matter of days, whereas sometimes they were more insidious. Participants agreed that once they experienced "the Crash," thereby descending into the acute depressive episode, it was too late to initiate preventive activities. All participants reported the occurrence of a prodromal phase of symptom onset with specific signs and symptoms in patterns that were unique to them. Many of these early signs and symptoms were different from the DSM diagnostic criteria. On the basis of the study results, the researchers theorized that persons with recurrent depression could often identify the signs and symptoms of their prodromal phase, learn to monitor for and recognize these early signs, make judgments about their depression, and initiate strategies to prevent or minimize the oncoming episodes.

Other Interventions

In positive psychotherapy, the therapist focuses on building strengths and emphasizing the positive rather than correcting negative thinking. The patient completes exercises that are designed to promote positive thinking. There are early indications that this approach can be helpful for the treatment of depression (Seligman, 2006).

Nurses have used interventions to treat depression that include exposing the patient to a healing environment or to activity such as gardening, guided imagery, and exercise (McCaffrey, 2007; Brown and Shirley, 2005). Approaches such as Internet interventions are now being investigated. Such interventions can educate patients about their disorders, improve and maximize patient communication with peers and therapists, and track symptom improvement (Allen et al, 2008) (Also see Chapters 26 and 27.)

Intervention for Adjustment Disorders

The keys to the treatment of adjustment disorders are support and normalization. Patterns of treatment often follow the guidelines that are available for use with crisis intervention. Patients need to feel that support is available to help sort out their feelings, options, and resources. At the same time, they need to learn that it is normal for people to have difficulty dealing with stressful situations and that they have the capacity to learn new ways of coping more effectively.

The treatment of adjustment disorders among children and adolescents includes additional methods. Family therapy addresses tension between family members. Some parents need assistance to understand the child's view of the stressor. Individual therapy helps to identify the meaning of the stressor for the child or adolescent. Brief, focused, and time-limited therapy concentrates on teaching relaxation techniques and cognitive problem solving, and group or classroom interventions are also helpful. The purpose of treatment for children and adolescents is to support existing coping strategies and to teach new ones that are appropriate to the developmental stage of the patient.

The use of medications for the treatment of adjustment disorders is controversial. Many clinicians believe that adjustment disorders will remit on their own or with only brief supportive psychotherapy. Some maintain that medicating the problem deprives people of the opportunity to learn how to cope with stressful situations.

EVALUATION

Nurses evaluate patients' progress by measuring their achievement of identified outcomes. Nurses collect data that support or refute the achievement of outcomes from personal observations, patients, patients' families and friends, and other health care providers. Evaluation occurs throughout hospitalization and during community care. Nurses working in community settings (e.g., psychiatric home care) sometimes evaluate outcomes for patients who have never been admitted to an inpatient setting.

With decreasing lengths of hospital stays, nurses in inpatient psychiatric units do not always see dramatic changes in patients' symptoms. However, they do see some clear progress related to priority short-term outcomes, such as the absence of imminent suicidal intent, a plan for addressing the potential return of suicidal ideation after discharge, and the ability to conduct self-care activities. Nurses also observe some alleviation of the neurovegetative symptoms of depression (i.e., sleep, loss of appetite, fatigue, psychomotor retardation); the alleviation of the severe hyperactive behavior of mania; improvements in cognitive functioning and communication; and an initial understanding of the disorder and its treatment, including necessary self-care management. In this setting, nurses make referrals to therapists, psychiatrists, psychiatric nurse practitioners, home care and community mental health agencies, and partial hospitalization programs for the patient's continued care in the community.

Nurses who work with patients in the community see improvements in longer-term outcomes such as improved socialization, return to usual activities, reduction in negative thinking, increased self-esteem, and the use of new coping strategies. Nurses also see improvement in areas such as the resumption of family and work roles, continued improvement in cognitive processes (e.g., attention, concentration), decreased fatigue, and adherence to treatment plans. For some patients, these outcomes become evident within weeks of starting psychotherapy or somatic treatment regimens. For others, improvement requires months before patients achieve longer-term outcomes. Data suggest that a return to previous levels of functioning after an episode of depression takes longer than previously thought, particularly if patients have had multiple episodes (Greden, 2001).

Patients with mania present a unique evaluative situation, because episodes of mania are often followed by episodes of depression. Therefore, although patients have returned to a hypomanic or euthymic state at the time of hospital discharge, nurses remain alert for any indications of depression. Careful follow-up monitoring after discharge into the community is imperative for patients with bipolar disorders.

⊚ CONCEPT MAP CASE STUDY 12-1

Kaitlyn is a 28-year-old married woman and the mother of two toddlers. She has had seven previous episodes of major depression, with the most recent occurring 2 years ago. She comes to an appointment with the nurse practitioner in the mental health clinic with the following signs and symptoms: frequent crying, sad mood, irritability, inability to concentrate that interferes with her work as a third grade teacher, extreme fatigue, self-blame for being a "bad mother," the inability to meet some of her children's needs (especially when they are very active), loss of appetite, inability to make meals, lying on the couch for hours at a time, and the loss of 12 pounds in the past 6 weeks. She has not showered in 10 days, and her hair appears unbrushed and greasy. Kaitlyn sleeps only 3 hours each night. She is having continuing thoughts of driving her car off of a bridge, and this frightens her. She has had two previous suicide attempts, one of which occurred during her last episode of depression when she overdosed on aspirin.

Kaitlyn was initially prescribed Prozac, and she reported that it "helped slightly." During her previous episode with depression, she was placed on 200 mg of venlafaxine (Effexor) daily. This medication was helpful, and she was able to return to parenting effectively and teaching her class of 15 students. Six months after starting the Effexor, she stopped the medication because she felt better and was functioning well in all aspects of her life.

Kaitlyn and her husband began to have conflict over their different parenting styles, and this conflict preceded Kaitlyn's current episode of depression. Kaitlyn expresses feeling "hopeless" and states that her family would be "better off" if she were "no longer in the picture."

DSM-IV-TR Diagnoses

Axis I   Major depressive disorder: recurrent, severe
Axis II   Deferred
Axis III   History of migraine headaches
Axis IV   Problems with support system, marital difficulties and occupational difficulties due to decrease in concentration
Axis V   GAF = 30 (current); GAF = 70 (past year)

Nursing Diagnosis *Risk for suicide. Risk factors: past suicide attempts, current suicidal thoughts, self-depreciating thoughts, severely depressed mood, hopelessness, marital conflict, issues related to parenting, blaming self for being a "bad mother," reduction of appetite, verbalizing not wanting to live*

NOC Risk detection, Risk control, Impulsive self-control, Suicide self-restraint, Depression level, Mood equilibrium, Social support, Will to live

Nursing Diagnosis *Ineffective coping related to suicidal thoughts, depressed mood, fatigue, sleep deprivation, and inability to concentrate as evidenced by inability to work or care for self, home, and family*

NOC Suicide, Self-restraint, Depression, Self-control, Coping, Decision-making, Sleep, Knowledge, Health resources, Role performance, Self-esteem, Quality of life
NIC Behavior management: self-harm; Mood management; Coping enhancement; Decision-making support; Sleep enhancement; Support system enhancement; Therapy group

Nursing Diagnosis *Self-care deficit (bathing/hygiene, dressing/grooming) related to depressed mood and fatigue secondary to major depression as evidenced by disheveled appearance and lack of attention to appearance*

NOC Self-care: bathing; Self-care: hygiene; Self-care: dressing; Self-care: activities of daily living; Psychomotor energy; Motivation; Patient satisfaction: physical care
NIC Bathing, Dressing, Caregiver support, Energy management, Self-responsibility facilitation, Self-esteem enhancement

GAF, Global Assessment of Functioning; NIC, Nursing Interventions Classification; NOC, Nursing Outcomes Classification.

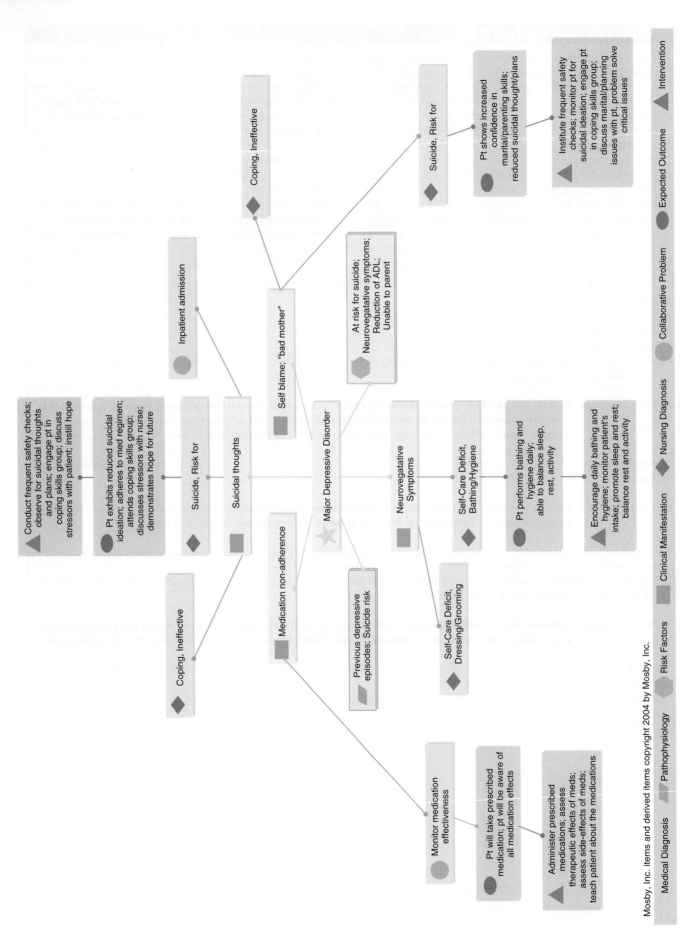

FIGURE 12-3. Concept map: major depression.

Mosby, Inc. items and derived items copyright 2004 by Mosby, Inc.

Medical Diagnosis Pathophysiology Risk Factors Clinical Manifestation Nursing Diagnosis Collaborative Problem Expected Outcome Intervention

CONCEPT MAP CASE STUDY 12-2

Ryan is a 40-year-old insurance salesman. He has recently separated from his wife, and he has two preteen children. Ryan was diagnosed with bipolar disorder when he was 21 years old, right after he graduated from college with a degree in business administration. He functions well between episodes of his illness, especially when his condition is stabilized with his medication (lithium). During the past month, Ryan has become increasingly hyperactive, starting new projects every day without completing any of them, including painting the inside of the house in loud, garish colors; searching for business opportunities on the Internet; and buying one gadget after another that he does not need. He has been calling his friends to urge them to buy additional insurance policies, and he becomes angry when they decline. He plans to invest all of his savings in a risky business venture, and wants to hire 10 to 15 employees, although he has already spent a lot of his savings. Ryan sleeps only 3 hours a night, and he is unable to sit still for a full meal or even to stand still to drink a beverage. He has been complaining of a dry mouth and increased thirst, with some dizziness and nausea. He speaks at a rapid rate, and he gets annoyed when people say that they cannot understand him. He feels that he has important things to say, but his thoughts are moving so quickly that it makes his verbalizations difficult to follow. When his wife left him, she cited his irritability, his pacing at all hours of the night, his grandiose ideas, and his lack of financial responsibility. He stopped taking his lithium 2 months ago. He was ultimately taken to the psychiatric emergency department by his parents and a close friend.

DSM-IV-TR Diagnoses

Axis I   Bipolar I disorder: manic episode
Axis II   Deferred
Axis III   Rule out deficient fluid volume
Axis IV   Marital stress; consequences of impulsive behavior
Axis V   GAF = 25 (current); GAF = 75 (past year)

Nursing Diagnosis *Disturbed thought processes related to ineffective processing and synthesis of stimuli (secondary to brain chemistry changes in bipolar mania) and exaggerated responses to psychosocial stressors (secondary to bipolar mania) as evidenced by flight of ideas, grandiosity, initiating multiple simultaneous projects, poor judgment and insight, and intrusion in others' lives*

NOC Personal safety behavior, Impulse self-control, Cognition, Information processing, Communication, Medication response, Safe home environment
NIC Environmental management: safety; Behavior management: overactivity/inattention; Reality orientation; Delusion management; Mood management; Medication management

Nursing Diagnosis *Noncompliance related to personal abilities and motivational forces (unable or unwilling to comply secondary to biochemical imbalance of mania) as evidenced by hyperactive and disorganized behavior indicating failure to adhere to medication regimen, evidence of exacerbation of manic symptoms, failure to progress toward normal behavior patterns, lack of family support in medication regimen*

NOC Compliance behavior: prescribed medication; Symptom control; Motivation; Acceptance: health status; Knowledge: treatment regimen; Patient satisfaction: communication; Family coping; Family participation in professional care; Social support
NIC Behavior management: Overactivity/inattention; Impulse control training; Medication management; Mood management; Self-awareness enhancement; Health literacy enhancement; Family involvement promotion; Support group; Therapy group

Nursing Diagnosis *Risk for deficient fluid volume: Risk factors: factors influencing fluid needs (e.g., hypermetabolic state); Deviations affecting access to fluids (patient's rapid thought processes and disorganized behaviors result in inability to access sufficient fluids on a regular basis); Deviations affecting intake of fluids (patient is too hyperactive to drink sufficient fluids to maintain normal fluid volume); Knowledge deficiency (patient's awareness of fluid needs is interrupted by rapid and disorganized thoughts secondary to mania); Medication (lithium) mismanagement*

NOC Hydration; Fluid balance; Electrolyte and acid-base balance; Nausea and vomiting severity; Agitation level; Appetite; Nutritional status: food and fluid intake; Knowledge: disease process; Knowledge: medication; Compliance behavior: prescribed diet; Self-care status
NIC Fluid/electrolyte management; Vital signs monitoring; Nausea management; Hypovolemia management; Medication management; Fluid monitoring; Acid-base management; Nutritional monitoring; Teaching: disease process; Teaching: prescribed medication; Decision-making support; Family involvement promotion

Nursing Diagnosis *Ineffective role performance related to responses to mental illness (bipolar disorder, mania), neurological deficits (biochemical imbalance), inappropriate linkage with the health care system (failure to seek*

Continued

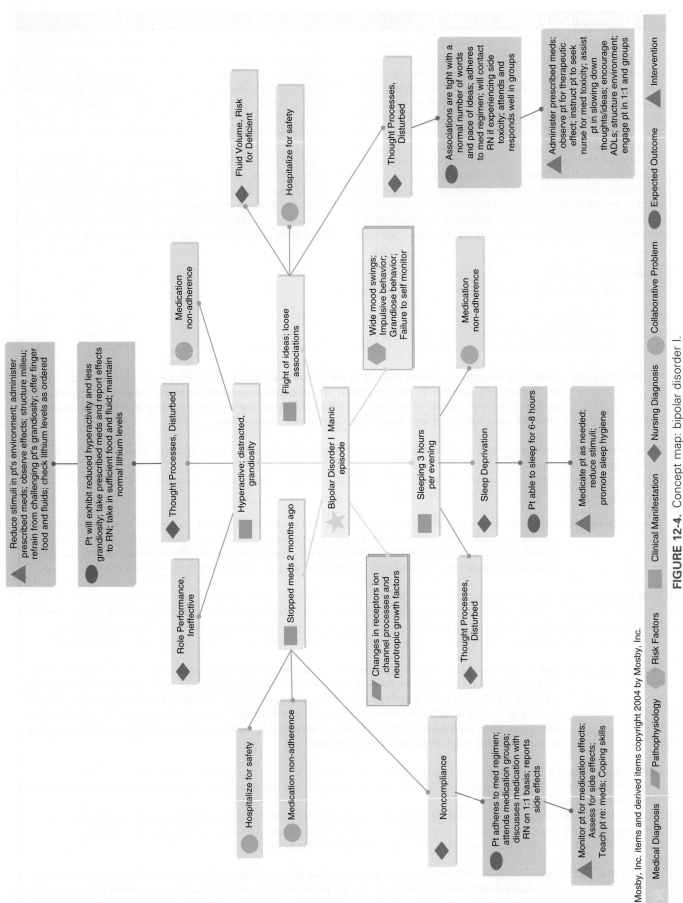

FIGURE 12-4. Concept map: bipolar disorder I.

⊙ CONCEPT MAP CASE STUDY 12-2—cont'd

medical or psychiatric help), and inadequate support system (separated from wife and lives alone); Inadequate role socialization (alienated coworkers and friends with intrusive behaviors) as evidenced by inadequate self-management (unable to manage illness and medication), deficient knowledge (lack of insight into grandiose behaviors resulting from mental illness), and inadequate role competency (failure to perform age-appropriate roles as husband, father, son, and coworker)

NOC Role performance, Agitation level, Psychomotor energy, Cognition, Information processing, Motivation, Depression self-control, Family functioning

NIC Anxiety reduction; Medication management; Mood management; Delusion management; Behavior management: overactivity/hyperactivity; Coping enhancement; Cognitive restructuring; Family involvement promotion; Support group; Therapy group

Nursing Diagnosis *Sleep deprivation related to biochemical imbalance affecting normal sleep patterns secondary to mania and hyperactivity (pacing during the night) as evidenced by agitation; irritability; inability to concentrate on role performance, medication regimen, and fluid and food intake; and sustained environmental stimulation (multitasking throughout the day)*

NOC Agitation level; Fatigue level; Mood equilibrium; Psychomotor energy; Concentration; Distorted thought self-control; Comfort status: environment; Rest; Sleep; Energy conservation

NIC Anxiety reduction, Medication management, Mood management, Calming technique, Progressive muscle relaxation, Relaxation therapy, Self-awareness enhancement, Environmental management, Health education, Self-awareness enhancement, Family involvement promotion, Energy management, Emotional support, Music therapy

CHAPTER SUMMARY

- Mood disorders are a major public health problem, and depression is a leading cause of the condition's burden (including morbidity and mortality) in the world.
- Major depression is currently occurring at younger ages, and those most at risk are women with a family history of mood disorders.
- Mood disorders are usually recurrent and require lifelong management. Manifestations and treatment concerns vary across the life span.
- Two broad types of mood disorders include unipolar depressive and bipolar disorders.
- Multiple theories, including biologic and psychosocial, attempt to explain mood disorders. Theories regarding the etiology of mood disorders are multiple, including a genetic and biologic predisposition for risk.
- Mania and depression are manifested by symptoms that involve the affective, cognitive, physical, social, and spiritual aspects of the individual.
- Mania and depression occur in any health care setting and not only in psychiatric units.
- Comorbid (co-occurring) medical conditions are frequently seen in patients with mood disorders.
- The nursing care of individuals who are experiencing depression or mania consists of a thorough assessment and subsequent planning and interventions for a range of nursing diagnoses related to physical, psychosocial, and spiritual needs.
- Nurses collaborate with other mental health care providers for care related to somatic, family, and group interventions.
- Adjustment disorders are passing episodes of clinically significant emotional or behavioral nonpsychotic symptoms in response to identifiable psychosocial stress or stressors. Symptoms develop within 3 months after the stressful event.
- The diagnosis of adjustment disorder means that the patient's behaviors or symptoms are different from his or her usual patterns of response and that the symptoms have persisted for less than 6 months (acute), unless the symptoms are in response to an ongoing stressor or stressors (chronic).
- The severity of the reaction to a stressor is not predictable in relation to the stressor, and the reaction is unique to each individual.
- Patients with adjustment disorder are often treated as outpatients, because the severity of their symptoms or subjective distress does not require inpatient hospitalization.
- Attempting to understand the patient's experience from his or her point of view fosters the therapeutic process.

REVIEW QUESTIONS

1. A patient says to the nurse, "I had my first depression after my father died about 10 years ago, but I didn't get any treatment. Now it seems even little life events cause me to get depressed again." Which theory of neurotransmission may explain the patient's complaint?
   1. Stress increases the activity of monoamine oxidase.
   2. Dysfunctional grieving inhibits metabolism of serotonin.
   3. Prolonged grief depletes neuronal supplies of G-proteins.
   4. Kindling may alter neuronal cell structure and function.

2. Which individual has the highest risk for major depression?
   1. 8-year-old girl
   2. 16-year-old boy
   3. 35-year-old woman
   4. 60-year-old man

3. A nurse assesses an elderly person for depression. Select the best question for the nurse to ask?
   1. "How do you compare your activities and health now to 6 months ago?"
   2. "Would you say you are currently having a major depressive episode?"
   3. "What is your family history related to depressive illnesses?"
   4. "Are you having crying spells every day?"

4. A nurse prepares the plan of care for a person having a manic episode. Which nursing diagnosis is most likely to apply? You may select more than one answer.
   1. Imbalanced nutrition: more than body requirements
   2. Sleep deprivation
   3. Risk for deficient fluid volume
   4. Social isolation
   5. Disturbed thought processes

5. A patient says to the nurse, "Life doesn't have any joy in it anymore. Things I once did for pleasure aren't fun." How would the nurse document this complaint?
   1. Dysthymia
   2. Anhedonia
   3. Euphoria
   4. Psychomotor retardation

6. A patient with an adjustment disorder participates in a series of outpatient therapy sessions. The goals of the therapy are stress inoculation and assisting the patient with self-management. Place these statements by the nurse in the correct sequence for this treatment modality.
   1. "Let's talk while you make a list of the biggest problems in your life and discuss some possible solutions for each problem."
   2. "Choose one problem-solving technique to decide how to handle arguments with your spouse."
   3. "The purpose of our group today is to understand stressful events and how they affect one's abilities to manage life."

REFERENCES

Abramson LY et al: Learned helplessness in humans: critique and reformulation, *Abnorm Psychol* 87:49, 1978.

Allen M et al: Improving patient-clinician communication about chronic conditions: description of Internet-based nurse E-coach interventions, *Nurs Res* 57:102, 2008.

Bailey MK et al: Patterns of depressive symptoms in children, *J Child Adolesc Psychiatr Nurs* 20:86, 2007.

Barnow S et al: The importance of psychosocial factors, gender, and severity of depression in distinguishing between adjustment and depressive disorders, *J Affect Disord* 72:71, 2002.

Beck AT: *Depression: clinical, experiential, and theoretical aspects*, New York, 1967, Hober.

Beck CT: State of the science on postpartum depression: what researchers have contributed—part 1, *Am J Matern Child Nurs* 33:121, 2008.

Beesdo K et al: Mood episodes and mood disorders: patterns of incidence and conversion in the first three decades of life, *Bipolar Disord* 11:637, 2009.

Brown GW, Harris T: *Social origins of depression*, New York, 1978, The Free Press.

Brown MA, Shirley JL: Enhancing women's mood and energy: a research-based program for subthreshold depression using light, exercise, and vitamins, *Holist Nurs Pract* 19:278, 2005.

Carota A et al: A prospective study of predictors of poststroke depression, *Neurology* 64:428, 2005.

Clement K et al: St. John's wort and the treatment of mild to moderate depression: a systematic review, *Holist Nurs Pract* 20:197, 2006.

Consensus Development Panel: Mood disorders: pharmacological prevention of recurrences, *Am J Psychiatry* 142:469, 1985.

Duman RS: Neuronal damage and protection in the pathophysiology and treatment of psychiatric illness: stress and depression, *Dialogues Clin Neurosci* 11:239, 2009.

Evans DL et al: Mood disorders in the medically ill: scientific review and recommendations, *Biol Psychiatry* 58:175, 2005.

Fitzgerald PB et al: A randomized, controlled trial of sequential bilateral repetitive transcranial magnetic stimulation for treatment-resistant depression, *Am J Psychiatry* 163:88, 2009.

Freud S: Mourning and melancholia. In *The complete psychological works of Sigmund Freud*, London, 1957, Hogarth.

Frodl T et al: Neuroimaging genetics: new perspectives in research on major depression? *Acta Psychiatrica* 118:363, 2008.

George MS et al: Vagus nerve stimulation and deep brain stimulation. In *Textbook of mood disorders*, Arlington, Va, 2006, American Psychiatric Association.

George MS et al: Noninvasive techniques for probing neurocircuitry and treating illness: vagus nerve stimulation (VNS), transcranial magnetic stimulation (TMS) and transcranial direct current stimulation (tDCS), *Neuropharmacology Reviews* 35:301, 2010.

Gillespie CF, Nemeroff CB: Early life stress and depression, *Curr Psychiatry* 4:15, 2005.

Golden RN et al: The efficacy of light therapy in the treatment of mood disorders: meta analysis of the evidence, *Am J Psychiatry* 162:656, 2005.

Gonzalez HM et al: Depression care in the United States: too little for too few, *Arch Gen Psychiatry* 67:37, 2010.

Greden JF: *Recurrent depression*, Washington, DC, 2001, American Psychiatric Publishing.

Hagerty BM et al: Prodromal symptoms of recurrent major depressive episodes: a qualitative analysis, *Am J Orthopsychiatry* 67:308, 1997.

Heim C et al: The link between childhood trauma and depression: insights from HPA axis studies in humans, *Psychoneuroendocrinology* 33:693, 2008.

Hirshfeld-Becker DR et al: Temperamental correlates of disruptive behavior disorders in young children: preliminary findings, *Biol Psychiatry* 51:563, 2002.

Holmes TH, Rahe RH: The social readjustment rating scale, *J Psychosom Res* 11:213, 1967.

Jones R et al: Readmission rates for adjustment disorders: comparison with other mood disorders, *J Affect Disord* 71:199, 2002.

Katon W et al: A randomized trial of relapse prevention of depression in primary care, *Arch Gen Psychiatry* 58:241, 2001.

Keltikangas-Jarvinen L, Salo J: Dopamine and serotonin systems modify environmental effects on human behavior: a review, *Scand J Psychol* 50:574, 2009.

Kendler KS: Twin studies of psychiatric illness: an update, *Arch Gen Psychiatry* 58:1005, 2001.

Kendler KS et al: Gender differences in the rates of exposure to stressful life events and sensitivity to their depressogenic effects, *Am J Psychiatry* 158:587, 2001.

Kendler KS et al: A Swedish national twin study of lifetime major depression, *Am J Psychiatry* 163:109, 2006.

Kessler RC et al: Prevalence, severity, and comorbidity of twelve-month DSM-IV disorders in the National Comorbidity Survey Replication (NCS-R), *Arch Gen Psychiatry* 62:593, 2005.

Malkoff-Schwartz S et al: Social rhythm disruption and stressful life events in the onset of bipolar and unipolar episodes, *Psychol Med* 30:1005, 2000.

Marshall AJ, Harper-Jaques S: Depression and family relationships: ideas for healing, *J Fam Nurs* 14:56, 2008.

McCaffrey R: The effect of healing gardens and art therapy on older adults with mild-moderate depression, *Holist Nurs Pract* 21:79, 2007.

Merikangas KR, Pato M: Recent developments in the epidemiology of bipolar disorder in adults and children: magnitude, correlates, and future directions, *Clin Psychol Sci Pract* 16:121, 2009.

National Institute of Mental Health: *Initial results help clinicians identify patients with treatment-resistant depression* (website): www.nimh.nih.gov/science-news/2006/initial-results-help-clinicians-identify-patient. Accessed April 15, 2010.

National Institute of Mental Health: *The numbers count: mental disorders in America* (website): www.nimh.nih.gov/health/publications/2008/the-numbers-count-mental-disorders-in-america. Accessed April 15, 2010.

Nesse RM: Evolution at 150: time for truly biological psychiatry, *Br J Psychiatry* 195:471, 2009.

Nomura Y et al: Family discord, parental depression and psychopathology in offspring: ten-year follow-up, *J Am Acad Child Adolesc Psychiatry* 41:402, 2002.

Olie E et al: Higher psychological pain during a major depressive episode may be a factor of vulnerability to suicidal ideation and act, *J Affect Disord* 129:226, 2010.

Pelkonen M et al: Suicidality in adjustment disorder: clinical characteristics of adolescent outpatients, *Eur Child Adolesc Psychiatry* 14:174, 2005.

Perlis RH et al: Clinical features of bipolar depression versus major depressive disorder in large multicenter trials, *Am J Psychiatry* 163:225, 2006.

Pittenger C, Duman RS: Stress, depression, and neuroplasticity: a convergence of mechanisms, *Neuropsychopharmacology* 33:88, 2008.

Post RM: Transduction of psychosocial stress in the neurobiology of recurrent affective disorders, *Am J Psychiatry* 149:999, 1992.

Ravindran AV et al: Stress, coping, uplifts, and quality of life in subtypes of depression: a conceptual frame and emerging data, *J Affect Disord* 71:121, 2002.

Regenold WT et al: Increased prevalence of type 2 diabetes mellitus among psychiatric inpatients with bipolar I affective and schizoaffective disorders independent of psychotropic drug use, *J Affect Disord* 70:19, 2002.

Rush AJ, et al: Comorbid psychiatric disorders in depressed outpatients: demographic and clinical features, *J Affect Disord* 87:34, 2005.

Sanchez-Gistau V et al: Atypical depression is associated with suicide attempt in bipolar disorder, *Acta Psychiatr Scand* 120:30, 2009.

Seligman ME: *Helplessness: on depression development and death*, New York, 1975, WH Freeman.

Seligman ME et al: Positive psychotherapy, *Am Psychol* 61:774, 2006.

Shin NM et al: Gender comparison in depressive symptoms and use of antidepressant medications after acute coronary syndrome, *Appl Nurs Res* 23:73, 2010.

Solberg LI et al: Follow-up and follow-through of depressed patients in primary care: the critical missing components of quality care, *J Am Board Fam Pract* 18:520, 2005.

World Health Organization: *The global burden of disease*, Switzerland, 2008, World Health Organization.

Yamada M et al: Antidepressant-elicited changes in gene expression: remodeling of neuronal circuits as a new hypothesis for drug efficacy: a review, *Prog Neuropsychopharmacol Biol Psychiatry* 29:999, 2005.

Yiend J et al: Long term outcome of primary care depression, *J Affect Disord* 118:79, 2009.

Online Resources

American Association of Suicidology: www.suicidology.org

American Foundation for Suicide Prevention: www.afsp.org

Child & Adolescent Bipolar Foundation: www.bpkids.org

Depression and Bipolar Support Alliance: www.dbsalliance.org

National Alliance on Mental Illness: www.nami.org

National Institute of Mental Health: www.nimh.nih.gov

National Suicide Prevention Lifeline:
    www.suicidepreventionlifeline.org

Mental Health America: www.nmha.org

Suicide Prevention Resource Center: www.sprc.org

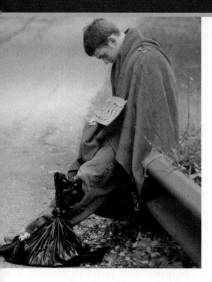

Schizophrenia and Other Psychotic Disorders

Judy A. Malone Cole

"Everything about you starts being attributed ... to the mental health diagnosis you have ... other things just get ignored; you're not seen as a whole person ... the separation between the systems that happens is really detrimental because you have this whole group of medically oriented people who feel like they don't know anything about the psychiatric stuff ... that it belongs to someone else, and there you are ... in a big gap in between."

Gaillard and colleagues, 2010

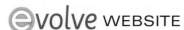

WEBSITE

http://evolve.elsevier.com/Fortinash/

OBJECTIVES

- Identify the various theories and models that explain schizophrenia that have evolved over time.
- Relate the significance of the biologic theory and its current role in the development of schizophrenia.
- Discuss advancements in research that link genetic factors to schizophrenia.
- Compare and contrast the course of illness, symptoms, and nursing interventions for the subtypes of schizophrenia and for associated disorders such as schizoaffective disorder.

- Apply the nursing process to patients who are experiencing the positive, negative, cognitive, and depressive symptoms of schizophrenia.
- Assess the situation of persons with schizophrenia and their families in the community.
- Develop nursing care plans for prevention, aftercare, and psychoeducation for patients with schizophrenia and their families.
- Evaluate the effectiveness of the various treatment modalities for schizophrenia in the clinical setting.

KEY TERMS

affect	delusion	heterogeneous	poverty of thought
ambivalence	depressive symptoms	loosening of associations	premorbid phase
anhedonia	derealization	negative symptoms	prodromal phase
apathy	dereism	neurotransmitter	psychotic phase
autistic thinking	echolalia	paranoia	residual symptoms
avolition	echopraxia	perseveration	thought blocking
cognitive symptoms	hallucination	positive symptoms	

Schizophrenia is a fairly common, chronic, debilitating, and often devastating mental disorder. It is not a single disorder but rather one of a group of related disorders with a wide range of severity and symptoms among individuals. Schizophrenia is heterogeneous, meaning it is comprised of dissimilar elements with variable patient outcomes. It is also a complex brain disease, therefore it is a neuropsychiatric disorder, because symptoms occur from a number of factors that affect the brain's neurotransmitter system and that result in impaired thoughts, perceptions, cognitive functions, moods, and motivations (Sadock et al, 2009). Schizophrenia is a universal disorder that exists in all cultures and among members of all socioeconomic groups (National Institute of Mental Health [NIMH], 2005). It is often called a *psychotic disorder*, which means that people with schizophrenia have periods when they lose touch with reality and exhibit various kinds of psychotic symptoms. All symptoms of schizophrenia are debilitating, but not all symptoms are psychotic. The symptoms seem to come from different mechanisms, perhaps because different brain regions or circuits are affected. Therefore, symptoms respond to a variety of psychosocial and psychopharmacologic treatments (Lieberman, 2006) which are discussed in this chapter and in Chapters 25 and 16.

Symptoms of schizophrenia are divided into four main groups:

1. Positive symptoms are psychotic symptoms, which are often called *florid symptoms* because of their dramatic nature. They include the presence of unusual sensations and perceptions such as hallucinations (false perceptions), delusions (false beliefs), paranoia (irrational suspicion), bizarre (odd or eccentric) behavior, and confused or obsessive thoughts that seem to return periodically and that are usually provoked by a variety of stressors.

   Because of the acute (sudden) onset of positive symptoms and their obvious detachment from reality, they grab our attention the most. Long-term studies and treatments indicate that these florid and dramatic symptoms respond favorably to hospitalization, medication, reduced stimuli, and interactive therapy and that they may not be as debilitating as the negative symptoms described below. Positive symptoms generally present early in the illness, but tend to diminish in intensity in the fifth and sixth decades of life; however, research also suggests that each successive episode of psychosis may bring less resolution of positive symptoms and more prominent negative symptoms that often become more enduring. Both types of symptoms present unique challenges to patients, their families, and the community, and it is important for all health care personnel to focus on evidence based practices that provide the most effective outcomes for each patient. (Lieberman et al, 2008).

2. Negative symptoms as indicated above, are more complex and difficult to treat, and they are present during all phases of the illness. They include apathy (indifference), withdrawal, avolition (lack of motivation), blunted or flat affect (reduced emotional expression), loss of warmth or vibrancy, poverty of thought (absent or reduced thoughts), and anhedonia (loss of pleasure in things previously enjoyed).

   Negative symptoms are not as obvious as positive symptoms, and their onset is insidious (slow); however, they may be more debilitating in the long run because of their paralyzing effect on the person's thoughts, emotions, and motivation (Beng-Choon et al, 2004). The persistence of negative symptoms can immobilize these individuals by making it difficult for them to relate to others in normal social situations. They tend to miss common social cues that most of us take for granted (Lieberman, 2006). Negative symptoms have a poor response to the older typical antipsychotics, and in fact negative symptoms may worsen

when these drugs are used to treat the positive symptoms, thereby making medication adherence a significant issue for the patient and the family. In a recent study 74% of patients discontinued their medication within 18 months. Nonadherence often leads to remission of symptoms and possibly hospitalization. Atypical antipsychotics were initially thought to help with adherence because of a reduction in neurologic side effects and the promise of better results for negative symptoms; however, metaanalyses have found that drop-out rates are no better with atypical antipsychotics than with the older typical antipsychotics. Evidence suggests that delays in initiating antipsychotic therapy may result in a lifetime deleterious effect on psychotic episodes (Schultz et al, 2007) (see Chapter 25).

3. Cognitive symptoms, also termed *neuropsychologic* or *neurocognitive* deficits, are at the core of the disorganized and bizarre behaviors and confusion that result in functional disabilities and that affect 40% to 60% of individuals with schizophrenia. In patients with schizophrenia, the brain's working memory is impaired. Working memory is the capacity to sequence memories that are the foundations for daily living skills. This means that the brain loses its ability to access and process sensory stimulation and to integrate it with existing short- and long-term memories. Other disabling symptoms include confusion, inability to maintain attention, and disturbances in executive functioning (i.e., planning, organizing, reasoning, abstract thinking, and problem solving). The cognitive symptoms of impaired memory, inattention, and disturbances in executive functioning seem to be associated with the negative symptoms of apathy, poverty of thought, and avolition. Both sets of symptoms make it difficult for individuals to care for themselves, to live independently, to hold a job, or to maintain a social life. Individuals with good verbal memories are better able to learn and retain the cognitive and social skills necessary to live a more productive life within the limitations of their illness Most patients seem to sustain a further reduction in cognitive functioning at the time of the first psychotic episode, and there is little or no evidence that improvements in cognitive symptoms will occur naturally over time. In fact, some elderly persons gradually worsen over time (Lieberman et al, 2008) (see Chapter 16).

4. Depressive symptoms include anxiety, dysphoria (anguish), and irritability, and these often occur concurrently with schizophrenia (see Chapter 12). Suicide is a common cause of death in patients with schizophrenia, and the risk of suicide is strongly associated with depression, previous suicidal attempts, agitation or motor restlessness, fear of mental disintegration, poor adherence to treatment, and recent loss (Schultz et al, 2007). Depressive symptoms contribute to the 10% lifetime incidence of suicide among patients with schizophrenia; 20% to 40% of individuals with schizophrenia attempt suicide at least once during the course of their illness. Many suicides occur during periods of remission (when symptoms are reduced) and after 5 to 10 years of living with this devastating illness (American Psychiatric Association [APA],

2004) (see Chapter 22) In addition, 50% of patients with schizophrenia have a co-occurring substance use disorder, (e.g., alcohol, nicotine, cannabis, cocaine), most frequently alcohol and cannabis (see Chapter 15). Medical conditions such as obesity and type 2 diabetes mellitus also co-occur with schizophrenia. Mortality caused by natural and unnatural causes is considerable, and in the United States, people with schizophrenia die approximately 25 years earlier than others in the general population (Lieberman et al, 2008).

Symptoms of schizophrenia negatively affect all areas of the person's ability to function as a productive member of society, and the burden on the family and the community is enormous.

Schizophrenia is a disorder with "ebbs and flows," which means that there are periods of relapse when symptoms are most obvious, and periods of remission when symptoms are reduced. Therefore, individuals who are being treated may not demonstrate the obvious positive signs of the disorder, such as hallucinations and delusions. If negative symptoms are present others may view apathy as shyness, lack of motivation as laziness, withdrawal as rudeness, poverty of thought as ignorance, and poor grooming as sloppiness, all of which add to the stigma of schizophrenia. The stigma of schizophrenia works its ill effects in ways that cannot be completely measured, but it produces a major impact on opportunities for a normal life, healthy self-esteem, and good morale (Lieberman et al, 2008). The following examples describe behaviors that indicate the presence of schizophrenia among individuals in the community:

- The unkempt middle-aged woman talking to herself while pushing a shopping cart filled with objects that look like junk but that have special meaning for her
- The young man with a disheveled look who is cursing to himself and frantically searching for cigarettes in the gutter

These individuals may have other problems as well, including drug or alcohol abuse, mood disorders, and malnutrition. However, many of them are also struggling with untreated schizophrenia, and they represent that group of unfortunate individuals who cannot get the help they need to treat their mental illness. They are generally left alone to wander aimlessly until they commit a crime or social injustice that brings them to the attention of the psychiatric or legal system. They may then be hospitalized or jailed for a time, receiving treatment randomly, until they are once again released to the streets. Their families and friends have long since abandoned them, and, with no support system and no insurance, prospects for recovery present special challenges (see Chapter 30).

For the more fortunate individuals who receive treatment early during the course of schizophrenia and who have a strong support network, there is hope, if not yet a cure. For example, consider the young first-year college student with a strong familial history of schizophrenia who is experiencing his first psychotic break. He tried to kill both of his parents with a knife, because he believed that they were plotting against him. With newer medications and early interventions, this young adult will probably be able to manage his

symptoms of paranoid schizophrenia and possibly finish college. This is a very different outcome from what might have happened in the past, when people with schizophrenia were institutionalized for many years. Today, most people with schizophrenia are living in community settings.

Despite their prevalence, chronicity, and pervasive symptoms, the schizophrenic disorders did not have the benefit of a scientific, biologic approach until the middle of the 19th century. The research supporting the relationship of these complex disorders with the structure and function of the brain has produced more effective treatments and outcomes. Today, many long-term follow-up studies have supported the early research that some patients with schizophrenia have the capacity for symptomatic remission and functional improvement early in the course of illness, and even later in life. In addition, advancements in genetic and biologic research are helping scientists understand how specific genes, and neurodevelopmental and environmental stressors relate to the cause, pathophysiology, and treatment of schizophrenia, which offers even more promise for the coming decades (Lieberman et al, 2008)

HISTORIC AND THEORETIC PERSPECTIVES

Historically, schizophrenia has been described in the sciences and the literature as a complex, multifaceted disorder that goes beyond the hallucinations, delusions, and decreased motivation and drive that are most commonly associated with it (Sadock, et al 2009). Although the current understanding of the neurophysiology of brain and cognitive functioning is blossoming, there is much more mystery surrounding this syndrome that is only beginning to be appreciated.

The term *schizophrenia* emerged during the 1800s and was defined and described by two pioneers. Emil Kraepelin (1856–1926), a German psychiatrist, identified schizophrenia as *dementia praecox*, with its severe intellectual, cognitive, and memory deterioration (dementia), and premature (praecox) onset, which was characterized by hallucinations and delusions. Kraepelin viewed the illness as progressive and deteriorating, which was reinforced for many years by the limitations of existing treatments and more recently by research on brain abnormalities and neurodevelopmental theories of schizophrenia described later in this chapter. Eugen Bleuler (1857–1939), a Swiss psychiatrist coined the term *schizophrenia*, which means "split mindedness," and is a combination of two Greek words. *Schizein* means "to split" and *phren* means "mind." He equated the term with the "fragmented mind" characteristics of the disorder. The "split" refers to the inconsistencies among the patient's emotions, thoughts, and behaviors, although the essence of the individual's personality remained intact; therefore, schizophrenia should not be confused with the "split personality" related to "multiple personality disorder" now called dissociative identity disorder described in Chapter 14. Bleuler challenged Kraepelin's pessimistic view because he recognized that patients with dementia praecox constituted a heterogeneous "group of schizophrenias" with highly variable outcomes. He noted that

BOX 13-1 **BLEULER'S FOUR A'S: FUNDAMENTAL SYMPTOMS OF THE THOUGHT DISORDERS**

Affect: Observable outward bodily expression of emotions such as joy, sorrow, and anger. *Blunted affect*: Restricted expression of emotions. *Flat affect*: Lack of expression of emotions. *Inappropriate affect*: Affect that does not match the emotion being felt (e.g., laughing when sad). *Labile affect*: Rapid changes in emotional expression.

Ambivalence: Simultaneously holding two different attitudes, emotions, thoughts, or feelings about a person, object, or situation.

Autistic thinking: Disturbances in thought that result from the intrusion of a private fantasy world that is internally stimulated and that result in abnormal responses to people and events in the real world. A condition known as dereism is associated with autistic thinking. Dereism is a loss of connection with reality and logic, where thoughts become private and idiosyncratic (odd or peculiar).

Loosening of associations: Thought disturbance in which the speaker rapidly changes from one subject to another in an unrelated and fragmented manner.

From Sadock BJ et al: *Kaplan and Sadock's comprehensive textbook of psychiatry*, ed 9, 2009, Philadelphia, Lippincott Williams & Wilkins.

some patients' symptoms subsided or remitted completely, which enabled them to return to normal functioning. an observation that has stood the test of time. (Lieberman et al, 2008). Bleuler laid out the conceptual foundation for thought disorders, which more accurately describes schizophrenia. He also identified the four As of schizophrenia: (1) *a*utism; (2) *a*mbivalence; (3) disturbances in *a*ffect; and (4) disturbances in *a*ssociations (Sadock et al, 2009) (Box 13-1).

Throughout the 20th century and into the 21st century, the etiology and physiology of psychosis and schizophrenia have remained elusive. Theoretically, from a social perspective, research has touched upon "schizophrenogenic mothers" and social isolation (Sullivan, 1953) as causative agents; these have fueled stigma, isolation, and health care policies that have disenfranchised individuals with mental illnesses.

Thought disorders begin with the misinterpretation of internal or external stimuli that is manifested as behaviors that appear irrational, that are not grounded in reality, or that are frankly bizarre. The thought disorder symptoms may be mild disruptions in the ability to think or act, or they may be very dramatic. For example, some individuals may simply not be able to think; their thought processes are slowed down or are "blocked" a symptom known as "thought blocking." The person may appear preoccupied, or inattentive, and he or she is not able to sequence words or to follow conversations or directions. These individuals may not physically move. If a person comes to believe that the tap water is poisoned and the government is attempting to kill him or her, then he or

she may refuse to eat or drink any water or refuse to leave his or her apartment or bedroom. These symptoms tend to build on intense emotions or concepts that involve many social rules. Delusions (false fixed beliefs) and hallucinations (false perceptions) typically have political or religious themes or involve issues of authority. A few examples include the following:

- A woman believes she is the Queen of England and is waiting for the palace guards to return her to the throne. She does not recognize her husband or her children.
- A young man believes that he is the devil incarnate and that he is the new emerging messiah who controls the destiny of all nonbelievers.
- A teenager believes that the FBI is out to kill him as part of a plot by a Columbian drug cartel and that the CIA is collaborating to make sure that he is silenced, because he knows the government's secrets and that the government is run by the drug cartels.

When these symptoms interfere with functional capacity, the family and society usually take note and may intervene. Throughout history, there have been a wide variety of responses to psychotic symptoms. Some societies respond with reverence for the wisdom and "visions," whereas others react fearfully and exclude the "insane." Regardless, the contributions of these individuals continue to amaze and challenge modern perceptions of schizophrenia.

Consider the genius of Dutch painter Vincent van Gogh (1853–1890), who created one of his most noted paintings, *The Starry Night*, while institutionalized with a serious mental illness. More recently, John Nash, a mathematician who won the Nobel Prize in 1994, was diagnosed with paranoid schizophrenia; his story was the basis of the movie *A Beautiful Mind*, which starred Russell Crowe. The complexity of the syndrome of schizophrenia is abundantly apparent, and it defies simple explanation.

ETIOLOGY

Research into the etiology of schizophrenia has never been more exciting or challenging, particularly with regard to the roles that heredity, genes, and neurodevelopmental factors play in this complex disorder of the mind and brain as described below.

Heredity Genetic Factors

Since the early 20th century, both schizophrenia and bipolar disorder have been observed to run in families. This link was conclusively determined to be partly due to genes in a number of twin and/or adoption studies. Dozens of whole-genome linkage studies clearly implicated a few genomic regions in each disorder, and provoked many debates on the issue. Since 2002, genes have been identified in schizophrenia samples and subsequently replicated in independent samples. Since 2007, whole-genome association studies have been performed in even larger samples. The identification of numerous copy-number variants on a genome-wide scale in independent samples highlighted commonalities between schizophrenia

TABLE 13-1	SCHIZOPHRENIA AND GENETIC RISKS
RELATIONSHIP TO PERSON WITH SCHIZOPHRENIA	**GENETIC RISK OF DEVELOPING SCHIZOPHRENIA (%)**
Identical twin (monozygotic)	50
Fraternal twin (dizygotic)	17
Child (both parents have schizophrenia)	35
Child (one parent has schizophrenia)	15
First degree relative (e.g., parent, sibling)	6–17
Second degree relative (grandparents, aunt, uncle, nephew, niece)	2–6
Third degree relative (e.g., first cousin)	2
No affected relative (e,g., general population)	1

Adapted from Schultz SH, North SW, Shields, CG, Schizophrenia: A Review, *Am Fam Physician* 75(12): 1821–1829, 2007.

and developmental and learning disorders. At the present time, large-scale sequencing and investigations of genetic development, gene-to-gene, and gene-to-environment interactions, and other sources of complexity are in very early stages but are likely to contribute substantially in the future (Fanous, 2010). Studies also show that a number of factors interact to produce schizophrenia. These include heredity; events that occur during fetal development that affect the developing brain, such as viruses passed on to the fetus during pregnancy; environmental stressors, such as exposure to pollutants, toxins; and other substances, and stress (Lieberman, 2008).

Numerous studies of families, twins, and adopted children demonstrate that the tendency to develop schizophrenia is at least 60% inherited. A person has a 6% to 17% chance of developing schizophrenia if a parent or sibling has schizophrenia. For the general population, the chance is only 1%. If an identical (monozygotic) twin has schizophrenia, the probability rises to 50%. Because monozygotic twins share 100% of their genes, and there is only a 50% chance of developing schizophrenia, this suggests that other factors may predetermine the development of schizophrenia, such as the environmental factors, viruses, and stress mentioned above, In nonidentical (dizygotic) twins, the incidence is 17%. Studies have shown that adopted children raised in an environment away from their birth parents who have schizophrenia have a much higher chance of developing the disorder themselves. (Schultz et al, 2007). Research suggests a possible link to an infectious agent in the human genome that may play a role in schizophrenia (Mortensen et al, 2010) (Lencz et al, 2007) (see Immunologic factors later in this chapter). Some genes associated with schizophrenia code for enzymes and proteins that help the cells in the brain to communicate. These enzymes

and proteins are involved in neurotransmitter systems such as dopamine, glutamate, and gamma-aminobutyric acid. Other genes code for proteins that are involved in brain development (NIMH, 2005). Whatever results new research brings, nurses are continuously challenged to treat the person with schizophrenia as a whole human being by combining the biologic sciences with the caring and interpersonal concepts of the psychosocial models. Table 13-1 lists the genetic risks for schizophrenia, although these vary slightly, depending on the study. Figure 13-1 reveals structural changes in twins with schizophrenia.

Dopamine Hypothesis

Researchers believe that dopamine, which is a catecholamine-type neurotransmitter, acts within certain brain cells and nerve tracts to help regulate both movement and emotions. Therefore, dopamine affects mood, affect, thoughts, and motor behavior. The dopamine hypothesis, which is a major hypothesis regarding the etiology of schizophrenia, suggests that persons with schizophrenia have an increased level of dopamine in certain areas of the brain such as the nigrostriatal tract, which runs from the substantia nigra to the basal ganglia. Figure 13-2 illustrates the four main dopamine pathways or tracts (nigrostriatal, tuberoinfundibular, mesocortical, and mesolimbic) and some critical functions. The nigrostriatal pathway is a main dopamine tract responsible for the normal execution of motor and cognitive functions. A certain amount of dopamine is thus necessary for smooth motor movements and clear thought processes. However, excess dopamine causes symptoms of psychosis (e.g., hallucinations, delusions), because it disrupts cognition and thought. Postmortem data support this theory by having demonstrated a 66% increase in the number of dopamine receptors in persons with schizophrenia. Thus, researchers think that schizophrenia results from too much dopamine-dependent neuronal activity in the brain. This means that there is an abundance of nerve cells that crave dopamine and that overreact in a way that produces psychotic symptoms. Researchers also believe that, in patients with schizophrenia, there is excess production or release of dopamine at nerve endings, increased receptor sensitivity, or decreased activity of dopamine antagonists (i.e., drugs or substances that block or counteract dopamine) (Figure 13-3). Some studies suggest that abnormalities in dopamine storage, vesicular transport, and release or uptake by presynaptic neurons may be the proximal cause of psychotic symptoms and that this may contribute to the risk for schizophrenia (Gaur et al, 2008).

Dopamine Hypothesis and Illicit Drugs

Cocaine and amphetamines are dopaminergic compounds, which means that their chemical structure is similar to that of dopamine; therefore, they are dopamine agonists. They also induce psychosis in healthy individuals, and at very low doses, they can provoke psychotic symptoms in persons with schizophrenia. This supports the dopamine hypothesis that too much dopamine produces psychosis. Individuals with Parkinson's disease have reduced levels of dopamine.

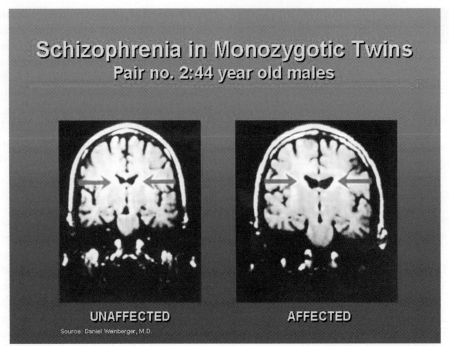

FIGURE 13-1. Loss of brain volume associated with schizophrenia is clearly shown by magnetic resonance imaging scans that compare the size of the ventricles (the butterfly-shaped, fluid-filled spaces in the midbrain) of identical twins, one of whom has schizophrenia *(right)*. The ventricles of the person with schizophrenia are larger, which suggests structural brain changes associated with the illness. Note that such scans cannot be used to diagnose schizophrenia in the general population because of normal genetic variation in ventricle size; many unaffected people have large ventricles. (Courtesy of Daniel R. Weinberger, MD, Chief Researcher, Clinical Brain Disorders Branch, National Institute of Mental Health, Bethesda, MD.)

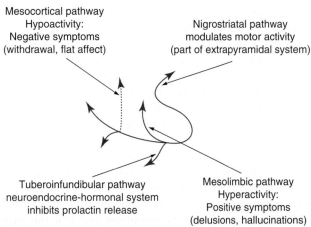

FIGURE 13-2. The four main dopaminergic tracts. (Adapted from Genetic Science Learning Center, *Beyond the reward pathway.* Learn Genetics, 2010. http://learn.genetics.utah.edu/content/addiction/reward/pathways/html)

Sometimes these individuals take levodopa (L-dopa) which is a type of dopamine, and they experience psychosis as a side effect (Gaur et al, 2008).

Another hypothesis states that lysergic acid diethylamide causes or increases hallucinations by its effects on serotonin.

This indicates that the newer-generation antipsychotics achieve a synergistic therapeutic effect by blocking both dopamine and serotonin. Persons with schizophrenia who take street drugs are at risk because of the unpredictable effects caused by these illicit substances. Consciousness-altering drugs (e.g., marijuana) tend to counteract the effects of antipsychotic medications by inducing the effects of the illness again (Gaur et al, 2008).

Other Neurotransmitters Associated with Schizophrenia

Six other neurotransmitters that are also relevant by themselves or in conjunction with dopamine are serotonin, acetylcholine, norepinephrine, cholecystokinin, glutamate, and gamma-aminobutyric acid (Table 13-2).

Neurodevelopmental Hypothesis

The neurodevelopmental theory indicates that etiologic and pathogenic factors occur long before the onset of the illness (probably in gestation). These factors or stressors disrupt the course of normal neural development in the fetus, and produce alterations of specific neural circuits that cause vulnerability and ultimately lead to biological and psychosocial malfunction. According to this theory, once the neurodevleopmental diathesis of schizophrenia is established (meaning

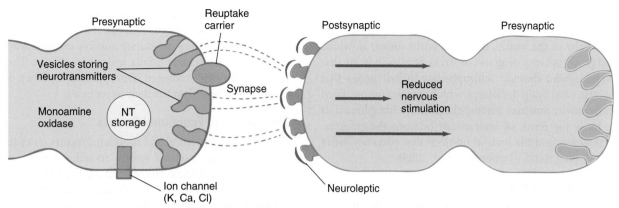

FIGURE 13-3. Neuroleptic (antipsychotic) action. Neurotransmitter action at the synapse is modified by neuroleptics, which block postsynaptic receptor sites to reduce nervous stimulation, thereby reducing the symptoms of schizophrenia. NT, neurotransmitter.

TABLE 13-2	NEUROTRANSMITTERS IN SCHIZOPHRENIA	
NEUROTRANSMITTER	**TYPE**	**FUNCTION**
Dopamine	Catecholamine	Regulates motor behavior in extrapyramidal nerve tracts and also transmits in the cortex
		Increases vigilance and may increase aggression
		Too much produces psychosis; too little causes movement disorders (extrapyramidal symptoms)
Serotonin	Indolamine	Brainstem transmitter that modulates mood and lowers aggressive tendencies
		Deficiency likely responsible for some forms of schizophrenia
Acetylcholine	Cholinergic	Transmits at nerve–muscle connections (central nervous system and autonomic nervous system)
		Controls extrapyramidal symptoms
		Deficiency increases confusion and acting out behavior
Norepinephrine	Catecholamine	Transmits in the sympathetic nervous system
		Induces the flight-or-fight response (hypervigilance)
		Sometimes insufficient in patients with schizophrenia who display anhedonia (loss of pleasure)
Cholecystokinin	Peptide	Excites limbic neurons
		Deficiency is related to avolition (lack of motivation) and a flat affect
Glutamate	Amino acid	Excitatory neurotransmitter.
		Impairment in the N-methyl-D-aspartate, or NMDA, affects glutamate, which leads to problems in cognition, delusions, and possibly some negative symptoms of schizophrenia.
Gamma-aminobutyric acid	Amino acid	Inhibitory neurotransmitter; predominantly a brain transmitter
		Promotes a balance between dopamine and glutamate and thus inhibits impulsive behaviors

the brain has been disposed to schizophrenia), the illness then runs its inevitable course. (Lieberman et al, 2008)

Most people who develop schizophrenia do not show symptoms until later in their adolescence. Studies of teens who develop schizophrenia provide clues about the neurodevelopmental process. Normally, teens lose some unused neural connections as their brains mature. However, magnetic resonance imaging (MRI) reveals that teens with schizophrenia lose these connections at an accelerated rate (NIMH, 2005)

Faulty wiring is possibly responsible for genes creating too many or too few of the proteins that are needed to help

neurons develop and migrate in the developing brain. Viruses or parasites that the pregnant mother catches also possibly affect these processes. Toxin exposure as a result of breathing (pollutants), eating, drinking, and smoking are also perhaps responsible. Birth complications and psychoactive drug use can also adversely affect neurodevelopment. (Lieberman et al, 2008).

Environmental Factors

Environmental factors associated with schizophrenia include toxins, pollution, infections, and viral exposure; malnutrition; being born in winter; being born in a city; and childhood brain injury. Some researchers define environment as everything from the nutritional environment, viruses that affect a baby in the womb, the social environment in which a child grows up, teen drug use, or stress. Studies indicate that individuals who develop schizophrenia inherit genes that cause structural brain deviations, which may be compounded by early environmental insults; therefore, schizophrenia is most likely the result of interactions between the environmental factors and the brain conditions that adversely affect the developing mind. (Lieberman et al, 2008).

Other Biologic Research

Extensive research regarding the neuroendocrine mechanisms that underlie the stress response influenced psychiatrists to research these mechanisms for their possible involvement in several forms of psychotic states and mental disorders. An example is the research related to oxytocin, a pituitary hormone that stimulates the uterus to contract. Oxytocin also reduces the stress responses of the hypothalamic–pituitary–adrenal axis (HPA). Researchers studied the role oxytocin plays in maternal bonding and theorized that diminished plasma oxytocin activity could be attributed to specific symptoms of schizophrenia, such as emotional deficits, impaired cognitive and behavioral functions, poor social interactions, agitation, and trust issues (Goldman et al, 2008). Researchers agree that increased knowledge is needed about the role the neuroendocrine system plays in influencing the complex symptoms of schizophrenia. Because our knowledge of the neurobiology, pathophysiology, and heterogeneity of schizophrenia is incomplete, research must be continued in these areas as well if we are to provide effective evidence-based interventions for the majority of patients with schizophrenia and related disorders (Lieberman et al, 2008).

Immunologic Factors

Viral exposure—particularly exposure to influenza during pregnancy—is a risk factor for the development of schizophrenia in later life. Scientists theorize that the influenza virus creates maternal antibodies that become autoantibodies in the developing fetus and are an external source of developmental change. Early exposure to other viruses has also been associated with the development of schizophrenia. These include polio, measles, varicella-zoster, rubella, and herpes simplex virus type 2, as well as exposure to unspecified central nervous system (CNS) viruses during childhood. Two recent studies assessed in utero or early postnatal exposure to the infectious agent *Toxoplasma gondii*. In one study of 63 individuals who developed schizophrenia spectrum disorders (disorders with similar characteristics of schizophrenia), maternal serum obtained during pregnancy showed an increased risk of having antibodies associated with *T. gondii*. Similar findings were seen in another study involving 71 patients. These studies indicate possible direct effects of maternal antibodies on the CNS of the developing fetus; however, the precise cause that links these mechanisms are speculative, prompting further research in this area

(Mortensen et al, 2007). Periconceptional maternal genital infections are also possible risk factors. The mother's exposure to a virus during pregnancy possibly explains why some siblings develop schizophrenia and others do not. There are few immunologic studies of schizophrenia, and they depend on epidemiologic data for their hypotheses.

Structural and Functional Factors

The theory of structural and functional factors states that the structure of the nervous system includes both gross and microanatomic defects. Studies that are used to examine the structural and functional impairment of the brain are discussed in the next paragraphs.

Magnetic Resonance Imaging. MRI is a brain imaging technique that is available today and that is used at the time of diagnosis to rule out structural causes of psychosis in patients with schizophrenia. MRIs are internal snapshots of the brain taken slice-by-slice with the use of magnets instead of radiation. These snapshots or images are transmitted over a time sequence onto a monitor screen, where they can be examined in depth. A review of 193 MRI studies taken from 1988 to 2000 showed some consistent structural abnormalities in patients with schizophrenia, including ventricular enlargement; abnormalities of the medial and superior temporal lobes; and frontal, parietal, and cerebellar abnormalities (Lieberman et al, 2008) (see Figure 13-1).

Positron Emission Tomography. Unlike MRI scans, positron emission tomography (PET) scans make use of radioactively labeled probes to track blood flow changes or metabolic or other chemical changes in the brain. Researchers study these brain functional changes to find information about cognitive functioning in patients with schizophrenia.

PET studies are also useful for tracking the action of various medications that are used to treat schizophrenia. By binding a radioactive tracer with a medication, researchers are able to study the specific sites that the medications affect (Lieberman, 2006)

Disease and Trauma

Some studies support the idea that schizophrenia is developmentally related to disease and trauma that occur during the prenatal period or during early childhood Complications that possibly increase risk for schizophrenia include viral infections during pregnancy, rhesus incompatibility, maternal preeclampsia, anemia, and diabetes mellitus. Other stressors include malnutrition and infection, birth complications, and psychoactive drug use. (Lieberman, 2006)

Substance Abuse

Substance abuse is a common concurrent condition in patients with schizophrenia. More than 75% of this population is addicted to nicotine, 30% to 50% is addicted to alcohol, 15% to 25% is addicted to cannabis, and 5% to 10% is addicted to cocaine and amphetamines Research suggests that substance use disorders among patients with schizophrenia are especially common among men with a history of childhood conduct disorder problems (Swartz et al, 2006). Thirthalli and Benegal (2006) cited studies that demonstrated an association between the adolescent use of cannabis and the later development of schizophrenia or schizophreniform disorder. Depending on a person's genes, there is an increased vulnerability to psychosis after cannabis use. Cocaine initiates neurochemical changes in the brain by substituting for the natural endorphins, thus creating an intense craving for the drug. Eventually the long-term user experiences apathy, depression, and anhedonia, which are also often seen in patients with chronic schizophrenia. It is widely published that persons with schizophrenia often indulge in substances such as nicotine, caffeine, and cocaine to self-medicate and perhaps to help improve their attention spans as they attempt to deal with the competing stimuli that are constant disruptions in their lives. According to several studies, 90% of hospitalized patients with schizophrenia smoke cigarettes, and they smoke at a rate of 2 to 4% greater than the general population and more than other patients (Schultz et al, 2007). In addition, there is accumulating evidence that certain drugs used during pregnancy are linked with later schizotypal illnesses during childhood and adolescence.

Psychologic and Psychosocial Theories

Many biologic factors predispose an individual to schizophrenia; however, psychosocial considerations are significant as well. Most models indicate that a person's vulnerability interacts with stressful environmental influences to produce the symptoms of schizophrenia (Sadock et al, 2009). Psychosocial stressors include stressful life events such as interpersonal losses, sociocultural stresses such as poverty or homelessness, or a stressful emotional situation where the patient lives (APA, 2004). Before the explosion in biologic theories, many thought schizophrenia was partially the result of individual or family faults. Some of these flaws included personality characteristics of the patient's mother or father, marital discord, hostile dependency traits of the mother or other caregivers, poor infant–mother bonding, and interpersonal communication problems. With advances in biology, these theories have lost some credibility. However, outcomes related to family climate studies have been defined only in terms of rehospitalization frequency and symptom intensity. Family treatments have the most empiric support for improving symptoms and reducing hospitalizations. Multiple studies have shown that family treatments reduce relapse rates and improve symptoms, adherence to medications and functioning. Several psychosocial rehabilitative interventions have been shown to improve the quality of life in patients with schizophrenia (Schultz et al, 2007).

Cultural and Environmental Theories

Although schizophrenia exists in all socioeconomic groups, persons with schizophrenia more commonly inhabit the lower socioeconomic group. There are various explanations for this condition, one of which has to do with a downward drift hypothesis. According to this hypothesis, the patient with schizophrenia who possesses a low level of social skills either moves into a lower socioeconomic group or fails to rise to a higher group (Sadock et al, 2009). People with schizophrenia also tend to be more numerous in urban and selected immigrant populations There are also racial differences in the diagnosis of schizophrenia. For example, African Americans are more likely to have symptoms attributed to schizophrenia than other racial groups; whereas Hispanics are more likely to be diagnosed with major depression even though they present with psychotic symptoms. History and assessment of the development of signs and symptoms of schizophrenia is critical (Schultz et al, 2007) (see Chapters 3 and 8). Homeless persons with schizophrenia often have additional stressors, such as abject poverty, hunger, sleep deprivation, substance abuse or dependency, violence, posttraumatic stress, infectious diseases, and social isolation (APA, 2004) (see Chapter 30). Individuals with schizophrenia are strongly affected by environmental supports, opportunities, stimulation, and stigma. People who are given opportunities to develop in social and vocational ways are more optimistic and experience better functional outcomes (Lieberman et al, 2008).

EPIDEMIOLOGY

In the United States, schizophrenia has a lifetime prevalence of 0.7 years, and it affects 1% of the population worldwide. It is equally prevalent in males and females, and more common in people living in urban areas (Box 13-2). Men typically present with the disease in their late teens or early 20s, whereas women present in their late 20s or early 30s (Schultz et al, 2007). Although equal numbers of males and females are affected, some data suggest that males may have more severe manifestations of schizophrenia, including an earlier age of onset (by 2 to 4 years), more marked neuropathologic abnormalities, poorer response to treatment, and less favorable outcomes. Mental health research shows that

---

BOX 13-2 EPIDEMIOLOGY OF SCHIZOPHRENIA

New diagnoses of schizophrenia occur in between 0.3 and 0.6 individuals per 1000 persons per year in the United States.

1% of the U.S. population has schizophrenia.

The age of onset is later in females than in males.

Paranoid-type schizophrenia occurs earlier in males than in females.

Disorganized-type schizophrenia occurs earlier in females than in males.

Prevalence is equal for males and females (some sources say males are more affected).

Childhood-onset is rare and affects 1 in 40,000 children (generally occurs prior to age 12).

The oldest age-of-onset group is after the age of 60 years.

A female fetus who is exposed to influenza has a higher risk for schizophrenia than a male fetus.

Males show significantly more structural brain abnormalities from perinatal or early childhood trauma than females do.

patients with schizophrenia report worse quality of life than the general population and than those with physical illnesses; that younger, female, married, and less educated patients report a higher quality of life; that length of illness correlates with lower quality of life; and that more symptoms, especially negative and cognitive symptoms, are related to a lower quality of life. In the United States, people with schizophrenia die approximately 25 years earlier than others in the general population (Lieberman et al, 2008). Accelerated heart disease is the most common cause of death in patients with schizophrenia, possibly influenced by heavy smoking and drug use (Schultz et al, 2007). The incidence of schizophrenia or the frequency of newly diagnosed cases in a specified population during a certain time period is between 0.3% and 0.6% per 1000 persons per year in the United States. The prevalence and prognosis of the disease vary according to socioeconomic, geographic, and cultural factors. Although symptoms of the disorder have common universal characteristics, schizophrenia presents itself in different ways, depending on the patients' situations and demographic backgrounds (Sadock et al, 2009).

Schizophrenia accounts for 20% of all hospital bed days and 50% of all psychiatric beds in the United States. Schizophrenia is the most costly mental illness, and it accounts for roughly 2.5% of annual health care cost in the United States. It is estimated that the economic burden of schizophrenia in the United States is over $65 billion (APA, 2004). Much of this cost was a result of the relapse of psychosis and rehospitalization, because most patients experience a chronic course, although this varies from patient to patient. Loss of work and productivity is also a reason for the high cost.

Child Onset Schizophrenia

Schizophrenia affects approximately 1 in 40,000 children as compared with 1 in 100 adults. The diagnostic criteria are the same as for adults, except symptoms appear before the age of 12 years. Like adults, children experience psychotic symptoms such as hallucinations and delusions, and irrational, paranoid, or bizarre thoughts. They demonstrate withdrawal, difficulty in paying attention, problems carrying out routine daily tasks such as bathing, and an increased risk for suicide (Mayo Clinic Foundation, 2008). Impairments in memory, reasoning, speech, social skills, and emotional expression along with depressed mood are present. Children with prepuberty psychosis show abnormal brain development. MRI scans reveal-fluid filled cavities in the middle of the brain enlarging abnormally between the ages of 14 and 18 years. This increase in fluid-filled cavities coincides with brain tissue volume shrinkage. These children lose gray matter beginning in the rear brain structures, which are involved in attention and perception. This loss of gray matter spreads to the frontal areas of the brain that are responsible for executive functions (planning, organizing, problem solving). Causes of this illness include genetic predisposition, prenatal factors, and stressful life events discussed previously in this chapter (National Institutes of Health, 2005). (see Clinical Alert #1)

❖ CLINICAL ALERT #1

Suicide is the leading cause of premature death among people who have been diagnosed with schizophrenia. Up to 30% attempt suicide and 4% to 10% die as a result of suicide. Suicide is most common within the first 6 years after the initial hospitalization and then again during periods of remission after 5 years of illness (APA, 2004).

Specific risk factors for suicide among individuals with schizophrenia include young age and a high socioeconomic status background. In addition, the person who is experiencing schizophrenia sometimes considers suicide if he or she has a high intelligence level and a high level of achievement and if he or she has set goals high before symptoms occurred and is aware of perceived future losses. Earlier onset and multiple relapses add to suicide risk. People with severe depression who feel hopeless are at risk. People who have expressed suicidal thoughts are also at risk. Despite the identification of these risk factors, it is often difficult to predict whether an individual will attempt suicide. Professionals need to evaluate these patients for suicide risk during all stages of the person's illness (APA, 2004). Overdose of prescribed medications as a method of suicide is not common because antipsychotics have a high therapeutic index and lethal doses are much higher than the doses that produce a therapeutic effect (Schultz et al, 2007).

Late-Onset Schizophrenia

Persons who first experience schizophrenia later in life have better outcomes in all areas. This is possibly because the person was able to be productive and to acquire coping skills before the onset of schizophrenia; better outcomes depend in part on their premorbid functioning (i.e., how they functioned before the illness). For example, if a patient developed good social skills, had a satisfying sex life, and succeeded in academic or vocational achievements before the onset of schizophrenia, the chances for a successful outcome after the illness improve significantly. With the overall increase in longevity, there will be more older patients with schizophrenia in the community. Approximately 80% of people with schizophrenia had an early onset, whereas 20% have a late onset (after the age of 40 years) or a very late onset (after the age of 60 years).

Diagnostic and Statistical Manual of Mental Disorders, fourth edition, text revision (DSM-IV-TR) (APA, 2004).

Course of Illness

The course of illness generally includes recurrent and acute exacerbations of psychotic symptoms (i.e., hallucinations and delusions). Preventing relapse is critical, because each time relapse occurs there is an increased risk for the deterioration of the individual's functions. Schizophrenia develops through premorbid, prodromal, and psychotic phases and follows a stereotypic pattern (APA, 2004).

The **premorbid phase** involves features that contribute to the later development of the illness and includes mild deficits in social, motor, and cognitive functions that occur during childhood and adolescence, such as subtle motor abnormalities during infancy and deficits in social functioning, organizational ability, and intellectual functioning around the ages of 16 to 17 years. In addition, some minor physical anomalies such as variations in limb length and angle and fingerprint patterns may be present in a subgroup of individuals, but these have a low predictive validity. Some people have premorbid functioning in the normal range, whereas others show prolonged poor functioning levels or severe deterioration in functioning before the onset of overt illness. These differences were the basis for the theory of good and poor prognosis, and more recently for concepts of deficit and nondeficit schizophrenia (Lieberman et al, 2008). Researchers have examined the possibility of preventive treatment (premorbid screening), but currently no treatment has been attempted before the onset of the definitive symptoms to avoid the high risk of false-positive results. Premorbid screening is not yet accurate enough to warrant the stigma and cost related to a misdiagnosis (Schultz et al, 2007).

The prodromal phase includes symptoms and behaviors that signal the approaching onset of the illness. This phase may last 2 to 5 years, with the psychotic symptoms that emerge late during this phase marking the beginning of the psychotic phase. Symptoms include the following:

- Mood symptoms (e.g., anxiety, irritability, dysphoria, anguish)
- Cognitive symptoms (e.g., distractibility, concentration difficulties, disorganized thinking)
- Obsessive behaviors
- Social withdrawal and role functioning deterioration
- Sleep disturbances
- Attenuated (weaker) positive symptoms, such as illusions (misinterpreting actual stimuli), ideas of reference (the belief that all events refer to the patient [e.g., "the man on TV is speaking to me"]), magical thinking (the belief that one's thoughts produce outcomes [e.g., "my bad thoughts were responsible for her illness"]), and superstitiousness

The psychotic phase progresses through an acute phase, a recovery or maintenance phase, and a stable phase (APA, 2004):

- *Acute phase.* Individuals experience florid positive symptoms such as delusions and hallucinations as well as negative symptoms such as apathy, withdrawal, and avolition. They are unable to perform self-care activities, and they may require brief hospitalization for their own safety and treatment.
- *Recovery or maintenance phase.* This occurs 6 to 18 months after acute treatment. Symptoms are present, but they are less severe than during the acute phase. By 5 to 10 years after onset, most patients have a leveling off of their illness and functioning. They are generally able to care for themselves with some supervision.
- *Stable phase.* This is the time during which symptoms are in remission, although some symptoms may persist or remain present in milder forms (residual symptoms).

Some people are able to live independently in the community during this time (see Chapter 30).

In most Western countries, 1 to 2 years elapse between the onset of psychotic symptoms and the first treatment. The long-term outcome varies widely from incapacitation to recovery. Approximately 10% to 15% of patients remain free of future episodes, whereas another 10% to 15% remain both chronically and severely psychotic. Better outcomes are associated with the following characteristics (APA, 2004):

- Female gender
- Lack of family history of schizophrenia
- Good pre-illness social and academic functioning
- Higher intelligence
- Married status
- Later age of onset
- Fewer comorbid factors
- Predominately positive symptoms

Socioeconomic Class

The portion of schizophrenia that is attributed to the social problems of the underprivileged class remains controversial (Fortinash and Holoday Worret, 2008; Sadock et al, 2009). The overcrowded poor neighborhoods and the homeless mentally ill persons who are receiving inadequate follow-up care are burdens on this vulnerable population and on society (see Chapter 30)

Culture and Geographic Influences

The manifestations of schizophrenia and its prognosis varies in different cultures. In less-developed nations, the prognosis for schizophrenia is better than in technologically advanced cultures, although severe cognitive impairment is rare in Western nations. Patients in developing countries tend to have a more acute onset, fewer episodic occurrences, and less frequent problems with affect. In addition, cultures in developing countries are more accepting of the illness, because persons with schizophrenia are more readily welcomed back into the family and into the community after an acute episode (Sadock et al, 2009)(see Chapter 8).

CLINICAL DESCRIPTION

According to the DSM-IV-TR classification, a diagnosis of schizophrenia must meet the following criteria: (1) it lasts at least 6 months, at least 1 month of which includes active-phase symptoms; and (2) the active-phase symptoms include at least two of the following manifestations: hallucinations, delusions, disorganized or catatonic behavior, or disorganized speech (see the DSM-IV-TR Criteria box).

Subtypes and Related Disorders

There are five major subtypes of schizophrenia and eight closely related disorders. The five subtypes of schizophrenia are as follows:
1. Paranoid
2. Disorganized (formerly called *hebephrenic*)

DSM-IV-TR CRITERIA

Schizophrenia

A *Characteristic symptoms.* Two (or more) of the following, each present for a significant portion of time during a 1-month period (or less if successfully treated):
1 Delusions
2 Hallucinations
3 Disorganized speech (e.g., frequent derailment or incoherence)
4 Grossly disorganized or catatonic behavior
5 Negative symptoms (i.e., affective flattening, alogia, or avolition)

NOTE: Only one criterion A symptom is required if delusions are bizarre or hallucinations consist of a voice keeping up a running commentary on the person's behavior or thoughts, or two or more voices conversing with each other.

B *Social/occupational dysfunction.* For a significant portion of the time since the onset of the disturbance, one or more major areas of functioning, such as work, interpersonal relations, or self-care, are markedly below the level achieved before the onset (or when the onset is in childhood or adolescence, failure to achieve expected level of interpersonal, academic, or occupational achievement).

C *Duration.* Continuous signs of the disturbance persist for at least 6 months. This 6-month period must include at least 1 month of symptoms (or less if successfully treated) that meet criterion A (i.e., active-phase symptoms) and may include periods of prodromal or residual symptoms. During these prodromal or residual periods, the signs of the disturbance may be manifested by only negative symptoms or two or more symptoms listed in criterion A present in an attenuated form (e.g., odd beliefs, unusual perceptual experiences).

D *Schizoaffective and mood disorder exclusion.* Schizoaffective disorder and mood disorder with psychotic features have been ruled out because either (1) no major depressive, manic, or mixed episodes have occurred concurrently with the active-phase symptoms; or (2) if mood episodes have occurred during active-phase symptoms, their total duration has been brief relative to the duration of the active and residual periods.

E *Substance/general medical condition exclusion.* The disturbance is not due to the direct physiologic effects of a substance (e.g., a drug of abuse, a medication) or a general medical condition.

F *Relationship to a pervasive developmental disorder.* If there is a history of autistic disorder or another pervasive developmental disorder, the additional diagnosis of schizophrenia is made only if prominent delusions or hallucinations are also present for at least a month (or less if successfully treated).

Classification of longitudinal course (can be applied only after at least 1 year has elapsed since the initial onset of active-phase symptoms):

Episodic with interepisode residual symptoms (episodes are defined by the reemergence of prominent psychotic symptoms); also specify if it presents with prominent negative symptoms

Episodic with no interepisode residual symptoms

Continuous (prominent psychotic symptoms are present throughout the period of observation); also specify if it presents with prominent negative symptoms

Single episode in partial remission; also specify if it presents with prominent negative symptoms

Single episode in full remission

Other or unspecified pattern

From American Psychiatric Association: *Diagnostic and statistical manual of mental disorders*, ed 4, text revision, Washington, DC, 2000, American Psychiatric Association.

3. Catatonic
4. Undifferentiated
5. Residual

The closely related disorders include the following:
- Schizophreniform disorder
- Schizoaffective disorder
- Delusional disorder
- Brief psychotic disorder
- Shared psychotic disorder (*folie a deux*)
- Psychotic disorder due to a general medical condition
- Substance-induced psychotic disorder
- Psychotic disorder not otherwise specified

Subtypes

Paranoid Schizophrenia

Paranoid schizophrenia results in less neurologic and cognitive impairment and a better prognosis for the individual.

However, during the active phase of the disorder, the afflicted individual is extremely ill, and the symptoms often make the person a danger to himself or herself or to others.

Delusions tend to be persecutory or grandiose and to have a consistent theme. The persecutory delusions generate anxiety, suspiciousness, anger, hostility, and violent behavior. Auditory hallucinations are common, and they are related to the delusionary theme. Interactions with others are rigid, intense, and controlled (Fortinash and Holoday Worret, 2008; Sadock et al, 2009).

According to the DSM-IV-TR criteria for schizophrenia, a diagnosis of paranoid schizophrenia must meet two of the symptoms in criterion A: the presence of delusions and hallucinations. The other diagnostic criteria for paranoid schizophrenia (i.e., disorganized speech, behavior, and other negative symptoms) are not prominent. The delusions and hallucinations must be present for a significant portion of time over a period of 1 month. This period is shorter if the condition is successfully treated. In addition, if the delusions are unusually bizarre or if the hallucinations involve commanding or commenting voices, only one of the criteria needs to be met. Paranoid schizophrenia often has a sudden onset, and it is sometimes triggered by severe stressors (APA, 2004; Fortinash and Holoday Worret, 2008).

Prognosis. The course of paranoid schizophrenia is varied, but it tends to be more hopeful than the courses of the other subtypes. Of all of the schizophrenias, paranoid schizophrenia often has a better prognosis, particularly in the areas of occupational function and independent living (APA, 2004).

Disorganized Schizophrenia

The disorganized type of schizophrenia was formerly known as *hebephrenic schizophrenia* because of its early dangerous onset and its resulting silly and childish affect. Severe disintegration of the personality characterizes this form of schizophrenia. Speech is disorganized and includes word salad (communication that includes both real and imaginary words in no logical order), incoherent speech, and clanging (rhyming). The associated behavior is odd, and it encompasses grimacing, grunting, sniffing, posturing, rocking, stereotypic behaviors, and uninhibited sexual behaviors (e.g., masturbating in public). Socially, the patient with disorganized schizophrenia is withdrawn and incompetent. There are many cognitive and psychomotor defects, such as concrete thinking, the literal interpretation and use of language, the inability to abstract, and poor coordination. Primary process thinking or prelogical thought that aims for wish fulfillment associated with the pleasure principle characteristic of the id portion of the personality is also a common defect (Fortinash and Holoday Worret, 2008).

The patient with disorganized schizophrenia has poor personal grooming and is often unable to complete activities of daily living without constant structural reminders, because the behavior is aimless and without goals (Sadock et al, 2009). Many negative (type II) symptoms are also present.

Prognosis. Prognosis for the patient with disorganized schizophrenia is poor as a result of an early premorbid history of impaired adjustment that continues after the active phase of the disorder.

Of all the subtypes, paranoid schizophrenia and disorganized schizophrenia have the most clearly defined clinical criteria and have been studied the most. Studies have indicated a wide interest in the cognitive symptoms of schizophrenia, which include memory impairment and a lack of problem-solving skills. Negative symptoms such as emotional blunting, apathy, withdrawal, and avolition (lack of motivation) also remain a focus of concern. After all, it is the residual negative symptoms and the cognitive impairment that prevent individuals with this type of schizophrenia from holding jobs and forming lasting and satisfying relationships. Continued research, new medications, and innovations in therapy all offer hope for a brighter prognosis.

BOX 13-3 POSITIVE (TYPE I) AND NEGATIVE (TYPE II) SYMPTOMS OF SCHIZOPHRENIA

Positive

Delusions, persecutory or grandiose
Delusions of being controlled
Mind-reading or thought-insertion ideas
Hallucinations, auditory or other sensory modes
Bizarre dress and behavior
Thought disorganization and tangential (superficial) speech
Aggressive and agitated behavior
Pressured speech
Presence of suicidal ideation
Ideas of reference

Negative

Flat or inappropriate affect
Poor eye contact
Anhedonic attitude (loss of pleasure) and asocial behavior; withdrawal
Poverty of speech; blocking and lack of inflection
Poor grooming and hygiene
Decreased spontaneity in behavior
Lack of expressive gestures
Avolition (lack of motivation); apathy
Severely disturbed relationships with family, friends, and peers
Inattentiveness

Box 13-3 lists the positive and negative symptoms of these conditions.

Catatonic Schizophrenia

Catatonic schizophrenia has as its predominant feature intense psychomotor disturbance. This disturbance often takes the form of stupor (psychomotor retardation) or excitement (psychomotor excitation). Manifestations of psychomotor disturbance include posturing, immobility, catalepsy (waxy flexibility), mutism, and negativism. There is sometimes automatic obedience followed by excessive and purposeless movement. Other symptoms include echopraxia (imitating the movements of others), echolalia (repeating what was said by another), grimacing, and stereotypic movements. Often there is rapid alteration between these extremes; (Fortinash and Holoday Worret 2008; Sadock et al, 2009).

The onset of catatonic schizophrenia often occurs with dramatic suddenness. An earlier withdrawal sometimes precedes catatonic stupor, which reflects the individual's reduced neurologic ability to filter out stimuli. There is no significant difference in age, sex, or education with regard to the incidence of catatonic schizophrenia. To meet the DSM-IV-TR criteria for catatonic schizophrenia, the patient must exhibit two of the following behaviors: motor immobility or excessive motor activity; extreme negativism (resistance to all instructions and attempts to be moved); peculiar voluntary movements, such as grimacing, stereotypic movements, or posturing; and echolalia or echopraxia (APA, 2004).

The person with catatonic schizophrenia presents a nursing challenge. While in a state of psychomotor excitement, the patient develops hyperpyrexia or collapses from extreme exhaustion. Close watching is necessary to prevent the patient from harming himself or herself or others. Conversely, while the patient is in a stuporous state, the disease is life threatening, because the person approaches a vegetative condition, will not eat, and is in danger of malnutrition or even starvation. Other complications include pressure ulcers from lack of mobility or strange posturing, constipation, or even stasis pneumonia in the older patient.

Delusions often persist throughout the withdrawn state. For example, a patient may believe that he has to hold his hand out flat in front of him because the forces of good and evil are warring on the palm of his hand and he will upset the balance of good and evil if he moves his hand. Oddly enough, although this individual does not seem to attend to the environment around him, when he later returns to a normal state of consciousness, he will remember in detail what has occurred. Nurses need to be aware of this factor and not say or do anything within the stuporous patient's hearing that they would not say or do when the patient is in a normal state of consciousness.

Prognosis. The prognosis for catatonic schizophrenia varies depending on the age of onset, which is often during the early 20s to 30s. It tends to begin with an acute episode that has an identifiable precipitating factor. If the patient has developed a good support system before the illness, he or she will probably recover from the acute phase and have a partial or complete remission. More research is needed for this particular type of illness, especially because it seems to have decreased in Western nations. However, it is more prevalent in developing nations, where remission is usually complete.

Undifferentiated Schizophrenia

Undifferentiated schizophrenia meets criterion A for schizophrenia, but it cannot be classified as paranoid, disorganized, or catatonic. It does not clearly meet the criteria necessary for a diagnosis in any of these conditions, but it has some aspects of each type. The psychotic manifestations are extreme, including fragmented delusions, vague hallucinations, bizarre and disorganized behavior, disorientation, and incoherence; (Fortinash and Holoday Worret, 2008; Sadock et al, 2009). Affect is usually inappropriate rather than flat, and catatonic symptoms are not present.

The onset is usually acute, with excited behaviors such as aggressive hitting or biting. Some patients have chronic schizophrenia, with behavior that no longer fits a specific type but that is a mixture of positive and negative symptoms. Usually the prodromal symptoms have developed over a period of years, and growth and development milestones have often been delayed. Thought processes are fragmented and involve a high level of fantasy content (primary process

thinking). The individual has few or no friends, and family relationships are strained because of the patient's odd and restless behaviors. Dress and grooming are careless, and the individual seems bored with life. Nightmares and early morning awakening disturb the patient's sleep patterns.

Prognosis. The prognosis for the patient with undifferentiated schizophrenia is generally poor, and the course is usually chronic. There are periods of exacerbation and remission; however, the presence of many negative symptoms prevents the patient from doing productive work, pursuing normal relationships, and enjoying life (Sadock et al, 2009).

Residual Schizophrenia

If an individual has had at least one acute episode of schizophrenia and is now free of prominent positive symptoms but has some negative symptoms, then he or she is diagnosed with residual schizophrenia or residual symptoms. In some patients, this pattern continues for years, with or without exacerbations; in others, it seems to decrease to a complete remission. The usual signs of the illness that persist for the individual with chronic or subchronic disease are the mild loosening of associations, illogical thinking, emotional blunting, social withdrawal, and eccentric behavior. Diagnostic criteria for the patient with residual schizophrenia are as follows: (1) the absence of prominent delusions, hallucinations, disorganized speech, and disorganized or catatonic behavior; and (2) continuing evidence of the presence of negative symptoms or reduced positive symptoms.

Prognosis. Prognosis is varied and unpredictable. It depends largely on the patient's premorbid history and the adequacy of his or her support system (Sadock et al, 2009).

Related Disorders
Schizophreniform Disorder

The defining characteristics of schizophreniform disorder are the same as those of schizophrenia, with two exceptions. The first is the duration, and the second is the impairment of function. The duration is at least 1 month but less than 6 months. If symptoms persist for 6 months or longer, then the diagnosis changes to schizophrenia. Social or occupational functioning impairment sometimes does not occur with this disorder, unlike the diagnosis of schizophrenia, with which functional disturbance (e.g., relationships, school, work, self-care) will be present.

Prognosis. Because schizophreniform disorder as a diagnosis involves a shorter onset of symptoms (although many believe it to be a provisional diagnosis for schizophrenia), the functional capacity of the individual is generally higher. In other words, the person is likely to be taking care of himself or herself, to be engaged in relationships, and to be working or going to school.

Schizoaffective Disorder

Schizoaffective disorder is closely related to schizophrenia, but the onset of illness generally occurs later in life. It presents with severe mood swings of either mania or depression, and it also involves some of the psychotic symptoms. Most of the time, mania or depression coexists with the psychotic symptoms, but there must be at least one 2-week period during which there are only psychotic episodes. Researchers still do not know the cause of schizoaffective disorder, but most believe that the etiology is related to a combination of biologic, genetic, and environmental factors. (see Schizoaffective Symptoms box)

SYMPTOMS OF SCHIZOAFFECTIVE DISORDER

SYMPTOMS OF SCHIZOAFFECTIVE DISORDER WITH MANIA	SYMPTOMS OF SCHIZOAFFECTIVE DISORDER, DEPRESSIVE TYPE
• Marked increases in social, work, or sexual activity	• Not eating, weight loss, or both
• Rapid and pressured speech	• Inability to sleep
• Increased risk behaviors, alcohol and drug use, and impulsiveness	• Agitation
	• Loss of interest in usual activities
• Irritability and aggression	• Lack of energy and motivation; fatigue
• Poor judgment	• Low self-esteem and feelings of worthlessness
• Binge spending sprees	• Feeling guilty
• Feelings of invulnerability and grandiose sense of self-importance	• Inability to think or concentrate
• Distractibility	• May perseverate regarding suicide and death
• Inability to sleep	• Hallucinations
• Delusions	• Delusions
• Hallucinations	• Grossly disorganized
• Disorganized thinking	• Immobile
• Bizarre behaviors	• Lack of speech or incoherent speech

Delusional Disorder

The most defining characteristic of delusional disorder is that the fixed false belief is not bizarre, that it may seem plausible, and that it lasts more than a month without causing obvious impairment in functioning. The individual may make decisions that are not obviously irrational. Themes of the disorder may be romantic attachment or spiritual connection to someone, usually of a higher status; efforts to contact the thought-about individual are common and may increase to stalking behaviors. Alternatively, the focus may be more grandiose in that the patient believes that he or she has a great destiny to fulfill. A more troubling type of delusional disorder is rooted in jealousy without evidence that is resistant to logic and that often leads to intense conflict in relationships. Sadness, grief, irritability, and legal problems are common as the delusion persists. It is important to know the culture and religious beliefs of the individual as reference points for determining whether the belief is truly bizarre.

Brief Psychotic Disorder

The chief characteristic of brief psychotic disorder is that it lasts less than a month, after which the individual returns to his or her prior level of functioning. During this time, there may be delusions, hallucinations, incoherent speech, or grossly disorganized and confusing dysfunctional behaviors. The symptoms are not related to substance abuse or medication; however, they can be associated with stressors, and they may include postpartum onset within 4 weeks of delivery. Individuals with this disorder are usually young adults who are at high risk for suicide as a result of grossly impaired judgment, perceptual disturbances, and cognitive disorganization. Care must focus on safety and attention to the basic needs of nutrition and hygiene. The clinician may also specify if there were major life stressors or events preceding the psychosis.

Shared Psychotic Disorder *(Folie a Deux)*

Within the context of a close relationship, an individual may "share" the same delusion with another person. However, aside from the shared delusion (e.g., the FBI is targeting the apartment with radiation), the functional levels of the individuals are intact. Other examples include patients believing that they have won millions of dollars, that they are being followed by the authorities, or that they are being slowly poisoned. If the primary person is a parent, the affected children may literally grow up with the delusions. In such situations, diagnosis and treatment are not sought and may go undetected until there is a problem that is brought to the attention of authorities or social service agencies.

Psychotic Disorder Due to a General Medical Condition

Physical illnesses and their treatments can provoke psychotic symptoms. In some instances, the psychosis may be the first clinical symptom. For example, a high fever caused by a kidney infection may induce hallucinations, confusion, disorganization, or aggressive or bizarre behavior. Other medical conditions that may present as psychosis include strokes, fluid and electrolyte imbalances, systemic lupus erythematosus, hypoxia, encephalitis, and hypoglycemia. The best philosophic approach for clinicians is to assume that psychosis is a manifestation of an underlying and undiagnosed medical problem until it is proven otherwise.

Substance-Induced Psychotic Disorder

Given the prevalence of drugs and alcohol abuse across all age groups, comprehensive histories, family assessments, and laboratory screenings are necessary to rule out a psychosis triggered by reactions to drugs or withdrawal symptoms from long-term abuse. Clinically, hallucinations and delusions are prominent. Tactile hallucinations (e.g., of insects crawling over the skin) are particularly characteristic of alcohol and drug abuse. However, persons with psychosis may use drugs and alcohol as a method of self-medicating. With substance-induced psychoses, the symptoms usually resolve within a month. Although drugs and alcohol are the usual agents, exposure to toxins, carbon monoxide, carbon dioxide, nerve gases, fuel fumes, paint fumes, and other environmental exposures should be considered.

Psychotic Disorder Not Otherwise Specified

Psychotic behaviors (i.e., hallucinations, delusions, confusion, and disorganization) with inadequate information about the related factors may be labeled as *not otherwise specified*. Generally, this type of psychosis cannot be categorized by timeframe, the etiology is unclear, or there are residual symptoms that linger. In addition, the clinical course may be highly complex, with multiple variables that cannot be clearly delineated. Obviously, because this diagnosis provides little information and direction, the clinical staff needs to invest in a more thorough exploration of causes that may have been missed.

Treatment. The following methods are useful for the treatment of schizoaffective disorder and other related disorders:

- *Psychotherapy.* The nurse and the patient work together to establish goals.
- *Medications.* Antipsychotics, antidepressants, lithium, and other mood stabilizers may be given. Often several medications are used in combination.
- *Skills training.* This treatment focuses on interpersonal skills, grooming, hygiene, budgeting, grocery shopping, job seeking, cooking, and other similar activities.

Self-management. Give the following instructions to the patient to help maximize the prognosis:

- Recognize that this is a prolonged illness.
- Identify strengths and limitations.
- Set clear and realistic goals.
- Develop a set of wellness strategies to help with daily living.
- Identify several people who will offer support as needed.
- Plan a regular, consistent, and predictable daily routine.
- Identify external stressors that possibly trigger illness.
- Identify internal symptoms that possibly trigger illness.
- Develop an action plan to deal with external and internal stressors.
- Make only one change in your life at a time.
- Work toward an active and trusting relationship with nurses and other treatment staff.
- Take your medication regularly, as prescribed.
- Identify early signs of relapse, and develop an early warning list.
- After a relapse, slowly and gradually return to your responsibilities.
- Avoid street drugs.
- Discuss any intake of alcoholic beverages with your physician.
- Eat a well-balanced diet.
- Get sufficient rest.
- Exercise regularly.
- Check reality with a trusted individual if you are unsure about the nature of your thoughts or feelings.
- Contrast your behavior with that of others if you are unsure about the nature of your actions.
- Accept that there will be occasional setbacks.

Managing relapse. Give the following instructions to the patient for managing a relapse:

- Develop a plan of action with your nurse or therapist if your relapse signs appear. (Do this during well periods.)
- Involve a friend, family member, or other trusted individual to help you during times of relapse.

The patient's plan should include specific warning signs of relapse, an agreement to notify the nurse or therapist as soon as relapse warning signs appear, an agreement to contact those individuals who will help to reduce stress and stimulation, and a list of specific ways to decrease stress and stimulation and to increase structure.

Prognosis. The prognosis for the diagnosis of schizoaffective disorder is considered guarded because of the duration of the symptoms and their complex emotional highs and lows. Both ends of the emotional spectrum increase the risk of suicide or other impulsive behaviors. The bipolar subtype of schizoaffective disorder with manic symptoms, depressive symptoms, or both, is more common among young adults. The schizoaffective disorder with depressive features only is more common among older adults. However, symptoms may begin at any time during the lifespan. The challenges of recovering and managing the illness are to learn the vulnerabilities for relapse and to recognize exacerbations early during their course.

Symptoms of the Schizophrenias

Neuropsychiatrists have tried to find common threads that link the schizophrenias as well as areas of differentiation that separate them. There is a common underlying theme in schizophrenic disorders that is connected to certain symptom profiles of a perceptual, thought, emotional, cognitive, behavioral, or social nature (see the Clinical Symptoms box).

Perceptual

Hallucinations occur in any of the five receptive senses (auditory, visual, tactile, olfactory, or gustatory), but the auditory area is the most common, with more than 50% of patients with schizophrenia reporting auditory hallucinations (i.e., the hearing of voices that are troubling for the patient) (Lieberman, 2006). Researchers believe that a left hemisphere brain abnormality causes these hallucinations, because the left hemisphere contains the Broca area, which is the language-processing center. From assessment procedures, researchers have determined that the left hemisphere responds to hallucinations as if it were hearing real voices, which may be an indication that the hallucinations are a reflection of the actual delusional thinking of the person with schizophrenia (Hugdahl, 2008).

Patients and families must recognize that hallucinations are symptoms of the illness and that they are real to the patient. Because of this, family attempts to force the truth on the patient are not therapeutic, and they are sometimes even demeaning. Hallucinations respond to a reduction in stress and an increase in antipsychotic medication. They often become less troubling when patients are distracted with

CLINICAL SYMPTOMS

Schizophrenia

Perceptual

Hallucinations
Auditory: may be commanding; content matches delusions
Visual: may see images that are not actually present
Tactile: for example, may feel like he or she is surrounded by spiderwebs
Olfactory and gustatory: may refuse to eat because food seems to smell or taste bad

Illusions
False perceptions caused by misinterpretations of real objects

Altered Internal Sensations
Formication: sensation of worms crawling around inside one's body
Chill: feeling of chills in the marrow of one's bones

Agnosia
Perceptual failure to recognize familiar environmental stimuli, such as sounds or objects seen or felt; sometimes called *negative hallucinations*

Distortion of Body Image
With respect to size, facial expression, activity, amount and nature of detail, or exaggeration or diminution of body parts

Negative Self-Perception
With respect to abilities and competence

Thought

Delusions
Unusual ideas that are not reality based:
  Omnipotence: perception of unrealistic power
  Persecution: perception that someone is out to harm or kill the individual
  Controlling or being controlled: with respect to an outside force or entity

Derealization
Loss of ego boundaries; cannot tell where his or her own body ends and the environment begins; feeling that the world around one is not real or is distorted

Ideas of Reference
Perception that other people or the media are talking to or about the individual

Incorrect Use of Language
Neologisms: invented words
Incoherence: nonsensical thoughts
Echolalia: imitating others' words
Word salad: mixed-up words
Concrete and restricted vocabulary: unable to use abstract reasoning or to conceptualize
Perseveration: persistent repetition of the same ideas

Obsessive Thoughts
Recurring thoughts

Poverty of Thought
Reduction in amount of thoughts

Thought Blocking
Abrupt disruption of flow of thoughts or ideas

Loosening of Associations
Fragmented thoughts noted in incoherent speech

Flight of Ideas
Abrupt change of topic in a rapid flow of speech

Emotional

Labile Affect and Range of Emotions
Apathy: indifferent or dulled response
Flattened affect: restricted facial expressions
Reduced responsiveness
Exaggerated euphoria
Rage

Inappropriate Affect
Laughing at sad events or crying about joyous ones

Disruption in Limbic Functioning
Inability to screen out disruptive stimuli and a loss of the voluntary control of responses

Cognitive
Errors in memory recall and retention, especially working memory
Difficulty with comprehending, processing, and categorizing information
Difficulty sustaining attention: unable to complete tasks and committing errors of omission
Lack of judgment: unable to assess or evaluate situations or to make rational choices
Lack of insight: unable to perceive or to understand the cause and nature of his or her own and others' situations (e.g., his or her own illness)
Difficulty with executive functioning (e.g., planning, decision making, problem solving)

Behavioral

Little Impulse Control
Sudden screaming as a protest of frustration
Self-mutilation to substitute physical pain for emotional pain
Injury to a body part that is believed to be offensive
Responding to command hallucinations

Inability to Cope With Depression
Depressed patient has a 50% risk for suicide
Frequent exacerbations and remissions in a patient who has insight
Lack of social support for help

CLINICAL SYMPTOMS—cont'd

Inability to Manage Anger
Anger and lack of impulse control lead to violence: verbal aggression, destruction of property, injury to others, and homicide

Substance Abuse As Coping
Dulls painful psychologic symptoms

Noncompliance with Medication
May feel it is not needed or has too many side effects

Social
Poor Peer Relationships
Few friends as a child or adolescent
Preference for solitude

Low Interest in Hobbies and Activities
Daydreamer
Not functioning well in social or occupational areas

Preoccupied and detached
Behavioral autism: marked impairment in social and behavioral functioning

Loss of Interest in Appearance
Careless grooming
Introversion

Not Competitive in Sports or Academics
Poor adjustment to school
Withdrawal from activities

May Suffer from the Following:
Attention deficit disorder
Somatic symptoms (i.e., multiple physical problems)
Schizoid or schizotypal traits: solitary, detached, self-absorbed, and socially anxious

---

other activities or strategies. For example, some time-proven methods that are effectively used by mental health personnel include keeping the patient busy, using competing stimuli to drown out the voices (e.g., whistling, clapping, shouting the word *stop*), and teaching the patient not to wait for the voices to occur, but instead engage in some other task or activity that fills idle time. These methods help the patient to occupy the mind with some other activity, or strategy, and tend to reduce agitation. (Fortinash and Holoday Worret, 2007).

Thought

Even adults have a tendency to personalize and misinterpret events, most notably during times of stress or fatigue. It is self-fulfilling to occasionally escape from reality and to imagine ourselves as more powerful or successful than we really are. For those of us without schizophrenia, however, these periods of fantasy are generally short lived and well within our control. What is different in the patient with schizophrenia who is experiencing a delusion during an acute period is that the conviction is fixed, and that person will reject any attempt by well-meaning individuals to explain reality during this time. Arguing with a patient who is experiencing a delusion leads to further mistrust or anger. Families and friends need to realize that delusions are a result of the illness and not stubbornness or stupidity on the part of the patient. Avoid emotional reactions, sarcasm, and threats. An empathetic response is always possible, no matter what the delusion or conviction is.

For example, a patient may believe that he is at the center of a government plot and cannot sleep at night. There are possibly underlying feelings of worthlessness or fear, and the delusion fills the need to be important and protected. An empathetic response is, "It must be difficult not to be able to get some sleep at night and to feel afraid. You are safe here in the hospital, and the care you get will help you feel better." This type of response builds trust, rapport, and, possibly, adherence to the treatment plan that will help the patient to improve (Fortinash and Holoday Worret, 2007). Implications for the psychoeducation of persons with schizophrenia include the following:

- Teaching at times when symptoms are relatively stable
- Simplifying instructions and reducing distractions (or providing distractions to offset symptoms, as necessary)
- Providing both visual and verbal information
- Using direct and clear terms rather than abstractions or concepts
- Teaching in small segments with frequent reinforcement
- Not offering choices, which often confuse the individual; offering more choices as the patient improves

As a result of thought disturbance, speech is affected. Subtle forms of speech disorders are circumstantiality, with which the person digresses to unnecessary details, and tangentiality, which involves responding in a manner irrelevant to the topic at hand. If the person is less impaired, listening for themes helps to identify patient concerns (Sadock et al, 2009).

Thought processes in schizophrenia change with the individual's clinical status. As the clinical status worsens, sometimes thoughts evolve into a world of fantasy or are expressed as autistic thinking (internally stimulated thoughts that are not based in reality), perseveration (persistent repetition of the same idea in response to different questions), poverty of thought (lack of ability to produce thoughts), and loosening of associations (fragmented and incoherent thoughts) (Sadock et al, 2009).

It is difficult to communicate with the patient during these acute phases, and this is frustrating to family and friends. Sometimes nonverbal communication (e.g., writing) is an effective way for these patients to communicate, because thoughts are usually more organized in writing. Concerned individuals should not force themselves to listen to the patient, because this will only frustrate both the patient and the listener. In addition, the patient should not be spoken about as if he or she were not there. Determine where the patient's interests and strengths are, and use music, art, exercise, and movement to communicate during this period (see Chapter 26). Even if the language side of the brain is not functioning, the patient is still able to focus on other activities. For the patient with chronic disease, there is a general decline in intellectual functioning over the years, which presents a real challenge to nurses, families, and caregivers (Lieberman et al, 2008). Patients with chronic schizophrenia have little insight into their illness, and, as such, they experience impaired judgment. Patience, empathy, and understanding are critical factors when caring for patients with chronic schizophrenia.

Emotional

Emotional blunting and a lack of displaying emotions are examples of negative symptoms in patients with schizophrenia. Some people show few emotions, whereas others demonstrate a total lack of facial expression. Some patients also avoid eye contact and have reduced verbal and nonverbal contact with others. The person's speech also lacks inflection, so he or she speaks in a monotone. Some have a lack of gestures (Lieberman, 2006). This decrease in expressed emotions coupled with a monotone and a lack of gestures when speaking makes it difficult to fully appreciate the interaction with the person.

Cognitive

Cognitive disturbances in people with schizophrenia affect everyday functioning. One area that is affected is vigilance. Vigilance is the ability to maintain attention over time. People who are unable to maintain this attention have difficulty following instructions that are critical to their care. Not being able to maintain attention along with having difficulty with verbal fluency also has a negative impact on social and work-related interactions. Other cognitive deficit areas include learning, reasoning, and problem solving. Difficulties in these areas hinder the person's ability to adapt to a rapidly changing everyday world (Lieberman, et al, 2008).

Behavioral

The behavioral disturbance of greatest concern in schizophrenia is the possibility of violence. The risk of violence increases if the patient also has coexisting alcohol abuse, substance abuse, an antisocial personality, or neurologic impairments (APA, 2004). However, these factors do not identify persons who will actually become violent. The challenges for nursing are to note changes in patient behavior, to read the situation accurately, to interact according to the patient's level of crisis, and to intervene at a level that meets the patient's needs (Johnson, 2004). It is important to ask about thoughts of violence and to determine who the intended victim is.

Setting limits and using the behavioral approach are two strategies that are used to manage persistently violent patients. Patients in the community who are more likely to be violent with relapses require mandatory outpatient treatment programs. Mandatory outpatient treatment is court-ordered treatment for those patients with mental illness who may not use services without a court order. Mandatory outpatient treatment should be considered a last resort (American Psychiatric Nurses Association, 2004) (see Chapters 26 and 30).

Social

Poor social competence is one of the hallmarks of schizophrenia, as evidenced by many of the negative symptoms described earlier in this chapter. Typically, people with schizophrenia have a history of a schizoid or schizotypal personality, which includes solitary behaviors, detachment, constricted or inappropriate affect, passive or indifferent responses, and a lack of strong emotions. It is difficult for them to respond to normal social cues, to initiate conversations, to develop relationships with others, and to become productive members of society (see Chapter 14).

Despite research into the biologic causes of schizophrenia, the issue of nature versus nurture still poses questions. There is speculation that children raised by parents with schizophrenia may emulate the parent's poor social behaviors. In addition, the parents of children with schizophrenia may be turned off by their child's inability to relate or display normal emotions. Although many of the older theories of mother and child detachment and poor bonding have lost credibility, these factors linger as a result of mental health's strong affinity for the psychosocial therapies as a viable method of treatment (see Chapters 14 and 26). Studies show that individuals with good verbal memories are better able to learn and retain social skills and therefore have more hope for a productive life within the limitation of their illness. (Sadock and colleagues 2009) state that, of all the diagnostic profiles used to describe schizophrenia, the early works of Bleuler (described earlier in this chapter), and Schneider are the most common. Kurt Schneider (1887–1967) was a German psychiatrist and researcher who followed Bleuler's interest in identifying and classifying the fundamental features of the schizophrenia. He developed "The Schneiderian System" of finding the correlations or commonalities of patients' symptoms. Schneider developed a set of "First Rank Symptoms" specific to diagnosis of schizophrenia's psychotic phase (NIMH, 2005) (Box 13-4).

Biologic Profiles

Neurologic examinations, neuropsychologic tests, and various brain-scanning techniques (neuroimaging) support symptom profiles and are relevant for patients with schizophrenia. Table 13-3 presents some of these examinations. In general, these tests verify findings that schizophrenia involves diffuse and nonlocalizable areas of dysfunction. Evidence of generalized impairment is present in persons with a first episode as well as those with chronic schizophrenia, although

TABLE 13-3	BIOLOGIC PROFILES IN SCHIZOPHRENIA
TEST	**FUNCTION**
Neurologic Examinations	
Apgar rating of the newborn	To rate the functioning of the newborn's nervous system
Physiologic and anatomic testing of the nervous system (general)	To discover infections, lesions, or metabolic problems that affect the nervous system
Neuropsychologic Tests	
Halstead–Reitan battery	To test higher cortical functioning
	To detect early signs of memory and cognitive dysfunction
	To design and evaluate remediation programs (Osmon, 1991)
Luria–Nebraska test battery	To predict behavior by examining neurologic functioning (Meador and Nichols, 1991)
	To assess patient progress in various areas
Eye tracking and auditory tests	To discover information-processing deficits (Perry and Braff, 1994)
Neuroimaging Studies	
Magnetic resonance imaging	To determine structural and functional changes in the brain, which confirm specific anomalies in the brains of individuals who have been diagnosed with schizophrenia
Positron emission tomography	To determine the effects of antipsychotic medications on certain neurotransmitter receptor sites and their various rates of occupancy by studying sections of the brain
Bioelectron activity measure	To measure activity of the brain in patients with schizophrenia with the use of colorized topography

BOX 13-4	DIAGNOSTIC PROFILES DESCRIBED BY BLEULER AND SCHNEIDER

Bleuler

Characteristics of Schizophrenia
Incongruence between feelings and thoughts
Incongruence in the behavioral expression of feelings and thoughts

Four Primary Symptoms of Schizophrenia (see Box 13-1)
Affect is disturbed.
Ambivalence is common.
Associations are loosened.
Autism is present.

Accessory Symptoms
Delusions
Hallucinations

Schneider

First-Rank Symptoms of Schizophrenia
Delusions
Hallucinations
Somatic experiences
Thought broadcasting (i.e., the belief that one's thoughts are broadcast from one's head)
Thought withdrawal (i.e., the belief that one's thoughts have been removed from one's head)

Second-Rank Symptoms of Schizophrenia
Feelings of emotional impoverishment
Mood changes
Perceptual disorders
Perplexity

the degree of impairment usually differs with subtypes. Individuals with schizophrenia seem to have impairments in the stimulus inhibition (gating) circuitry of the brain, which sometimes leads to stimulus overload. Thus, these individuals are handicapped with regard to sorting out and paying attention to the information necessary to solve a problem. Neuroimaging research has demonstrated decreased gray matter volume in the cerebral cortex, reduced volumes of the hippocampus and thalamus, and enlarged lateral and third ventricles and subarachnoid space (Lieberman et al, 2008) (see Figure 13-1).

Modern brain-scanning technology has enabled scientists to assemble not only a structural image of the brain but also a functional image that indicates activity in various areas (Figure 13-4). Forthcoming functional MRI studies, as mentioned previously, will improve this contemporary area of research, because modern technology enables the rapid transmission of information via the Internet.

DISCHARGE CRITERIA

For the patient with schizophrenia to be discharged to the community, the following criteria need to be met. The patient will do the following:

- Demonstrate an absence of suicidality.
- Verbalize the control of hallucinations.

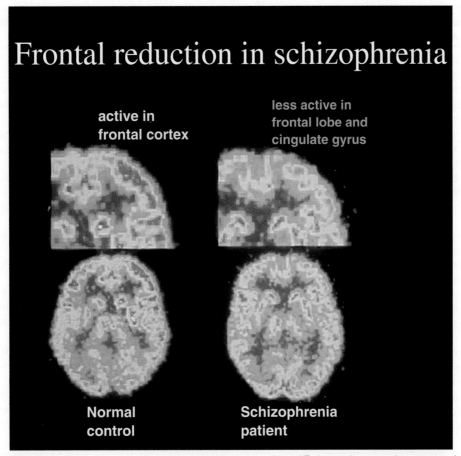

FIGURE 13-4. Positron emission tomography scan with 18F-deoxyglucose shows metabolic activity in a horizontal section of the brain in a control subject *(left)* and in an unmedicated patient with schizophrenia *(right)*. Red and yellow indicate lower activity in the white matter areas of the brain. The frontal lobe is magnified to show reduced frontal activity in the prefrontal cortex of the patient with schizophrenia. (Courtesy of Monte S. Buchsbaum, MD, Mt. Sinai School of Medicine, New York.)

- Identify events or episodes of increased anxiety that worsen symptoms.
- Have a family member or a significant other who is willing to serve as a support network.
- Accept the referral of himself or herself or of a significant other to a physician, therapist, or agency for help and monitoring.
- Accept responsibility for his or her own actions and self-care.
- Verbalize ways of coping with anxiety, stress, and problems encountered in the community.
- Have access to a safe living environment in the community (e.g., own home, board-and-care facility, halfway house).
- Use known community resources, such as support groups, day care centers, and vocational or rehabilitation programs.
- Explain the following about medication: its importance, its expected effects, its adverse effects, the prescribed dosage and the times for taking the medication, and the effects of the interaction of the medication with other substances (e.g., food, alcohol).

THE NURSING PROCESS
ASSESSMENT

The assessment of the individual with schizophrenia is complicated because of the different symptom profiles of the various subtypes of the condition. Nurses obtain subjective data through symptom reporting and by the descriptions of behavior provided by significant others. Nurses perform objective assessment observation by using rating scales and by checking biologic indicators as described in earlier sections. For psychiatric mental health nurses, it is important to not lose sight of the biologic focus that is so prevalent in the other specialties. For nurses, one of the critical components of assessment is what the patient says during the interview. However, for people with psychotic disorders, there is impaired processing of perceptual information. As a result, physical symptoms such as pain are misperceived or misread. Likewise, for the nurse, it can be difficult to tell the difference between a genuine complaint and a delusion (Reeves and Torres, 2003). For example, the patient who tells you she is pregnant and about to deliver a baby

NURSING ASSESSMENT QUESTIONS

Schizophrenia and Other Psychotic Disorders

1 What problems have you been having recently? How do you feel differently now than before? *To determine the patient's perception of the problem*

2 Do you now or have you ever used alcohol or drugs? If so, when and how often? *To determine the patient's use of substances*

3 Have you heard (sounds, voices, or messages), seen (lights or figures), smelled (strange, bad, or good odors), tasted (strange, bad, or good tastes), or felt (touching, warm, or cold sensations) anything that others who were present did not? *To determine if the patient is having hallucinations*

4 What are the voices like that you hear? What do they say? Are they troubling for you? *To determine if they instruct the patient to harm himself or herself or others*

5 It sounds like you're very scared right now. Can you focus on my voice?

6 I don't hear any other voices but yours and mine. What are the voices saying? *To screen for possible risk factors or messages*

7 What helps to make the voices go away or get quieter? *To reinforce the patient's ability to control or dampen the hallucinations when they occur*

8 Let's see if doing something (crafts, walking, singing, listening to music, or reading out loud) helps with the hallucinations. Sometimes distractions really help them to go away.

Questions to Determine if the Patient is Experiencing Delusions

1 Do you believe that someone or something outside of you is controlling you in some way? Are you able to control other people?

2 Do you believe that you are being watched or followed?

3 Are people talking about you? If yes, explain how you know this.

4 Are you experiencing guilt? Do you believe that you have anything to be guilty about? Do you think that you are a bad person? If yes, what makes you believe this?

Examples of What to Say if the Patient is Delusional

1 I know that you believe the CIA has you under surveillance. Let's go play a game and see if you can teach me to play Euchre.

2 I know that you believe there are aliens in your body. I see that you and sometimes people with schizophrenia have beliefs and experiences others do not because of chemical imbalances. Let's go take a walk.

3 You seem to get more scared in the afternoon and to hear more voices then. Let's talk about your niece who's coming to visit tomorrow.

4 Since I don't see the bugs on your skin, let's apply some lotion and see if that provides some relief.

---

may have menstrual cramps, endometriosis, a sexually transmitted disease, constipation, or any number of ailments that she interprets as a pregnancy. Likewise, a patient who tells you that his heart is broken could have angina, acid reflux, or other real complaints. Listening attentively to the patient and completing a physical assessment are necessary for an adequate assessment. Furthermore, paying attention to vital signs as well as nutrition, exercise, and sleep patterns is necessary.

Patients with schizophrenia are at increased risk for metabolic syndrome, and nurses need to assess for this syndrome. The metabolic syndrome is a cluster of findings that include increased visceral adiposity, which the nurse measures by waist circumference; hyperglycemia; hypertension; and dyslipidemia (Meyer, 2005). *PHATS* is a mnemonic that helps the nurse to monitor metabolic syndrome risk factors quickly (Box 13-5). The symptoms come from the National Cholesterol Education Program criteria.

In addition to the biologic components, the nursing assessment needs to include psychologic ratings (e.g., the mental status examination rating scale) to organize data (see Chapter 3). The mental status examination considers the categories of appearance, behavior, orientation, memory, thought processes, perceptual processes, intellectual functioning, feelings (mood) and affect, insight, and judgment.

BOX 13-5	PHATS*
Blood pressure	>130/85 mm Hg
High-density lipoprotein cholesterol level	<40 mg/dL in men <50 mg/dL in women
Abdominal obesity	Waist circumference: >102 cm in men >88 cm in women
Triglyceride level	≥150 mg/dL
Sugar level	Fasting blood glucose: ≥110 mg/dL

From Grove GA: Beware of PHATS in metabolic syndrome, *Current Psychiatry*, Vol 4(5):98, 2006.
*Three of five positive criteria indicate the presence of metabolic syndrome.

Four of these categories are particularly important for patients with schizophrenia: disturbances in perception, thought, feelings, and behavior (see the Nursing Assessment Questions box).

For children and adolescents, take into consideration the developmental status of the individual when assessing the positive and negative symptoms. Remember that, in children, normal patterns of thinking are concrete rather than abstract. Likewise, consider the patient's age when assessing impulse control, because it is not normally fully developed until adolescence.

NURSING DIAGNOSIS

Nursing diagnoses are formulated from the information that is obtained during the assessment phase of the nursing process. The accuracy of each diagnosis depends on a careful in-depth assessment. Nursing diagnoses are prioritized according to patient needs, from urgent to least urgent. Some of the more common diagnoses that are applicable to schizophrenia include the following:

- Risk for suicide
- Risk for self-directed violence
- Risk for other-directed violence
- Disturbed sensory perception
- Disturbed thought processes
- Impaired verbal communication
- Ineffective coping
- Interrupted family processes
- Self-care deficit (bathing/hygiene, dressing/grooming, feeding, toileting)
- Social isolation
- Risk-prone health behavior

OUTCOME IDENTIFICATION

Outcome identification is an estimate of the behavioral changes that are anticipated after interventions occur. The severity of the symptoms, the cultural setting, and the prognosis for the particular diagnosis all influence a patient's outcomes. The outcomes of schizophrenia therefore result from complex interactions. Outcomes are prioritized according to patient needs, from most urgent to least urgent. The patient will do the following:

- Demonstrate an absence of suicidal behaviors or violent behaviors toward others.
- Demonstrate an absence of self-mutilating behaviors.
- Demonstrate a significant reduction in hallucinations and delusions.
- Demonstrate reality-based thinking and behavior.
- Engage in his or her own hygiene and grooming and perform activities of daily living.
- Socialize with peers and staff and participate in all groups.
- Adhere to the prescribed medication regimen and verbalize an understanding of the role of medications in reducing psychotic symptoms.
- Demonstrate more functional coping and problem-solving methods.
- Participate in discharge planning with his or her family and significant others.

PLANNING

Planning nursing interventions and treatment that is geared toward the whole person and his or her social environment, including the family, is challenging. Because behavioral problems come from many sources and range from less serious to extremely serious, nurses need to consider interventions at a variety of levels and prioritize according to patient needs, from the most urgent to the least urgent. Medical interventions generally focus on underlying biologic factors and involve diagnostic procedures such as neuroimaging, somatic strategies, and treatment with medication. The nurse's role at this level is to prepare the patient and his or her family by explaining the rationale for the interventions and assisting with treatment adherence. The nurse also uses nursing measures at this level that are based on his or her knowledge of basic biologic functions and needs.

Interpersonally and socially, patients with schizophrenia are disadvantaged by being unable to view things from the perspective of others. Because of the inability to abstract and correctly interpret things, the individual with schizophrenia sees others as unpredictable and often misinterprets others' words and actions. Role-playing scenarios, which help patients to see things from another person's perspective, are helpful. Socialization is often a focus of the treatment plan, because it includes the patient in activities that are supportive and nonthreatening and provide helpful feedback about how the patient presents himself or herself to others. Social skills groups are useful for helping the individual build interpersonal skills. Nurses need to avoid power struggles (see the Case Study).

Family interactions are particularly difficult for the patient with schizophrenia. If the treatment team does not involve the family or significant supporters during the treatment planning for services after discharge, the family will be unable to help the patient to maintain community support, which will likely lead to relapses and rehospitalizations.

IMPLEMENTATION

It is important to involve the patient and family in the treatment process and to explain all interventions and reasons for care. Well-planned interventions will still be challenging for the nurse if there are misunderstandings about what to expect or if there is resistance from patient, family, or others. Financial and environmental limitations will also be problematic for such interventions. As much as possible, patients need to set their own goals and pace for treatment and progress.

In the beginning, some patients are so ill that they cannot understand or accept an appropriate effort to help. In that case, the nurse needs to work on establishing a therapeutic relationship first before the patient will accept the well-intended interventions.

An existing therapeutic relationship between the patient and the nurse will be expanded later to include the patient's family or significant others to increase the lasting effectiveness of the interventions. In some cases, the nurse will need to make interventions at yet another level: the school or the workplace. All involved individuals need to be aware of the what, why, and how of the therapeutic plan so that they are able to work as a team.

CASE STUDY

Lance, a 35-year-old man with chronic schizophrenia, was living in a single room in a downtown hotel that houses people with mental illness. Lance was never able to budget his minimal income to last the whole month. He had a fixed delusion that he owned the hotel where he lived but that the manager and the government were defrauding him of his rent money. When Lance was short of cash at the end of the month, he became abusive and aggressive. When Lance was assaultive, the manager called the police, and Lance was readmitted to the psychiatric hospital involuntarily for danger-ousness to others. After about 10 days, he was discharged to the same hotel, where he would live quietly for a while and help the manager with tasks until the next delusional episode. This was a repetitive pattern for Lance, who had no support from relatives or friends.

Critical Thinking

1 What is the significance of Lance's delusion?
2 Lance received good care at the psychiatric hospital, and standard outcome criteria for discharge were always met. If this pattern continued, what would the chances be that Lance would hold onto his delusion?
3 Why might a nurse's attempt to challenge the delusion be risky? What are some teaching strategies that nurses could use with Lance? In what form would they best be implemented? When Lance is stable, can he identify any early warning signs that things are starting to break down for him? Is Lance willing to accept or identify someone as a supporter who can help him?
4 If you were a community mental health nurse, how would you perform follow-up care for Lance? Consider his money-management issues and how these may affect his ability to obtain his medications, food, and other necessities at the end of each month.
5 What signs of escalating anxiety would you look for in Lance's behavior? How would you manage his anxiety?

When patients are in the most acute phase of their illness, choices are more limited, and the structured interventions are the most helpful. However, as the patient's condition improves, he or she can take advantage of more options, and nurses are able to develop a recovery model of hope and care.

The family's economic situation also deserves attention. Health care personnel are not usually thinking about the cost of implementing a care plan that involves therapy, medication, diet, transportation access to outpatient care, or other factors that involve unplanned expenses. It is important to assess for such expenses, to problem solve for related issues, and to include some solutions with the plan. Interventions are prioritized as much as possible according to patient needs, from most urgent to least urgent.

Nursing Interventions

On the basis of the overall nursing assessment, nursing inter-ventions do the following: (1) supplement the individual's activities of daily living (ADL) and instrumental activities of daily living (IADL); (2) manage the environment; (3) provide protection of the patient, others, family members, and sig-nificant other; (4) encourage self-management; and (5) manage relapse. Most care settings (e.g., hospital inpatient units, residential facilities, group homes, subacute care set-tings) require nurses to manage or direct the care of a group of patients (see Chapters 26 and 30).

Supplement Activities of Daily Living, Instrumental Activities of Daily Living, and Self-Care

- Assist with personal hygiene, appropriate dress, and grooming until the patient is able to function indepen-dently. *This helps to prevent physical complications and to preserve self-esteem.*
- Establish routine times and goals for self-care, and add more complex tasks as the patient's condition improves. *Routine and structure tend to organize and promote reality in the patient's world.*
- Spend intervals of time with the patient each day to engage in nonchallenging interactions. *This helps to ease the patient into the community by first developing trust, rapport, and respect.*

Manage the Environment. Caregivers need to carefully monitor the environment and actively monitor the noise, light, and aesthetic surroundings of the patient to promote calmness and order. From a neurologic perspective, the exter-nal stimulation is critical if not requisite for the appropriate processing of information and stimuli.

- Observe and monitor risk factors, specifically with regard to the potential for suicide or violence toward others. *This promotes the safety of the patient and others and reduces the risk for violence.*
- Minimize environmental stimulation. *This promotes a quiet and soothing setting that will lessen the patient's impulsivity and agitation and prevent accident or injury.*
- Provide frequent timeouts or brief, low-key interactions. *This calms the patient by providing opportunities for rest, relaxation, and the ventilation of impulsive feelings, which reduces the risk of acting-out behaviors.*
- Accompany the patient to group activities, beginning with the more structured and less threatening ones and gradu-ally incorporating more informal and spontaneous activi-ties. *This promotes the patient's socialization skills and expands the reality base in a nonthreatening way.*
- Act as a role model for social behaviors in interactions by maintaining good eye contact, appropriate social distance, and a calm demeanor. *This helps the patient to identify appropriate social behavior.*
- Keep all appointments for interactions with the patient. *This promotes patient trust and self-esteem.*
- Hold onto hope for patients until they are able to have hope for themselves. Increase the patient's level of partici-pation in his or her care as the patient's condition improves to the extent that the patient is able. Allow the patient to have choices within the limits of the setting. Identify the patient's strengths and assets, and incorporate these into his or her treatment plans. Focus on activities and tasks

that the patient can perform versus focusing on the patient's limitations. *These interventions promote the patient's hope and strengths and empower the patient as he or she strives to achieve mental and emotional health.*

Provide Protection for the Patient, Others, Family Members, and Significant Others. Hallucinations and sensory stimulation may exhaust an individual who is struggling for control. Monitoring the content of what is said is often helpful when trying to recognize themes that can help keep people safe, and it can alert caregivers to triggers or the escalating potential for patient violence towards himself or herself or others. Removing the stimuli or reducing access to the person or object often alleviates anxiety and helps to promote self-control.

- If the individual is impulsive or hyperactive with poor judgment, monitor for safety, and use distraction and redirection. As the individual experiences problems with thinking and perception, caregivers need to be very vigilant and use their interpersonal skills to channel energy and distract the patient from his or her hallucinations.
- If the patient is confused, paranoid, or acting bizarrely, remove potential weapons from the environment; this ensures the safety of all. However, family members may be defensive, so the nurse needs to be culturally sensitive.
- If the individual is scared or acting frightened, increase the physical space around him or her, and approach him or her calmly, with no surprises. The struggle to interpret stimulation increases the time that the patient needs to cognitively process the environment; by not provoking a closed-in or trapped feeling, the patient feels safer and is less impulsive.

Self-management. Most patients—particularly if their illness has been long term—have developed self-care strategies for coping with their confusion, hallucinations, and delusions. Asking what works to block or quiet hallucinations often reveals strategies that the person has used before; the nurse can then prompt the patient to use these skills when needed.

- If the patient is experiencing auditory hallucinations, encourage him or her to use headphones to listen to music, hum, whistle, or talk to others. Moving the vocal cords structures the stimulation within the brain and dampens or mutes auditory hallucinations. Headphones literally focus the attention on a louder source of stimulation that is more appealing than accusatory or paranoid delusions.
- Support and monitor prescribed medical and psychosocial interventions. This encourages the patient and the family to participate in the treatment plan, and it prevents the patient's behavior from escalating into violence.
- Use clear, concrete statements rather than abstract, general statements. The patient is not always able to understand complex messages, and, as such, the patient sometimes will develop misperceptions or hallucinations. Individuals with schizophrenia generally respond better to concrete messages during the acute phase.
- Attempt to determine factors that worsen the patient's hallucinatory experiences (e.g., stressors that trigger

sensory-perceptual disturbances). Although hallucinations have a biochemical etiology, outside stressors sometimes intensify hallucinations in a vulnerable patient. Identifying such stressors will help to prevent the severity of the hallucinatory experience.

- Praise the patient for reality-based perceptions, the reduction or cessation of aggressive or acting-out behaviors, and appropriate social interaction and group participation. Warranted praise reinforces the repetition of functional behaviors when given at appropriate times during the treatment plan, such as when medication has begun to take effect.
- Distract the patient from delusions that tend to exacerbate aggressive or potentially violent episodes. Engaging the patient in more functional and less anxiety-provoking activities increases the reality base and decreases the risk for violent episodes that troubling delusions cause.
- Focus on the meaning and look for themes of the patient's delusional system rather than focusing on the delusional content itself. This helps to meet the patient's needs, it reinforces reality, and it discourages false beliefs without challenging or threatening the patient.
- Assess the patient's self-concept. A low self-concept results from social isolation.
- Listen actively to the patient's family members and significant others, and allow them to express their fears and anxieties about mental illness. Give them support and empathy, and emphasize the patient's strengths. This helps the patient to express emotions, and it assists with calming the patient's irrational fears while acknowledging realistic concerns. It also promotes hope and bonding between the family members or significant others and the patient.

Managing Relapse. Give the following instructions to the patient for managing a relapse:

- Encourage and explore support groups for patients with mental illnesses. Most self-help groups are organized and facilitated by other patients, which provides a role model for hope and recovery as well as practical information about what works to manage symptoms.
- Educate the patient and family members and significant others about the patient's symptoms, the importance of medication compliance, and the continued use of therapeutic support services after discharge. This facilitates learning; increases the knowledge base of patients, family members, and significant others; ensures the patient's continued therapeutic support; and possibly prevents relapse after discharge from the hospital.
- Refer the patient to a patient network. For example, Wellness Recovery Action Planning is a patient curriculum that takes the patient step by step through the development of a plan for relapse prevention on the basis of that patient's strengths, social network, and preferences.

Additional Treatment Modalities

It is important that the mental health interdisciplinary treatment team members work together to manage each patient's mental and emotional disorders and symptoms.

Consequently, team meetings are common in the psychiatric setting. Psychiatric mental health nurses, psychiatrists, psychologists, social workers, occupational therapists, recreational therapists, pharmacologists, nutritionists, primary care providers, special education teachers (for children and adolescents), and other support staff come together to communicate their expertise regarding the patient's diagnosis, problems, and treatment plans. Briefly described in the Additional Treatment Modalities box are the various goals and activities of these collaborative professionals in their respective disciplines.

ADDITIONAL TREATMENT MODALITIES

Schizophrenia

Therapeutic methods to prevent and manage violence:
  Psychopharmacology
  Somatic therapy
  Milieu therapy
  Behavior modification
Specific psychosocial rehabilitation interventions:
  Assertive community treatment
  Family interventions
  Supported employment
  Cognitive behavioral therapy
  Social skills training
  Early intervention programs
Personal therapy
Group therapy
Patient education
Case management
Guided imagery
Assertiveness training
Exercise, movement therapy, and dance therapy
Occupational and recreational therapy
Community patient and family programs

Psychopharmacology

Psychopharmacology is the somatic treatment of choice for schizophrenia. The pharmacist gives medications to patients with psychiatric disorders according to the physician's prescription and stays informed about new developments in psychotropic drugs. In addition, the pharmacist—in collaboration with the physician and advanced practice nurses—educates the staff regarding the actions and side effects of the newer neuroleptic drugs. The pharmacist also consults with the psychiatrist about the chemical properties of the medications and their interactions with food and other drugs. In many institutions, the pharmacist also takes some responsibility for patient and family education.

Antipsychotic drugs are indicated for schizophrenia. Typical or first-generation antipsychotic drugs are high-affinity antagonists of dopamine D2 receptors, and they are most effective for reducing the positive psychotic symptoms (e.g., hallucinations delusions). However, these same medications have high rates of neurologic side effects (e.g., extrapyramidal symptoms (EPS); tardive dyskinesia), because they block dopamine, which is a neurotransmitter that is responsible for smooth muscle movement in the extrapyramidal nerve tracts. These are serious movement disorders that must be assessed and treated as soon as possible. The second-generation or atypical antipsychotics drugs promise increased efficacy and safety. The atypical drugs generally have a lower affinity for dopamine D2 receptors, so they may not produce the severe movement disorders that occur with the typical antipsychotics. The atypical drugs also have greater affinity for other neuroreceptors (e.g., serotonin, norepinephrine), and they target negative symptoms more effectively (Leiberman et al, 2008; Schultz et al, 2007).

Psychotropic drugs often have serious side effects (see the Research for Evidence-Based Practice box and Medication Key Facts box). Three of the most serious are akathisia (extreme restlessness), tardive dyskinesia (late-occurring EPS,

---

RESEARCH FOR EVIDENCE-BASED PRACTICE

Swanson JW, et al: Comparing antipsychotic medication effects on reducing violence in persons with schizophrenia. *Br J Psychiatry* 193:37-43, 2008.

Clinical Antipsychotic Trials of Intervention Effectiveness (CATIE) compared the newer atypical medications quetiapine (Seroquel), olanzapine (Zyprexa), risperidone (Risperdal) and ziprasidone (Geodon) with the older antipsychotic perphenazine (Trilafon). Results that were previously reported showed that perphenazine was just as effective in treating symptoms of schizophrenia symptoms than the newer atypical types. This new analysis examined whether any of the medication reduced the frequency of violence, a rare symptom associated with the disorder. Researchers from Duke University examined data from the 1445 CATIE participants for which baseline information on violent behaviors was available. They found that among the 653 participants who completed six months of treatment on their initially assigned medication, the frequency of violent acts declined from 16% to 9% overall. None of the atypical medications performed better than perphenazine, and quetiapine particularly appeared to be less effective than perphenazine. Those who took the medication as directed were less likely to be violent, except for those who had a history of childhood conduct problems. Those who lived with others, had substance use problems, had been victimized in the past, and were of lower socioeconomic status, were more likely to have problems with violent behavior regardless of the medication usage. The researchers concluded that contrary to some previous studies, the atypical antipsychotics have no advantage over the older medication in reducing violence. Also, violence associated with situations unrelated to the disorder, such as a history of conduct problems, are unlikely to be treated effectively with antipsychotics alone. Participants with these risk factors would require more intensive psychosocial or family-based treatments in order to reduce violent behavior.

Schizophrenia

Antipsychotics (Neuroleptics)

Weight, body mass index, fasting blood glucose, and lipid levels should be obtained at baseline and periodically during the course of treatment.

Conventional Antipsychotics

Chlorpromazine (Thorazine), fluphenazine (Prolixin), perphenazine (Trilafon), and thioridazine (Mellaril)

The use of conventional agents has dropped dramatically with the advent of atypical (second- and third-generation) antipsychotic agents, although recent studies have concluded that the use of low to moderate doses of mid-potency first-generation antipsychotics should be considered more frequently.

There is a high incidence of tardive dyskinesia* and agranulocytosis (marked decrease in number of granulocytes).

These drugs may cause seizures, NMS[†], cardiac arrest, tachycardia, and respiratory depression.

Alcohol and other central nervous system (CNS) depressants may increase these drugs' hypotensive effects as well as CNS and respiratory depression.

Lithium and epinephrine may increase neurologic toxicity.

Monoamine oxidase inhibitors, tricyclic antidepressants, and anticholinergic agents may increase anticholinergic effects.

Smoking decreases plasma levels.

Children are more susceptible to dystonias.

Elderly female patients have a greater risk of developing extrapyramidal side effects (EPSEs).[‡]

Herbal considerations: Betel palm and kava kava may increase the risk for EPSE.[‡]

Dietary considerations: Caffeine may increase akathisia and agitation.

Second-Generation (Atypical) Antipsychotics

Clozapine (Clozaril), olanzapine (Zyprexa), quetiapine (Seroquel), risperidone (Risperdal), and ziprasidone (Geodon)

Agranulocytosis may occur with clozapine.

Alcohol and other CNS depressants may increase CNS depression.

Extrapyramidal symptom-producing medications may increase EPSEs,[‡] especially with olanzapine and risperidone.

EPSEs may occur; TD* and NMS[†] are rare. NMS[†] is greater with quetiapine, and EPSE[‡] is greater with higher doses of Risperdal.

Herbal considerations: Betel palm and kava kava may increase the risk for EPSE.[‡]

Dietary considerations: Caffeine may decrease the clozapine level.

Third-Generation (Atypical) Antipsychotics

- Aripiprazole (Abilify)
- EPSE[‡] and NMS[†] occur rarely.
- Lithium and other antipsychotics increase EPSE.[‡]
- *Herbal considerations:* Cola tree, hops, nettle, and nutmeg increases neuroleptic effects. Betel palm and kava kava increase EPSEs.[‡]

Medication For EPSE And NMS

Dopamine Agonist

Amantadine (Symmetrel)

Its use is indicated for EPSE[‡] and NMS.[†]

Anticholinergics, antihistamines, phenothiazine, and tricyclic antidepressants may increase the anticholinergic effects of amantadine.

Hydrochlorothiazide may increase the amantadine blood concentration and risk for toxicity.

Herbal considerations: Belladonna and henbane increase the anticholinergic effect.

Antihistamine

Diphenhydramine (Benadryl)

Anticholinergics: Use of this drug may increase their anticholinergic effects.

Monoamine oxidase inhibitors may increase the anticholinergic and CNS depressant effects of diphenhydramine.

This drug is not recommended for children, neonates, or premature infants because of the increased risk for paradoxic reactions. Overdosage in children may result in hallucinations, seizures, and death.

Herbal considerations: Corkwood and henbane leaf increase anticholinergic effects.

β-Blocker

Propranolol (Inderal)

Abrupt withdrawal may result in sweating, palpitations, headache, and tremors.

Diuretics and other antihypertensives may increase the hypotensive effect.

Nonsteroidal anti-inflammatory drugs may decrease the antihypertensive effect.

Selective serotonin reuptake inhibitors decrease metabolism and increase propranolol effects.

Herbal considerations: Aconite may increase toxicity and lead to death.

Benzodiazepines

Diazepam, lorazepam, and clonazepam

These drugs have a beneficial effects for akathisia and acute dyskinesia.

Anticholinergic Agents

Benztropine (Cogentin)

This drug may produce severe paradoxic reactions that are marked by hallucinations, tremor, seizures, and toxic psychosis.

Amantadine, anticholinergics, and monoamine oxidase inhibitors may increase the effects of benztropine.

Antacids and antidiarrheals may decrease the absorption and effects of benztropine.

Elderly patients are more sensitive and are thus more likely to develop anticholinergic delirium.

Herbal considerations: Kava kava, jaborandi, and pill-bearing spurge decrease benztropine's effects.

---

*Tardive dyskinesia is a neurologic syndrome that consists of abnormal, involuntary, irregular choreoathetoid movements of the muscles, the head, the limbs, and the trunk that are caused by the long-term use of neuroleptic drugs. This condition is manifested as tongue protrusion, puffing of the cheeks, and chewing or puckering of the mouth; it occurs rarely, but it may be irreversible.

[†]NMS is a life-threatening neurologic disorder caused by an adverse reaction to antipsychotic drugs; it includes high fever, sweating, unstable blood pressure, stupor, muscle rigidity, and autonomic dysfunction. (Adapted from Schultz, et al, Schizophrenia: A Review. *Am Fam Physician* 15;75(12): 1821-1829, 2007.)

[‡]EPSEs are serious reactions that appear to be related to high dosages of neuroleptics. They are divided into three categories: (1) akathisia, which is the subjective feeling of muscular discomfort that causes patients to become agitated, to pace, to alternately sit and stand, and to feels a lack of control; (2) Parkinsonian symptoms, which present as muscle stiffness, cogwheel rigidity, shuffling gait, perioral tremor, hypersalivation, and mask-like facial expression; and (3) acute dystonias, which are spasmodic movements caused by slow, sustained, and involuntary muscle contractions such as torticollis, opisthotonos, and oculogyric crisis and can involve the neck, the jaw, the tongue, or the entire body.

which may be irreversible), and neuroleptic malignant syndrome (NMS), which can be potentially fatal. Acute dystonic reaction (neck or nuchal rigidity) is another troubling side effect that is commonly seen in the clinical setting (see Chapter 25).

Future Directions in Pharmacology. The National Institute of Mental Health (NIMH) established the Measurement and Treatment Research to Improve Cognition in Schizophrenia (MATRICS) program. MATRICS program researchers look at the brains of both healthy people and people with schizophrenia to see how they function. The information obtained during problem-solving tasks identifies potential molecular targets for new cognition-enhancing medications. In addition, the MATRICS program supports the development of a new test to measure cognition in people with schizophrenia. The results of the new tests will help to determine whether the cognition-enhancing medications are working (NIMH, 2005).

The Role of the Nurse in Pharmacotherapy. The role of the nurse in collaboration with the physician and pharmacist is to support or participate in drug research that leads to effective treatment outcomes for patients with schizophrenia but with minimal or no debilitating side effects. Although the newer atypical antipsychotic medications show promise for improving positive symptoms and an even greater advantage for the improvement of negative symptoms, there are still many challenges when treating patients with schizophrenia and helping their families to understand and cope with the illness. These challenges include encouraging ongoing adherence to drug therapy, promoting medication education, and providing lifelong skills for reintegration into the community (see Chapter 30).

Quality-of-life issues are also important with the long-term drug treatment of patients with schizophrenia. Nurses, the health care team, and families need to consider and manage potential adverse effects, such as weight gain, diabetes mellitus, sexual dysfunction, cardiac effects, cognitive impairment, and—first and foremost—risk for suicide). As drug research continues to evolve, most nurses, clinicians, and researchers agree that the best treatment practice consists of medication in combination with other treatment modalities and ongoing community involvement. Older adults often require special consideration regarding their medication regimen, especially those with compromised physical health. They should be provided with the lowest dose of medication that can provide the desired therapeutic effect and minimal side effects. Drug to drug combinations should also be monitored carefully in older adults (see Clinical Alert #2).

When a patient is discharged to the family and community, one important criterion is that he or she accepts responsibility for self-care, particularly with respect to medication. This has important implications for health teaching by nurses (Patient and Family Teaching Guidelines box).

Interventions for Agitation Symptoms. Research indicates that the rapid control of acute agitation in schizophrenia is achieved with the use of certain atypical antipsychotics and involves a low incidence of extrapyramidal symptoms.

❖ CLINICAL ALERT #2
Antipsychotics and the Elderly

For older individuals, the use of antipsychotic medications must be carefully managed. Among elderly patients who are taking conventional or atypical antipsychotic medications, there is an increase in cardiac complications that result in death. Since 2005, the U.S. Food and Drug Administration has required all manufacturers of atypical antipsychotic to add a black box warning to their labels that describes an increased risk of 1.6 to 1.7 related to cardiac events or infections. Diagnostic clarity is critical with these drugs: the response for mania symptoms occurs within a few days, and, for schizophrenia symptoms, it occurs within 1 week. There is also an additional risk for metabolic syndrome (weight gain, hyperlipidemia, adult-onset diabetes, diabetic ketoacidosis) and cerebral vascular accidents (stroke) (see Chapter 25).

However, studies also indicate that more clinical experience is necessary to ensure safety and efficacy in medication administration, especially with the older population and patients with renal or hepatic impairment (Schultz et al, 2007).

Pharmacotherapy is used in conjunction with physical or behavioral restraints for assaultive or combative patients when verbal interventions fail and when the patient refuses to take oral medications. Health care providers apply restraints according to the guidelines set forth by The Joint Commission (TJC), in conjunction with other accrediting bodies, such as the Department of Health Services and the Centers for Medicare & Medicaid) (see Chapter 9).

Somatic Therapy

Electroconvulsive therapy in combination with atypical antipsychotic medications can be beneficial. This combination is useful for patients with schizophrenia or schizoaffective disorder who also have severe symptoms that have not responded to antipsychotic medications alone. Furthermore, patients with catatonic features also respond to this treatment (APA, 2004). Nursing implications for the patient who is receiving electroconvulsive therapy are a clear explanation of the procedure, patient and family education, renegotiation of the patient's consent, nurturance, monitoring, orientation, support, and analgesics for headache after treatment. Chapter 26 discusses electroconvulsive therapy in more detail.

Milieu Therapy

Milieu therapy is a 24-hour environmental therapy that shelters, protects, supports, and enhances the patient with mental illness within the psychiatric setting. This is the model that is currently in use on psychiatric units today. The model involves the use of individualized treatment programs, self-governance, humanistic attitudes, an enhancing environment, and links to the family and the community. The purpose of milieu therapy is to assist the patient with learning to manage and cope with stress as well as understanding how to correct maladaptive behaviors (see Chapter 26).

Behavior Modification

Behavior modification is a precise approach to bringing about behavioral change. Health care providers make use of several types of behavior modification for patients with schizophrenia. For example, operant conditioning is widely used in child and adolescent units, and it is useful for anyone who requires behavioral controls. It operates on the principle of reinforcing desirable behaviors so that they will recur and ignoring negative behaviors. Techniques include relaxation and self-control procedures. Results from the use of this form of therapy indicate that intolerable behaviors such as withdrawal, screaming, incontinence, and incoherence will lessen (Lieberman et al, 2006).

Specific Psychosocial Rehabilitation Interventions

Rehabilitative efforts have become increasingly important in the management of long-term schizophrenia. Individuals whose disease is well controlled by their medications but who have difficulty with daily activities are excellent candidates for rehabilitative interventions. When these interventions are properly timed during the course of the illness, they often mean the difference between a good outcome and a poor outcome. Research has shown that there are several psychosocial rehabilitative interventions that are effective in improving the quality of life for individuals with schizophrenia. The Intensive Psychiatric Rehabilitation Treatment, which is a program that teaches living, job, and social skills to patients, has resulted in improvements in functioning. Social skills training has improved independent living skills; supported employment programs have shown improvements in the number of hours worked and wages earned; and in-home crisis intervention shows promise by reducing treatment dropout rates. Studies have shown that individual cognitive behavior therapy for schizophrenia reduces positive and negative symptoms, but currently there is no evidence that it reduces relapse rates (Schultz et al, 2007).

PATIENT AND FAMILY TEACHING GUIDELINES

Medications for the Treatment of Schizophrenia

TEACH THE PATIENT AND FAMILY	STRATEGIES	RATIONALE
Right to informed consent and disclosure regarding benefits, side effects, anticipated prognosis with and without medication, and alternatives	Initially and any time that the medication or dosage is changed, written permission is obtained from the patient, and the following points are discussed with the patient about his or her medication: Right to informed consent and disclosure regarding benefits, side effects, anticipated prognosis with and without medications, and alternatives. The nurse consults with the physician regarding disclosure that is beneficial to the patient as compared with disclosure that may be harmful.	The patient has the right to choose how much society intervenes. The patient experiences independence, self-esteem, and self-control. The patient develops trust because of others' regard for his or her concerns.
Correct storage and administration of medications	Explain, demonstrate, and request a return demonstration of the handling and administration of medications. Work with the patient to prepare a check chart for his or her medications, dosages, and times. Take control of the environment: reduce distractions, simplify instructions, teach in small segments, and reinforce teaching often.	The safety of the patient and others is ensured. The patient who is involved develops ownership of the process and adherence to the treatment plan. The patient will be able to better focus, minimize frustration, and feel successful.
Action of the medication as well as the symptoms that are reduced or eliminated by the use of the medication	Encourage the patient's own desire to prevent relapse; explain in a matter-of-fact way that many people have various illnesses and take medication to treat them.	This offers the patient hope and reinforcement and informs him or her of the rationale for treatment.
Side effects that may be experienced	Show the patient how to use a journal to record feelings, thoughts, and behaviors over time.	This helps the patient to assume responsibility for self-care and documents treatment effects.
Food and drug interactions to be avoided	Inform the patient about symptoms and events to report and who to tell.	This keeps side effects from getting out of control and causing complications.
How to use the support of family and friends	Include significant others in teaching sessions. Offer thorough education, answer questions, and engage in discussion.	This elicits the support of significant others, decreases family anxiety, and allows the nurse to be a patient advocate.

Assertive Community Treatment. With assertive community treatment, each program is designed specifically for the individual's strengths and deficits. Treatment teams work 24 hours a day and 7 days a week to deliver care on an outpatient basis. The staff helps the person with his or her activities of daily living, such as shopping, grooming, budgeting, and taking medications. Teams also help with job-seeking skills and placement and with offering support. This treatment is most beneficial for people with schizophrenia who have a low level of functioning or who have difficulty with treatment compliance (APA, 2004).

Family Interventions. With family interventions, the main goal is to reduce the risk of patient relapse through education, support, and training to all people whom the patient broadly considers "family." Effective family interventions include educating concerned family members about mental illness and the expected course of the illness; teaching family members effective coping, stress reduction, and problem-solving skills; and helping all family members to improve their communication so that they can effectively participate in the treatment planning process. Multiple studies have shown that family interventions reduce relapse rates and improve symptoms, adherence to medications, and functioning. Research suggests that there are weaknesses in many family intervention studies, which warrants additional investigation (Schultz et al, 2007).

Supported Employment. Supported employment focuses on helping the patient to improve vocational functioning with the goal of working toward competitive employment. The person helps to choose his or her job while the health care team offers ongoing and individualized support for his or her mental health issues. Studies have shown that people with schizophrenia have difficulty keeping the jobs that they obtain because of cognitive impairments, therefore, more research is needed in this area (APA, 2004).

Cognitive Behavioral Therapy. Aaron T. Beck, an American psychiatrist born in 1921, developed cognitive therapy in the early 1960s. It is based on the premise that distorted or dysfunctional thinking cause psychologic disturbances in mood and behavior. This type of therapy helps patients to explore the connection between distorted thinking and negative behavior. For example, the patient who engages in all-or-nothing type thinking does not participate in a craft session because the distorted thought—"I can never do anything right"—prevents the person from attempting to engage in therapy for fear of failure. For high-functioning patients, homework is assigned to separate negative thoughts from negative feelings. As an example, the patient is asked to challenge negative thoughts by recalling past successes and accomplishments with the goal of changing negative thoughts to more rational or realistic ones. Cognitive behavioral therapy involves helping the person to use his or her coping skills and supporting the patient as he or she rationally works on addressing the symptoms (APA, 2004) (see Chapter 26).

Social Skills Training. Social skills training focuses on teaching patients the specific behaviors that are necessary for success in social interactions. The therapist teaches these skills by demonstrating social skills or through role-playing. Research has shown that patients with schizophrenia are able to learn social skills and independent living skills and to use these skills even if their psychiatric symptoms are unchanged (APA, 2004).

Early Intervention Programs. Intervening early when symptoms indicate relapse occurrence has helped to prevent patient rehospitalizations. Health care providers teach patients and their families to recognize the early signs of relapse before the crisis occurs (APA, 2004). Interventions during the early phase of psychosis aim to eliminate symptoms completely (full remission), and prevent future episodes of psychosis. For the majority of first-episode patients, antipsychotic medications and evidence-based psychosocial treatments can achieve full or substantial remission of positive symptoms. Elimination of negative symptoms is much less certain. Future episodes of psychosis can be prevented, but only if patients continue to receive treatment. Approximately 90% of patients will have at least one psychotic relapse within 5 years, partially because of high attrition rates from treatment, failure to implement evidence-based interventions, and the limitations of available therapeutic modalities (Lieberman et al, 2008).

Limited Evidence-Based Strategies

In addition to evidence-based treatments, there are also some limited evidence-based strategies that have time-proven effectiveness. These treatment strategies include personal therapy, group therapy, programs to treat schizophrenia before the onset of illness, patient education, case management, cognitive remediation and cognitive behavioral therapy.

Personal Therapy. Personal therapy usually occurs weekly within a larger treatment program that includes medications, family involvement, and psychologic support. The primary purpose is to help the patient to achieve and maintain clinical stability. The person with schizophrenia meets with the therapist, and the focus is the patient's current level of functioning. As such, the therapist individualizes the therapy to meet the person's current needs (APA, 2004) (see Chapter 26).

Group Therapy. The typical goals of group therapy include helping the patient with problem-solving skills, setting goals, social interactions, and medication education and management. However, there is very weak evidence to support this therapy, and most of it is from the 1970s. Generally these groups consist of six to eight patients, and they are made for patients with enough awareness of reality to participate in a meaningful manner (APA, 2004).

The types of group therapy that are suitable for patients with schizophrenia vary according to the patients' levels of functioning. Nurses generally use the Rogerian model, which is also known as *patient-centered therapy;* this was developed by Carl Rogers (1902–1987), an American psychologist, during the 1940s. This is a humanistic therapy that helps patients to express and clarify their feelings and that promotes acceptance by the therapist. This therapy involves the use of the technique of reflection, and it is not confrontational. It also allows the patient to try out behaviors in a safe setting (Rogers, 1951) (see Chapter 26).

Patient Education. Researchers have not studied patient education enough to determine how to best provide this service to most effectively meet patients' needs. In addition, studies have not yet consistently shown that providing education improves patients' knowledge or changes their behavior. However, there are indications that this approach improves patients' social functioning (APA, 2004).

Case Management. A common problem with outpatient management is that patient care is disorganized. Patients have multiple needs that result from mental illness and physical illness needs, to financial, employment, social, and housing needs. Case management coordinates these various needs. However, this approach has been difficult to study in a controlled manner and therefore does not have a strong evidence base of support (APA, 2004) (see Chapter 30).

Self-help Groups. Persons with schizophrenia are becoming increasingly active in their own care with the intent of decreasing dependence on professionals, decreasing the stigma associated with mental illness, and having an increased adequate support network. Patient models focus on recovery. Recovery models support more patient involvement in care and focus on the patient's strengths rather than only on their symptoms. Individuals attempt to integrate their different life roles rather than seeing themselves as the illness. This movement fosters hope that change is possible. The person is able to make choices, thus feeling respected and self-directed. Empowerment and peer support are critical elements of success. (APA, 2004).

Guided Imagery. Guided imagery is a therapy during which the patient pictures past pleasant memories. Therapists often combine this with relaxation therapy and use it with role-playing. However, it is not for patients who are experiencing psychosis, because it confuses the patient who is out of touch with reality and can add to the patient's perceptual or thought disorder (see Chapter 26).

Assertiveness Training. Assertiveness training reduces the anxiety that can arise from interpersonal relationships, which is usually a problem for the patient with schizophrenia. This training promotes expressive, spontaneous, goal-directed, and self-enhancing behavior, such as learning to say "no" when necessary, rejecting unwanted behavior, and initiating conversations (see Chapter 4).

Occupational and Recreational Therapy. Occupational therapy is a diagnostic tool that assesses the functional level and progress of the patient with schizophrenia. The occupational therapist uses crafts as a tool to check hand–eye coordination, perception, and fine muscle tone. Some occupational therapists visit the patient's home to provide special equipment or needed therapy. In fact, today's psychosocial rehabilitation programs depend on active and directive learning principles that have been designed to help the patient regain or improve skills or to develop alternate compensatory skills that are useful for community living.

The recreational therapist's emphasis is on body kinesics, movement therapy, and resocialization through recreation; therapeutic interventions include exercise, movement therapy, and dance therapy. These physical therapies promote body image through kinesthetic stimulation, and they provide ways to cope with stress. The emphasis is on cooperation rather than competition, especially for patients with schizophrenia. The therapist also works on patient motivation, planning trips and outings, and arts and crafts. For a more detailed description of occupational and recreational therapy, see Chapter 26.

Community Patient and Family Programs. The National Alliance for the Mentally Ill (NAMI) is an example of an effective community organization that conducts family-to-family and peer-to-peer education programs that train members to teach others about mental illness and its effects on day-to-day living. NAMI also offers strategies for moving forward while coping with mental illness (see Chapter 30).

Therapeutic Methods to Prevent and Manage Violence. The possibility of violent behaviors exists in seriously ill patients with schizophrenia, although there is no way to accurately predict who will become violent. Nurses and other clinicians need to be aware of the ways that anger, aggression, and violence are reinforced and take steps to prevent assault. Violence in interpersonal relationships happens as a result of differing expectations regarding therapeutic rules and their enforcement. Because of the nature of the illness, a patient will misinterpret another person's intent, which will sometimes cause a violent response. A person in the acute stages of schizophrenia sometimes exaggerates another's irritation and misreads it as anger, or the patient may misinterpret laughter as ridicule and strike out in defense. Substance abuse can also trigger violence.

De-escalation skills are effective techniques in interpersonal relationships in any context, but they are especially important for the psychiatric mental health nurse. De-escalation consists of less intrusive interventions, such as using nonthreatening verbal and nonverbal messages, and it requires a more hands-on method to safely disengage and control the aggressor physically. The choice to use the techniques set forth in Table 13-4 depends on the stage of the threat, the speed of escalation of the impending violence, and the feedback received from the patient, which illustrates the effectiveness of the technique.

However, sometimes these strategies fail, and medication may be the most effective treatment for managing the emergency situation. Practitioners and experts in psychiatric emergencies have identified oral types as the preferred alternate medications for acutely aggressive or agitated patients, because of the traumatic effects of involuntary medication, especially when coupled with restraint. However, practitioners also agree with regulatory standards that, if it is not possible to administer oral medications and the danger of the emergency situation exceeds the patient's ability to demonstrate safe behaviors, intramuscular medications used in a limited manner (only for the emergency) are the safest choice. The risk of side effects was identified as the most important factor with the use of intramuscular medications. Emotional trauma experienced by the patient and the risk of compromising the patient–physician relationship were also important considerations (Allen et al, 2001) (see Chapter 9).

TABLE 13-4	DE-ESCALATION OF AGGRESSIVE BEHAVIOR	
CONCEPT	**BEHAVIOR**	**RATIONALE**
Managing the environment	Persuade the agitated or angry patient to move to another area. Get help from colleagues to remove other patients, but have one colleague near you.	Prevents anxiety transference and protects others
Showing confidence and leadership	Hold regular drills with staff to practice strategies. Give clear instructions. Be brief and assertive. Negotiate options. If the patient has a weapon, instruct him or her to put it on the floor.	Prevents panic when crises occur Avoids misunderstandings and not knowing what to do. Allows the patient to feel that he or she has some room to exercise options
Maintaining safety	Give the signal to staff to call an assault team or the police per policy (if verbal negotiations fail).	Protects the patient and others from harm or injury as a result of a possible lethal attack
Encouraging verbalization	Ask questions that are open ended and nonthreatening. Use the words *"How?" "What?"* and *"When?"* to get details, but not the word *"Why?"* Keep your voice calm and controlled.	Refocuses on the patient's problem and not on his or her intent to act out the anger Stops anger from escalating (*"Why?"* questions challenge patient)
Using nonverbal expressions	Allow the patient to have enough body space; do not stand closer to him or her than about 8 feet. Keep your body at a 45-degree angle with respect to the patient. Have an open posture with your hands at your sides and your palms facing outward.	Sends a nonthreatening message and expresses your willingness to listen to and accommodate the patient
Personalizing yourself and showing concern	Remind the patient who you are. Say words things as, "The world seems terrible now, but you haven't done any harm to him or her." Use words such as *we* and *us*. Use general leads such as "go on."	Shows empathy Encourages and reflects cooperation Shows that you are listening
Using disengagement breakaways	Manage hair pulls, choke holds, grabs, and hugs according to safety instructions, videos, and return demonstrations.	Prevents injury to yourself, the patient, and others
Using removal, seclusion, and restraints	Rehearse these procedures regularly.	Allows the patient to regain self-control
Accurately documenting the event and holding a debriefing session with staff	Keep a detailed record of the time, place, and circumstances of the situation. Review and discuss the event.	Keeps an accurate account (e.g., for legal aspects) Helps staff to debrief, to talk about feelings, and to learn what went right and how to improve such situations in the future

Modified from *Assault response training and education manual*, San Diego, CA, 2010, Sharp Behavioral HealthCare.

To prevent violence, it is important to avoid blame, ridicule, confrontation, teasing, and insulting. Give the individual privacy, and respect his or her emotional boundaries. Be aware of your feelings and emotions, and try to keep them neutral, as patients are generally sensitive to others' emotions. Maintain a calm and moderate demeanor with a nonthreatening physical stance with arms unfolded, and remain a reasonable distance from the patient. Keep your voice tone low to moderate, and refrain from whispering or laughing with others in the setting, especially within view of a patient with paranoid tendencies.

Do not allow yourself to be cornered in the room of a patient with a known history of violence or with one who has threatened others; always have another staff member with you, and make sure that there is an easy exit from the room. Try not to be intimidated by violent outbursts, but take whatever measures necessary to secure the safety of everyone concerned. In the hospital, this sometimes involves calling the assault response team, hospital security, or the local police department. In the community, try to secure help from friends or neighbors, and call the police if needed. The best way to prevent dangerous situations is to anticipate them and to be prepared with an effective plan of action per hospital or community procedure (Flowers, 2002) (see Chapter 23).

EVALUATION

Evaluation follows specific intervention statements and behavioral objectives, and it incorporates the concepts of

Mark, a 30-year-old man, was estranged from his parents since the age of 18 years, when he was diagnosed with chronic undifferentiated schizophrenia (Figure 13-5). The illness resulted in his unpredictable and disruptive behavior at home, which finally became intolerable. Mark was sent to live in a board-and-care facility, where he was maintained as long as he took his medications and complied with the program at the day treatment center that he attended. The day treatment program provided Mark with the predictable structure, support, and guidance from staff that he needed as well as some affiliation and socialization with other patients. Because of his disorder, other patients easily influenced Mark. One day a group of patients that he considered his friends persuaded him to take the government assistance check he had just received to "go party." Mark stopped taking his medications, took various street drugs, and did not return to the board-and-care facility or the day treatment center for a week. He showed up at the center one morning disheveled, dirty, incoherent, and frightened, stating, "I am really scared. Everybody left me. I'm hearing voices saying that I'm stupid and hopeless and that no one will help me because I'm not worth saving." Mark was admitted to the acute care unit in a psychiatric hospital for evaluation and treatment.

DSM-IV-TR Diagnoses

Axis I   Chronic, undifferentiated schizophrenia

Axis II   None

Axis III   None

Axis IV   Moderate to severe = 6 or 7; negative influence of friends, rejection by peers, ingestion of illicit drugs, lack of adequate support system (family, friends), economic issues (misuse of government assistance check)

Axis V   GAF = 10 (current); GAF = 30 (past year)

Nursing Diagnosis *Disturbed sensory perception related to auditory hallucinations (biologic factors) as a result of the diagnosis of schizophrenia, stopping prescribed medication, and briefly taking "street drugs"; isolation and loneliness and lack of adequate support system as evidenced by the patient stating that he hears derogatory voices telling him that he is stupid and worthless; he feels that others are rejecting him; he admits that he stopped taking his prescribed medications and took "street drugs" for a time.*

NOC Sensory function: hearing; Acute confusion level; Agitation level; Concentration; Cognitive orientation; Communication: receptive

NIC Suicide prevention, Medication administration, Hallucination management, Reality orientation, Environmental management, Emotional support, Cognitive restructuring

Nursing Diagnosis *Disturbed thought processes related to inability to process cognitive information (biologic factors) as a result of the diagnosis of schizophrenia, stopping medication, and briefly taking "street drugs"; isolation and loneliness and lack of adequate support system as evidenced by the patient believing that he is stupid and worthless and rejected by his peers; he admits that he stopped taking his medications and took "street drugs"*

NOC Personal safety behavior; Cognitive orientation; Distorted thought self-control; Information processing; Communication: expressive

NIC Suicide prevention, Medication administration, Delusion management, Cognitive restructuring, Reality orientation, Environmental management, Emotional support

Nursing Diagnosis *Ineffective coping related to situational crisis (symptoms of schizophrenia), inability to form a valid appraisal of stressors (lack of insight into illness), inadequate level of confidence in coping abilities (feels worthless and stupid), and inadequate social support created by characteristics of relationships (behaviors tend to alienate peers and isolate patient) as evidenced by difficulty with organizing information as a result of hallucinations and delusions, verbalizing an inability to cope, and the use of coping that impedes adaptive behavior (stopped medication and took "street drugs") Inadequate problem solving (easily influenced by others)*

NOC Coping, Stress level, Impulse self-control, Concentration, Information processing, Social support, Role performance, Decision making

NIC Suicide prevention, Coping enhancement, Calming technique, Impulse control training, Reality orientation, Active listening, Substance use prevention, Support group, Therapy group, Family involvement promotion

Nursing Diagnosis *Risk for loneliness: risk factors: physical isolation, social isolation, affectional deprivation (estrangement from parents; sent to board-and-care facility, rejection by peers who influenced patient toward wrongful behaviors), feelings of aloneness, auditory hallucinations (voices telling patient that he is stupid and worthless)*

NOC Loneliness severity, Neglect cessation, Risk detection, Risk control, Communication, Social involvement, Social support, Social interaction skills, Family functioning, Family social climate, Personal resiliency

NIC Suicide prevention, Active listening, Milieu therapy, Support group, Therapy group, Family involvement promotion, Self-esteem enhancement

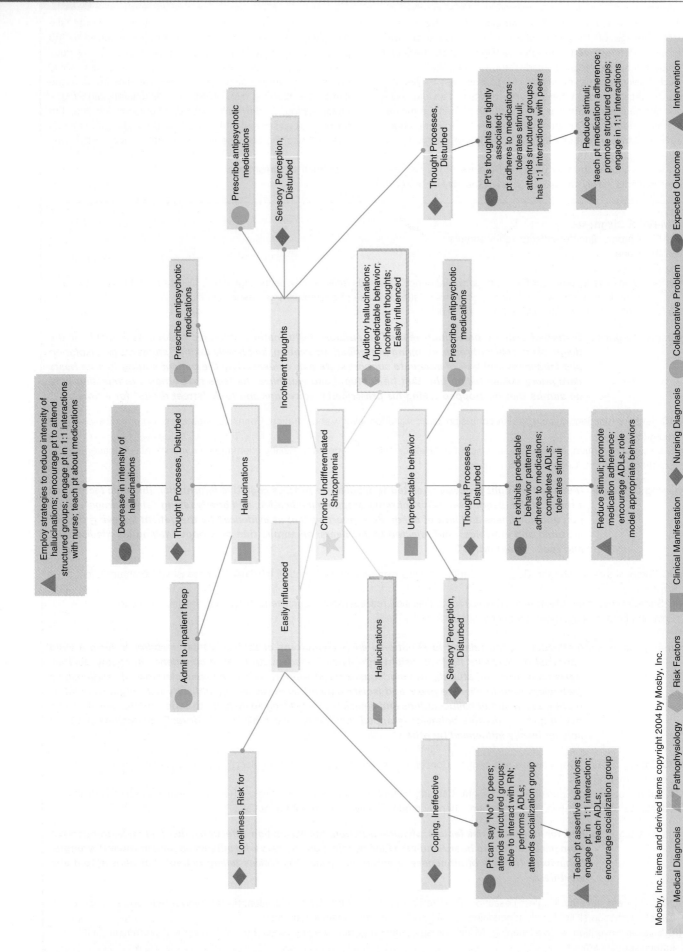

Mosby, Inc. items and derived items copyright 2004 by Mosby, Inc.

FIGURE 13-5. Concept map: schizophrenia.

Medical Diagnosis   Pathophysiology   Risk Factors   Clinical Manifestation   Nursing Diagnosis   Collaborative Problem   Expected Outcome   Intervention

CONCEPT MAP CASE STUDY 13-2

Luke is a 45-year-old stockbroker who works in a busy office in the financial district. Luke has always been a high achiever with lots of energy and ambition, and he enjoys the challenges of his job. He mingled well with friends and coworkers, and he was often the center of conversation. He is married to a busy lawyer, and they have two beautiful daughters, ages 10 and 13, who are also high achievers. During the past month, Luke's family and friends have commented that he has not been himself lately. He is less upbeat and more despondent, and his conversations are morbid, with themes of death. He has been missing work lately, and he says that his boss intends to fire him anyway. He rarely socializes with his friends and coworkers, and his wife has trouble getting him out of the house. He isolates himself in his room for long periods of time. He admits that he has a hard time coping with his high-paced work situation, and he cannot seem to shake off feelings of doom and

despair. His boss insisted that Luke see the company counselor, who advised him to see a psychiatrist who could prescribe medication for his symptoms before things got worse. The psychiatrist diagnosed Luke with schizoaffective disorder (Figure 13-6) and prescribed a combination of the antipsychotic medication risperidone (Risperdal, 2 mg in the morning and 2 mg at bedtime) for his disturbed thoughts of death and doom and the antidepressant medication sertraline (Zoloft, 50 mg per day in the morning) for his depressed mood. However, Luke abruptly stopped taking the medications, and, as a result, his symptoms worsened, and he experienced 2 weeks of psychotic symptoms such as delusions of persecution, immobility, and hallucinations telling him that death was his only hope. At his wife's insistence, Luke agreed to enter a mental health facility for treatment.

DSM-IV-TR Diagnoses

Axis I Schizoaffective disorder, depressed type

Axis II None

Axis III None

Axis IV Moderate to Severe = 6 or 7; high-stress work place; over achiever; high achieving family/coworkers

Axis V GAF = 30 (current); GAF = 90 (past year)

Nursing Diagnosis *Risk for suicide: risk factors: depressed mood, delusional thoughts of death, hallucinations telling him that "life is not worth living," refusal to take prescribed medication, unable to cope at work, isolating self from friends and coworkers*

NOC Risk control, Suicide self-restraint, Depression level, Stress level, Symptom control, Mood equilibrium, Social support, Social involvement, Will to live

NIC Suicide prevention, Medication administration, Mood management, Cognitive restructuring, Reality orientation, Coping enhancement, Family involvement promotion, Support group

Nursing Diagnosis *Disturbed thought processes related to biochemical imbalance resulting from mental illness (schizoaffective disorder) as evidenced by paranoid thoughts that his coworkers are against him and that his boss is planning to fire him*

NOC Cognitive orientation, Distorted thought self-control, Agitation level, Information processing

NIC Suicide prevention, Reality orientation, Medication management, Delusion management, Anxiety reduction, Mood management, Family involvement promotion, Support group

Nursing Diagnosis *Social isolation related to alterations in mental status (schizoaffective disorder) and inability to engage in satisfying personal relationships (rejects coworkers and friends); the patient remains isolated in his room for hours at a time and refuses to get out of bed and go to work.*

NOC Depression level; Social support; Mood equilibrium; Social involvement; Social interaction skills; Patient satisfaction: communication

NIC Delusion management 7, Hallucination management, Medication management, Reality orientation, Active listening, Calming technique, Family involvement promotion, Support group

Nursing Diagnosis *Ineffective coping related to situational crisis (symptoms of schizoaffective disorder), inadequate level of perception of control (he perceives that he is unable to function at pre-illness level) as evidenced by verbalization of inability to cope, poor concentration (depressed mood, disturbed thoughts), sleep disturbance (paces all night), and inability to meet role expectations (refuses to go to work, rejects coworkers and friends)*

NOC Stress level, Depression self-control, Sleep, Fatigue level, Concentration, Information processing, Coping, Social support, Social interaction skills, Decision making, Role performance

NIC Anxiety reduction, Medication management, Reality orientation, Mood management, Delusion management, Coping enhancement, Family involvement promotion, Support group

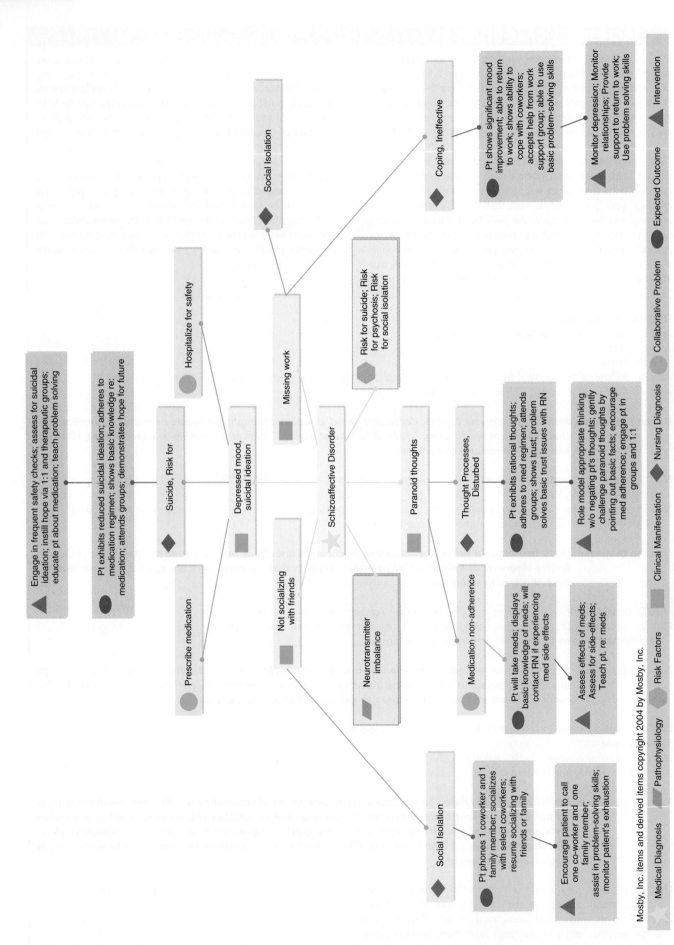

Mosby, Inc. items and derived items copyright 2004 by Mosby, Inc.

FIGURE 13-6 Concept map: schizoaffective disorder.

quality, quantity, and time. For example, if the goal is to resocialize a patient who has been isolating herself while on the unit, the intervention may consist of having the patient join the community meeting along with other patients on the unit. To evaluate the effectiveness of this intervention, nurses state specific behavioral patient outcomes in measurable terms. For example, a beginning behavioral objective may be the following: "On her second day on the unit, Kayla will accompany the nurse to the community meeting, and she will remain with the group for 15 minutes."

Note that the outcome has specific criteria regarding time (on the second day), quality of experience (going to the community meeting with the nurse), and quantity (for 15 minutes). These criteria are measurable. If all of these criteria are met, the minimal acceptable level of performance will progress so that, by the third day, the patient outcome will read, "Kayla will go to the community meeting on her own, remain for 30 minutes, and make at least one comment."

The nursing process is dynamic and always changing. It is an ongoing design for interaction with the environment, and it is evaluated as such. For example, if the nurse evaluates a criterion and finds that it is not met on the second day, then the nurse will reconsider the patient outcomes and nursing interventions and perhaps rewrite them at a level closer to the patient's ability to perform. If a nurse revises the outcomes and they are still not met, then the nurse needs to examine the rest of the nursing process in total. Thus, eventual success with the nursing process demands patience and persistence. Improvements occur in small steps, especially among patients with chronic schizophrenia (see Chapter 3).

CHAPTER SUMMARY

- Schizophrenia is one of the most complex and debilitating mental disorders.
- Schizophrenia is a not a single disorder but rather a syndrome (group of diseases) known as *the schizophrenias.*
- The schizophrenias are the largest group of mental disorders.
- Biologic factors are the primary focus of the research regarding the etiology and treatment of schizophrenia.
- The five biologic models that are currently being considered are as follows: (1) heredity/genetic; (2) neuroanatomic/neurochemical; (3) neurotransmitter function (specifically the dopamine hypothesis); (4) immunologic; and (5) stress/disease/trauma/drug abuse.
- Advancements in genetic research hold promise for the more effective treatment of schizophrenia during the next decade.
- The five major subtypes of schizophrenia are paranoid, disorganized, catatonic, undifferentiated, and residual.
- The diagnostic criteria for schizophrenia include two or more of the following symptoms being evident for at least

1 month: hallucinations, delusions, disorganized or catatonic behavior, and disorganized speech.
- Involving the patient with schizophrenia and the patient's family or significant others in the patient's treatment plan, as appropriate, is important and contributes to more effective treatment.
- Many practitioners use psychopharmacology as an intervention for many symptoms of schizophrenia. New medications with fewer side effects offer hope and more effective treatment outcomes for the complex symptoms of schizophrenia.
- Milieu therapy, psychosocial rehabilitation, patient and family education, and behavior modification are some treatments that are used with patients with schizophrenia.
- Community resources are critical for rehabilitating patients with schizophrenia and reintegrating them back into the community.

REVIEW QUESTIONS

1. A nurse plans a series of psychoeducational groups for persons with schizophrenia. Which topic would take priority?
   1. How to complete an application for employment
   2. The importance of taking your medication correctly
   3. The ways to dress and behave when attending community events
   4. How to give and receive compliments
2. A young adult is hospitalized with undifferentiated schizophrenia. The parents are distraught and filled with guilt. Which of the following would be an appropriate nursing response?
   1. "There are many theories about the cause of schizophrenia, but this illness is not your fault."

   2. "Does anyone in your family have mental illness? Schizophrenia is a genetically transmitted disease."
   3. "Look on the bright side. With the right medications and treatment, this disease can be cured."
   4. "I'll recommend some excellent Web sites with information about schizophrenia and other mental illnesses."
3. A person with disorganized schizophrenia participates in a rehabilitative outpatient program. Select the most appropriate initial outcome for this individual.
   1. The individual will identify environmental triggers that produce feelings of fear.
   2. The individual will have increased organization of thought patterns.

3. The individual will report the absence of auditory and visual hallucinations.

4. The individual will set lunch tables correctly and fill cups with ice daily.

4. Which statement by a person with paranoid schizophrenia most clearly indicates that the antipsychotic medication that he or she is taking is effective?

1. "I used to hear scary voices, but now I don't hear them anymore."

2. "My medicine is working fine. I'm not having any problems."

3. "Sometimes it's hard for me to fall asleep, but I usually sleep all night."

4. "I think some of the staff members don't like me. They're mean to me."

5. Select the nursing diagnosis that is most likely to apply to a person with an acute exacerbation of schizophrenia, paranoid type.

1. Social isolation related to impaired ability to trust others

2. Deficient diversional activity related to unstable control of hostile impulses

3. Impaired social interaction related to inadequately developed superego

4. Fear related to lack of confidence in significant others

6. A patient with catatonic schizophrenia has been sitting mute and rigid for 2 hours. Which nursing intervention would be the most appropriate?

1. Encourage the patient to participate in a group sporting activity.

2. Put the patient's extremities through passive range-of-motion exercises.

3. Seclude the patient until voluntary movement is observed.

4. Offer short but frequent verbal phrases to communicate caring.

REFERENCES

American Nurses Association: *Psychiatric mental health nursing: Scope and standards of practice.* Silver Springs, MD, 2007. American Nurses Association.

American Psychiatric Association: *Diagnostic and statistical manual of mental disorders*, ed 4, text revision, Washington, DC, 2000, American Psychiatric Association.

American Psychiatric Association: *Practice guidelines for the treatment of patients with schizophrenia*, ed 2, Washington, DC, 2004.

American Psychiatric Nurses Association: Position statement: mandatory outpatient treatment (MOT), *J Am Psychiatr Nurses Assoc* 10:247-253, 2004.

Allen MH et al: *The expert consensus guideline series: treatment of behavioral emergencies, a postgraduate medicine special report*, New York, 2001, McGraw Hill.

Beng-Choon H et al: Schizophrenia and other psychotic disorders. In Hales RE, Yudofsky SC, editors: *Essentials of clinical psychiatry*, ed 2, Washington, DC, 2004, American Psychiatric Publishing, p. 200.

Fanous, AH: Genetic studies of schizophrenia and bipolar disorder, American Psychiatric Association, *Focus* 8:323-338, 2010.

Flowers CJ: *Antipsychotic polypharmacy in schizophrenia: eighth annual psychopharmacology update*, sponsored by Sharp HealthCare, San Diego, Calif, September 21, 2002.

Fortinash KM, Holoday Worret PA: *Psychiatric mental health nursing*, ed 4, St. Louis, 2008, Mosby-Elsevier.

Fortinash KM, Holoday Worret PA: *Psychiatric nursing care plans*, ed 4, St. Louis, 2007, Mosby.

Gaillard LM et al: Mental health patient's experiences of being misunderstood, *J Am Psychiatr Nurses Assoc* 15:191-199, 2010.

Gaur N, et al: The biochemical womb of schizophrenia: a review. *Indian J Clin Biochem* 23:307-327, 2008.

Genetic Science Learning Center, *Beyond the reward pathway, Learn Genetics*, 2010 (website): http://learn.genetics.utah.edu/content/addiction/reward/pathways.html

Goldman M, et al: Diminished plasma oxytocin in schizophrenic patients with neuroendocrine dysfunction and emotional deficits, *Schizophr Res* 9(1-3):247-255, 2008.

Grove GA: Beware of PHATS in metabolic syndrome. *Current Psychiatry* (5) 2006, page 98.

Hugdahl, K et al: Auditory hallucinations in schizophrenia: the role of cognitive, brain structural and genetic disturbances in the left temporal lobe, *Front Hum Neurosc* 1:1-6, 2008.

Johnson ME: Violence on inpatient psychiatric units: state of the science, *J Am Psychiatr Nurses Assoc* 10:119, 2004.

Lencz T et al: Converging evidence for a pseudoautosomal cytokine receptor gene locus in schizophrenia, *Mol Psychiatry* 12(6):572-580, 2007.

Lieberman JA et al: *The American Psychiatric Publishing textbook of schizophrenia*, Arlington, Va, 2006, American Psychiatric Publishing.

Lieberman JA et al: Science and recovery in schizophrenia, *Psychiatr Serv* 59:487-496, 2008.

Mayo Clinic Foundation for Medical Education and Research: *Childhood Schizophrenia*: 2010 (website): www.mayoclinic.com/health/childhood-schizophrenia/DS00868. Accessed November, 2010.

McEvoy J et al: Effectiveness of clozapine versus olanzapine, quetiapine, and risperidone in patients with schizophrenia who did not respond to prior atypical antipsychotic treatment, *Am J Psychiatry* 163:600-610, 2006.

Meyer JM: *Schizophrenia and the metabolic syndrome*: Medscape Psychiatry Mental Health, 2005 (website): www.medscape.com/viewarticle/506136. Accessed January 3, 2010.

Mortensen PB et al: Early infections of toxoplasma gondii and the later development of schizophrenia. *Oxford Journals of Medicine, Schizophrenia Bulletin* 53(3):741-744, 2007.

Murphy MC: The agitated, psychotic patient: guidelines to ensure staff and patient safety, *J Am Psychiatr Nurses Assoc* 8(Suppl 4):S2-S8, 2002.

National Institute of Mental Health: *Schizophrenia research at the National Institute of Mental Health, 2005* (website): www.nimh.nih.gov/publicat/schizresfact.cfm. Accessed April 5, 2006.

Reeves RR, Torres RA: Medical disorders among psychiatric patients, *Psychiatr Serv* 54:748, 2003.

Rogers CP: *Client-centered therapy*, Boston, 1951, Houghton Mifflin.

Sadock BJ, Sadock VA, Ruiz P: *Kaplan and Sadock's comprehensive textbook of psychiatry*, ed 9, Philadelphia, 2009, Lippincott Williams & Wilkins.

Schultz H et al: Schizophrenia: A Review. *Am Fam Physician* 75(12):1821-1829.

Selye H: *Stress of life*, ed 2, New York, 1978, McGraw-Hill.

Sullivan H: *The interpersonal theory of psychiatry*, New York, 1953, WW Norton. (classic)

Sullivan PF: The genetics of schizophrenia, *PLoS Medicine*, 2(7):e12, 2005. doi:10.1371/journal.pmed.00202212.

Swanson JW et al: Newer antipsychotics no better than older medications in reducing schizophrenia-related violence. *Science Update of the National Institutes of Mental Health*, 2008 (1 page).

Swartz MS et al: Substance use in persons with schizophrenia: baseline prevalence and correlates from the NIMH CATIE study, *Journal of Nerv Ment Dis* 194(3) 2006.

Thirthalli J, Benegal V: Psychosis among substance users, *Curr Opin Psychiatry* 19:239-249, 2006.

Online Resources

Mental Health America(NARSAD): www.nmha.org

NARSAD, the Brain and Behavior Research Fund: www.narsad.org

National Alliance on Mental Illness: www.nami.org

National Institute of Mental Health: www.nimh.nih.gov

14

Personality Disorders

Pamela E. Marcus

"Or was there something else hidden in the boy, some fiery-eyed wolf that would occasionally creep out to hurt and destroy, only to crawl back into the shell of innocence that the boy had created? He was cruel. There was no question about that. But what moved him, what drove him to these acts of cruelty, this apparent lack of caring for another soul?"

Ronald A. Williams (Four Saints and an Angel)

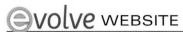 WEBSITE

http://evolve.elsevier.com/Fortinash/

OBJECTIVES

- Identify three elements of personality development as described by Freud in the psychosexual stages of development.
- Discuss two contributions that Margaret Mahler and Otto Kernberg made to object relations theory.
- Name two biologic indices that are often abnormal in patients with a personality disorder.
- Briefly explain the behaviors that differentiate Clusters A, B, and C of Axis II in the *Diagnostic and Statistical Manual of Mental Disorders,* ed 4, text revision.
- Recognize two nursing diagnoses for each cluster of the personality disorders.

- Describe splitting behaviors, and list two nursing interventions that effectively challenge the patient's black-or-white view of the world.
- Apply the nursing process to the management of patients with personality disorders.
- Develop a nursing care plan for an individual with antisocial personality disorder.
- Develop a concept map for the care of the individual with borderline personality disorder.

KEY TERMS

devaluation	object constancy	projective identification	trait disorders
idealization	object relations	splitting	transitional objects
milieu therapy	personality traits	state disorders	

Personality disorders, as classified by the *Diagnostic and Statistical Manual of Mental Disorders,* fourth edition, text revision (DSM-IV-TR), are longstanding, pervasive, maladaptive patterns of behavior when relating to others that are not caused by Axis I disorders. According to the DSM-IV-TR, a personality disorder is an "enduring pattern of inner experience and behavior that deviates markedly from the expectations of the individual's culture, is pervasive and inflexible, has an onset in adolescence or early adulthood, is stable over time, and leads to distress or impairment" (American Psychiatric Association, 2000). All human beings have a personality that is made up of one's definition of self, skills that are used to relate to others, and a defense structure. When studying personality disorders, the nurse has to determine to what degree an individual compromises these qualities. Nurses determine these behaviors by observing how individuals relate to others, their perception of surroundings, and their ability to problem solve.

When reviewing the diagnostic criteria for the various personality disorders (Axis II), it is important to differentiate personality traits from personality disorders. DSM-IV-TR has defined six general diagnostic criteria for a personality disorders; these are listed in the DSM-IV-TR Criteria box.

DSM-IV-TR CRITERIA

Personality Disorder

A An enduring pattern of inner experience and behavior that deviates markedly from the expectations of the individual's culture. This pattern is manifested in two (or more) of the following areas:
1 Cognition (i.e., ways of perceiving and interpreting self, other people, and events)
2 Affectivity (i.e., the range, intensity, lability, and appropriateness of emotional response)
3 Interpersonal functioning
4 Impulse control
B The enduring pattern is inflexible and pervasive across a broad range of personal and social situations.
C The enduring pattern leads to clinically significant distress or impairment in social, occupational, or other important areas of functioning.
D The pattern is stable and of long duration, and its onset can be traced back at least to adolescence or early adulthood.
E The enduring pattern is not better accounted for as a manifestation or consequence of another mental disorder.
F The enduring pattern is not due to the direct physiologic effects of a substance (e.g., a drug of abuse, a medication) or a general medical condition (e.g., head trauma).

From the American Psychiatric Association: *Diagnostic and statistical manual of mental disorders*, ed 4, text revision, Washington, DC, 2000, American Psychiatric Association.

Personality traits are those behaviors and those patterns of perceiving, relating to others, and thinking about the environment and oneself that are exhibited in a wide range of social and personal contexts (American Psychiatric Association, 2000). These traits are either adaptive or maladaptive **trait disorders**, depending on whether the trait is inflexible or causes significant functional impairment or subjective distress. When a person demonstrates inflexible and maladaptive methods of problem solving and relating to others that cause difficulty with functioning, this individual can be described as having a personality disorder. The symptoms of a personality disorder are longstanding, enduring, and not responsive to short-term psychotherapy or pharmacologic measures. These symptoms may intensify during a crisis, but the maladaptive behavior continues after the crisis is resolved. Several researchers have studied functional impairment in individuals with several different types of personality disorders. They found that patients with schizotypal personality disorder and borderline personality disorder consistently had

either moderate or poor functioning across several levels of psychosocial functioning, such as marital status, completion of school, and the ability to maintain employment. People who have avoidant personality disorder demonstrated an intermediate functional impairment (Choi et al, 2010; Skodol et al, 2000; VanLuyn et al, 2007; Zanarini et al, 2009).

Diagnoses made on Axis I are state disorders. These diagnoses constitute behavior patterns that are not as long in duration. Often health care providers are able to alleviate the symptoms of these disorders with the use of medication, psychotherapy, and milieu therapy for severe symptoms. Personality disorder diagnoses are listed on Axis II of the DSM-IV-TR in a cluster format as follows:
- *Cluster A:* Paranoid, schizoid, and schizotypal make up the odd or eccentric cluster. These diagnoses are more likely to be concurrent with psychotic disorders.
- *Cluster B:* Antisocial, borderline, histrionic, and narcissistic constitute the dramatic and emotional cluster. Disorders from the Cluster B group are often concurrent with affective disorders and some anxiety disorders, such as posttraumatic stress disorder (Goldstein et al, 2010).
- *Cluster C:* Avoidant, dependent, and obsessive-compulsive compose the anxious and fearful cluster. These diagnoses are often associated with anxiety disorders (American Psychiatric Association, 2000).

Individuals with personality disorder diagnoses in each cluster are at risk for developing concurrent specific Axis I diagnoses.

HISTORIC AND THEORETIC PERSPECTIVES

Individuals who have the symptoms of personality disorders are unable to identify a sense of self and therefore are unable to determine their own likes, dislikes, needs, and values. Often the person who has a personality disorder has problems relating to others and sustains difficulty with functioning at school or work as a result of this difficulty. The use of theoretic concepts is helpful to promote an understanding of the individual's pattern of emotional reaction and behavior. Theoretic frameworks assist the nurse with planning nursing care and setting realistic goals for the patient's care.

Freudian Theories

Sigmund Freud (1856–1939), the noted psychoanalyst, was one of the early published students of human development and inner psychologic conflict. Freud (1905) describes the psychosexual stages of development in his *Three Essays on the Theory of Sexuality*. The first stage he describes is the oral stage. The traits associated with the successful completion of this stage include the ability to relate to others without excessive dependency or jealously. Trust begins to develop, and, with trust, comes a sense of self-reliance and trust of self. Individuals who have difficulty with this stage often lack trust and are self-centered, dependent, and jealous. This may be evident with individuals who have a paranoid personality disorder, a borderline personality disorder, or a histrionic personality disorder.

The anal stage is the second stage described by Freud. This takes place from approximately the ages of 1 to 3 years. Adults demonstrate the successful completion of this stage with their ability to manage ambivalence (uncertainty) by making decisions without shame or self-doubt. They show a sense of self-autonomy and independence. A person who finds it difficult to successfully complete this stage of development is unable to make decisions, withholds friendships or cannot share with others, is full of rage, is stubborn, and may have sadomasochistic tendencies (i.e., the desire to hurt others or to be hurt by others). Examples of these behavioral patterns can be seen in individuals who have antisocial personality disorder, borderline personality disorder, histrionic personality disorder, and dependent personality disorder.

The phallic stage is the next stage that was identified by Freud. It is the period of development when the child becomes interested in his or her genitals. Freud understood this stage in terms of male development. According to his theory, the phallus (penis) is the principal organ of concern for both boys and girls. This stage occurs from the age of 3 years through the age of 6 or 7 years. The child who successfully completes this stage masters his or her internal processes and impulses and gains a beginning sense of relating to other people in the environment. Individuals who are unable to resolve the conflict inherent in the phallic stage can experience multiple psychiatric disorders, particularly those that involve the superego function of guilt. Individuals with antisocial personality disorder do not have a well-developed superego.

According to Freud, the antisocial, borderline, histrionic, and narcissistic personality disorders involve individuals who experienced problems identifying with their sexual identity during the critical phallic stage. For example, an individual with a histrionic personality disorder who acts sexually provocatively but denies that this behavior is sexually driven has experienced an internal conflict with his or her sexual identity.

The next stage of psychosexual development is the latency stage. During this stage, the child represses the libidinal (sexual) drives and turns his or her attention toward learning and industry. This stage takes place from the sixth or seventh year of life until puberty.

With this stage comes the exploration of the environment and play, when the child learns how to do things and to enjoy life and have fun while continuing to develop inner control over instinctive drives and emotions. This stage is important for later adult functioning, because the child with a sense of industry is able to delay gratification, which helps in areas of learning, work, and relating to others. Individuals who have problems successfully completing this stage have either too much or too little ability to develop inner control. Those who lack inner control have difficulty relating to others, because their emotions rule their interactions and problem-solving abilities, which is seen in individuals with borderline personality disorder. Individuals who have an excess of inner control have isolated their emotions and are more regulated, and they use the repetition of thoughts or behavior to relate or problem solve. Individuals with obsessive-compulsive personality disorder demonstrate these behavioral patterns.

The genital stage is the last stage in an individual's psychosexual development described by Freud. This stage takes place during puberty. The importance of this stage is that there is an opportunity to rework earlier issues that the individual has not resolved in the service of achieving a healthy and mature sense of sexual and adult identity. With the ability to work and learn, individuals establish goals and values within the context of their own unique personal identities.

If individuals have difficulty during the genital stage, this will compromise their sense of self and their ability to relate to others. They will therefore be unable to attain their identified goals or to form values. They will also experience difficulty identifying their strengths and weaknesses, their likes and dislikes, and the types of skills that they want to acquire. Some individuals who have difficulty resolving the genital stage manifest symptoms and behaviors that are within the whole range of the personality disorders.

OBJECT RELATIONS

Object relations is a theoretic framework that studies the ability of individuals to relate to one another. As theorists studied human behavior further, particularly observing the development of personality structure and relatedness, the theory of object relations began to develop. Many have contributed to this theory, and it is being reevaluated and expanded as the study of human relations and personality development.

Separation–Individuation Phase

Approaching object relations from a developmental standpoint, Margaret Mahler (1897-1985), a Hungarian physician, identified and studied the separation–individuation phase of development, which occurs between ages of 3 and 25 months. Mahler's theory of separation and individuation evolved from a longitudinal study during which she observed normal mothers and their babies during the child's first 3 years of life. The term *separation* in this context refers to the child's gradually developing self that is distinct and separate from that of the mother. The term *individuation* in this context means to recognize the infant's attempts to form a distinctive identity and to develop characteristics that are unique to that individual (Mahler, 1963).

Mahler (1963, 1972) described four stages of the process of separation and individuation: differentiation, practicing, rapprochement, and object constancy. These stages are presented in Box 14-1.

Kernberg's Theories

Otto Kernberg (1928-), a psychoanalyst, identified two essential tasks that the early ego has to accomplish for the internalization of object relations. The first task involves the ability of the child to distinguish between the self and other people to formulate healthy feelings about the self and to identify with the other person; this is similar to Mahler's

BOX 14-1 MAHLER'S STAGES OF SEPARATION AND INDIVIDUATION

1. **Differentiation:** Differentiation occurs when the child is between 3 and 8 months old. During this stage, the child begins to differentiate his or her own image from that of the mother or another significant nurturer.
2. **Practicing:** Practicing occurs when the child is between 8 and 15 months old. The task of this stage is for the child to actively explore his or her world in a manner in which the child seems oblivious to the mother. This occurs when the child begins to walk and is able to explore the environment around him or her as locomotion becomes more stabilized.
3. **Rapprochement:** Rapprochement occurs when the child is between 15 and 22 months old. The child begins to return to the mother for emotional needs after completing the exploration of the surroundings (which occurred during the practicing phase). During this time, the toddler becomes moody, is in distress, and exhibits temper tantrums, even when the mother is with the child. The child wishes to have things his or her way, which is not always what the mother had planned. The task is for the child to deal with the conflict between his or her wish for independence and individuation and with that of wanting love and comfort from the mother.
4. **The beginning of object constancy:** This phase occurs at about the age of 25 months. Object constancy involves the ability to maintain a relationship regardless of frustration and changes in the relationship. The toddler at 25 months is able to think about the mother even when the mother is not close to the child and therefore comforts himself or herself with the use of the mother's representation. This comfort sometimes includes a blanket or a stuffed toy that reminds the child of the mother.

Modified from Mahler MS: Thoughts about development and individuation, *Psychoanal Study Child* 18:307-324, 1963; and Mahler MS: On the first three subphases of the separation-individuation process, *Int J Psychoanal* 53:333-338, 1972.

differentiation stage. The second task that Kernberg discussed is that there is an integration of "good" and "bad" self-images as well as an integration of "good" and "bad" object (i.e., the other person's) images. This task helps the person to be able to identify strengths and weaknesses in the self and others. In people who have healthy relationships with others, there is an ability to tolerate both the "good" and "bad" in the self and others. Kernberg identified splitting as a primary defense of the individual with borderline personality disorder.

Splitting is the inability to synthesize the positive and negative aspects of the self and others. The person with borderline personality disorder exhibits splitting by his or her difficulty with perceiving that he or she and other people have both good and bad aspects. There is a tendency to idealize persons or groups when those persons meet the needs of the individual with borderline personality disorder. This process is called *idealization*. At the other extreme, a person with

borderline personality disorder devalues persons or groups when he or she perceives that his or her needs are not being met. This process is called *devaluation*. The person with borderline personality disorder views the self and others as either all good or all bad and is unable to reach a state of object constancy, which means that one is unable to hold the memory of significant others in mind. This individual is unable to use transitional objects that represent the significant other and that help him or her remember the other person. For example, an individual with object constancy thinks of his or her loved one when experiencing something that reminds him or her of the other person, such as a favorite song or a tangible object (e.g., a wedding ring representing the marital bond). An individual who is unable to obtain object constancy cannot picture his or her loved one when that individual is away from him or her. Therefore, the person views the absence of the significant other as abandonment.

James Masterson (1926-2010) identified, in 1976, four defenses that block the patient's developmental growth from the stages of individuation and separation to autonomy: projection, clinging, denial, and avoidance. According to Masterson, the patient with borderline personality disorder becomes stuck in the subphases of the individuation–separation stage. This leads to the patient's failure to achieve object constancy.

A patient with borderline personality disorder does not relate to people as wholes but as parts. He or she is unable to maintain a relationship through the frustration of everyday living and tends to experience anger and rage when feeling rejected or ignored. This individual is unable to evoke the images of significant others when they are not present. If a significant person in the patient's life dies, the patient with borderline personality disorder cannot mourn but often exhibits one or more of the six constituent states: (1) depression; (2) anger and rage; (3) fear; (4) guilt; (5) passivity and helplessness; and (6) emptiness and void.

Another defense against the patient's anxiety that is important for understanding the individual with a Cluster B personality disorder is projective identification. This defense is a primitive type of projection. Kernberg (1984) described this defense as having the following characteristics:

- The tendency to continue to experience the impulse that is simultaneously being projected onto the other person
- Fear of the other person under influence of that projected impulse
- The need to control the other person under the influence of this mechanism

For example, Danielle is angry with her mother because her mother disapproves of her taste in clothes. She views her mother as having old-fashioned views. Danielle begins to yell at her mother, telling her that she dresses like a little old lady *(projection)*. Danielle's mother feels hurt and angry at her daughter and raises her voice, telling Danielle that her dress is provocative and that it will bring unwanted attention *(mother reacts to the projection)*. Danielle tells her mother that she refuses to talk to her anymore about how she feels unless the mother shows that she cares about Danielle *(controlling mother's response)*.

ETIOLOGY

As researchers addressing the biologic aspects of behaviors began to study some of the physiologic markers that were consistent with Axis I diagnoses, they used some of the same studies with individuals with personality disorders, and they obtained consistent results. There have been family studies, including twin studies, that demonstrate a strong genetic influence, thereby suggesting some ties between biologic factors and personality organization (Coryell and Zimmerman, 1989; Kavoussi and Siever, 1991; Marin et al, 1989; Siever, 1992; Siever and Davis, 1991).

Research that involves individuals with schizotypal personality disorder has focused on the biologic similarities between this disorder and schizophrenia. Studies were conducted on tasks that measure the person's ability to correctly interpret information in the environment, such as eye-tracking behavior and backward masking. Individuals with schizophrenia demonstrate difficulty with smooth-pursuit eye movements, and many researchers believe that this reflects the disrupted neurointegrative functioning of the frontal lobes. The impaired eye-tracking studies are associated with the "deficit" traits of schizophrenia, namely the social isolation, detachment, and inability to relate to others. Individuals with schizotypal personality disorder demonstrated deficits similar to those of individuals with schizophrenia, but the deficits were not as severe (Kavoussi and Siever, 1991; Siever, 1985).

Modinos and colleagues (2010) recently compared brain magnetic resonance images of normal subjects with subjects who scored high on a psychometric (paper-and-pencil) test for schizotypy experiences. The images of the individuals who had subthreshold psychotic signs (according to the psychometric tests) were similar to those of individuals who have schizophrenia.

There are some neurochemical measures that are important indicators of the biologic manifestations of the schizotypal personality disorder. Siever (1992) reported that cerebrospinal fluid homovanillic acid levels were increased in preliminary studies of schizotypal patients and that this correlated with positive psychotic-like criteria for schizotypal personality (but without the negative or deficit symptoms). He also reported that plasma homovanillic acid levels were increased in patients with schizotypal personality disorder as compared with controls (Kavoussi and Siever, 1991).

For patients who have difficulty with affective regulation (mood), some biologic indices or tests are important to consider. Several early studies have demonstrated disturbances in central serotonergic neurotransmission, which indicates that aggressive and suicidal behaviors in individuals with a personality disorder correlate with reduced levels of the cerebrospinal fluid 5-hydroxyindoleacetic acid. This acid is a major metabolite of serotonin, so the lower level indicates a reduction in serotonin activity (Brown and Linnoila, 1990; Kavoussi and Siever, 1991; Leyton et al, 2001; Marin et al, 1989). Low 5-HT synthesis capacity was found in the corticostriatal pathways, which is possibly a factor that affects the development of impulsive behaviors in individuals with borderline personality disorder.

There is also a possible dysfunction of the brain system's ability to modulate and inhibit aggressive responses to environmental stimuli. Some data indicate that electroencephalogram slow-wave activity and a low threshold for sedation distinguish individuals with antisocial personality disorder from individuals with long-term depression (Siever and Davis, 1991).

Recent research is concentrating on the role of opioid receptors as they relate to emotional regulation. In recent studies by Prossin and colleagues (2010) and New and Stanley (2010), the researchers looked at individuals with borderline personality disorder who self-injure by cutting, and hypothesized that the reason for the self-mutilation is to facilitate self-medicating to reduce the effects of an intense affective state. This is the result of a decrease of μ-opioid receptors in the brain of the individual with borderline personality disorder. With the decrease of this important neurotransmitter receptor, the individual is not able to regulate intense emotions, so self-mutilation is used by the individual to assist with this regulation (Prossin et al, 2010; New and Stanley, 2010).

The fact that individuals with personality disorders manifest some biologic markers is exciting for researchers and clinicians, because this information provides some suggestions that will be useful when treating this population. There is a need for future research in this area as the functions of the brain and the neurotransmitters become better known and understood.

EPIDEMIOLOGY AND CLINICAL DESCRIPTION

Cluster A Personality Disorders

Cluster A is often described as the "odd" or "eccentric" cluster. This cluster consists of the following personality disorders: paranoid, schizoid, and schizotypal. Patients with disorders in this cluster all have difficulty relating to others, they isolate themselves, and they are unable to socialize comfortably. Box 14-2 and the Clinical Symptoms box provide epidemiology and summaries of the clinical symptoms of each disorder.

Cluster B Personality Disorders

Cluster B personality disorders have components of dramatic behavior, which is a description that is widely used when describing individuals with these types of personality disorders. The four diagnostic categories that make up this cluster are antisocial, borderline, histrionic, and narcissistic. Each personality disorder has unique features, but each shares a dramatic quality in the way that the individual lives his or her life. Box 14-3 and the Clinical Symptoms box on page 303 provide epidemiology and summarize the key clinical symptoms of these disorders.

Cluster C Personality Disorders

Cluster C personality disorders are in the anxious or fearful cluster. These include avoidant personality disorder,

CLINICAL SYMPTOMS
Cluster A Personality Disorders

Paranoid Personality Disorder
Distrust and suspicion
Difficulty adjusting to change
Sensitivity and argumentation
Feelings of irreversible injury by others, often without evidence
Anxiety and difficulty relaxing
Short temper
Difficulty with problem solving
Lack of tender feelings toward others
Unwillingness to forgive even minor events
Jealousy of spouse or significant other, often without evidence

Schizoid Personality Disorder
Brief psychotic episodes in response to stressful events
Lack of desire to socialize; enjoys solitude
Lack of strong emotions
Detached and self-absorbed affect
Lack of trust in others
Difficulty expressing anger
Passive reactions to crises

Schizotypal Personality Disorder
Incorrect interpretation of external events and belief that all events refer to self
Superstition and preoccupation with paranormal phenomena
Belief in possession of magical control over others
Constricted or inappropriate affect
Anxiety in social situations

BOX 14-2 EPIDEMIOLOGY OF CLUSTER A PERSONALITY DISORDERS

Paranoid Personality Disorder
Families who have one or more members that have already been diagnosed with paranoid personality disorder are at increased risk.
Males are diagnosed more often than females.
Substance abuse is common.

Schizoid Personality Disorder
Males are diagnosed slightly more often than females.
Families with members who have schizophrenia or schizotypal personality disorder have increased prevalence.

Schizotypal Personality Disorder
Individuals with schizotypal personality disorder seek treatment for anxiety or depression and not generally for the personality disorder features.
First-degree relatives of individuals with schizophrenia are at increased risk.
Males are diagnosed slightly more often than females.

CLINICAL SYMPTOMS
Cluster B Personality Disorders

Antisocial Personality Disorder
Irresponsibility
Failure to honor financial obligations, plan ahead, or provide children with basic needs
Involvement in illegal activities
Lack of guilt
Difficulty learning from mistakes
Initial charm dissolves into coldness, manipulation, and blaming others
Lack of empathy
Irritability
Abuse of substances

Borderline Personality Disorder
Suicidal ideation
Self-mutilation
Impulsivity
Tendency to engage in impulsive acts (e.g., bingeing, spending money, reckless driving, unsafe sex)
Negative or angry affect
Feelings of emptiness and boredom
Difficulty being alone or feeling of abandonment
Difficulty identifying self
Perception of people as all good or all bad
Intense and stormy relationships

Histrionic Personality Disorder
Use of suicidal gestures and threats when feeling abandoned
Fluctuation in emotions
Attention-seeking and self-centered attitude
Sexual seduction and flamboyance
Attentiveness to own physical appearance
Dramatic and impressionistic speech style
Vague logic; a lack of conviction in arguments, often switching sides
Shallow emotional expression
Craving for immediate satisfaction
Complaints of physical illness; somatization

Narcissistic Personality Disorder
Grandiose view of self
Lack of empathy toward others
Need for admiration
Preoccupation with fantasies of success, brilliance, beauty, and ideal love

---

dependent personality disorder, and obsessive-compulsive personality disorder. Box 14-4 and the Clinical Symptoms box on page 304 provide epidemiology and summarize the key clinical symptoms of these disorders.

Unspecified Personality Disorders

The category of unspecified personality disorders describes individuals whose personality pattern meets the general criteria for a personality disorder but not the criteria for any specific personality disorder. It is also for an individual whose

BOX 14-3   **EPIDEMIOLOGY OF CLUSTER B PERSONALITY DISORDERS**

Antisocial Personality Disorder
This is usually diagnosed in an individual by the time he or she is 18 years old.
Individuals have a history of conduct disorders before the age of 15 years.
Males are diagnosed more often than females.
Characteristics are evident by early childhood in males and by puberty in females.
A high percentage of diagnosed individuals are in substance abuse treatment settings and prisons.
Incidence is more common in the lower socioeconomic classes.
Substance abuse is common.
Impulsive behavior is common.
Approximately 1% of individuals 18 years old or older in the United States are diagnosed with antisocial personality disorder.

Borderline Personality Disorder
This condition is diagnosed in 1.6% of the general population in the United States who are 18 years old or older.
Diagnosed individuals often have a history of physical and sexual abuse, neglect, hostile conflict, and early parental loss or separation.
Females are diagnosed more often than males.

Histrionic Personality Disorder
Females are diagnosed more often than males.

Narcissistic Personality Disorder
Males are diagnosed more often than females.

BOX 14-4   **EPIDEMIOLOGY OF CLUSTER C PERSONALITY DISORDERS**

Avoidant Personality Disorder
The diagnosis is equal for males and females.
It is diagnosed in 5.2% of individuals 18 years old or older in the United States.

Dependent Personality Disorder
More females are diagnosed than males.
Symptoms are demonstrated early during life.
Children or adolescents with chronic physical illness or separation anxiety disorder may be predisposed to this condition.

Obsessive-Compulsive Personality Disorder
Males are diagnosed twice as often as females.

References: American Psychiatric Association: *Diagnostic and statistical manual of mental disorders*, ed 4, text revision, Washington, DC, American Psychiatric Association, 2000; and the National Institute of Mental Health: *The numbers count: mental disorders in America* (website): www.nimh.nih.gov/health/publications/the-numbers-count-mental-disorders-in-america/index.shtml. Accessed November 21, 2010.

CLINICAL SYMPTOMS
Cluster C Personality Disorders

Avoidant Personality Disorder
Fearful of criticism, disapproval, or rejection
Avoidance of social interactions
Tendency to withhold thoughts and feelings
Negative sense of self and low self-esteem

Dependent Personality Disorder
Submissiveness and tendency to cling
Inability to make decisions independently
Inability to express negative emotions
Difficulty following through on tasks

Obsessive-Compulsive Personality Disorder
Preoccupation with perfection, organization, structure, and control
Procrastination
Abandonment of projects because of dissatisfaction
Excessive devotion to work
Difficulty relaxing
Rule-conscious behavior
Self-criticism and inability to forgive own errors
Reluctance to delegate
Inability to discard anything
Insistence on others' conforming to own methods
Rejection of praise
Reluctance to spend money
Background of stiff and formal relationships
Preoccupation with logic and intellect

personality pattern meets the general criteria for a personality disorder; however, the person has a personality disorder that is not in the current classification, such as passive-aggressive personality disorder.

The DSM-V is due to be published and implemented in 2013. The definitions of personality disorders in this text will be organized differently. The study group for this edition of the DSM is proposing a method to assist clinicians with making more definitive diagnoses without overlap between personality disorder diagnoses. Further research will occur before publication in the form of field studies (Skodol and Bender, 2009).

PROGNOSIS

When providing nursing care to patients with personality disorders, it is important to consider the prognosis for improvement. This is especially important during the planning and evaluating phases of the nursing care plan. By definition, individuals with personality disorders have demonstrated pervasive and inflexible behaviors and thoughts that differ from cultural expectations (American Psychiatric Association, 2000). These patterns first begin during adolescence or early adulthood, and they are stable over time. The symptoms of a personality disorder lead to distress as well as functional and relationship impairments. With this definition in mind, the prognosis for individuals with personality disorders is guarded as a result of the ingrained and pervasive nature of these disorders (Choi et al, 2010; Zanarini et al, 2010) (see Research for evidence-based practice on this page).

Realistic expectations for improvement include a commitment by the patient to explore and evaluate his or her thoughts and behaviors, especially when under stress. The nurse plays a powerful role by providing support, tools for this exploration, and patient teaching. If the patient is able to use the knowledge of his or her dysfunctional patterns to predict how he or she will respond when faced with a stressor, the nurse is able to plan innovative options for problem solving. In this way, the individual learns new responses and improves functioning. This process often needs to be repeated over time before behavioral and thought patterns change. Therefore, long-term treatment aimed at problem solving and cognitive reframing is indicated for these patients.

Marsha Linehan (1943-) identified, in 1993, the repeating behavioral patterns of individuals with borderline personality disorder. She then began to study what interventions decrease the most destructive behavioral patterns, such as parasuicidal behavior, splitting, and intense emotional reactivity. This research yielded a treatment strategy called *dialectical behavioral therapy*. The principal assumption is to use dialogue to assist the patient with reworking destructive ways of dealing with crises. Dialectical behavioral therapy teaches the patient that there are choices when working through the crisis that decrease suicidal thoughts or emotionally reactive patterns. This type of therapy focuses on the patient learning new patterns of thoughts and behaviors. Current research suggests that individuals who are treated with dialectical behavioral therapy have a decrease in hospitalizations because of a decrease in suicidal drive and a higher level of interpersonal functioning (Osborne and McCornish, 2006) (see Chapter 26).

DISCHARGE CRITERIA

Patients with personality disorders present in both inpatient and outpatient settings, such as day treatment facilities, partial hospital units, clinics, and private office practices. To determine when to discharge a patient from an inpatient hospital setting, it is important to consider the risk factors of safety for the patient and others. Some patients with personality disorders have suicidal ideas that are part of their day-to-day thought process. When evaluating patients with this ongoing theme, it is important to determine whether the patient has a suicidal plan and if he or she intends to implement that plan (see Chapter 22).

Individuals with a personality disorder who are hospitalized often have more than one psychiatric diagnosis. Their lives are complex and chaotic. Psychiatric follow-up care—whether in a partial hospitalization program, a day treatment center, or with an outpatient psychotherapist—is important to help the patient to work through some of the issues that contributed to the crisis that culminated in the hospital stay. Before discharge from the hospital, it is important for the

RESEARCH FOR EVIDENCE-BASED PRACTICE

Zanarini MC et al: Prediction of the 10 year course of borderline personality disorder, *Am J Psychiatry* 163(5):827-834, 2006.

Zanarini MC et al: Time to attainment of recovery from borderline personality disorder and stability of recovery: a 10-year prospective follow-up study, *Am J Psychiatry* 167(6):663-667, 2010.

Zanarini and colleagues studied 290 individuals in a 10-year longitudinal research study to determine if symptoms of borderline personality disorder (BPD) are able to show remission. All of the original research participants were hospitalized in an inpatient unit at a New England psychiatric hospital for symptoms related to BPD. Researchers gave the individuals several tools to verify the diagnosis of BPD. Subjects were excluded from the research if they had a history of schizophrenia, schizoaffective disorder, bipolar I disorder, or an organic condition. Two interviewers determined the diagnosis. The individuals in the research were followed for 10 years, with interviews occurring every 2 years. Researchers defined remission as no longer meeting the criteria for BPD in accordance with the DSM-IV-TR and the *Revised Diagnostic Interview for Borderlines*.

Of the 275 participants who were initially enrolled in the research, 242 reached remission from the symptoms of BPD. The individuals who were able to achieve remission were younger when they were first diagnosed with BPD, and they had no psychiatric hospitalizations before the hospitalization that occurred when the initial research took place. These individuals had no history of childhood sexual abuse, and they had experienced less severe childhood abuse or neglect. Their family history was negative for mood and substance abuse. There was an absence of posttraumatic stress disorder and symptoms of the anxious Cluster C personality disorders. The individuals who achieved remission had low neuroticism (i.e., a predisposition toward negative affective states, such as depression, anxiety, and anger), high extroversion, high agreeableness, high conscientiousness, and a good vocational record. The remission of symptoms was described as a patient having good social and vocational functioning for 2 years.

The statistics showed that, over the entire 10 years of the study, 50% of the individuals showed recovery from the symptoms of BPD for 2 years. However, of these individuals, 34% were unable to sustain the recovery. Ninety-three percent of the study participants showed some remission of the symptoms of BPD for 2 years, with 86% demonstrating a continuous remission for 4 years. Of the individuals who had a remission of some of their symptoms over 2 years, 30% had a symptomatic recurrence, and 15% of the individuals who had a remission for 4 years demonstrated a recurrence of symptoms. The research highlights the enduring symptoms of this personality disorder. It is often difficult for individuals with BPD to sustain the remission. If the person was able to achieve a recovery, this was described as being able to maintain that recovery for the 10 years of the study.

This research is useful to therapists who provide care for individuals with BPD. It is helpful to be able to anticipate that a patient can achieve remission if there is a combination of the characteristics mentioned here with psychotherapy.

patient to have a plan for outpatient follow-up care and the first posthospital appointment established.

Patient teaching is a powerful tool to help the patient understand the psychiatric problems that he or she is experiencing as well as to help prevent a relapse of symptoms. Before discharge from the hospital, each patient needs to receive education in the following areas:

- The need for follow-up care in an outpatient setting
- The psychiatric symptoms that indicate a need for emergent treatment
- An understanding of any medications that the patient is receiving

This patient teaching takes place in a group setting or on an individual basis. If one of the location activities is a relapse prevention group or a medication group, it is helpful for the nurse to review the material specific to each patient before his or her discharge.

If the patient is in an outpatient setting, the nurse needs to consider the following issues before discharge from treatment:

- The patient no longer has active thoughts of wanting to harm himself or herself or others.
- The patient controls self-destructive impulses such as substance abuse when feeling upset or shoplifting when feeling empty.
- The patient has an understanding of the symptoms that caused the need for psychotherapy.
- The patient understands the types of symptoms that indicate a need for further treatment in the future.
- The patient is able to use community 12-step groups if this is relevant to his or her problems, such as Alcoholics Anonymous, Narcotics Anonymous, Co-Dependents Anonymous, Incest Survivors Anonymous, and Overeaters Anonymous.

THE NURSING PROCESS
ASSESSMENT

When the nurse assesses a patient for a personality disorder, the interview needs to take place in a comfortable, quiet, private, and safe environment. Make sure that there are no interruptions during the assessment. Individuals with these disorders are often withdrawn, defensive, guarded, and impulsive; alternatively, they can be charming and friendly.

Do not be judgmental or confrontational during the interview. If the patient demonstrates an escalation of anger or makes hostile or threatening comments in response to the assessment questions, a break will help the patient to regain composure. Do not threaten the patient with a coercive intervention, such as early discharge, because this will provoke him or her to impulsively lose control as a result of abandonment anxiety.

The Nursing Assessment Questions box represents a comprehensive evaluation for patients who have a personality disorder. The five domains of human behavior examined are the physical, emotional, cognitive, social, and spiritual domains (see Case Study #1 on page 308).

NURSING DIAGNOSIS

Nurses develop a diagnosis on the basis of the in-depth assessment of the patient's health status. The nursing diagnosis is a statement that defines the problem, its characteristics, and its contributing factors and that guides the development of the nursing care plan (see Nursing Assessment Questions #1 and #2). Nursing diagnoses are prioritized according to patient needs and safety issues. The following nursing diagnoses (North American Nursing Diagnosis Association International, 2007) are the most common when caring for patients with personality disorders.

Paranoid, Schizoid, and Schizotypal Personality Disorders (Cluster A)

- Anxiety
- Ineffective coping
- Social isolation
- Disturbed thought processes

Antisocial, Borderline, Histrionic, and Narcissistic Personality Disorders (Cluster B)

- Risk for suicide
- Risk for other-directed violence
- Risk for self-mutilation
- Risk for self-directed violence
- Ineffective coping
- Disturbed personal identity
- Chronic low self-esteem
- Impaired social interaction
- Complicated grieving

Avoidant, Dependent, and Obsessive-Compulsive Personality Disorders (Cluster C)

- Anxiety
- Ineffective coping
- Chronic low self-esteem
- Impaired social interaction

OUTCOME IDENTIFICATION

An individual with a personality disorder has disturbances in self-image and relationships throughout life. Identifying outcomes includes the patient's ability to demonstrate an understanding of problem areas and to display healthy and effective adaptive behaviors. The focus is on helping the individual to find patterns of maladaptive behaviors, thoughts, and emotions that produce distress. The nurse and patient will work together to explore options to change these maladaptive patterns to more effective coping strategies.

The outcome criteria come from the nursing diagnoses and are the expected patient responses or behaviors that occur as a result of the plan of care. Nurses state outcomes in clear and measurable terms.

NURSING ASSESSMENT QUESTIONS #1

Personality Disorders

Physical Domain

1 Is there evidence of appropriate activities of daily living?
2 Is the patient neatly groomed?
3 Is the patient dressed appropriately?
4 Does the patient appear to be adequately nourished?
5 Is there evidence of a regular exercise program in his or her life?
6 Is there evidence of any physical illnesses?
7 Does the patient concentrate on somatic concerns?
8 Is the patient able to maintain eye contact?
9 Is the patient experiencing tension?
10 Does the patient demonstrate sympathetic stimulation, cardiovascular excitation, superficial vasoconstriction, or pupil dilation?
11 Does the patient report trouble sleeping?
12 Is the patient glancing about in a suspicious manner?
13 Is the patient demonstrating extraneous movements, such as foot shuffling or hand and arm movements?
14 Does the patient show facial tension?
15 Is his or her voice quivering?
16 Does the patient report increased wariness?
17 Is the patient having an increase in perspiration?
18 Does the patient have a history of any of the following physical conditions?
Temporal lobe epilepsy
Progressive central nervous system disorder
Head trauma
Hormonal imbalance
Mental retardation
Abuse of alcohol or drugs
19 Is the patient dressed inappropriately or in a seductive manner?
20 Does the patient have a high incidence of accidents?
21 Is the patient overly concerned with physical attractiveness?

Emotional Domain

1 Does the patient indicate having thoughts of harming himself or herself or others?
2 Does the patient demonstrate demanding or hostile behavior?
3 Does the patient have a history of aggressive actions?
4 Is the patient emotionally volatile?
5 Does the patient have poor impulse control?
6 Is the patient suspicious of others?
7 Is the patient fearful or highly anxious?
8 Does the patient express feelings of helplessness?
9 Does the patient appear to be apprehensive?
10 Does the patient's thought pattern include feelings of uncertainty?
11 Does the patient discuss concerns about unspecified consequences?
12 Does the patient have persistent worries?
13 Does the patient demonstrate critical behavior toward himself or herself and others?
14 Does the patient have low self-esteem?
15 Is the patient concerned about how others will evaluate him or her?
16 Does the patient inflate his or her importance?

17 Does the patient describe feelings of guilt or regret?
18 Does the patient lack remorse and use excuses to justify hurting another person?
19 Does the patient lack empathy?
20 Is the patient vindictive?
21 Does the patient demonstrate a low frustration tolerance?
22 Does the patient show a lack of motivation?
23 Is the patient dependent on others to meet his or her needs?
24 Is the patient's behavior passive?
25 Does the patient discuss feelings of inadequacy?
26 Does the patient deny strong emotions, such as anger and joy?
27 Does the patient describe feelings of hopelessness?
28 Does the patient demonstrate inappropriate sexually seductive behavior?
29 Does the patient manifest a constricted affect?
30 Does the patient exhibit an inappropriate affect?
31 Does the patient display lability of his or her mood?

Cognitive Domain

1 Does the patient demonstrate inaccurate interpretation of stimuli, both internal and external?
2 Does the patient have difficulty understanding abstract ideas?
3 Is the patient able to identify problem areas?
4 Is the patient able to identify options for solving his or her problems?
5 Does the patient's identification of the problem area involve blaming others or himself or herself?
6 Is the patient vindictive with regard to his or her problem solving?
7 Does the patient lie?
8 Is the patient able to identify both good and bad traits in others?
9 Is the patient able to distinguish positive and negative options in the area of problem solving?
10 Does the patient reflect too much on issues of concern?
11 Is the patient's thought pattern redundant?
12 Is the patient able to tolerate a delay in gratification?
13 Is the patient able to identify his or her value system?
14 Does the patient have difficulty learning from his or her mistakes?
15 Is the patient impulsive?
16 Does the patient manifest any deficits in long-term or short-term memory?
17 Is the patient preoccupied?
18 Does the patient have a lack of consensual validation?
19 Does the patient describe any delusions?
20 Does the patient experience any hallucinations? If so, are they auditory, visual, tactile, gustatory, or olfactory? What is the content of the hallucinations?
21 Does the patient reveal any perceptual experiences?
22 Does the patient confirm that he or she has any ideas of reference?
23 Does the patient discuss any odd beliefs or magical thinking that influence his or her behavior?
24 Is the patient's speech impoverished, digressive, vague, or inappropriately abstract?

Continued

NURSING ASSESSMENT QUESTIONS #1—cont'd

Social Domain

1 Does the patient prefer to be alone?
2 Does the patient express a desire to socialize but have concerns that others will not accept him or her?
3 Is the patient dependent on others for meeting his or her needs?
4 Does the patient participate in family activities?
5 Does the patient have any friends?
6 Does the patient have unstable relationships that consist of conflict and concerns about abandonment?
7 Is the patient able to identify the dynamics of relationship problems?
8 Is the patient using manipulative behavior as a means of getting his or her needs met?
9 Does the patient show evidence of splitting? Does the patient place great value on relating with one person while becoming critical and angry with another? Does the patient devalue and complain about one individual to another person with whom the patient has a positive relationship?
10 Does the patient identify his or her sense of self by indicating membership in a relationship?
11 Does the patient often want to be the center of attention?
12 Is the patient preoccupied with how others view him or her?
13 Is this patient extremely sensitive to the praise and criticism of others?
14 Is the patient reluctant to give time, gifts, and support to his or her friends unless he or she will profit?
15 Does the patient choose solitary activities?
16 Does the patient engage in any social activities?
17 Does the patient feel increasingly anxious when in a social situation?
18 Does the patient express no desire to have a sexual experience with another person?
19 Does the patient have multiple sexual partners?
20 Is the patient indifferent to the praise and criticism of others?
21 Does the patient expect others to exploit him or her?
22 Does the patient exploit others to meet his or her needs?
23 Does the patient question the loyalty or trustworthiness of friends or associates? Does the patient question the loyalty of his or her spouse or sexual partner?
24 Does the patient read hidden meanings into the harmless remarks of others?
25 Does the patient have grudges against others?
26 Is the patient reluctant to confide in others?
27 Is the patient preoccupied with himself or herself to the exclusion of others?
28 Does the patient fail to honor financial obligations?
29 Does the patient fail to plan ahead, such as traveling without a clear plan or quitting work without plans to begin another job?
30 Does the patient provide his or her children with the basic needs for their health?
31 Does the patient engage in illegal activities?
32 Does the patient abuse drugs or alcohol?
33 Does the patient demonstrate a sense of entitlement?

Spiritual Domain

1 Does the patient have a belief in a higher power?
2 Is the patient able to state a meaning and purpose for his or her life?

CASE STUDY #1

Nicholas, a 32-year-old single man, was evaluated by a nurse in an outpatient clinic at the recommendation of his father because of an increase in his isolative behavior. Nicholas did not want to come in for the interview, because he did not consider "being alone" a problem. He was oriented three times, but he was not spontaneous with answers to the nurse's assessment questions. His affect was flat, he averted his eyes, and his leg was shaking. He was unkempt, with a disheveled appearance and mismatched clothing. He had a vague, wandering, and nonspecific way of discussing his problem and his lifestyle.

His mother had been recently hospitalized with pneumonia; however, Nicholas did not see that as part of his problem. He was able to hold a job cleaning offices for a small firm, but perceived that his boss and the office staff disliked him, because they believed he was "weird." However, Nicholas made no attempt to initiate conversation with his coworkers, or join in the usual office activities. Nicholas said that he had no friends, that he found socializing difficult, and that he tended to withdraw further when forced to interact with others. He was suspicious of the interviewer and of his father's motives for asking him to seek psychiatric intervention.

The problem that he identified was that he felt he had to "do more around the house" in his mother's absence. That seemed "unfair and like a burden" to Nicholas. "She just got sick so she wouldn't have to cook supper or do the laundry," Nicholas stated. "The doctors put her in the hospital so that they will make more money off of her. Dad is in on it; he sent me here so you could make money."

Nicholas had not visited his mother in the hospital because he was afraid he would get germs there. Although he saw no reason for this interview, he consented to return to the clinic to "help" his father.

Critical Thinking

1 What questions should the nurse ask Nicholas to determine the presence of symptoms in the physical domain?
2 How could the nurse assess the emotional domain?
3 How could the nurse assess Nicholas's problems in the cognitive domain?
4 What information about Nicholas helps to determine his functioning in the social domain?
5 What questions could the nurse ask Nicholas to assess how he functions in the spiritual domain?

The patient will do the following:
- Demonstrate the absence of active suicidal ideation.
- Interrupt and not respond to thoughts about harming others.
- Use mindfulness meditation to reduce impulsive behaviors and to reduce intense emotional states (Gaines and Barry, 2008).
- Refrain from self-mutilation.
- Reach and maintain the highest functioning possible as demonstrated by the ability to function at home, work, and in the community and to interact with others in an appropriate manner.
- Identify two impulsive behavior patterns that take place during times of stress.
- Recognize when he or she is experiencing cognitive distortions during a stressful period of time.
- Identify a cognitive distortion that is used most often during times of stress.
- Identify one new method of problem solving.
- Reward himself or herself as part of self-soothing, both with an item (e.g., flowers, going to a movie) and a positive thought, when he or she is able to successfully identify and change a cognitive distortion.
- Identify some patterns of isolative behavior.
- Tolerate short interactive periods with the nurse, family members, and peers (see Case Study #2).
- Identify with positive role models.
- Contribute one statement in a group setting that is directed toward facilitating increased socialization.

PLANNING

When planning interventions with a patient who has a personality disorder, it is important for the nurse to recognize that changes in behavior or thoughts often occur slowly. These changes are a result of the patient's perception of the need for that change. Individuals with a personality disorder have disturbed interpersonal relationships and values that do not reflect the views held by the general population. Because of these disturbances, the nurse needs to collaborate with the patient regarding the goals that are identified during treatment.

IMPLEMENTATION

The implementation of the plan of care for patients with personality disorders includes interventions that are focused on modifying lifelong disruptive and dysfunctional behaviors and thoughts while promoting safety.

Nursing Interventions

1. Assess the patient for suicidal ideation and to determine the level of lethality *to prevent suicide, harm, or injury.*
2. If warranted, place the patient on suicide precautions, depending on his or her level of lethality (e.g., a patient who has verbalized plans to hang himself or herself while on the unit requires close individual observation, even

---

NURSING ASSESSMENT QUESTIONS #2

Personality Disorders

These questions involve the nurse's observations of the patient's appearance, general nutritional status, and level of observable anxiety manifestations:

1. Does the patient appear to be appropriately dressed? Does the patient maintain eye contact? Does he or she appear to be properly nourished? Does the patient exhibit signs of anxiety, such as pacing, foot tapping, sighing, or facial tension? Does the patient appear to be hypervigilant (overly watchful)? Does the patient appear to be withdrawn?

   The following questions will help the nurse to determine if there are disturbances in the patient's relationships, thought processes, and behaviors:

2. How would you describe yourself? What do you like about yourself? What would you like to change about yourself?
3. Describe your relationships with your spouse or your significant other, your children, your parents, and your other family members. Describe your relationships with your friends. What do you talk about? What types of activities do you do together?
4. How do you feel about your job? Do you get along with your boss and your coworkers?
5. If you have a personal problem, who do you trust to help you with it?
6. What are your main worries? How often do you think about them? Do you talk to anyone about these worries? Does that help?
7. Do you ever feel like hurting yourself or anyone else? Have you ever been suicidal? Have you ever hurt yourself by cutting your skin or burning yourself? If yes, how often does this occur?
8. Have you ever felt hopeless, helpless, worthless, and like a burden? Do you feel this way now? Are you getting any support from friends or family?
9. Do you ever use alcohol or illegal drugs? Have you ever gone to the doctor to get tranquilizers to reduce your nervousness? What did the doctor give you? What are you taking now?
10. What are your religious beliefs and practices?

---

with no means or provisions to carry out the intent) *to prevent suicide.*

3. Encourage the patient to attend all unit group sessions *to receive support from peers and to provide opportunities for problem solving.*
4. Assess the patient for an escalation of anger to rage and possible impulsive actions against others (obtain a history of violence, if possible) *to prevent harm or injury to others.*
5. Teach the patient other options for managing angry and impulsive feelings and behaviors, such as leaving the room in which the conflict is occurring or using a quiet area (e.g., an unlocked seclusion room) until the impulse to do harm passes. *Removing the patient from a*

CASE STUDY #2

Olivia, a 30-year-old outpatient has a pattern of unlawful behaviors usually stemming from relationship issues. She has been working on these issues with a nurse for the past 3 years in outpatient psychotherapy. She was recently arrested for stealing some candy and lipstick at a local department store after an argument with her boyfriend. During the session after the arrest, the nurse suggested to Olivia that she explore the dynamics of the incident and how this related to the argument with her boyfriend. Olivia became angry and then scared, expressing concern that she might lose the respect of the nurse which could end their therapeutic relationship. She ran out of the room, yelling that the nurse did not understand her pain, and slammed the door. Several minutes later, Olivia returned, apologized, and asked the nurse to forgive her.

Critical Thinking

1 Which of Olivia's responses indicate that she had some insight into the dynamics of her impulsive stealing behaviors?
2 What changes in behavior are anticipated as a result of Olivia's gaining understanding about her impulsive behavior?
3 What two outcomes would be realistic for Olivia?
4 How should the nurse respond to Olivia's anger and subsequent apology?

stimulating and provocative environment will decrease his or her angry impulses.

6. Discuss angry feelings in a group setting that is focused on exploring alternative problem-solving options. *Alternative actions will distract the patient from angry feelings and help to focus energy on constructive activities.*

7. Assess the patient for evidence of self-mutilation. *Patients who are self-destructive are likely to repeat such acts and may require further intervention.*

8. Place the patient on individual close watch until the urge to harm himself or herself passes or until the patient is able to identify another way to obtain emotional relief (e.g., wrapping up in a sheet [Dresser, 1999] or participating in a movement therapy group) *to protect the patient from harmful impulses and to redirect the impulses toward alternative and constructive methods.*

9. If self-mutilation occurs, attend to the wounds in a matter-of-fact manner *to provide the patient with safe care in a nonjudgmental manner.*

10. Encourage the patient to keep a journal of the thoughts and feelings that he or she had before experiencing the urge to self-mutilate *to help the patient to acknowledge feelings and thoughts and to help decrease impulsivity.*

11. Medicate the patient with an anxiolytic or antipsychotic medication as ordered *to help the patient to control his or her intense anxiety or rage rather than self-mutilating.*

12. Use a timeout period, a seclusion room, and physical restraints if all attempts of least restrictive measures

have been unsuccessful. Document this intervention as per Joint Commission requirements *to protect the patient.*

13. Assist the patient with recognizing thought patterns that contribute to impulsive behavior. Nurses are able to do this by helping the patient understand the role that intense feelings (e.g., abandonment, anger, rage, anxiety) play in precipitating impulsive behavior or distorted thinking (Gabbard and Horowitz, 2009). The use of a journal to document such feelings and thoughts and receiving feedback during group sessions can be helpful and instructive methods. *Nurses teach patients to manage their impulsive behaviors and distorted beliefs through a variety of methods within the setting.*

14. Suggest alternative behaviors to deal with the intense feelings, such as the following:
    a. Recognizing the intense emotional state and writing in a journal or thinking about an action that helps to relieve the intensity of the feeling without resorting to impulsive or self-destructive acts
    b. Using mindfulness meditation to reduce the intense feelings and to prevent impulsive responses to these feelings (Gaines and Barry, 2008)
    c. Talking about the intense feelings while looking into a mirror and telling the mirror what the patient would like to express to the object of anger
    d. Identifying healthy options for dealing with the anger, such as discussing the issue with the person who is involved in the interaction
    e. Role-playing with the nursing staff different ways to approach the problem that precipitated the intense feelings
    f. Introducing the issue in a problem-solving setting or group meeting to receive feedback from peers
    g. Rewarding the self by self-soothing with something that is pleasant and healthful, such as buying flowers, going to a movie, playing a video game, or reading a novel
    h. Learning alternative ways to cope with intense feelings to thereby reduce anger and anxiety and to provide constructive ways of managing life stressors

15. Help the patient to explore behavior that relates to the community, such as safe driving and responsibility for the environment, *to help the patient to focus on changes that he or she can make to live in a more healthy and responsible way.*

16. Evaluate the patient's family system by observing the family dynamics and determining the patient's role within the family. *How the patient interacts within the family system and the role that the patient takes (e.g., victim, placater) offer the nurse insight into the patient's self-perception.*

17. Engage the patient in frequent short interactions several times during the shift *to illustrate the value of interacting with others.*

18. Make use of problem-solving groups and other groups that concentrate on self-care and community

responsibilities *to help the patient to understand the value of interacting with others* (see Chapter 26).

19. Teach the patient assertiveness techniques *to improve the patient's ability to relate to others* (see Chapters 4 and 26).

20. Provide the patient with direct feedback about his or her interaction with others in a nonjudgmental fashion *to facilitate the patient's ability to learn new social skills.*

❖ CLINICAL ALERT

Patients with personality disorders have difficulty relating to others. As a consequence, these individuals have difficulty defining boundaries between themselves and others. Part of nursing care is to define boundaries within the therapeutic relationship in order to develop safe, patient-centered therapeutic relationships. This is particularly important for the nurse to think about when he or she is feeling vulnerable, perhaps because of other personal or professional stressors. It is important that nurses assess their feelings toward the patients who are in their care as well as toward their own current stressors. Nurses need to ask themselves the following questions: "Are the stressors interfering with my functioning on the job?" "In what ways can I deal with these issues without becoming vulnerable to the patients under my care?" If nurses recognize that they are experiencing special feelings for a particular patient, they need to discuss these feelings with a colleague or obtain clinical supervision or assistance from the employee assistance program (Bland et al, 2007).

Additional Treatment Modalities

A team approach that involves many disciplines provides the most comprehensive interventions for a patient with a personality disorder in an inpatient, partial hospitalization, or day treatment setting (see the Additional Treatment Modalities box and Chapter 26).

Nurses are in a position to encourage and participate in research (see Online Resources). The more information that the patient and the patient's family have, the more the choices regarding the use of treatment services and medication adherence make sense. Research will assist the nurse with providing more comprehensive care, and will help the nurse to answer questions that will drive clinical practice.

Occupational Therapy

The occupational therapist assesses a patient's abilities and disabilities and helps the patient to increase his or her functioning and independent living skills in areas such as self-care, work, and leisure activities. The occupational therapist teaches adaptive skills for home, school, and job functioning. The occupational therapist often plans and leads groups that focus on areas such as stress management, enhancing parenting skills, conflict resolution, time management, money management, budgeting, feeling, and self-awareness.

Art Therapy

The art therapist uses art as a means of helping the patient to express thoughts and feelings that he or she is not able to verbalize. This intervention helps the patient to understand problem areas from a symbolic standpoint. The art therapist also teaches the patient an alternative means of expression and self-soothing. For example, a patient who is feeling intense rage and who wants to self-mutilate will use art to express these feelings rather than acting on them.

ADDITIONAL TREATMENT MODALITIES
Personality Disorders

- Occupational therapy
- Art therapy
- Music therapy
- Movement therapy
- Recreational therapy
- Medication therapy
- Individual therapy
- Cognitive behavioral therapy
- Dialectical behavioral therapy
- Group therapy
- Family therapy
- Milieu therapy

Music Therapy

The music therapist uses music to help the patient to express feelings and thoughts that are not easy to verbalize. Music helps the patient to relax and learn alternative self-soothing strategies.

Movement Therapy

Movement therapy teaches patients how to move their bodies when they are stressed, and it helps them to learn about methods of relaxation. Movement therapy is helpful for patients who become numb when experiencing intense feelings (e.g., abandonment, anger) to teach them to use methods of self-touching to reestablish a feeling state rather than self-mutilating.

Recreational Therapy

Recreational therapy helps patients with personality disorders to explore ways to enjoy themselves without the use of self-destructive behaviors, such as abusing alcohol or drugs. This modality is helpful for patients who have difficulty socializing, because recreation strengthens social skills.

Medication Therapy

Medications often play a major role in helping the patient with a personality disorder. Patients who are demonstrating violence against others sometimes require medications to gain emotional and behavioral control over their impulses. The practice guidelines for the treatment of individuals with borderline personality disorder (American Psychiatric

Association, URL update, 2005). suggest that patients who have affect dysregulation show a reduction in symptoms with the use of a selective serotonin reuptake inhibitor. If there is an anxiety component along with the affective dysregulation, this usually indicates the need for a benzodiazepine such as clonazepam (Klonopin) along with the selective serotonin reuptake inhibitor. Mood stabilizers such as lithium carbonate, carbamazepine (Tegretol), and valproate (Depakote) have been successful adjunctive treatments for affective dysregulation. For individuals who are demonstrating anger and impulsivity, a selective serotonin reuptake inhibitor is the treatment of choice. The clinical practice guideline recommends the use of fluoxetine (Prozac) as the first line of treatment for this symptom. Patients who are very agitated or who have psychosis sometimes respond to the use of a low-dose neuroleptic or an antipsychotic class medication. Patients with extreme violence who are unable to control this impulse sometimes receive intravenous or intramuscular sedative-hypnotics such as barbiturates, benzodiazepines such as diazepam (Valium), or antipsychotics such as haloperidol (Haldol). Monitoring side effects is an important nursing function (see Chapter 25).

Individual Therapy

Individual therapy helps the patient to explore problem areas, to define new options, and to discuss how the new behavior will help to solve the original problem. With the emphasis in the health care system on short-term therapy, individual therapy is now problem-solving oriented as opposed to explorative with regard to early trauma. The use of Linehan's dialectical behavioral therapy, which was described earlier, has an excellent rate of symptom reduction with the borderline individual (American Psychiatric Association, URL update 2005); Osborne and McCornish, 2006).

✏ MEDICATION KEY FACTS

Personality Disorders

- Pharmacologic interventions are symptom oriented, regardless of the type of personality disorder.
- Medications include the short-term use of benzodiazepines and antipsychotics for aggressiveness and impulsivity.
- Mood stabilizers are used for rage, violence, impulsivity and feelings of losing control.
- Other medications include antidepressants and antianxiety agents.

Group Therapy

Group therapy is also problem-solving oriented. The work in group therapy is based on the repeated dynamics of the individuals in the group. This is especially beneficial for patients with a Cluster B personality disorder who are dramatic and require a lot of attention. The group members help the patient to understand the effects that his or her behavior have on each of them so that the patient is able to use this information when relating to significant people in his or her everyday life.

Family Therapy

Family therapy is helpful for patients with a personality disorder because the dynamics of the family system are often repeated in other relationships in the patient's life, such as with his or her boss or spouse. The family sessions consist of an assessment of the family system and an exploration of how the current problems that caused the patient to seek care affect family dynamics. Because of the current philosophy of short-term therapy, the exploration of earlier dynamics or trauma focuses on the current issue.

Milieu Therapy

When a patient is hospitalized in an inpatient psychiatric setting or participates in a partial hospitalization program or a day treatment facility, the patient becomes part of that milieu (environment). The purpose of milieu therapy is to recreate a community setting on these units so that the patient is able to interact with other patient peers to identify and problem-solve issues that occur when relating to others. Such relationship issues are discussed in community meetings or other problem-solving groups (e.g., a coping skills group).

The community meetings are for delegating the tasks of the unit, such as cleaning off the tables at the end of the meal. This meeting is often used to ask each member to think through a daily goal for therapy and to discuss how he or she plans to meet that goal. If something happens on the unit (e.g., if someone becomes aggressive or brings in drugs or alcohol), then the group discusses these concerns during the community meeting.

Problem-solving groups, such as coping skills groups, often pick a common area of concern, and the group works together to explore the issues and options that are necessary to solve the dilemma.

As in any other community, socializing is an important part of the interaction. In an inpatient partial hospitalization program or day treatment milieu, socialization groups discuss problems with socializing. For example, the socialization group uses the discussion of a movie that the group has just seen or current events read from a magazine or a newspaper to enrich the discussion.

EVALUATION

The evaluation stage of the nursing process is ongoing and takes place to ensure accountable, respectful, and nonjudgmental nursing practice. There are two steps to the evaluation stage:

1. The nurse compares the patient's current functioning with the identified outcome criteria.
2. The nurse asks questions to determine possible reasons for the outcome criteria not being met (Fortinash and Holoday Worret, 2007).

CONCEPT MAP CASE STUDY 14-1

Jared was admitted to the psychiatric unit directly from the emergency department because he was involved in a fight with another man at a bar. He was under the influence of both phencyclidine (PCP) and alcohol while at the bar. The emergency department staff assessed him as medically stable, but they suggested admission because of his potential for violence.

When Jared arrived on the unit, he was angry. He loudly stated that he had been treated unfairly in the emergency department and that he did not need to be admitted to the psychiatric unit "with all those nuts!" He demanded a television in his room and a cigarette. When the staff denied his requests, he became louder and threatening. He told the charge nurse that he would get his way, that he had friends on the hospital board, and that there would be an investigation into the hospital treatment of his case if he was not allowed to smoke or to watch television in private. He reminded the nurse that he was admitted for fighting in a bar, and he stated, "I know how to get my way."

DSM-IV-TR Diagnoses

Axis I   Substance abuse: alcohol and PCP

Axis II   Antisocial personality disorder

Axis III Medically stable, monitor for intoxication and withdrawal symptoms

Axis IV   Problems related to the social environment

Axis V   GAF = 40 (current); GAF = 60 (past year)

Nursing Diagnosis *Risk for other-directed violence: risk factors: a perception that others are denying him his rights and his control over his environment; a history of violence against others; recent ingestion of PCP and alcohol; impulsivity; and an increase in verbal demands, a loud voice, and verbally threatening behavior*

NOC Aggression self-control; Abusive behavior self-restraint; Impulse self-control; Stress level; Risk detection; Risk control: alcohol use, Risk control: drug use

NIC Anger control assistance; Environmental management: violence prevention; Anxiety reduction; Behavior management; Surveillance: safety; Security enhancement; Medication management

Nursing Diagnosis *Ineffective coping related to intoxication and withdrawal from alcohol and PCP as evidenced by the patient's loud and threatening behavior, impulsivity, and loss of control*

NOC Anxiety self-control; Aggression self-control; Impulse self-control; Coping; Social support; Knowledge: health resources; Decision making

NIC Anxiety reduction; Anger control assistance; Coping enhancement; Substance use prevention; Teaching: individual; Support system enhancement; Decision-making support

Nursing Diagnosis *Chronic low self-esteem related to long-term negative feedback and the patient's belief that he is unable to deal with problems as evidenced by self-destructive behavior (drinking, using PCP, and physical fighting in the bar), inability to accept constructive limit setting from the nursing staff, and the tendency to demean others to increase his own feelings of self-worth*

NOC Self-esteem, Motivation, Role performance, Social interaction skills, Hope, Quality of life

NIC Self-esteem enhancement, Support system enhancement, Socialization enhancement, Emotional support, Counseling

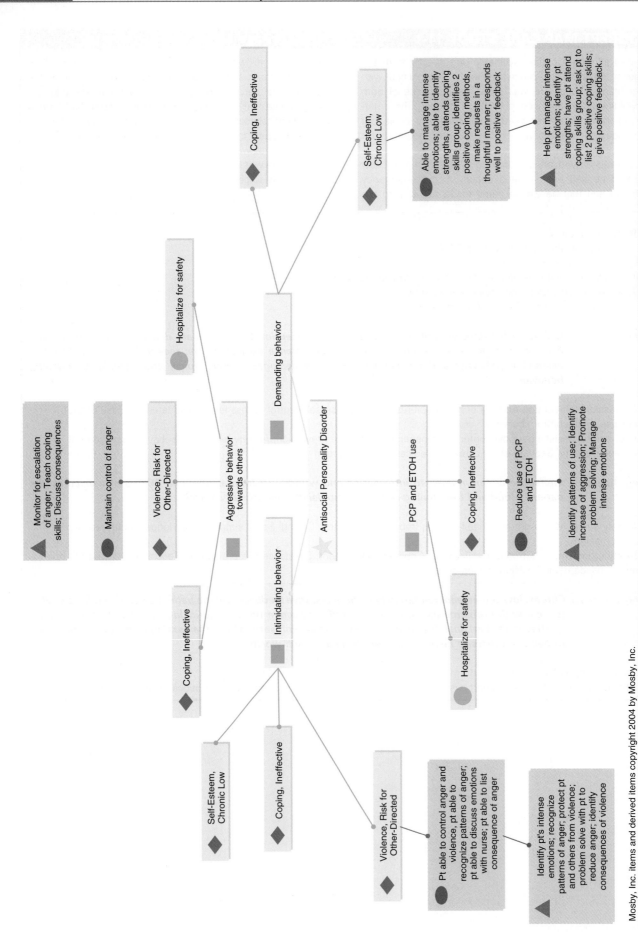

Mosby, Inc. items and derived items copyright 2004 by Mosby, Inc.

FIGURE 14-1. Concept map: antisocial personality disorder.

⊚ CONCEPT MAP CASE STUDY 14-2

Joanna is a 29-year-old single woman who became suicidal after her boyfriend, Evan, told her that their relationship was over. She started to drink and use diazepam (Valium) to calm down after Evan left her. The relationship had become stormy, with frequent threats from Evan that he would stop seeing her. Joanna became vengeful, went to Evan's parents' house where he was staying, and threw a rock into their living room window, shouting that she loved Evan and could not live without him. She shouted, "I don't want to hurt anyone. I just want to die!" and ran into the street in front of an oncoming car. The driver slammed on the brakes and hit Joanna hard enough to knock her down and cause a pelvic fracture. She was admitted to the local hospital, and she was still vowing to harm herself if Evan did not return to her.

DSM-IV-TR Diagnoses

Axis I   Substance abuse: alcohol and diazepam (Valium)
Axis II   Borderline personality disorder
Axis III   Pelvic fracture
Axis IV   Problems with primary support groups (breakup with boyfriend)
Axis V   GAF = 30 (current); GAF = 60 (past year)

Nursing Diagnosis *Risk for suicide: risk factors: intense feelings of abandonment, increased anxiety level, impulsivity, and a history of suicidal attempts*

NOC Suicide self-restraint, Depression level, Impulse self-control, Risk control, Personal well-being, Social support
NIC Suicide prevention; Mood management; Surveillance: safety; Impulse control training; Patient contracting; Support group

Nursing Diagnosis *Ineffective coping related to boyfriend ending a significant relationship as evidenced by the patient's vengeful behavior toward the boyfriend, her impulsive behavior to do self-harm, and her use of drugs and alcohol*

NOC Suicide self-restraint; Impulse self-control; Coping; Information processing; Social support; Psychosocial adjustment: life change; Personal well-being
NIC Coping enhancement; Impulse control training; Teaching: individual; Support system enhancement; Decision-making support; Therapy group

Nursing Diagnosis *Complicated grieving related to boyfriend ending a significant relationship as evidenced by the patient's use of drugs and alcohol, vengeful behavior, suicidal ideation, and impulsive behavior to do self-harm*

NOC Grief resolution; Coping; Communication; Depression self-control; Self-esteem; Psychosocial adjustment: life change
NIC Suicide prevention, Grief work facilitation, Hope instillation, Coping enhancement, Support group, Support system enhancement

GAF, Global Assessment of Functioning; NIC, Nursing Interventions Classification; NOC, Nursing Outcomes Classification.

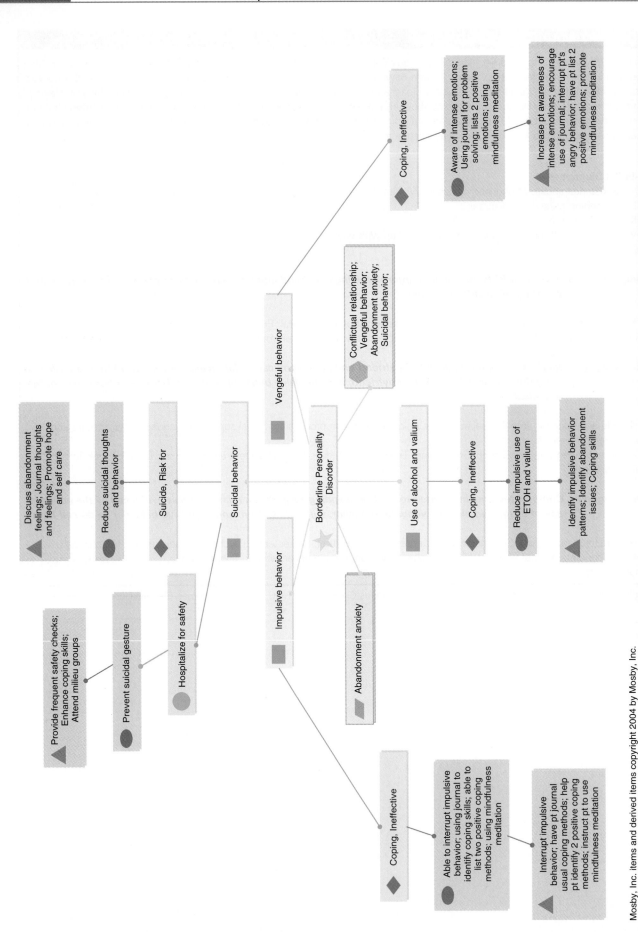

Mosby, Inc. items and derived items copyright 2004 by Mosby, Inc.

FIGURE 14-2. Concept map: borderline personality disorder.

CHAPTER SUMMARY

- A personality disorder is a longstanding, pervasive, and maladaptive pattern of behavior and relating to others that is not caused by an Axis I disorder.
- In psychodynamic theory, there is a belief that an individual who develops a personality disorder has deficits in his or her psychosexual development or has failed to achieve object constancy.
- Research has hypothesized several biologic considerations as possible causal factors for individuals who have developed personality disorders.
- The DSM-IV-TR Axis II is set up in a three-cluster format.
- Patients with personality disorders have difficulty relating to others at home, at work, and in the community.

- When working with individuals with personality disorders, it is most important to assess each patient for the risk of violence toward himself or herself or others.
- Patients with personality disorders often exhibit self-destructive behaviors such as self-mutilation, shoplifting, alcohol or substance abuse, and eating disorders (see Chapters 15 and 18).
- Realistic expectations for improvement include a commitment by the patient to explore and evaluate his or her thoughts, relationships, and behaviors, especially when under stress.

REVIEW QUESTIONS

1. The nurse explains to a patient with a borderline personality disorder that the patient's former psychiatrist resigned and that a new psychiatrist has been hired. Which reaction is most likely?
   1. Silence
   2. Withdrawal
   3. Rage
   4. Anxiety

2. A nurse manages the care of an individual with a personality disorder. Select the most attainable outcome for this patient.
   1. Within 2 weeks, the patient will establish a satisfying intimate relationship with another adult.
   2. Within 5 days, the patient will identify factors that led to the development of the personality disorder.
   3. Within 1 week, the patient will make a permanent commitment to never self-mutilate.
   4. Within 4 weeks, the patient will describe the personal characteristics of his or her reactions to stress.

3. An individual with an obsessive-compulsive personality disorder is consistently late for outpatient appointments as a result of writing and rewriting the list of topics to

bring up during the session. Which nursing diagnosis applies?
   1. Anxiety
   2. Social isolation
   3. Disturbed personality identity
   4. Situational low self-esteem

4. An adult patient with a borderline personality disorder vomits immediately after drinking 1 ounce of dishwashing soap in a suicide gesture. What should the nurse do first?
   1. Assess and record the patient's vital signs.
   2. Promptly place the patient on suicide precautions.
   3. Immediately notify the attending psychiatrist.
   4. Sit quietly with the patient until the vomiting subsides.

5. A nurse assesses an individual with schizotypal personality disorder. Which characteristics are most likely? You may select more than one answer.
   1. Male gender
   2. Complaints of depression
   3. Charges pending for assault
   4. Chronic physical illness
   5. Sibling diagnosed with schizophrenia

REFERENCES

American Psychiatric Association: *Diagnostic and statistical manual of mental disorders*, ed 4, text revision, Washington, DC, 2000, American Psychiatric Association.

American Psychiatric Association: *Practice guideline for the treatment of patients with borderline personality disorder, 2001*, URL update, 2005 (website): www.psych.org/psych_pract/treat//pg/prac_guide.cfm.

Bland AR et al: Nursing care of inpatients with borderline personality disorder, *Perspect Psychiatr Care* 43(4):204-213, 2007.

Brown GL, Linnoila MI: CSF serotonin metabolite (5-HIAA) studies in depression, impulsivity, and violence, *J Clin Psychiatry* 51(Suppl):31-41, 1990.

Choi LW et al: A longitudinal study of the 10-year course of interpersonal features in borderline personality disorder, *J Pers Disord* 24(3):365-376, 2010.

Coryell WH, Zimmerman M: Personality disorder in the families of depressed, schizophrenia, and never-ill probands, *Am J Psychiatry* 146:496-502, 1989.

Dresser J: Wrapping: a technique for interrupting self-mutilation, *J Am Psychiatr Nurses Assoc* 5(2):67-70, 1999.

Fortinash KM, Holoday Worret PA: *Psychiatric nursing care plans*, ed 4, St. Louis, 2007, Mosby.

Freud S: Three essays on the theory of sexuality, *Standard Edition of the complete works of Sigmund Freud*, 7:125-243, 1905.

Gabbard GO, Horowitz MJ: Insight, transference, interpretation, and therapeutic change in the dynamic psychotherapy of borderline personality disorder, *Am J Psychiatry* 166(5):517-522, 2009.

Gaines T, Barry LM: The effect of a self-monitored relaxation breathing exercise on male adolescent aggressive behavior, *Adolescence* 43(170):291-303, 2008.

Goldstein RB et al: Antisocial behavioral syndromes and additional psychiatric comorbidity in posttraumatic stress disorder among U.S. adults: results from wave 2 of the National Epidemiologic Survey on Alcohol and Related Conditions, *J Am Psychiatr Nurses Assoc* 16(3):145-165, 2010.

Kavoussi RJ, Siever LJ: Biologic validators of personality disorders. In Oldham JM, editor: *Personality disorders: new perspectives on diagnostic validity*, Washington, DC, 1991, American Psychiatric Press.

Kernberg OF: *Severe personality disorders: psychotherapeutic strategies*, New Haven, Conn, 1984, Yale University Press.

Leyton M et al: Brain regional alpha-{11C} methyl-L-tryptophan trapping in impulsive subjects with borderline personality disorder, *Am J Psych* 158:775-782, 2001.

Linehan MM: *Cognitive-behavioral treatment of borderline personality disorder*, New York, 1993, Guilford Press.

Mahler MS: Thoughts about development and individuation, *Psychoanal Study Child* 18:307-324, 1963.

Mahler MS: On the first three subphases of the separation-individuation process, *Int J Psychoanal* 53:333-338, 1972.

Marin D et al: Biological models and treatments for personality disorders, *Psychiatr Ann* 19:143, 1989.

Masterson JF: *Psychotherapy of the borderline adult: a developmental approach*, New York, 1976, Brunner/Mazel.

Modinos G et al: Schizotypy and brain structure: a voxel-based morphometry study, *Psychol Med* 40(9):1423-1431, 2010.

New AS, Stanley B: An opioid deficit in borderline personality disorder: self-cutting, substance abuse and social dysfunction, *Am J Psychiatry* 167(8):882-885, 2010.

North American Nursing Diagnosis Association International: *NANDA nursing diagnoses: definitions and classification, 2007-2008*, Philadelphia, 2007, North American Nursing Diagnosis Association International.

Osborne LL, McCornish, JF: Working with borderline personality disorder: nursing interventions using dialectical behavioral therapy, *J Psychosoc Nurs Ment Health Serv* 44:40-48, 2006.

Prossin AR et al: Dysregulation of regional endogenous opioid function in borderline personality disorder, *Am J Psychiatry* 167(8):925-1011, 2010.

Siever LJ: Biologic markers in schizotypal personality disorder, *Schizophr Bull* 11(4):564-574, 1985.

Siever LJ: Schizophrenia spectrum personality disorders. In Tasman A, Riba MB, editors: *American Psychiatric Press review of psychiatry*, vol 11, Washington, DC, 1992, American Psychiatric Press.

Siever LJ, Davis KL: A psychobiological perspective on the personality disorders, *Am J Psychiatry* 148:1647-1658, 1991.

Skodol A et al: Functional impairment in patients with schizotypal, borderline, avoidant, and obsessive-compulsive personality disorder, *Am J Psychiatry* 159:276-283, 2000.

Skodol AE, Bender DS: The future of personality disorders in DSM-V? *Am J Psychiatry* 166(4):388-391, 2009.

VanLuyn B et al, editors: *Severe personality disorders: everyday issues in clinical practice*, New York, 2007, Cambridge University Press.

Zanarini MC et al: Defense mechanisms associated with borderline personality disorder, *J Pers Disord* 23(2):113-122, 2009.

Zanarini MC et al: Time to attainment of recovery from borderline personality disorder and stability of recovery: a 10-year prospective follow-up study, *Am J Psychiatry* 167(6):663-667, 2010.

Online Resources

Borderline Personality Disorder Research Foundation: www.borderlineresearch.org

International Society for the Study of Personality Disorders: www.isspd.com

Mental Health America: www.nmha.org

National Alliance on Mental Illness: www.nami.org

National Institute of Mental Health: www.nimh.nih.gov

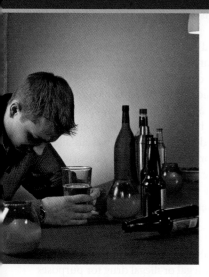

Substance-Related Disorders and Addictive Behaviors

Merry A. Armstrong

"Obsessed by a fairy tale, we spend our lives searching for a magic door and a lost kingdom of peace."

Eugene O'Neill

evolve WEBSITE

http://evolve.elsevier.com/Fortinash/

OBJECTIVES

- Identify major theories related to substance use disorders and impulse control disorders.
- Identify a multisystem approach to the etiology of addiction.
- Describe the neurobiology of chemical addiction.

- Define levels of substance use and abuse.
- Apply the nursing process for patients with chemical use disorders.
- Describe treatment options for patients with substance-related disorders.

KEY TERMS

addiction
alcoholic blackouts
alcoholism
comorbid
craving
cross-tolerance
detoxification

drug of choice
dual diagnosis
eating disorders
fetal alcohol syndrome
gateway drugs
harm reduction
Internet addiction

pathologic gambling
prevention
pseudoaddiction
relapse prevention
screening
sexual addiction
substance abuse

substance dependence
substance use disorder
substance misuse
tolerance
withdrawal

Addiction is a term that is often applied to chemical or substance use disorders (SUDs), eating disorders, or impulse control disorders (e.g., gambling). The term *addiction* is better replaced with more precise descriptions of substance or behavioral disorders. Current literature refers to SUDs, which include abuse and dependence. Disorders of abuse and dependence are defined and described in the *Diagnostic and Statistical Manual of Mental Disorders*, fourth edition, text revision (DSM-IV-TR) (American Psychiatric Association, 2000), and they are therefore within the domain of psychiatric mental health practice. Nurses need to be aware of the stigma and importance of these disorders to assess and intervene appropriately with many patients. For a variety of

reasons, SUDs are significant factors in the health status and life satisfaction of patients, from tiny neonatal infants to elderly individuals. Substance use is a significant factor in dollars spent for illness care, loss of productivity, and disruption in family systems. According to the Robert Wood Johnson Foundation, addiction is the largest health care problem in the United States. Addictions occur in all ethnicities, socioeconomic strata, ages, and groups; it is an equal opportunity problem.

Nurses and other health care professionals are instrumental in providing effective treatment to patients. The overall goals for patients with substance disorders are treatment, remission, and healing. Depending on the setting, the nurse's ideal role is to be actively involved in the assessment, treatment, and prevention of substance misuse—the use of a psychoactive substance (drug or alcohol) for a purpose other than that for which it was intended and that causes physical, social, and psychologic harm. Addiction is described by Bickel and Potenza (2006, p. 9) as a self-organizing system that "… emerges from the interaction of evolutionarily old behavioral processes and their associated brain regions." These authors state that addiction is the result of many interdependent brain processes, and this phenomenon is increasingly noted in SUD research.

The nurse is often the first health care professional to become aware of a patient's problematic substance use, to share this information with other members of the health care team, and to coordinate subsequent nursing care or integrated care. The nurse's role is often instrumental in making referrals to or working with rehabilitation and recovery programs and to assessing and treating symptoms of physical illness of chemical dependence.

The American Nurses Association, in conjunction with the International Nurses Society on Addictions, published the *Scope and Standards of Addictions Nursing Practice* (American Nurses Association, 2004). These standards are statements of competencies for basic and advanced-level practitioners. The International Nurses Society on Addictions supports evidenced-based practice and the care of persons with addictive disorders. Generalist and specialized practice nurses join this organization, attend annual conventions, become certified in the treatment of addiction at either basic or advanced levels, and read the organization's publication *The Journal of Addictions Nursing*. The organization has several publications, including the *Core Curriculum for Addictions Nursing*; information about publications and organization activities are on the organization's website at www.intnsa.org.

Is substance dependence (i.e., addiction) a disease or a disorder? Substance dependence, like alcoholism, cannot be transmitted from one person to another like a condition such as tuberculosis, thus some argue that the term *disorder* is more accurate, and it is actually becoming more commonly used. The new DSM-V, which is to be published in 2013, proposes a continuum approach to abuse and dependence and refers to specific SUDs (e.g., alcohol use disorder, cocaine use disorder); hence, the term *disorder* will be used in this chapter. The use of this term does not ignore that disease sometimes occurs as the result of addiction (e.g., cirrhosis of the liver). Addiction is, according to the National Institute of Drug Abuse (NIDA, 2002a), a "… complex, neurobehavioral disorder characterized by impaired control, compulsive use, dependency, and craving for the activity, substance, or food." In addition, "… addiction is often (but not always) accompanied by physiological dependence, consisting of a withdrawal syndrome, and/or tolerance" (NIDA, 2002b). The spectrum of addictions covers SUDs, impulse control disorders such as pathologic gambling, Internet addiction, sexual addiction, and process disorders, including eating disorders such as bulimia and anorexia. The purpose of this chapter is to discuss chemical use disorders and SUDs. Chapter 18 addresses eating disorders.

Addictions are classified as psychiatric issues for the reasons that have been outlined in the preceding paragraph. The spectrum of addictive disorders is increasingly understood to have its base in biology, with psychologic dimensions. One of the founders of Alcoholics Anonymous (AA), Dr. Silkworth, thought that, because of the unique effect that alcohol had on some individuals, alcoholism was an allergy to alcohol. In 1939, Silkworth was found to be correct in suspecting a physical cause for alcoholism and addiction. Although alcoholism is not an allergy, it is recognized as a partially brain-based disorder and that some brains are more susceptible than others.

For ease of reading, the terms addiction and *SUD* and references to other chemical dependencies are interchangeable. Misuse is the use of any legal or illegal drug for purposes other than that for which it was intended or in excess (e.g., using alcohol beyond the legal limit). Misuse, abuse, and dependence are different magnitudes of the same behavior.

Individuals become addicted in various ways and over varied periods of time, and addiction is a complex process. Therefore, recent thinking related to addiction does not place responsibility solely with the individual. Although all people share certain life experiences (e.g., developmental milestones, physical health or illness, psychologic health or illness), variations of individual responses are endless. Researchers believe that those with a predisposition to SUDs have brains that are different before, during, and after exposure. However, acknowledging this does not account for responses to those differences or to variations in coping abilities. Human brain chemistry is unique to each person, as is life experience. It is incorrect to say that, because a person has alcoholic parents, he or she will or will develop alcoholism later in life; life is too complex for such broad statements. Scientists and researchers assess probability, which is different from certainty. The association of conditions does not prove causality.

The statistical manipulation of data provides information that forecasts trends or probabilities relative to groups of individuals, but this kind of calculation does not apply to each person in the group. Scientists do not have adequate longitudinal data (i.e., data collected over many years of a person's life) to predict with any confidence which individual will develop an SUD. Many studies that describe characteristics of persons with SUDs are conducted after the person has had an SUD, so their functioning and characteristics before the problem existed are unknown. Were the measured characteristics a product of addiction, or did they exist before the addiction? To date, there is little longitudinal data to contribute to the identification of individual risk factors. However, there is group data that sorts out some of the factors that put people at risk for SUDs. These risk factors are addressed in a later section of this chapter.

Some habit-forming substances that are very addicting are legal, such as nicotine and alcohol. Using substances is not illegal, but possessing or selling illicit substances is illegal.

Of course, a person must possess a drug, if even briefly, before using it, so many gray legal areas exist with regard to the interpretation of possession. State laws vary widely regarding drug possession and whether possession is a misdemeanor or a felony. State laws differ for different drugs, although federal standards apply everywhere, and Mexico and Canada have different regulatory restrictions regarding the sale and distribution of substances. The legally endorsed medical use of marijuana varies from state to state; it is the basis of a current interesting story about a formerly illegal drug now being accepted by some as having legitimate use. Patients Out of Time is an organization that supports the use of marijuana for patients with medical problems (www.medicalcannibis.com/), and Law Enforcement Against Prohibition (www.leap.cc) is an organization of retired or former law enforcement officers and others involved in the legal system who observe that inordinate amounts of resources are dedicated to the interdiction and control of marijuana and are now in favor of treatment.

HISTORIC PERSPECTIVES

Some theorists believe that the relief of suffering is a basic human need and that relief from stress is often the initial goal of the use of substances. This opinion is reflected in the reality that people in most cultures have used intoxicating substances for various reasons, including pain relief, ceremony, and healing. During the 1700s and the 1800s, armies and other paramilitary efforts (e.g., the Lewis and Clark expedition) had to guarantee their recruits a specific amount of alcohol each day, and a great deal of effort went into ensuring its availability under difficult circumstances.

The development of psychoactive substances began far before recorded history (Westermeyer, 2006). For example a 3500-year-old Sanskrit text mentioned a mushroom (*Amanita muscaria*) as a plant that was used for intoxication, which was thought to be named *soma*. Early peoples in the Americas crafted hundreds of stimulant or hallucinogenic concoctions, including tobacco, cocaine, coffee, peyote, and others. In early Greek and Roman societies, as in many countries today, alcohol was routinely an important element of meals, celebrations, and religious ceremonies, and the Bible mentions that ark-building Noah was fond of alcohol. Before 1800 in the United States, alcohol and opium were readily available and used in combination for calming and sedating effects. In the 1800s and the early 1900s, unregulated patented medicines contained cocaine, opium, morphine, and (after 1898) heroin. Hemp was grown in the American colonies, and smoking hemp became popular during the early 1900s; it was not deemed illegal until 1937. It is interesting to note that inhaling a substance is the fastest way for the drug to enter the circulatory system.

The development of synthetic drugs during the 19th century resulted in powerful habit-forming substances. Like many developments in health care, war stimulated the need for the development of new substances to enhance performance, relieve pain, and combat infection. In 1887, German scientists synthesized amphetamines, but research for practical use did not occur until the 1920s. The use of amphetamines was common during World War II by the military of various countries for increased vigilance and decreased need for sleep; the military still dispenses amphetamines for these purposes.

By 1900, there was a significant population with SUDs in the United States. Contributing to this problem was the development of the hypodermic needle, which permitted the direct injection of powerful purified substances, such as heroin and, later, morphine. This situation led to state and federal antinarcotics laws to regulate the sale and prescription of narcotics, the most important of which was the Harrison Narcotic Act of 1914 (Nace and Crowder, 2006). The Harrison Narcotic Act removed individual physician choice for the treatment of patients and essentially put the federal government in control of one aspect of medical practice. Over the years, some prescribed substances (e.g., amphetamines, Talwin, heroin) were not thought to be habit forming; however, as more people used these drugs, data indicated otherwise, and the drugs were reclassified.

To date, regulations, law enforcement, and many other efforts have not eliminated the use of illegal substances or the misuse of legal substances. People who use and abuse substances continue to actively search for new substances or new uses for existing substances. In an often-repeated pattern, as the use of a substance gains popularity and momentum, law enforcement initiates efforts to address that problem. Subsequently, users find a new substance, which results in social dysfunction, addiction, and significant physical impairment. Drug sales are lucrative, and drugs are amazingly available, which makes the control of these substances very difficult.

Cigarettes and brands of distilled alcohol are widely advertised. Cigarette companies target adolescent and preteen populations (Centers for Disease Control and Prevention, 2009), whereas marketing research heavily targets women (Carpenter et al, 2005). A quick review of the ads in teen magazines demonstrates this effort in subtle and obvious ways; the ads portray smoking and drinking alcohol as attractive behaviors. A recent study reported by the Center for Disease Control (2009) found that three heavily advertised cigarette brands were preferred by 81% of U.S. youth between the ages of 12 and 17 years. Curiously, each of the three biggest tobacco companies owns one of those brands; this is obviously an important shared niche market that these companies wish to maintain. The drop in rates of smoking among high school students stalled in 2003, and, in 2007, a slow rate of quitting was noted (Reinberg, 2009).

The U.S. Drug Enforcement Administration (DEA) Schedule of Controlled Substances lists restricted substances. The entire schedule is presented on the DEA website at www.dea.gov, and a summary of the schedules appears in Box 15-1. Debate continues about placing various compounds on this list, because listing every substance or combination of chemicals that has addictive or possibly addictive properties is not practically possible. Some drugs have no medical use and therefore are placed in the absolutely restricted category,

BOX 15-1 UNITED STATES DRUG ENFORCEMENT ADMINISTRATION SCHEDULE OF CONTROLLED SUBSTANCES

Schedule I

Drug/substance has a high potential for abuse and has no currently accepted medical use in treatment in the United States.

Examples: Heroin, ibogaine, mescaline, marijuana

Schedule II

Drug/substance has high potential for abuse but has currently accepted medical use with severe restrictions; abuse of the drug may lead to psychologic or physical dependence.

Examples: Cocaine, codeine, hydrocodone, methadone, morphine, meperidine

Schedule III

Drug/substance potential for abuse less than for schedules I and; II and is currently accepted in medical practice, abuse of drug/substance leads to moderate or low physical dependence or high psychologic dependence.

Examples: Anabolic steroids, ketamine, thiopental

Schedule IV

Drug/substance has low potential for abuse, is in current medical use, and abuse may lead to limited physical dependence or psychologic dependence, less than schedule III.

Examples: Benzodiazepines, Stadol, Darvon, Ambien, Sonata, Meridia, chloral hydrate

Schedule V

Only contains cough preparation with codeine up to 200 mg/100 mL, or 100 g.

From the U.S. Drug Enforcement Administration: *Drug Enforcement Administration home page* (website): www.dea.gov. Accessed November 23, 2010.

which means that there is no legal access to that substance in the United States unless it is for research purposes. Readers are encouraged to visit the DEA website to view changes to the schedule and to see what the DEA considers to be its priority concerns.

Neurobiologic Basis of Addiction

Drugs of dependence are categorized as depressants, stimulants, opiates, hallucinogens, inhalants, and nicotine. Nicotine and alcohol, although they are extremely high in addictive potential, are legal and thus researchers have extensively studied them. Virtually all drugs of abuse evoke a rapid release of neurochemicals that is followed by a reduced-from-baseline level of neurotransmitter when the effect of the drug wears off, thereby creating an elevated reward threshold and a biologic need or craving for more of the drug (Koob and Volkow, 2010). The drug serves as a reinforcer that increases the probability of a repeat behavior and the use of that substance. The three stages of use are as follows: (1) preoccupation/anticipation; (2) binge/intoxication; and (3) withdrawal/negative effect. Impulsivity characterizes the early stages and the compulsivity in the later stages. During the shift from impulsivity to compulsivity, there is also a shift in motivation to use: during the early stages, use is equated with pleasure; during the later stages, use is equated with avoiding pain (withdrawal) (Koob, 2006).

Recently, the two sides of addiction (beginning use and end use) have been referred to as the *light side* and the *dark side*, respectively, of addiction (Koob, 2006 and 2010); they are driven by different reward and avoidance systems, and the neurochemicals that are active during these two processes are different. During beginning use (i.e., the light, pleasurable side) the "feel good" neurotransmitters dopamine, serotonin, opioid peptides, and other neurochemicals predominate. As the individual becomes habituated to the drug, tolerance and withdrawal symptoms develop; this constitutes the dark side. At this point, the neurotransmitters norepinephrine and corticotropin-releasing factor (CRF) as well as the stress circuits are activated, which results in withdrawal symptoms; the individual then uses the substance not to feel good but to prevent the physical and psychologic stress and discomfort of withdrawal. After an individual has used a substance over time, the "high" that was initially experienced becomes harder and harder to find, if not impossible. One author (Miller & Armstrong 2006) hypothesizes that there is only so much pleasure potential in the human brain and that when it's gone, it's gone.

Knowledge of the effects of substances—both the light and dark sides—are a result of research technology (e.g., positron emission tomography, single photon emission tomography, functional magnetic imaging resonance scans) that allows researchers to actually visualize the neurobiologic effects of drugs. Other researchers have developed "knockout mice" in which they remove a particular genetic component. For example, mice have been developed without glutamate receptors (implicated in spatial learning and memory). These genetically altered mice do not become addicted to cocaine. These kinds of studies support the acceptance of genetic influences on addiction. For example, an individual with genetically greater neuroplastic potential for glutamate and dopamine production and activation may be more prone to addiction (Begley, 2007).

At least four interdependent and overlapping circuits in the brain comprise the neural network of addiction: (1) reward, which involves the nucleus accumbens and ventral palladium; (2) memory and learning, which involve the amygdala and the hippocampus; (3) cognitive control, which is located in the prefrontal cortex and the dorsal anterior cingulated cortex; and (4) motivation, drive, and salience, which are located in the orbital frontal cortex (Baler and Volkow, 2006). All of these functions contribute to the initiation and continuation of substance use.

Dopamine that is located in the mesolimbic system is the primary neurotransmitter that is associated with reward (i.e., the light side). Dopamine levels normally increase during pleasurable sensory activities (e.g., eating, sex) and mediate an approach response to this stimulation (Navqui and Bechara, 2008). Drugs artificially stimulate this same response, without the physical experience or cue, thereby creating an incentive for the individual to seek the same sensation (Robinson and Berridge, 2008). Somewhere during the course of addiction, the goal of substance use changes from pleasure seeking to preventing the discomfort of withdrawal. Over the course of millennia, human brains have served to keep humans alive, and they have efficiently evolved to specifically "remember" what is pleasurable. Behaviors that evoke dopamine release and that subsequently strengthen approach mechanisms evolve into compulsive behaviors.

The process of memory formation involves sensation plus thought. The limbic system, which is a part of the brain that contains a great deal of dopamine, is associated with emotion and memory. The limbic system that mediates pleasure is located deep within the brain, where it is protected from external harm; it is a critical survival center. Dopamine and other neurotransmitter-releasing activities activate this part of the brain. The mesolimbic dopamine system includes the amygdala, and it extends into the frontal region of the brain, which is responsible for prioritization, organization, and decision making. Because this portion of the brain is activated during addictive behavior, this greatly affects reasoning ability and the act of making responsible choices. In a sense, the drug "hijacks" the brain. This pathway is a one-way street from the amygdala to the frontal cortex. Unfortunately, the frontal cortex does not have reciprocally direct communication with the amygdala. If it did, it might say, "Stop that, it's not good for you!" Thus, those who have been addicted over a long period of time have particular difficulty with making logical and insightful decisions about their health or that involve the seeking of treatment (Goldstein et al., 2009).

Situational, individual, and environmental factors interact to sustain or restrain behavior. Researchers are still seeking a universal theory of addictions, and, although key elements of the brain are involved, there will always be variances in individual neurologic functioning. A recently implicated portion of the brain, the insula, functions in conscious emotional experience and feeling. When this portion of the brain is impaired as a result of trauma or other mechanisms, the affected organism (i.e., a laboratory animal) seems to lack motivation to continue to use a particular drug (Navqui and Bechara, 2008). Although drug use is not completely outside of voluntary control, the longer that one uses a drug or repeats a behavior, the more strongly entrenched the behavior/memory becomes and the less volition the individual has with regard to that behavior (Childress et al, 2008; Goldstein et al, 2009). Some hypothesize that the same neural pathways are involved for impulse-control disorders such as gambling, sex addiction, and eating disorders. The person with an SUD is like a passenger in a car without a conscious driver. Science promises advances in drug treatments that block the effects of drugs.

The development of immunization against nicotine and amphetamines is made possible by advancements in the knowledge of neurophysiology. Issues of informed consent, effectiveness of immunization techniques, and many other aspects of immunization are debated. Many arguments exist on all sides of these issues, including reimbursement for these vaccines (Harwood and Meyers, 2004). This type of immunization involves the administration of a substance to which the molecules of a drug (e.g., nicotine) will adhere. This molecular attraction renders the substance unavailable to brain receptors. Research to study the effectiveness and safety of a vaccine for nicotine (NicVAX) is currently in phase III trials (www.drugabuse.gov/pdf/news/NR103009.pdf), and these studies show promise. Two other compounds for nicotine immunization are in testing, as are agents to block cocaine, phencyclidine, morphine, and methamphetamine (Kinsey and Orson, 2009). However, it is possible that individuals might override the blocking effect by using extreme quantities of the substance; this would obviously be potentially lethal. An implant that contains long-acting naltrexone is used during rapid opiate withdrawal, although, as of this writing, it is not approved by the U.S. Food and Drug Administration. The implant is sutured subcutaneously into abdominal fat, and it slowly releases the blocking agent over a 2-month period of time. Sudden withdrawal occurs, and these symptoms are then treated. Some patients return for another implant, receive a long-acting injection, or continue to take oral naltrexone.

THEORETIC PERSPECTIVES

Understanding brain function has taken science a long way toward understanding addiction. Early theorists focused on individuals who were dependent on or who abused drugs. During the 1930s—and long before the DSM-IV-TR criteria were developed—Jellinek was a premier researcher in the field of alcoholism, and he was a strong believer of alcoholism as a disease. He proposed that addictive processes had a biochemical basis and noted that people with alcoholism progress through four stages, with the two more severe stages resulting in dependence. The stages were as follows: (1) the prealcoholic symptomatic phase; (2) the prodromal phase; (3) the crucial phase; and (4) the chronic phase. These phases correspond with the three evolving phases of addictive use mentioned previously: (1) preoccupation/anticipation; (2) binge/intoxication; and (3) withdrawal/negative affect. Blackouts occur when so much alcohol has been ingested that the hippocampus is anesthetized, and memory is temporarily erased. Blackouts are considered part of the prodromal phase; at this point, the individual begins to sneak drinks, minimize use, and typically ignore healthy behaviors such as normal eating in favor of drinking. The condition then becomes chronic.

Despite scientific knowledge about addiction, today—as at the turn of the century—alcoholism and other drug dependences are often considered moral problems. Considering alcoholism or drug addiction to be a sign of moral corruption or poor willpower is not useful. Many prominent and respected people—including musicians, politicians, clergy, military, celebrities, students, professionals, and next-door neighbors—develop drug problems. Another erroneous view is that drug addiction is related to a lack of intelligence. Historically, some very bright people have been dependent on drugs. No one is too smart to become dependent or to abuse drugs; it's not that simple. Individual factors (but not intelligence) contribute to addiction and are identified in this chapter. Importantly, no single theory adequately explains substance abuse or addiction. Although scientists are unable to predict which person will develop alcoholism, genes and social and cultural factors interact in ways that place a person at high risk for the development of the disease. As the relationship between these factors is further defined, researchers hope to take action to prevent the disease from occurring.

ETIOLOGY

Researchers have investigated multiple and intersecting causes of SUDs and other addictions. Data yielded from this research contributes to understanding the vulnerability factors that predispose groups of persons to developing an SUD. **Prevention** efforts focus on factors that are known to affect vulnerability. These efforts focus on one of three domains that influence the development of addiction: individual, situational, and environmental. No one factor is generally adequate to explain addiction phenomena, and overlapping areas exist among factors and categories; however, they are useful groupings when considering contributing influences. Some researchers hypothesize that patterns begun during childhood to deal with stress lead to choices regarding substances or behaviors in later life. These three main patterns are seeking satiety (e.g., eating, alcohol consumption), thrill seeking (e.g., gambling, sex addiction), and fantasizing (e.g., preferred use of hallucinogens) (Milkman and Sunderwirth, 2010). These authors hypothesize that drugs and activities of choice are substitutes for soothing and coping behaviors; that they are "antidotes for psychic pain" (Milkman and Sunderwirth, 2009, p. 19); and that people become addicted to the experiences achieved through the use of substances. A drug that a particular person prefers is known as his or her **drug of choice**.

Individual Factors

Age, gender, ethnicity, and other demographic descriptors fall into this category. The individual's history of drug use, qualities of decision making, positive beliefs about the effects of drugs, availability of drugs and the money to purchase them, and an individual's physiologic response are all factors that contribute to the development of an SUD. In addition, the person's appraisal and belief systems are considered, as is his or her perceived risk of use and the availability of friends who purchase drugs.

An individual's genetic predisposition toward the use of alcohol is supported by research. A threefold to fourfold risk exists for alcoholism among primary family members of individuals who are alcohol dependent; it is 50% for men whose fathers were alcoholic. Twin studies performed among women indicate 50% to 60% concordance (i.e., one twin being alcoholic predicts that the other will) (Kendler et al, 1992), thereby indicating a significant genetic contribution to susceptibility to alcoholism. The rate of problems with alcohol increases with the number of relatives with alcoholism, the severity of the disease, and the closeness of the genetic relationship to the person at risk. Genetic theories continue to evolve, and researchers are testing them primarily in animal models. The gene alleles *ALDH2* and *ALDH3* influence an individual's predisposition to alcoholism (National Institute on Alcohol Abuse and Alcoholism, 2000), because these genes influence the metabolism of alcohol, which is genetic and varies among individuals. Dopamine and glutamate are neurotransmitters that occur in various concentrations in different parts of the brain. Genetics influence the production and regulation of these and other neurotransmitters and play an important role in addiction.

Studies of children of parents with alcoholism have led to predictions about who will develop alcoholism on the basis of a lower level of response to alcohol. The lower level of response refers to tests that indicate that some individuals are more sensitive to the effects of alcohol than others (Schuckit, 1984 and 2000; Schuckit et al, 2004). A reduced subjective response to alcohol is a risk factor for the development of alcoholism. People with a reduced subjective response have to drink more alcohol than others to feel the same effects. Researchers have reported the results of the first genome scan for drug abuse. The study provided evidence that specific regions of the human genome differ between abusers of illegal drugs and nonabusers. This study was an important step in identifying individuals who are at high risk for addiction. This knowledge makes it possible to direct appropriate preventive efforts and treatments toward those individuals (NIDA, 2002). People in some ethnic groups have particular genetic risks for addiction as a result of inherited metabolic patterns.

Comorbid (co-occurring) mental illness is associated with greater rates of addiction and abuse. Posttraumatic stress disorder creates a risk for substance use or relapse. Some individuals begin to abuse substances after exposure to trauma. A total of 30% to 60% of persons with SUDs meet the criteria for comorbid posttraumatic stress disorder. Persons with bipolar disorder also have increased risk for SUDs, as do patients with anxiety, depression, or schizophrenia disorders.

Along with the predisposition to addiction, researchers have also demonstrated a strong neurobiologic correlation between stress and drug use, especially in relation to relapse. For example, smokers who are experiencing stress sometimes relapse, even after long periods of abstinence. Prolonged or chronic stress also fosters the continuation of addiction behaviors. Stress increases the hormone production of CRF, which in turn initiates the body's biologic response to stressors. After exposure to stress, CRF is in areas of the brain in increased amounts. Almost all drugs of abuse also increase CRF levels, which possibly indicates a neurobiologic connection between stress and substance abuse (Koob, 2006 and 2010). Withdrawal induces rises in CRF. Various psychologic theories explain SUDs. Although researchers have studied addictive personality attributes carefully, no one unique personality profile is more prone to addiction than another. However, early aggressive behavior and poor social skills are individual factors that may predispose a person to drug abuse (NIDA, 2008). Theories of psychologic causation alone are insufficient to adequately explain the development of substance use.

Situational Factors

Situational factors include peer influence, social norms, family influences, and social supports (Holder, 2000). Again, in real life, these factors overlap with other situational, environmental, and individual influences.

Family systems theory is useful as a conceptual model to help promote an understanding of emotional family functioning. Bowen's use of interrelated and interdependent concepts characterizes what happens in families when a member abuses substances (Bowen, 1978; Kaufman and Brook, 2006; Steinglass and Kutch, 2006). Children from these families tend to become enmeshed in the family system. Their boundaries become blurred within the family, and they live solely for each other. Family members use family secrets and myths as survival measures. These family members tend to cut off communication with those outside of the family structure. The multigenerational transmission process traces the recurrence of the disease in the family in subsequent generations. The family conspires to maintain a system that supports addiction. The term *codependent* describes a person who helps another person to maintain his or her addiction by caring for that person, handling that person's problems, and running interference. On the surface, these efforts appear to be helpful, but they do not permit the affected individual the opportunity to experience the consequences of their behavior, which is an important agent for change. The term *codependent* is confusing and suggests the notion of blame for someone else's problems, thereby creating a double-victim situation. The terms *co-alcoholic* and *co-addict* have also been used. Because addiction carries stigma, the current thinking is to refrain from labeling individuals on the basis of these behaviors.

Research about family influences on substance abuse led to interventions that strengthen the family unit. The social ecology model data suggest that parents have an early influence on the development of the drug-use patterns of their children (McCrady, 2006). Crespi and Sabatelli (1997) identified a connection between the developmental implications of parental alcoholism and achieving one's own independence. Some families tend to restrict the process of individuation and separation.

Healthy parental support is a strong predictor of decreased drug use in youth (NIDA, 2008). Researchers have looked at family dynamics related to problem behaviors (e.g., academic failure, antisocial behavior, high-risk sex, substance abuse). They designed treatment measures to improve family involvement, parenting skills, and parental monitoring, with the goal of reducing adolescent drug use and associated behaviors. Involved parents are known to be a protective factor.

Peer-group pressures and the need to belong to the group are powerful positive reinforcers for youth (NIDA, 2008). Prevention efforts that target situational influences include changing perceptions in groups, promoting positive peer influences, bonding with nonusing peers, and improved parenting skills. Modeling theory suggests that adolescents reared in homes in which substances are readily available often repeat the behavior of adults and other role models who use substances to feel good. This is an example of overlapping areas, because modeling theory also applies to the environmental area of influence.

A related issue is the age at which an individual begins drinking. The risk for developing an alcohol use disorder increases for those who start drinking before the age of 17 years (24.5%) as compared with those who start drinking at the age of 21 or 22 years (10%) or the age of 25 years (<4%) (Grant and Dawson, 1997). A group of researchers developed subtypes of alcoholism on the basis of the age at which individuals began drinking and their progression into alcoholism (see www.niaaa.nih.gov/NewsEvents/News Releases/alcoholism_subtypes.htm) These subtypes are presented in Box 15-2.

Environmental Factors

Environmental factors include an individual's access to and the cost of the desired substance; policies and policy enforcement; and the severity of the punishment of those who engage in illegal behavior to obtain substances or who sell to minors (Holder, 1999; NIDA, 2008). Researchers in community and public health disciplines determine the extent to which environmental factors influence addiction.

Community health researchers assess communities for risk factors with the use of several available models. One model is available through NIDA. Researchers use maps and the mapping of neighborhoods to identify problem areas within communities and to then form action agendas for prevention and intervention.

Reimbursement is often poor for drug and alcohol treatment. The impression that addictions are self-created is partially true. However, so are some forms of diabetes, heart disease, and respiratory disease. There are no limits regarding the treatment for chronic obstructive pulmonary disease, although these patients have smoked for years. Reimbursement is available for the consequences of addiction, but prevention and treatment are expensive and not well funded. Some states have insisted on parity for policies sold in their individual states.

Researchers conduct descriptive and analytic epidemiology studies in communities and across the nation to track alcohol and drug use trends. Drug availability and poverty are known community factors that influence drug use (NIDA, 2008). With the goal of prevention, these researchers implement strategies to help individuals and communities.

BOX 15-2 ALCOHOLISM SUBTYPES

Young adult subtype: 31.5% of U.S. alcoholics; young adult drinkers with relatively low rates of co-occurring substance abuse and other mental disorders, a low rate of family alcoholism, and who rarely seek any kind of help for their drinking

Young antisocial subtype: 21% of U.S. alcoholics; tend to be in their mid-20s and had an early onset of regular drinking and alcohol problems; more than half come from families with alcoholism, and about half have a psychiatric diagnosis of antisocial personality disorder; many have major depression, bipolar disorder, and anxiety problems; more than 75% smoke cigarettes and marijuana, and many also have cocaine and opiate addictions; more than one third of these alcoholics seek help for their drinking

Functional subtype: 19.5% of U.S. alcoholics; typically middle aged and well educated, with stable jobs and families; about one third have a multigenerational family history of alcoholism, about one quarter have had major depressive illness sometime in their lives, and nearly 50% are smokers

Intermediate familial subtype: 19% of U.S. alcoholics; middle aged, with about 50% coming from families with multigenerational alcoholism; almost half have had clinical depression, and 20% have had bipolar disorder; most of these individuals smoke cigarettes, and nearly one in five have problems with cocaine and marijuana use; only 25% ever seek treatment for their problem drinking

Chronic severe subtype: 9% of U.S. alcoholics; comprised mostly of middle-aged individuals who had early onset of drinking and alcohol problems, with high rates of antisocial personality disorder and criminality; almost 80% come from families with multigenerational alcoholism; this group has the highest rates of other psychiatric disorders, including depression, bipolar disorder, and anxiety disorders, as well as high rates of smoking and marijuana, cocaine, and opiate dependence; two thirds of these alcoholics seek help for their drinking problems, which makes them the most prevalent type of alcoholic found in treatment

Intervention before dependence occurs is a secondary goal. The majority of adolescents who use drugs do not develop SUDs. The culture of early adulthood often includes alcohol use and drug experimentation; however, most people stop these behaviors when they enter the workforce and have families and financial obligations.

EPIDEMIOLOGY

Federal and individual state agencies concerned about drug use conduct many surveys to estimate drug use trends. Box 15-2 illustrates consumption standards for alcohol and classifications for different types of drinkers. The National Survey on Drug Abuse and Health is a data set that helps researchers to track the use of various substances in the United States.

The 2008 Substance Abuse and Mental Health Service Administration (SAMHSA) study revealed that 20.1 million Americans (8% of the population) 12 years old or older used at least one illicit drug during the month before taking the survey (SAMHSA, 2009), which was the same percentage that was found in 2007. The following discussion is taken from the SAMHSA 2009 study. Between 2002 and 2008, there was no significant change in the number of persons with substance dependence or abuse (i.e., 22.0 million in 2002 and 22.2 million in 2008).

Marijuana, which is classified as a hallucinogen, was the most common illicit drug used in 2008 among those aged 12 years old and older, with 15.2 million (5.8%) people using it during the month before the study, which was similar to the use seen in 2007. There were 1.9 million cocaine users, approximately 1.1 million people used hallucinogens (0.4%), and there were an estimated 800,000 heroin users. The number of current users of ecstasy had decreased between 2002 and 2003, but the number did not change between 2003 and 2004 (450,000 people). In 2008, 6.2 million people were current users of psychotherapeutic drugs taken nonmedically. Most of these drugs were pain relievers.

Researchers noted significant increases in the lifetime prevalence of use in 2008 in several categories of pain relievers among individuals between the ages of 18 and 25 years. Specific pain relievers with statistically significant increases in lifetime use were Vicodin, Lortab, or Lorcet; Percocet, Percodan, or Tylox; hydrocodone products; OxyContin; and oxycodone products.

Among youth between the ages of 12 and 17 years, rates of current illicit drug use varied significantly among major racial and ethnic groups in 2008. The rate was highest among those who said that they identified as two or more races, followed by African Americans, Native Americans/Alaska Natives, whites, Hawaiians or other Pacific Islanders, and Latinos (see Figure 15-1). Approximately 51.6% of the responders (129 million people) said that they were current alcohol drinkers. Heavy drinking (i.e., binge drinking on 5 or more days during the previous month) was reported by 6.9% (17.3 million people), which was the same rate as 2007. These numbers are similar for both 2002 and 2003. The highest prevalence (41%) of binge and heavy drinking in 2008 was for young adults between the ages of 18 and 25 years, with a peak at the age of 21 years. In 2004, young adults between the ages of 18 and 22 years who were in college full time were more likely than their peers who were not enrolled in school full time to use alcohol, to binge drink, and to drink heavily.

Approximately 28.4% of respondents reported currently using tobacco products. Young adults between the ages of 18 and 25 years continued to have the highest rate of cigarette use during the previous month (39.5%). The rate of cigarette use among youth between the ages of 12 and 17 years declined from 9.8% in 2007 to 9.1% in 2008. The 2008 estimate averages out to approximately 6600 new cigarette smokers every day. Most new cigarette smokers in 2008 were younger than 18 years old when they first smoked cigarettes (58.8%).

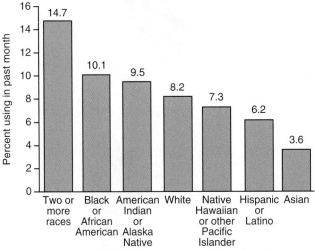

Past month illicit drug use among persons aged 12 or older, by race/ethnicity: 2008 (SAMHSA 2009)

FIGURE 15-1. Drug use by population density.

Smokeless tobacco is also popular among youth, and smoking with the use of a water pipe (i.e., a hookah) is a trend in some areas and is discussed later in this chapter.

Trends and the initiation of use are another category to use when considering this data. From the same study and on the basis of a new approach to estimating incidence, the 2008 National Survey on Drug Abuse and Health shows that the illicit drug category with the largest number of new users was that of the nonmedical use of pain relievers. In all, 2.4 million persons used these pain relievers for the first time within the previous 12 months. The average age at first use among these new initiates was 21.2 years, which was down from that seen 2007. The average age at first use among the 2.1 million recent marijuana initiates was 18.0 years in 2004 and 17.8 years in 2008. In 2008, 4.4 million persons had used alcohol for the first time within the previous 12 months. Most (84.6%) of the 4.5 million alcohol initiates were younger than the age of 21 years at the time of initiation. Young adults between the ages of 18 and 22 years who were enrolled full time in college were more likely than their peers who were not enrolled full time (i.e., part-time college students and persons not currently enrolled in college) to use alcohol during the past month, to binge drink, and to drink heavily. Among full-time college students in 2008, 61.0% were current drinkers, 40.5% binge drank, and 16.3% were heavy drinkers. Among those who were not enrolled full time in college, these rates were 54.2%, 38.1%, and 13.0%, respectively. Rates of current alcohol use and binge use for full-time college students decreased from 2007, when they were 63.7% and 43.6%, respectively. Among underage drinkers who did not pay for the alcohol the last time they drank, the most common source was an unrelated person who was 21 years old or older (37.4%). Other underage persons provided the alcohol on the last occasion 21.1% of the time. Parents, guardians, or other adult family members provided the alcohol 21.0% of the time. Other

sources of alcohol for underage drinkers included taking the alcohol from their own home (5.8%), taking it from someone else's home (3.2%), and getting it some other way (6.9%).

The White House Office of National Drug Control Policy and others have studied the total economic cost of alcohol, tobacco, and other drugs since 1985. According to estimates, the economic cost of substance abuse each year is about $400 billion, although others disagree with this figure. This estimate includes premature deaths, treatment and prevention costs, crime, social welfare programs, destruction of property, and costs associated with the loss of jobs and earnings (SAMHSA, 2002).

In this area, the U.S. government primarily funds research into addiction. Resources developed by the Drug Abuse Warning Network, the Community Epidemiology Work Group, the DEA, and multiple other nongovernmental groups (e.g., Erowid [www.erowid.org]) provide nurses and other health care providers with databases and information about trends that influence the direction of education, prevention, and treatment. Regardless of their chosen practice area, nurses have a responsibility to update their information about drug use trends by using resources that are readily available on the Internet. Nurses should know what the major drugs of abuse are in their geographic area, the signs of use, and the resources that will be helpful for users.

Substance Abuse in Special Populations

Substance use disorders have a negative impact on all populations, and researchers who study addiction recognize that, for some people, substance abuse results in particularly negative consequences. Everyone is at risk, but some groups are more vulnerable, including women, adolescents, older adults, and professionals.

Women

Although men are twice as likely as women to meet lifetime DSM-IV-TR criteria for any drug use disorder, women are at higher risk than men for problems related to alcohol use, including organ damage and other problems (Blume and Zilberman, 2006), and they are less likely to be assessed for SUDs (Vandermause, 2007). Women begin problem drinking later in life than men (i.e., late 20s or early 30s), and they develop significant physical and psychosocial problems in a shorter period of time, often during their childbearing years; this phenomenon is known as *telescoping*. Women more often than men cite an event such as divorce or separation that preceded drinking. Alcohol abuse also renders women more vulnerable than men to domestic violence and completed suicide. Even lower rates of drinking predispose women to work-related problems, interpersonal relationship problems, and parenting problems. Treatment programs and 12-step programs were originally developed to treat men because social norms did not acknowledge women's addiction. However, as times change, gender-specific programs have been developed and are being evaluated (Armstrong, 2008).

Perinatal Conditions

Despite general knowledge about the danger of drinking alcohol while pregnant, binge drinking or frequent drinking is a problem in this population. The use of any drug during pregnancy requires medical scrutiny. Research through the years has shown that substances affect the mother and fetus in different ways when they are used during pregnancy. Many of the substances that are used by pregnant women are teratogens to the fetus, which cause developmental malformations. Because some women abuse more than one drug, it is difficult to predict the damage that will occur to their babies. The effects of specific substances on fetuses are dependent on a number of factors, including the type of drug, the amount, the pattern of maternal consumption, and the timing of exposure. According to the 2008 SAMHSA survey, 5.1% of pregnant women between the ages of 15 and 44 years old used illicit drugs during the past month on the basis of data averaged for 2007 and 2008. This rate was significantly lower than the rate seen among women in this age group who were not pregnant (9.8%). The rate of current illicit drug use in the combined 2007 and 2008 data was lower for pregnant women than for nonpregnant women among those between the ages of 18 and 25 years (7.1% and 16.2%, respectively) and among those between the ages of 26 and 44 years (3.0% and 6.7%, respectively). Among women between the ages of 15 and 17 years, however, those who *were* pregnant had a higher rate of use than those who *were not* pregnant (21.6% and 12.9%, respectively). Among pregnant women between the ages of 15 and 44 years, an estimated 10.6% reported current alcohol use, 4.5% reported binge drinking, and 0.8% reported heavy drinking. These rates were significantly lower than the rates for nonpregnant women in the same age group (54.0%, 24.2%, and 5.5%, respectively). Binge drinking during the first trimester of pregnancy was reported by 10.3% of pregnant women between the ages of 15 and 44 years. All of these estimates by pregnancy status are made on the basis of data averaged for 2007 and 2008. The 2007 and 2008 estimate for first-trimester binge drinking was higher than it was for 2005 and 2006, when it was 4.6%.

Smoking during pregnancy accounts for an estimated 20% to 30% of low birth weight babies, up to 14% of preterm deliveries, and 10% of all infant deaths. Infants also have an increased risk of congenital abnormalities. Even healthy full-term babies of mothers who smoke have been born with narrowed airways and curtailed lung function. Children of mothers who smoke during pregnancy sometimes exhibit hyperactivity and have an increased risk of cancer later in life. Studies show that babies born to marijuana users were shorter, weighed less, and had smaller head sizes than those born to mothers who did not use the drug. In addition, research has revealed that children born to mothers who used marijuana also have difficulty concentrating when they are older (NIDA, www.drugabuse.gov/ResearchReports/Marijuana/Marijuana4.html#pregnancy).

Opioids present special problems in pregnant women and their offspring. Fetal damage is a result of genetic changes caused by these drugs. Other medical problems include

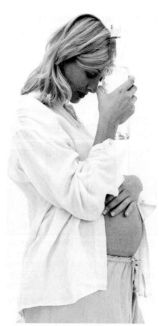

FIGURE 15-2. Alcohol and drug use during pregnancy interfere with normal fetal development.

elevated rates of intrauterine death, low birth weight in infants, premature delivery, and a 2% to 5% risk of infant death. Newborns of opioid-dependent mothers exhibit withdrawal symptoms. At birth, children exposed to cocaine prenatally exhibited more abnormal reflexes, less motor maturity, and a decreased ability to regulate their state of attentiveness as compared with unexposed children (Bauer, 2005).

Prenatal alcohol consumption continues to be a major concern. Drinking during pregnancy is the leading known cause of preventable birth defects and learning difficulties (Figure 15-2). These difficulties and defects are 100% preventable. Drinking rates among pregnant women, although they are substantially lower than the rates among nonpregnant women of similar ages, highlight a major concern because of the effects of alcohol on the fetus. Fetal alcohol syndrome (FAS) is part of a continuum of disorders called *fetal alcohol spectrum disorders* (FASDs) (for more information, see www.fasdcenter.samhsa.gov). The term *FASDs* refers to a spectrum of conditions that include FAS, fetal alcohol effects, alcohol-related neurodevelopmental disorder, and alcohol-related birth defects. Although disorders within the spectrum can be diagnosed, the term *FASDs* itself is not intended for use as a clinical diagnosis. The effects of these disorders include physical, mental, behavioral, and learning disabilities with possible lifelong implications. Each year in the United States, as many as 40,000 babies are born with an FASD. The cost to the nation for FAS alone is about $6 billion a year. The most severe effects of alcohol on the fetus are fetal alcohol syndrome (Figure 15-3). The diagnosis of FAS has three criteria: (1) growth retardation; (2) central nervous system involvement that results in mental retardation and other learning difficulties; and (3) facial and other

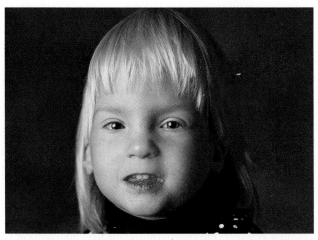

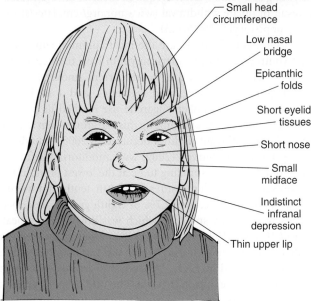

- Small head circumference
- Low nasal bridge
- Epicanthic folds
- Short eyelid tissues
- Short nose
- Small midface
- Indistinct infranal depression
- Thin upper lip

FIGURE 15-3. Fetal alcohol syndrome. Milder forms of alcohol-induced effects on the fetus and the infant are known as *fetal alcohol effects.*

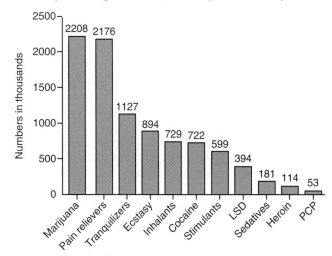

Past year initiates for specific illicit drugs among persons aged 12 or older: 2008 (SAMHSA 2009)

Marijuana 2208
Pain relievers 2176
Tranquilizers 1127
Ecstasy 894
Inhalants 729
Cocaine 722
Stimulants 599
LSD 394
Sedatives 181
Heroin 114
PCP 53

(Numbers in thousands)

FIGURE 15-4. Initiation of drugs.

abnormalities (Bowden and Rust, 2000). FAS occurs in 1 to 3 per 1000 live births. Surviving infants exhibit any mixture of signs of the syndrome, which may include a small head; a small physical stature; mild to severe mental retardation; facial abnormalities, including a flat bridge of the nose, an absent philtrum (i.e., the median groove between the upper lip and the nose), and an epicanthal eye fold (i.e., a vertical skinfold over the angle of the inner canthus of the eye); an atrial or ventricular septal heart defect; syndactyly (i.e., malformations of the hands and feet with the fusion of fingers or toes); and disorders of the temporomandibular joint.

Other signs of FASDs include hearing loss or other developmental delays. As children reach school age, they have problems with reading, spelling, and arithmetic. As they grow older, they have an increased risk for developing alcohol abuse and dependence, and some develop antisocial personality disorders and other psychiatric conditions.

Developments in the creation of maternal or neonatal biomarkers to detect alcohol use during pregnancy assist health care providers with detecting exposure (Savage, 2006). Many of these tests are not practical for routine use, but they help researchers to study the effect of alcohol on developing fetuses and children. Nurses need to avoid victimizing women with substance use issues (Armstrong, 1992). It may be difficult to believe in the age of information and the Internet that women sometimes do not know the facts about using drugs or alcohol while they are pregnant or that they do not know where to find these facts. Several states legislated mandatory incarceration for women who use substances while pregnant, but these programs have failed because they were found to be unconstitutional.

Adolescents

Adolescents often experiment or use drugs in conjunction with specific events such as parties, developmental or emotional crises, and peer group influences and pressures. The criteria presented in the DSM-IV-TR for symptoms of psychologic dependence or physical dependence may not apply to teenagers. Although the peak use of alcohol and drugs occurs during the late teens or the early 20s, most people return to normal drinking patterns and do not progress to alcoholism or chronic abuse. Some adolescents go on to develop pervasive and recurrent patterns of use that then result in serious consequences and diagnosable substance-related disorders (see Figure 15-4). Studies of vulnerability factors help researchers to design prevention programs for at-risk youth. For example, one factor is age, because those who begin drinking before the age of 17 years are more likely to develop an alcohol use disorder (24.5%) than those who begin drinking at the age of 21 or 22 years (10%) or the age of 25 years (<4%) (Spoth et al, 2009). Society considers experimenting with substances to be normative behavior for young adults. Many high school students drink or smoke cigarettes before the age of 13 years. Knight and colleagues (2007) screened adolescents in primary care and found that 15% were positive for substance abuse.

The popularity of substances rises and falls, with the use of hallucinogens declining among high schoolers (SAMHSA, 2009). The same data suggest that adolescent drug use is ubiquitous and that it is found in rural, urban, and suburban populations. Of interest—and contrary to popular notions—is that the researchers who performed this survey noted that the use of crack and heroin does not always occur in urban areas. A significant number of adolescents continue to use inhalants. Unfortunately, 6.9% of 12 year olds have "huffed," whereas 1.4% have used pot, 0.7% have used hallucinogens, and 0.1% have used cocaine. The report found that 5.2% of adolescents smoked cigarettes. The increased use of inhalants among preteens is concerning.

Boys in this age group have somewhat higher rates of illicit drug use than girls, and they have much higher rates of smokeless tobacco and steroid use (NIDA, 2009). Students who are not college bound are more likely to use illicit drugs, to drink heavily, and to drink alcohol while in high school. In the lower grades, the college-bound students showed a greater increase in cigarette smoking during the mid-1990s as compared with their non–college-bound peers. A variety of smokeless tobacco products are available; Snus (pronounced "snoos") is a newer smokeless and spitless tobacco product that originated in Sweden. It comes in a pouch that is placed between the upper lip and the gum. It is left there for about 30 minutes, during which time the user does not have to spit; the pouch is then discarded. Other forms of tobacco are lozenges (these are not the same thing as nicotine lozenges), twists, and smokeless types that require spitting. Yet another form of tobacco smoking involves a hookah or water pipe, and this is gaining popularity in some areas. Unfortunately, more nicotine per inhalation is produced with this kind of device (Eissenberg and Shihadeh, 2009). The 2009 SAMHSA study revealed that, in 2008, among persons with substance dependence or abuse, the proportion of individuals with dependence on or abuse of illicit drugs was also associated with age: 60.6% of youth between the ages of 12 and 17 years were dependent on or abused illicit drugs as compared with 37.4% of young adults between the ages of 18 and 25 years and 24.3% of adults 26 years old or older. In addition, the rate of alcohol dependence or abuse among youth between the ages of 12 and 17 years was 4.9% in 2008, which was down from 5.4% in 2007 and from 5.9% in 2008. The use of any illicit drug during the previous year was down by more than a third among eighth graders, down by under a quarter among tenth graders, and down by only 10% among twelfth graders. Half of American secondary school students have tried an illicit drug by the time that they reach graduation. Marijuana is the most prevalent of illicit drugs, and the 2008 survey indicated no significant decline in the use of this substance. The annual use of ecstasy is declining since it peaked in 2001. Amphetamine use declined in upper the grades but not in the eighth grade. Tranquilizer use increased steadily from 1992 until 2000, but it is now in decline.

Prevalence rates for tranquilizer use was reported to be 2.8% in grade 8 and 6.8% in grade 12.

Among drugs that showed almost no change in 2008 were cocaine, crack, and heroin. Crystal methamphetamine prevalence is 2.3% among twelfth graders. Heroin use peaked in 2001, and it is now slightly below 1% in all three grades. Narcotics other than heroin are reported only for the twelfth grade, with the annual prevalence rate at 9%; Vicodin and OxyContin are the most common of these. A type of heroin called "cheese heroin" is gaining popularity in some parts of the country. "Cheese" is heroin that is mixed with Tylenol and water and then dried, with the resulting substance looking like parmesan cheese. It is sold for about $8, often to elementary school children. This substance is snorted, and children as young as 9 years old have required medical intervention as a result of opiate withdrawal (www.npr.org/templates/story/story.php?storyId=89070113).

Alcohol and cigarettes are the most common substances that youth use. Half of American youth have tried cigarettes by the twelfth grade, and 23% are current smokers. By the eighth grade, 26% have tried cigarettes, and 1 in 11 has become a current smoker. Cigarette use reached its peak in 1996. Declines in smoking among this age group seem to have leveled; no significant declines occurred in 2005. The Monitoring the Future Survey (2009; www.monitoringthefuture.org) found cigarette smoking to be at the lowest point in the survey's history on all measures for eighth, tenth, and twelfth graders. For example, only 2.7% of eighth graders described themselves as daily smokers, which was down from a peak rate of 10.4% in 1996. Similarly, 11.2% of high school seniors stated that they smoked daily, which was less than half of the 24.6% rate found in 1997. However, one area of concern is the rate of smokeless tobacco use. The rate of tenth graders using smokeless tobacco during the previous month was 6.5%, which was up from the previous year and the same as it was in 1999.

Seventy-five percent of high school seniors have tried alcohol (more than just a few sips), and 41% have done so by the eighth grade. More than half (58%) of high-school seniors and 20% of eighth graders reported being drunk at least once, which causes concern given the fact that alcohol disorders develop faster when drinking begins early.

Researchers believe that "generational forgetting" contributes to drug use; this occurs when drugs are reintroduced to young people who do not know about the dangers of particular substances. Researchers believe that, when the adverse effects of certain drugs become known (e.g., lysergic acid diethylamide [LSD], methamphetamine), these particular drugs fall out of use. Both of these drugs had very bad reputations during the 1960s and the 1970s. Over time, this information is forgotten, and young people begin to use these drugs again, only to rediscover unfortunate or fatal outcomes. Persons who are interested in preventing adolescent drug use focus on the "grace period" between when a drug becomes popular and when use falls off because of these negative consequences. Information campaigns to educate and publicize adverse effects are helpful during these times.

Of particular concern are widely abused prescription drugs. The use of these drugs is increasing, and the trend is rising among younger adolescents. Researchers believe that this is partially the result of the general practice of prescription drug advertising, which imparts the idea that drugs are safe. Prescription drugs have become gradually more popular, and adolescents obtain them from friends, relatives, parents, or others who have usually obtained them legally. According to the SAMHSA 2009 literature, among persons 12 years old or older in 2007 and 2008 who used pain relievers nonmedically during the past 12 months, 55.9% got the pain relievers that they used most recently from a friend or relative for free. Another 8.9% bought them from a friend or relative, and 5.4% took them from a friend or relative without asking. Nearly one fifth (18.0%) indicated that they got the drugs that they used most recently through a prescription from one doctor. About 1 in 20 users (1.6%) got pain relievers from a drug dealer or another stranger, and 0.4% bought them on the Internet. These percentages are similar to those that were reported in 2006 and 2007. In 81.7% of the instances in which nonmedical users of prescription pain relievers who were 12 years old or older obtained the drugs from a friend or relative for free, the individuals indicated that their friend or relative had obtained the drugs from just one doctor. Nurses need to encourage everyone to dispose of their medications when the medications are no longer in use. To avoid introducing these substances into the water supply by flushing or dissolving them in the sink, one recommendation is to wrap them in moist paper and put them in the trash, where they will likely be incinerated. Several states are considering legislation to authorize pharmacies to accept unused medications and dispose of them safely.

Research conducted since the 1970s has produced a convincing body of evidence that the use of cigarettes, alcohol, and marijuana by children and adolescents is especially dangerous. These drugs impede social and intellectual development, cause disease or brain damage, and ruin or destroy lives. They often lead to dangerous activities such as driving under the influence, premature or unprotected sex, and violence. Eating disorders and impulse disorders occur more frequently with substance abuse disorders. The Parents and Teens Attitude Tracking Study (Partnership for a Drug-Free America, 2009) discovered that high school students' perceptions of risk from marijuana use declined in 2009. Decreased perceived risks included resulting depression, impaired judgment, or putting themselves or others in danger. Researchers think that factors that may have influenced teens are publicity about medical marijuana and the many movies, videos, and television programs that portray marijuana use as normal behavior without consequences. Figure 15-4 illustrates the most recent study results regarding ethnicity and drug use.

Researchers at the Center on Addiction and Substance Abuse (CASA) at Columbia University analyzed the use of alcohol, cigarettes, and marijuana as entry or gateway drugs that lead to the subsequent use of other illicit drugs, regardless of the age, ethnicity, or race of those involved. The highlights of their report emphasize the dangers that gateway

drugs present to youth. They found that age at first use, frequency of use, and number of drugs used increase the probability of a youth becoming a regular drug user and addict. The implications of this comprehensive report are clear. If a child or adolescent makes it through the teenage years without smoking cigarettes and without repeatedly drinking beer or other types of alcohol, then the odds are overwhelming that the child will not develop an alcohol use disorder or smoke marijuana. The Patient and Family Teaching Guidelines box lists signs of substance abuse in children or adolescents and strategies to prevent substance abuse.

PATIENT AND FAMILY TEACHING GUIDELINES

Signs of Adolescent Drug Use and Abuse
- Bloodshot, red eyes; droopy eyelids
- Wearing sunglasses at inappropriate times
- Changes in sleep patterns (e.g., napping, insomnia)
- Unexplained periods of moodiness, depression, anxiety, or irritability
- Decreased interaction and communication with family
- Loss of interest in previous hobbies, sports, and so on
- Change in friends; will not introduce new friends
- Decline in academic performance; drop in grades
- Loss of motivation and interest in school activities
- Change in peer group
- Disappearance of money or items of value
- Use of eye drops and mouthwash
- Unfamiliar containers or locked boxes
- Money missing from the house

Prevention of Adolescent Substance Use and Abuse
- Ensure positive role modeling by parents and adults in the adolescent's world.
- Reinforce the dangers of substance use, and teach positive behaviors.
- Provide support in coping with the social pressure exerted by peers.
- Establish limits, structure, and house rules for the adolescent's behavior.
- Help the adolescent to anticipate pressures, and reinforce positive coping behaviors.
- Engage the adolescent in life skills training programs in which the emphasis is on positive skills training, resistance training, and group support.
- Monitor the adolescent's use of television, computer, movies, and video games, because the media may portray legal and illegal substances as a part of daily life.

From The Clean Foundation, San Diego, Calif.

Developmentally, adolescents and children do not clearly understand what addiction means. When nurses interact with younger patients, they need to determine what the child knows to provide effective care and teaching. Children are afraid of addiction; they worry about their family members who smoke, and they also worry that they will become addicted themselves (Miller and Armstrong, 2006).

BOX 15-3 **TYPE OF ILLICIT DRUGS USED DURING THE PAST YEAR AMONG ADULTS 50 YEARS OLD OR OLDER WHO USED ILLICIT DRUGS DURING THE PAST YEAR: 2006 TO 2008**

TYPE OF DRUG USE	PERCENTAGE
Marijuana use	44.9%
Nonmedical use of prescription-type drugs	33.4%
Other illicit drug use	6.1%
Marijuana and nonmedical use of prescription-type drugs	6.1%
Marijuana and other illicit drug use	5.5%
Nonmedical use of prescription-type drugs and other illicit drug use	0.8%
Marijuana, nonmedical use of prescription-type drugs, and other illicit drug use	3.2%

Source: 2006 to 2008 SAMHSA national surveys on drug use and health (NSDUHs).

Older Adults

By 2030, Americans 65 years old and older will comprise 20% of the population. Older adults are an at-risk population for substance abuse (see Box 15-3) Estimates about drug and alcohol abuse and gambling problems among older adults (i.e., those >60 years old) probably underrepresent the true numbers. In one study, approximately 70% of individuals older than 60 years of age admitted to hospitals had experienced health problems or accidents related to alcohol consumption (Colleran and Jay, 2002). Men in this age group have increased rates of drinking, and females who are older than 60 years of age have a 1% to 8% chance of having problem drinking patterns (Blow and Barry, 2003). The physiologic effects of aging intensify the effects of alcohol and other drugs (Goldberg, 2008) because of decreased volume of body water, decreased body mass, central nervous system sensitivity, and decreased rate of metabolism of alcohol in the gastrointestinal tract. Relatively low levels of alcohol aggravate chronic health problems. Brennan and colleagues (2006) studied alcohol use by older adults and discovered that many adults between the ages of 55 and 65 use alcohol to manage chronic pain. Higher levels of pain were associated with the increased use of alcohol for all drinkers, but problem drinkers used alcohol 31% of the time to manage mild pain and 56% of the time to manage moderate to severe pain. Nonproblem drinkers' rates were 18% for mild pain and 21% for moderate to severe pain.

Caregivers need to carefully assess patients for these problems and to be alert for the possibility that alcohol disorder or another SUD is creating some of the patient's physical problems. For example, alcohol-induced cognitive changes mimic Alzheimer disease, and falls, assaults, and suicides are also correlated with alcohol use. According to estimates and because of the growing number of older adults, the number of adults 50 years old and older who use illicit drugs will increase from 1.6 million in 1999 to 2001 to 3.5 million in 2020 (Box 15-3).

Alcohol abuse can be triggered by the multiple losses that older adults experience: jobs, income, spouses, physical vitality, and other challenges. Since a third of alcohol abusers began drinking after middle age, this is definitely an at-risk population. Interaction with medications is another issue, because many people in this group take medications. Aspirin and nonsteroidal anti-inflammatory medications may raise alcohol levels and increase bleeding times; benzodiazepines, narcotics, and antihistamines increase sedation and impair psychomotor function. Tricyclic antidepressants are strictly contraindicated with alcohol consumption because of their potential effect on cardiac function. Nurses who are entering the profession need to be cognizant of these issues.

Health Care Professionals

Health care professionals have the same prevalence of alcoholism and illicit drug use as the general population. Exact numbers are elusive because studies are limited, and underreporting is common. One estimate is that approximately 9% of physicians use drugs or alcohol and that 10% to 15% of all health care providers will misuse drugs or alcohol at some point during their careers (Baldiserri, 2007). About 10% to 20% of nurses are identified as having substance abuse problems, and 6% to 8% of registered nurses have impaired practice as a result of their abuse of alcohol and drugs (Griffith, 1999). High-stress jobs (Trinkoff et al, 2000; Trinkoff and Storr, 1998), frequent contact with illness and death, and accessibility to prescription and controlled medications result in susceptibility to drug use, abuse, or dependence by those in the health care field. Two books by Simeca (2008, 2010) detail one nurse's experience. An exception to the overall estimate is that physicians and nurses who practice in particular specialties such as anesthesiology have higher rates of substance abuse disorders than those who practice in other specialties (Wilson and Compton, 2009). Some researchers hypothesize that repeated passive exposures to minute amounts of anesthetic agents sensitize the brain pathways of workers in operating rooms to opiates (Center for Substance Abuse Research, 2005). The rate of addiction to opiates is high among anesthesiologists and surgeons. However, more research is needed in this important area (Wilson and Compton, 2009).

Each state has programs to monitor and treat health care professionals with SUDs. It is a professional obligation to report suspected impaired practice. Signs that a coworker may be abusing drugs and reporting information can be found at www.deadiversion.usdoj.gov/pubs/brochures/drug_hc.htm.

Dual Diagnosis

Dual diagnosis, *comorbidity*, and *co-occurring disorders* are terms that describe concurrent mental illness and drug abuse or dependence. These disorders occur at the same time, or one follows the other; eventually it is difficult to tell which came first. The symptoms of one condition often mask or conceal the symptoms of the other, and either condition assumes priority at any given time. Even though *dual* is common terminology, it is important to recognize that many individuals suffer from *two or more* disorders concurrently (e.g., severe psychosis, depression, and cocaine dependence). In 2008, it was found that serious mental illness during the past year was associated with substance dependence or abuse during that same year (SAMHSA, 2009). Among adults 18 years old or older with serious mental illness in 2008, 25.2% (2.5 million) were dependent on or abused illicit drugs or alcohol. The rate among adults without serious mental illness was 8.3% (17.9 million). The most prevalent psychiatric disorders among those with a history of substance abuse are antisocial personality disorder, bipolar disorder, and schizophrenia. The substances that individuals most often abuse are alcohol, marijuana, and cocaine. Many patients with severe and persistent chronic mental illness are addicted to nicotine as well. Depression and bipolar disorder are also associated with increased rates of substance abuse.

As it is with the general population, substance abuse or dependence complicates almost every aspect of life. However, people with dual diagnoses are difficult to diagnose and to engage in treatment. Often they have lost their support systems and suffer from repeated relapses, hospitalizations, and involvement in the criminal justice system. National statistics indicate that a high percentage of forensic populations have dual diagnoses. In these settings, treatment for drug dependency (other than detoxification) is often absent. Comprehensive and repeated assessments are required to meet the needs of this population (Mueser et al, 2006).

Co-occurring Physical Conditions

Sharing and reusing needles, syringes, and other types of drug-injection equipment exposes individuals to the risk of multiple infectious processes. Contact with injecting drug users often results in the transmission of human immunodeficiency virus (HIV), hepatitis B virus (HBV), hepatitis C virus (HCV), and tuberculosis. There are no clear boundaries among the members of major risk groups that engage in multiple types of drug abuse, unsafe sex practices, and contaminated equipment use. The increase of heterosexual HIV transmission among women—especially young women—has been linked to the mixing of drugs, alcohol, and unprotected sex. Injecting drug users have one of the highest HBV rates among all risk groups and account for at least half of all new HCV cases. Prevalence rates are as high as 50% for HBV and as high as 65% for HCV among people who have injected drugs for less than a year. Coinfections of HBV and HCV often cluster in injecting drug users (http://tie.samhsa.gov/topics/infectious_wictn.html). Professionals are encouraged to screen patients with known SUDs for other morbidities.

CLINICAL DESCRIPTION

Caffeine, tobacco products, and alcohol are the three most frequently used substances by many Americans, and most

---

BOX 15-4 CLASSES OF SUBSTANCE ABUSE

- Alcohol
- Amphetamines or similar-acting drugs
- Caffeine
- Cannabis
- Cocaine
- Hallucinogens
- Inhalants
- Nicotine
- Opioids
- Phencyclidine or similar-acting substances
- Sedatives, hypnotics, and anxiolytics

From the American Psychiatric Association: *Diagnostic and statistical manual of mental disorders*, ed 4, text revision, Washington, DC, 2000, American Psychiatric Association.

Americans try or use at least one substance that sometimes results in further use, abuse, or eventual addiction during their lifetime. Many people learn from negative experiences and do not continue to use the substance, or engage in a lifestyle that often results in negative consequences of substance abuse. The substance-related disorders described in DSM-IV-TR include disorders related to the following:

- Drugs of abuse
- Medications
- Toxin exposures that may be accidental or intentional

There are 11 different classes of substances (Box 15-4). The DSM-IV-TR also addresses polysubstance dependence and other substance-related disorders.

The DSM-IV-TR divides substance-related disorders into two groups. One group contains the SUDs, and the other contains the substance-induced disorders. Each of these groups contains criteria for substance abuse, dependence, intoxication, and withdrawal that apply to the different classifications. The criteria for substance abuse and substance dependence are listed in the DSM-IV-TR Criteria box.

Specific Substances
Alcohol

Alcohol Use. Alcohol is the most widely used and most abused substance. About 9.6% of American males and 3.2% of American females are alcohol dependent (American Psychiatric Association, 2000). When those in good health use it sparingly, any changes in body function that occur are usually reversible. Likewise, some data reveal that alcohol under certain circumstances has beneficial effects. In limited amounts, alcohol increases socialization, stimulates the appetite, and decreases the risk for macular degeneration and gallstones. Research also indicates that it decreases the risk of cardiovascular disease by increasing high-density lipoproteins and decreasing platelet adhesion (Schuckit, 2000). When alcohol consumption exceeds two drinks daily or when those in poor physical health drink, damage to body systems is more rapid and pervasive. Any amount of alcohol is considered harmful to developing fetuses, children, adolescents, and recovering alcoholics. It is also harmful to people who are taking medications that interact adversely with alcohol and for those with certain medical conditions or psychiatric disorders. A telephone survey conducted between 2002 and 2003 revealed that 15% of U.S. workers (19.2 million people) reported using or being impaired by alcohol at work at least once during the preceding year. Impairment included being hungover (i.e., morning-after effects) at work (9.2%) and using alcohol during the workday (7.1%). Seventy percent of workers reported using or being impaired by alcohol less than monthly, 19% reported monthly impairment, and 11% reported weekly impairment (Frone, 2006). Among persons 12 years old or older, white individuals in 2008 were more likely than other racial and ethnic groups to report the current use of alcohol (56.2%). The rates were 47.5% for persons reporting two or more races, 43.3% for American Indians or Alaska Natives, 43.2% for Hispanics, 41.9% for blacks, and 37.0% for Asians.

Numerous studies document the relationship between violence and drugs. Persons who are in treatment for domestic violence and criminal offences have high rates of substance abuse problems. The severity of violence escalated when persons with higher drinking levels added other drugs (Chermack and Blow, 2002).

Genetics partially determines the rate of metabolism of the substance, the physiologic reactions, the level of tolerance, and the rates of elimination (Keltner and Folks, 2005; Schuckit, 2004). The liver metabolizes alcohol, where the enzyme alcohol dehydrogenase converts alcohol first to acetaldehyde. Then the enzyme aldehyde dehydrogenase converts acetaldehyde to acetate, and alcohol is ultimately metabolized into carbon and water.

Japanese, Chinese, and Korean men and women are more likely than Caucasians to have an inactive form of alcohol dehydrogenase, which metabolizes alcohol in the liver. Another 40% of this population has active enzymes with decreased activity, which results in an exaggerated response to alcohol (Li, 2000); this produces flushing, nausea, dizziness, and rapid heartbeat. The lack of this enzyme is protective against alcoholism. Native Americans, who are possibly genetically related to people of central Asian ancestry, do not lack this enzyme, so they do not have the benefit of protection.

The alcohol-deterrent drug Antabuse (disulfiram) also produces a flush reaction. Disulfiram inactivates aldehyde dehydrogenase in a person who carries the normal gene for that enzyme, thereby in effect producing the same situation as in the Asians who have the inactive form of the enzyme. Acetaldehyde increases in the blood quickly, and the resulting discomfort serves as an effective deterrent to further drinking.

Alcohol Intoxication. Alcohol intoxication as defined by the DSM-IV-TR criteria is based on evidence of clinically significant psychologic or maladaptive changes that occur during or shortly after the ingestion of alcohol. These changes include such behaviors as inappropriate sexual or aggressive actions, lability of mood, impaired judgment, and impaired

---

BOX 15-5	**STANDARD DRINK AND CONSUMPTION LEVELS**

A Standard Drink*
12 oz of beer
5 oz of wine
8 oz of malt liquor
1.5 oz of 80-proof spirits

Consumption Definitions
Abstinence
No drinking

Light Drinking
<5 g of alcohol per day

Moderate Drinking
Women: 1 drink or 15 g of alcohol per day
Men: 2 drinks or 30 g of alcohol per day

Heavy or At-Risk Drinking
Women: >7 drinks per week or >3 drinks per occasion
Men: >14 drinks per week or >4 drinks or more per occasion
Any drinking by a minor
Any drinking by a pregnant woman
>15 g of alcohol per day in an individual who is older than 65 years old

Data from the U.S. Department of Health and Human Services: *Frequently asked questions* (website): www.cdc.gov/alcohol/faqs.htm. Accessed November 23, 2010.
*All of these contain about 15 g of alcohol.

---

social or work-related functioning. Associated signs related to these changes include slurred speech, lack of coordination, unsteady gait, nystagmus, the breath smell of alcohol, impaired attention and memory, and coma or stupor. Other medical or mental disorders must be ruled out (see Box 15-5).

Effects on the Neurologic System

Cellular damage and the loss of brain tissue have been documented as a result of alcohol use. Some individuals experience symptoms such as intense anxiety, psychoses, depressed mood, auditory hallucinations, or paranoia with intoxication after ingesting alcohol. Most individuals show a clearing of clouded consciousness within a few hours. However, those with a previous history of severe alcohol abuse, brain damage, or trauma remain confused for days or weeks. This sometimes affects older individuals similarly.

Nurses should assess alcohol use in all cases of rapidly developing confusion. Assessment is imperative in the case of persons with known mental disorders so that providers do not confuse an alcoholic delirium with dementia or with a worsening mental disorder such as schizophrenia. Temporary or permanent signs of confusion are also associated with the direct effects of alcohol and with specific vitamin deficiencies. Korsakoff's syndrome symptoms include a severe form of amnesia that is much more profound than that which usually

DSM-IV-TR CRITERIA

Substance Abuse and Substance Dependence

Substance Abuse

A A maladaptive pattern of substance use leading to clinically significant impairment or distress, as manifested by one (or more) of the following and occurring within a 12-month period:

1 Recurrent substance use resulting in a failure to fulfill major role obligations at work, school, or home (e.g., repeated absences or poor work performance related to substance use; substance-related absences, suspensions, or expulsions from school; neglect of children or household)

2 Recurrent substance use in situations in which it is physically hazardous (e.g., driving an automobile or operating a machine when impaired by substance use)

3 Recurrent substance-related legal problems (e.g., arrests for substance-related disorderly conduct)

4 Continued substance use despite having persistent or recurrent social or interpersonal problems caused or exacerbated by the effects of the substance (e.g., arguments with spouse about consequences of intoxication; physical fights)

B The symptoms have never met the criteria for substance dependence for this class of substance.

Substance Dependence

A maladaptive pattern of substance use, leading to clinically significant impairment or distress, as manifested by three (or more) of the following and occurring at any time in the same 12-month period:

1 Tolerance, as defined by either of the following:

a Need for markedly increased amounts of the substance to achieve intoxication or desired effect

b Markedly diminished effect with continued use of the same amount of the substance

2 Withdrawal, as manifested by either of the following:

a The characteristic withdrawal syndrome for the substance

b The same (or a closely related) substance is taken to relieve or avoid withdrawal symptoms

3 The substance is often taken in larger amounts or over a longer period than was intended

4 There is a persistent desire or unsuccessful efforts to cut down or control substance use

5 A great deal of time is spent in activities necessary to obtain the substance (e.g., visiting multiple doctors or driving long distances), use the substance (e.g., chain-smoking), or recover from its effects

6 Important social, occupational, or recreational activities are given up or reduced because of substance use

7 The substance use is continued despite knowledge of having a persistent or recurrent physical or psychologic problem that is likely to have been caused or exacerbated by the substance (e.g., current cocaine use despite recognition of cocaine-induced depression or continued drinking despite recognition that an ulcer was made worse by alcohol consumption)

Specify if:

With physiologic dependence: evidence of tolerance or withdrawal or both (i.e., either item 1 or item 2 is present)

Without physiologic dependence: no evidence of tolerance or withdrawal (i.e., neither item 1 nor item 2 is present)

From American Psychiatric Association: *Diagnostic and statistical manual of mental disorders*, ed 4, text revision. Washington, DC, 2000, American Psychiatric Association.

occurs during early dementia. The person also exhibits an inability to learn new skills. Korsakoff's syndrome can progress to Wernicke-Korsakoff syndrome, which occurs as a consequence of a thiamine deficiency after many years of excessive alcohol consumption. Symptoms of Wernicke-Korsakoff syndrome related to this condition involve neurologic abnormalities, including inflammatory hemorrhagic degeneration of the brain. Wernicke-Korsakoff syndrome has a mortality rate of more than 15% (Schuckit, 2000).

Marchiafava-Bignami disease also occurs as a result of alcohol abuse. The identification of this condition was rare before the routine use of neuroimaging. Atrophy of the corpus callosum and impaired cerebral blood flow characterize this disease. Studies suggest that there are possibly subtypes of this disease. Clinical presentation is acute or chronic (Heinrich et al, 2004). The acute presentation includes dysarthria, impaired consciousness, tetraparesis, and symptoms of interhemispheric dysregulation; the acute presentation is associated with poor outcomes.

Alcoholic blackouts (also called *anterograde amnesia*) occur in individuals who have consumed sufficient alcohol such that the substance interferes with the acquisition and storage of new memories in the hippocampus portion of the brain. The information is lost from memory within minutes of its occurrence. About one third of drinkers report having had at least one alcoholic blackout. Approximately 40% of teenage and young adult males have blackouts (Galanter and Kleber, 2006). The history of a blackout experience probably indicates at least one episode of a rapidly consumed excessive amount of alcohol. If there are no other symptoms of alcohol-related problems, a blackout is not indicative of alcohol dependence. Persons who have been alcohol dependent for many years have had blackouts after consuming only a small amount of alcohol. Blackouts are frightening and unpleasant, regardless of how long the person has been drinking.

Peripheral Neuropathy. Peripheral nerve deterioration in both hands and feet result from chronic alcohol intake.

Peripheral neuropathy occurs in about 10% of alcoholics after years of heavy drinking. Symptoms include numbness of the hands and feet that is often bilateral and that is often accompanied by tingling and paresthesias. Damage does not always improve with abstinence. Ulcerations develop from co-occurring circulatory problems related to alcohol use.

Effects on the Liver. Alcohol metabolism occurs primarily in the liver. As a result, excessive use of alcohol may cause liver damage. Increased alcohol use results in the accumulation of fats and proteins in liver cells, which produces a (usually) reversible condition called *fatty liver*. The inflammation of liver cells along with an elevation of some liver function tests and other signs of alcoholic hepatitis such as fever, chills, nausea, abdominal pain, and jaundice result in excess deposits of hyaline and collagen near blood vessels, which signals the early signs of cirrhosis of the liver. As damage progresses, normal blood flow through the liver decreases, dilated veins or varices develop, and fluid seeps from the liver and accumulates in the abdomen as ascites. As liver failure progresses, cognitive impairment also develops as a result of hepatic encephalopathy (Galanter and Kleber, 2006).

Effects on the Gastrointestinal Tract. Alcohol is associated with ulcers and gastritis or inflammation of the stomach. Alcohol stimulates gastric secretions and promotes the colonization of a bacterium identified in the development of ulcers. Inflammation of the pancreas occurs as a result of the blockage of pancreatic ducts along with the simultaneous stimulation of the production of digestive enzymes. The result is either acute or chronic pancreatitis (Schuckit, 2000). Esophageal varices occur in cases of severe alcoholism and result from impaired liver circulation. These dilated and congested veins sometimes rupture and produce a fatal hemorrhage.

Nutrition. Alcohol has a profound effect on an individual's metabolism of carbohydrates, because it impairs the function of the liver and pancreas to respond normally to insulin. This impairment results in very high or low levels of insulin in the blood and has a negative effect on the control of blood sugar in diabetics. Alcohol also interferes with the absorption, storage, and distribution of vitamins such as B1, B6, D, and E. Vitamins B2, A, and K are often deficient in alcoholics (Schuckit, 2000).

Effects on the Cardiovascular System. Heavy consumption of alcohol increases blood pressure and elevates both low-density lipoprotein cholesterol and triglycerides. These changes in turn increase the risk for myocardial infarction and thrombosis. Alcohol at high doses also produces a non-reversible deterioration of the heart muscle. Wasting of the heart muscle results in cardiac arrhythmias and congestive heart failure or alcoholic cardiomyopathy (Galanter and Kleber, 2006). Higher levels of alcohol consumption are related to an increased risk for hemorrhagic stroke.

Effects on the Immune System. Researchers estimate that, for some people, alcohol intake of between 4 and 8 drinks per day decreases the production of white blood cells and interferes with the ability of these cells to get to sites of infection. That amount of alcohol also interferes with red blood cell production, significantly increases the average size of red blood cells (i.e., the mean corpuscular volume), and impairs the production and efficiency of clotting factors and platelets (Galanter and Kleber, 2006). A less-effective immune system contributes to an increased risk of contracting HIV and tuberculosis as well as to the potential for developing other infectious and noninfectious disease processes.

Sleep Disturbance. Alcohol intoxication often interferes with sleep. Persons under the influence fall asleep more quickly, but they have depressed levels of rapid eye movement and less stage 4 sleep. Interruptions between sleep stages, called *sleep fragmentation*, also occur (Galanter and Kleber, 2006). Although some people say that they use alcohol to fall asleep, alcohol often interrupts their sleep architecture, which means that they do not experience the normal pattern of light and deep sleep. The excitatory neurotransmitter glutamate increases as the initial depressant effect of alcohol wanes, thereby causing irritability and an inability to sleep. Glutamate rebound is also responsible for many hangover symptoms.

Hormonal Changes. Hormonal changes occur as a result of heavy alcohol consumption. Acute intoxication sometimes results in changes in amounts of prolactin, growth hormone, adrenocorticotropic hormone, and cortisol. It also produces a reduction in parathyroid hormone, which is associated with lowered levels of blood calcium and magnesium. Some of these changes result in symptoms of menstrual irregularity, decreased sperm production and motility, decreased ejaculate volume, decreased production of testosterone, and impotence.

Accidents. Accident rates that result from alcohol consumption dramatically influence mortality and morbidity rates in the United States. In the year 2000, more than 1 in 10 Americans 12 years old and older (22.3 million persons) stated that they drove under the influence of alcohol at least once during the previous 12 months (SAMHSA, 2007). There is evidence that a blood alcohol level as low as 15 mg/dL (0.01), or that which results from about one drink, significantly impairs a person's ability to drive an automobile. Alcohol also significantly contributes to bicycle and pilot errors and to accidents in the home and workplace, and this is exclusive of age. Researchers have discovered significant discrepancies in the attention levels of college-aged binge drinkers (Crego et al, 2009).

Prescription Drugs

Taken for nonmedical reasons, prescription opiates or other scheduled medications cause addiction, overdose, and death. Four categories of prescription drugs were researched in the 2007 SAMHSA study: pain relievers, tranquilizers, stimulants, and sedatives. In 2007, 2.1% persons 12 years old and older (5.2 million) reported using prescription pain relievers nonmedically during the previous month: 2.7% of youth (670,000), 4.6% of young adults (1.5 million), and 1.6% of adults 26 years old or older (3 million). Prescription drug use is designated as follows: pain relievers (2.8 million users), tranquilizers (1 million users), stimulants (0.8 million users), and sedatives (0.2 million users).

Some trends of concern are occurring among older adults, women, and adolescents. Misuse of prescription medications is the most common form of drug abuse among older adults. This population is especially vulnerable because of the multiple drugs that are often prescribed for medical conditions. Cognitive impairment and physical instability result in or from alterations of medication ingestion causing increased risk for automobile accidents and falls. Risks increase because older adults have a decreased capability for metabolizing many medications and often need a fraction of what a middle-aged person requires.

Because the frequency of adolescent prescription drug use is increasing, it is wise for parents and grandparents to be aware of prescription medications in their homes and to dispose of them properly when they are no longer needed.

Anxiolytic Drugs

Central nervous system (CNS) depressants work in different ways, but they all produce drowsy, calming, and sedating effects to help with sleep disorders and symptoms of anxiety. If an individual uses them over a long period, the body develops tolerance because of the brain's adaptive mechanism called *neuroplasticity*. Many of these medications are lethal in overdose situations. Patients obtain them either by prescription or through other sources "on the street." As noted previously, substances that are shorter acting with rapid onset (e.g., lorazepam) have higher addictive potential. When these are used as drugs of abuse, individuals often take them to reduce subjective unpleasant anxiety or to manage withdrawal symptoms from other drugs (e.g., alcohol, cannabis, heroin, methadone, cocaine, amphetamines).

Medications in the hypnotic class include the carbamates, the barbiturates, the barbiturate-like hypnotics, all prescription sleeping medications, and almost all prescription antianxiety medications, with the exception of a nonbenzodiazepine antianxiety agent such as buspirone (Buspar). Some medications in this class are anticonvulsants (see Chapter 25). Carbamates include medications such as meprobamate (Miltown, Equanil) and tybamate (Salacen, Tybatran), which are not common in the United States. They are lethal when taken in overdose amounts. The carbamates also seem to have a higher potential for dependence.

The names of barbiturates all end in *-al* in the United States. Examples include phenobarbital (Luminal) and secobarbital (Seconal). Barbiturate-like hypnotics include medications such as methaqualone (Quaalude, which is now no longer available legally because of its history of abuse), ethchlorvynol (Placidyl), and glutethimide (Doriden). The class of hypnotics also includes chloral hydrate (Noctec). Benzodiazepines used as hypnotics include flurazepam (Dalmane), temazepam (Restoril), and triazolam (Halcion).

γ-Hydroxybutyric acid (GHB) is an illegal CNS depressant that relaxes or sedates the user. Individuals often use it in combination with alcohol, and it is known as a *designer drug*. It has been involved in date rapes, poisonings,

overdoses, and deaths. Individuals abuse GHB either for its intoxicating, sedative, or euphoria-producing properties or for its growth-hormone–releasing effects, which build muscles. The effects last up to 4 hours, depending on the dose. In high doses, GHB depresses respirations and heart rates until death occurs. Overdose occurs quickly, with nausea, vomiting, headache, and loss of consciousness and reflexes. The body metabolizes GHB rapidly, so the drug is difficult to detect in emergency departments.

Benzodiazepines include chlordiazepoxide (Librium), diazepam (Valium), lorazepam (Ativan), clonazepam (Klonopin), and alprazolam (Xanax). Benzodiazepines are relatively safe with regard to the potential for overdose as compared with most other types of sedatives and hypnotics. When they are used in high doses, benzodiazepines disturb sleep patterns and cause changes in affect. Withdrawal from benzodiazepines is lengthy, and rapid discontinuation after the habitual use of large amounts often causes seizures. Versed is a popular benzodiazepine that is used for anesthesia induction. The following link is a good resource to use to explore this class of medications: www.pharmacorama.com/en/Sections/Gaba_4_1.php.

Rohypnol is a benzodiazepine that is illegal in the United States, although it is used in Europe, Mexico, and more than 60 other countries for the treatment of insomnia, for sedation, and as a preoperative anesthetic. It is tasteless and odorless, and it dissolves easily in carbonated beverages, creating a blue hue that can be disguised in dark-colored liquid. When it is used as a drug of abuse, alcohol accelerates its toxic and sedative effects. Rohypnol causes anterograde amnesia or blackouts. When it is used to victimize others, such as in cases of sexual assault or date rape, as little as 1 mg will impair a person for 8 to 12 hours (www.justice.gov/ndic/pubs6/6074/index.htm).

Stimulants

This category of substances includes caffeine, ephedrine, propanolamine, amphetamines, and amphetamine-like substances. It also includes substances that are similar in action but with a different chemical structure (e.g., diet pills). Stimulants are popular drugs of abuse because of their effects on the brain. People become addicted to the sense of high energy, alertness, and well-being that these drugs produce. These drugs act centrally, which means that their effect is on the CNS mechanisms that control heart rate and respiration. Methamphetamine not only creates an immediate surge in dopamine, but it also blocks the reuptake of dopamine, thereby creating more available neurotransmitter in the synaptic spaces. The efficiency of this drug to produce a stimulating high is also responsible for the eventual depletion and destruction of the neurons that produce dopamine.

Individuals ingest stimulants orally, intranasally, by smoking, or by injection. "Ice" is a very pure form of methamphetamine that individuals smoke to produce an immediate and strong stimulant effect. Abusers of this stimulant have recovered from the damage to dopamine receptors substantially after 9 months of abstinence, but they do not recover from impairments in motor skills and memory (Mathias and Zickler, 2001). In 2004, 51% of methamphetamine treatment admissions came from the criminal justice system (SAMHSA, 2009).

Stimulants such as methylphenidate (Ritalin) and dextro-amphetamine (Dexedrine) are used for the treatment of medical disorders such as narcolepsy, attention-deficit/hyper-activity disorder, and obesity. The effects of the stimulants are similar to those of cocaine, but these drugs do not cause local anesthetic effects. In some instances, individuals take them on a regular schedule, similar to what is done for other medi-cations, even when the drugs are being abused. Users some-times binge and have brief drug-free times. These drugs raise the blood pressure and the body temperature to dangerous levels and elevate the heart and respiration rates. Aggressive or violent behavior occurs with high-dose use, and anxiety, paranoia, and psychotic episodes occur with the abuse of and dependence on stimulants.

Caffeine-related disorders are in the DSM-IV-TR. Caffeine is the most widely consumed psychoactive stimulant in the world. It is a methylxanthine, and so are theobromine (in chocolate) and theophylline (Theo-Dur). More than 80% of adults in the United States consume this substance regularly. Caffeine produces a wide variety of symptoms, depending on the individual and the level of consumption. Tolerance some-times develops. Caffeine is in many beverages, including coffee, tea, chocolate, sodas, and as an additive in some brands of bottled water. Caffeine is also in some medications. Some people who ingest large amounts of caffeine develop delir-ium. The cessation of caffeine use causes withdrawal symp-toms, including headaches, but because a person's lifestyle is generally not focused on obtaining and using caffeine, it is not typically considered a drug of abuse. However, it is important to ask mental health patients how much caffeine they take, because too much can cause anxiety.

Cocaine

Cocaine is an alkaloid stimulant that is similar in clinical pattern, intoxication, and treatment approaches to that of other stimulants, such as the amphetamines. Cocaine is sold on the street as an impure powder that is mixed with glucose, mannitol, or lactose. Individuals usually inject the powder intravenously or snort it nasally. Individuals often sprinkle freebase cocaine (which has a lower melting point) over tobacco or smoke it in pipes designed for that purpose. The crystallized form of cocaine, also called *crack*, has a relatively low melting point, and it is readily soluble in water. Freebase or crack cocaine is usually 40% or more pure cocaine, whereas powdered cocaine is less pure. Intranasal use has a time to onset of about 3 to 5 minutes, with peak effects occurring in 10 to 20 minutes. The high begins to fade in 45 minutes or less. Intravenous use gives a high that lasts 10 to 20 minutes or less. Peak blood levels usually develop quickly, within 5 to 30 minutes. The cocaine effects disappear relatively quickly over 2 hours, although some effect will remain for about 4 hours. Traces of cocaine are in the urine for at least 3 days, and they may be in the urine for up to 14 days if high doses

were used. As with all drugs with high abuse potential, toler-ance develops quickly.

Changes such as euphoria, affective blunting, hypervigi-lance, agitation, anger, impaired judgment and social func-tioning, and anxiety characterize cocaine intoxication. Depressant effects such as sadness, decreased blood pressure, and psychomotor retardation occur with long-term, high-dose use. The course of intoxication is usually self-limiting to approximately 24 hours, after which withdrawal symptoms occur. These withdrawal symptoms are often referred to as the *crash*, when the person is depressed; this stimulates a repeat cycle of use, withdrawal, and using again.

Opioids

Opioids include natural substances such as morphine, syn-thetics with morphine-like action, and semisynthetic drugs such as heroin. People have used opioids for at least 3500 years. Codeine and related medications such as oxycodone (OxyContin), hydrocodone (Vicodin), and hydromorphone (Dilaudid) are synthetics with morphine-like action. Fentanyl is a synthetic medication that individuals inject or use transdermally. Other opioids are either injected or taken orally. Other manufactured synthetic opioids include meperi-dine (Demerol), methadone, and propoxyphene (Darvon). Opioids are anesthetic agents, antidiarrheal agents, cough suppressants, and pain relievers. Heroin is the most widely abused opiate alkaloid. It used to be prescribed in the United States to treat pain until its abuse potential was realized, but other countries still use it for pain control. Individuals either inject or smoke heroin, and it may be snorted when a very pure form of the drug is available. Trends in the abuse of prescription opioids are rising, as has been previously men-tioned. OxyContin abuse is rampant. These pills can be dis-solved and injected intravenously, or they may be crushed and snorted or swallowed.

Those with opioid SUDs have lives that center on acquir-ing and using drugs. Individuals who are dependent on morphine and heroin consume huge amounts (as much as 5000 mg) of the drug each day. Fatal overdose is not unusual, and it is often caused by mistakes involving the strength of the drug or the quantity required for the desired effect. Signs of opioid intoxication include maladaptive behavioral or psychologic changes, which develop during or shortly after use, and pinpoint pupils. Euphoria is fol-lowed by apathy, dysphoria, psychomotor retardation or agitation, and impaired judgment or functioning. Cognitive changes such as drowsiness, coma, and slurred speech are also evident.

Because opioids are pain-numbing analgesic drugs, indi-viduals who use them routinely are often unaware of their own serious health problems. Intravenous drug users are at risk for subacute bacterial endocarditis and other circulatory compromise created by foreign substances introduced during the process of intravenous use. Infection with methicillin-resistant *Staphylococcus aureus* is endemic among intrave-nous drug users; rates of HIV, HBV, and HCV are also increased. Regardless of the setting, nurses need to ask about intravenous drug use whenever a patient presents with fever of unexplained origin.

Steroids

Among the often-abused drugs are anabolic androgenic steroids, which are generally manufactured substances related to male sex hormones. The term *anabolic* refers to muscle building, and *androgenic* refers to increased masculine characteristics (www.drugabuse.gov/infofacts/steroids.html). Since the 1950s, athletes have used these types of steroids to boost their athletic performance. Individuals take anabolic steroids orally or by injection, usually in cycles of weeks or months rather than continuously. This type of schedule, called *cycling*, involves taking multiple doses of anabolic steroids over a specific period of time, stopping for a time, and then starting again. Users also combine several types of steroids to maximize effectiveness while minimizing negative effects; this is called *stacking*. With the process called *pyramiding*, a person starts with low doses of stacked drugs and then gradually increases the doses for 6 to 12 weeks. During the second half of the cycle, the individual gradually reduces the doses to zero.

The abuse of anabolic steroids is associated with higher risks for heart attacks and strokes and an increased risk of liver problems among those who ingest oral doses. Physical changes include breast development and genital shrinking in men plus increased risk for prostate cancer, infertility, and reduced sperm count. Women experience masculinization of their bodies, as evidenced by the growth of facial hair, male-pattern baldness, changes in the menstrual cycle, enlargement of the clitoris, and a deepened voice. Effects on adolescents are changes in growth hormones, which result in arrested physical development. For all individuals, extreme mood swings occur, and these may be accompanied by violent behaviors. Depression, paranoid jealousy, delusions, and impaired judgment all occur as a result of anabolic steroid abuse (NIDA, 2002). Previous-month use of these substances among twelfth-grade males has remained stable for several years, and overall use has dropped (SAMHSA, 2009).

Hallucinogens

The use of hallucinogens among teenagers between the ages of 12 and 17 years increased from 0.07% in 2007 to 1.0% in 2009 (SAMHSA, 2009). Overall use is stable according to statistics from recent years. Many different compounds are in this class of drugs. Hallucinogens alter perception, cognition, and mood. LSD, which is one of the primary drugs in this class, was discovered in 1943. The widespread use of this semisynthetic drug, which was developed by the military for possible use as a chemical warfare agent, led to the widespread use and abuse of hallucinogenic drugs. These drugs were made more cheaply and distributed more easily than the botanical versions, such as psilocybin mushrooms and mescaline (peyote cacti). LSD is illegal, but it is available in various forms.

Other drugs in this class include 3,4-methylene-dioxy-methamphetamine (MDMA; also called *ecstasy*); 3,4-methy-lenedioxyamphetamine (MDA); and 3,4-methylenedioxy-*N*-ethylamphetamine (MDEA). These are considered "club drugs" or "designer drugs," and they are neurotoxic. Individuals usually take MDA and MDMA orally. The effects of these drugs last between 3 and 6 hours, although confusion, depression, sleep problems, and paranoia often last for weeks.

The use of MDA and MDMA sometimes results in death caused by neurotoxicity or serotonin syndrome. Symptoms include drug-induced anxiety or panic, hyponatremia, and hyperthermia (i.e., oral temperatures of >103°F). Autopsies show signs of rapid muscle destruction with massive hepatic necrosis, kidney failure, and heat stroke. Ecstasy causes neurons to release serotonin, which leads to euphoria. Some individuals couple the use of ecstasy with the use of antidepressants that block the reuptake of serotonin from the synaptic space, thereby creating a substantial increase of serotonin in the brain; this can result in a potentially fatal condition called *serotonin syndrome*. Individuals manufacture hallucinogenic drugs illegally in unregulated labs, so purchasers are never certain about the substances that they are ingesting. An analysis of ecstasy has yielded amphetamines, ketamines, and other substances.

Clinical symptoms of hallucinogen use include altered vital signs, panic attacks, flashbacks (i.e., the unwanted recurrence of drug effects), psychosis, delirium, altered moods, and states of anxiety. Tolerance and dependence occur occasionally. Hallucinogens are different from other drugs of abuse in that the cessation of use after long-term use does not result in a distinct withdrawal syndrome. Hallucinogens also place a person at higher risk for suicide and trigger psychiatric disorders from as little as one dose.

Phencyclidine and Ketamine

Phencyclidine (PCP) is a hallucinogen, but it has its own set of CNS reactions. PCP interacts with uniquely high-affinity binding potentials. It was initially an anesthetic, but providers discontinued its use because of severe reactions. It has a long duration of action, and, because of its potency, it carries a high risk of toxicity. Individuals usually inhale or smoke it, although there are other routes of administration. Individuals often use PCP with other substances, such as tetrahydrocannabinol (THC), cocaine, methamphetamine, or LSD. Clinical indications of significant neuronal hyperexcitability, hypertension, and hyperthermia are potential medical emergencies. As concentrations of PCP change, mixtures of symptoms of intoxication, delirium, psychosis, confusion, paranoia, hallucinations, and violent outbursts occur. The use of this drug has been popular in the southern United States and in Washington, DC (NIDA, 2002).

Ketamine, which is also known as *special K* or *vitamin K*, is an agent that is sometimes used illegally instead of PCP because it is less potent and has a shorter duration of action. Individuals often smoke it with marijuana or tobacco products for its effects of dreamlike states and hallucinations; sometimes it is injected intramuscularly. At low doses, ketamine impairs attention, learning, and memory. In high doses, it causes delirium, amnesia, impaired motor function, elevated blood pressure, depression, and potentially fatal respiratory problems. Like propofol, ketamine is legally used in surgery before the administration of anesthetic agents.

Nicotine

Nicotine dependence is the most deadly and costly of all substance dependencies. Approximately 50% of smokers die of smoking-related illnesses. An estimated 70.9 million Americans reported the current use of a tobacco product in 2009. More than 6000 children die each year primarily as a result of sudden infant death syndrome and respiratory infections that are linked to parental smoking and low birth weights associated with smoking during pregnancy. The rate of current use of any tobacco product among persons 12 years old or older remained steady from 2007 to 2008 (28.6% and 28.4%, respectively). Rates of current use of cigarettes, smokeless tobacco, cigars, and pipe tobacco also did not change significantly during that period. However, between 2002 and 2008, previous-month use of any tobacco product decreased from 30.4% to 28.4%, and previous-month cigarette use declined from 26.0% to 23.9%.

One hopeful trend is the increased recognition of the need for the treatment of tobacco dependence. Individuals with other substance-abuse problems, especially alcohol abuse, are typically heavy smokers, as are people with psychiatric illnesses, including those with dual diagnoses.

Recent findings about the neurobiology of nicotine are interesting, because nicotine has been found to suppress craving. This suggests that nicotine does not cause pleasure. DiFranza (2008), when studying how nicotine addiction develops in novice smokers, observed that the brain can be remodeled after the first cigarette, which creates a neurobiologic craving for the drug. The most likely time for addiction to occur, according to the same author, is within a month after having smoked the first cigarette.

Dependence on nicotine occurs within a relatively short time period, and usually after the fifth exposure to the drug (DiFranza, 2008). Brain activity is intense and widespread in response to the nicotine. The reinforcement of smoking and the desire to continue using nicotine results from increases of dopamine, norepinephrine, epinephrine, and serotonin. The body rapidly absorbs nicotine into the circulation, and it reaches the CNS is less than 15 seconds. Nicotine has both stimulant and depressive qualities. Smoking is also socially reinforcing for some individuals, particularly youth. The body metabolizes nicotine at variable times, which is why some people need cigarettes often but can also go quite a while without nicotine. Because of this property, the mechanism of nicotine depletion in the brain acts as an intermittent reinforcer, which, according to behavioral theory, is the most compelling. Scientists do not yet know the mechanisms for the variable times of the metabolism of nicotine.

Cannabis

Marijuana and hashish come from the Indian hemp plant. Marijuana typically comes from the upper leaves, the flowering tops, and the stems of the plant, whereas hashish comes from the dried resinous exudates from the tops and backs of the leaves of some plants. Cannabis, which is the bioactive substance that is extracted from the plant, remains the world's most commonly used illicit drug; it ranks fourth in the world after caffeine, nicotine, and alcohol. The active ingredient in these substances is THC, which produces most of the effects that lead to continued use. Hashish contains about 10% THC, whereas most marijuana purchased on the street contains from 1% to 5% THC. Some forms available today, however, contain up to 40% THC (Bennett and Bennett, 2002). Two species are of interest. *Cannabis sativa* is generally between 8 and 12 feet tall. The leaves have long, thin fingers and are light green. The more equatorial varieties have more yellow pigments to protect the plant from intense light. Sativa buds are long and thin, and they turn red as they mature in a warm environment. In cooler environments, the buds may be slightly purple. Sativa plants smell sweet and fruity, and their smoke is generally quite mild. It is a source of fiber for rope and other products, and it contains THC, which gives smokers the psychic effects that they seek. The leaves of this plant are smoked, but the most highly prized part of the plant is the top.

Cannabis indica is plentiful in the Mideast, India, and Central Asia, especially Afghanistan, Kashmir, and Pakistan. It is a short plant that is generally between 3 and 6 feet tall, and its leaves have short, broad fingers. The leaves are generally dark green, and they are sometimes tinged with purple. As they near maturity, the leaves may become significantly more purple. It is a strong-smelling plant with a "stinky" or "skunky" smell. The smoke of this plant is generally thick and more prone to cause coughing when inhaled. Indicas are the traditional source of hashish (www.erowid.org).

Individuals usually smoke cannabis in cigarettes or pipes, although some ingest it in food. Others combine it with other drugs, such as opium, cocaine, and PCP. Symptoms of intoxication vary and include a "high" feeling of euphoria accompanied by inappropriate laughter; feelings of grandiosity, sedation, lethargy, and impaired cognition; distorted sensory perceptions; impaired motor skills and performance; and a sensation of prolonged time sequences. The psychoactive effects are followed by other signs within 2 hours of use, such as conjunctival injection (i.e., bloodshot eye appearance), increased appetite, tachycardia, and dry mouth. If the individual smokes cannabis, the effects develop within minutes and usually last 3 to 4 hours. The intensity of symptoms is related to several factors that include the dose, the method of ingestion, and the individual characteristics of the user. Cannabis is fat soluble, and high-dose effects sometimes persist for 12 to 24 hours as the drug is released from the tissues. Dependence and tolerance can develop over time.

In 1972, the federal government declared cannabis to be a class I drug; however, 14 states have medically legalized its use, and 16 are debating legislation. The use of cannabis is endorsed for a variety of medical conditions, including chronic pain, neurodegenerative diseases, glaucoma, and many other conditions; information may be found at www.medicalcannabis.com. Ongoing clinical trials are useful for evaluating the use of cannabis for particular medical disorders. The use of any substance has risks, and any drug abuse is particularly harmful to the developing brain.

Inhalants

Products with breathable chemical vapors that produce psychoactive effects are included in this classification. More than a million people used inhalants to get high in the year 2000. For young people especially, these substances are cheap and easily accessible. Inhalants fall into three categories:

1. Solvents (e.g., paint thinners, degreasers, gasoline, glues) include toluene, gasoline, ketones, chlorofluorocarbons, and others.
2. Gases (e.g., refrigerant gases and aerosol gases for whipping cream, spray paints, hair or deodorant sprays, and fabric protectors) include ether, chloroform, nitrous oxide (sold as "poppers"), butane, propane, gasoline, ketones, chlorofluorocarbons, ethyl chloride, and others. A common method of ingestion is the use of "whippets," which are balloons that are filled with an inhalant; the contents of these balloons are breathed in for intoxicating effects.
3. Nitrites (e.g., aliphatic nitrites, including cyclohexyl nitrite, amyl nitrite, and butyl nitrite [now illegal]).

Inhalants cause effects similar to those of anesthesia, and they slow body functions. Depending on the dose, users experience slight stimulation, decreased inhibition, or loss of consciousness. Sniffing high concentrations induces heart failure, suffocation, and death. Other irreversible effects include hearing loss, peripheral neuropathies or limb spasms, CNS damage, and bone marrow damage. Reversible effects include liver and kidney impairment and blood oxygen depletion. Amyl and butyl nitrites have been associated with Kaposi's sarcoma. Long-term use leads to diffuse abnormalities in white brain matter (Rosenberg, 2002). Few formal human studies exist in this area, because researchers cannot ethically conduct studies in which they ask a participant to do something injurious. In 2008, there were 729,000 persons 12 years old or older who had used inhalants for the first time within the previous 12 months; 70.4% were younger than 18 years old when they first tried these drugs (SAMHSA, 2009). There was no significant change in the number of inhalant initiates from 2007 to 2008, but the number in 2008 was significantly lower than the 2005 estimate of 877,000.

Club Drugs and Designer Drugs

As described previously in this chapter, young adults at all-night parties called *raves* or *trances* are using club drugs (designer drugs). MDMA, GHB, Rohypnol, ketamine, methamphetamine, and LSD are some of the drugs that are ingested at these events. All club drugs have potential lethal effects or produce long-lasting or permanent brain or other physical damage. Uncertainties about drug sources, the chemicals used, and possible contaminants make it difficult if not impossible to determine the symptoms, toxicity, and consequences of the use of these club drugs in any given community.

Other Substances of Concern

Several substances are known for their abuse potential but do not fit any other classification; they have limited use and are not currently on the DEA schedule. For example, propofol (Diprivan) is widely used intravenously for anesthesia induction or procedures that require light sedation. Propofol abuse is a major problem with frequent fatal outcomes; several deaths have been reported after self-administration, and one researcher stated that, of 110 sampled certified registered nurse anesthetists in recovery, 4% identified propofol as their drug of choice (Stocks, 2009). Ease of access was the main reason given. However, 33% had abused propofol at least once. Propofol is an example of a drug that would not appear on a routine screening test for substance use; another is Vistaril. Professional groups are working with the DEA to have some of these substances declared schedule I drugs.

K2 and Spice (Spice Gold, Spice Silver, and Spice Diamond) are currently legal substances that are marketed as substitutes for cannabis. These compounds consist of chemicals that are thought to be cannabinoid agonists. Several states have banned synthetic cannabis.

Pseudoaddiction

An important distinction to note is differences between people who become addicted because of voluntary abuse and those who become medically addicted because they take large amounts of opiates or other addicting drugs over a long period of time for legitimate medical reasons, which results in **pseudoaddiction**. Although the second group also becomes dependent on the drug, their lifestyles do not resemble those of typical drug addicts. Those with chronic pain conditions fall into this category, which is not in the DSM-IV-TR. In addition, some people with an addiction have physical problems that require pain relief. Some are anxious about obtaining the medication required for pain and are in psychologic and physical distress if the medication is not available. The undertreatment of pain sometimes leads to this phenomenon. Individuals with inadequate pain control sometimes horde medications to use when they are in severe pain and have escalating anger and frustration when they are unable to obtain the needed medication. Thus, they appear to be drug seeking. These individuals need a pain-management plan and access to medications to relieve their pain. Careful assessment is necessary to determine patient needs (Freeman, 2005b).

Non–Dependence-Producing Drugs of Abuse

The *International Classification of Diseases*, tenth edition, has a category for medications or substances that patients continue to use (sometimes very excessively) although they are medically unnecessary. Medications in this category include antidepressants, analgesics, antacids, vitamins, steroids, hormones, laxatives, specific herbal or folk remedies, and diuretics. Usually the patient has a strong motivation to take these drugs and to continue taking them, but no dependence or withdrawal symptoms develop. Ephedrine (which is contained in some cold medicine) is an example of this type of drug, and its use is now monitored. Before legislation, energy and sports supplements often contained ephedrine. Negative reactions to this drug include irregular or rapid heartbeat, chest pain, severe headache, shortness of breath, dizziness, loss of consciousness, sleeplessness, and nausea. Another reason for limiting the distribution of this substance is that it is an ingredient that is used to make methamphetamine.

Polysubstance Abuse and Dependence

Many people who use drugs try a variety of substances and settle on a "drug of choice"; however, the use of multiple substances by those who use drugs is most common. Multiple drug use or abuse, which commonly referred to as *polysubstance use or abuse*, is also likely to occur among individuals who progress through use or dependence on a variety of drugs over time. For example, some people start their use or abuse with nicotine, caffeine, or alcohol. If they continue on to use other drugs, they often try cannabis, and this may be followed by stimulants, hallucinogens, or other CNS depressants. This differs from young people who consume any drug that is readily available at a party. The ingestion of multiple substances at the same time creates additional risks as a result of chemical drug interactions or potentiating effects.

Although individuals may mix any combination of substances, some drug mixtures are more likely to occur. Those individuals with alcohol dependence are more likely to use or develop nicotine dependence. Those who are cocaine dependent are more likely to become dependent on alcohol. Some people who use opioids combine heroin and cocaine in a mixture called a *speedball*; this combination enhances the effects and decreases the side effects of both drugs. Other combinations of multiple drugs exist (Galanter and Kleber, 2006).

PROGNOSIS

The development of substance dependency is usually gradual and insidious. As mentioned previously, individual, environmental, and situational factors influence this process. The same is true of the recovery process. One of the most prominent factors that leads an individual to recovery is the patient's recognition that substance use has caused or influenced his or her life's problems and interrupted his or her functioning. The recognition of serious problems takes a long time, partially as a result of impaired frontal lobe function in individuals with addiction, as mentioned previously. Treatment professionals refer to the recognition of serious problems as *hitting bottom*, which means that the individual is often without options for basics such as shelter and food or is unwilling to tolerate his or her lifestyle any longer because of its negative consequences.

The steps that individuals take differ in detail, but ultimately the goal is to change patterns of functioning to maintain sobriety. Sobriety is the goal of complete abstention from drugs, alcohol, and addictive behaviors. The patient has to learn how to prevent or minimize relapses and to get back on course toward achievement and the maintenance of abstinence. Most people who seek recovery from SUDs succeed. Sobriety often involves several attempts, and many patients relapse nine or ten times before achieving and sustaining sobriety. A relapse or slip is not a failure but an expected part of the recovery process. Compare the recovery process to the commitment to exercise or dieting; it is difficult for most people to maintain these activities without lapses. Addiction is not an intellectual process; some people are intellectually brilliant and still become addicted. Addiction is insidious and puzzling. It is a difficult challenge, and people who have addictions are opposing a powerful force.

The course of substance use, intoxication, dependence, abuse, and withdrawal varies with the class of substance, the route of administration, other factors as discussed previously with regard to specific substances and internal and external factors. Nevertheless, there are some generalizations about prognosis and recovery. Intoxication usually develops rapidly after use and continues as long as the individual uses the substance. When use declines or stops, withdrawal develops and continues for varying lengths of time, depending on the half-life of the substance and related factors. Because developing a dependency takes time, persons whose use of substances is recent are diagnosed as having *substance abuse*. For many, the trajectory of abuse unfortunately progresses to *substance dependence* involving the same substances.

The trajectory of substance dependence varies. It is usually chronic and lasts 6 months or more, with periods of heavy intake that are sometimes stress related and periods of partial or full remission. During the first year after patients achieve sobriety, they are particularly vulnerable to relapse. Individuals with a history of earlier onset of use, higher levels of substance intake, and greater numbers of substance-related problems who also exhibit a history of tolerance or withdrawal have a more difficult course of recovery. In a similar way, persons who exhibit serious comorbid mental disorders such as conduct disorders, antisocial personality disorder, untreated major depression, and bipolar disorder are more likely to experience ongoing impairments and, ultimately, a poorer outcome. A supportive community that includes family and friends—who are often lost during an individual's time of addiction—take a while to recreate or replace. Recovery groups and their members frequently become the recovering addict's primary social support, at least during the early recovery phases and often for years.

RECOVERY AND DISCHARGE CRITERIA

The following are examples of outcome criteria that determine a patient's willingness to live drug-free. The patient will do the following:

- Maintain abstinence or reduce harm (this is more applicable to some substances than others) from substance use.
- Admit to potential or actual lifelong dependence on psychoactive substances.

- Express knowledge of the continual process of recovery (i.e., "one day at a time").
- Verbalize realistic goals.
- Maintain attendance in a support group (e.g., AA, Narcotics Anonymous).
- Express increased self-esteem.
- Demonstrate new and constructive coping mechanisms and strategies to manage anxiety, stress, frustration, and anger.
- Engage in the use of substitutes to replace drug-seeking and drug-taking behaviors, such as hobbies, school, employment, spiritual support, volunteer work, and social relationships.
- Express the feeling of being in control of one's life.
- Express hope for the future.
- Abandon people and situations that influence and contribute to drug-taking behaviors.
- State the consequences of psychoactive substance use on one's biopsychosocial, cultural, and spiritual well-being.
- State the names and phone numbers of resources to contact when unable to cope or when experiencing a desire to relapse to substance-taking behaviors.
- Investigate substance abuse assistance programs in the workplace, such as the employee assistance program.
- Ask family or significant others to attend Al-Anon or Alateen support groups.

THE NURSING PROCESS
ASSESSMENT

Persons who abuse substances often have negative experiences with judgmental health care professionals. Although it is understandable, this type of judgmental or negative approach discourages the patient's involvement in the health care system. Nurses have the choice to reinforce the stereotype of the rejecting health care professional or to form a new relationship with the patient on the basis of insight into and an understanding of the patient's situation. The development of a beginning trusting nurse–patient relationship is a priority with any patient, but particularly for patients with SUDs, because patients often hide, deny, or minimize substance abuse even when they are desperately in need of treatment. Because of the social stigma associated with SUDs, the nurse needs to be skilled in gathering information and building trust by firmly and gently questioning the patient about potential substance use problems.

The identification of substance-related symptoms is usually based on self-report. The nurse's awareness of what the patient does *not* say as well as what the patient says is important. The nurse makes decisions about when to ask questions, what questions to ask, and when to seek more information from those who know the patient (see the Case Study). In many instances—and with the patient's expressed consent—the nurse confirms the patient's history with family members, significant others, and previous treatment facilities.

The nurse also assesses the patient's readiness for change, because motivation plays a key role in the success or failure of treatment efforts. By remembering that assessment is an ongoing process, the nurse will obtain critical assessment data, even when the patient limits disclosure.

CASE STUDY

Christy is a 32-year-old woman who is admitted to the emergency department in a local hospital at 0200 hours after an assault near a tavern where she had spent the evening drinking. Although she never drank as a young adult, vowing that she would never be an alcoholic like many in her family, Christy began drinking heavily at age 29 and was in a treatment program after driving under the influence 1 year ago. Her drinking began after a divorce. Christy is now a single parent of two children, ages 10 and 7.

She presented with facial lacerations and possible other blunt trauma head injuries, and she states that a man she did not know assaulted her when she did not want to go home with him. She was incoherent and confused. The nurse noted that Christy's temperature was 99°F, her blood pressure was 160/60 mm Hg, and her respirations were 28 breaths per minute. A packet of white powder found in Christy's pocket was sent to the laboratory for analysis.

Critical Thinking
1. What is Christy's most immediate problem?
2. What would you assess first?
3. What physical findings (other than alcohol) might indicate drug use?
4. What drug screening tests would be appropriate, if any?
5. What nursing diagnoses would be relevant at this time?
6. What complications might exist if Christy requires medical or surgical procedures?

When gathering information about drug use, the nurse uses a systematic approach by integrating questions about legal and illicit substances into the general history. The nurse also assesses the patient's age, ethnicity, and demographic factors related to drug use at this time. In addition, the nurse obtains information about the use of drugs from other categories listed in Box 15-6. A patient's positive response regarding any drug use alerts the interviewer to obtain further information about the specific drug or drugs used. The nurse focuses on the patient's age at first use, the period of heaviest lifetime use, patterns of use, the presence or absence of binges, and any occurrence of blackouts. The nurse assesses use during the immediate past to determine the possibility of withdrawal symptoms or toxicity. The other components of a complete health history include a psychosocial history, a family history, a determination of the risk for suicide or violence (toward self or others), and a mental status examination.

Collaboration among the nurse, the patient, the family, and treatment team is essential to the assessment, planning, and implementation of the plan of care. For the patient who

---

BOX 15-6 DRUG CATEGORIES CONSIDERED DURING AN ASSESSMENT

Nicotine: Cigarettes, chewing tobacco, pipe smoking, snuff, and so on
Alcohol: Beer, wine, whiskey, gin, and so on
Cannabis: Marijuana, pot, and hashish
Cocaine: Crack and freebase
CNS depressants: Sedatives, hypnotics, and anxiolytic-related drugs
CNS stimulants: Caffeine, Ephedra, amphetamines, diet pills, and Benzedrine inhalers
Opioids: Heroin, codeine, methadone, oxycodone (OxyContin), hydrocodone (Vicodin), and morphine
Hallucinogens: LSD, mescaline, PCP, mushrooms, and peyote
Inhalants: Solvents (glue, paint, gasolines), aromatic hydrocarbons (aerosols, gases, hair spray), and nitrites
Anabolic-androgenic steroids
Synthetics: Meperidine hydrochloride (Demerol) and propoxyphene hydrochloride (Darvon)
Over-the-counter drugs: Antihistamines, cough syrups, sleeping pills, hormones, laxatives, and herbal products
Designer and club drugs: MDMA, MDEA, MDA, GHB, Rohypnol, and ketamine

---

BOX 15-7 CAGE SCREENING TEST FOR ALCOHOLISM

1 Have you ever felt that you ought to **C**ut down on your drinking?
2 Have people **A**nnoyed you by criticizing your drinking?
3 Have you ever felt **G**uilty about your drinking?
4 Have you ever had a drink first thing in the morning to steady your nerves or to get rid of a hangover (an **E**ye-opener)?

From Ewing JA: Detecting alcoholism: the CAGE questionnaire, *JAMA* 252:1905-1907, 1984.

---

abuses or is dependent on substances, the path to treatment and recovery requires hope, realistic outcome criteria, and a comprehensive plan of care; see the Research for Evidence-Based Practice box.

RESEARCH FOR EVIDENCE-BASED PRACTICE

Vandermause R: Assessing for alcohol use disorders in women: Experiences of advanced practice nurses in primary care settings, *J Addict Nurs* 18(4):187-198, 2007.

Alcohol use disorders among female patients are frequently missed in primary care settings. This study explores common assessment practices by advanced practice nurse prescribers in one Midwestern state. Transcribed in-depth interviews with 23 advanced practice nurse prescribers were analyzed with the use of Heideggerian hermeneutic research methods. Two patterns emerged from an overarching idea of "becoming aware": 1) recognizing alcohol in everyday life and 2) attending to her story. The first pattern revealed ways that nurses approach and think about assessing for alcohol use disorders in women. The second pattern revealed practices of listening and responding to women's unique and complex stories. These findings inform education and practice by raising new questions and suggesting possibilities for education and research.

Physical Examination

On examination, the identification of specific physical health findings associated with alcohol or drug dependence suggests the possibility of a substance abuse problem. For alcohol abuse, signs and symptoms include the following:

- Jaundice
- Arcus senilis (an opaque ring that is gray to white in color that surrounds the periphery of the cornea)
- Acne rosacea (facial redness)
- Palmar erythema
- Enlarged liver
- Cigarette burns and stains on the fingers
- Upper abdominal pain that results from the inflammation of the pancreas
- Decreased sensation in the feet or hands as a result of peripheral neuropathy
- Positive stool guaiac test that demonstrates gastrointestinal bleeding
- Hypertension
- Tremor
- Tachycardia

For drug abuse, signs and symptoms may include the following:

- Cardiac arrhythmias
- Needle tracks
- Cellulites
- Conjunctivitis
- Poor dentition
- Rapid weight loss
- Changes in pupil size
- Changes in nasal mucosa (if the drug is taken intranasally)

In addition, signs of withdrawal or intoxication specific to each drug class are sometimes present. During the assessment process, the nurse observes for and questions the patient about the incidence of accidents and injuries that are related to substance use.

Screening Instruments

A wide variety of instruments are available for screening for substance-related or induced disorders. The CAGE questionnaire is a well-validated and brief screening instrument that is easy to memorize and use (Box 15-7). A positive response to two of the four items of the CAGE questionnaire indicates a potential problem with alcoholism. The Drug Abuse Screening Test (DAST) contains 28 self-reported items and is easy to answer. The Alcohol Use Disorders Identification Test (AUDIT) is useful for identifying both drug and alcohol abuse disorders. If screening test scoring shows that problems possibly exist, the nurse should follow up with questions about withdrawal symptoms, tolerance, legal and social complications, and work history. The diagnostic criteria for substance abuse and dependence are in the DSM-IV-TR Criteria box on p. 335. Screening instruments should be a routine part of a health care visit. An impediment to the identification of patients with SUDs is the reluctance of health care professionals to ask about SUDs (Armstrong and Holmes, 2005).

Laboratory Tests

Laboratory tests for SUDs are part of a routine assessment. Ethical issues continue to be a concern with drug testing as a result of issues such as the potential infringement of civil rights and the need to obtain the patient's informed consent. The use of laboratory tests for diagnosing substance abuse continues to become more complex and sophisticated. A large number of variables affect the results, including the type of drug, the dosage ingested, the frequency of use, the type of body fluid tested (urine, blood, stool), differences in drug metabolism, the half-life of the drug, the sample collection time and its relationship to the time of use, and the sensitivity of the test itself. A negative drug test may not mean that the metabolites of the drug are not present but that the levels are not sufficient for reporting. For example, a person who is physically proximate to someone else who is smoking marijuana inhales some of the product. That person's laboratory test may be positive for THC, but it will not be at the level that the government sets for reportability.

Laboratory tests do not always detect alcohol or the presence of substances; relying solely on the results of laboratory tests is therefore misleading. However, abnormal laboratory test results often suggest substance abuse or dependence problems. They are also useful for the tracking of relapses or compliance successes of individuals who are in treatment or recovery. Blood tests are clinically useful for determining light or heavy alcohol or drug use. These are quantitative measures because they measure serum levels of intoxication. The disadvantages of blood testing include increased expense, the use of an invasive procedure, a narrow window of time for the detection of drugs, and a lack of usable veins in intravenous drug users. One of the most commonly used laboratory tests is the blood alcohol level. In most states, the blood alcohol level determines legal intoxication. Table 15-1 provides information about blood alcohol levels and the associated extent of impairment.

Other laboratory test results that are used as markers include elevated liver enzymes and macrocytic anemia. Elevation of the liver enzyme γ-glutamyl transpeptidase is the most sensitive marker; an increase in the level indicates recent alcohol use. However, γ-glutamyl transpeptidase is rarely elevated in persons who are younger than 30 years old, and it is a less-sensitive marker in women than in men. More than half of alcoholic patients tracked have elevated levels of γ-glutamyl transpeptidase, red blood cell mean corpuscular volume, uric acid, triglycerides, aspartate aminotransferase,

TABLE 15-1	ALCOHOL INTOXICATION
BLOOD ALCOHOL LEVEL	**CONSEQUENCES**
20–50 mg alcohol/dL blood (0.02–0.05)	No legal consequences; some impaired coordination and potential changes in behavior
80–100 mg alcohol/dL blood (0.08–0.1)	Legal intoxication; impaired ability to drive, slurred speech, staggered gait, and impaired sensory function
100–150 mg alcohol/dL blood (0.1–0.15)	Markedly uncoordinated balance and gross cognition and judgment distortions
>200 mg alcohol/dL blood (0.2–0.3)	Notable impairment in all sensory and motor functions
>300 mg alcohol/dL blood (≥0.3)	Potential for cardiovascular and respiratory collapse; coma and death can occur if lifesaving measures are not initiated

Data from Schuckit MA: *Drug and alcohol abuse: a clinical guide to diagnosis and treatment*, ed 5, New York, 2000, Kluwer Academic/Plenum.
Note: States may differ with regard to defining blood levels for legal intoxication and traffic violations. For example, Colorado has defined a blood alcohol level of 0.02 to 0.05 as a traffic violation if the driver is younger than 21 years old (2000).

and urea. Another indicator of recent heavy drinking (i.e., five or more drinks) is an elevated level of carbohydrate-deficient transferrin (CDT). The presence of hepatitis C antibody raises questions about substance use, although individuals can acquire hepatitis C in many ways other than intravenous drug use.

Urine drug screens provide help with detecting the presence of drug and alcohol consumption within a specified time frame. Urine testing is qualitative and notes the presence or absence of the substance. Many report a significant number of false-positive and false-negative findings. Urine specimen tests vary, but most are low cost and have well accepted and monitored standards, and the samples can be retested or saved, if necessary. Typical urine drug screens that an emergency department performs include morphine, codeine, amphetamine, methamphetamine, cocaine metabolite (benzoylecgonine), THC metabolite, benzodiazepines, barbiturates, and alcohol. Many of these tests are also available for job testing or for home or private use. Shortcomings of urine samples include privacy issues surrounding the sample collection and possibilities of sample dilution, substitution, or alteration by deceptive patients. Many drugs are not included in either blood or urine laboratory detection measures. To determine heroin or cocaine abuse, many recommend collecting a urinalysis three times weekly. However, random intermittent interval screening also works and is less expensive. Table 15-2 provides guidelines regarding the length of time that a substance remains detectable in urine. However,

TABLE 15-2	SUBSTANCE DETECTION IN URINE	
SUBSTANCE	**DAYS SINCE LAST USE**
Alcohol	0.5
Amphetamine	1–2
Barbiturates (short acting)	3–5
Barbiturates (long acting)	10–14
Benzodiazepines (diazepam)	2–4
Cocaine	0.3
Opioids (codeine and morphine)	1–2
Opiates (heroin)	2–3
Phencyclidine (PCP)	2–8
Cannabis (THC)	2–8 (acute); 14–22 (chronic)

Data from Withers NW: Deceptions in addiction psychiatry, *Am J Forensic Psychiatry* 22:7-28, 2001.

rates of excretion depend on multiple variables, so some figures vary from those presented in the table.

NURSING DIAGNOSIS

Information obtained during the assessment phase of the nursing process is assessed and evaluated by the nurse who applies a nursing diagnosis. The accuracy of diagnoses depends on a careful in-depth assessment. Therefore, input from the patient, the family, significant others, and treatment team members is often critical for determining which nursing diagnoses are most relevant to treatment planning. It is the nurse's responsibility to prioritize nursing diagnoses for each patient in accordance with patient needs. Frequently-used nursing diagnoses when caring for patients with substance-related disorders generally address orientation, level of anxiety, limitations in function (either mental or physical) as a result of substance use, social limitations, and diagnoses related to altered family relationships. A current list can be obtained at the North American Nursing Diagnosis Association website (www.NANDA.org). The "At Risk For" nursing diagnoses relate to withdrawal, trauma, and relapse, among other things. Because SUDs are damaging to the individual as well as to his or her immediate relationships, the list is long. An axiom when working with patients who have SUDS is to be aware of difficulties with the "4 Ls": love, livelihood, liver (health), and legal (problems).

OUTCOME IDENTIFICATION

Expected responses that the patient will achieve are stated as outcome criteria. Nurses direct outcomes toward short- or long-term changes in behaviors and lifestyle. Nurses select outcomes depending on the particular characteristics of the substances abused, the degree of dependence, the patient's age, and other relevant demographic characteristics of the user. Outcomes provide the nurse and patient with definitive

and measurable steps to achieve before attaining desired discharge criteria. Examples of outcome criteria are listed here. The patient will do the following:
- Maintain safety and health.
- Maintain sobriety.
- Maintain his or her vital signs within the normal range.
- Maintain normal fluid hydration.
- Remain free of seizure activity.
- Verbalize the ability to sleep without sedation.
- State that there is a reduction in symptoms of withdrawal (although this may occurs weeks or months after the last use).
- Verbalize a reduction in delusional thinking, an absence of hallucinations or illusions, and an absence of suicidal or homicidal ideation.
- Verbalize the desire to stop drinking or using drugs or, in some instances, to decrease or limit use.
- Verbalize that he or she feels safe in his or her environment.
- Maintain a well-balanced diet of sufficient calories to meet prescribed nutritional needs.
- Participate in the therapeutic activities of the treatment plan (i.e., individual, group, and family activities).
- Express a need to contact family members or significant others regarding support.
- Explore factors that interfere with the treatment plan (e.g., lack of social or family support, lack of financial resources, seeking old drinking buddies or drug-using peers).
- Verbalize that recovery is a lifelong process that occurs one day at a time.
- Express the desire to establish relationships with sober friends and to avoid situations that previously invoked alcohol or drug use.
- Identify realistic goals for rehabilitation (e.g., continue with the 12-step program, participate in random urine drug screens).
- Use community resources to establish and maintain recovery.
- Reestablish structure in his or her lifestyle that limits opportunities for drug or alcohol use (e.g., work, school, and family activities).
- Substitute healthy coping mechanisms and activities for drug use behavior.

PLANNING

Although basic needs such as housing, employment, and nutrition are the focus of the care plan, nurses address many aspects of care when planning for the patient with an SUD. If the patient is hospitalized, discharge plans include sobriety support as well as resources to help the patient obtain and sustain housing and income. Many have debated the topic of addiction being a disability, and, because addiction is such a complex situation, there has been no lasting or complete answer. Patients in early recovery clearly need a great deal of assistance, but, as with any chronic disorder, stability is achievable.

Relapse is part of recovery, and the nurse and the patient need to develop a plan of care that meets the individual's ongoing needs. As in any nursing situation, the nurses' judgment about necessary care is based on data gathered during the assessment process. Nurses consider the patient's immediate needs, which are often of an emergent nature, as well as the long-range goals of treatment and aftercare. Collaboration with patients and others who care for them is essential to developing, revising, and evaluating the plan of care. For the patient who abuses substances or who has an impulse control disorder such as gambling, the road to abstinence and recovery requires realistic outcome criteria and a consistent plan of care.

IMPLEMENTATION

When implementing any plan, patient safety and health are always the first priorities, so the nurse focuses on treating and supporting the patient through the drug withdrawal process called *detoxification*. Nutritional support, including protein-rich diets and supplementation with vitamin B, occurs during this first stage. If violence or threats toward the self or others are a problem, then the nurse and the staff intervene to provide safety for patients and the environment.

During subsequent stages of recovery, the nurse and the health team members focus on education regarding the drug abuse and dependence process; the physical, psychologic, and psychosocial consequences of continuing to use drugs; relationship skills training; anger management; and self-esteem building. The nurse assists the patient with identifying healthy supports and developing a new support system that does not include drug-taking activities or friends. Abstaining from the substance is often the least complicated part of recovery; the final stage focuses on the patient's life after drugs. To attain and maintain sobriety, people in recovery often must give up acquaintances and friends who regularly use drugs. They also frequently have to change their living situations, get new clothing, learn to manage money, reconcile longstanding issues such as outstanding debts and warrants, and, most especially, deal with the emotional realities of life as a sober person. Without the buffering effects of substances, even small problems seem like major crises until the individual has been sober long enough to gain perspective and stability. This is a very hard-won position. Students who are interested in gaining more insight into this process could attend an AA meeting. Meetings are advertised in local communities, and meetings that are noted to be "open" welcome visitors. Participants welcome health care personnel, because an educated workforce will provide better services.

Nurses assist patients with developing short-term goals and with addressing vocational rehabilitation. It is essential to provide some sort of posttreatment contact with the patient to monitor progress and to provide ongoing support. Twelve-step programs such as AA, Narcotics Anonymous, and Cocaine Anonymous can provide the individual with a framework and network of support for ongoing recovery, with the hope that sobriety is achievable, and with contacts who understand the process of withdrawal and recovery. Other groups such as Rational Recovery are also available. For families, Al-Anon and Alateen are 12-step model programs that are available to provide support to those who are affected by addiction.

Acute Treatment: Withdrawal and Detoxification

The response to drugs varies greatly depending on situational, individual, and environmental factors and of course on the drug itself. The amount of drug that creates withdrawal symptoms in one person is sometimes different for another person. These variations are the result of individual neurochemistry, tolerance, and many other factors. Predicting exactly what amount of drug will cause an overdose is also dependent on the individual, although there are limits. In addition, because street drugs vary in strength and purity, it is difficult to know the exact amounts that a person has taken.

Sudden withdrawal or rapid decreases in the amounts of certain substances in an individual who is physically dependent often require immediate medical intervention. Withdrawal states related to depressants such as alcohol and stimulants are the most likely to lead to emergency treatment situations. Withdrawal from opiates is unpleasant, but it is not usually life threatening. As with other types of emergencies, the initiation of life-support measures is a first priority. These measures include the maintenance of respirations and cardiac function as well as control of hemorrhaging and seizures. A patient who is debilitated before going through withdrawal is more at risk for complications of the withdrawal processes.

If a patient requires medication during withdrawal, health care providers often administer adequate doses to prevent the dangerous or problematic effects of withdrawal. Nurses who lack experience sometimes fail to give adequate doses of medication when a dosage range is prescribed. During the process of detoxification, the nurse gives enough of the drug (or one to which the person has cross-tolerance) to relieve the withdrawal symptoms. This substance (e.g., Librium, Ativan) is then decreased gradually over a period of days. Benzodiazepines such as lorazepam (Ativan) have a cross-tolerance with alcohol, so they are used to manage withdrawal symptoms. Providers also use barbiturates. After stabilization has occurred, accurate history taking, physical evaluation, and laboratory testing will help to identify additional priorities for care. If an individual is withdrawing from multiple substances, he or she is at increased risk for serious outcomes. The Clinical Indicators for Withdrawal Scale—(Box 15-8) is used in many institutions to guide the amount of medication needed. The provider assesses the patient on a variety of criteria and medicates the person on the basis of a total score. This scale is typically used for alcohol withdrawal with a revised version for use with opiate withdrawal. The individual may require intravenous support to remain hydrated or to correct electrolyte imbalances. Drugs to curtail the effects of

BOX 15-8   CLINICAL INSTITUTE WITHDRAWAL ASSESSMENT FOR ALCOHOL SCALE

Pulse or heart rate, taken for 1 minute: _____ Blood pressure: _____ / _____ mm Hg

NAUSEA AND VOMITING — Ask "Do you feel sick to your stomach? Have you vomited?" Observation.
0 No nausea and no vomiting
1 Mild nausea with no vomiting
2
3
4 Intermittent nausea with dry heaves
5
6
7 Constant nausea with frequent dry heaves and vomiting

TREMOR — Arms extended and fingers spread apart. Observation.
0 No tremor
1 Not visible but can be felt fingertip to fingertip
2
3
4 Moderate with patient's arms extended
5
6
7 Severe even with patient's arms not extended

PAROXYSMAL SWEATS — Observation.
0 No sweat visible
1 Barely perceptible sweating with moist palms
2
3
4 Beads of sweat obvious on forehead
5
6
7 Drenching sweats

ANXIETY — Ask "Do you feel nervous?" Observation.
0 No anxiety; at ease
1 Mildly anxious
2
3
4 Moderately anxious or guarded, so anxiety is inferred
5
6
7 Equivalent to acute panic states as seen with severe delirium or acute schizophrenic reactions

AGITATION — Observation.
0 Normal activity
1 Somewhat more than normal activity
2
3
4 Moderately fidgety and restless
5
6
7 Paces back and forth during most of the interview or constantly thrashes about

TACTILE DISTURBANCES — Ask "Do you have any itching, pins and needles sensations, burning sensations, or numbness? Do you feel bugs crawling on or under your skin?" Observation.
0 None
1 Very mild itching, pins and needles sensations, burning sensations, or numbness

2 Mild itching, pins and needles sensations, burning sensations, or numbness
3 Moderate itching, pins and needles sensations, burning sensations, or numbness
4 Moderately severe hallucinations
5 Severe hallucinations
6 Extremely severe hallucinations
7 Continuous hallucinations

AUDITORY DISTURBANCES — Ask "Are you more aware of the sounds around you? Are they harsh? Do they frighten you? Are you hearing anything that is disturbing to you? Are you hearing things that you know are not there?" Observation.
0 Not present
1 Very mild harshness or ability to frighten
2 Mild harshness or ability to frighten
3 Moderate harshness or ability to frighten
4 Moderately severe hallucinations
5 Severe hallucinations
6 Extremely severe hallucinations
7 Continuous hallucinations

VISUAL DISTURBANCES — Ask "Does the light appear to be too bright? Is its color different? Does it hurt your eyes? Are you seeing anything that is disturbing to you? Are you seeing things that you know are not there?" Observation.
0 Not present
1 Very mild sensitivity
2 Mild sensitivity
3 Moderate sensitivity
4 Moderately severe hallucinations
5 Severe hallucinations
6 Extremely severe hallucinations
7 Continuous hallucinations

HEADACHE, FULLNESS IN HEAD — Ask "Does your head feel different? Does it feel as if there is a band around it?" Do not rate for dizziness or lightheadedness. Otherwise, rate severity.
0 Not present
1 Very mild
2 Mild
3 Moderate
4 Moderately severe
5 Severe
6 Very severe
7 Extremely severe

ORIENTATION AND CLOUDING OF SENSORIUM — Ask "What day is this? Where are you? Who am I?"
0 Oriented and can do serial additions
1 Cannot do serial additions or is uncertain about date
2 Disoriented for date by no more than 2 calendar days
3 Disoriented for date by more than 2 calendar days
4 Disoriented for place, person, or both

Total score: _____
Rater's initials: _____
Maximum possible score: 67
This scale is not copyrighted and may be used freely.

withdrawal are given as needed; symptom severity is individual and varied.

Central Nervous System Depressants

As with stimulants, symptoms of withdrawal from depressants are usually the opposite of the acute effects of the associated drug. The length of the withdrawal period is the half-life of the drug of abuse. Many individual variables influence this as well. Withdrawal symptoms from CNS depressants include insomnia; high levels of anxiety; elevated body temperature; elevated pulse and respiratory rates; fine tremors; gastrointestinal upset; muscle aches; diaphoresis; and labile blood pressure. Confusion and other cognitive changes such as delirium, hallucinations, and delusions may occur in some clinical cases of depressant drug withdrawal. With alcohol and barbiturates especially, grand mal seizures sometimes develop. Withdrawal from depressants lasts from 3 to 7 days for short-acting drugs and up to 3 to 6 months for longer-acting drugs. Withdrawal from benzodiazepines results in characteristic symptoms similar to those that occur during alcohol withdrawal.

Alcohol

For 95% of those experiencing withdrawal from alcohol, symptoms are mild to moderate in severity and are similar to those of opiate withdrawal. Withdrawal symptoms include two or more of the following: autonomic hyperactivity (i.e., a pulse rate of >100 bpm or sweating); increased hand tremor; insomnia; psychomotor agitation; anxiety; nausea or vomiting; and, occasionally, grand mal seizures and transient visual, auditory, or tactile hallucinations or illusions. Alcohol withdrawal begins within 12 hours of stopped or decreased alcohol consumption, peaks in 48 to 72 hours, and usually decreases by 4 to 5 days. Some symptoms last several weeks or months longer. These symptoms cause clinically significant impairment or distress in areas of the individual's life that are important to usual functioning. The mortality rate is typically low for those experiencing alcohol withdrawal. As with intoxication, other disorders need to be ruled out. Alcohol withdrawal delirium (delirium tremens) occurs in less than 10% of those who experience the alcohol withdrawal syndrome. Alcoholic hallucinosis occurs more frequently and often includes frightening visual hallucinations, such as of worms or bugs. Although the affected individual has perceptual disturbances, he or she is generally oriented to time, place, and person. Disorientation characterizes impending delirium tremens. Adequate and rapid medical intervention in patients who are withdrawing from alcohol should eliminate these more severe symptoms. Patients who are experiencing severe withdrawal symptoms from alcohol usually require B vitamins, including thiamine (vitamin B1), folic acid, and vitamin B12 as a result of inadequate dietary intake and malabsorption. If alcohol withdrawal delirium is diagnosed, other general medical conditions such as liver failure, pneumonia, or recent head trauma may exist. If the person has been drinking heavily, withdrawal symptoms can start within 4 hours after stopping alcohol intake.

Pharmacologic intervention is not necessary for all cases of alcohol withdrawal. In some instances, general support measures will improve comfort. Although any depressant medication works, providers most often use the benzodiazepines, because they are less likely to cause neurotoxicity and decreases in vital signs, and they are consistently effective. Short-acting benzodiazepines such as oxazepam (Serax) and lorazepam (Ativan) are given to patients with severe liver failure or to those patients with severely impaired cognition. Longer-acting drugs such as chlordiazepoxide (Librium) are for most others who are experiencing severe withdrawal symptoms (Schuckit, 2000). If the patient has had withdrawal seizures before, antiseizure medication such as clonidine is necessary. The history of withdrawal seizures is an important part of an intake assessment for an individual who is withdrawing from alcohol.

Acamprosate (Campral) is a medication that is used to treat cravings that occur during early sobriety. Clinical studies are in progress, and patients report mixed results. Other medications are in the development stages. Naltrexone is used in conjunction with antidepressants and Campral is used during early recovery, both with mixed results.

Opioids

Beginning withdrawal from the last dose ranges from 4 to 12 hours for heroin and up to 1 to 3 days for methadone. Peak intensity occurs within 48 to 72 hours. Acute withdrawal symptoms from heroin last about 5 days, and those for methadone last several weeks. Sometimes withdrawal symptoms last longer, and sometimes they do not completely end for several months. Symptoms of morphine and heroin withdrawal include craving and irritability, lacrimation (tearing of the eyes), rhinorrhea (runny nose), diaphoresis, and yawning. As withdrawal progresses, the following occur: restless sleep, involuntary leg movements, restlessness, hypertension, tachycardia, temperature irregularities, dilated pupils, loss of appetite, gooseflesh, back and other muscle or bone pain, and tremors. Finally, insomnia, yawning, and a flulike syndrome also occur. Clonidine (Catapres) is the most commonly used nonopioid medication for the treatment of withdrawal symptoms from opioid use. Side effects from clonidine include sedation and hypotension, so nurses need to monitor patient blood pressure. Methadone has been the treatment of choice for morphine and heroin addicts. L-α-acetylmethadol (LAAM) is another drug that is used during opioid withdrawal. It is longer acting, and it is useful in communities that are far from methadone clinics. Suboxone (buprenorphine; known on the street as *boop*) is a long-acting medication that is used in maintenance therapy, and people can obtain this at a qualified physician's office rather than at a clinic; it has a high street value and abuse potential. Methadone, buprenorphine, and LAAM are synthetic opioids that are given to addicts to suppress withdrawal symptoms, and they are continued until the person withdraws from these substitute drugs. All three of the replacement drugs are addicting, but individuals withdraw from them by gradually decreasing the total daily dose until they are symptom free. Overdose of these substances leads to cardiovascular collapse and death. They are all sold illegally. These drugs may also be used as detoxification agents and not just as replacement agents.

Providers often give naltrexone (Narcan is the intravenous form, Revia is the oral form) to people in recovery to block opioids from reaching receptors in the brain. New forms have been developed that deliver a steady dose of the drug. Two forms of long-acting naltrexone are available: Vivitrol, which is a depot injection that lasts about a month, and a naltrexone implant that lasts 2 months. Implants are sometimes used as part of rapid opiate withdrawal protocols.

Stimulants

For cocaine, amphetamines, and other CNS stimulants, the physical signs of withdrawal are limited. Because of tolerance, withdrawal may develop while the person is still taking the drug and include nonspecific aches and pains. The clinical syndrome includes intense craving and drug-seeking behaviors, agitation, temporary intense depression, and a loss of appetite that gives way over time to fatigue, with associated insomnia, continued depression, and a decrease in craving. Sometimes cocaine-related stimuli, such as seeing a white powder substance, trigger cravings for cocaine. These conditioned responses probably contribute to relapse, and they are difficult to eliminate. Symptoms related to the final phase of withdrawal from stimulants include exhaustion, a rebound in appetite, and a need to sleep; these occur during the first 9 hours to 14 days. The normalization of sleep patterns, decreases in cravings, and a more normal mood follow. Withdrawal then progresses to a recurrence of fatigue, anhedonia, and anxiety. Treatment focuses on the symptoms, and providers generally avoid the use of medications. An inherent danger is that patients will seek other mood-altering substances, including alcohol and benzodiazepines, to fill the void that they experience as a result of giving up stimulants.

Emerging data suggest that it is best to treat persons with methamphetamine addiction for at least 3 months to a year in an intensive, comprehensive, and highly structured living environment. Patients also participate in a long-term and intensive outpatient program that provides information about structure and life skills as well as instruction and education focused on managing triggers and cravings. Relapse prevention includes providing educational, vocational, and employment opportunities and involvement in 12-step programs, with the recommendation of lifetime enrollment in such programs. No one treatment or protocol works for everyone (SAMHSA; retrieved July 2006 from www.nida.nih.gov/Infofacts/methamphetamine.html).

Caffeine

Caffeine is the most popular psychoactive substance in the world, and 80% of the U.S. population consumes it each day (Reissig et al, 2008). Recently, popular drinks like Jolt, AMP, and Monster have become popular with adolescents and young adults. Producers and retailers earned $744 million in the sales of these drinks between June 2006 and June 2007 (International Food Information Council, 2008). Drinks with

caffeine and high sugar levels will produce decreased alertness after 15 to 20 minutes as a result of the metabolism of glucose (Anderson and Horne, 2006).

The development of energy drinks that include alcohol are dangerous, because the caffeine may mask symptoms of alcohol intoxication while, at the same time, having a stimulant effect. Both alcohol and caffeine are dehydrating agents, and alcohol metabolism is disturbed by dehydration. Withdrawal symptoms in the form of a "hangover" might be the result. Some states have prohibited the sale of these beverages.

Caffeine withdrawal occurs around 12 to 24 hours after consumption ends, and it usually resolves in 2 to 7 days. Symptoms include headache, fatigue, yawning, and nausea or more disturbing symptoms, such as muscle tension, irritability, anxiety, and cognitive changes. Because the symptoms of caffeine withdrawal often overlap with other medical conditions, psychiatric disorders, and drug withdrawal states, a careful assessment of recent caffeine use is an important consideration. If a patient consumes caffeine and this relieves the symptoms, this will clarify the diagnosis. Withdrawal from caffeine-related disorders usually occurs with relatively low doses of caffeine in both adults and children.

Nicotine

Nicotine withdrawal has characteristic features of dysphoric or depressed mood, insomnia, irritability, frustration, anger, anxiety, difficulty concentrating, restlessness, impatience, decreased heart rate, and increased appetite or weight gain. Craving is a common occurrence after quitting. Most withdrawal symptoms peak in 1 to 3 days, but withdrawal symptoms often last 4 to 6 weeks or more. Craving and weight gain continue even longer. Symptoms are most acute among those who smoke cigarettes. Nicotine replacement therapies (e.g., gum, patches, sprays, inhalers) help to lessen the impact of withdrawal symptoms and double the cessation rates of tobacco use. Non-nicotine medications such as bupropion (Zyban or Wellbutrin), clonidine (Catapres), and varenicline (Chantix) can reduce craving. Without medical assistance, 80% of smokers who quit will relapse within the first 2 years. Studies indicate that remaining in a smoking cessation program for at least a year significantly improves success rates. These programs involve phoning the patient or having him or her check in online, with the patient always having the option to return to a cessation class when necessary.

Hallucinogens and Inhalants

There is no clinically significant withdrawal syndrome for hallucinogens or inhalants. Treatment facilities for inhalant users are difficult to find. Research suggests that chronic users are the most difficult to treat, and they exhibit numerous social and psychologic problems. Users often suffer withdrawal symptoms such as hallucinations, nausea, excess sweating, hand tremors, muscle cramps, headaches, chills, and delirium tremens. Relapse is common (Rosenberg, 2002).

Other categories of both illicit and legal drugs are generally associated with mild to moderate withdrawal symptoms.

Symptoms of cannabis withdrawal, such as irritability, tremor, perspiration, nausea, appetite change, and sleep disturbances, have been documented with high doses, but the clinical significance is uncertain. Therefore, withdrawal is not a criterion in the DSM-IV-TR. Treatment is supportive.

Nursing Interventions

In *acute situations*, nurses will do the following:

1. Maintain a patent airway in the patient, monitor the patient's vital signs, and intervene in situations that involve patient hemorrhage, seizures, or cardiac arrest *to address the patient's life-threatening problems.*

   For all patients, nurses should do the following:

2. Maintain the safety of the patient and others (chemical or mechanical restraint is sometimes necessary), *because some patients exhibit unanticipated, out-of-control, violent, or assaultive behaviors.*

3. Observe for additional signs and symptoms of substance overdose, withdrawal, and drug–drug interactions *to prevent complications.*

4. Assess the physiologic and psychologic symptoms of withdrawal and the effects of the medications prescribed during the withdrawal process *to provide safe and effective treatment during withdrawal.*

5. Initiate therapeutic interventions to treat withdrawal symptoms, including anxiety and other complications, *to help the patient to safely withdraw from the addictive substance.*

6. Provide emotional support to the patient, the family, and significant others *to establish trust and to include those people who are important to the patient in the treatment process.*

7. Support the patient in meeting nutritional and metabolic needs either orally or intravenously, depending on the patient's ability to take and retain fluids, *to provide adequate hydration and food as needed.*

8. Refer to a nutritionist as needed or engage the family in identifying and meeting the patient's personal, cultural, or spiritual preferences *to offer holistic and interdisciplinary care.*

9. Increase the patient's carbohydrate intake and offer straws or other edible or nonedible but safe objects or foods for the patient to chew on (e.g., sugar-free hard candies, trail mix, toothpicks, straws, gum) *to decrease some of the patient's cravings for illicit substances and to satisfy the patient's oral needs.*

10. Initiate a vitamin and mineral replacement therapeutic regimen as prescribed, *because low levels of vitamin B and other vitamins and minerals such vitamins A, C, D, E, and K, iron, magnesium, and zinc are common with chronic alcohol ingestion.*

11. Provide support to the patient and the family by acknowledging the patient's deception and denial. *A variety of psychotherapeutic techniques are useful for the patient and the family. Interventions that involve support and empathy, while not enabling the patient, assist the individual and the family with working through the denial process and developing awareness that many life problems are related to substance abuse (see Chapter 26).*

12. Intervene with secondary medical complications or residual effects of substance use exhibited by the patient, *because the prolonged use or abuse of alcohol or other drugs sometimes causes a variety of complications and temporary or permanent damage to major body systems.*

13. Establish a trusting, caring, and empathic yet firm therapeutic relationship with the individual *to help the patient improve self-esteem and deal with thoughts of guilt and remorse.*

14. Encourage the patient's efforts to establish, reestablish, or strengthen the support of family and significant others through a variety of measures, such as role-playing and providing a quiet and private environment for the patient to meet with or telephone family, *because patients who abuse substances frequently have lost meaningful contact with their family and significant others.*

15. Teach the patient, the family, and significant others about substance abuse, symptoms, management, treatment, and prevention, both individually and as group members. Assess the style of learning that works best for the patient to meet learning needs (i.e., verbal, visual, or written). Use materials in the language the patient is most comfortable with, if possible. Provide factual information about prevention measures that work. *The nurse acts as an advocate and a resource person regarding successful treatment and prevention efforts and the need for a healthy lifestyle for patients and their families and significant others.*

16. Support the patient and family in maintaining active involvement with 12-step or alternative support groups, such as AA, Al-Anon, Alateen, Narcotics Anonymous, and Rational Recovery. *Experience with patients with substance abuse issues indicates that lifelong membership in a 12-step or alternative recovery program is, for many individuals, the key to remaining sober. Families also benefit from groups that help them to change previous patterns of relating to the patient and others.*

17. Encourage the family to be flexible and supportive regarding the patient's participation in support groups, *because establishing a new lifestyle, such as engaging in a support group network, takes time, effort, and motivation.*

18. Assist the patient with establishing a new social support system by putting him or her in touch with community organizations in which the patient will find alternative housing, make new friends, and experience opportunities to build inner strength and to develop drug-free coping measures. *The patient often faces the enormous task of establishing a new social network that is drug free; knowledge and guidance regarding resources and recovery programs will provide invaluable assistance for making the patient's efforts successful.*

Additional Treatment Modalities

Rehabilitation for substance disorders is a vital part of treatment. Now more than ever before, researchers are evaluating treatment outcomes with the use of funded studies. In 2002, SAMHSA launched a new program called "Changing the Conversation: The National Treatment Plan Initiative to Improve Substance Abuse Treatment." The goal of this program was to ensure that quality treatment services and programs were available to all who needed them. In this initiative, five key guidelines were identified:

1. There is "no wrong door" to treatment (i.e., anyone who needs treatment is identified and receives it).
2. Invest for results (i.e., use treatment and services wisely to produce desired results).
3. Commit to quality (i.e., continually strive to improve treatment).
4. Change attitudes (i.e., challenge stigma and misinformation regarding addiction treatment and the nature of the recovery process).
5. Build partnerships (i.e., work together to make needed changes).

Treatment programs offer a wide variety of services and goals. Likewise, patients have different motivations and reasons for seeking treatment. It is important to recognize that there will be no perfect match of patient and program. Instead, it is the genuineness, interest, and preparation of the staff and the approaches that they use that will help the patient to achieve recovery. Collaborative team interventions enhance successful treatment and rehabilitation outcomes. Providers need to use all available resources. Ultimately, it will be the patient's decision and responsibility to achieve and maintain a life of sobriety and recovery. The following principles were published in 1999 by NIDA and thus far are reliable:

- Treatments are aimed at reducing the prevalence of a disorder.
- No single treatment is effective for all individuals.
- Effective treatment focuses on multiple needs.
- Remaining in treatment for an adequate time is critical for treatment effectiveness.
- An individual's treatment plan requires continual assessment and modification as necessary.
- Multiple types of treatment are necessary for most people and include medication; individual, group, and family therapies; and other treatment modalities.
- The majority of individuals who require alcohol and drug treatment are likely to have a co-occurring psychiatric disorder (i.e., dual diagnosis).
- Recovery from addiction is a long-term process that frequently requires multiple episodes of treatment.

Psychotherapy

Therapy has to comprehensively address patient needs. Psychotherapy for individuals with addictions is usually successful, and it addresses the patient's addiction as well as any comorbid (co-occurring) disorders or life-interfering behaviors that are present. For example, therapy models and interventions for individuals with personality disorders will be different from therapies for persons with depression or anxiety. In general, patients with addictions are actively involved in a recovery program in addition to participating in individual or group therapies. Categories of behavioral therapies are generally brief motivational, contingency management, cognitive behavioral, and family and social network (Carroll and Rounsaville, 2006). These therapies can be used in a variety of settings, which are discussed as follows.

Individual Therapy. One type of individual psychotherapy is for patients who have high levels of anxiety, inadequate coping mechanisms, and a low tolerance for frustration. The primary focus is on the here and now of the patient's life as he or she learns to relate to others and to adjust to a life without reliance on drugs. Some patients communicate more effectively in a one-on-one relationship as compared with a group setting. Cognitive behavioral therapy is an evidence-based approach to therapy for substance using and abusing patients (Freeman, 2005a). Dialectic behavioral therapy (DBT) is also research based, and it has been adapted for use with SUDs. Research has also found motivational interviewing techniques to be effective with persons with addictions (Miller and Rollnick, 2002). Providing therapy to adult children of alcoholics on the basis of developmental theories has also been described (Brown, 1988).

Therapists need to address the patient's protective patterns of denial and deception during the course of therapy. Like many other patients, these individuals often test the therapeutic bond between the patient and the therapist. These therapists often address issues such as relapse, onset of depression, and resistance to continuation of therapy.

Group Therapy. Most therapies conducted on an individual basis are also adaptable to a group mode. Group therapy is typically more cost effective, and it reaches greater numbers of people. Group therapy has certain advantages for patients with substance-related disorders that are difficult to achieve in individual therapy. In a group setting, patients with similar experiences and problems confront or support each other in a relatively safe environment. The role of the nurse or therapist is to facilitate group members' participation and to assist with clarifying interpersonal interactions within the group. In addition to discussions, the group also shares didactic or educational information about substance use and recovery. Patients in recovery who have maintained sobriety share experiences and serve as role models for newly admitted patients.

Family Therapy. Family therapy has gained credibility in treatment programs designed for both adults and adolescents. Family therapy is based on family systems theory. The genogram (Bowen, 1978) is a useful instrument for tracing the intergenerational use of substances. Researchers are scanning genomes to identify which members in a family are more likely to use illicit drugs. Recently, researchers working with teenagers isolated a particular gene that influences susceptibility to smoking. If the teen is also depressed, this increases the genetic effect. Other genetic and environmental research studies are under way to link family members with specific types of substance use. Some researchers believe that from 60% to 80% of addiction is related to genetic susceptibility.

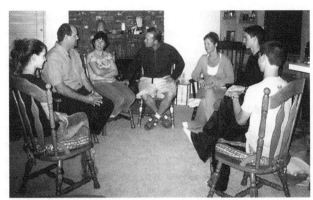

FIGURE 15-5. Family therapy is an important factor when one member is in recovery for substance abuse.

Recognition and acceptance of alcoholism as an illness that affects all members of the family supports a need for family therapy (Figure 15-5). When the family member who abuses alcohol suddenly attains sobriety, the dynamics of the entire family change. Some patients experience relapse if the family does not know how to relate to the person when he or she is sober. Family members in alcoholic families often have a tendency to lack trust for one another, to feel unloved and unwanted, and to carry a heavy burden of guilt.

Behavioral Therapy. Some programs use behavioral approaches such as relaxation therapy or biofeedback to teach patients how to manage everyday stressors and insomnia. Usually behavioral modification approaches are used in addition to other forms of education and counseling. Approaches include assertiveness training and aversive conditioning.

Aversive conditioning is used with nicotine-dependent patients to develop learned negative associations with cigarettes. Aversive conditioning with disulfiram (Antabuse) is one technique of behavior therapy that is used for alcoholics. This treatment is not used extensively in the United States. Claims for lasting success are questionable because long-term studies are rare and the therapy is not considered evidence-based, but it is still used. The patient is conditioned by pairing the sight, smell, and taste of alcohol with an emetic. Induced nausea and vomiting subsequently result in aversion to alcohol. After the conditioning experience, the patient is given disulfiram, which inhibits the enzyme aldehyde dehydrogenase; even a small amount of alcohol causes a toxic reaction as a result of acetaldehyde accumulation in the blood.

Patients in treatment for aversive conditioning need to be in good health, highly motivated, and cooperative. Providers warn them about the consequences of using the drug disulfiram if and when even small amounts of alcohol are ingested. If ingestion occurs, patients experience flushing and feelings of heat in the face, chest, and upper limbs. Other symptoms include pallor, hypotension, nausea, general malaise, dizziness, blurred vision, palpitations, air hunger, and numbness of the upper extremities.

Contingency management is a form of behavioral therapy that is based on operant conditioning in which the patient is given a reward for abstinence (Shoptaw et al, 2009). Examples of rewards are vouchers for inexpensive prizes, coupons for goods or services, or money. The hope is that an interruption in substance use provides patients with relief from addictive behavior and allows them to create new behaviors. There is evidence that contingency management works relatively quickly, although relapse is certainly possible in the absence of incentive.

Medications

The one magic bullet drug to cure craving and prevent relapse is elusive. The best way to cure addiction is to avoid addictive substances altogether. However, as this chapter has demonstrated, avoidance does not always work.

No one drug guarantees recovery. Therefore, medications are typically an adjunct to other therapies. These include acamprosate (Campral), a promising medication that has been used in Europe to calm the withdrawal effects of alcohol and to lessen the preference for it, and naltrexone (Revia, Trexan, Vivitrol), which has a clinical usefulness that has been demonstrated in some studies.

Methadone and L-α-Acetylmethadol Treatment Programs. Methadone is a long-acting opioid that has similar properties to those of heroin. LAAM is an analog of methadone that has a 72- to 96-hour half-life. Providers give these drugs for similar reasons: to serve as substitutes for other opioids such as heroin, to reduce criminal activity, and to decrease drug craving.

Methadone and LAAM maintenance for opioid dependence are administered only in facilities that are licensed; that offer counseling services, including outreach; and that have security measures in place to minimize the illegal use of opioids. The patient must have been opioid dependent for a year or more and must not have benefited from drug-free treatment approaches. Some patients stay on these substitutes for 10 years or more.

❖ **CLINICAL ALERT**

All patients who are taking naloxone (Revia) need to carry a card or wear a metal bracelet stating that they are taking the drug and that, if they are injured, they will not respond with analgesia from narcotics. This information is critical in the event of a traumatic injury, and it is important for emergency personnel to know.

Opiate antagonists such as naloxone (Narcan) and naltrexone (Trexan, Revia, Vivitrol) block the effects of heroin and other opioids during rehabilitation and overdose. Most patients are then tested periodically for the resumption of opioid use. Treatment occurs along with other approaches and has varying degrees of success (Galanter and Kleber, 2006).

Rapid Detoxification Procedures

One form of rapid detoxification lasts about 3 days and involves heavy sedation to shorten opiate withdrawal; this is usually accomplished in a hospital under the continual supervision of an anesthesiologist. Ultra-brief detoxification lasts approximately 4 to 6 hours or less. This is sometimes performed in a physician's office, and health care providers have used the ultra-rapid anesthesia detoxification method in the United States since 1995. Both procedures include administering naltrexone to the patient, sometimes in combination with midazolam. As previously mentioned, naltrexone blocks the drug from the receptor sites in the brain and nervous system, thereby ending the effect of opiate drugs. A subcutaneous time-released naltrexone implant can be inserted in a small incision in the abdominal fat, and this lasts for about 2 months. A timed-release injection that lasts a month is also available (Vivitrol); however, because the lifestyle of addiction has not been addressed with these rapid methods, patients return home to their previous situations without other supports in place. Although the patient is in fact detoxified from the substance, he or she is still in active addiction, because the person's behaviors have not changed. Postprocedure follow up is encouraged with the use of a 12-step program or another route.

Oral naltrexone has few side effects, and it is the treatment of choice for highly motivated patients, such as addicted professionals and individuals in the criminal justice system. Revia, which is the oral form of naltrexone, prevents any effect of opiates. Some clinical trials suggest that patients in early sobriety who are depressed have a better response to treatment and remain sober longer if they also take oral naltrexone. Providers need to warn patients that, if they are taking this medication and they injure themselves, they will not respond to a narcotic analgesic agent until the naltrexone is cleared.

Relapse Prevention

Principles of relapse prevention are used throughout the rehabilitation process to help patients avoid or take control of situations in which relapse is possible. The patient practices what to do if relapse occurs and develops a comprehensive plan to follow. The individual identifies situations in which he or she is most likely to relapse or use drugs and makes lifestyle changes, including in living areas, shopping, and selection of friends and family who will support a life of abstinence.

Harm Reduction

Harm reduction techniques help an individual to change patterns of use to decrease the risk of harm and to adapt a healthier lifestyle. For example, acknowledging that some persons are addicted and that they will use intravenous drugs, needle-exchange programs were created to reduce the rates of acquired immunodeficiency syndrome (AIDS) and HCV. In addition, providing opiate replacements (e.g., methadone, LAAM, buprenorphine) eliminates the necessity of illegal activities such as burglary to fund an addiction. Does this exchange one addiction for another? Yes, but harm-reduction techniques allow addicts to work, live relatively stable lives, and create support systems to improve the probability that they will be able to live without illegal drugs. Other examples of risk reduction include designated driver programs, cigarettes with lower levels of tar and nicotine, and HBV programs for drug users who inject drugs (Miller and Carroll, 2006).

12-Step Support Groups

For decades, AA and similar groups were the only widely available treatment programs. These groups still provide support and reinforcement during recovery for a large number of individuals. More recently, other programs of treatment based on other principles and research have become available. For those who benefit from groups, options are available to meet a wide variety of needs. Individuals who have been active in a 12-step program or in Al-Anon serve as sponsors (mentors) for those who are involved in the earlier stages of recovery. Help is available 24 hours a day, every day of the week. Although the 12-step programs do not keep statistics because they do not see that as their role, anecdotal information suggests that the greater the level of participation in the group and the greater the intensity of exposure, the more successful the outcome. Participants in these programs see recovery as a lifetime process. They do not promote harm reduction; sobriety is the accepted goal. Contrary to popular opinion, AA has never supported aggressive confrontation. The goal has been to establish a safe and welcoming community with many resources where individuals who abuse alcohol are able to turn.

AA is the original self-help group for recovering alcoholics. AA was founded in 1935, and it was built on the foundation that support and encouragement from others with alcoholism help other persons who are on the road to recovery. AA encourages new members to work with a sponsor (a recovering alcoholic), who negotiates with the newcomer about working the 12 steps (this is sometimes a yearlong process) and other goals of the sponsor–sponsee relationship. Women sponsor women, and men sponsor men. Relationships during early recovery are not recommended, for a variety of reasons. The goal of sobriety is to create a life outside of addiction and to give back to the recovery community through service. The Twelve Steps of AA are listed in Box 15-9.

AA groups are available in each community. Meetings are open or closed. During open meetings, anyone with an interest—including spouses, friends, and significant others—are able to attend. Closed meetings are only for individuals in the recovery process. Groups are available for specific populations, such as women, nonsmokers, businesspeople, and professionals. Some groups use American Sign Language, and many provide access for the handicapped. Many AA groups now accept the need for those with dual diagnoses to take prescribed psychotropic medications to keep their illnesses stabilized. AA is an international organization with a growing presence in many countries.

Narcotics Anonymous embraces a philosophy that is similar to that advocated by AA. It is a support group for individuals who are addicted to narcotics. Because many

BOX 15-9 THE TWELVE STEPS OF ALCOHOLICS ANONYMOUS

1 We admitted we were powerless over alcohol, that our lives had become unmanageable.
2 Came to believe that a Power greater than ourselves could restore us to sanity.
3 Made a decision to turn our will and our lives over to the care of God as we understood Him.
4 Made a searching and fearless moral inventory of ourselves.
5 Admitted to God, to ourselves, and to another human being the exact nature of our wrongs.
6 Were entirely ready to have God remove all these defects of character.
7 Humbly asked Him to remove our shortcomings.
8 Made a list of all persons we had harmed, and became willing to make amends to them all.
9 Made direct amends to such people wherever possible, except when to do so would injure them or others.
10 Continued to take personal inventory, and when we were wrong promptly admitted it.
11 Sought through prayer and meditation to improve our conscious contact with God as we understood Him, praying only for knowledge of His will for us and the power to carry that out.
12 Having had a spiritual awakening as the result of these steps, we tried to carry this message to alcoholics and to practice these principles in all our affairs.

The Twelve Steps are reprinted with permission of Alcoholics Anonymous World Services, Inc. Permission to reprint this material does not mean that AA has reviewed or approved the contents of this publication. AA is a program of recovery from alcoholism *only*—use of the Twelve Steps in connection with programs and activities that are patterned after AA, but that address other problems, does not imply otherwise.

individuals are polysubstance abusers or dependent on multiple drugs, attendees often have problems with one or more substances. Cocaine Anonymous is another variant. Sometimes persons with multiple addictions attend AA, acknowledging that they are addicted to alcohol; persons who exclusively use alcohol are in the minority, although many people recognize that alcohol was their first problem substance.

Al-Anon and Alateen self-help groups operate independently from AA groups. Al-Anon is a support group for spouses and friends of individuals with alcoholism. There are opportunities to learn about alcohol as a disease and to share common problems and solutions with other spouses. These groups also discuss behaviors and issues that are common to the disease process, such as boundary setting, avoidance, enabling, self-inflicted guilt, and shame. Alateen is a nationwide support group for children 10 years old and older who have alcoholic parents. Similar to Al-Anon, the group helps children to realize that they are not the cause of their parent's drinking. Sharing experiences and feelings normalizes experiences that children think are theirs alone.

Adult Children of Alcoholics is a support group for adults who were raised in alcoholic homes. Adult children of alcoholics manifest behaviors of control, enabling, making excuses for others' behaviors (especially the behavior of alcoholic individuals), inability to trust one's self, and feelings of inadequacy and insecurity. Individuals learned these patterns during childhood, often from parents who themselves were products of alcoholic households. Individuals in these situations develop constant patterns of assuming responsibility for and taking care of others' needs. The support groups provide opportunities to discuss problems and to feel acceptance from others with similar experiences. Sometimes people with these patterns are drawn to the helping professions.

Some people object to the faith orientation of traditional 12-step programs, which asks that members identify a "higher power." Although this power is defined in whatever terms the individual chooses, the inclusion of Christian prayer in most meetings suggests support for a traditional Christian orientation. Alternative groups to AA include Rational Recovery, which uses more behavioral approaches, Secular Organization for Sobriety, and Women for Sobriety.

Inpatient Care

Inpatient hospitalization provides a structured treatment program for those who are severely impaired or debilitated, those who fail in outpatient treatment efforts, and those who have serious medical or psychiatric problems or who are in an acute state of crisis. The hospital stay is typically short term (about 2 to 4 weeks), and it is most effective when it is followed by extended aftercare for 6 to 12 months.

Outpatient Care

Program personnel in outpatient treatment centers teach the patient to change and adjust to life without drugs while living in a real-life situation. It is less expensive than inpatient hospitalization, and it is just as effective in many cases. Outpatient care generally continues until the patient is ready for a less-intensive level of care.

Halfway Houses

Sober living environments known as *halfway houses* provide shelter as well as support, group therapy, and direct access to AA meetings. These living situations provide opportunities for gradual reentrance into the family, the work environment, and society. Halfway house placement is for patients who have been alienated from their families or who are homeless. Oxford House is an independent organization that rents homes for the purpose of housing people in recovery. These homes are found in most mid to large cities in the United States. Prospective residents must apply and be interviewed by the residents before they are accepted, and they can be asked to leave if they violate sobriety.

Day or Night Hospitalization

Partial hospitalization is for patients who need additional professional support and who may be at some risk for the physical sequelae of chemical use. Some patients resume

---

MEDICATION KEY FACTS

Substance-Related Disorders

Alcohol Dependence

Acamprosate calcium (Campral) for abstinence and disulfiram (Antabuse) as a deterrent to alcohol use and abuse

- Cyclic antidepressants may cause neurotoxicity.
- Monoamine oxidase inhibitors may cause delirium and psychosis with combination use.
- Acamprosate is not recommended for children.
- Herbal considerations: St. John's wort may cause alcohol-like reactions.

Alcohol and Opioid Dependence

Naltrexone (Revia, Trexan, Vivitrol) to work as an adjunct in the treatment of alcohol dependence and opiate addiction by decreasing cravings

- The patient must be drug-free before beginning treatment.

Opioid Dependence

Buprenorphine/naloxone (Narcan, Suboxone) and levomethadyl acetate (LAAM, ORLAAM)

- Methadone is a substitute drug for narcotic analgesic dependence therapy and the treatment of severe pain.
- Methadone has a high physical and psychologic dependence liability, and withdrawal symptoms will occur with abrupt discontinuation.
- Alcohol and other CNS depressants may increase CNS or respiratory depression, and hypotension may cause fatal reactions with high doses.
- Monoamine oxidase inhibitors may produce a severe or sometimes fatal reaction; these should not be used together.

- Children are more prone to experience paradoxic excitement. Naloxone and LAAM are not recommended for children who are younger than 16 years old.
- These medications are not recommended for elderly adults.
- Herbal considerations: Valerian, chamomile, kava kava, and poppy may increase CNS depression.

Nicotine Dependence

Bupropion (Zyban) and varenicline (Chantix) for smoking cessation

Other Drugs for the Treatment of Alcoholism

Diazepam (Valium), clonazepam (Klonopin) for alcohol intoxication or withdrawal, and chlordiazepoxide (Librium) for alcohol withdrawal and anxiety

- These drugs are contraindicated with acute alcohol intoxication and acute angle-closure glaucoma.
- Abrupt or too-rapid withdrawal may result in pronounced restlessness, irritability, insomnia, and seizures.
- Alcohol and CNS depressants increase CNS depression.
- These medications are not indicated for children who are younger than 6 years old.
- Herbal considerations: Cowslip, kava kava, and valerian may increase CNS depression.

---

employment and spend the night in the hospital, whereas others spend the day at the treatment center and go home at night. As with the halfway house, partial hospitalization provides additional therapeutic support during early or difficult phases of rehabilitation.

Previous research has shown that a minimum of 90 days of treatment for residential and 21 days for short-term inpatient programs is predictive of positive treatment outcomes for adults. Unfortunately, many long-term treatment programs have been cut or eliminated as a result of managed care. In the first large-scale study that focused on drug abuse treatment outcomes for 1167 adolescents, researchers found that longer stays in treatment programs effectively reduced substance abuse, symptoms of mental illness, and criminal activity (Hser et al, 2001).

Community-Based Organizations and Faith and Spiritual Communities

Social support from outside influences can moderate the effects of a family history of drug and alcohol problems. Many communities have developed after-school programs, mentoring activities, sports and educational programs, and other funded or nonfunded programs to provide opportunities for healthy relationships and activities.

Spirituality is an important part of recovery for many individuals. For 6 out of 10 Americans, religious faith is the most important influence in their lives; for 8 out of 10, religious beliefs provide comfort and support (*Alcohol, tobacco and other drugs*, 1995). Teens who never attend religious services are at above-average risk for drug and alcohol problems, whereas those who attend at least weekly have a lower-than-average risk (*National survey of American attitudes*, 2001). Factors that foster teens' ability to resist drugs include positive peer affiliations, bonding in school activities, relationships with caring adults, opportunities for school success and responsible behavior, and the availability of drug-free activities.

EVALUATION

What outcomes has the patient achieved? The purpose of evaluation in the nursing process is to determine the changes and outcomes that occur as a result of nursing and other interdisciplinary interventions. The nurse observes for changes in the patient's behaviors and responses to treatment and interventions with the use of the outcome criteria. It is important to recognize that the resolution of the acute phase is merely the first step in treatment. The success for the

NURSING CARE PLAN

Andre is a 45-year-old Bosnian immigrant who was recently separated from his wife and his two grown children. He was admitted to a psychiatric acute care unit with recurring symptoms of major depression (feeling sad and hopeless) and the possible abuse of alcohol and hydrocodone (Vicodin). Andre sustained a back injury 5 years ago before leaving Bosnia, when his family was forced to quickly abandon their home and he tried to carry his valued objects with him. He took pain medication (Vicodin) as prescribed, but sometimes it was not effective, and he had trouble sleeping. He then began drinking alcohol to alleviate the pain and to help him sleep. He is requesting more pain medication. Since admission, Andre reports insomnia, nervousness, and loss of appetite. He expresses despair about his constant back pain. This is his second hospital admission in the past year. The first admission was 3 months ago for suicidal depression. He was discharged on antidepressants, but he has stopped taking them because he could not afford the prescription. He denies any suicidal plans or intentions now. Andre says he drinks "a pint or so" of vodka a day and more when he can afford it. He is afraid of what happens to him when he tries to stop drinking, and he admits that he needs help to withdraw from alcohol. He thinks he might have had a seizure in the past when he tried to withdraw on his own. He would also like to stop taking Vicodin, but his work stocking shelves is hard on his back, and he is often in pain at the end of the day. He was an electrician in Bosnia, but he does not have the credentials to work as a licensed electrician in the United States. His wife also works, and she does not want a divorce. There is some hint of domestic violence, but Andre will not talk about it. Both he and his wife are employed full time, but they have no insurance. They have been active in a local church, which Andre says is important to him and his family.

DSM-IV-TR Diagnoses

Axis I Recurrent major depression, alcohol dependence, and opioid dependence (with physiologic dependence)
Axis II None
Axis III Chronic back pain
Axis IV Severity of psychosocial stressors (extreme = 4) inadequate finances, no health insurance, disruption in relationship, situational stressors secondary to immigration
Axis V GAF = 15 (current); GAF = 45 (past year)

Nursing Diagnosis *Risk for injury related to alcohol and opiate withdrawal as evidenced by altered electrolytes and history of seizure disorder*

NOC Seizure control; Aspiration prevention; Fall prevention behavior; Knowledge: personal safety; Risk control
NIC Seizure management; Fall prevention; Medication management; Teaching: disease process; Risk identification; Health education

PATIENT OUTCOMES	NURSING INTERVENTIONS	EVALUATION
Andre will verbalize symptoms of withdrawal from alcohol (rapid heart rate, sweating, tremors, insomnia, agitation) and Vicodin (craving, irritability, restlessness). He will comply with the prescribed medication protocol to manage these symptoms, especially withdrawal from alcohol, which can be life threatening.	Administer prescribed medication according to Andre's mental and physical status *to relieve initial signs of withdrawal and to prevent or limit the development of life-threatening withdrawal symptoms.*	The patient verbalizes his willingness to go through withdrawal to stop feeling "so sad and hopeless." He also acknowledges the need for help managing his back pain other than with the use of Vicodin, which he knows is an addictive substance.
Andre will be free from episodes of life-threatening symptoms related to substance withdrawal, such as seizures, aspiration, or falls, which can lead to head injury and death. He will trust the staff and the treatment protocol used to maintain his safety.	Reassure the patient that he will be safe and free from harm or injury *to develop trust and to decrease feelings of anxiety by explaining that he will be monitored continually and that his symptoms can be controlled with appropriate treatment interventions.*	The patient states that he is able to verbalize withdrawal symptoms and to ask for support as soon as they occur. He expresses trust in the staff and the treatment protocol used to control his symptoms safely.
Andre and his wife will verbalize knowledge of the following: Alcohol and narcotic dependence and withdrawal symptoms The risk for injury or death The need for medical intervention, especially for alcohol withdrawal Available community support networks The importance of their church and their faith	Educate the patient and his spouse about alcohol and drug dependence, risks for injury or death, symptoms of withdrawal, the importance of medication for safe withdrawal, and aftercare support *to help prevent relapse, injury, or death and to empower the patient and his spouse through education.*	Andre and his wife are able to verbalize knowledge of alcohol and narcotic dependence and withdrawal symptoms, the risk for injury or death, and the need for medical intervention at the first signs of alcohol withdrawal. They are able to list available community support networks, and they have made plans to attend a meeting of one of them and to continue attending their church.

Continued

◎ **NURSING CARE PLAN—cont'd**

Nursing Diagnosis *Ineffective coping related to chronic pain as evidenced by dependence on alcohol and narcotic pain medication*

NOC Risk control: alcohol use; Risk control: drug use; Impulse self-control; Coping; Anxiety self-control; Depression self-control; Decision-making; Quality of life

NIC Substance use treatment: alcohol withdrawal; Substance use treatment: drug withdrawal; Medication management; Coping enhancement; Anxiety reduction; Impulse control training; Mood management; Emotional support; Decision-making support

PATIENT OUTCOMES	NURSING INTERVENTIONS	EVALUATION
Andre will verbalize the following: (1) that has a problem with escalating narcotic drug use; (2) that he will comply with efforts to control pain with non-narcotic analgesia; and (3) that he will identify problems created by alcohol and narcotic pain medications.	Support the patient's statement that he is dependent on drugs for pain control, and offer hope that he can withdraw safely while symptoms are managed. *Additional support by the nurse can help the patient to achieve the first step toward abstinence.*	The patient verbalizes that he is frightened and depressed and that he wants help from his family and the health care system.
Andre will practice effective coping skills that were previously used during difficult times and learn new skills to manage problems related to pain control.	Evaluate the patient's usual coping style by using interview and counseling techniques *to establish attainable goals and to determine coping methods that can be used to achieve them.* Help the patient to explore his strengths and areas for growth *to assist with the development of new coping skills and to build on previously effective coping methods while discarding ineffective ones.*	The patient is effectively integrating existing coping skills with newly acquired coping methods at the time of discharge. Andre identified the following effective coping methods: Perform exercises to reduce back spasms (with a physician's approval). Use only non-narcotic pain treatments. Find work that does not contribute to back pain or injury. Participate in alcohol and drug support groups (e.g., AA, Narcotics Anonymous). Meet with a trusted clergy member or therapist regularly. The patient and the staff are meeting to discuss pending discharge goals and to contact resources for the patient's reintegration with his family and the community. The patient is actively seeking alternative work that will not result in pain or injury to his back. The patient will participate in community support groups for alcohol and drug abuse and continue with church activities. Collaborate with other health care professionals to explore the continuation of the patient's non-narcotic pain treatment after discharge and to pursue a work evaluation for skills that the patient may have for nonphysical labor *to ensure that the patient continues to pursue effective coping skills and to prevent relapse.*

*Further assessment is necessary to detect if Andre has a pseudoaddiction, although the nurse suspects this when the patient is admitted. Because of his limited financial resources and lack of health care insurance, Andre's back injury may not have been pursued as aggressively as possible, although alternative non-narcotic pain relief measures were included in his treatment regimen. When his pain is adequately controlled, it is likely that Andre's need for alcohol would be eliminated, because there is no history of a drinking problem before his back injury. It is important for the nurse to ensure that arrangements are made for Andre to receive outpatient care, which is challenging in a no-insurance situation. In this case, nurses need to collaborate with social workers who may be able to find low-cost insurance or to arrange for temporary public assistance until Andre's problems are stabilized. This would prevent readmission and further difficulties with depression and pain control. Andre should always be assessed for recurring depression, risk for suicide, and the need for antidepressant therapy given his history, although he denied suicidality on this admission. (See Chapter 11 for more information about depression and suicide.)

recovery process and rehabilitation depends on many factors, including access to treatment programs, 12-step or other support groups, continuing health care, the support of family members and significant others, vocational rehabilitation, and community support.

Many patients relapse during the rehabilitation process. For this reason, it is difficult to predict the time at which patients will be sufficiently motivated to change their lifestyles and to accept their illnesses. Evaluation is an ongoing process. As people attain sobriety, they internalize a commitment to change their lifestyle, which often affects their relationships with family, significant others, and coworkers. Many patients develop a lifetime commitment to their 12-step program or to another program that best meets their needs.

CHAPTER SUMMARY

- Substance abuse causes more deaths, illnesses, and disabilities than any other preventable health condition.
- The use of alcohol, tobacco, and illicit drugs changes in response to shifts in public tolerance of the behaviors and with various political, economic, and social events.
- Assessment for substance misuse and dependence needs to be a part of every patient history and physical examination.
- Alcohol is the number one drug of choice in American society today among adolescents and adults, and it is the most widely available legal drug.
- Nicotine use is a major health problem.
- Fetal alcohol syndrome is 100% preventable if the pregnant woman abstains from alcohol use.

- The treatment of SUDs requires patient perseverance.
- Situational, individual, and environmental factors influence substance abuse.
- Dual diagnosis and comorbidities require in-depth assessment followed by the concurrent treatment of both the substance abuse and the psychiatric diagnoses.
- Current DSM-IV-TR diagnoses of abuse and dependency do not adequately describe substance use in the adolescent population. It is preferable to use terms such as *problematic drinking* or *excessive substance use*.
- Secondary complications of drug use are often causative factors related to physical illnesses and health concerns.

REVIEW QUESTIONS

1. An emergency department nurse assesses a patient who is suspected of drug abuse. Assessment findings reveal the following vital signs: temperature, 103°F; blood pressure, 178/104 mm Hg; extreme anxiety; and a serum sodium level of 138 mEq/L. Which problem will the nurse suspect?
   1. Steroid-induced psychosis
   2. Marchiafava-Bignami disease as a result of alcohol abuse
   3. Wernicke-Korsakoff syndrome as a result of alcohol dependence
   4. Serotonin syndrome as a result of MDA or MDMA use
2. A nurse assesses a 15-year-old boy for substance abuse and dependence. Abuse of which of the following substances would be most likely? You may select more than one answer.
   1. Alcohol
   2. Cocaine
   3. Heroin
   4. Methaqualone
   5. Nicotine
3. A patient describes an experience of having a blackout. The nurse would suspect the use of which of the following substances? You may select more than one answer.
   1. Alcohol
   2. Caffeine
   3. Ephedrine
   4. Lorazepam
   5. Rohypnol

4. A nurse directs the nursing assistant to offer fluids to a patient who is being detoxified from alcohol. The nursing assistant responds, "That patient doesn't deserve my help. Will power and faith could have avoided this situation." What is the nurse's best response?
   1. "You always help our other patients. Why are you making such unkind comments about this one?"
   2. "It sounds like you're being judgmental, but we accept alcoholism as a disease and provide compassionate care."
   3. "In addition to giving oral fluids, maybe you would pray with the patient for relief from this problem."
   4. "Regardless of the reasons, the patient still needs our help. Offer the fluids as I have instructed."
5. A nurse cares for a patient with gastrointestinal bleeding who was admitted to a medical unit 3 days ago. Today, the patient is irritable and restless, and she says to the nurse, "There are roaches everywhere in this hospital. They've been crawling on me. I'm scared of bugs." The admission assessment shows that the patient drinks socially. How would the nurse analyze this situation?
   1. The patient may have minimized her use of alcohol and is experiencing withdrawal symptoms.
   2. The facility's infection control nurse should be consulted about the insect infestation.
   3. The patient probably has dementia, which was inadequately assessed at admission.
   4. Caring behaviors by nursing staff have been inadequate, and the patient is lonely.

REFERENCES

Alcohol, tobacco and other drug abuse: challenges and responses for faith leaders, DHHS Publication No. (SMA) 95-3074, Washington, DC, 1995, ES, Inc., for the U.S. Department of Health and Human Services, Substance Abuse and Mental Health Services Administration, Center for Substance Abuse Treatment (Contract No. 270-91-0016).

American Nurses Association: *Scope and standards of addictions nursing practice*, Washington, DC, 2004, American Nurses Publishing.

American Psychiatric Association: *Diagnostic and statistical manual of mental disorders*, ed 4, text revision, Washington, DC, 2000, American Psychiatric Association.

Anderson C, Horne J: A high sugar content, low caffeine drink does not alleviate sleepiness but may worsen it, *Hum Psychopharmacol* 21(5):299-303, 2006.

Armstrong M: *Being pregnant and using drugs: a retrospective phenomenological inquiry*, unpublished doctoral dissertation, 1992.

Armstrong M: Foundations of gender based treatment model for women in recovery from chemical dependency, *J Addict Nurs* 19(2):77-82, 2008.

Armstrong M, Holmes E: Frequency of nurse practitioner screening for substance use disorders, *J Addict Nurs* 2005.

Baldiserri M: Impaired health care professional, *Crit Care Med* 35(2):106-116, 2007.

Baler R, Volkow N: Drug addiction: the neurobiology of disrupted self-control, *Trends Mol Med* 12:559-566, 2006.

Bauer C: Perinatal effects of prenatal drug exposure, *Arch Dis Child* 90(1), 2005.

Begley D: Structure and function of the blood-brain barrier. In Touitou E, Barry B, editors: *Enhancement in drug delivery*, pp. 571-590, Boca Raton, Fla, 2007, CRC Press.

Bennett SS, Bennett WM: Potency matters, *Drug Watch World News* VII:3, 2002.

Bickel W, Potenza M: The forest and the trees: addiction as a complex self-organizing system. In Miller WR, Carroll KM, editors: *Rethinking substance abuse*, 2006, Guilford Press.

Blow F, Barry C: Use and misuse of alcohol among older women, *Alcohol Res Health* 26:308-315, 2003.

Blume S, Zilberman M: Addiction in women. In Galanter and Kleber, editors: *Textbook of substance abuse treatment*, 2006, American Psychiatric Association Publishing.

Bowden R, Rust D: A review of fetal alcohol syndrome for health educators, *J Health Educ* 26:231-237, 2000.

Bowen M: *Family therapy in clinical practice*, New York, 1978, Jason Aronson.

Brennan P et al: Pain and use of alcohol to manage pain: prevalence and 3 year outcomes among older problem and non-problem drinkers, *Addiction* 100:777-786, 2006.

Brown S: *Treating adult children of alcoholics: a developmental perspective*, New York, 1998, John Wiley and Sons.

Carpenter et al: Cigarettes for women: new findings from the tobacco industry documents, *Addiction* 100:837-851, 2005.

Carroll K, Rounsaville B: Behavioral therapies: the glass would be half full if only we had a glass. In *Rethinking Substance Abuse* pp. 223-239, New York, 2006, The Guilford Press.

Center for Substance Abuse Research (CESAR): Anesthesiologists' high rate of opiate abuse and dependence may be related to passive exposure in the operating room, *CESAR FAX* 14:1-2, 2005.

Centers for Disease Control and Prevention: Cigarette brand preference among middle and high school students who are established smokers—United States, 2004 and 2006, *Morb Mortal Wkly Rep* 58(5):112-115, 2009.

Chermack ST, Blow FC: Violence among individuals in substance abuse treatment: the role of alcohol and cocaine consumption, *Drug Alcohol Depend* 66:29-37, 2002.

Childress AR et al: Prelude to passion: limbic activation by "unseen" drug and sexual cues, *PLoS ONE* 3(1):e1506, 2008.

Colleran C, Jay D: *Aging & addiction: helping older adults overcome alcohol or medication dependence*, Center City, Minn, 2002, Hazelden Foundation.

Crego et al: Binge drinking affects attentional and visual working memory processing in young university students, *Alcohol Clin Exp Res* 33(11):1870-1879, 2009.

Crespi TM, Sabatelli RM: Children of alcoholics and adolescence: individuation development and family systems, *Adolescence* 32:407, 1997.

DiFranza J: Hooked from the first cigarette, *Scientific American* May 3:84-87, 2008.

Eissenberg, Shihadeh: Waterpipe tobacco and cigarette smoking: direct comparison of toxicant exposure, *Am J Prev Med* 37(9):518-523, 2009.

Freeman S: Substance misuse disorders. In Freeman SM, Freeman A, editors: *Cognitive behavior therapy in nursing practice*, New York, 2005a, Springer.

Freeman S: Taxonomies of addiction. In *Core curriculum of addictions nursing*, 2005b, International Nurses Society on Addictions.

Frone M: Prevalence and distribution of alcohol use and impairment in the workplace: a U.S. National Survey, *J Stud Alcohol* 67:147-156, 2006.

Galanter M, Kleber HD: *Textbook of substance abuse treatment*, Washington DC, 2006, American Psychiatric Publishing.

Goldberg R: Substance abuse and the aging brain: screening, diagnosis, and treatment, *Brown University Geriatric Psychopharmacology Update* 12(4):1-6, 2008.

Goldstein R et al: The neurocircuitry of impaired insight in drug addiction, DOI:10.1016/jtics, 2009.

Grant BF, Dawson DA: Age at onset of alcohol use and its association with DSM-IV alcohol abuse and dependence: Results from the National Longitudinal Alcohol Epidemiologic Survey, *J Subst Abuse* 9:103-110, 1997.

Griffith J: Substance abuse disorders in nurses, *Nurs Forum* 34:4, 1999.

Harwood HJ, Myers TG: *New treatment for addictions: behavioral, ethical, legal, and social questions*, Washington, DC, 2004, National Academy Press.

Heinrich A et al: Clinicoradiologic subtypes of Marchiafava-Bignami disease, *J Neurology* 251:1050-1059, 2004.

Holder H: Prevention aimed at the environment. In McCrady B, Epstein E, editors: *Addictions: a comprehensive guidebook*, New York, 1999, Oxford University Press.

Holder, HD: Community prevention of alcohol problems, *Addictive Behaviors* 25, 843-859, 2000.

Hser Y-I et al: An evaluation of drug treatment for adolescents in four US cities, *Arch Gen Psychiatr* 58:689-695, 2001.

International Food Information Council: August 4, 2008.

Kaufman E, Brook D: Family therapy: other drugs. In Galanter and Kleber, editors: *Textbook of substance abuse treatment*, Arlington, Tex, 2006, American Psychiatric Publishing.

Keltner NL, Folks DG: *Psychotropic drugs*, ed 4, St. Louis, 2005, Mosby.

Kendler K et al: A population-based twin study of alcoholism in women, *J Am Med Assoc* 268:1877-1882, 1992.

Kinsey, Orson: Anti-drug vaccines to treat substance abuse, *Immunol Cell Biol* 87(4):309-314, 2009.

Knight J et al: Prevalence of positive substance abuse screens results among adolescent primary care patients, *Arch Pediatr Adolesc Med* 161:1035-1041, 2007.

Koob G: The neurobiology of addiction. In Miller W, Carroll K, editors: *Rethinking substance abuse*, 2006, Guilford Press.

Koob G: The role of CRF and CRF-related peptides in the dark side of addiction, *Brain Res* 16:1314:3-14, 2010.

Koob G, Volkow N: Neurocircuitry of addiction, *Neuropsychopharmacology* 36:317-328, 2010.

Li T: Pharmacogenetics of responses to alcohol and genes that influence alcohol drinking, *J Stud Alcohol* 61:5-12, 2000.

Mathias R, Zickler P: NIDA congerence highlights scientific findings on MDMA/ecstasy, *NIDA Notes* 16:1,5,6-8,12, 2001.

McCrady B: Family and other close relationships. In Miller W, Carroll K, editors: *Rethinking substance abuse*, 2006, Guilford Press.

Milkman H, Sunderwirth S: Craving for ecstasy and natural highs: a positive approach to mood alteration, 2010, Sage Publications.

Miller K, Armstrong M: Developmental concepts of nicotine addiction, *J Pediatr Nurs* 21:108-114, 2006.

Miller W, Rollnick S: *Motivational interviewing: preparing people for change*, ed 2, New York, 2002, Guilford Press.

Miller WR, Carroll KM: *Rethinking substance abuse: what the science shows, and what we should do about it*, ed 1, New York, 2006, The Guilford Press.

Mueser K et al: Comorbid substance use disorders and psychiatric disorders. In Miller W, Carroll K, editors: *Rethinking substance abuse*, 2006, Guilford Press.

Nace E, Crowder J. In Galanter and Kleber, editors: *Textbook of substance abuse treatment*, 2006, American Psychiatric Publishing.

National Institute on Alcohol Abuse and Alcoholism: *Alcohol and the brain: Neuroscience and neurobehavior*, ed 10, Special report to Congress on alcohol and health, p. 67, National Institutes of Health Publication No. 99-1180, Rockville, Md, 2000, National Institute on Alcohol Abuse and Alcoholism.

National Institute on Drug Abuse: Anabolic steroids, *Community Drug Alert Bulletin* (1-3), retrieved May 27, 2002a, from www.drugabuse.gov.

National Institute on Drug Abuse: Club drugs, *Community Drug Alert Bulletin* (1-5), retrieved May 27, 2002b, from www.drugabuse.gov.

National Institute on Drug Abuse: *Diagnosis and treatment of drug abuse in family practice*, 2002, Public Health Service, National Institutes of Health and Human Services, U.S. Department of Health and Human Services, 2002.

National Institute on Drug Abuse: Dopamine may play role in cue-induced craving distinct from its role regulating reward effects (May 28, 2002), *News Scan* (1-4); retrieved June 22, 2002, from www.drugabuse.gov.

National Institute on Drug Abuse: *Frequently asked questions* (website): www.drugabuse.gov. Accessed July 4, 2002.

National Institute on Drug Abuse: *Drug Abuse Prevention*, 2008, Public Health Service, National Institutes of Health and Human Services, Department of Health and Human Services, 2008.

National Institute on Drug Abuse: *Drug Abuse Prevention*, 2009, Public Health Service, National Institutes of Health and Human Services, Department of Health and Human Services, 2009.

National survey of American attitudes on substance abuse VI: teens, New York, 2001, National Center on Addiction and Substance Abuse, Columbia University.

Navqui N, Bechara A: The hidden island of addiction: the insula, *Trends Neurosci* 1(32):56-67, 2008.

Partnership for a Drug-Free America. *Parents and teens attitude tracking study report*, 2009

Reinberg S: Tobacco companies targeting teens, study says, *HealthDay News*, www.healthfinder.gov, 2009, Accessed January 10, 2010.

Reissig C et al: Caffeinated energy drinks—a growing problem, *Drug Alcohol Depend* 165(10):1256-1260, 2008

Robinson T, Berridge K: The incentive sensitization theory of addiction: some current issues, *Philos Trans R Soc Lond B Biol Sci* doi:10.1098/rstb.2008.0093, 2003.

Rosenberg M: Neurophysiologic impairment and MRI abnormalities associated with chronic solvent abuse, *J Toxicol Clin Toxicol* 40:21-34, 2002.

Savage C: Screening for alcohol use in women of childbearing age, *J Addict Nurs* 17:67-69, 2006.

Schuckit et al: The search for genes contributing to the low level of response to alcohol: patterns of findings across studies, *Alcohol Clin Exp Res* 28:1449-1458, 2004.

Schuckit M: Acetaldehyde and alcoholism: methodology. In Hesselbrock V, et al, editors: *Biological and genetic markers of alcoholism*, pp. 23-48, 1984.

Schuckit MA: *Drug and alcohol abuse: a clinical guide to diagnosis and treatment*, ed 5, New York, 2000, Kluwer Academic/Plenum.

Shoptaw et al: Psychosocial and behavioral treatment of methamphetamine dependence. In Roll et al, editors: *Methamphetamine addiction: from basic science to treatment*, 2009, Guilford Press.

Simeca P: *Unbecoming a nurse: bypassing the hidden chemical dependency trap*, 2008.

Simeca P: *From unbecoming a nurse to overcoming addiction: candid self-portraits of nurses in recovery*, 2010.

Spoth R et al: Further clear examples of the need for more reasonable conclusions and critiques about prevention. *Addiction* 104:54-155, 2009.

Steinglass P, Kutch S: Family therapy: alcohol. In Galanter and Kleber, editors: *Textbook of substance abuse treatment*, 2006.

Stocks G: *A survey of recovering nurse anesthetists*. Peer Assistance Update, North Carolina Association of Nurse Anesthetists, General Session Presentation, October 2009.

Substance Abuse and Mental Health Services Administration (SAMHSA), Office of Applied Studies: *Emergency department trends from the drug abuse warning network, preliminary estimates January-June 2001 with revised estimates 1994 to 2000*, DAWN Series D-20, U.S. Department of Health and Human Services Publication No. (SMA) 02-3634, Rockville, Md, 2002, SAMHSA.

Substance Abuse and Mental Health Services Administration (SAMHSA): *Results from the 2006 National Survey on drug use and health: national findings*. U.S. Department of

Health and Human Services Publication No. SMA 07-429, Rockville, Md, 2007, SAMHSA.

Substance Abuse and Mental Health Services Administration (SAMHSA): *Results from the 2008 National Survey on drug use and health: national findings.* Department of Health and Human Services Publication No. SMA 07-429, Rockville, Md, 2009.

Trinkoff AM et al: Workplace access, negative proscriptions, job strain, and substance use in registered nurses, *Nurs Res* 49:83-90, 2000.

Trinkoff AM, Storr CL: Substance use among nurses: differences between specialties, *Am J Public Health* 88:581-585, 1998.

Vandermause R: Assessing for alcohol use disorders in women: experiences of advanced practice nurses in primary care settings, *J Addict Nurs* 18(4):187-198, 2007.

Westermeyer J. In Galanter and Kleber, editors: *Textbook of substance abuse treatment*, Washington DC, 2006, American Psychiatric Publishing.

Wilson H, Compton M: Reentry of the addicted certified nurse anesthetist, *J Addict Nurs* 20:177-184, 2009.

Online Resources

Al-Anon/Alateen: www.al-anon.alateen.org

Alcoholics Anonymous: www.aa.org

CASA: The National Center on Addiction and Substance Abuse: www.casacolumbia.org

Center for Substance Abuse Research: www.cesar.umd.edu

Centers for Disease Control and Prevention: www.cdc.gov

Erowid: www.erowid.org

International Nurses Society on Addictions: www.intnsa.org

Join Together: www.jointogether.org

Law Enforcement Against Prohibition: www.leap.cc

MADD: Mothers Against Drunk Driving: www.madd.org

Marijuana Anonymous: www.marijuana-anonymous.org

Medical Cannabis: www.medicalcannabis.com

Monitoring the Future Study: www.monitoringthefuture.org

NAADAC: The Association for Addiction Professionals: www.naadac.org

National Asian Pacific American Families Against Substance Abuse: www.napafasa.org

National Association for Children of Alcoholics: www.nacoa.org

National Clearinghouse for Alcohol and Drug Information: www.ncadi.samhsa.gov

National Institute on Alcohol Abuse and Alcoholism: www.niaaa.nih.gov

National Institute on Drug Abuse: www.nida.nih.gov, www.drugabuse.gov, www.clubdrugs.gov, www.steroidabuse.gov

National Youth Anti-Drug Media Campaign (Freevibe): www.freevibe.com

Office of National Drug Control Policy: www.whitehousedrugpolicy.gov

Partnership for a Drug-Free America: www.drugfree.org

Patients Out of Time: www.medicalcannabis.com

QuitNet: www.quitnet.org

Research Institute on Addictions: www.ria.buffalo.edu

Smoke-Free Families: www.smokefreefamilies.org

Substance Abuse and Mental Health Services Administration: www.samhsa.gov

Substance Abuse Librarians and Information Specialists: www.salis.org

U.S. Drug Enforcement Administration: www.dea.gov, www.deadiversion.usdoj.gov

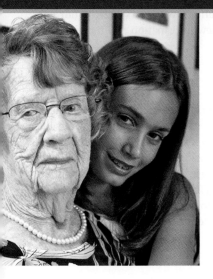

Cognitive Disorders: Delirium, Dementia, and Amnestic Disorders

Russell Kelley

"A place in thy memory, dearest,
Is all that I claim;
To pause and look back when thou hearest
The sound of my name."

Gerald Griffin

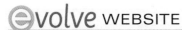

evolve WEBSITE

http://evolve.elsevier.com/Fortinash/

OBJECTIVES

- Analyze the various theories of the nature and development of the dementias and other cognitive disorders.
- Discuss the most currently accepted theories of the dementias and other cognitive disorders.
- Describe the pathophysiologic changes in the brain related to Alzheimer's disease and other dementias.
- Classify the progressive symptoms of Alzheimer's disease into three stages: mild, moderate, and severe.

- Differentiate between the different types of dementia: reversible and irreversible.
- Apply the nursing process to the management of patients with cognitive disorders.
- Describe current trends in psychopharmacology for the treatment of dementia.
- Explain and plan therapeutic activities for patients who are experiencing dementia.

KEY TERMS

agnosia	aphasia	delirium	neologism
agraphia	apraxia	dementia	neurofibrillary tangles
Alzheimer's disease	catastrophic reaction	disorientation	paranoia
amnestic disorders	cognition	dysarthria	perseveration
amyloid plaques	confabulation	mild cognitive impairment	sundowning

The term *cognition* is derived from the Greek word *gnosis*, which means "knowledge"; it refers to the human ability to think, perceive, and reason. A deficit in cognition represents a change in a person's previous level of functioning (American Psychiatric Association, 2000). A cognitive disorder refers to any one of several disorders that either permanently or temporarily interferes with the ability to think, perceive, and reason. The cognitive disorders range from mild memory loss to full (pervasive) dementia. This chapter discusses dementia, delirium, and amnestic disorders.

Dementia is a global disorder that develops over a relatively slow period of time and that causes multiple changes in an individual's ability to think, perceive, and reason. It is a progressive and degenerative central nervous system disorder. Alzheimer's disease (AD) is the predominant type in this category. The *Diagnostic and Statistical Manual of Mental Disorders,* fourth edition, text revision (DSM-IV-TR), categorizes the dementias as follows: (1) dementia of the Alzheimer's type; (2) vascular dementia; (3) dementias as the result of a general medical condition; (4) dementias that result from substances; and (5) dementias with either mixed or unknown etiologies (American Psychiatric Association, 2000).

Delirium is an acute state of confusion, attention, and perception. The cognitive changes of delirium develop over a short period of time and are usually the result a medical condition, substance abuse, or both (American Psychiatric Association, 2000). The cause of delirium is often unknown.

Amnestic disorders are impairments of memory that occur without delirium and dementia (American Psychiatric Association, 2000). An amnestic disorder is a condition with which a person has difficulty learning new information or with remembering previously learned information. The disorder may be the result of a general medical condition, substance use, of an unknown etiology. Amnestic disorders do not include the dissociative type of amnesia (e.g., dissociative fugue), which is described in Chapter 11.

HISTORIC AND THEORETIC PERSPECTIVES

Dementia was fairly common at the turn of the nineteenth century because of a condition called *general paresis* (a type of paralysis) that indicated the neurologic complications of syphilis, a venereal disease that manifested dementia during its late (tertiary) stages (Katzman, 2004). In 1898, Redich identified the presence of neuronal plaques in the brains of people with dementia. He called them *miliary bodies* because of their similarity in size to miliary or millet seeds. Redich thought that these bodies or lesions were glial or neuroglia cells (nerve cells) (Venes et al, 2005). The discovery of AD occurred after new staining techniques and microscope technology enabled Alois Alzheimer (1864-1915), a neurologist, to more accurately identify the neuronal lesions associated with the disease. In 1907, Alzheimer published his description of the lesions in the brain of a 51-year-old woman suffering from dementia and paranoia, and he identified the plaques and neurofibrillary tangles within the neurons in the brains of people with dementia (Katzman, 2004).

In an early psychiatric text published in 1910, Kraepelin referred to cases similar to Alzheimer's as *presenile dementia*. Now, however, when dementia occurs before the age of 65 years, it is called *dementia of the Alzheimer's type, with early onset* (American Psychiatric Association, 2000). The inclusion of AD in Kraepelin's classic text categorized it as a psychiatric process rather than a neurologic one, and thus, for many decades, it was the responsibility of specialists in psychiatry.

The state of delirium has existed throughout history. Sutton used this word in 1813 to describe delirium tremens, the most severe expression of alcohol withdrawal syndrome marked by hallucinations and disorientation, which indicate a state of delirium. Greiner also specifically described delirium in 1817 as a "clouding of consciousness" (Clary and Krishnan, 2001).

Korsakoff's syndrome is a form of amnestic (memory) disorder caused by a deficiency in thiamine, a B-complex vitamin, and it is the result of chronic alcohol abuse (National Institute of Neurological Disorders Cond Stroke, 2010f). Sergei Korsakoff, a Russian neurologist, discovered this condition in 1889 (Kopelman, 2002). Patients with Korsakoff's syndrome have difficulty acquiring new information and forming new memories.

ETIOLOGY

AD is the most common form of dementia. However, many other forms of dementia exist, including both the irreversible and potentially reversible types. The irreversible dementias include vascular dementia, Parkinson's dementia, and dementias caused by Pick's disease (frontotemporal dementia), Creutzfeldt-Jakob disease, Huntington's disease, progressive supranuclear palsy, and Down's syndrome. Box 16-1 lists etiologic factors of the potentially reversible or secondary dementias.

Irreversible Dementias
Alzheimer's Disease

Alzheimer's disease (AD) is an irreversible and progressive disease that ultimately leads to death. It is usually diagnosed

---

BOX 16-1   ETIOLOGIC FACTORS OF THE REVERSIBLE OR SECONDARY DEMENTIAS

Toxic Causes
Alcoholism
Barbiturate intoxication
Metabolic disorders
Polypharmacy
Potassium loss from self-purgation

Other Electrolyte Disturbances
Hepatic disease
Porphyria

Nutritional Causes
Undernutrition by prolonged neglect or self-isolation
Chronic malabsorption syndrome
Vitamin B12 deficiency
Nicotinic acid encephalopathy

Infective Causes
Chronic respiratory infection with cardiac decompensation
Pulmonary tuberculosis
Bacterial endocarditis
Endocrine disease
Myxedema
Pituitary insufficiency
Addison's disease

Cerebral Disease
Slow-growing cerebral tumor (e.g., frontal meningioma)
Multiple cerebral emboli
Normal-pressure hydrocephalus*

*Normal-pressure hydrocephalus is a disorder that is characterized by dementia, gait disorder, and urinary incontinence. Dilation of the ventricles in the absence of increased cerebrospinal fluid is a prominent manifestation. A shunt is usually effective treatment for this condition.

after ruling out other etiologies (see the DSM-IV-TR Criteria box). AD is not a normal part of aging. It affects approximately 5.3 million people in the United States (Alzheimer's Association, 2010f). Factors that contribute to the development of the late-onset form of AD include the following: (1) socioeconomic status; (2) lifestyle choices, such as smoking and obesity; (3) environmental factors; (4) medical conditions and illnesses, including high blood pressure and dyslipidemia; and (5) medical treatments for these conditions, such as coronary artery bypass surgery (National Institutes of Health, 2009a). The less common early-onset form of AD that occurs before the age of 60 years may be the result of an inherited mutated gene. The late-onset form of AD develops in 40% of people who carry an altered form of the apolipoprotein E (Apo-E) gene (National Institute on Aging, 2010). However, not all people with the altered gene develop the disease, and not all people with the disease have that altered gene.

Several factors described in the following sections are associated with the development of AD. These include the accumulation of abnormal proteins, genetic mutations, neurotransmitter deficiency, and diminished blood-brain barrier competence.

Abnormal Proteins and Their Products

Amyloid Plaques. The classic characteristics of AD are the accumulation of amyloid plaques outside of and between neurons and the development of neurofibrillary tangles within the cells.

Amyloid plaques, which are also called *senile plaques* or *neuritic plaques*, are made of amyloid proteins, and they surround affected neuronal cells. The degree of mental deterioration is related to the amount of plaque formation. Amyloid plaques interfere with cell-to-cell communication and result in the decreased availability of acetylcholine (ACh), which is a neurotransmitter and chemical messenger of the central nervous system that plays a role in learning and memory. The plaques accumulate as a result of too much production or too little destruction of the protein, thereby destroying ACh-producing neurons (Stahl, 2008). A decrease of ACh is associated with Alzheimer's and Parkinson's diseases.

A major theory is that amyloid plaques are formed by the faulty processing of amyloid precursor protein (APP). The errors may be the result of abnormalities in the genes that code for either APP or the genes that code for APP enzymes (Stahl, 2008). APP is a transmembrane protein that may be cleaved by certain enzymes to form shorter peptide chains. One enzyme, α-secretase, cleaves the APP and leaves an 83-amino-acid peptide in the membrane until it is cleaved again by γ-secretase. This produces two nontoxic peptides. However, another enzyme, β-secretase, cleaves APP in such a way that a slightly longer 91-amino-acid peptide is left in the membrane along with a soluble fragment, β-APP. The 91-amino-acid peptide is cleaved by γ-secretase, which releases toxic peptides that are 40, 42, or 43 amino-acid-molecules long. The 43-amino-acid chain, called $A\beta42$, is particularly toxic, and it forms the amyloid plaques (Stahl, 2008).

Inflammation. Inflammatory processes are involved in AD. Proinflammatory cytokines (i.e., signaling proteins secreted by cells) are increased in patients with AD. Also increased are major histocompatibility complex (MHC) II and macrophage inhibitor factor (MIF). MHC II is found in the microglia of the brain, whereas MIF is found in both the microglia, and in neurons of the hypothalamus, hippocampus, and cortex areas of the brain. MIF mediates lymphocytes and is also a pituitary factor with endocrine properties. (Bryan et al, 2008). With mild to moderate AD, fewer T cells are found in the hippocampus and the cortex. The increased gene expression of MHC II in the hippocampus has an inverse correlation with cognitive ability (Parachikova et al, 2007). A membrane protein called *CD74*, acts as both a chaperone for MHC II molecules as well as a receptor binding site for MIF. CD74 is increased in patients with AD, and increased in the microglia of patients with AD, and it is associated with a significant increase in neurofibrillary tangles and amyloid plaques (Bryan et al, 2008).

Neurofibrillary Tangles. Microtubules determine cell shape and movement and help to transport nutrients within the cell.

Neurofibrillary tangles are formed when the τ protein, which is an abnormal part of the microtubule structure, causes the microtubule structure to collapse (Alzheimer's Disease Research, 2010).

Lewy Bodies and Lewy Body Disease. Frederic Lewy, a German neurologist (1885-1950), first described Lewy bodies in 1913 in association with Parkinson's disease. Lewy bodies are neuronal cells or lesions with colored bodies that are found in the substantia nigra (i.e., the nuclei of the midbrain that help to regulate unconscious muscle activity) (Lewy Body Dementia Association, 2010). Although Lewy bodies are present in the gray matter of patients with Parkinson's disease, the location of the lesions and the neurodegenerative process of Lewy body disease (LBD) are different (see the information about Parkinson's dementia later in this chapter).

Diffuse LBD is a late-life primary degenerative dementia that affects mostly men. Pure dementia caused by LBD is quite rare; most people with LBD have both LBD and AD. In these individuals, the onset is at about 60 years of age, and autopsy generally indicates that Lewy bodies, senile plaques, and neurofibrillary tangles are all present.

Genetic Mutations. Researchers estimate that 10% to 40% of AD cases are genetic. Some scientists believe that eventually all cases of AD will show a genetic determination. The identification of the abnormal proteins and neurofibrillary tangles associated with AD helped researchers to identify the respective genes associated with the disease's development. Early-onset AD has been frequently associated with mutations in one of three genes: (1) APP on chromosome 21; (2) presenlin-1 on chromosome 14 caused by APP formation; and (3) a mutation on chromosome 1 that leads to the production of presenlin-2 on chromosome 1. Chromosome 19, which codes for the Apo-E type 4 allele, is a common susceptibility gene that is associated with late-onset AD. This gene possibly accounts for up to 40% of the cases of late-onset dementia (National Institute on Aging, 2009). However, not all cases of AD are associated with Apo-E. Recently, polymorphisms (i.e., genetic variations) of the neuronal sortilin-related receptor have been identified as predisposing genes for AD (Webster et al, 2008).

Neurotransmitter Deficiencies. Cholinergic neurons normally decrease in number as people age, which makes less ACh available. Neurons that produce ACh are destroyed early during the course of AD (Stahl, 2008). The structures of the basal forebrain that are responsible for producing ACh include the diagonal band, the medial septum, and the substantia innominata (Memory Loss, 2010). Part of the substantia innominata is the nucleus basalis of Meynert, which is the major brain center for the cholinergic neurons that project throughout the cortex of the brain (Stahl, 2008). ACh conducts impulses between the neurons of the frontal cortex, which is responsible for complex thought,

and the hippocampus, which is responsible for memory and cognition. Cholinergic cell loss and a decrease in available ACh are directly associated with memory and cognitive impairment, and it is believed that the degeneration of neurons in the nucleus basalis of Meynert causes the short-term memory loss that is seen in patients with AD (Stahl, 2008).

Angiopathy and Blood-Brain Barrier Incompetence. The neurovascular model of AD development describes a compromised blood-brain barrier that results in the dysregulation of brain interstitial fluid and injury to neurons. On autopsy, capillary wall changes are often found in the brains of persons with AD. These changes, which are caused by atherosclerotic plaques, lead to nodular vessels with a lumpy thickening of the basement membrane that is accompanied by the thinning of the endothelium and a loss of the fine network that normally covers the surfaces that come in contact with blood. The result is the destruction of the barrier that prevents many blood serum components from entering the brain (i.e., the blood-brain barrier). Consequently, amyloid proteins are deposited in the walls and blood vessels of the cerebral cortex (Stahl, 2009).

Vascular Dementia (Multi-infarct Dementia)

Vascular dementia (VaD), which was formerly called *multi-infarct dementia*, is a change in cognition that is caused by the effects of one or more strokes on cognitive function. Nutrients are not able to nourish the brain because of the occlusion or obstruction of small arteries or arterioles in the cerebral cortex (see the DSM-IV-TR Criteria box below).

Parkinson's Dementia

Parkinson's disease (PD) is a neurologic disorder that causes tremors, rigidity (inflexibility), bradykinesia (slow motor movements), abnormalities of posture, a grave or mask-like facial expression, and a shuffling gait. Dopamine-producing nerve cells in the substantia nigra develop the pigmented Lewy body lesions that are a sign of this disease. As mentioned previously, although Lewy bodies are present with both PD and LBD, the dementia of PD is a direct physiologic consequence of PD, and it occurs in 20% to 60% of individuals with PD.

The amyloid lesions of AD are found in approximately 30% of PD cases. Similarly, about 50% of patients with AD demonstrate typical symptoms of PD.

Frontotemporal Lobar Degeneration

Frontotemporal lobar degeneration (FTLD), which was formerly called *frontotemporal dementia* or *Pick's disease*, includes a group of degenerative disorders of nerve cells that usually affect the frontal and temporal lobes of the brain. Associated disorders include primary progressive dementia, semantic dementia, corticobasal degeneration, progressive supranuclear palsy, and frontal lobe degeneration associated with PD (National Institutes of Health, 2009b). Changes in personality occur early during the course of the disease. Social skills decline, emotions are dull, patients are unable

Vascular Dementia

A The development of multiple cognitive deficits manifested by both of the following:
  1 Memory impairment (impaired ability to learn new information or to recall previously learned information)
  2 One (or more) of the following cognitive disturbances:
    a Aphasia (language disturbance)
    b Apraxia (impaired ability to carry out motor activities despite intact motor function)
    c Agnosia (failure to recognize or identify objects despite intact sensory function)
    d Disturbance in executive functioning (i.e., planning, organizing, sequencing, abstracting)
B The cognitive deficits in criteria A1 and A2 each cause significant impairment in social or occupational functioning and represent a significant decline from a previous level of functioning.
C Focal neurologic signs and symptoms (e.g., exaggeration of deep tendon reflexes, extensor plantar response, pseudobulbar palsy, gait abnormalities, weakness of an extremity) or laboratory evidence indicative of cerebrovascular disease (e.g., multiple infarctions involving cortex and underlying white matter) that is judged to be etiologically related to the disturbance.
D The deficits do not occur exclusively during the course of a delirium.

From the American Psychiatric Association: *Diagnostic and statistical manual of mental disorders*, ed 4, text revision, Washington, DC, 2000, American Psychiatric Association, 2000.

to control impulses (behavioral disinhibition), and language abnormalities occur. Pick's bodies, which are the neuronal inclusions that gave the disease its previous name, are not always present on autopsy (Graff-Radford and Woodruff, 2007).

Creutzfeldt-Jakob Disease

Creutzfeldt-Jakob disease (CJD) is a rare condition that leads to dementia. In CJD, prions cause a spongiform encephalopathy. These proteins act as infective agents that cause cognitive losses, involuntary movements, and electroencephalogram changes. CJD typically develops at about the age of 60 years. CJD is not contagious, but corneal grafts, infected electrodes, and injected crude growth hormone from human pituitaries are able to transmit CJD. Some cases have shown that genetics possibly plays a role in this disease, and some health care workers have contracted the disease. Although autoclaving can destroy the causative agent, it is resistant to boiling, formalin, alcohol, and ultraviolet irradiation. CJD begins with the onset of confusion, depression, and altered sensation, and it progresses in weeks or months to dementia, ataxia, palsy, and sometimes cortical blindness.

CJD usually is not associated with bovine spongiform encephalitis, which is commonly known as *mad cow disease.*

However, there is strong evidence that a different form of CJD, called *variant CJD* [vCJD], is the same agent that is responsible for the spongiform encephalopathy that is transmitted by the consuming of affected cattle. Variant CJD is rare, and there is a low risk of an individual becoming infected after the ingestion of contaminated cattle (Centers for Disease Control and Prevention, 2007).

Huntington's Disease

The dementia of Huntington's disease (HD) is a direct consequence of that disease, which is the result of a single faulty autosomal-dominant gene on chromosome 4 (MedlinePlus, 2010). The disease results in the progressive degeneration of cognition, emotion, and movement. It usually occurs in susceptible people during their late 30s or 40s; however, HD has occurred as early as the age of 4 years and as late as the age of 85 years.

Progressive Supranuclear Palsy

Progressive supranuclear palsy (PSP) is a degenerative process that is associated with frontotemporal lobar degeneration, and it affects the nuclei of neurons. It is defined by the presence of neurofibrillary tangles in the neurons (Williams and Lees, 2009). People with PSP present clinically with dementia, progressive paralysis of downward and vertical gaze (supranuclear gaze), dysarthria (i.e., difficulty with articulating words), ataxic (unsteady) gait, and bradykinesia with muscular rigidity, which is most common in the neck area. Men are affected more than twice as often as women. Diminished cognition and changes in personality are present, but usually these changes are not as pronounced as they are with other dementias (Eggenberger et al, 2010).

Down's Syndrome Dementia

Down's syndrome dementia is difficult to diagnose, despite the extensive AD-type lesions seen in the cortex of the brain on autopsy of patients with this condition. Persons with Down's syndrome have three copies of chromosome 21, which is a condition called *trisomy 21*, and they often develop amyloid plaques and AD at an early age. About 50% of individuals with Down's syndrome who are older than 40 years of age have dementia. It usually begins manifesting as memory loss. The low percentage of dementia diagnoses among patients with Down's syndrome is probably a result of the difficulty ascertaining the presence of dementia in patients who have mental deficiencies, particularly if the degree of mental retardation is severe.

Cerebrovascular Accidents

Cerebrovascular accidents are stroke-like episodes that occur in approximately 20% of patients with AD. Cerebrovascular amyloid deposits either block a vessel or cause a vessel to rupture and produce a cerebral hemorrhage. These lesions occur predominantly in the gray matter, which will not result in paralysis. However, if a vessel ruptures in the leptomeninges that covers the brain's surface, severe hemorrhage will result in paralysis and death.

Reversible Dementias

Reversible or secondary dementias are a group of processes that represent about 10% of cases of dementia; however, after treatment, less than 1% of cases may actually reverse (Dennis, 2008). The vast majority of these conditions are treatable if treatment is instituted before irreversible damage occurs. The etiologic factors of secondary dementia are listed in Box 16-1. Secondary dementias are similar to delirium, which is described later in this chapter, but they involve less fluctuation of sensorium (consciousness).

Depression is commonly associated with reversible dementia, and is seen among older adults who do not always have the usual signs and symptoms of depression, and may present with memory loss only. Depression may be treated easily with the newer antidepressant medications, and it sometimes coexists with dementia. Holtzer and colleagues (2005) found that 40% of the patients with AD that they initially studied had symptoms of depression but that, over time, fewer subjects exhibited depressive symptoms. During the fourth year of study follow up, 28% of the participants had symptoms of depression, and this number decreased to 24% by the fifth year. The authors concluded that the study participants' level of functioning in daily activities was more of a determinant of depression than was their cognitive status.

Other Cognitive Disorders
Mild Cognitive Impairment

Mild cognitive impairment (MCI) refers to memory loss that does not interfere with activities of daily life. It is recognizable by other people and by cognitive screening tests, but, because it does not disrupt the person's life, it is not dementia (Alzheimer's Association, 2010c). There are several subtypes of MCI, one of which is amnestic impairment. Amnestic MCI does not meet the criteria of amnestic disorders. A recent study (Shaw et al, 2009) found biologic markers in cerebrospinal fluid that predicted whether or not subjects with MCI would go on to develop AD. Triebel and colleagues (2009) found that the financial skills of people with MCI declined approximately 1 year before their symptoms advanced to AD.

Studies have identified the active regions of the brain in both normal subjects and those with MCI. With the use of functional magnetic resonance imaging, researchers measured the changes in metabolic activity in different regions of the brain in subjects with MCI and in those without cognitive difficulties. Functional magnetic resonance imaging measures increased metabolic activity in parts of the brain with increased neuronal activity (Radiology Info, 2006). By comparing the activity in areas of the brain associated with encoding (learning) new information and memory, the researchers found that the memory deficits of MCI are related to areas of the brain that have not previously been identified. The temporal lobe (hippocampus) was identified as the area of the brain associated with the atrophy that begins early during the AD process. This study found differences in the activation of the frontal lobe during both learning and memory as well as changes in activity in the temporal lobes. This suggests that changes in MCI occur early during the disease process. A study by Devanand and colleagues (2007) found that combining magnetic resonance imaging measures of volumes of the hippocampus and the entorhinal cortex with age and cognitive measures leads to a high degree of predictive accuracy for the conversion of MCI to AD. Smaller volumes are indicative of AD.

Disorders such as delirium and amnestic disorders may easily be confused with dementia, because patients often have some of the same symptoms. Treatment for each of these disorders varies widely, thus making recognition and accurate diagnosis important. Table 16-1 describes the differences among the types of memory loss.

Delirium

Delirium is a disturbance of consciousness and a change in cognition that develops over a short period and that tends to come and go during the course of a day. Of hospitalized elderly patients in the United States, 14% to 56% are found to be delirious (Kannayiram and Blanchette, 2010). Delirium is a syndrome with multiple causes that affects consciousness, perception, thought, memory, and behavior.

Disorientation to time, place, and situation; inability to focus or shift attention; incoherent speech; and continual and aimless physical activity characterize this condition. Delirium is a medical emergency that always has an organic basis that nurses need to carefully identify and assess.

Patients with AD often become delirious when a severe infection or another medical condition occurs. Delirium is also the first or only indicator of illnesses that range from pneumonia to myocardial infarction to drug toxicity. Failure to recognize delirium leads to significant morbidity and mortality, both from the underlying illness and from self-inflicted injuries. When delirium overlies dementia of the Alzheimer's type, differentiating between the conditions becomes more difficult yet more vital to positive patient outcomes. Criteria for delirium caused by multiple etiologies are listed in the DSM-IV-TR Criteria box on page p. 370. A comparison of delirium with dementia is presented in Table 16-2.

Amnestic Disorders

A disturbance in learning and memory in an alert and responsive person characterizes an amnestic disorder. Amnestic memory deficits are the result of either the direct physiologic effects of a general medical condition or the persisting effects of substance use or abuse or toxin exposure. The primary problem with this disorder is the disturbance of memory, which can last hours to days. Chronic amnesia lasts for more than a month (see the DSM-IV-TR Criteria box on p. 370).

A leading cause of amnestic disorders is a nutritional deficiency of thiamine (vitamin B1) that is usually the result of alcohol abuse and that leads to Korsakoff's syndrome or Wernicke's encephalopathy (National Institute of Neurological Disorders and Stroke, 2010f). People with Korsakoff's syndrome are able to think and reason, but they cannot remember beyond the short term. Wernicke's encephalopathy is also the result of deficiencies in thiamine. It is a

TABLE 16-1	DIFFERENCES IN TYPES OF MEMORY LOSS	
NORMAL AGE-RELATED MEMORY LOSS	**MEMORY LOSS WITH MILD COGNITIVE IMPAIRMENT**	**MEMORY LOSS WITH ALZHEIMER'S DISEASE**
Sometimes misplaces keys, eyeglasses, or other items	Frequently misplaces items	Forgets what an item is used for or puts it in an inappropriate place
Momentarily forgets an acquaintance's name	Frequently forgets people's names and slow to recall them	May not remember knowing a person
Occasionally has to search for a word	Has increasing difficulty with finding desired words	Begins to lose language skills and may withdraw from social interaction
Occasionally forgets to run an errand	Begins to forget important events and appointments	Loses the sense of time; does not know what day it is
May forget an event from the distant past	May forget recent events or newly learned information	Has seriously impaired recent memory and difficulty learning and remembering new information
When driving, may momentarily forget where to turn, but quickly orients self	Becomes temporarily lost more often; may have trouble understanding and following a map	Becomes easily disoriented or lost in familiar places, sometimes for hours
Jokes about memory loss	Worries about memory loss; family and friends notice lapses	May have little or no awareness of cognitive problems

From the National Institute of Aging: *New research illuminates memory loss and early dementia* (website): www.nia.nih.gov/Alzheimers/Researchinformation/Newsletter/Spring2009/feature01.htm. Accessed December 8, 2010.
Adapted from Rabins PV: Memory. In *Johns Hopkins White Papers*, Baltimore, Md, 2010, Johns Hopkins University. Medical Education Services.

TABLE 16-2	DIFFERENCES IN TYPES OF MEMORY LOSS		
TYPE OF MEMORY LOSS	**AGE RELATED**	**MILD COGNITIVE IMPAIRMENT**	**ALZHEIMER'S DEMENTIA**
Losing Things	Sometimes misplaces familiar items	Frequently misplaces common items	Forgets an item's purpose
Recalling Names	May briefly forget a friend's name	Often forgets names of acquaintances	Does not recognize people
Finding Words	Sometimes needs to search for a word	Increased difficulty finding a word or words	Loses ability to express self
Remembering Errands	Occasionally forgets to complete a task	Forgets important appointments and errands	Does not know the day, is not aware of important events
Recalling the Past	Forgets the distant past	May forget the recent past	Seriously impaired memory of recent past, difficulty learning
Driving	Momentarily gets lost	More frequently gets disoriented	Easily lost in familiar places for longer periods of time
Managing the Loss	Jokes about memory loss	Worries about memory loss	No longer aware of memory loss

Adapted from: National Institute of Aging: http://www.nia.nih.gov/Alzheimers/Researchinformation/Newsletter/Spring2009/feature01.htm

degenerative brain disorder that is caused by alcohol abuse, dietary deficiencies, prolonged vomiting, eating disorders, and chemotherapy (National Institute of Neurological Disorders and Stroke, 2010f). Patients with Wernicke's encephalopathy experience confusion, amnesia of recent events, confabulation, disorientation, attention deficit and vision impairment. Wernicke's encephalopathy and Korsakoff's syndrome may be considered two phases of the same disorder, with Wernicke's representing the acute phase and Korsakoff's being the chronic stage (National Institute of Neurological Disorders and Stroke, 2010f).

Other causes of amnestic disorders are herpes encephalitis, hypoxia, vascular disorders, head injury (Kopelman, 2002), and medications such as the benzodiazepines (see Chapter 15).

EPIDEMIOLOGY

Sixty to 80% of all cases of dementia are the result of AD, and some estimate that more than 5.3 million people in the United States have AD (Alzheimer's Association, 2010f). One person in America develops AD every 70 seconds, and it is anticipated

DSM-IV-TR CRITERIA

Delirium Due to Multiple Etiologies

A Disturbances of consciousness (i.e., reduced clarity of awareness of the environment) with reduced ability to focus, sustain, or shift attention.

B A change in cognition (such as memory deficit, disorientation, language disturbance, perceptual disturbance) that is not better accounted for by a preexisting, established, or evolving dementia.

C The disturbance develops over a short period (usually hours to days) and tends to fluctuate during the course of the day.

D There is evidence from the history, physical examination, or laboratory findings that the delirium has more than one etiology (e.g., more than one etiologic general medical condition: a general medical condition plus substance intoxication or medication side effect).

From the American Psychiatric Association: *Diagnostic and statistical manual of Mental Disorders*, ed 4, text revision, Washington, DC, 2000, American Psychiatric Association.

that, by the middle of the century, an American will develop AD every 33 seconds (Alzheimer's Association, 2010a). Unless ongoing research leads to medical breakthroughs for the treatment or prevention of AD, experts project that between 11 and 16 million people older than the age of 65 years will live with AD (Alzheimer's Association, 2010a).

DSM-IV-TR CRITERIA

Amnestic Disorder

1 The development of memory impairment as manifested by impairment in the ability to learn new information or the inability to recall previously learned information.

2 The memory disturbance causes significant impairment in social or occupational functioning and represents a significant decline from a previous level of functioning.

3 The memory disturbance does not occur exclusively during the course of a delirium or a dementia.

4 There is evidence from the history, physical examination, or laboratory findings that the disturbance is the direct physiologic consequence of a general medical condition (including physical trauma).

Transient: If memory impairment lasts for 1 month or less

Chronic: If memory impairment lasts for more than 1 month

From the American Psychiatric Association: *Diagnostic and statistical manual of mental disorders*, ed 4, text revision, Washington, DC, 2000, American Psychiatric Association.

The age of onset of AD depends on its etiology. The highest incidence of dementia occurs after the age of 85 years, and nearly half of individuals who are older than 85 years old have AD (Alzheimer's Association, 2010b). It is estimated that, as of 2010, nearly 36 million people in the world will be living with dementias of all types, and this number is expected to double every 20 years (World Alzheimer Report, 2009).

VaD is responsible for 15% to 20% of dementias. In addition, patients have mixed dementias, such as a combination of both VaD and AD (Alzheimer's Association, 2010d); 45% of the autopsied brains of people with dementia show a combination of these two conditions.

LBD is the cause of 20% to 25% of all dementias, as shown by autopsy (Lewy Body Dementia Association, 2010). As previously noted, however, cases of pure LBD are rare, and most dementias are the result of mixed LBD and AD.

The frequency of dementia associated with PD increases with age, and it is estimated to be between 20% and 40%. In one study, PD was present in approximately 99 of 100,000 people, and 44% of those with PD had dementia (Swanberg and Kalapatapu, 2010).

The onset of FTLD usually occurs between the ages of 40 and 60 years. FTLD has a strong genetic association. It is believed that as many as 10% of all cases of dementia are caused by FTLD (National Institutes of Health, 2009b).

CJD is rare, and it affects 1 person in a million per year worldwide. Three major categories of CJD have been identified: (1) sporadic CJD, which accounts for 85% of cases; (2) a hereditary form that is responsible for 5% to 10% of cases of CJD; and (3) an acquired form that accounts for less than 1% of cases of CJD (National Institute of Neurological Disorders and Stroke, 2010a).

HD is an inherited disease that is found all over the world. It affects 1 out of every 10,000 people. Approximately 30,000 people in the United States have the disease, and an estimated 150,000 people have a 50% chance of developing it (National Institute of Neurological Disorders and Stroke, 2010c). PSP is also rare and occurs in about 1 out of every 100,000 people (Warren et al, 2005).

It is estimated that delirium occurs in 10% to 30% of hospitalized patients, and up to 40% of elderly ill patients experience delirium at a given time (American Psychiatric Association, 2000). Alternatively, researchers do not know how often amnestic disorders occur. Individuals with a predisposing medical condition, who take certain medications (e.g., benzodiazepines), or who abuse alcohol are at risk for an amnestic disorder.

CLINICAL DESCRIPTION

Dementia results in multiple cognitive deficits. These deficits include memory impairment and one of the following:

- Aphasia The individual exhibits deficits in language functioning. In severe forms, the person may not speak at all.
- Apraxia The person is unable to perform motor activities despite intact function.
- Agnosia The individual experiences difficulties with object identification, usually with common household items.
- A disturbance in executive functioning

Executive dementias impair functioning more than memory. Problems with executive functioning include difficulties with abstract thinking, reasoning, planning, and starting and stopping complex behavior.

The memory impairment of dementia includes difficulty learning new information and problems with forgetting. Other characteristics of dementia include the following:

- Spatial disorientation
- Poor judgment and disinhibition
- Poor insight
- The potential for violence
- Loss of motor skills
- Possible mood and sleep disturbances

Alzheimer's Disease

During the early stages of AD, neurofibrillary tangles attack the hippocampus, which leads to the loss of recent memory. After this, the temporoparietal regions usually deteriorate, which produces cognitive deficits in learning, attention, judgment, orientation, and speech and language use. To further complicate matters, other regions of the brain are occasionally affected, which results in a variety of symptoms. The onset of the disease makes the situation worse, because many often perceive it as inattention, restlessness, mild forgetfulness, and depression. Patients grow progressively more confused and unaware of their surroundings. They later become incapable of caring for their basic activities of daily living (ADLs), such as feeding, grooming, and toileting (Figure 16-1).

Patients with AD do not present a uniform or coherent history, and the time of onset is not clearly definable. This presents a serious problem with regard to differential diagnosis (i.e., distinguishing AD from other diagnoses). Caregivers seek medical care for a loved one after observing specific behavioral difficulties, such as difficulty shopping, driving, managing finances, or performing common household tasks. Frequently, family members who have not seen the person for a while fail to notice the subtle changes that have occurred. Hasty judgments that are based on a short visit often lead to conflict between the family caregiver and the relatives of the patient, particularly when institutionalization comes into question. Unfortunately, the loss of a job or a serious auto accident is the most convincing evidence of serious cognitive loss and usually motivates the family members to act on behalf of their loved one.

Although patients themselves often notice the early signs of cognitive impairment, many will use one or more of the defense mechanisms of denial, repression, projection, aggression, regression, or rationalization to defend against their memory and cognitive deficits. Some will succeed in deceiving their family, friends, and employers for a time. Distinguishing these behaviors from actual cognitive deficits further complicates the diagnostic process.

A careful history reveals many or all of the following symptoms:

- Altered thought processes, specifically **paranoia** (i.e., fear-based delusions of being persecuted)
- Confused or disoriented state
- Impaired intellect and memory (especially short-term memory during the early stages)
- Sensory and perceptual alterations (i.e., hallucinations)

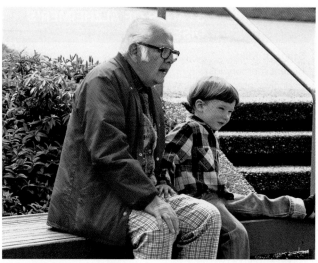

FIGURE 16-1. A grandson brings comfort to his grandfather, who is experiencing a loss of faculties as a result of Alzheimer's disease. Image © 2007 JupiterImages Corporation.

- Decreased sensorium
- Loss of body functions
- Self-care deficit
- Fear, anxiety, and depression
- **Catastrophic reactions** (i.e., patient may impulsively act out in anger or panic)
- Self-concept disturbance or feelings of powerlessness
- Compromised physical abilities
- Social isolation and apathy
- Impaired verbal communication
- Emotional lability
- Sleep disturbances
- **Confabulation** (i.e., patient fabricates stories to fill in memory gaps; this occurs in mild to moderate stages and is not considered lying

Stages of Alzheimer's Disease

Several staging systems for AD are available. The most commonly used system is a three-stage system that defines the early, mid, and late stages of dementia. It assesses cognitive, functional, and behavioral symptoms. Determining the stage helps to identify the individual's needs and the potential response to treatment. The stages of AD are listed below and also in Box 16-2. Each stage brings with it additional physical and psychoemotive losses as well as increasing dependency needs.

Stage 1: Mild. The most distinguishing characteristic of the first stage of AD is memory loss. Sensory and motor functions are not usually affected at this stage. Memory impairment is often so mild that the patient, family, and caregivers attribute it to normal aging. As this disease progresses, however, the patient often recognizes that there is a problem. Recent memories about the previous day's events are lost, yet the patient is able to remember events from long ago. Patients have problems naming common items, they repeat things often, they lose things easily, and they get lost frequently. The

---

BOX 16-2 STAGES OF ALZHEIMER'S DISEASE

Stage 1: Mild
Recent memory loss
Cognitive loss in the following areas:
  Communication
  Calculation
  Recognition
Anxiety and confusion
Mild behavior problems, such as the inability to initiate and
  complete a task

Stage 2: Moderate
Stage 1 symptoms increase
Behavior problems increase, which may include the
  following:
  Catastrophic reactions
  Sundowning (confusion and irritation due to reduced
    stimulation and tiredness)
  Perseveration (repetitive verbalizations or motions due
    to thought disturbances)
  Aimless pacing
  Wandering
Confusion
Incontinence, mild
Hypertonia

Stage 3: Severe
Stage 2 symptoms increase
Incontinence, total
Choking
Emaciation
Total care required
Progressive gait disturbances that lead to nonambulatory
  status

- Perseveration: Repetitive verbalizations or motions, or persistent repetition of the same idea in response to different questions. Also seen in patients with schizophrenia.
- Sundowning or sundowner's syndrome: Increased negative behavioral disturbances such as irritation or confusion occurring during the afternoon or evening. This may be related to reduced stimulation and routine, and tiredness from struggling to interpret the environment during the day.
- Sleep disturbances: Characterized by restlessness and wandering during the night, which may be related to sundowning.
- Catastrophic reactions: A sudden or gradual negative change in behavior caused by the inability to understand and cope with environmental stimuli. Individuals may react excessively, out of proportion to the situation, or panic and act out violently (see Box 16-3).

Stage 2 lasts approximately 2 to 10 years. Patients in this stage of AD have trouble with simple daily tasks, such as remembering how to perform ADLs. During this stage, patients often hallucinate and become depressed. They also become argumentative and wander, and they require close supervision.

Stage 3: Severe. Late dementia lasts from approximately 1 to 3 years. During this stage, patients cannot use or understand words, and they cannot recognize themselves or others. They can no longer care for themselves, and they are totally dependent on others.

There is a loss of meaningful communication with the patient. Patients often lose weight and bladder control, and they often develop secondary illnesses and conditions. Immobility leads to pneumonia, urinary tract infections, and the development of pressure ulcers, which often require hospitalization. The progressive loss of neurons leads to the loss of the ability to swallow, and death is usually a result of aspiration pneumonia. The caregiver makes all decisions about the patient's medical and social needs.

Vascular Dementia

The cognitive deficits that result from VaD are similar to those described previously. The onset of VaD is sudden, and deficits occur in steps, although sometimes the deficits will seem to appear and then disappear for a while between steps. With VaD, there is evidence of cerebrovascular disease and focal neurologic signs, such as gait abnormalities, the exaggeration of deep tendon reflexes, and the weakness of an extremity. Changes are rapid rather than slow, and, depending on the areas of the brain that are affected, patients exhibit a patchy and uneven pattern of deficits.

Other Dementias

The course of LBD is similar to that of AD, but it also involves PD-like movement disorder. LBD involves a significant cognitive decline with later memory deficits, the presence of visual hallucinations, ataxic gait, and motor changes like those associated with PD (Lewy Body Dementia Association, 2010). However, the dementia that accompanies PD occurs

---

inability to find words and the use of inappropriate words when unable to remember is common.

Neologisms, which are invented and meaningless words, are also common. Patients lose interest and spontaneity, and they begin to show signs of personality changes. It is during this time of self-awareness of loss that many patients suffer profound depression. Approximately 40% of patients with AD experience depression at some point during their illness (Holtzer, 2005). Stage 1 lasts for approximately 2 to 4 years. The patient's needs during this stage are primarily for support and guidance.

Stage 2: Moderate. During stage 2, intellectual decline continues to increase and includes amnesia, disorientation, apraxia, aphasia, and depression. Memory and cognitive impairment gradually lead to the loss of the ability to care for oneself. Patients have difficulty making decisions as a result of decreased concentration, and they lack the cognitive skills to make appropriate judgments. Some patients develop delusions that are paranoid in nature. As the disease progresses toward the terminal stages, both short- and long-term memory are affected. The patient displays agnosia, apraxia (described above), and the following manifestations:

| BOX 16-3 | **CATASTROPHIC REACTIONS** |

Catastrophic reactions are overexaggerated emotional responses that are initiated as a result of a perceived failure at a task or a change in the environment (Webster and Grossberg, 1996).

Often patients with dementia are unjustly labeled as non-compliant, disruptive, uncooperative, or threatening. Patients are not trying to annoy, get attention, or hurt the caregiver; rather, they are trying their best to understand a world that they can no longer comprehend. Patients display a catastrophic reaction as verbal or physical aggression, verbal outbursts, worry, anger, tension expressed in body language, labile mood swings, pacing, paranoia, crying, or hysteric laughter.

Analysis of a Catastrophic Reaction
Was the person doing the following?
- Trying unsuccessfully to comprehend more than one or two sensory messages at once
- Feeling insecure (e.g., being in new surroundings or surrounded by unfamiliar staff)
- Having a minor accident (e.g., spilling a drink or dropping something) or failing at a task
- Asked to reason, make a judgment, or perform a multistep or complex task
- Experiencing negative interactions such as scolding, arguing, anger, frustration, or irritation
- Experiencing a hallucination, delusion, or illusion

Interventions for a Catastrophic Reaction
- Reassure the patient that he or she is safe.
- Use positive and therapeutic behavioral interactions.
- Maintain the patient's personal space; do not touch the patient without asking his or her permission.
- Eliminate or reduce all outside stimulation.
- Identify and remove either the source of the problem or the patient.
- Redirect the patient to a less demanding activity.
- Be patient and allow sufficient time for the patient to calm down. This will take only a few minutes or hours, and it varies with each patient and situation.
- If the nurse cannot stop or minimize the reaction:

Leave the patient alone for a while in a quiet, safe place within view of staff or family.

When readdressing the patient, act as if nothing has happened. Redirect conversations to familiar topics.

Have one person address the patient. Minimize hand gestures, and be aware of facial expressions. Speak in a soft and nonthreatening voice while redirecting the conversation or task.

later during the course of the disease. Approximately 20% to 60% of patients with PD will develop dementia.

Changes in behavior and personality characterize FTLD. Behavioral changes include socially inappropriate behavior, agitation, and apathy. Language difficulties include problems speaking and understanding speech (National Institute of Neurological Disorders and Stroke, 2010b). Unusual behaviors may include sexually inappropriate behaviors and unusual verbal or physical behaviors. Some patients with FTLD develop amyotrophic lateral sclerosis, which is also known as *Lou Gehrig's disease* (University of California, San Francisco Medical Center, 2009).

CJD causes a progressing dementia that develops over weeks to months. Initially, problems with muscular coordination and vision as well as personality changes develop. As the disease progresses, myoclonic ataxia, severe mental impairment, and possibly blindness occur (National Institute of Neurological Disorders and Stroke, 2010a).

The symptoms of HD include cognitive impairment, motor disturbances, and psychiatric changes. Behavior may change before movement problems occur. Cognitive changes include memory loss and a loss of planning and decision-making abilities. Motor changes include both choreatic (involuntary dancing or writhing of the limbs and facial muscles) and nonchoreatic movements and the slowing of voluntary motor actions. The condition may progress to ataxia, dysphagia, and incontinence. Psychiatric disturbances include depression, irritability, paranoia, hallucinations, and agitation (MedlinePlus, 2010).

PSP is similar to PD, and it is caused by a gradual degeneration of the brain cells in the brainstem. The first symptom of PSP is a loss of balance that progresses to stiffness and unexplained falls. Symptoms are similar to those of PD, because damage to the substantia nigra occurs in both disorders. Other symptoms are personality changes, apathy, and irritability. Later, vision problems develop, including blurred vision and difficulty with controlling eye movement. Patients with PSP have difficulty looking downward and are not able to maintain eye contact. PSP is not a direct cause of mortality, but it does predispose patients to death by pneumonia, choking, or head injury (National Institute of Neurological Disorders and Stroke, 2010e).

Delirium and Amnestic Disorders

Delirium is a change in consciousness, cognition, attention, and perception that develops rapidly over the course of hours to days. It is an outcome of other underlying conditions. Although delirium is sometimes confused with dementia, the changes of delirium are rapid and have a changing course (American Psychiatric Association, 2000). Although delirium is reversible, in hospitalized patients, it is responsible for significantly increased occurrences of complications and mortality (Twedell, 2005). Mortality rates rise with an increase in the severity of symptoms of delirium (McCusker, 2004). The clinical course and treatment of delirium depends on the underlying cause of the precipitating condition.

Symptoms of delirium include a fluctuating consciousness with a reduced ability to sustain attention, memory impairment, disorientation, language disturbances, and delusions (Alagiakrishnan and Blanchette, 2010).

One study identified four subtypes of delirium: (1) hypoactive/mild; (2) hypoactive/severe; (3) mixed with hyperactive features/severe; and (4) normal/mild. The authors identified the hypoactive mild group as having the highest mortality rate (Yang et al, 2009). Hyperactive delirium is the most familiar form to nurses, because patients with this condition are aroused and hyperactive. Hypoactive delirium is less familiar and presents as depression. Patients with hypoactive delirium are lethargic, inactive, and indifferent. Because of inactivity, hypoactive delirium patients are more likely to develop further complications, including decubiti, aspiration, and pulmonary embolism. The mixed type of delirium involves sudden shifts in behavior from the hypoactive form to the hyperactive form; this is the most common form of delirium.

The cause of delirium must quickly be identified and corrected. Conditions that disrupt structural or metabolic integrity will cause delirium (Alagiakrishnan, 2010). Risk factors for delirium include sensory impairment, neurologic disease, comorbid illnesses, drugs, surgery, and environmental influences (Tardiff, 2009) One of the simplest ways to manage delirium is to ensure that glasses, hearing aids, and other sensory assistance devices are available. Similarly, the clinical course and treatment of amnestic disorders depend on the underlying condition responsible for their development.

PROGNOSIS

The duration of AD averages 10 years, with a range from 3 to 20 years (Sanders et al, 2008). There is no medical treatment that will prevent, arrest, or modify the course of AD. Medications to modify and lessen some of its symptoms exist. Positive interventions by the caregiver will result in behavioral modification and help to reduce anxiety, avoid incontinence, and eliminate sleep disturbances and depression. A planned therapeutic activity program will increase the patient's awareness, verbal and physical responses, and level of functioning.

Although patients with VaD may improve for a time, they usually plateau and decline again. Managing the patient's blood pressure helps to prevent further progression (National Institute of Neurological Disorders and Stroke, 2010d).

Mortality is higher among patients with PD with dementia than among those without dementia. People who develop PD when they are younger than 50 years old have a reduced likelihood of developing PD-related dementia (Swanberg and Kalapatapu, 2010).

The prognosis for FTLD is poor, because the disease steadily progresses over a period of 2 to 10 years (National Institute of Neurological Disorders and Stroke, 2010b). As with other dementias, death among patients with FTLD is usually the result of pneumonia or other infections.

CJD carries an extremely poor prognosis. Approximately 90% of patients die of CJD within 1 year of diagnosis (National Institute of Neurological Disorders and Stroke, 2010a). Alternatively, HD progresses relatively slowly over a period of 10 to 30 years, and patients with HD usually die from an infection (usually pneumonia) (National Institute of Neurological Disorders and Stroke, 2010c). Suicide is a common cause of death among these patients (MedlinePlus, 2010).

PSP alone is not directly life threatening, but it is a progressive neurodegenerative disease with no known cure. Symptomatic treatment with antiparkinson drugs, cholinesterase inhibitors, and antidepressants has demonstrated some success with helping to control symptoms. Swallowing difficulties predispose patients to pneumonia (National Institute of Neurological Disorders and Stroke, 2010e).

The prognoses for delirium and the amnestic disorders depend on the nature and treatment of the condition that is causing the disorder. The progression of the amnestic symptoms associated with Korsakoff's syndrome is delayed for the patient who does not drink alcohol and who has a healthy diet. Approximately 25% of patients with Korsakoff's syndrome who follow this plan improve significantly, about 50% improve somewhat, and 25% do not recover. The disease progresses among patients who continue to drink (Alzheimer's Association, 2010f).

DISCHARGE CRITERIA

AD and other primary dementias are progressive and chronic diseases that require discharge planning on the basis of individual patient needs and the stage of the illness. As the patient and his or her primary caregiver progress through the stages of dementia, the health care team and the caregiver work together to continually make adjustments in care. The patient's prognosis depends on the severity of the dementia and how the patient responds to treatment. The following indications of success in specific areas are should be considered:

- The patient has an absence of risk of self-harm and harm of others.
- The patient accomplishes ADLs and instrumental ADLs (IADLs) with minimal assistance.
- The patient is free from catastrophic reactions.
- The patient participates in a therapeutic activity program that has been individualized to assess and meet his or her needs.
- The primary caregiver has satisfactory knowledge of AD and related disorders.
- The primary caregiver has used positive and therapeutic behavioral interactions during caregiving.
- The primary caregiver has instituted plans and developed resources for his or her own self-care.
- The primary caregiver has appropriate legal and financial plans in place for the patient and for himself or herself.
- The primary caregiver has appropriate backup systems in place in case of emergency (e.g., the sudden illness or death of the patient or the caregiver).

The family and the primary caregiver deserve special attention because, without support, the burdens of caring for someone with dementia are overwhelming. Placement in a long-term care facility is usually the final step in the caregiver's commitment to the ill family member. Many years of care and concern generally precede the decision for out-of-home care. Emotional stresses as well as financial expenses become significant. Health care and in-home services, special equipment and foods, and loss of income for the patient and the caregiver are only a few of the cost factors. More than 50% of nursing home care costs are paid from the private funds of patients and their families. Family education and counseling will help to ease the demands of caring for a patient with AD (see the Case Study).

CASE STUDY

Simon, who is 70 years old, has been brought to the emergency department by his 66-year-old wife, Ann, for the treatment of an extensive skin tear on his right forearm, which is bleeding and wrapped in a large gauze roller bandage. During treatment of Simon's wound, the nurse interviews Ann and notices that her appearance is gaunt and that she has dark circles under her eyes. Ann also appears disheveled, with uncombed hair and poor grooming. Simon has been retired for 5 years, but Ann is still working part time as a receptionist for a busy insurance company. Ann would like to retire, but she feels that she has to supplement their income. Ann says that Simon has been "acting crazy," that he "has accidents in the bathroom," that he "never sits still," and that he has kept her up for the last four nights. She tells the nurse that she feels "exhausted" and "frustrated," and she says, "if I don't get some sleep, I'm afraid I may hit Simon or do something I'll regret." Further questioning reveals that Simon lost his job as an accountant because of errors in mathematics and low productivity. Simon's affect is flat, and he speaks in a slow, monotone voice. His gait is unsteady, and his movements are slow. He states, "I can't remember how I hurt my arm; I just saw the blood." Simon's untidy appearance, soiled clothes, and strong body odor reveal that his hygiene and grooming are poor. Ann admits to the nurse that she and Simon have not seen a doctor for several years, because Simon believes that "all doctors are useless." Ann claims to be too busy working and caring for Simon to take him to the doctor.

Critical Thinking

1 What are the primary immediate and long-term needs of Simon and Ann?
2 What therapeutic approach should the nurse use to gain their trust and confidence?
3 Which assessment tools might be useful for determining their special needs and psychosocial statuses?
4 What questions might elicit information regarding Ann's knowledge of Simon's behavior?
5 What teaching approaches might be successful for getting this couple to seek future help?

THE NURSING PROCESS

ASSESSMENT

The assessment of patients with cognitive disorders is often difficult, because it depends on information from several sources, and the assessment of patients with AD poses a particular challenge. For example, the first symptom that is generally reported with AD is recent memory loss. However, recent memory loss also adversely affects the patient's remote memory as a result of the symptoms of disorientation,

depression, delusions, and hallucinations. A comprehensive assessment should include a thorough history, a physical assessment, a functional assessment, and a mental status evaluation (see Chapter 3).

No screening guidelines for dementia exist. Because there are no therapies for AD that alter the course of the disease, screening should be targeted for those patients who have risk factors for the disease (Moorhouse, 2009). Patients who have experienced a stroke, who have delirium, or who have signs of depression should be screened. Screening should also be considered for patients with changes in the performance of ADLs or with changes in their behavior or levels of cognition (Mulhausen, 2010).

Assessment Environment

When interviewing the patient or administering an assessment test, it is critical to have a positive physical and emotional environment. Make sure that the room is free from distractions and that it is quiet and away from the noise of any activity. Visual and auditory deficits are often present in these patients, and the evaluator needs to maintain eye contact and speak clearly and directly to the patient in a low-frequency range, because high tones are usually less discernible. If the patient usually wears hearing aids or glasses, make sure that they are in place and in working condition. Any printed material that requires a patient response needs to be in large, heavy type that is easy to read. If English is not the patient's native language, someone who speaks the patient's primary language needs to administer the test or translate for the patient and the interviewer for valid results. Paraphrasing questions is permissible to clarify an item. Patients will need sufficient time to process the information and to form a correct response. In general, the attitude of the evaluator needs to be friendly, nonthreatening, and nonjudgmental. Giving positive feedback to the patient by saying, "You're doing fine," "That was good," or "This is a really hard one" helps to relieve the stress of testing. Avoid indications that a response is correct or incorrect.

Also include the same courtesies in interviews with the caregiver that you would use with the patient. Conduct these interviews separately and in private; this will ensure honest responses and avoid the danger of talking about the patient in the patient's presence.

Cognitive Assessment Tools

Because of the lack of biologic indicators, health care professionals rely on clinical criteria to make a diagnosis of probable or possible AD. A variety of tools will reveal a person's cognitive status. Administering a test in sections is permissible if the patient has become too fatigued, has too short of an attention span, or shows signs of anxiety. It is best to test the patient alone, without an informant or caregiver, so that the responses are entirely the patient's own and not influenced by hints or responses from someone else.

Many cognitive assessment tools are available to assess orientation, intellectual functioning, memory, and reading and math skills. Among the most common are the mini-mental state examination (MMSE), the Dementia Severity Rating Scale, the Geriatric Depression Scale, the Memory Impairment Screen, and the Mini-Cog. In addition, the Functional Assessment Staging Tool (FAST) helps to identify specific stages of dementia.

Mini-Mental State Examination

The MMSE (Folstein et al, 1975) is a frequently used and cited test that is actually a proprietary test owned by Psychological Assessment Resources (2010a), although it is available online on multiple Web sites. Psychological Assessment Resources requires that examiners meet credentialing requirements before administering the MMSE. The MMSE allows health care professionals to measure global cognitive performance, to follow the course of an illness, and to monitor patients' responses to treatment. The test includes a series of 30 questions that assess orientation, registration, attention span, calculation, language recall, and perception. It can be administered in as short a time as 5 to 10 minutes. It provides standardized methods of data collection, scoring, and interpretation in specific areas of cognitive impairment. Scores that are less than or equal to 24 indicate cognitive impairment. An expanded version, the MMSE-2, is available to test people with milder forms of cognitive deficits (Psychological Assessment Resources, 2010b). The cost and credentialing requirements may be prohibitive for some potential examiners.

Dementia Severity Rating Scale

The Dementia Severity Rating Scale assesses the elderly patient's ability to function in the home (Clark and Ewbank, 1996). The 11-item scale assesses memory, orientation, judgment, knowledge of community affairs, home activities, personal care, speech and language recognition, feeding, incontinence, and mobility. This functional assessment is most often used as a long-term assessment throughout the course of a disease (Cotter et al, 2003).

Geriatric Depression Scale

The Geriatric Depression Scale is a 30-item questionnaire that asks patients simple yes-or-no questions (Yesavage et al, 1983). When an elderly patient attains a score of 11 or higher, further assessment and diagnostic evaluation are necessary. This assessment is for patients with AD when they are able to comprehend the questions being asked of them (Cotter et al, 2003).

Memory Impairment Screen

The Memory Impairment Screen is a four-item test that takes approximately 4 minutes to administer (Buschke et al, 2007). Because the test does not show educational or language bias, it is recommended for patients who belong to ethnic minorities.

Mini-Cog

The Mini-Cog is a rapid three-item test for the screening of dementia. It combines the clock drawing test, which requires the patient to draw a specific time, with tests of executive functioning, visuospatial functioning, and object recall. The entire test takes less than 3 minutes to administer, and it is a screening test rather than a diagnostic test (Doerflinger, 2007).

Functional Assessment Staging Tool

The FAST (Reisberg et al, 1985) is a 16-item ordinal inventory that measures a person's stage of dementia on the basis of his or her functional abilities. The results of the FAST involve seven stages: stage 1 indicates no dementia; stages 2, 3, and 4 indicate progressive memory loss; and stages 5, 6, and 7 are roughly equivalent to early, middle, and late dementia. The FAST is particularly useful for providing individualized care on the basis of the needs of a person during a specific stage.

Neurologic Deficits

Pathologic changes in the brain—including amyloid (neuritic) plaques, neurofibrillary tangles, and fibrillary deposits in cerebral vessels—result in neurologic deficits with ensuing behavioral changes. Determining the status of a patient with AD or another related dementia involves the assessment of neurologic deficits that can be remembered with the use of the mnemonic *PALMER:* *p*erception and organization, *a*ttention span, *l*anguage, *m*emory, *e*motional control, and *r*easoning and judgment. These areas are described in detail in the following sections.

Perception and Organization

How well does the patient interpret the following?
- Sensory cues
- The relationships between objects and between himself or herself and the environment
  How well does the patient organize the following?
- Movement, such as sitting, standing, and transferring
- Tasks, such as dressing in proper sequence
- Solutions to simple puzzles

Attention Span

How well does the patient do the following?
- Initiate an activity
- Sustain an activity (i.e., does he or she have a shortened attention span or a loss of interest?)
- Terminate an activity when it is completed or in an established pattern (i.e., does the patient demonstrate perseveration [excessive repetition]?)

Language

How well does the patient do the following?
- Express thoughts verbally (an inability to do this is called *expressive aphasia*)
- Comprehend the spoken word (an inability to do this is called *receptive aphasia*)
- Read and comprehend the written word (an inability to do this is called *alexia*)
- Express thoughts in writing (an inability to do this is called *agraphia*)

Memory

How well does the patient remember the following?

- Recent events immediately after their occurrence (immediate recall)
- Recent events within a matter of minutes (recent memory)
- Events from months or years ago (remote or long-term memory)

Emotional Control

- Is the patient's emotional control consistent with and appropriate to the situation?
- Is the patient's emotional control sustained for an appropriate length of time?
- Does the patient's emotional control represent a change from his or her previous behavior?

Reasoning and Judgment

How well has the patient done the following?

- Made appropriate decisions on the basis of good advice or facts
- Followed social conventions
- Reacted appropriately in an emergency situation

Emotional Status
Mood and State of Mind

Each time that a nurse approaches a patient, the nurse makes an informal assessment of the patient's mood and state of mind. The Omnibus Budget Reconciliation Act of 1987 requires a more formal psychiatric assessment of a patient before admission to a skilled nursing facility and before the administration of any psychotropic medications or physical restraints (see the Nursing Assessment Questions box). In documentation, the consistent use of significant quoted statements and regular documented mental status examinations will assist professional staff with communicating information in a systematic way.

Depression

Preexisting depression has been identified as a risk factor for dementia and secondary depression that often occurs in the patient with dementia. The presence of depression with cognitive impairment may lead to increased mortality (Gellis et al, 2010). Nurses need to assess signs and symptoms thoroughly and develop treatment plans that address this condition. The Geriatric Depression Scale is useful as an assessment tool during the mild stages of dementia, when language ability is present. The patient will sometimes communicate feelings of sadness, guilt, and suicidal ideation.

Functional Ability

The determination of a patient's functional ability is essential to developing nursing diagnoses. Excess disability occurs when the caregiver responds verbally or physically with more assistance than is necessary, because this diminishes the patient's speaking or activity skills. Maintaining independence in ADLs and IADLs is vital if patients with dementia

---

NURSING ASSESSMENT QUESTIONS
Cognitive Disorders

The following questions may be helpful for attaining a thorough nursing history:

1. Has the onset been rapid or insidious?
2. Has the progression of cognitive decline fluctuated (delirium), or has there been a continuous decline (dementia)?
3. What is the duration of the following symptoms?
   a. Difficulty learning and retaining new information
   b. Difficulty completing multiple-step tasks (e.g., driving, cooking, financial management)
   c. Problem-solving difficulties
   d. Disorientation
   e. Word-finding problems
   f. Difficulty participating in conversation
   g. Changes in baseline behaviors (e.g., irritability, passivity, suspiciousness)
4. Does the patient have a history of the following?
   a. Known psychiatric disorders (e.g., depression)
   b. Neurologic disorders (e.g., head injury, stroke, PD)
   c. Alcohol or drug use
   d. Endocrine disorders (e.g., diabetes mellitus, hypothyroidism)
   e. Renal disorders
   f. Infections (e.g., pneumonia, urinary tract infections)
5. Ask the patient, the family, or the caregiver to tell you all of the medications that the patient is taking (i.e., prescribed, over-the-counter, and herbal preparations).
6. Inquire if there is a family history of dementia, Down's syndrome, or any familial diseases that may lead to dementia (e.g., HD).

---

are to retain their self-esteem and engage in worthwhile activities.

Behavior

Because people with dementia have difficulty understanding and expressing themselves, they often manifest their needs and discomfort with behaviors. Behaviors often found in patients with AD and other cognitive disorders are grouped in the following manner:

Behaviors related to mood:

- Pacing, wandering, and rummaging (these indicate anxiety)
- Decreased or inappropriate socialization (these signify apathy)
- Refusal to eat, bathe, or groom (these result from depression)
- Hoarding or accusations of thievery (these are caused by paranoia)

Behaviors that result from perceptual or cognitive deficits:

- Day/night reversal
- Inappropriate eating (e.g., eating too rapidly or too much, eating nonfood items)

- Falls and accidents (e.g., walking into walls or furniture, not being aware of hazards)
- Delusions, hallucinations, and paranoia
  Behaviors that result from the loss of impulse control:
- Inappropriate toileting activities
- Inappropriate sexual behavior (e.g., display of penis or breasts, sexually explicit comments or language)
- Disinhibited social behavior (e.g., inappropriate jokes, neglecting personal hygiene, exhibiting undue familiarity with strangers)

When any change in behavior from previous observations occurs, reassess the patient. The patient often cannot communicate to others about the distressing signs or symptoms of an illness. Determining how a patient feels requires the use of seasoned observation skills, especially with regard to the assessment of body language.

Physical Manifestations

Alteration in nutritional status is a problem that involves many factors. Related reasons include an inability to physically purchase and prepare food, a lack of financial resources to buy food, medical conditions that decrease the older patient's appetite, or cognitive dysfunction that prevents the patient from remembering to eat. Nurses need to note any weight changes of 3 to 5 pounds or more and make an assessment for treatable problems unrelated to the illness of dementia. If no other clinical signs or symptoms are present, examine the patient's immediate environment. During mealtimes, the nurse observes for and corrects distracting lighting, provides seating arrangements that are compatible, provides for low noise levels, and ensures the physical comfort of the table and chairs.

The family or caregiver needs to keep a food diary and to monitor the patient's food intake, being alert for dehydration. Often older persons significantly decrease their oral intake to prevent incontinence. Dehydration and malnutrition lead to multiple medical diagnoses, including hypoalbuminuria, hypoproteinemia, anemia, hypoglycemia, and other vitamin and mineral deficits (see Physical and Laboratory Examinations later in this chapter).

People with cognitive deficits often have difficulty reporting their pain. Performing a baseline pain assessment and identifying potential pain indicators with the use of a standard pain assessment tool will enable caregivers to identify characteristic behaviors of the patient who is experiencing pain and to observe changes in these characteristic behaviors. The Pain Assessment in Advanced Dementia Scale (Horgas, 2007; Warden et al, 2003) is one such tool. On a 0 to 2 scale, it measures nonlanguage behaviors, including breathing, negative vocalization, facial expression, body language, and the ability of the patient to be consoled.

Aspiration is a critical risk factor, particularly during stage 3 of AD, and the resulting aspiration pneumonia is often the immediate cause of death. The caregiver who is monitoring the patient's feeding needs to watch for a swallow after each bite, which is indicated by the larynx rising and returning to the resting position. If possible, patients should sit at a

> ❖ **CLINICAL ALERT #1**
>
> **Signs of Silent Aspiration (Choking)**
> - Watering eyes
> - Reddening of the face
> - Rhonchi on pulmonary auscultation
> - Variable rates of respiration
> - Grimacing
> - Coughing
> - Gagging
> - Throat clearing
> - Pocketing of food in the oral cavity

> ❖ **CLINICAL ALERT #2**
>
> **Types of Urinary Incontinence**
> - Stress: The involuntary loss of small amounts of urine associated with coughing, sneezing, laughing, and so on
> - Urge: The loss of larger amounts of urine that results from an inability to delay voiding after feeling the sensation of a full bladder
> - Overflow: The loss of small amounts of urine that results from stresses on an overly full bladder
> - Functional: The loss of large amounts of urine that results from cognitive deficits that lead to not recognizing cues from the bladder, the inability to find the bathroom, or increasing apraxia

90-degree angle and keep the chin toward the chest when swallowing rather than hyperextending the chin. Thickened liquids are often easier for the patient to swallow. As patients become more dependent, they should be left in a sitting position for 30 minutes after the meal. The nurse checks the oral cavity for pocketed food and removes any food that is found. These nursing activities prevent silent aspiration when the patient is in a lying position. (see Clinical Alert #1)

When a patient has changes in gait, be alert for other possible disease processes: (1) vision problems, inner ear disturbances, pain from osteoarthritis, or an injury that the patient is not able to identify; (2) neuropathy that results from vascular or diabetic problems; and (3) the general decrease of the righting reflex (i.e., the reflex that enable one to maintain the body in alignment with the head and thus keep the body in an upright position). Treating underlying problems will usually help the patient to maintain a more effective gait during the early stages of AD. As the disease progresses, however, decreases in sensory interpretation, neurologic deficits, and hypertonia will require increased awareness and interventions by the caregiver to prevent falls.

Some patients complain of feeling cold, even on the warmest summer days. The level of activity and the amount of body fat present are among several factors that influence body comfort with regard to heat or cold. The best way to judge a patient's response to environmental temperature is to actually feel his or her skin. If perspiration is present, reduce the amount of clothing. Conversely, if the skin feels cold to the touch, the patient needs additional layers of clothing, even if such layers appear to be excessive.

Incontinence usually occurs during the later stages of AD. As a result of physical and cognitive changes, the patient no longer has the ability to maintain bowel and bladder control. Functional incontinence is associated with cognitive impairment. The loss of urinary control is directly related to physical and cognitive functioning or environmental barriers and constraints. Incontinence can also be a physical sign of a urinary tract infection or benign prostatic hypertrophy in older men. A thorough assessment of premorbid bladder and bowel function is essential, and so is the continuous assessment of medications, fluid and food intake, and potential environmental constraints, including side rails, poor lighting, and wheelchair seatbelts. (see Clinical Alert #2)

Physical and Laboratory Examinations

Additional information is available to help determine the cause and needs of the person with dementia. These include laboratory tests, neuroimaging, and neuropsychologic testing.

Nurses need to conduct a physical examination carefully and thoroughly to rule out neoplasia (e.g., brain tumors), metabolic disorders, systemic illnesses (e.g., hypertension, human immunodeficiency virus infection [HIV]), and polypharmacy. Physical examination, mental status assessment, and functional assessment are imperative to begin to develop a list of differential diagnoses.

No laboratory test exists to confirm AD. As previously noted, signs of some metabolic conditions appear to be dementia, but they are reversible with proper treatment. Laboratory tests that help with determining possible metabolic causes include tests to assess thyroid function (thyroid-stimulating hormone and thyroxine); liver function tests; B12 and folate levels; a complete blood cell count including differential and erythrocyte sedimentation rate; serum blood chemistries for electrolytes and glucose; and blood urea nitrogen and creatinine levels (Lab Tests Online, 2010). Evidence suggests that, in the absence of risk factors, testing for syphilis is not necessary (American Academy of Neurology, 2010).

Computed tomography scanning and magnetic resonance imaging may be useful for the diagnosis of vascular disease or for obtaining evidence of trauma or tumors. Less commonly, an Aβ42 and τ protein correlation test of the cerebrospinal fluid may be helpful for differentiating AD from other dementias. A decreased Aβ42 level and an increased level of τ protein indicate a higher probability of AD as compared with other dementias in symptomatic patients. Other less often used tests include the Apo-E genotype test, which is associated with late-onset AD, and the presenelin-1 test, which is associated with half of the cases of early-onset AD (Lab Tests Online, 2010).

Neuropsychologic testing is helpful for making the diagnosis of AD and for differentiating AD from other forms of dementia. In addition, neuropsychologic testing can help to differentiate AD from other psychiatric problems (Alzheimer's Research Forum, 2007)

NURSING DIAGNOSIS

Nurses make diagnoses from information obtained during the assessment phase of the nursing process. The accuracy of diagnosis depends on a careful, comprehensive, and in-depth nursing assessment. Diagnoses are prioritized according to patient needs, from most urgent to least urgent.

Safety or health risks include the following:
- Risk for aspiration
- Risk for imbalanced body temperature
- Risk for infection
- Risk for injury
- Impaired physical mobility
- Bathing/hygiene self-care deficit
- Dressing/grooming self-care deficit
- Feeding self-care deficit
- Toileting self-care deficit
- Insomnia
- Wandering

Perceptual/cognitive disturbances include the following:
- Anxiety
- Impaired verbal communication
- Acute confusion
- Chronic confusion
- Grieving
- Disturbed personal identity
- Impaired memory
- Risk for powerlessness
- Ineffective role performance
- Impaired social interaction
- Disturbed thought processes

Disruption in coping abilities (patient or family) may be demonstrated by the following:
- Caregiver role strain
- Risk for caregiver role strain
- Impaired verbal communication
- Compromised family coping
- Interrupted family processes
- Hopelessness
- Ineffective therapeutic regimen management

OUTCOME IDENTIFICATION

Outcome criteria come from nursing diagnoses and are the expected patient responses to be achieved. In actual clinical situations, outcomes have time frames for attainment and are prioritized according to patient needs, from most urgent to least urgent. Outcomes considered for patients with cognitive disorders include those listed here.

The patient will do the following:
- Maintain health and safety with caregiver help.
- Reach and maintain the highest functional level possible within his or her capacity.
- Maintain the best possible physical status.
- Participate in a therapeutic activity program for cognitive stimulation and socialization and to meet other psychosocial needs.

- Participate in planning for care within his or her capacity, especially with regard to making legal and financial decisions while the ability for decision making is still intact. The caregiver will do the following:
- Maintain the best personal physical and mental health status.
- Initiate contacts with support services for legal and financial planning, support groups or individual counseling, case management, and respite services.
- Increase his or her knowledge base regarding the disease process, positive behavior interactions, and therapeutic activities.

PLANNING

The nurse needs to address a few common issues to achieve appropriate planning for the patient with a cognitive disorder. Care planning is prioritized according to patient needs, from most urgent to least urgent.

Short-Term and Long-Term Goals

Nurses in diverse roles will have contact with patients and their families for varying lengths of time. Acute care nurses often have only hours or days to formulate and implement a treatment plan, so their opportunities to assess, diagnose, identify outcomes, plan, implement, and evaluate focus on the resolution of immediate problems (e.g., trauma crisis; preoperative or postoperative care; the stabilization of medical, health, and safety needs).

Nurses who specialize in chronic care, psychiatry, and geriatrics focus on maintaining the patient's highest functional level, educating the caregiver about effective and realistic outcomes and interventions, and referring the patient and family to available options for care in the home and in the community.

Flexibility and Change

Care plan documentation is not permanent, because care plans change as often as assessment indicates. Acute care nurses need to adapt the care plan to fit the patient's needs as each shift changes, whereas nurses in long-term care need to set routine times (e.g., every 3 months) to closely examine the patient's needs and adjust care accordingly.

Collaboration

Collaboration by both acute care and long-term care nurses as well as other members of the health care team is critical; the collective knowledge and experience at all levels ensure more effective and realistic patient outcomes as well as caregiver gratification.

IMPLEMENTATION

The care and treatment of patients with cognitive disorders present the nurse or caregivers with a variety of situations that are both challenging and gratifying. Each plan of care needs to reflect the unique qualities of the individual and give

special consideration to the family as well as the patient. It is the nurse who keeps the health care team focused on both short- and long-term goals that address patient problems that result from dementia and delirium.

Caregiver and support system integrity will be maintained by involving the family and significant others in planning, intervention, and evaluation. As Sanders and colleagues (2008) revealed, nurses need to be acutely aware of how much their knowledge, compassion, and expression of concern can affect the experience of grief by caregivers (see the Research for Evidence-Based Practice box on p. 382). The Patient and Family Teaching Guidelines box lists issues to address with regard to caregiver involvement. Nurses need to address advance directives, living wills, and treatment options early. The patient needs a realistic knowledge base regarding the patient's diagnosis, treatment, and prognosis. As the therapeutic relationship between the nurse, the patient, and the family and caregivers develops, the nurse will be able to introduce these sensitive and often painful topics while preserving hopefulness and family integrity. Types and levels of care are listed in Box 16-4, p. 381.

Nursing Interventions

Nursing interventions are prioritized according to patient needs, from most urgent to least urgent.

Structure

1. Inform all caregivers (i.e., family and nursing) about the nursing care plan *to maintain a consistent physical and cognitive approach that ensures patient safety and integrity.*
2. Identify the patient's current functional state, and encourage the patient to use his or her skills *to promote independence as long as possible.*
3. Set up fairly structured routines. *This helps to overcome short-term memory losses, to promote independence, and to reduce anxiety.*
4. Allow the patient time to himself or herself. Do not overstimulate and fatigue the patient *to ensure the patient's privacy, to demonstrate respect, and to conserve the patient's energy.*
5. Remain flexible with the daily schedule *to promote the patient's feelings of security and to reduce frustration.*

Approach

1. Keep all interactions with the patient pleasant, calm, and reassuring *to decrease anxiety, because patients with cognitive disorders copy the emotional climate around them.*
2. Do not ask the patient to participate in ADLs when he or she is agitated, *because this will only increase the patient's frustration.*
3. Attempt to understand the patient's feelings *to decrease frustration and meet patient needs.*
4. Respond to the patient's feelings and validate them with words, body language, and actions *to help the patient to feel understood and to increase his or her feelings of self-worth.*

BOX 16-4   TYPES AND LEVELS OF CARE FOR COGNITIVE DISORDERS

Acute Care

Nurses who work in clinics, physicians' offices, emergency departments, urgent care units, and acute care facilities need to be alert to the signs and symptoms of cognitive impairment. It is critical that nurses understand the differences between dementia, delirium, and depression and that they plan accordingly. Nursing care needs to be holistic, with assessments and interventions designed to meet the needs of the caregiver as well.

Day Care

Adult day health care licensing regulations throughout the country vary, but, in general, the focus of these centers is on education, rehabilitation, training, the maintenance of physical function, and mental status. Dementia day care provides specialized respite, education, and support for the caregivers of patients with dementia. These programs offer therapeutic activity groups and appropriate behavior management approaches for the patient with dementia.

In-Home Care

As the disease progresses, an increasing amount of physical and emotional support will be necessary. The role of nurse case managers is to coordinate and provide appropriate care for the patient and the caregiver in the home. This enables the patient to stay at home longer, thus increasing the quality of life, conserving financial and emotional resources, and postponing institutionalization.

Residential Care Facility

There are many residential care options, and state regulations vary. The services offered generally include housekeeping and communal meals, which are sufficient during the early stages of AD. However, as deficits in memory and decision making increase, more supervision will be necessary. A residential care facility is an appropriate placement during the moderate stage of dementia, because physically the patient is sometimes active and otherwise well. Residential care staff members are usually specially trained in dementia care and interact positively for successful outcome achievement.

Skilled Nursing Facility

Skilled nursing facilities provide 24-hour professional nursing care. Patients with late-stage AD are admitted as a result of their extensive physical care needs. Financing this phase of the long-term care continuum is becoming increasingly problematic. The financial resources of the patient, the family, and the state and federal governments all become involved.

Hospice Care

Patients with late-stage AD are terminally ill and eligible for hospice care services. Hospice care for both the patient and the family focuses on quality-of-life issues. Lifesaving measures are not used. Instead, hospice care makes patients comfortable and supports families during the final stage of illness.

---

5. Help the patient to maintain his or her self-esteem by keeping interactions on an adult level. Use proper names *to avoid infantilizing or patronizing the patient. Remember that, despite their cognitive losses, patients do not lose their sense of being an adult.*

Communication

1. Simplify the verbal message, and use no more than five or six words at a time. Accompany words with visual or tactile clues *to decrease confusion and to increase the clarity of the message.*
2. Break down each task into separate components *to avoid confusion and frustration.*
3. Repeat the message, if needed, and allow time for the patient to respond. Use the same words. Do not go on to another message until you are sure that the patient understands the first one; do not leave and return to explain it in a different way. *Using these techniques will avoid or lessen such common behavior problems as catastrophic reactions (see Box 16-3) and sundowning, and they will prevent excess disability.*

Choices

1. Provide the patient with an opportunity to make simple choices. *Choosing offers the patient some control and helps him or her to maintain a sense of independence.*

2. Avoid questions for which the answer could be "no." *The opportunity for the patient to say "no" creates roadblocks to providing care and promoting activities.*
3. Present choices or situations that promote success *to increase the patient's self-esteem.*
4. Praise successes and facilitate the use of the patient's remaining strengths *to increase the patient's self-esteem and to reduce his or her sense of failure.*
5. If errors or failures occur, assure the patient that no harm has been done, and avoid any criticism. Avoid negative responses and commands, and avoid "why" questions. *Patients with dementia are often aware that there is something wrong with their performance, and they do not totally comprehend their environment. They are sensitive to criticism, and they are not always able to respond to "why" questions, which may provoke a sense of failure.*
6. Involve the patient in activities in which he or she wants to participate. Arrange the activity to be a one-to-one or small-group activity for a short period *to decrease resistance and to promote success.*

Additional Treatment Modalities
Interdisciplinary Team

The purpose of the interdisciplinary team is to provide comprehensive holistic care to a patient with measurable outcomes (see the Additional Treatment Modalities box). Older

RESEARCH FOR EVIDENCE-BASED PRACTICE

Sanders S et al: The experience of high levels of grief in caregivers of persons with Alzheimer's disease and related dementia, *Death Stud* 32:495-523, 2008.

In this qualitative study, the authors wanted to describe the lived experience of spouses and adult children who are caregivers of people with dementia and who are experiencing high levels of grief. The study is part of a larger mixed-method descriptive study. The authors' search of the literature demonstrated that individuals who experience intense and prolonged grief symptoms are at risk for physical and mental health consequences. Because the progression of this disease can last from 3 to 20 years, these symptoms are of great concern. Participants in the study were required to be a spouse or an adult child and a primary or secondary caregiver of a person with dementia. All participants completed questionnaires and interviews. The lived experience of caregivers who scored high on the Marwit and Meuser Caregiver Grief Inventory, Short Form (MM-CGI-SF), was described. Three subscales were identified that included the burden of personal sacrifice, sadness and longing, and worry and isolation. Seven main themes were identified: (1) yearning for the past; (2) regret and guilt; (3) isolation; (4) restricted freedom; (5) life stressors; (6) systemic issues; and (7) coping strategies. The researchers found that there was a significant difference between members of the high-grief group and the moderate- and low-grief participants with regard to each of the seven themes. High-grief participants yearned for normalcy in their lives; they felt guilt, particularly with regard to the relationship with the person with dementia; they felt alone, and they identified the person with dementia as their primary source of support; and they felt that there was no escape from their situation. They experienced more life stressors, such as deaths in the family and financial difficulties. They felt that they had many more obstacles to care than did those in the moderate- and low-grief group. They were more likely to believe that professionals who provide clinical services to caregivers did not understand the needs of the person with dementia and that these professionals adversely affected the care of the person with dementia by creating more anguish and grief with their actions. In addition, nurses were identified as being neglectful, and case managers were thought of as being unavailable and unresponsive. Professionals were identified as being inept and rude. Coping strategies used by members of the high-grief group were identified as spiritual faith, social supports, and animals and pets. Participants believed that they would not be doing as well as they were without their faith, their friends, their family members, their support groups, and their pets. Spouses expressed more yearning for the past and isolation, whereas adult children spoke of guilt and regret as well as systemic barriers. The strengths of the study were its multimethod design and its use of qualitative methods. Limitations include that the study may not be generalizable. The authors concluded that professionals need to be sensitive to patient and caregiver needs and to know what to do to help caregivers with their feelings. They suggested that the MM-CGI-SF is a tool that could be used to help to identify caregivers with high levels of grief and to provide a focus for future work. The researchers identified support groups, educational programs, and meetings of family members as ways to help caregivers learn and connect. The authors stated that, although grief needs to be addressed, experiencing times when the consequences of caregiving are not the primary focus is beneficial. Professionals need to help caregivers to develop their coping skills of faith, social supports, and pets. The authors concluded that professionals need to be educated about the needs of caregivers to provide needed services without magnifying the grief that the caregivers experience.

PATIENT AND FAMILY TEACHING GUIDELINES

Cognitive Disorders

- A strong professional and family support network is important for the caregiver who has to carry out exhausting tasks.
- Psychiatric intervention for the caregiver will help him or her adjust and cope with difficulties that arise.
- The caregiver needs the time and opportunity to mourn and complete the grieving process.
- Verbalizing concerns and feelings is important for coping.
- Action regarding finances need to be taken while the patient still retains the capacity to make decisions.

patients, especially those with cognitive disorders, have complex health, social, and economic problems that necessitate a comprehensive approach. The most important member of the interdisciplinary team is the patient (and, if appropriate, the family members). The following professionals are also part of the team: the nurse practitioner, the clinical nurse specialist, the gerontologist, the geropsychiatrist, the social worker, the dietitian, the pharmacist, and the rehabilitation specialists (e.g., speech, physical, occupational), each with a special knowledge of gerontology.

Pharmacologic Interventions

Decreased cholinergic functioning leads to disruptions in memory (Stahl, 2008). ACh mediates thinking and memory, and it is reduced in patients with AD and in those with some other dementias (e.g., PD, LBD). Because acetylcholinesterase (AChE) is responsible for the breakdown of ACh within the synaptic spaces of the neurons, cholinesterase inhibitors (i.e., drugs that inhibit the action of AChE) have improved the symptoms of AD by increasing the availability of ACh in the synapses. The goal of treatment is to improve symptoms and to stop the progression of the disease. Interventions provided earlier during the course of dementia will possibly lead to clinically meaningful improvements in function, behavior, and cognition (American Academy of Neurology, 2010). However, AChE inhibitors are more often shown to prevent or slow the decline in function in Alzheimer's for several months rather than to improve their functioning above baseline (Stahl, 2008).

Four cholinesterase inhibitors are currently available for the treatment of mild to moderate AD: (1) tacrine (Cognex); (2) donepezil (Aricept); (3) rivastigmine (Exelon); and (4) galantamine (Razadyne). A fifth drug, memantine (Namenda), has a different mechanism of action, and it is for the treatment of moderate to advanced AD (Stahl, 2008).

Tacrine (Cognex) was the first cholinesterase inhibitor available. It is rarely used now because of its side effect profile, its potential hepatic toxicity, and the need to take four doses per day (Stahl, 2008). Some patients who responded well to it may still be taking it.

Donepezil (Aricept) was the next of these drugs to be developed. It is usually well tolerated, and it requires only once-per-day dosing. It is believed that donepezil enhances cholinergic function by the reversible inhibition of the hydrolysis of ACh by AChE. It is effective when cholinergic neurons are intact. Over time, the degeneration of neurons occurs, and the effect may lessen. Donepezil may produce gastrointestinal side effects by inhibiting AChE in the periphery (Stahl, 2008).

Rivastigmine (Exelon) is indicated for the treatment of mild to moderate AD and PD (Novartis, 2006). It is possible that the drug inhibits AChE selectively in the cortex and the hippocampus more than in other parts of the brain (Stahl, 2008). Exelon is available in tablet, oral solution, and patch forms. The oral form requires twice-per-day dosing. According to Stahl (2009), this drug is advantageous for patients who do not respond to other anticholinergic drugs or who are in the later stages of AD. Side effects of rivastigmine include nausea, vomiting, and dizziness (Novartis, 2006). The transdermal form of rivastigmine is effective and has fewer peripheral side effects as compared with the oral form.

Galantamine (Razadyne) is the fourth and newest AChE inhibitor, and it is a reversible inhibitor of AChE. It is indicated for the treatment of mild to moderate AD (Ortho-McNeil, 2008). Like the other AChE inhibitors, it increases the availability of ACh; it also affects nicotinic cholinergic receptors in such a way that AChE inhibition can theoretically be enhanced (Stahl, 2008). Galantamine has been shown to decrease agitation and to increase cognition. The immediate-release form requires twice-daily dosing, and the extended-release form allows for once-daily dosing (Ortho-McNeil, 2008).

ADDITIONAL TREATMENT MODALITIES
Dementia and Alzheimer's Disease

- Interdisciplinary team
- Pharmacologic interventions
  - Drugs used to modify behavior and increase function
  - Drugs used in the therapy of AD
- Therapeutic activity programs

Memantine (Namenda) is indicated for moderate to severe AD (Forest Laboratories, 2007). It is the newest drug for AD that has a different mechanism of action from the AChE inhibitors in that it is an N-methyl-D-aspartate receptor

MEDICATION KEY FACTS
Alzheimer's Dementia

Mild to Moderate Alzheimer's Dementia
Cholinesterase Inhibitors
Donepezil (Aricept), tacrine (Cognex),* rivastigmine (Exelon), and galantamine (Razadyne)
- Do not use in children or in patients with conduction abnormalities, bradyarrhythmias, or sick sinus syndrome.
- Antipsychotics may exacerbate extrapyramidal symptoms.
- Anticholinergic agents produce antagonism effects.
- Nonsteroidal anti-inflammatory drugs may increase gastric acid secretion.
- Herbal considerations: Pill-bearing spurge (euphorbia) may increase the effects.

Moderate to Severe Alzheimer's Dementia
N-Methyl-D-Aspartate Antagonist
Memantine (Namenda)
- Alkaline agents (antacids) increase levels of memantine.
- No age-related precautions have been noted among elderly patients, but memantine is not recommended for elderly patients with severe renal impairment.
  First-line agents for delirium are atypical antipsychotics. See Chapter 13 for Medication Key Facts related to antipsychotics.

*Tacrine is rarely used because of the required frequency of dosing (four times daily) and the increased incidence of liver toxicity.

antagonist that blocks the effects of excess glutamate. Glutamate, which is an excitatory neurotransmitter, is the most abundant neurotransmitter. It is important for memory and learning, but it is toxic in excess amounts. Memantine blocks the excitotoxic effects of glutamate while allowing normal glutamate neurotransmission to occur (Stahl, 2008). It requires once-per-day dosing. (see Medication Key Facts box).

The therapeutic plan is individualized on the basis of presenting behavioral problems. Before initiating pharmacologic management for behavioral problems, it is important to exhaust all behavioral management techniques as well as environmental and social strategies.

After all other attempts have failed, medication is the most appropriate intervention for the agitated person with dementia, both for safety and quality of life. When intervening with behavior problems, it is important to remember that patients often communicate pain through behaviors other than words. If a patient in pain is medicated with a psychotropic drug, the behavior sometimes diminishes while the person continues to experience pain (Kovach et al, 2006).

Drug therapies need to be individualized for the patient, but several approaches to the treatment of agitation exist. Typical antipsychotics such as haloperidol have been used in the past, but, because of their side effect profile, other approaches are safer. The U.S. Food and Drug Administration (FDA) has issued black box warnings about the dangers of using typical and atypical antipsychotic drugs to treat agitation in elderly persons with dementia. Studies have revealed higher mortality rates when these drugs are used (U.S. Food and Drug Administration, 2008). Agitation and aggression are preferably treated with selective serotonin reuptake inhibitors such as citalopram (Celexa) and sertraline (Zoloft) or with serotonin norepinephrine reuptake inhibitors such as venlafaxine (Effexor) and desvenlafaxine (Pristiq) rather than with typical or atypical antipsychotic drugs (Stahl, 2008). Other pharmaceutic approaches include the administration of anticonvulsants such as divalproate sodium and carbamazepine; these may be helpful, and they do not carry black box warnings (Bronson, 2007). In addition, medications such as trazodone, which is a tricyclic-like serotonin reuptake inhibitor; buspirone, which is a nonbenzodiazepine anxiolytic; β-blockers, such as propranolol; and small doses of benzodiazepines may given (Alzheimer's Association, 2010e). The latter is especially effective in the presence of other problems, such as extrapyramidal symptoms and sleep disturbances, but it often creates an increased risk of falls and paradoxic agitation.

Some dementias result from the destruction of ACh neurons (e.g., in the nucleus basalis of Meynert), whereas other dementias that involve τ pathology do not. The dementias caused by alcohol, vascular damage, LBD, and PD are caused by the degeneration of acetylcholine neurons and may respond to AChE inhibitors. Alternatively, the frontal lobe and temporal lobe changes of FTLD, which does not involve ACh neurons, do not respond to AChE inhibitors (Stahl, 2008).

The results of studies of vitamin E for the prevention of AD are mixed, and, at this time, there is no convincing evidence that vitamin E slows the progression of AD (Stahl, 2008). Stahl also points out that there is concern about the health effects of long-term high doses of vitamin E. Researchers are investigating other antioxidants, and many other drug research studies are currently happening to find a drug that will slow or reverse the cognitive decline in persons with AD. For example, inflammation is implicated in the development of AD, and several studies have suggested that nonsteroidal anti-inflammatory drugs reduce the destructive effects of inflammation and the risk of the development of AD (Stahl, 2008).

Other pharmacologic agents that researchers are investigating for the treatment of cognitive symptoms include selegiline (Eldepryl), which is an antioxidant that may slow the progression of AD; vaccines, to decrease the production of β-amyloid protein; and statins, to lower cholesterol to reduce protein-related risks (Stahl, 2008).

For patients with hallucinations and paranoia, low-dose antipsychotics (most frequently risperidone [Risperdal]) may be necessary and helpful. Antipsychotic medications are frequently prescribed for patients with AD and other related dementias who demonstrate delusions and aggressive behaviors that pose dangers to the patients themselves or to others. Findings from a study sponsored by the National Institute of Mental Health (Schneider et al, 2006) confirm the potential lethal adverse effects of several newer antipsychotic drugs (e.g., olanzapine [Zyprexa], quetiapine [Seroquel], risperidone [Risperdal]) for elderly patients with heart problems and pneumonia. Again, the FDA has issued a black box warning that all antipsychotics—both first and second generation—carry an increased risk of death for elderly patients with dementia. Research in this area continues (see Chapter 25).

Multisensory Experience

Multisensory environments (MSEs) were developed during the 1970s in Holland, and they were originally named *Snoezelen*. The word *snoezelen* is derived from two Dutch words that mean "to seek out or explore" and "to relax" (Snoezelen, n.d.). The concept of the MSE has grown in popularity since then, and MSEs are now used in a variety of settings for people with a broad range of difficulties, including dementia. An MSE is a controlled, safe, and comfortable environment that is designed to provide a multitude of sensory experiences for therapeutic benefit. It is nondirective, and participants choose the activities in which they wish to participate (Fowler, 2008). MSEs make use of a broad range of materials to create multisensory experiences for all of the senses, including sight, hearing, taste, smell, touch, and balance (Snoezelen, n.d.). Staal and colleagues (2007) found that MSEs in combination with behavioral therapy for patients with moderate to severe dementia provided the following: (1) a greater decrease in the level of agitation as compared with the control group; (2) a decrease in apathy as compared with the control group, which had no change, and (3) a greater increase in general independence.

Therapeutic Activity Program

An activity is any project that a person enjoys and that produces a positive feeling. A therapeutic activity program is part of a total plan of care that is developed on the basis of an assessment of the patient's needs and the history of his or her previous activities. The activity program for persons with cognitive disorders is specifically designed to meet identified needs and to prevent or lessen problematic behaviors caused by unmet needs. An accurate and thorough assessment leads to the identification of these needs. Understanding how dementia-related changes influence the way that activities are structured will help caregivers to meet these needs (Smith et al, 2009). The goal is to keep the person functioning at the highest possible level. Programs that make use of a structured, comprehensive, and holistic approach that includes all daily activities and behaviors show the greatest success with regard to caring for individuals with dementia.

Building on strengths (e.g., retained remote memory, the use of habitual skills, preserved gross and fine motor skills, intact emotional responses) is the basis of success. It is exceedingly difficult if not impossible for the person with AD to learn new skills. "Use it or lose it" is a relevant motto when working with patients with dementia. After a patient loses a skill, it is usually gone forever, and the patient is not able to relearn it.

A therapeutic program is a primary treatment for persons with dementia, because often the first neurologic losses in these patients result in the inability to plan, initiate, carry out activities in ordered steps (sequence), or remember activities by themselves. Thus, it is the role of the caregiver to guide or assist the patient throughout the activity, from beginning to end. Use positive reinforcement each step of the way.

Nurses measure the success of a therapeutic activity program with regard to some objective terms by addressing the following questions:

- Has the number of times per day or week that the patient is actively involved increased or decreased?
- Have incidents of catastrophic reactions or sundowning decreased?
- Have incidents of the patient aimlessly pacing or wandering and getting lost decreased?
- Has the level of functioning in ADLs and IADLs remained stable, or is it decreasing at a slower pace than before the program was initiated?
- Are caregivers feeling less stress, which is indicated by fewer incidents of anger or crying, improved sleep patterns, or enhanced feelings of physical and mental well-being?

EVALUATION

Evaluating the patient's progress and determining how much nurses have achieved satisfactory patient and caregiver outcomes are especially challenging when working with patients with AD and other cognitive disorders. Factors that influence success vary greatly with each person. Here are some questions that the nurse needs to clearly answer and understand before addressing specific topics:

- Is the cognitive impairment reversible or irreversible?
- For reversible dementias, has the underlying medical condition or substance use been identified and resolved?
- Is the patient experiencing delirium, depression, dementia, an amnestic disorder, or a combination of these?
- What is the setting (i.e., acute care, long-term care, home)?
- Is the living situation adequate for the patient's needs?
- Are ADLs, nutrition and safety concerns, and emotional and activity needs adequate for the patient's condition or stage of progression?
- What is the caregiving situation?
- Are caregiver resources, knowledge, and understanding adequate? Are additional resources or training sessions needed?
- What medical and psychiatric problems have been identified during the nursing assessment and history taking?
- What is the patient's current medication profile?
- Is medication adherence a problem?
- Have medications for the treatment of AD been ordered? If so, are side effects a problem?
- Are there difficulties obtaining adequate medical supervision?
- What behavioral problems have been identified?
- What behavioral interventions have been effective?
- What is the patient's functional status?
- What is the interdisciplinary plan of care?

When the nurse has answered these questions satisfactorily, the interdisciplinary team will be better able to determine how the specifics of the patient outcomes have been achieved.

◎ NURSING CARE PLAN

Anita, a 71-year-old married woman, was referred to a home health nurse by her primary physician for evaluation for home care. Anita was diagnosed with probable AD with a secondary diagnosis of controlled type 2 diabetes. Anita's husband of 49 years, Karl, is a 69-year-old part-time pharmacy representative who travels occasionally. When he is gone, Anita's widowed sister, Alma, stays with Anita both day and night. The sisters are very close, but it is becoming more difficult for Alma to manage Anita. After an interview with Anita, Karl, and Alma, the following information about Anita's condition was determined:

- Anita has a 2-year history of recent memory loss, which is getting progressively worse.
- Anita appears to understand the spoken language only if thoughts are stated slowly and in simple, concrete terms.
- Anita's expressive language lacks the correct grammar, and there is evidence of word searching and parroting words used by the interviewer.

- Anita's recent episodes of crying, negativity, and angry verbal outbursts have caused the family and their community of friends concern and fear.
- Anita has a history of being well-groomed, but she now refuses to bathe and change clothes; she also dresses inappropriately, putting on clothes in the wrong sequence.
- Karl has been staying away more on his business trips and leaving the care of his wife to Alma, who is also in charge of checking Anita's blood sugar.
- Alma is not eating well, she is losing weight, and she has been dropping out of her personal and social activities; her friends in the community are becoming concerned about her.
- Anita is also frustrated with her condition, and she is occasionally aware that "things are not the same."

DSM-IV-TR Diagnoses

Axis I   Dementia of the Alzheimer's type with cognitive-perceptual disturbances
          Dementia of the Alzheimer's type with behavioral disturbances

Continued

◎ NURSING CARE PLAN—cont'd

Axis II   Rule out dependent personality disorder (traits)
Axis III   Diabetes type 2, controlled
Axis IV   Patient is occasionally aware of her decline and expresses frustration.
           Patient misses her husband whenever she can remember their life together.
Axis V   GAF = 35 (current); GAF = 45 (past year)

Nursing Diagnosis   *Disturbed thought processes related to the inability to process and synthesize information as evidenced by recent memory loss (becoming progressively worse), decreased ability to reason and form judgments, and interruption in logical stream of thought*

NOC Safe home environment; Cognitive orientation; Concentration; Memory; Information processing; Communication: expressive; Communication: receptive; Medication response,
NIC Environmental management: safety, Cognitive stimulation, Memory training, Dementia management, Reminiscence therapy, Medication management, Family support

PATIENT OUTCOMES	NURSING INTERVENTIONS	EVALUATION
Anita will use her intellect and judgment to the best of her ability with the help of family and caregivers.	Develop a stimulating therapeutic activities program. *Cognitive stimulation in deficit areas and positive reinforcement promote self-esteem and encourage Anita to attain the highest functional level possible.*	Karl and Alma find that Anita enjoys walks, and they establish routines. Anita recognizes some previously familiar birds and indicates that she wants birdseed to feed them. She also enjoys simple puzzles and assisting Alma with laundry tasks.
Anita will retain some control in her life by exercising her right to choose.	Monitor Anita's environment and activities and collaborate with all caregivers to do the following: Simplify her choices of food, clothes, colors, and activities. Use multiple sensory cues—especially auditory, visual, and tactile—to indicate choices. *Choices, even simple ones, give control back to Anita and improve her self-esteem, thereby making her more willing to try to participate in daily activities.*	Anita is responding to the use of multiple cues by increasingly exercising her right to choose. During the first week, Anita makes independent choices five times. During the second week, she makes seven choices.
Anita will be oriented to place, time of day, scheduled activities, and family members.	Develop simple calendars with daily routines, and provide easy-to-read clocks. Encourage family members to repeat their names and relationships often during conversations with Anita. *These actions assist with overcoming recent memory loss. Establishing routine decreases the stress of making decisions; verbal cues reinforce recognition and eliminate the need to chat.*	After 2 weeks, Anita knows the time for her walks with Karl and indicates that she wants her supply of birdseed. She is less frequently confused regarding the identification of persons, and she never fails to recognize Karl and Alma.
Anita will use remote memory during periods of reminiscence.	Make time each day for periods of reminiscence with the use of old photos, specially designed picture books, and rummage boxes. *The use of multiple sensory cues to stimulate remote memory builds on the retained strength of habitual skills to stimulate the use of remote memory.*	Anita looks at old photographs with Karl and Alma and indicates her recognition with short phrases and smiles. She independently finds a box of various colors and textures of yarns and handles them with satisfaction, indicating that she remembers knitting when she was well.
Anita will have decreased catastrophic reactions (see Box 16-3).	Analyze with all caregivers what the previous causes of catastrophic reactions have been. Simplify the environment; evaluate furniture, objects, colors, and noise level. *Analyzing and simplifying the environment maximizes the patient's safety and reduces the stressors that may cause catastrophic incidents. Collaborative planning ensures consistent successful approaches to tasks and reduces patient and caregiver stress.*	Anita has had two catastrophic reactions during the past 2 weeks. Karl and Alma analyze each incident and discover that the underlying causes were (1) increased noise from street repairs in front of the house and (2) being rushed to leave for a dental appointment.

◎ NURSING CARE PLAN—cont'd

Nursing Diagnosis *Self-care deficit (bathing/hygiene, dressing/grooming) related to perceptual and cognitive alterations secondary to neurologic damage in the brain as evidenced by the inability to recognize the need for self-care (bathing, changing clothes), the inability to dress in the right order, and the inability to reason and judge (inappropriate choice of clothing)*

NOC Self-care: bathing; Self-care: hygiene; Self-care: oral hygiene; Self-care: dressing; Coordinated movement; Self-direction of care; Self-care: activities of daily living; Patient satisfaction: physical care

NIC Dementia management: bathing; Self-care assistance: bathing/hygiene; Oral health maintenance; Self-care assistance: dressing/grooming; Teaching: individual; Self-care assistance: instrumental activities of daily living; Self-responsibility facilitation; Body image enhancement

PATIENT OUTCOMES	NURSING INTERVENTIONS	EVALUATION
Anita will bathe three times a week with prompting from family or caregivers.	Determine Anita's habitual time and manner of bathing. *Establishing a pattern on the basis Anita's previous habits will make use of her retained remote memory.* Ensure privacy *to preserve Anita's dignity and self-esteem.* Determine Anita's preferred room and water temperature. *Comfort and safety will encourage a positive patient response.* Reduce sensory stimulation (i.e., noise from the television, radio, other people) to enable the patient to attend to the task at hand. Mirrors need to be covered if the patient incorrectly interprets the reflection to be an observer. *Limiting the number of responses required by Anita facilitates her cooperation and independence.* Provide a home health aide three times a week for 2 weeks. *The caregivers Alma and Karl will increase their knowledge and skills and thus enhance their confidence and ease with regard to assisting Anita. The home health aide will teach the caregivers ways to maintain Anita's skin integrity and general health. The supervising nurse will check on Anita's general health status and her type 2 diabetes.*	The home health aide (HHA) successfully bathes Anita twice during the first week with Alma's help. During the second week, Alma is successful on two occasions with the HHA assisting. Extend HHA assistance for 1 more week, and then reevaluate.
Anita will be well groomed with the assistance of family and caregivers, and she will comply with dental and hygiene care.	Determine Anita's areas of dysfunction in grooming. Set adequate routines that involve visual and verbal cues to assist with grooming routines. Assist directly only as necessary to help Anita to complete a task. Use positive reinforcement. Refer Anita for dental prophylaxis, and assist the family with preplanning with the dentist and hygienist for a successful visit. Assist Karl and Alma with formulating a follow-up plan for Anita's daily oral hygiene. *These interventions reduce stress for both the patient and her caregivers, provide a positive environment, avoid unnecessary physical disabilities, and promote physical well-being.*	Alma and Karl are successful on 5 out of 7 successive days with cueing Anita to complete her dental hygiene and with helping her to comb her hair. An appointment is made with the dentist who previously cared for Anita, and Karl informs the dentist of the present situation. Evaluate the success of the visit later.

Continued

◎ NURSING CARE PLAN——cont'd

PATIENT OUTCOMES	NURSING INTERVENTIONS	EVALUATION
Anita will dress herself appropriately with assistance from family and caregivers as needed.	Check Anita's clothing supply. Simplify dressing choices for Anita by doing the following: Remove clothes that are not currently being worn. Assemble coordinated outfits on one hanger, and limit these to six to eight choices. Stack clothes in the order in which they are to be put on. Sort clothes and assist the family with choosing those that are appropriate yet easy for Anita to put on (e.g., eliminate buttons, buckles, and pantyhose, and provide clothes with elastic waistbands, snaps, Velcro fasteners, and knee- or thigh-high hose). *Anita will retain control and independence by making some simple clothing decisions, and she will be socially appropriate in her attire, thus increasing her self-esteem and reducing stress for all.*	The family, the nurse, and the HHA see improvements in Anita's appearance, and Anita is responding to compliments about her appearance by smiling. Karl is having some problems adjusting to the changes in Anita's dress style (i.e., not putting on pantyhose and high-heeled shoes, as she often had) and with moving out of the closet some of Anita's outfits that he especially likes. Alma comments favorably on the ease of dressing Anita now and on Anita's increased comfort, which is evidenced by Anita's willingness to participate in activities and her calmer interactions.

CHAPTER SUMMARY

- The prevalence of dementia increases with age.
- AD is the most common form of dementia.
- The cause of AD is unclear. Current theories include genetics, abnormal proteins and their products, neurotransmitter and receptor deficiencies, angiopathy, and blood-brain barrier incompetence.
- The key pathologic process of dementia is abnormal amyloid in the brain, which alters the brain's metabolism and results in neuronal death.
- The pathologic process of cognitive disorders results in neurologic deficits such as the reduced ability to perceive the environment and to organize appropriate responses, a decreased attention span, language deficits, memory loss, changes in emotional responses, and a decline in the ability to reason and form judgments.

- AD has three stages: mild, moderate, and severe.
- A variety of cognitive assessment tools are used to determine medical and nursing diagnoses.
- The nurse plans and supervises therapeutic activity programs to achieve the highest possible functional status for the patient and to prevent excess disability.
- Caring for a person with a cognitive disorder is a significant physical and emotional burden for caregivers.
- All nursing care for patients with cognitive disorders occurs in collaboration with the patient's caregivers.
- Nurses formulate care plans that are based on the assessment of both the patient's needs and the caregiver's needs.
- Successful care plans are developed on the basis of attaining a successful functional status and not on a curative basis.

REVIEW QUESTIONS

1. A nurse assists a patient with moderate stage AD at mealtime. Which statement should the nurse use?
   1. "Would you like beans or potatoes?"
   2. "Why aren't you eating your dinner, honey?"
   3. "Your food is getting cold. Eat your dinner now."
   4. "If you don't eat, you could get dehydrated."

2. A nurse counsels family members of a patient with early AD regarding the stages of the disease. Order these symptoms in the sequence that they are most likely to occur.
   1. Urinary incontinence
   2. Neologisms
   3. Apraxia

3. An elderly patient is hospitalized with pneumonia and treated with multiple antibiotics. After 2 days, the patient becomes irritable and restless, and he says to the nurse, "My pet parakeet flew across the room." A family member says that the patient has been healthy and living independently but that he does not own a pet. Select the most likely analysis of this scenario.
1. The patient is delusional and likely experiencing depression.
2. The patient is experiencing illusions as a result of delirium.
3. Dementia has emerged as a result of the stress of the physical illness.
4. The antibiotic doses have been inadequate to treat the patient's infection.

4. A nurse prepares the plan of care for a 79-year-old patient with late-stage AD. Which nursing diagnoses would be priorities to include? You may select more than one answer.
1. Risk for infection
2. Acute confusion
3. Risk for aspiration
4. Impaired verbal communication
5. Hopelessness

5. A nurse administers medications to four patients with AD. Which medication would be expected to interfere with glutamate rather than with cholinesterase?
1. Donepezil (Aricept)
2. Rivastigmine (Exelon)
3. Galantamine (Razadyne)
4. Memantine (Namenda)

REFERENCES

Alagiakrishnan K, Blanchette P: *Delirium*, 2010 (website): http://emedicine.medscape.com/article/288890-overview. Accessed December 9, 2010.

Alzheimer's Association: *2010 Alzheimer's disease facts and figures*, *Alzheimers Dement* 6:158-194, 2010a.

Alzheimer's Association: *Alzheimer's facts and figures*, 2010b (website): www.alz.org/documents_custom/report_alzfactsfigures2010.pdf. Accessed December 9, 2010.

Alzheimer's Association: *Mild cognitive impairment*, 2010c (website): www.alz.org/alzheimers_disease_mild_cognitive_impairment.asp. Accessed December 9, 2010.

Alzheimer's Association: *Mixed dementia*, 2010c (website): www.alz.org/alzheimers_disease_mixed_dementia.asp. Accessed December 9, 2010.

Alzheimer's Association: *Related dementias*, 2010d (website): www.alz.org/alzheimers_disease_related_diseases.asp. Accessed December 9, 2010.

Alzheimer's Association: *Standardized treatments*, 2010e (website): www.alz.org/alzheimers_disease_standard_prescriptions.asp. Accessed December 9, 2010.

Alzheimer's Association: *What is Korsakoff's syndrome?* 2010f (website): www.alzheimers.org.uk/factsheet/438. Accessed December 9, 2010.

Alzheimer's Disease Research: *Plaques and tangles*, 2010 (website): www.ahaf.org/alzheimers/about/understanding/plaques-and-tangles.html. Accessed December 9, 2010.

Alzheimer's Research Forum: *Tests*, 2007 (website): www.alzforum.org/dis/dia/tes/default.asp. Accessed December 9, 2010.

American Academy of Neurology: *Detection, diagnosis and management of dementia*, 2010 (website): www.aan.com/professionals/practice/pdfs/dementia_guideline.pdf. Accessed December 9, 2010.

American Psychiatric Association: *Diagnostic and statistical manual of mental disorders*, ed 4, text revision, Washington, DC, 2000, American Psychiatric Association.

Bronson B: *Clinical correlations: how should you treat agitation in patients with dementia?* 2007 (website): www.clinicalcorrelations.org/?p=102. Accessed December 9, 2010.

Bryan KJ et al: Expression of CD74 is increased in neurofibrillary tangles in Alzheimer's disease, *Mol Neurodegener* 3:13-24, 2008.

Buschke H et al: Screening for dementia with the memory impairment screen. *Neurology* 52:231-238, 2007.

Centers for Disease Control and Prevention: *vCJD (Variant Creutzfeldt-Jakob disease)*, 2007 (website): www.cdc.gov/ncidod/dvrd/vcjd/. Accessed December 9, 2010.

Clark CM, Ewbank DC: Performance of the dementia severity rating scale: a caregiver questionnaire for rating severity in Alzheimer disease, *Alzheimer Dis Assoc Disord* 10:173-178, 1996.

Clary GL, Krishnan KR: Delirium: diagnosis, neuropathogenesis and treatment, *J Psychiatr Pract* 7:310-323, 2001.

Cotter VT et al: Cognitive function assessment in individuals at risk for Alzheimer's disease, *J Am Acad Nurse Pract* 15:79-86, 2003.

Devanand DP et al: Hippocampal and entorhinal atrophy in mild cognitive impairment: prediction of Alzheimer disease, *Neurology* 68(11):828-836, 2007.

Dennis MS: Other causes of dementia, *Psychiatry* 7(1):33-35, 2008.

Doerflinger DM: How to try this: the mini-cog, *Am J Nurs* 107(12)62-71, 2007.

Eggenberger ER et al: *Progressive supranuclear palsy*, 2010 (website): http://emedicine.medscape.com/article/1151430-overview. Accessed December 9, 2010.

Folstein MF et al: "Mini-mental state": a practical method for grading the cognitive state of patients for the clinician, *J Psychiatric Res* 12:189-198, 1975.

Forest Laboratories: *Namenda prescribing information*, 2007 (website): www.frx.com/pi/namenda_pi.pdf. Accessed December 9, 2010.

Fowler S: *Multisensory rooms and environments: controlled sensory experiences for people with profound and multiple disabilities*, Philadelphia, 2008, Jessica Kingsley.

Gellis ZD et al: *Treatments for depression in older persons with dementia* (website): www.annalsoflongtermcare.com/content/treatments-depression-older-persons-with-dementia. Accessed December 9, 2010.

Graff-Radford NR, Woodruff BK: Frontotemporal dementia, *Semin Neurol* 27(1):48-57, 2007.

Holtzer R et al: Depressive symptoms in Alzheimer's disease: natural course and temporal relation to function and cognitive status, *J Am Geriatr Soc* 53:2083-2089, 2005.

Horgas A: *Assessing pain in older adults. Alzheimer's Association Try This: best practices in nursing care to older adults*, 2007 (website): consultgerirn.org/uploads/File/trythis/try_this_d2.pdf. Accessed December 9, 2010.

Kannayiram A, Blanchette P: *Delirium*, 2010 (website): http://emedicine.medscape.com/article/288890-overview. Accessed December 9, 2010.

Katzman R: A neurologist's view of Alzheimer's disease and dementia, *Int Psychogeriatr* 16:259-273, 2004.

Kopelman MD: Disorders of memory, *Brain* 125:2152-2190, 2002.

Kovach J et al: The serial trial intervention: an innovative approach to meeting needs of individuals with dementia, *J Gerontol Nurs* 32:18-25, 2006.

Lab Tests Online: *Alzheimer's disease*, 2010 (website): www.labtestsonline.org/understanding/conditions/alzheimers-2.html. Accessed

Lewy Body Dementia Association (LBDA): *Lewy body dementia by Jane Kaiser*, 2010 (website): www.lbda.org/category/4336/lewy-body-dementia-by-janet-kaiser.htm. Accessed December 9, 2010.

McCusker J: The delirium index, a measure of the severity of delirium: new findings on reliability, validity, responsiveness, *J Am Geriatr* 52:1744-1749, 2004.

MedlinePlus: *Huntington's disease*, 2010 (website): www.nlm.nih.gov/medlineplus/ency/article/000770.htm. Accessed December 9, 2010.

Memory loss and the brain: Memory Disorder Project, The newsletter of the memory disorder project at Rutgers University, 2010; Gluck M, editor (website): www.memorylossonline.com/glossary/basalforebrain.html.

Moorhouse P: Screening for dementia in primary care, *Can Rev Alzheimers Dis Other Demen* 12(1):8-12, 2009.

Mulhausen P: *Geriatric lecture series: screening for dementia*, 2010 (website): www.healthcare.uiowa.edu/igec/e-learning/geriatric-lecture-series/assets/03_2010_presentation.pdf. Accessed December 9, 2010.

National Institute of Neurological Disorders and Stroke: *Creutzfeldt-Jakob fact sheet*, 2010a (website): www.ninds.nih.gov/disorders/cjd/detail_cjd.htm. Accessed December 9, 2010.

National Institute of Neurological Disorders and Stroke: *Frontotemporal dementia information page*, 2010b (website): www.ninds.nih.gov/disorders/picks/picks.htm. Accessed December 9, 2010.

National Institute of Neurological Disorders and Stroke: *Huntington's disease: hope through research*, 2010c (website): www.ninds.nih.gov/disorders/huntington/detail_huntington.htm. Accessed December 9, 2010.

National Institute of Neurological Disorders and Stroke: *Multi-infarct dementia information page*, 2010d (website): www.ninds.nih.gov/disorders/multi_infarct_dementia/multi_infarct_dementia.htm. Accessed December 9, 2010.

National Institute of Neurological Disorders and Stroke: *Progressive supranuclear palsy information page*, 2010e (website): www.ninds.nih.gov/disorders/psp/psp.htm. Accessed December 9, 2010.

National Institute of Neurological Disorders and Stroke: *Wernicke-Korsakoff syndrome information page*, 2010f (website): www.ninds.nih.gov/disorders/wernicke_korsakoff/wernicke-korsakoff.htm. Accessed December 9, 2010.

National Institute on Aging: *Alzheimer's disease genetics fact sheet*, 2009 (website): www.nia.nih.gov/alzheimers/publications/geneticsfs.htm. Accessed December 9, 2010.

National Institute on Aging: *Alzheimer's disease fact sheet*, 2010 (website): www.nia.nih.gov/Alzheimers/Publications/adfact.htm. Accessed December 9, 2010.

National Institutes of Health: *Cognitive and emotional health project: the healthy brain*, 2009a (website): http://trans.nih.gov/cehp/ReviewDocs.htm. Accessed December 9, 2010.

National Institutes of Health: *Frontotemporal dementia fact sheet*, 2009b (website): www.nih.gov/about/researchresultsforthepublic/Dementia.pdf. Accessed December 9, 2010.

Novartis: *Exelon prescribing information*, 2006 (website): www.pharma.us.novartis.com/product/pi/pdf/exelon.pdf. Accessed December 9, 2010.

Ortho-McNeil: *Razadyne prescribing information*, 2008 (website): www.ortho-mcneilneurologics.com/sites/default/files/shared/pi/razadyne.pdf#zoom=100. Accessed December 9, 2010.

Parachikova A et al: Inflammatory changes parallel the early stages of Alzheimer disease, *Neurobiol Aging* 28:1821-1833, 2007.

Psychological Assessment Resources: *Mini-mental state exam (MMSE)*, 2010a (website): www4.parinc.com/Products/Product.aspx?ProductID=MMSE. Accessed December 9, 2010.

Psychological Assessment Resources: *Mini-mental state exam, 2nd edition (MMSE-2)*, 2010b (website): www.minimental.com. Accessed December 9, 2010.

Rabins, PV: Memory. In *Johns Hopkins White Papers*, Baltimore MD, 2007, Johns Hopkins University, Medical Education Services.

Radiology Info: *Functional MR imaging—brain*, 2006 (website): www.radiologyinfo.org/en/info.cfm?pg=fmribrain. Accessed December 9, 2010.

Reisberg B et al: Practical geriatrics: an ordinal functional assessment tool for Alzheimer's type dementia, *Hosp Community Psychiatry* 36:593-595, 1985.

Sanders S et al: The experience of high levels of grief in caregivers of persons with Alzheimer's disease and related dementia, *Death Stud* 32:495-523, 2008.

Schneider LS et al: Effectiveness of atypical antipsychotic drugs in patients with Alzheimer's disease, *N Engl J Med* 355:1525-1538, 2006.

Shaw LN et al: Cerebrospinal fluid biomarker signature in Alzheimer's disease neuroimaging initiative subjects, *Ann Neurol* 65(4):403-413, 2009.

Smith M et al: Beyond bingo: meaningful activities for persons with dementia in nursing homes, *Ann Longterm Care* 17(7):22-30, 2009.

Staal JA et al: The effects of Snoezelen (multi-sensory behavior therapy) and psychiatric care on agitation, apathy, and activities of daily living in dementia patients on a short term geriatric psychiatric inpatient unit, *Int J Psychiatry Med* 37(4):357-370, 2007.

Stahl SM: *Stahl's essential pharmacology: neuroscientific basis and practical applications*, ed 3, New York, 2008, Cambridge University.

Stahl SM: *Essential psychopharmacology: the prescriber's guide*, ed 3, New York, 2009, Cambridge University.

Swanberg MM, Kalapatapu RK: *Parkinson disease dementia*, 2010 (website): http://emedicine.medscape.com/article/289595-overview. Accessed December 9, 2010.

Tardiff K: Delirium in older adults: deciphering this complex condition, *Adv Nurse Pract* 17(9):31-35, 2009.

Triebel KL et al: Declining financial capacity in mild cognitive impairment: a 1-year longitudinal study, *Neurology* 73:928-934, 2009.

Twedell D: Clinical updates: delirium, *J Cont Educ Nurs* 36:102-103, 2005.

University of California, San Francisco Medical Center: *Frontotemporal dementia*, 2009 (website): www.ucsfhealth.org/adult/medical_services/memory/fronto/conditions/ftd/signs.html. Accessed December 9, 2010.

U.S. Food and Drug Administration: *Information for professionals*: *conventional antipsychotics*, 2008 (website): www.fda.gov/Drugs/DrugSafety/PostmarketDrugSafetyInformationforPatientsandProviders/ucm124830.htm. Accessed December 9, 2010.

Venes D et al, editors: *Taber's Cyclopedic Medical Dictionary*, ed 20, Philadelphia, 2005, FA Davis Co.

Warden V et al: Development and psychometric evaluation of the pain assessment in advanced dementia (PAINAD) scale, *J Am Med Dir Assoc* 4:9-15, 2003.

Warren NM et al: Cholinergic systems in progressive supranuclear palsy, *Brain* 128:239-249, 2005.

Webster J, Grossberg GT: Strategies for treating dementing disorders, *Nurs Home Med* 6:161, 1996.

Webster JA et al: SORL1 as an Alzheimer's disease predisposition gene? *Neurodegener Dis* 5(2):60-64, 2008.

Williams DR, Lees AJ: Progressive supranuclear palsy: clinicopathological concepts and diagnostic challenges, *Lancet Neurol* 8(3):270-279, 2009.

Yang FM et al: Phenomenological subtypes of delirium in older persons: patterns, prevalence, and prognosis, *Psychosomatics* 50:248-254, 2009.

Yesavage JA et al: Development and validation of a geriatric depression screening scale: a preliminary report, *J Psychiatr Res* 17:37-49, 1983.

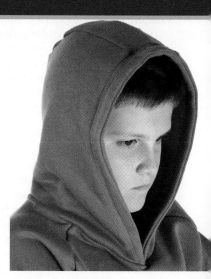

CHAPTER
17

Disorders of Infancy, Childhood, and Adolescence

Chantal M. Flanagan

"The potential possibilities of any child are the most intriguing and stimulating in all creation."

Ray L. Wilbur

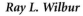 WEBSITE

http://evolve.elsevier.com/Fortinash/

OBJECTIVES

- Describe the symptomatology of infants, children, and adolescents for each of the following: autism, separation anxiety disorder, attention-deficit/hyperactivity disorder, intermittent explosive disorder, oppositional defiant disorder, and conduct disorder.
- Differentiate the symptoms that a child or an adolescent exhibits as compared with an adult for major depressive disorder, bipolar disorder, schizophrenia, and anxiety.
- Describe the methods that the interviewer will use to build trust and foster open communication with the child or adolescent patient.

- Discuss the components of a thorough nursing assessment and the application of the nursing process for infants, children, or adolescents.
- Identify five nursing interventions that are relevant for children and adolescents with behavioral disorders.
- Identify three effective ways to include the family in the treatment process for infants, children, and adolescents.

KEY TERMS

assent	consent	palilalia
behavior modification	coprolalia	stereotypic motor activities
behavioral contract	echolalia	therapeutic play
catastrophic reaction	echopraxia	tic

Changes within the family unit and advancing technologies have produced new challenges for the maturing child and adolescent. School-aged children are more adept than their parents with regard to surfing the Internet; engaging with communication media, such as Twitter; texting on cell phones; and using social networking services such as MySpace. This leaves the average parent at a loss regarding how to monitor and prevent unsafe behaviors, but the challenges that are seen and unseen are far greater for the children.

The family system has dramatically altered from two-parent homes to homes where single parents, same-sex parents, or grandparents serve as the primary caregivers.

Youth violence is widespread, with gang activities occurring and children bringing weapons to school. Supervision by parents and school personnel is diminishing as both parents work away from the home and schools become overcrowded. These factors make it difficult for the child to achieve the expected developmental, cognitive, and emotional milestones required to succeed later in life. The inability of a child to achieve these milestones impairs the child's ability to function at home or in school, and it hinders the child from developing healthy peer relationships, which often results in truculent behavior, drug and alcohol abuse, and mental disorders.

Mental disorders are increasing among children and adolescents. According to the U.S. Surgeon General's Report (1999), approximately 20% of children and adolescents suffer from some impairment as a result of a mental disorder. According to this report, from 5% to 9% of children and adolescents between the ages of 9 and 17 years have "serious emotional disturbances." Anxiety disorders are the most prevalent, with social phobia being the most common. Major depression is the second most commonly occurring disorder. The National Institute of Mental Health (2005) identified that 1 out of every 10 children in the United States suffers from a mental disorder that affects their ability to function in at least one environmental setting, such as school. Only half of these children are receiving professional mental health services.

Cultural values and beliefs may impede mental health treatment even further; African Americans and Mexican Americans are significantly less likely to seek mental health treatment as compared with Caucasians (National Institute of Mental Health, 2005).

Nurses have the opportunity to assess and treat infants, children, and adolescents in diverse health care settings. They play a key role in assessing for potential risk factors that occur before the appearance of a mental disorder. By listening to parental concerns and assisting parents with understanding normal developmental milestones and behaviors during the infancy and toddler stages, problematic behaviors and concerns can be prevented or identified early. Nurses then support the family and initiate access to multidisciplinary treatment modalities.

Some infants will present with colicky behavior, feeding and sleeping problems, and failure to thrive. Some toddlers will require treatment for behavioral problems such as aggression and impulsivity (Thomas et al, 1977). Children and adolescents often present symptoms differently from adults and frequently present with presumed medical problems when in fact the underlying problem is a mental disorder. Infants, children, and adolescents are often treated by their pediatricians. Consequently, symptoms are often misdiagnosed.

Nurses treat children and adolescents within the context of the family system; one cannot be separated from the other. It is important for the nurse to understand the mental health problems and needs that infants, children, and adolescents face and the effect that these issues will have on the growth and development of these young patients. This chapter discusses the major mental disorders that affect infants, children, and adolescents, and it provides direction for applying the nursing process to the assessment, diagnosis, and treatment of this population.

HISTORIC AND THEORETIC PERSPECTIVES

Child and adolescent emotional and behavioral issues were rarely discussed before the eighteenth century. Children with emotional problems were viewed as being possessed by evil spirits. There was no individualized treatment, because children were seen as miniature adults and treated the same way.

The beginning of the twentieth century marked the reform of child welfare. The Children's Bureau was founded in 1912 to protect the rights and welfare of children, and this included the introduction of child labor laws. Public school systems were also developed to guarantee education for all children. The first psychologic clinic for children was opened in 1896, but its focus was primarily on school-related issues (Silk et al, 2000).

President Harry Truman signed the National Mental Health Act on July 3, 1946. The National Institute of Mental Health was formed in 1949. At this time, many believed that mothers were responsible for their child's emotional and psychologic well-being. Psychiatrists and pediatricians started to train as child psychiatrists, and the American Academy of Child Psychiatry was formed in 1953. The National Institute of Mental Health funded programs for advanced education in infant, child, and adolescent psychiatric mental health nursing during the early 1950s (Schowalter, 2005).

SPECIFIC MENTAL DISORDERS

Note: some names of specific mental disorders and criteria that define them will change in the fifth edition of the *Diagnostic and Statistical Manual of Mental Disorders* (DSM5), due for publication in 2013.

Currently, the infant, child, and adolescent mental disorder classifications are as follows.

Mental Retardation
Etiology and Epidemiology

Mental retardation is listed under Axis II of the *Diagnostic and Statistical Manual of Mental Disorders,* fourth edition, text revision (DSM-IV-TR), and it is described as an intelligence quotient below 70 that impairs the individual's social adaptation and development in at least two areas, such as self-efficacy, interpersonal interactions, and cognition. The onset occurs before the age of 18 years (American Psychiatric Association, 2000).

Despite extensive evaluations, no definitive cause can be found in 58% to 78% of individuals with mild mental retardation and in 23% to 43% of individuals with severe or profound mental retardation. When it is found, the etiology is genetic, medical, environmental, or a combination of these. Researchers estimate the prevalence of mental retardation at 1% among the U.S. population (Szymanski et al, 1999).

Clinical Description

Subtypes. Approximately 85% of individuals with mental retardation have *mild retardation.* Children with mild retardation typically develop social and communication skills during the preschool years, have only minimal sensorimotor problems, and often are not identified until a later age. They generally acquire academic skills up to approximately the sixth-grade level. In adulthood, they generally achieve social and vocational skills that are adequate for minimum self-support. They usually require some level of supervision, guidance, and assistance (American Psychiatric Association, 2000).

Approximately 10% of the population with mental retardation has *moderate retardation*. Most individuals with moderate mental retardation acquire some communication skills during early childhood and benefit from vocational training, but they seldom advance academically beyond the second-grade level. With moderate supervision, they are usually able to provide for their own personal care and to learn to travel in familiar areas. Peer relationships often decline during adolescence because of problems with recognizing and acquiring socially correct interactions. During adulthood, these individuals generally perform unskilled or semiskilled work and live and function in the community in supervised settings (American Psychiatric Association, 2000).

About 3% to 4% of individuals with mental retardation have *severe retardation*. They typically acquire little if any communicative speech during early childhood, but they sometimes learn to use basic communication and to develop elementary self-care skills in the school-aged period. They may benefit from learning to sight read some "survival" words. As adults, some are able to perform simple skills in closely supervised settings. They generally live in some protected environment within the community, such as a group home or with their families, unless some other handicaps require specialized nursing or other care (American Psychiatric Association, 2000).

Only 1% to 2% of mentally retarded individuals suffer from *profound retardation*. Most also have identified neurologic conditions such as cerebral palsy, sensory deficits, epilepsy, and other neurologic disorders that cause the retardation. These individuals have considerable sensorimotor problems that are recognized during early childhood such as poor head control, feeding problems, and the inability to roll over. They require a highly structured setting with constant monitoring and assistance for the best possible development. With this level of care, some of these patients develop sufficient motor skills, self-care skills, and communication abilities to perform simple tasks in a closely supervised and sheltered setting (American Psychiatric Association, 2000).

Prognosis

The prognosis reflects the interaction of biomedical, psychologic, and environmental factors. Studies show that individuals with mild mental retardation may live reasonably satisfying and productive lives; on the other hands, those individuals with severe to profound mental retardation have a shortened life expectancy as a result of medical conditions such as epilepsy and feeding problems as well as limitations of self-care and communication (Szymanski et al, 1999).

PERVASIVE DEVELOPMENTAL DISORDERS

The onset of pervasive developmental disorders is usually observed before the age of 3 years as a result of parental concerns that the child has not achieved language skills and other developmental skills as expected. However, other children may not be identified until later during their school years. Impairments may be seen in language, cognition, behavior, and social interactions (American Psychiatric Association, 2000).

Autistic Disorder
Etiology

The exact cause of autism remains undetermined. Scientists offer several theories regarding the cause of this disorder. Possible causes include genetic, neurologic, metabolic, immunologic, and environmental factors as well as complications during birth. Most researchers agree that the etiology of autism is multifaceted and cite the combination of complex genetic factors with environmental exposures (Plauche et al, 2007). Excessive sugar, food sensitivity, food additives, vaccines, and allergies do not cause autism (Valente, 2004).

Epidemiology

Currently, studies suggest that the rate of autistic disorder is as high as 1 in 500 or fewer, whereas other sources such as the DSM-IV-TR report 5 cases per 10,000 children. According to the Autism Speaks Organization (2009), 1 in 110 children is affected, with 1 in 70 of these children being male. Rates are three to four times higher among males as compared with females. However, females with autism tend to have more severe mental retardation. Siblings of individuals with autism have an increased risk of developing autistic disorder (American Psychiatric Association, 2000; Volkmar, 1999). Family members of the autistic child sometimes have other behavioral and developmental disorders, such as attention-deficit disorder or Asperger's disorder (Valente, 2004). The American Academy of Pediatrics recommends that all children between the ages of 18 and 24 months be screened for autism (Plauche et al, 2007).

Clinical Description

A variety of behavioral symptoms are often present in these children, including any of the following: hyperactivity, short attention span, impulsivity, aggressiveness, self-injurious behaviors, and temper tantrums. Abnormal eating patterns (e.g., limiting intake to a few foods or eating non-nutritious objects) or sleeping patterns (e.g., recurrent awakenings with rocking) are present as well. These patients are often unable to tolerate even minor changes in their environment, and they may have an intense or catastrophic reaction to minor changes such as a new chair or a new seating arrangement at dinner. Some children demand the maintenance of nonfunctional and unreasonable adherence to rituals and routines.

Autistic children often demonstrate stereotypic motor activities (e.g., clapping or flapping of hands, spinning, rocking, swaying) and postures (e.g., walking on tiptoes, odd postures, strange hand movements). Their play cannot be disrupted, and these children often show intense preoccupation with objects such as buttons or zippers. They are frequently fascinated with the movement of such things as fans and revolving objects, the opening and closing of doors or drawers, or turning the light switch on and off. Some become attached to unusual objects, such as a piece of string or a rubber band, and they ignore typical items to which children usually become attached, such as a blanket or a teddy bear.

Individuals with autistic disorder typically lack emotional reciprocity, and they do not actively participate in simple social play or games. Instead, they prefer solitary activities, or they only attempt to involve others as objects of their play (e.g., an autistic child may position another child as bench to sit on). Mood or affective abnormalities are often present, such as giggling or weeping for reasons that are not apparent to the observer or showing no emotional reaction when a situation normally calls for a reaction. Sensory processing disorder is often seen in children with autism. This is a growing area being studied in which sensory signals are inappropriately organized and cause an abnormal response. In the future, this may be included as a separate diagnosis in the DSM-V. These children may have inappropriate responses to danger, such as showing no fear of real danger or excessive fear of harmless objects. Some also injure themselves by head banging or biting various body parts. Some have a high pain threshold, an oversensitivity to sound or touch, or an exaggerated response to light or color. Others have a fascination with a particular sensory stimulation, such as constantly rubbing a hard surface or a specific piece of furniture (Miller et al, 2007).

Approximately 80% of individuals with autistic disorder function in the mental retardation range; approximately 50% have severe or profound retardation, and 30% have mild retardation (Volkmar, 1999). Autism also affects other cognitive areas, such as insight, reasoning, and judgment.

Communication problems may present so severely in both verbal and nonverbal areas that spoken language is often absent. Individuals who do speak are not always able to begin or keep up a conversation with others, or they use such stereotyped and repetitive language that others find it difficult to continue a conversation. Speech often contains abnormal pitch, intonation, rate, and rhythm (e.g., a monotonous or inappropriate sing-song pitch and rhythm or question-like raises of tone at the end of declarative sentences). Grammar is often immature, stereotyped, and repetitive (e.g., the inappropriate repetition of jingles or commercials, regardless of meaning). Sometimes grammar is idiosyncratic so that only those familiar with the individual's use of language understand what the autistic child is communicating. Some individuals are not able to understand simple questions, directions, or jokes, whereas others develop excellent long-term memory of insignificant data such as train schedules, baseball statistics, songs, or dates (American Psychiatric Association, 2000; Volkmar, 1999) (see the DSM-IV-TR Criteria box). Some individuals with autistic disorder develop exceptional but circumscribed skills that are commonly referred to as "islands of genius." For example, a person may not be able to count appropriate change in a store but is able to quote and solve complicated mathematic formulas. Another example is when the individual with autism may not be able to read sheet music but can play complex symphonic pieces after hearing them only once.

DSM CRITERIA FOR AUTISM

A A total of six (or more) items from criteria 1, 2, and 3, with at least two from criterion 1 and one each from criteria 2 and 3:

1 Qualitative impairment in social interaction, as manifested by at least two of the following:

   a Marked impairment in the use of multiple nonverbal behaviors such as eye-to-eye gaze, facial expression, body postures, and gestures to regulate social interaction

   b Failure to develop peer relationships appropriate to developmental level

   c A lack of spontaneous seeking to share enjoyment, interests, or achievements with other people (e.g., by a lack of showing, bringing, or pointing out objects of interest)

   d Lack of social or emotional reciprocity

2 Qualitative impairments in communication as manifested by at least one of the following:

   a Delay in, or total lack of, the development of spoken language (not accompanied by an attempt to compensate through alternative modes of communication such as gesture or mime)

   b In individuals with adequate speech, marked impairment in the ability to initiate or sustain a conversation with others

   c Stereotyped and repetitive use of language or idiosyncratic language

   d Lack of varied, spontaneous make-believe play or social imitative play appropriate to developmental level

3 Restricted repetitive and stereotyped patterns of behavior, interests, and activities, as manifested by at least one of the following:

   a Encompassing preoccupation with one or more stereotyped and restricted patterns of interest that are abnormal either in intensity or focus

   b Apparently inflexible adherence to specific, nonfunctional routines or rituals

   c Stereotyped and repetitive motor mannerisms (e.g., hand or finger flapping or twisting, or complex whole-body movements)

   d Persistent preoccupation with parts of objects

B The client shows delays or abnormal functioning in at least one of the following areas, with onset before age 3 years: (1) social interaction, (2) language as used in social communication, or (3) symbolic or imaginative play

C The disturbance is not better accounted for by Rett's disorder or childhood disintegrative disorder

From the American Psychiatric Association: *Diagnostic and statistical manual of mental disorders,* ed 4, text revision, Washington, DC, 2000, American Psychiatric Association.

Prognosis

There is no cure for autism. Language skills and overall intellectual level are the strongest factors related to the ultimate prognosis. Earlier studies suggested a bleaker prognosis, with only a small percentage of individuals with this disorder living independently as adults. However, a recent study by Dawson and colleagues (2009) offers a more optimistic prognosis. In this randomized, controlled study, children from 18 to 30 months old who had been diagnosed with autism and who received early intervention demonstrated improvements in their intelligence quotient, language, and adaptive behaviors 2 years later to the degree that 30% of the population no longer met the criteria for autism but were then diagnosed with pervasive developmental disorder, not otherwise specified. In about a third of the autistic patients, some degree of partial independence is possible. The highest-functioning adults with autistic disorder typically continue to exhibit problems with social interaction and communication together with restricted interests and activities. Evidence demonstrates that early interventions help the patient achieve the highest level of functioning in social, communication, and cognitive skills.

Asperger's Disorder

Unlike autism, language and cognition are unaffected in patients with Asperger's disorder. However, many features are similar to those of autistic disorder, such as behavioral problems, underdeveloped or impaired social interactions, and restricted repetitive patterns (American Psychiatric Association, 2000). This disorder follows a continuous course, and the duration is usually lifelong. There is a better long-term outcome for individuals with Asperger's disorder than there is for those with autism. The prognosis for these patients is best if treatment begins by the time they are 24 to 36 months old (Tanguay, 2000; Volkmar, 1999).

DISORDERS OF INFANCY OR CHILDHOOD

Reactive Attachment Disorder
Etiology and Epidemiology

Reactive attachment disorder is a disorder that may occur in some children who experience pronounced parental physical and emotional abuse or neglect, or who are institutionalized, or who are exposed to extreme poverty. There is a disturbance in the way that these children relate to others, as described in the following sections. The prevalence rate is unclear, but the number of maltreated children in foster care is estimated at 12 per 1000 (U.S. Department of Health and Human Services, 2005).

Clinical Description

Reactive attachment disorder usually begins within the first few years of life and typically results from abusive or neglectful caregiving. This disorder has two subtypes: *inhibited* and *disinhibited*.

With the inhibited type, the child is unable to socially interact in accordance with his or her developmental level. Because of the lack of early healthy bonding and intimacy, the child fails to initiate or respond to social cues (e.g., fails to seek being comforted or to engage in social interactions). Some children are even fearful of accepting comfort from others. With the disinhibited type, the child lacks appropriate

DSM-IV-TR CRITERIA

Reactive Attachment Disorder

A Markedly disturbed and developmentally inappropriate social relatedness in most contexts, beginning before age 5 years as evidenced by either of the following:
   1 Persistent failure to initiate or respond in a developmentally appropriate fashion to most social interactions, as manifest by excessively inhibited, hypervigilant, or highly ambivalent and contradictory responses (e.g., the child may respond to caregivers with a mixture of approach, avoidance, and resistance to comforting, or he or she may exhibit frozen watchfulness)
   2 Diffuse attachments as manifest by indiscriminate sociability with a marked inability to exhibit appropriate selective attachments (e.g., excessive familiarity with relative strangers or lack of selectivity in choice of attachment figures)
B The disturbance in criterion A is not accounted for solely by developmental delay (as in mental retardation) and does not meet criteria for a pervasive developmental disorder.
C Pathogenic care is evidenced by at least one of the following:
   1 Persistent disregard of the child's basic emotional needs for comfort, stimulation, and affection
   2 Persistent disregard of the child's basic physical needs
   3 Repeated changes of primary caregiver that prevent formation of stable attachments (e.g., frequent changes in foster care)
D There is a presumption that the care in criterion C is responsible for the disturbed behavior in criterion A (e.g., the disturbances in criterion A began following the pathogenic care in criterion C).
   Specify type:
Inhibited type: if criterion A1 predominates in the clinical presentation
Disinhibited type: if criterion A2 predominates in the clinical presentation

From the American Psychiatric Association: *Diagnostic and statistical manual of mental disorders*, ed 4, text revision, Washington, DC, 2000, American Psychiatric Association.

boundaries and is unable to differentiate between strangers and safe attachment relationships. For example, these children may inappropriately seek comfort and attention from unknown adults (e.g., they may run up to strangers in a public place and hug them), or they may become distressed when they are separated from strangers (American Psychiatric Association, 2000; Boris et al, 2005) (see the DSM-IV-TR Criteria box).

Often the caregiver brings the child to the pediatrician and reports problems of severe colic or feeding difficulties, failure to gain weight, detached and unresponsive behavior, difficulty being comforted, or avoidance of social interactions (Maldonado-Duran et al, 2005).

Prognosis

Children may learn to develop healthy emotional attachments if they are placed in a stable, nurturing environment and receive necessary treatment (Maldonado-Duran et al, 2005).

Separation Anxiety Disorder
Etiology and Epidemiology

Separation anxiety disorder may be experienced by infants who are younger than 1 year old who are separated from their mothers. Children who are entering school for the first time may also exhibit symptoms. The disorder is more common among first-degree relatives, and it is possibly more common among children whose mothers have panic disorder. It usually develops after a stressful event (e.g., the death of a close and valued relative or pet, an illness in the child or parent, or a major change in the environment [e.g., a move to a new neighborhood]). This disorder occurs in approximately 4% of children and adolescents, and it is more common among females. Patients with the disorder typically present before late adolescence (American Psychiatric Association, 2000).

Clinical Description

The child exhibits at least three symptoms: excessive worry about being separated from the caregiver; significant distress when separated; and fear of being alone, which may include refusal to attend school, after-school activities, and camps. Academic difficulties result from a refusal to attend school and thus increases the problem with social avoidance. School refusal occurs in about 5% of all school-aged children, primarily between the ages of 5 and 6 years and 10 and 11 years (King, 2001) (see the DSM-IV-TR Criteria box).

Children with separation anxiety disorder demonstrate clinging behavior when in the presence of the caregiver, some to the point of following the caregiver to the bathroom. Bedtime is difficult, with the child or adolescent insisting that the parent remain with him or her until he or she falls asleep. During the night, these individuals often try to get into bed with parents or other significant figures. Some will even sleep outside the parent's door if they are unable to enter the room. Nightmares often contain elements of the child's fears, such as family death as a result of fire, murder, or another catastrophe.

Other symptoms of anxiety may also be present, including physical complaints such as stomachaches, headaches, nausea, and vomiting. Older children and adolescents experience a racing or pounding heart, dizziness, and faintness. These somatic complaints may lead to numerous trips to physicians and subsequent medical procedures.

Individuals with this disorder often experience recurrent and excessive distress when they are away from home or major attachment figures, and they are extremely fearful that imagined harm will happen to the significant others. Some become preoccupied with reunion fantasies. Fears about danger to themselves or their families sometimes present as fears of animals, monsters, the dark, muggers, burglars, kidnappers, accidents, or plane or train travel. Some fears also present as concerns about death and dying. These children show various moods, such as excessive worry that no one loves them and they therefore want to die; or unusual anger when someone tries to separate them from their parent or a significant other. At times, the depressed mood justifies a diagnosis of major depression. When these patients reach adulthood, some will develop panic disorder with agoraphobia.

Comorbidities are not uncommon and include other anxiety disorders, such as generalized anxiety disorder and social phobia, as well as major depressive disorder. Approximately 60% will have one of the other anxiety disorders, whereas 30% will have all three (Sadock and Sadock, 2007).

DSM-IV-TR CRITERIA

Separation Anxiety Disorder

A Developmentally inappropriate and excessive anxiety concerning separation from home or from those to whom the individual is attached, as evidenced by three or more of the following:
  1 Recurrent excessive distress when separation from home or major attachment figures occurs or is anticipated
  2 Persistent and excessive worry about losing or possible harm befalling major attachment figures
  3 Persistent and excessive worry that an untoward event will lead to separation from a major attachment figure (e.g., getting lost or being kidnapped)
  4 Persistent reluctance or refusal to go to school or elsewhere because of fear of separation
  5 Persistent and excessive fear or reluctance to be alone or without major attachment figures at home or without significant adults in other settings
  6 Persistent reluctance or refusal to go to sleep without being near a major attachment figure or to sleep away from home
  7 Repeated nightmares with the theme of separation
  8 Repeated complaints of physical symptoms (such as headaches, stomachaches, nausea, or vomiting) when separation from major attachment figures occurs or is anticipated
B The duration of the disturbance is at least 4 weeks.
C The onset is before age 18.
D The disturbance causes clinically significant distress or impairment in social, academic (occupational), or other important areas of functioning.
E The disturbance does not occur exclusively during the course of a pervasive developmental disorder, schizophrenia, or other psychotic disorder and, in adolescents and adults, is not better accounted for by panic disorder with agoraphobia.

From the American Psychiatric Association: *Diagnostic and statistical manual of mental disorders,* ed 4, text revision, Washington, DC, 2000, American Psychiatric Association.

Prognosis

There may be periods of severity and periods of a reduction of symptoms. Both the anxiety about possible separation and the avoidance of situations that involve separation may persist for many years. Prognosis typically depends on the age of onset, the duration, and the coexistence of other disorders. Children who attend school and after-school activities and who have healthy peer and parental relationships do better than those who do not (Sadock and Sadock, 2007).

CASE STUDY

The mother of a 4-year-old boy is seeking an evaluation of her son. She reports that her son has no friends in preschool and that he is always playing alone. He says some words, but he does not speak in sentences. At times, he can be seen rocking back and forth, especially when he appears to be anxious. He enjoys looking at baby pictures of himself, and he will often organize them chronologically. He does not use eye contact when he speaks.
1 What questions will the nurse ask the mother?
2 What laboratory tests would be helpful?
3 How would you educate the mother about her son's behaviors and available resources?

TIC DISORDERS

Tourette's Disorder
Etiology and Epidemiology

Tourette's disorder is most often a genetic neurologic disorder, although other factors are responsible in 10% to 15% of children, including head trauma, carbon monoxide poisoning, and complications from pregnancy. Tourette's disorder occurs in approximately 5 to 30 of every 10,000 children and 1 to 2 of every 10,000 adults. It is approximately two times more common in males than in females. Other disorders associated with Tourette's disorder include attention-deficit/hyperactivity disorder (ADHD), obsessive-compulsive disorder, and learning disorders (American Psychiatric Association, 2000).

Clinical Description

With Tourette's disorder, the individual experiences multiple motor tics and at least one vocal tic many times a day for at least 1 year. The individual's ability to function is impaired. A tic is a sudden, rapid, involuntary, and repetitive movement or vocalization (American Psychiatric Association, 2000). Although tics are experienced as irresistible, some patients are able to suppress them for varying lengths of time. Stress typically exacerbates tics, while distracting activities such as reading or sewing may reduce them. Tics are often markedly decreased or absent during sleep.

Some simple motor tics include eye blinking, neck jerking, shoulder shrugging, facial grimacing, and coughing. Simple vocal tics include throat clearing, grunting, sniffing, snorting, and barking. Complex motor tics are expressed as facial gestures, grooming behaviors, jumping, touching, stamping, smelling an object, and echopraxia, which is the imitation of

another's movements. Complex vocal tics include coprolalia, palilalia, and echolalia.

Coprolalia is the repeating of socially unacceptable words, typically obscene words. Palilalia is the repeating of one's own sounds or words. Echolalia is the repeating of the last-heard words, sounds, or phrases of another person.

Common vocal tics include clicks, grunts, barks, sniffs, snorts, and coughs. Coprolalia occurs in less than 10% of the cases. Complex motor tics reported with Tourette's disorder include touching, squatting, deep knee bends, retracing steps, and twirling during walking. The most frequent initial tic is blinking. Other initial tics that have been reported include tongue protrusion, squatting, sniffing, hopping, skipping, throat clearing, stuttering, uttering sounds or words, and coprolalia. Other relatively common symptoms include hyperactivity, distractibility, and impulsivity. Obsessions and compulsions are common in a patient with Tourette's disorder. In some cases, these tics lead to physical injuries. For example, head banging sometimes results in retinal detachment, or knee and neck jerking lead to orthopedic problems. Some patients obsessively pick at their skin, and this potentially leads to infection or mutilation.

Shame, self-consciousness, and depressed mood occur as a result of the problems associated with Tourette's disorder. Various learning disabilities (e.g., dyslexia) are also common among individuals with this condition. Frequently reported associated symptoms include social discomfort and rejection by others that interfere with social, academic, and occupational functioning. In severe cases, tics interfere with activities of daily living (e.g., reading, eating) or cause medical complications (American Psychiatric Association, 2000) (see the DSM-IV-TR Criteria box).

DSM-IV-TR CRITERIA

Tourette's Disorder

A Both multiple motor and one or more vocal tics have been present at some time during the illness, although not necessarily concurrently. (A *tic* is a sudden, rapid, recurrent nonrhythmic, stereotyped motor movement or vocalization.)

B The tics occur many times a day (usually in bouts) nearly every day or intermittently throughout a period of more than 1 year, and during this period there was never a tic-free period of more than 3 consecutive months.

C The disturbance causes marked distress or significant impairment in social, occupational, or other important areas of functioning.

D The onset is before age 18.

E The disturbance is not due to the direct physiologic effects of a substance (e.g., stimulants) or a general medical condition (e.g., Huntington's disease or postviral encephalitis).

From the American Psychiatric Association: *Diagnostic and statistical manual of mental disorders*, ed 4, text revision, Washington, DC, 2000, American Psychiatric Association.

Prognosis

Tourette's disorder begins as early as 2 years of age, but patients typically present during childhood or early adolescence. Although it is almost always a lifelong disorder, in most cases, symptoms diminish during adolescence and adulthood (American Psychiatric Association, 2000).

ATTENTION-DEFICIT AND DISRUPTIVE BEHAVIORAL DISORDERS

Attention-Deficit/Hyperactivity Disorder
Etiology

Researchers do not know the etiology of ADHD, but studies suggest an interaction between psychosocial and biologic factors. There is a strong correlation between genetic factors and ADHD; concordance is 51% in monozygotic twins and 33% in dizygotic twins. Adoption studies also support genetics over environmental causes (Cantwell, 1996). ADHD occurs more often among the first-degree relatives of children with ADHD (American Psychiatric Association, 2000). There are no scientific studies that support sugar, food additives, colorings, or preservatives as possible causes of hyperactive behavior (Sadock and Sadock, 2007).

Epidemiology

ADHD occurs more frequently in males than females, with ratios from 2:1 up to 9:1. Rates of ADHD among school-aged children are estimated at 3% to 7% of the population. As many as two thirds of those diagnosed with ADHD also meet the criteria for another mental disorder, including up to 50% for oppositional defiant disorder (ODD) or conduct disorder. Other disorders that frequently occur with ADHD include mood disorders, anxiety disorders, Tourette's and chronic tic disorders, substance abuse, speech and language delays, and learning disorders.

Clinical Description

Behavioral manifestations include problems with attention, impulsivity, and hyperactivity. To meet the criteria, the child must have behavioral problems that occur before the age of 7 years and that are seen in at least two settings, such as in school and at home. The level of problems typically varies from time to time in the same or different settings. Symptoms generally worsen in situations that require sustained attention or that lack interest to the child or adolescent, such as listening to teachers, performing repetitive tasks, or reading lengthy materials. Symptoms actually disappear or become minimal when the child is under strict control, such as during a diagnostic interview or when receiving frequent rewards for appropriate behavior. Symptoms tend to worsen in unstructured group situations, such as the typical classroom and playground.

Hyperactivity presents in many forms: fidgeting or squirming in a seat, getting up when one is expected to remain seated, excessive running or climbing when it is dangerous or inappropriate, loud and disruptive play during quiet activities, and demonstrating a driven verbal or motor quality.

Although toddlers developmentally present with a lot of activity and inquisitiveness, toddlers with ADHD present qualitatively different. They are always moving, running, jumping, and climbing on furniture, or they are unable to remain still for the completion of simple tasks such as putting on a coat or listening to a simple story.

They stay focused for activities that they enjoy, such as watching TV or playing video games, but cannot maintain attention or focus for activities that they find boring or difficult. At home, they frequently do not finish meals or even finish activities that they have begun. They make excessive noise, interrupt others during quiet times, and talk constantly (e.g., they may provide a running commentary of a television show). Adolescents often express a subjective feeling of restlessness and report a preference to engage in active rather than sedentary activities.

Children with ADHD may act impulsively by blurting out the answers in class before being called on; taking someone else's turn in a game; grabbing others' clothing, limbs, or belongings; or touching things that do not belong to them. Accidents caused by the child's impulsivity and inattention may be demonstrated by knocking over objects, running into people, grabbing dangerous objects (e.g., a hot pan), or taking dangerous risks without considering the consequences (e.g., riding a bicycle at night without reflective lights). They may exhibit temper outbursts, bossiness, stubbornness, and excessive, frequent insistence that their requests to be met.

Inattention occurs in various settings. Schoolwork or other activities often contain careless errors that show a lack of attention to detail. Work is messy, with evidence of not thinking through the project or schoolwork. Often it appears that the child is daydreaming and not listening to what is being said or asked. Trivial stimuli such as household noises often distract these individuals, who then leave their assigned task to attend to the interrupting stimuli. The child moves from one unfinished task to another, leaving increasing clutter in his or her wake. Materials that are needed for specific tasks typically become scattered, lost, or carelessly handled and damaged. These children often forget and miss appointments, fail to meet schoolwork deadlines, or forget lunch money.

As a result, academic achievement is often low. Children with ADHD are often regarded as lazy and unmotivated, and they are believed to have below-average intelligence. Studies have demonstrated that 10% to 20% of children with ADHD also have a learning disorder and are, in fact, of normal intelligence (Nearns, 1997). Family members frequently develop resentment, particularly when the variability of symptoms leads parents to believe that their children's troublesome behavior is willful. Families of these children likely have more stress, experience feelings of inadequacy and parental incompetence, have marital discord and disruption, and experience increased social isolation (Dulcan et al, 1997). Because of their inattention, hyperactivity, and impulsivity, these children commonly experience a low frustration tolerance. They have difficulties with relationships with peers, they experience academic failures, and consequently, their self-esteem

Attention-Deficit/Hyperactivity Disorder

A Either criterion 1 or 2 is present:
1 Six (or more) of the following symptoms of inattention have persisted for at least 6 months to a degree that is maladaptive and inconsistent with developmental level:

Inattention
a Often fails to give close attention to details or makes careless mistakes in schoolwork, work, or other activities
b Often has difficulty sustaining attention in tasks or play activities
c Often does not seem to listen when spoken to directly
d Often does not follow through on instructions and fails to finish schoolwork, chores, or duties in the workplace (not the result of oppositional behavior or a failure to understand instructions)
e Often has difficulty organizing tasks and activities
f Often avoids, dislikes, or is reluctant to engage in tasks that require sustained mental effort (such as schoolwork or homework)
g Often loses things necessary for tasks or activities (e.g., toys, school assignments, pencils, books, or tools)
h Is often easily distracted by extraneous stimulus
i Often forgetful in daily activities

2 Six (or more) of the following symptoms of hyperactivity/impulsivity have persisted for at least 6 months to a degree that is maladaptive and inconsistent with developmental level:

Hyperactivity
a Often fidgets with hands or feet or squirms in seat
b Often leaves seat in classroom or in other situations in which remaining seated is expected
c Often runs about or climbs excessively in situations in which it is inappropriate (in adolescents or

adults, may be limited to subjective feelings of restlessness)
d Often has difficulty playing or engaging in leisure activities quietly
e Is often "on the go" or often acts as if "driven by a motor"
f Often talks excessively

Impulsivity
g Often blurts out answers before questions have been completed
h Often has difficulty awaiting turn
i Often interrupts or intrudes on others (e.g., butts into conversations or games)

B Some hyperactive-impulsive or inattentive symptoms that caused impairment were present before age 7 years.
C Some impairment from the symptoms is present in two or more settings (e.g., at school [or work] and at home).
D There must be clear evidence of clinically significant impairment in social, academic, or occupational functioning.
E The symptoms do not occur exclusively during the course of a pervasive developmental disorder, schizophrenia, or other psychotic disorder and are not better accounted for by another mental disorder (e.g., mood disorder, anxiety disorder, dissociative disorder, or personality disorder).

Code based on type:
• *Attention-deficit/hyperactivity disorder, combined type:* If both criteria A1 and A2 are met for the preceding 6 months
• *Attention-deficit/hyperactivity disorder, predominantly inattentive type:* If criterion A1 is met but criterion A2 is not met for the preceding 6 months
• *Attention-deficit/hyperactivity disorder, predominantly hyperactive-impulsive type:* If criterion A2 is met but criterion A1 is not met for the preceding 6 months

*The DSM-V, which is currently in development, is considering changing the age of onset to on or before the age of 12 years instead of the age of 7 years. There is also consideration of removing the subtypes of this disorder and only having one diagnostic code.
From the American Psychiatric Association: *Diagnostic and statistical manual of mental disorders,* ed 4, text revision, Washington, DC, 2000, American Psychiatric Association.

suffers (Sadock and Sadock, 2007) (see the DSM-IV-TR Criteria box).

Prognosis

Symptoms of hyperactivity diminish in 50% of children as they mature, whereas the remaining 50% of children and adolescents will continue to have problems with inattention and impulsivity throughout their lives (Sadock and Sadock, 2007). Many adults who were diagnosed with ADHD during childhood report a decrease of behavioral hyperactivity but a continuation of difficulty concentrating for long periods of time or attending to complex projects. Behavioral management is the best psychosocial intervention. Structure and

consistency in the home and at school is of particular importance for a positive outcome (Pliszka, 2000).

Oppositional Defiant Disorder
Etiology

Oppositional defiant disorder (ODD) can occur among children as young as 3 years old, but it is typically diagnosed in school-aged children. ODD occurs more often in families in which the childcare is disrupted by a succession of different caregivers or in which harsh, inconsistent, or neglectful child-rearing practices occur. The disorder occurs more commonly when serious marital problems are present (American Psychiatric Association, 2000).

Epidemiology

ODD occurs more frequently in males before puberty and with approximately equal frequency in both genders after puberty. Rates vary considerably, from 2% to 16%, on the basis of the nature of the population sample and method of assessment (American Psychiatric Association, 2000). No specific family patterns have been associated with parents of children with this disorder; however, parents commonly demonstrate the need for power, control, and autonomy (Sadock and Sadock, 2007).

Clinical Description

Manifestations of this disorder, which include negativism, defiance, disobedience, and hostility toward authority figures, are typically exhibited in the home and may not be seen in the school setting. Symptoms are usually directed toward those the child knows best, such as the parents. Evidence of defiance also presents as the deliberate and persistent testing of limits, typically by ignoring directions, arguing, and refusing to accept responsibility for misbehavior. Hostility is usually directed at adults or peers and includes deliberately annoying others verbally. Individuals with ODD do not regard themselves as troublesome; rather, they blame others for making unreasonable demands, or they blame the circumstances (American Psychiatric Association, 2000; Sadock and Sadock, 2007).

During the school years, the following problems often occur among children with this condition: low self-esteem, mood lability, and low frustration tolerance. Swearing and the use of alcohol, tobacco, or illicit drugs that affect peer relationships and that disrupt adult relationships are also common. Cognitive and perceptual symptoms are not usually present in children with ODD (American Psychiatric Association, 2000) (see the DSM-IV-TR Criteria box).

Prognosis

Some children with ODD may progress to conduct disorder, whereas 25% will not meet the diagnostic criteria several years later. The onset is typically gradual, usually occurring over the course of months or years (Loeber, 2000).

Conduct Disorder
Etiology

Children who experience continual parental neglect and rejection, harsh discipline practices, physical or sexual abuse, lack of supervision, frequent changes in caregivers or early institutionalization, and association with a delinquent peer group are at an increased risk for developing conduct disorder. Conduct disorder occurs more frequently when a biologic or adoptive parent has antisocial personality disorder; when a biologic parent has alcohol dependence, a mood disorder, schizophrenia, or a history of ADHD or conduct disorder; or when a sibling has conduct disorder. Although a definitive cause for conduct disorder has not been found, one current and widely accepted model proposes that the disorder is linked to genetic predisposition triggered by environmental risk and low stress tolerance coupled with inadequate coping

---

DSM-IV-TR CRITERIA
*Oppositional Defiant Disorder**

A A pattern of negativistic, hostile, and defiant behavior lasting at least 6 months, during which four or more of the following are present:
1 Often loses temper
2 Often argues with adults
3 Often actively defies or refuses to comply with adults' requests or rules
4 Often deliberately annoys people
5 Often blames others for his or her mistakes or misbehavior
6 Is often touchy or easily annoyed by others
7 Is often angry and resentful
8 Is often spiteful or vindictive
Note: Consider a criterion met only if the behavior occurs more frequently than is typically observed in individuals of comparable age and developmental level.
B The disturbance in behavior causes clinically significant impairment in social, academic, or occupational functioning.
C The behaviors do not occur exclusively during the course of a psychotic or mood disorder.
D Criteria are not met for conduct disorder, and, if the individual is aged 18 years or older, criteria are not met for antisocial personality disorder.

*The DSM-V, which is currently in development, is considering categorizing the above symptoms into three categories: (1) angry/irritable mood; (2) defiant/headstrong behavior; and (3) vindictiveness. For children who are younger than 5 years old, the behaviors must be seen for most days during a 6-month period. For children 5 years and older, the identified behaviors must be exhibited at least once a week during a 6-month period.
From the American Psychiatric Association: *Diagnostic and statistical manual of mental disorders,* ed 4, text revision, Washington, DC, 2000, American Psychiatric Association.

---

skills (American Psychiatric Association, 2000; Sadock and Sadock, 2007).

Epidemiology

There is a 4:1 ratio of boys to girls, and 1% to 10% of the general population is considered to have this disorder. Generally 10- to 12-year-old boys meet the criteria, whereas girls have a later age of onset at 14 to 16 years old (Sadock and Sadock, 2007). According to the DSM-IV-TR, rates appear to be higher in urban areas than in rural settings, and they vary depending on the nature of the population sampled and methods of research used (American Psychiatric Association, 2000).

Clinical Description

The defining symptom of conduct disorder is demonstrated when the child violates the basic rights of others. The child lacks empathy and shows no remorse for his or her actions. Children or adolescents with conduct disorder generally do not empathize with other people's feelings and are unconcerned with other's situations or needs. They exhibit uncaring behavior, but they will often express words of guilt or remorse because they have learned that it reduces or prevents punishment. This stated sense of remorse is usually fabricated and insincere (Loeber, 2000).

Patients with conduct disorder manifest aggressive behavior and react aggressively toward others. They bully, threaten, and intimidate; initiate physical fights, use weapons in ways that could lead to injury, act cruelly to people or animals, steal, and force sexual activity. The severity of these behaviors sometimes involves rape, assault, or (rarely) homicide. Deliberate destruction of property results in fire damage, vandalism, and the destruction of others' property for simple vengeance. In addition to engaging in theft or robbery, the child or adolescent is often deceitful, demonstrating frequent lying or breaking promises to obtain goods or favors or to avoid obligations or responsibilities. The behaviors typically are seen in a variety of settings, including home, school, and the community.

These patients also frequently attempt to avoid consequences by blaming others. The early onset of problematic behavior usually includes sexual activity, drinking, smoking, the use of illegal substances, and other acts that involve a high level of risk. These behaviors usually persist into adulthood, and they frequently lead to school suspensions, unplanned pregnancies, physical injuries, sexually transmitted diseases, legal problems, dismissals from work or other activities, and the inability to attend regular schools.

Although these individuals project an image of "toughness," they often experience low self-esteem with poor frustration tolerance, irritability, temper outbursts, and reckless behavior. There are two subtypes of conduct disorder: *overt* and *covert*. Overt behavior is confrontational and includes fighting and aggression; covert disruptive behaviors manifest as concealing and theft. The behaviors associated with conduct disorder often impair peer relationships (see the DSM-IV-TR Criteria box).

DSM-IV-TR CRITERIA

Conduct Disorder

A A repetitive and persistent pattern of behavior in which the basic rights of others or major age-appropriate norms or rules are violated, as manifested by the presence of three (or more) of the following criteria in the preceding 12 months, with at least one criterion present in the preceding 6 months:

Aggression to people and animals:

1 Often bullies, threatens, or intimidates others
2 Often initiates physical fights
3 Has used a weapon that can cause serious physical harm to others (e.g., a bat, brick, broken bottle, knife, gun)
4 Has been physically cruel to people
5 Has been physically cruel to animals
6 Has stolen while confronting a victim (e.g., mugging, purse snatching, extortion, armed robbery)
7 Has forced someone into sexual activity

Destruction of property:

8 Has deliberately set fires with the intention of causing serious damage
9 Has deliberately destroyed others' property (other than by setting fires)

Deceitfulness or theft:

10 Has broken into someone else's house, building, or car
11 Often lies to obtain goods or favors or to avoid obligations (i.e., cons others)
12 Has stolen items of nontrivial value without confronting a victim (e.g., shoplifting, but without breaking and entering; forgery)

Serious violations of rules:

13 Often stays out at night despite parental prohibitions, beginning before age 13 years

14 Has run away from home overnight at least twice while living in parental or parental surrogate home (or once without returning for a lengthy period)
15 Is often truant from school, beginning before age 13 years

B The disturbance in behavior causes clinically significant impairment in social, academic, or occupational functioning.
C If the individual is aged 18 years or older, criteria are not met for antisocial personality disorder.

Code based on age at onset:

Conduct disorder, childhood-onset type: Onset of at least one criterion characteristic of conduct disorder before age 10 years
Conduct disorder, adolescent-onset type: Absence of any criteria characteristic of conduct disorder before age 10 years
Conduct disorder, unspecified onset: Age at onset is not known

Specify severity:

Mild: Few if any conduct problems in excess of those required to make the diagnosis *and* conduct problems cause only minor harm to others
Moderate: Number of conduct problems and effect on others intermediate between mild and severe
Severe: Many conduct problems in excess of those required to make the diagnosis *or* conduct problems cause considerable harm to others

Prognosis

The prognosis is guarded for children with this condition who are diagnosed early, because they tend to exhibit more severe and frequent behaviors, and they also may develop coexisting diagnoses such as mood disorder or substance abuse later in life (Sadock and Sadock, 2007).

Intermittent Explosive Disorder
Etiology and Epidemiology

The cause of intermittent explosive disorder (IED) is unknown, but there are several postulated theories being researched. Biologically, there is some evidence that the neurotransmitter serotonin plays a role in the development of IED. First-degree relatives of patients with IED have higher rates of uncontrolled temper or explosive outbursts as compared with the general population. Children or adolescents with this disorder tend to be raised with harsh discipline, physical abuse, and alcohol dependence. This disorder is usually diagnosed from childhood through early adulthood, and it is underreported. IED is more common among males than females (Sadock and Sadock, 2007).

Clinical Description

The child is unable to resist aggressive impulses that result in severe acts of aggression. This includes destroying property, striking or hurting others, and threatening to harm a person. The degree of violence is disproportionate to the precipitating event. For example, the child destroys his room after being told to put his clothes in the hamper. The violence will last minutes or hours, and the child describes the aggressive acts as "spells" or "attacks." The child will feel an immediate tension release followed by feelings of remorse or embarrassment (American Psychiatric Association, 2000).

During the aggressive episode, the child experiences feelings of rage, racing thoughts, and increased energy. After the aggressive act, the child reports feelings of depression and fatigue. Some have reported tingling sensations, tremors, palpitations, chest tightness, pressure in the head, or hearing an echo that precedes the aggressive attack (American Psychiatric Association, 2000) (see the DSM-IV-TR Criteria box).

Prognosis

Children with IED often experience school problems such as suspension or detention, and they may have impaired relationships with their peers. They may also become physically injured as a result of their aggressive outbursts. There is limited data regarding the prognosis of IED, but the course appears to be chronic or episodic, lasting from the childhood years into the early 20s.

ADOLESCENT SUICIDE

Suicide is the third leading cause of death among adolescents after accidents and homicides, with rates doubling during the past 50 years. Risk factors include the following: previous suicide attempts, history of a current psychiatric disorder, history of physical or sexual abuse or exposure to violence in

---

DSM-IV-TR CRITERIA

Intermittent Explosive Disorder

A Several discrete episodes occur that suggest a failure to resist aggressive impulses that result in serious assaultive acts or destruction of property.
B The degree of aggressiveness expressed during the episodes is grossly out of proportion to any precipitating psychosocial stressors.
C The aggressive episodes are not better accounted for by another mental disorder (e.g., antisocial personality disorder, borderline personality disorder, a psychotic disorder, a manic episode, conduct disorder or attention-deficit/hyperactivity disorder) and are not due to the direct physiologic effects of a substance (e.g., a drug of abuse, a medication) or a general medical condition (e.g., head trauma, Alzheimer's disease).

From the American Psychiatric Association: *Diagnostic and statistical manual of mental disorders,* ed 4, text revision, Washington, DC, 2000, American Psychiatric Association.

---

the home, family history of suicidal behavior or mood disorders, and homosexual orientation. Factors associated with suicidal behaviors consist of substance abuse, access to firearms, interpersonal conflicts, legal problems, and feelings of hopelessness or helplessness (Ahluwalia, 2009).

Approximately 15% of high school students have seriously considered suicide, with 11% developing a plan and 7% attempting during the past year. Ninth and tenth graders are more likely to have attempted suicide during the past year than eleventh and twelfth graders (Hallfors et al, 2006). Hanging was the most common method used in the 10- to 15-year-old age group, whereas firearms were the most common method used during later adolescence. Fewer warning signs and fewer precipitating events preceded the suicides of children and young adolescents. Intoxication and romantic failure were not risk factors among those younger than 15 years old, although these are very common risks for older adolescents. Significant risk factors for suicide include the following: males with a prior attempt who are 16 years old or older with an associated mood or substance disorder and females with a mood disorder and a prior attempt. Patients with a diagnosis of major depression and agitation are at high risk for suicide (Shaffer, 2001).

YOUTH VIOLENCE

With the increased availability of drugs, the presence of gang activity, and diminished supervision at home, youth violence has become a common reaction to these pressures. Early childhood aggression has a relatively high likelihood of persistence over time (Vance et al, 2002). Students bringing guns and knives to school have prompted the school systems to have stricter "no tolerance" rules and higher security, such as metal detectors and on-site police officers.

The U.S. Surgeon General (2001) published a report about youth violence that summarized research studies that discussed possible risk factors, interventions, and prevention. Potential risk factors include the following: paranoia; low frustration tolerance; prejudicial attitudes; alienation, rejection, and being a victim of bullying or bullying others; negative or violent home life; poor emotional attachment to parents; gang affiliation; obsession with violence in video games, movies, music, and writings; poor academic performance; and substance abuse (Muscari, 2009).

Approximately 30% to 40% of males and 15% to 30% of females have committed a serious violent act at some point during their lives. There were more arrests for violent crimes committed by African Americans and Hispanics, but confidential surveys completed by adolescents demonstrated a more narrow racial disparity (Surgeon General, 2001).

SELF-INJURIOUS BEHAVIOR

Approximately 1% of the population engages in self-injurious behaviors. The act of self-injury involves damaging bodily tissue to alter one's mood. Types of injury include cutting, burning, biting, head banging, bruising, picking at the skin, and hair pulling. Teenagers learn this behavior from their peers as an immediate release of emotional tension. There are also websites that describe techniques for "cutting" as well as methods for hiding the wounds. Self-injurious behavior is not suicidal behavior, but it may be rehearsal behavior, and some teenagers accidentally commit suicide in the process. Repeated acts of self-injury also desensitize the individual, who may subsequently find it easier to commit suicide. The nurse needs to assess for signs of self-injurious behavior, educate the family, and help the teenager to develop adaptive strategies and techniques for coping with anxiety and stress.

Protective Factors

On the positive side, researchers have identified protective factors in association with self-injurious behaviors. These include positive parent–child relationships, positive and consistent parental discipline, daily structure, and family and church involvement. Children whose parents have a high school or higher education, who have family support, and who have good problem-solving abilities are less at risk for developing violent behaviors. Living at home, having an internal locus of control, using faith as a coping method, being competent in daily life, and having good interpersonal skills are also protective factors (Vance, 2002) (see the Research for Evidence-Based Practice box).

ADULT DISORDERS AMONG CHILDREN AND ADOLESCENTS

Anxiety Disorders

Anxiety disorders are the most common mental disorders among children and adolescents, and they affect up to 10% of the population. Epidemiologic studies in nonreferred 11-year-old children documented the following prevalences: separation anxiety, 3.5%; overanxious disorder, 2.9%; simple phobia, 2.4%; and social phobia, 1%. Risk factors for the

> ### RESEARCH FOR EVIDENCE-BASED PRACTICE
>
> A study by Johnson and colleagues (2008) compared urban, suburban, and rural adolescents across the country to investigate drug use and exposure to violence. Twenty-eight factors were studied, including violent activities (e.g., carrying a weapon, fighting), suicidal behavior (e.g., suicidal ideation, plans, attempts), and alcohol and drug use. Data was obtained from the 2003 Youth Risk Behavior Survey of 15,219 adolescents: 2394 in rural areas, 7027 in suburban areas, and 5798 in urban areas. The incidence of violent and suicidal behavior and drug use was comparable if not higher among rural teens as compared with suburban and urban teens. Violent behavior and victimization were higher among nonwhite adolescents in the suburban and urban groups, but racial differences were nonexistent in the rural group. The authors concluded that rural areas did not provide a strong protective factor against high-risk and violent behaviors and that programs and teaching should be provided to this community subtype.

development of anxiety disorders in children include behavioral inhibition, insecure attachment, cognitive factors, developmental events, traumatic events, and access to support systems (Bernstein et al, 1996).

Developmental differences exist with regard to the symptoms of anxiety. Children between the ages of 5 and 8 years old most commonly report unrealistic worry about harm to their parents and attachment figures as well as school refusal. Between the ages of 9 and 12 years, children report excessive distress during times of separation. Adolescents typically report somatic complaints and school refusal; school refusal is present in three quarters of those identified with separation anxiety disorder.

In a community sample, more than two fifths of youths met criteria for exposure to at least one major trauma by the age of 18 years, and 6% met the criteria for a lifetime diagnosis of posttraumatic stress disorder. Symptoms for children younger than 5 years old included excessive clinging, crying, and withdrawal. Children between the ages of 6 and 11 years old exhibited disruptive behavior, difficulty paying attention, loud outbursts, difficulties in school, feelings of depression and anxiety, and somatic complaints. Teenagers exhibited flashbacks, emotional numbing, sleep problems, substance abuse, risk-taking behaviors, suicidal thoughts, and isolation. After a natural disaster, separation from parents, ongoing maternal preoccupation with the event, and altered family functioning were greater predictors of symptom development than exposure alone (Cohen, 1998). Adolescents with panic attacks were three times as likely to verbalize suicidal thoughts and two times as likely to have attempted suicide in the past than adolescents without panic attacks (Pilowsky et al, 1999).

Obsessive-compulsive disorder has a 6-month prevalence of 1 in 200 children and adolescents. It has been reported in children as young as 5 years old, with the mean age being 10 years old. Children typically demonstrate normal age-dependent obsessive-compulsive behaviors, such as wanting things done "just so" and sometimes insisting on elaborate bedtime rituals. These behaviors usually stop by middle childhood and are replaced by collections, hobbies, and focused interests. Frequently observed symptoms in children and adolescents include obsessions (e.g., contamination fears); worry about harm to themselves or others; aggressiveness; sexual ideas; scrupulosity, religiosity, and forbidden thoughts; the need to tell, ask, or confess; and compulsions (e.g., washing, repeating, checking, touching, counting, ordering, arranging, hoarding, praying).

Factors that predict a more positive outcome for children and adolescents in whom anxiety disorders have been diagnosed include the ability of the child to continue attending school, a later onset of symptoms, the duration of the illness, and the absence of another psychiatric diagnosis (Sadock and Sadock, 2007).

Depression

Depression among children and adolescents tends to be episodic, and it may go unidentified for some time. Initial symptoms include declining academic functioning, impairment in peer relationships, and withdrawal from after-school activities. Population studies report a prevalence of major depression and dysthymia of approximately 0.4% to 2% of children and 4% to 8% of adolescents, with a lifetime prevalence of major depression among adolescents of 15% to 20%. Children with at least one depressed parent are three times as likely to develop major depression. Symptoms include changes in appetite, sleep, energy level, and concentration. Some children exhibit a depressed or irritable mood, behavioral problems (e.g., temper tantrums), and low frustration tolerance, and they may manifest anxiety symptoms accompanied with somatic symptoms. Adolescents with depression typically exhibit increased sleep and appetite disturbances, suicidal ideations and attempts, and difficulties functioning in relationships in school and at home (Birmaher et al, 1996).

Other problems often accompany depressive disorders, including substance abuse, suicidal tendencies, and behavioral problems. Children and adolescents with depression have a comorbid diagnosis in 40% to 70% of cases; those with dysthymic disorder or anxiety have a comorbid diagnosis in 30% to 80% of cases (Birmaher et al, 1996).

Bipolar Disorder

The incidence of children and adolescents diagnosed with bipolar disorder has increased, with 20% to 40% of adolescents previously diagnosed with depression being later diagnosed with bipolar disorder within 5 years. Health care providers often miss the diagnosis of pediatric bipolar disorder because of the overlapping of symptoms. Children frequently present with atypical symptoms that are often markedly labile and irregular; they are irritable, aggressive, or mixed rather than euphoric. Reckless behavior often leads to school failure, fighting, dangerous play, and inappropriate sexual activity. Youths who are diagnosed with bipolar disorder are more likely to have rapid cycling or mixed episodes, with a greater risk of suicide. These symptoms are different from common childhood phenomena of boasting, imaginary play, overactivity, and youthful indiscretions (Beiderman, 1998; McClellan et al, 1997).

Individuals may be impulsive as demonstrated by sexual promiscuity, excessive spending, or dangerous driving, and they may exhibit grandiose thinking, such as believing that they will be rap stars or that they are geniuses when they are failing school. According to the study conducted by Birmaher and colleagues (2006), children and adolescents had a poorer outcome if they were diagnosed early in life or had a longer duration, if they were of a lower socioeconomic group, or if they also experienced psychotic symptoms.

Distinguishing between ADHD and bipolar symptoms can be difficult even for the experienced clinician. Table 17-1 compares of the two disorders.

Psychosis

The onset of schizophrenia is rare, and the condition is often more severe if it is diagnosed before the age of 12. It is estimated that 1 in every 10,000 children has schizophrenia, whereas adolescents are 50 times as likely to have it, bringing

TABLE 17-1	COMPARISON OF BIPOLAR DISORDER AND ATTENTION-DEFICIT/HYPERACTIVITY DISORDER
BIPOLAR DISORDER	**ATTENTION-DEFICIT/HYPERACTIVITY DISORDER**
• Symptoms occur after the age of 7 years	• Hyperactive before the age of 7 years (i.e., since he or she "started walking")
• Symptoms are cyclical	• Symptoms always present
• Talkative with pressured speech	• Talkative but speech not pressured
• Extreme irritability and aggression that are uncontrollable	• Less extreme irritability and aggression
• Change in mood with change in cognition and behavior (i.e., crying; bossiness or cockiness; increased self-esteem; the affected person believes that he or she has special talents and is more important; silliness and euphoria cannot be redirected)	• Mood remains constant
	• Consistently distractible
	• Cognition not affected unless distractibility interferes with listening
• Distractibility and agitation increase as compared with the baseline level	

Stokowski L: Bipolar disorder and ADHD in children: confusion and comorbidity, *Advanced Practice Nursing eJournal* 9(4), 2009. Retrieved November 11, 2009, from www.medscape.com/viewarticle/711223.

the number to 2 per every 1000 (Sadock and Sadock, 2007). An onset before the age of 13 years (i.e., very early onset schizophrenia) is usually insidious and includes withdrawal, poor hygiene, odd behaviors (e.g., hoarding or storing food and other objects), and a decline in academic functioning. Other developmental delays occur as well, including delays in cognitive, motor, sensory, and social functioning. Communication and interaction with family members and peers are problematic.

The presence of psychosis in preschool-aged children presents an extremely difficult problem. Brief hallucinations under stress, imaginary friends, and fantasy figures are common. By the school-aged years, persistent hallucinations are associated with serious disorders. Delusional content and hallucinations are reflected in developmental problems. Hallucinations often include monsters, pets, or toys, and delusions typically revolve around identity issues and are usually less complex than adult hallucinations. After the age of 7 years, loose and illogical thinking does not usually occur among normal children (McClellan et al, 1997). Determining factors of prognosis include the child's level of functioning before the onset of schizophrenic symptoms, the age of onset, the intelligence quotient, the pharmacologic response, the level of functioning after the first episode, and the availability of healthy support systems (Sadock and Sadock, 2007).

Substance Abuse

Adolescent substance abuse continues to be a public health concern in the United States. In 1996, the annual Monitoring the Future Study found that nearly one third of high-school seniors reported having been drunk during the month before taking the survey; one fifth reported marijuana use during that period, and nearly 5% reported daily marijuana use (Weinberg et al, 1998). By the end of high school, approximately 90% of students have tried alcohol, and 40% have tried an illicit drug, typically marijuana (Bukstein et al, 1997).

Adolescents need to only look in their own medicine cabinets at home to get a high. The abuse of prescription and over-the-counter medications by adolescents continues to rise, and these are the third most abused drugs among teens. A study by Crouch and colleagues examined nonprescription drug abuse cases reported to the regional poison control center in Utah and found that 38% of drug abuse by children aged 6 to 19 years was intentional. Intentional abuse was defined as the "improper or incorrect use of a substance for the likely achievement of a euphoric or psychotropic effect" (Crouch et al, 2004). Nonprescription medications included products that contained dextromethorphan (e.g., cough and cold products), stimulants (e.g., ephedrine, phenylpropanolamine), and antihistamines. The most commonly used over-the-counter medications among children between 6 and 19 years old were antihistamines during the early- to mid-1990s. The use of dextromethorphan radically increased during the latter part of the study period. The use of dextromethorphan in high enough doses causes hallucinations, thus giving the drug its nicknames "poor man's PCP" and "over-the-counter ecstasy." Toxic symptoms include nystagmus, hallucinations,

ataxia, and central nervous system depression (Crouch et al, 2004). See Chapter 15 for more information.

Factors that contribute to the appeal of nonprescription medication abuse consist of the false assumption of safety, the availability and legality of the drugs, and the fact that they are inexpensive. They can be purchased at any age from any local grocery store or pharmacy as well as online. The use of automatic checkout lanes eliminates suspicion when large quantities are purchased (Crouch et al, 2004).

Factors that protect against substance use and abuse include adequate intelligence and problem-solving ability, positive self-esteem, intact affect regulation, supportive family relationships, and positive role models (Weinberg et al, 1998).

THE NURSING PROCESS

Before the nursing process begins, the nurse first develops a trusting relationship with the child or adolescent. This can prove difficult at times, because children are not forthcoming with information as a result of their developmental age, and adolescents may be guarded and difficult to reach. Although the nurse must maintain clear therapeutic boundaries, he or she may need to engage the child by conversing about things that are important in the child's life, such as friends, activities, and interests in music or sports. Most adolescents just want to be heard, and, by using silence with a nonjudgmental attitude, even the adolescent who refuses to talk initially will acquiesce after safety and trust are established.

The nursing process is applicable to children and adolescents in the psychiatric setting. Knowledge of growth and development is essential, as is the ability to perform a thorough clinical assessment that includes both medical and psychosocial aspects. The nurse assesses the child or adolescent within the context of the entire family structure and the family dynamics, including the associated cultural and socioeconomic situation.

Parents often seek treatment for the child or adolescent after being referred by the school system or after their own multiple attempts to change the child or adolescent have been unsuccessful. It is often difficult for adults to comprehend that children, especially young children, have mental disorders. As a result, parents delay treatment for years in the hope that the child will "grow out of it." Although it is common for a family to present a child or adolescent as the identified patient (i.e., the family member with the problem), it is important to remember that children will often act out the underlying family dynamics or family psychopathology. In addition, families are often in denial that the child may have a disorder that has been identified in other family members, such as a tic disorder, obsessive-compulsive disorder, a mood disorder, or psychosis.

Some families are skeptical of proposed treatment recommendations and discredit the therapeutic interventions. They continue to use unhealthy multigenerational parenting techniques. Families see initial improvement in a child or adolescent who is in treatment and then prematurely discontinue newly adopted interventions; this inevitably results in the relapse of the child's or adolescent's condition and a continuation of family dysfunction. Treatment success and outcome depend on the family's commitment to learning new skills and consistently applying them. Early assessment and intervention from all caregivers and educators is the most ideal treatment goal.

❖ CLINICAL ALERT #1

When working with children, the nurse is aware that the child or adolescent is a minor and that the primary caregiver or guardian has legal rights in addition to the child's rights. Children and adolescents are able to give assent, and caregivers and guardians give informed consent. This applies to all forms of treatment, including medications and research. In the inpatient setting, this applies to all patient rights, including admission to the mental health units, seclusion, and restraint. The nurse obtains the child's or adolescent's signature in addition to the caregiver's or guardian's signature in accordance with facility policy on all assent and consent forms.

ASSESSMENT

When assessing the child, it is important to have the parents present to evaluate interactions, limit-setting, and communication. Specific behaviors to observe include how the child engages in play; how the parent soothes the child, if required; and level of affection expressed between the parent and the child. Pay particular attention to the types of words used and the facial expressions. Interviewing the parents without the child present will enable an open dialog regarding parental concerns. Forms of discipline, the level of supervision and structure, the expectations of the child, and recent stressors or problems that the family has endured must also be determined (Thomas et al, 1977). A thorough physical assessment that involves all body systems and a thorough mental status examination help the nurse identify potential physical or emotional problems that contribute to the overall health and well-being of the child or adolescent (Box 17-1).

During the assessment, it is essential to obtain a thorough alcohol and drug history that includes the amount used, the length of use, and the dates and times of use. A drug history consists of questions that cover all potential methods of drug use, such as sniffing paint thinners and other similar intoxicating chemicals, glue, or the contents of aerosol cans; smoking; drinking; and injecting.

Developmental Stage

Because each child and adolescent has unique strengths and weaknesses, the patient's individual characteristics are considered and assessed in the context of the family, the culture, the socioeconomic circumstances, and phases of normal growth and development. Infants, children, and adolescents experience developmental delays as a result of family trauma,

---

BOX 17-1 — MENTAL STATUS EXAMINATION FOR AN INFANT OR TODDLER

Appearance: Level of nourishment, hygiene, and dress

Reaction to situation: Initial reaction to strangers and reaction to the transition of the nurse playing with the infant during assessment

Self-regulation: Level of alertness, including crying and the ability to be soothed and to soothe the self; reactions to sensory stimulation (e.g., sound, touch); unusual behaviors, such as head banging, hair pulling, spinning objects, flapping hands, and walking on toes; activity level, such as sitting quietly, climbing on furniture, and exploring the room; attention span (e.g., following an object with the eyes, exploring an object with the hands, playing with a toy); frustration tolerance, such as the ability to persist in a difficult task, crying, and tantrums; aggressiveness, including appropriate assertiveness or excessive aggressiveness

Motor: Muscle tone and strength, movement of face and tongue, swallowing, drooling, and unusual tics or seizures; gross motor, including picking the head up, rolling over, standing up, walking, running, and hopping; fine motor, including grasping with fingers, pincer grasp (i.e., thumb to index finger), stacking, scribbling, and completing puzzles

Speech and language: Vocalization and speech production, such as quality, rate, and volume; receptive language, including comprehension of language and responding to questions and commands appropriately; expressive language, including the child's effectiveness of communicating, babbling, imitation, vocalization of single words, and use of complete sentences

Thought*: Fear, such as a feared object or a fear of being separated from a caregiver; dreams, including nightmares; dissociative state, including sudden withdrawal and inattention, glazed eyes, and tuning out

*Taking into consideration the age and developmental level of the patient, this category may not apply; however, symptoms such as looseness of associations and echolalia may precede thought disorders later in life.

Modified from Thomas J et al: Practice parameters for the psychiatric assessment of infants and toddlers (0–36 months), *J Am Acad Child Adolesc Psychiatry* 37:127–132, 1998.

---

social deprivation, abuse, neglect, or complications from a major mental disorder.

Family Life

The child's or adolescent's family life and home environment are crucial aspects of assessment that lead to a comprehensive understanding of the presenting mental health problems. The nurse needs to have an understanding of the types of interactions that occur within the family relationships and each member's perception of the family dynamics, successes, and problems. It is important for the nurse to understand characteristics of the home environment, including the cleanliness and size of the home; where and with whom the child or adolescent sleeps; patterns of meals, pet care, chores, and homework; times and frequencies of recreational activities; and bedtime rituals.

NURSING DIAGNOSIS

All current North American Nursing Diagnosis Association International nursing diagnoses are applicable to children and adolescents (North American Nursing Diagnosis Association International, 2007). However, because of the tendency for children and adolescents to act out the many problems with which they struggle, some diagnoses are more important. Safety issues are most significant, and they are a first priority with any patient in the mental health setting.

In addition to the patient's individual needs and problems, family problems will always be considered relevant. Ineffective role performance, impaired parenting, and interrupted family processes are all important diagnoses for the nurse to consider. Always consider the needs of the family during the process of assigning nursing diagnoses.

OUTCOME IDENTIFICATION

Outcome criteria come from the nursing diagnoses that are developed during the nursing process. The nurse prioritizes outcomes and states them in simple terms. The outcome criteria for children and adolescents will consider and focus on the promotion of normal growth and development in an effort to improve areas of current developmental deficits in addition to improving any identified dysfunction. Outcome criteria include treatment goals of the child or adolescent, the nurse, the interdisciplinary team, and the caregivers. Children and adolescents are more likely to participate in the treatment process when they are included in decisions about their care and progress. Examples of outcome criteria are listed here. The client will do the following:

- Refrain from harm to self or others.
- Seek assistance and support from adults before losing self-control.
- Identify triggers that provoke negative behavioral responses.
- Demonstrate age-appropriate relationships with adults.
- Demonstrate age-appropriate relationships with peers.
- Use age-appropriate play and recreational activities to express himself or herself.

PLANNING

During the beginning phases of the nursing process, the nurse sets realistic expectations on the basis of the child's or adolescent's developmental level of ability and function. The nurse is aware that negative behavioral patterns have been part of the family dynamics and that often they have occurred for long periods of time. Ideally, the nurse plans for small incremental changes in behavior with obtainable goals. The nurse's effort for mutual goal setting will demonstrate respect and trust to the child or adolescent. The nurse explains the plan to the child or adolescent in simple

terms and asks for the patient's active participation and best effort, with the understanding that the nurse will work in a cooperative effort with the patient and family to obtain the stated treatment goals.

IMPLEMENTATION

As the nurse implements the individualized and prioritized care plan, his or her role is to support the child or adolescent and the family through the behavioral change process. The child or adolescent will continue to try to use previously established behaviors, many of which are negative. The nurse will demonstrate clear, consistent, and realistic expectations with the use of role-modeling and therapeutic communication skills. The nurse will set consistent boundaries and limits as the child or adolescent questions authority and struggles to learn adaptive age-appropriate functioning.

Nursing Interventions

1. Conduct a thorough assessment with the parents or guardians and the patient *to observe interactions,* and then assess them separately if appropriate.
2. Assess for the presence of suicidal ideation and for past aggressive behaviors including triggers of aggressive behavior *to ensure the patient's safety and to prevent harm to others.*
3. Maintain a safe environment by continually assessing for contraband (e.g., objects that are sharp, alcohol, illicit drugs) and being aware of any behavioral changes or signals that may indicate increasing anger or aggression *to prevent violence and to maintain a safe environment.*
4. Establish a therapeutic alliance and maintain appropriate boundaries *to ensure consistency and security.*
5. Help the patient to identify strengths and positive qualities *to foster self-esteem, self-assurance, and self-confidence.*
6. Demonstrate, teach, and reinforce cooperative, respectful, and positive behaviors *to assist the patient with developing and redefining successful and positive relationships.*
7. Set clear and consistent limits in a calm and nonjudgmental manner *to promote a safe environment and to develop trust.*
8. Redirect disruptive behavior with recreational activities *to channel excess energy and to prevent escalation.*
9. Inform the patient of the consequences of not adhering to the limits *to allow the patient to have the opportunity to respond, to express feelings, and to cognitively process his or her options.*
10. Use timeouts or quiet time when the patient does not respond to limits *to give the patient time to deescalate in a quiet environment and to process the event.*
11. Role-play situations that trigger aggressiveness or self-mutilation or that encourage alcohol or illicit drug use *to explore and reinforce alternative methods of coping.*
12. Teach anger management techniques *to lessen the patient's feelings of powerlessness and to prevent future escalation.*
13. For the younger child, initiate therapeutic play *to encourage the patient to express thoughts and feelings in*

alternative ways in the absence of adequate language and to reestablish healthy boundaries.

14. Establish a behavior modification program for the preschool-aged child and the school-aged child that rewards the patient for expressing the self safely *to reinforce positive behaviors, to enhance self-esteem, and to foster a sense of accomplishment.*

15. Involve the adolescent patient in developing a behavioral contract by identifying expected behaviors and privileges *to reinforce positive behaviors and to enhance self-esteem and independence.*

16. Engage the patient in group therapy and recreational activities *to assist the patient with developing positive peer communication and to improve social skills and motor skills.*

17. Provide positive feedback and recognition when the patient adheres to the behavioral program and treatment plan *to promote self-esteem and to reinforce positive behaviors.*

18. Teach the parents and guardians about the patient's disorder, the importance of consistency and structure, and the significance of medication compliance, if indicated, *to minimize guilt, to increase their knowledge base regarding the disorder, to help them to develop realistic expectations, and to reinforce the consequences of medication noncompliance.*

19. Assess the parents and guardians for available support systems and refer them to support groups and individual and family therapy as needed *to increase their ability to cope and to minimize feelings of isolation and guilt.*

Additional Treatment Modalities

Nurses use a variety of collaborative interventions with children and adolescents in the mental health setting. Recreational, occupational, music, and art therapies—in addition to school, group, family, and individual therapies—are treatment modalities that promote overall health and well-being for the child and the adolescent. Cognitive behavioral therapy groups have demonstrated effectiveness for teaching the adolescent to manage symptoms, to use problem-solving skills, and to change negative thought patterns and emotional reactions.

Pharmacologic Interventions

Many medications for adults are also used for children and adolescents. The predominant classifications include stimulants, antidepressants, antianxiety agents, anticonvulsants, and antipsychotics. The nurse plays a crucial role in administering the medication, monitoring for clinical effectiveness and adverse reactions, and assessing compliance. The nurse communicates his or her findings to the multidisciplinary treatment team and to the primary care provider. The nurse remains current with regard to the knowledge of medications and continually seeks education about newly developed medications and their clinical effects on this population. The Medication Key Facts box describes medications that are used for children and adolescents with ADHD and its nursing implications.

💊 MEDICATION KEY FACTS

Pharmacotherapy for Attention-Deficit/Hyperactivity Disorder

Pharmacologic therapy for ADHD includes psychostimulants (dextroamphetamine [Dexedrine], methylphenidate [Ritalin, Concerta], dextroamphetamine and amphetamine salts [Adderall]), and noradrenergic specific reuptake inhibitors (atomoxetine [Strattera]); adrenergic agents (clonidine [Catapres]); antidepressants (bupropion [Wellbutrin]); and selective serotonin reuptake inhibitors (citalopram [Celexa], fluoxetine [Prozac], fluvoxamine [Luvox], paroxetine [Paxil], sertraline [Zoloft], and venlafaxine [Effexor]).

Psychostimulants/Noradrenergic Specific Reuptake Inhibitors
- Hypertensive crisis may occur if these drugs are combined with or used within 14 days of monoamine oxidase inhibitors.
- Abrupt withdrawal after the prolonged use of high doses may produce lethargy that lasts for weeks.
- There is an increased risk of seizures with methylphenidate.
- The prolonged administration of these drugs to children with ADHD may inhibit their growth.
- Herbal considerations: St. John's wort may produce serotonin syndrome in individuals who are taking these drugs; this condition is characterized by a number of mental, autonomic, and neuromuscular changes.

Adrenergic Agents
- Abrupt withdrawal may result in rebound hypertension.
- Life-threatening elevations of blood pressure may occur with tricyclic antidepressants and β-blockers.
- Herbal considerations: Aconite increases the toxicity of these drugs and may lead to death.

New Agent (Modafinil)
- Central nervous system stimulants may potentiate the action of this drug.

❖ CLINICAL ALERT #2

The nurse will carefully observe the child or adolescent who has ADHD and who is taking medications. Children or adolescents who are taking stimulant medications such as methylphenidate hydrochloride (Ritalin) may demonstrate adverse changes in appetite, sleep, and levels of restlessness. In addition, children or adolescents sometimes develop new tics, or previously existent mild tics may exacerbate. Atomoxetine (Strattera) also increases suicidal thoughts in some children and adolescents. If this occurs, it is important that the nurse withhold the medication, ensure safety, document the findings, and notify the provider of the clinical observations. Changes in dosage or the discontinuation of the medication will often be required.

There is a U.S. Food and Drug Administration warning label of possible heart-related problems or mental health issues for all stimulants related to sudden cardiac death among patients taking stimulants who also had heart impairment. If there is any question of cardiac abnormalities, the child should receive an electrocardiogram before beginning the use of stimulants (Vetter et al, 2008). For additional pharmacological information, see Chapter 25.

Group Activities

Group play and recreational activities are important when assisting the child or adolescent to develop positive peer communication and to improve interpersonal relationships. Group play offers an excellent opportunity for the nurse to role-model and teach new age-appropriate skills, to reinforce positive behaviors, and to promote nurturing peer relationships. The nurse will set limits in group play to promote a safe environment and to demonstrate ways to show cooperation with and respect for peers. Children and adolescents have often learned to tease and to provoke their peers in group settings. The nurse will nonjudgmentally assist them with redefining successful relationships.

Interventions are often more difficult with adolescents than with children, depending on the clinical presentation. It is normal for adolescents to question authority and to test limits and rules. The nurse will establish rapport and a therapeutic alliance with the adolescent early during the course of treatment. Adolescents need and look for role models, so it is imperative that the nurse maintains appropriate boundaries and does not behave as an adolescent or a friend to gain acceptance.

Group activities provide an excellent opportunity for the nurse to interact with adolescents during treatment. Group activities enable the adolescent to develop interpersonal skills, to give and accept feedback during communication with peers, to practice more adult-like relationships, to listen with empathy, to achieve success, and to learn appropriate ways to interact with the world.

Behavior Modification Programs

For the child who is approximately 3 to 11 years old, a behavior modification program is frequently used as part of a treatment plan. Behavior modification involves a systematic and structured program that identifies developmental and age-appropriate goals that are observable and measurable within an established time frame. The goals often focus on activities of daily living, impulse control, and peer and sibling relationships. The child is rewarded for the accomplishment of each goal. A chart lists each goal, and the child is rewarded with stars, stickers, or colors to signify progress. Many programs use colored charts. Sometimes a behavior program is implemented in the home to correlate with the school program and thereby promote consistency. Behavior modification is often used in child and adolescent psychiatric treatment settings.

Preadolescents and adolescents often make use of a behavioral contract. These contracts emphasize one to three goals that are more complex in nature (e.g., will speak to others with respect, will actively participate in group activities). The nurse will usually place a checkmark after each goal to signify that the adolescent has accomplished that goal. Rewards in the form of increased privileges (e.g., a later bedtime or

curfew, an activity with a parent or friend) are outcomes of maintaining the contract. A sample behavioral contract appears in Box 17-2.

Therapeutic Play

For the younger child, nursing interventions frequently occur within activities of therapeutic play. Play is the work of children. Children are able to use recreational and creative play activities to form or facilitate relationships with peers and adults and to work to master new developmental tasks. Even when unable or unwilling to verbally communicate, children express their thoughts, feelings, frustrations, fears, and hopes through therapeutic play. The perceptive nurse observes and guides the child in play and interacts to modify distortions and to reestablish healthy boundaries and safe limits as the child redefines behaviors through play.

EVALUATION

The evaluation phase of the nursing process documents the treatment progress as evidenced by actual outcomes. The observant nurse objectively reviews the evaluation phase to determine the effectiveness of the treatment plan. In addition to outcomes, the nurse examines other factors. For instance, were the treatment goals cognitively and developmentally appropriate for the child or adolescent? Are there other stressors within the family or social support system that are adding to the presenting problems and thus contributing to unrealistic expectations for the child or adolescent (e.g., health, financial, or placement problems)?

The interdisciplinary team coordinates any care plan modifications in an effort to maintain cohesiveness within the implementation of the treatment. It is also important to continually communicate the treatment evaluation with the caregivers. This helps to reinforce treatment gains, to reinforce new methods of parental interventions, and to assist the caregivers with monitoring and reestablishing new and realistic expectations.

For inpatient hospitalization, it is important that the nurse begin, early during the course of treatment with the family, to prepare them for the potential and pending discharge. Work that initially begins in an inpatient setting is usually transitioned to home or other outpatient placements, such as day treatment, residential care, or a group home. During the evaluation phase, the nurse encourages the child or adolescent and the family to make healthy transitions to the ongoing therapeutic relationship with the next primary mental health provider (i.e., the nurse specialist, social worker, psychologist, or psychiatrist).

DISCHARGE CRITERIA

The patient will do the following:
- Demonstrate safe conduct toward the self and others.
- Engage in self-care within his or her level of capability.
- Demonstrate emotional and behavioral control within his or her capacity.

BOX 17-2   EXAMPLE OF A BEHAVIORAL CONTRACT

Contracts are effective tools for compliance with desired behaviors if they are (1) realistic; (2) age appropriate (i.e., younger children require simple, single-level expectations); (3) consistently maintained (i.e., the parent cannot make a change from the contract by telling the child that he or she can play first and then fulfill expected behaviors after play); and (4) valued by all parties involved.

Behavioral Contract Principles
- The criteria of the contract are determined as a result of negotiation among all parties.
- The contract is most effective if it is written.
- Short-range and attainable goals are defined.
- Behaviors are rehearsed before final commitment to the contract.

Procedure
1 Write a clear and brief but detailed description of the patient's desired behavior.
2 Set the time and frequency of expected behaviors.
3 Specify positive reinforcements that are dependent on the fulfillment of items 1 and 2.
4 Specify adverse consequences that are dependent on the nonfulfillment of items 1 and 2.
5 Add a bonus clause that includes additional positive reinforcements if the patient exceeds the initial minimal demands.
6 Specify how responses will be observed, measured, and recorded (e.g., a chart on the refrigerator), and specify the procedure for informing the patient about achievement.
7 Deliver reinforcement soon after the response (i.e., do not wait to give an earned reward).

Scenario
Steve is a 13-year-old boy who has been missing homework assignments, cutting class, and failing his English and math classes. He has also been smoking marijuana and drinking alcohol on the weekends with his friends. His free time is primarily spent on the computer playing video games. Steve

and his parents have been in family counseling, and they agree to write a behavioral contract.

Sample Contract

Behaviors
Steve will do the following:
1 Be on time for and attend every class
2 Complete each homework assignment as instructed by his teachers.
3 Refrain from using drugs or alcohol.

Procedures
1 Steve will check his school website for homework assignments each day.
2 Steve's parents will communicate with his English and math teachers via e-mail weekly to monitor Steve's progress to determine if a tutor is needed.
3 Steve will comply with random urine drug screens.
4 Steve's friends may come to the house to socialize for the next 2 weeks as specified below.

Rewards
When his homework is completed, Steve may play with one electronic device of his choice for 1 hour (e.g., video game, computer, iPod).

If the above procedures are followed, Steve will spend 2 hours with his friends on Saturday or Sunday doing an activity of their choice (e.g., seeing a movie, playing paintball, skateboarding).

Consequences
Any further truancy or failure to complete assignments will result in the following:
- The restriction of friends and electronics until missed homework assignments are completed.
- Daily tutor at the house after school to assist with homework assignments.

A positive urine drug screen will result in the following:
- Attendance at Narcotics Anonymous meetings twice a week in addition to all of the above criteria.

Signed (Steve) _____ Date _____
(Mom) _____
(Dad) _____

Adapted from Fortinash KM, Holoday Worret PA: *Psychiatric nursing care plans*, ed 5, St. Louis, 2007, Mosby

---

- Attend to tasks, schoolwork, and performance without unnecessary anger or frustration.
- Exhibit a healthy self-concept and self-esteem in words and actions.
- Use cognitive, communication, and language skills to make himself or herself understood and to get his or her needs met.
- Express his or her feelings safely without acting out aggressively toward the self or others.
- Demonstrate interactive skills that are appropriate for his or her level of development.
- Interact meaningfully with staff, peers, and family within his or her capabilities.
- Seek attention and assistance appropriately from significant persons, and refrain from unnecessary or aggressive interactions.

- Adhere to the treatment regimen, including medications, as needed.
- Play appropriately with peers in accordance with age and unit guidelines.
- Engage in educational and vocational programs as prescribed.
- Use adaptive coping techniques and stress-reducing strategies.
- Respond satisfactorily to others' attentions and requests.
- Use community resources to enhance his or her quality of life.
- Engage in ongoing individual and family therapy.
- State specific reasons that demonstrate readiness for discharge.

◎ NURSING CARE PLAN

Michael, a 9-year-old boy, was admitted to the children's unit after he attempted to stab his teacher with a pencil. He has a history of poor peer and sibling relationships and frequently is placed on detention at school for fighting with peers during recess. He has been taking Ritalin for the past year after he was diagnosed with attention deficit hyperactivity disorder. His mother complains that Michael continues to have a low frustration tolerance, often displaying temper outbursts when he does not get his way or when he is asked to do his homework or chores. He physically assaulted his 6-year-old sister when she was playing with his toy and then proceeded to break her toys. There are marital problems between Michael's parents related to his father's excessive drinking. Michael's mother acknowledges that she has difficulty being consistent and firm with Michael. She thinks that her husband is too strict and tries to compensate by being more flexible. The mother related that she has suffered from depression the past 2 years and has been taking Paxil. The family has recently started family therapy.

DSM-IV-TR Diagnoses

Axis I   Attention deficit hyperactivity disorder; rule out intermittent explosive disorder
Axis II   None
Axis III   Asthma
Axis IV   Severity of stressors = 3 (moderate): school detentions, alcoholism of biologic father, mother's depression
Axis V   GAF = 35 (current); GAF = 45 (past year)

Nursing Diagnosis ***Risk for other-directed violence. Risk factors: a positive history of aggression toward peers, sibling and teacher (e.g., attempted to stab his teacher with a pencil, detentions at school)***

NOC Abuse Protection, Abuse Cessation, Abuse Behavior Self-Restraint, Hyperactivity level, Impulse Self-Control, Fear Level
NIC Abuse Protection Support, Anger Control Assistance, Anxiety Reduction, Impulse Control Training, Behavior Modification: Social Skills, Support Group

CLIENT OUTCOMES	NURSING INTERVENTIONS	EVALUATION
Michael will demonstrate safe behaviors.	Provide close observation as indicated to *ensure the client's safety and to maintain a safe environment*. Set firm limits and consequences for aggressive behaviors. *Structure and clear expectations clarify boundaries for improved self-control.* Help Michael to identify situations that precipitate his aggressive outbursts *to help the client identify sources of frustration.*	Michael continues aggression, pushing peers and throwing objects when he is angry, requiring time out in his room.
Michael will demonstrate alternative behaviors to violent outbursts.	Help Michael to identify three alternative behaviors to use when he becomes frustrated or angry. Give Michael stickers for the star program every time he uses alternative behaviors *to reinforce appropriate behaviors and build self-esteem.* Encourage Michael to play nerf football when he is frustrated or angry *to promote socially acceptable and safe ventilation of negative feelings.* Encourage Michael to draw his feelings on a daily basis *to express his hostile feelings in safe manner.*	Michael identifies precipitants for his behavior only after aggressive acts and is working on recognizing triggers before he acts on feelings. Michael seeks staff when he is feeling angry and on the verge of losing control 75% of the time. Michael is currently on the silver level of the program, earning the use of his Game Boy and privilege of eating in the cafeteria with peers. Michael plays nerf football when he feels frustrated 80% of the time.
Michael will identify three situations that precipitate violent outbursts.	Encourage the patient to verbalize feelings in daily one-to-one conversations *to ventilate emotions and receive encouragement and reinforcement from staff.* Discuss possible situations that precipitate Michael's violent outbursts *to connect negative feelings with aggressive actions.*	Michael draws pictures to help identify his feelings daily. His insight is improving slowly. Michael verbalizes when he feels angry with peers and with staff 50% of the time. Michael identifies situations that cause him to get angry (when he doesn't win or a game, when peers make fun of him, and when he's told he's done something wrong).

NURSING CARE PLAN—cont'd

CLIENT OUTCOMES	NURSING INTERVENTIONS	EVALUATION
Michael will follow the unit rules and maintain the silver or gold level on the star program.	Explain the unit's rules and the star program *to clarify information and expectations for client.* Provide consistent staffing *to build a trusting relationship.* Set firm limits and consequences for breaking the unit rules. *Structure and clear expectations clarify boundaries for improved self-control.*	Michael demonstrates an understanding of the unit rules and the star program. Michael is beginning to respond positively to his designated staff. Michael continues to provoke peers, and he requires frequent timeouts during the shift. He continues to be on bronze level with no privileges.

GAF, Global Assessment of Functioning.

CHAPTER SUMMARY

- Of all mentally retarded individuals, 85% are mildly retarded, 10% are moderately retarded, 3% to 4% are severely retarded, and 1% to 2% are profoundly retarded.
- Children with autistic disorder present with repetitive movements, no emotional reciprocity, impaired communication (both verbal and nonverbal), and an indifference to affection. Seventy-five percent of these individuals have some degree of mental retardation.
- The most commonly diagnosed mental disorders are ADHD, mood disorder, and pervasive development disorder.
- Some children with ADHD have the following histories: child abuse or neglect, multiple foster placements, neurotoxin exposure, infections, drug exposure in utero, low birth weight, and mental retardation.
- ADHD causes problems in academics, social relationships, self-esteem, and occupation because of its demanding, impulsive, and seemingly lazy manifestations.
- Separation anxiety is a disruptive disorder that prevents children from engaging in normal activities because of a constant fear that their loved ones will be harmed in their absence.
- Like autistic disorder, Tourette's disorder involves repetitive movements, sounds, and actions; however, unlike autistic disorder, these symptoms diminish during adolescence and adulthood, and the disorder is not pervasive.
- One of the main characteristics of conduct disorder is the patient's violent or aggressive behavior and little concern for how this behavior affects others.
- Behavior modification programs are systematic structured plans with specific goals and time frames. The patient is rewarded for attaining stated goals.
- The early identification and treatment of problems in the child and adolescent are crucial to assisting the patient in the home, school, and social settings for both the short term and the long term.
- Nursing interventions with children and adolescents often are intense and challenging. The nurse works closely with the family and the interdisciplinary team to provide best practice and optimum care.

REVIEW QUESTIONS

1. A nurse assesses a 9-year-old girl for the risk of violence. School officials report that, although the patient is very intelligent, she was suspended for bringing illicit drugs onto the school campus. The child has lived with her mother since her parents were divorced 2 years ago, and her father is in prison. How many risk factors for committing a violent act are present for this child?
   1. One
   2. Two
   3. Three
   4. Four

2. A nurse prepares the plan of care for an adolescent with moderate mental retardation. Select the highest level of achievable outcomes for this patient. You may select more than one answer.
   1. Within 5 years, the patient will complete high school or pass a general educational development test.
   2. Within 5 years, the patient will safely use local public transportation.
   3. Within 5 years, the patient will live independently in an apartment.

REVIEW QUESTIONS—cont'd

4. Within 5 years, the patient will know how to correctly use a telephone.
5. Within 5 years, the patient will attain employment in a sheltered workshop.

3. A nurse counsels the parents of a child with autistic disorder. The parents say, "We are going to completely redecorate our child's room. We think that will help." Select the nurse's best response.
   1. "Children with autistic disorder usually prefer that things stay the same."
   2. "Bright colors are often stimulating for children with autistic disorder."
   3. "Remember to not use rugs so that your child will not slip and fall."
   4. "New toys and games will help develop your child's intellectual abilities."

4. A nurse suggests activities for a 7-year-old child with autistic disorder. Which activity is most likely to engage this child?
   1. Playing checkers with one other child
   2. Building with blocks alone
   3. Playing kickball with a small group of children
   4. Having a birthday party with six to eight other children
5. The parent of a child with Tourette's disorder says to the nurse, "I think my child is faking the tics, because they're absent during sleep." Select the nurse's accurate response.
   1. "Perhaps your child was misdiagnosed."
   2. "This finding indicates a worsening of the child's condition."
   3. "Your observation indicates that the medication is effective."
   4. "Tics are often reduced or absent during sleep."

REFERENCES

Ahluwalia J: *Suicidal behavior in adolescents: risk factor identification, screening, and prevention* (website): cme.medscape.com/viewarticle/702018. Accessed May 13, 2009.

American Academy of Child and Adolescent Psychiatry: *Children and watching TV, Facts for families #54*, Washington, DC, 2002, American Academy of Child and Adolescent Psychiatry. (website): www.aacap.org/page.ww?name=children+and+TV+violence&section=Facts+for+Families. Accessed February 18, 2010.

American Psychiatric Association: *Diagnostic and statistical manual of mental disorders*, ed 4, text revision, Washington, DC, 2000, American Psychiatric Association.

Autism Speaks Organization: *Top ten autism research findings of 2009: leading autism advocacy organization documents progress to discover causes and treatments for autism spectrum disorders* (website): http://www.autismspeaks.org/press/top_10_research_achievements_2009.php. Accessed February 9, 2011.

Bernstein GA et al: Anxiety disorder in children and adolescents: a review of the past 10 years, *J Am Acad Child Adolesc Psychiatry* 35:1110-1119, 1996.

Biederman J: Resolved: Mania is mistaken for ADHD in prepubertal children: affirmative, *J Am Acad Child Adolesc Psychiatry* 37:1091-1096, 1998.

Birmaher B et al: Childhood and adolescent depression: a review of the past 10 years, part I, *J Am Acad Child Adolesc Psychiatry* 35:1575-1583, 1996.

Birmaher B et al: Clinical course of children and adolescents with bipolar spectrum disorders, *Arch Gen Psychiatry* 63:175-183, 2006.

Boris N et al: Practice parameter for the assessment and treatment of children and adolescents with reactive attachment disorder of infancy and early childhood, *J Am Acad Child Adolesc Psychiatry* 44:1206-1219, 2005.

Bukstein O et al: Practice parameters for the assessment and treatment of children and adolescents with substance use disorders, *J Am Acad Child Adolesc Psychiatry* 44:609-621, 1997.

Cantwell DP: Attention deficit disorder: a review of the past 10 years, *J Am Acad Child Adolesc Psychiatry* 35:978-987, 1996.

Cohen J et al: Summary of the practice parameters for the assessment and treatment of children and adolescents with posttraumatic stress disorder, *J Am Acad Child Adolesc Psychiatry* 37:997-1001, 1998.

Crouch B et al: Trends in child and teen nonprescription drug abuse report to a regional poison control center, *Am J Health Syst Pharm* 61:1252-1257, 2004.

Dawson G et al: Randomized, controlled trial of an intervention for toddlers with autism: the early start Denver model, *Pediatrics* published online, 2009.

Dulcan M et al: Practice parameters for the assessment and treatment of children, adolescents, and adults with ADHD, *J Am Acad Child Adolesc Psychiatry* 36(10 Suppl):855-1215, 1997.

Hallfors D et al: Feasibility of screening adolescents for suicide risk in "real world" high school settings, *Am J Public Health* (96)2:282-287, 2006.

Johnson A et al: Violence and drug use in rural teens: the national prevalence estimates from 2003 youth risk behavior survey, *J School Health* 78(10):554-561, 2008.

King NJ: School refusal in children and adolescents: a review of the past 10 years, *J Am Acad Child Adolesc Psychiatry* 40:197-205, 2001.

Loeber R et al: Oppositional defiant disorder and conduct disorder: a review of the past 10 years, part I, *J Am Acad Child Adolesc Psychiatry* 39:1468-1684, 2000.

Maldonado-Duran M et al: *Child abuse and neglect: reactive attachment disorder* (website): http://emedicine.com/ped/topic2646.htm. Accessed January 9, 2006.

McClellan J et al: Practice parameters for the assessment and treatment of children and adolescents with bipolar disorder, *J Am Acad Child Adolesc Psychiatry* 36(10 Suppl):1775-1935, 1997.

Miller LJ et al: Concept evolution in sensory integration: a proposed nosology for diagnosis, *Am J Occup Ther* 61(2):135-140, 2007.

Muscari M: *How can I detect the warning signs of extreme violence in my patients?* (website): www.medscape.com/viewarticle/708159. Accessed September 9, 2009.

National Institute of Mental Health: *Child and adolescent mental health, 2005* (website): www.nimh.nih.gov/healthinformation/childmenu.cfm. Accessed October 17, 2005.

Nearns J: Attention deficit/hyperactivity disorder, *CME Resource* 1-28, 1997.

North American Nursing Diagnosis Association International: *NANDA nursing diagnoses: definitions and classifications, 2007-2008*, Philadelphia, 2007, North American Nursing Diagnosis Association International.

Pilowsky E: Panic attacks and suicide attempts in mid-adolescence, *Am J Psychiatry* 156:1545-1549, 1999.

Plauche Johnson C, Myers S: Identification and evaluation of children with autism spectrum reports, *Pediatrics* 120(5):1183-1215, 2007.

Pliszka S: The Texas children's medication algorithm project: report of the Texas consensus conference panel on medication treatment of childhood attention deficit/hyperactivity disorder: part II tactics, *J Am Acad Child Adolesc Psychiatry* 39:920-927, 2000.

Sadock BJ, Sadock VA: *Synopsis of psychiatry: behavioral sciences/clinical psychiatry*, ed 10, Philadelphia, 2007, Lippincott Williams & Wilkins.

Schowalter J: *A history of child and adolescent psychiatry in the United States* (website): www.psychiatrictimes.com/p030943.html. Accessed January 9, 2006.

Shaffer D et al: Practice parameters for the assessment and treatment of children and adolescents with suicidal behavior, *J Am Acad Child Adolesc Psychiatry* 40:24-51, 2001.

Silk J et al: Conceptualizing mental disorders in children: where have we been and where are we going? *Dev Psychopathol* 12:713-735, 2000.

Stokowski L: Bipolar disorder and ADHD in children: confusion and comorbidity, (website): www.medscape.com/viewarticle/711223. Accessed November 11, 2009.

Szymanski L et al: Practice parameters for the assessment and treatment of children, adolescents and adults with mental retardation and comorbid mental disorders, *J Am Acad Child Adolesc Psychiatry* 38:5-31, 1999.

Tanguay PE: Pervasive developmental disorders: a 10-year review, *J Am Acad Child Adolesc Psychiatry* 39:1079-1095, 2000.

Thomas A, Chess S: *Temperament and development*. New York, 1977, Brunner/Mazel.

U.S. Department of Health and Human Services: *Child welfare outcomes 2002-2005: report to Congress* (website): www.acf.hhs.gov/programs/cb/pubs/cwo05/chapters/chapter1.htm. Accessed January 6, 2010.

U.S. Surgeon General: *Mental health: a report of the Surgeon General* (website): www.surgeongeneral.gov/library/mentalhealth/chapter3/sec3.html. Accessed January 4, 2010.

U.S. Surgeon General: *Youth violence: a report of the surgeon general* (website): www.surgeongeneral.gov/library/youthviolence/youvioreport.html. Accessed April 24, 2002.

Valente S: Autism, *J Am Psychiatr Nurses Assoc* 10:236-243, 2004.

Vance JE et al: Risk and protective factors as predictors of outcome in adolescents with psychiatric disorder and aggression, *J Am Acad Child Adolesc Psychiatry* 41:36-43, 2002.

Vetter et al: Cardiovascular monitoring of children and adolescents with heart disease receiving medications for attention deficit/hyperactivity disorder, *Circulation* 120(7):55-59, 2008.

Volkmar FR: Practice parameters for the assessment and treatment of children, adolescents, and adults with autism and other pervasive developmental disorders, *J Am Acad Child Adolesc Psychiatry* 38:32-54, 1999.

Weinberg NZ et al: Adolescent substance abuse: a review of the past 10 years, *J Am Acad Child Adolesc Psychiatry* 37:252-261, 1998.

Online Resources

American Academy of Child and Adolescent Psychiatry: www.aacap.org

American Academy of Pediatrics: www.aap.org

Association of Child and Adolescent Psychiatric Nurses: www.ispn-psych.org/html/acapn.html

Attention Deficit Disorder Resources: www.addresources.org

Autism Society: www.autism-society.org

Child Abuse Prevention Association: www.childabuseprevention.org

Federation of Families for Children's Mental Health: www.ffcmh.org

Mental Health America: www.nmha.org

National Alliance on Mental Illness: www.nami.org

National Institute of Mental Health: www.nimh.nih.gov

National Youth Violence Prevention Resource Center: www.safeyouth.org

Substance Abuse and Mental Health Services Administration's National Mental Health Information Center: Caring for Every Child's Mental Health Campaign: www.mentalhealth.samhsa.gov/child

18

Eating Disorders: Anorexia Nervosa and Bulimia Nervosa

Anne Clarkin

"You gain strength, courage, and confidence by every experience in which you really stop to look fear in the face … you must do the thing you think you cannot do."

Eleanor Roosevelt

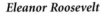 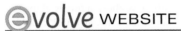 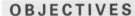

WEBSITE

http://evolve.elsevier.com/Fortinash/

OBJECTIVES

- Identify the behavioral and psychologic symptoms of anorexia nervosa and bulimia nervosa.
- Compare and contrast the medical complications of anorexic and bulimic behavior.
- Analyze the biologic, sociocultural, familial, and psychologic factors that contribute to the etiology of eating disorders.
- Explain the vicious cycle of eating disorder behavior.

- Discuss the psychologic issues associated with eating disorder behaviors.
- Describe the type of therapeutic relationship that is most effective with patients who have eating disorders, including the approach and attitude that the nurse should demonstrate to achieve this relationship.
- Apply the nursing process for patients with eating disorders.

KEY TERMS

alexithymia	body image disturbance	dichotomous thinking	interoceptive deficits
anorexia nervosa	bulimia nervosa	emotional dysregulation	purging
binge eating disorder	comorbidity	enmeshed families	secondary gains

Eating disorders are serious psychiatric illnesses with devastating and potentially fatal medical complications. Eating disorders have the highest mortality rate of all mental illnesses, and they often become chronic, lifelong conditions. With anorexia nervosa, a pathologic drive for thinness and a disturbed body image lead to self-starvation. With bulimia nervosa, a similar drive for thinness exists, but dietary restraint leads to cycles of binge eating and purging, usually with self-induced vomiting.

The epidemic of eating disorders during the late twentieth century happened at the same time as cultural trends in three major industries: the fashion industry, the diet and fitness industry, and the women's movement. A shift toward thinness in fashion, the emergence of the diet and fitness industry, and

changes in women's roles created a climate for an outbreak of eating disorders. Box 18-1 summarizes these cultural trends.

This epidemic of eating disorders got the public's attention. The media are still fascinated with eating disorders, which has helped to raise awareness about eating disorders worldwide. An explosion of literature since the 1980s includes medical and psychiatric research, sociocultural essays, autobiographies, and works from the popular press.

HISTORIC AND THEORETIC PERSPECTIVES

The drastic increase in eating disorders during the late twentieth century suggests that it is a fad or trend of modern,

BOX 18-1	CULTURAL TRENDS AND EATING DISORDERS

Fashion Industry

Cultural ideals of beauty have always been reflected in current fashion. The trend in fashion since the 1960s has been increasingly toward thinness. By the late twentieth century, fashion had become a huge industry fueled by advertising dollars and exerting great influence on the public, especially women. The media are full of images of the thin, fit, "perfect" body, and this represents an ideal that is unattainable for most people. Epidemiologic studies show that 0.1% of people have a natural body type that matches the ideal. This leads most people to believe that their normal, healthy shape is too fat. The pervasiveness of this trend is reflected in the dieting behavior and body dissatisfaction found among high school, elementary school, and middle school children.

Diet and Fitness Industry

The second trend that affects eating disorders is the diet and fitness industry. Weight management has moved out of the doctor's office and into multibillion-dollar businesses run by opportunistic, business-minded people who are not part of the health professions. The media flood the public with an array of products such as pills, powders, packaged food, diet books, videos, and a variety of health club and diet program memberships designed to help us attain the "perfect body." Men have become more obsessed with an ideal, lean, and muscular body, which is equally unattainable for the average guy, and this has led men to buy into the diet and fitness industry. Eating disorders have become much more common among males.

Women's Movement

A third trend is the ongoing women's movement. Although women's struggles for equality are not new, women's roles have changed dramatically since the early 1980s. Pressure to balance motherhood, marriage, and career has influenced women of all generations. The need for women to achieve success both academically and professionally while still fulfilling their traditional female roles creates conflicts, even as it affords women greater societal rights and freedom.

Professional women need to be aggressive to successfully compete in the business world, yet women are still socialized to be passive and accommodating. Some feminists view the drive for thinness as symbolizing a woman's attempt to destroy her femininity to compete in a man's world or as male society's reaction to the women's movement. Pressuring women to strive for an impossible ideal of thinness promotes feelings of inadequacy that drive women to constantly diet and exercise.

fashion-conscious young women and, more recently, of body-conscious young men. However, self-starvation, bingeing, and purging have existed for centuries. Throughout history, food has always been a compelling cultural symbol, so the denial of appetite and the rejection of food are always attention-getting behaviors. Earlier in history, cases of anorexia nervosa were rare and poorly understood.

Incidence in History

Brumberg, in *Fasting Girls* (1989), and Bell, in *Holy Anorexia* (1987), noted that medieval women commonly starved themselves in devotion to Christ. Both authors detail the case of Saint Catherine of Siena of Italy (1347-1380), who kept an extensive diary of her fasting and self-induced vomiting. Her piety also included self-flagellation and other self-punishing behaviors, which were not very different from the self-destructive behaviors that are common today among patients with anorexia and bulimia. This demonstrates the connectedness of anorexic and bulimic behaviors from the beginning of their known existence.

Few clinical accounts of normal-weight bulimia nervosa existed until case histories began to appear in psychoanalytic literature during the 1950s. In "The Case of Ellen West," American psychoanalyst Binswanger (1958) described a woman whom he treated in 1915 who starved herself, binged and purged with self-induced vomiting, exercised excessively, and used laxatives. Obsessed with food and clinically depressed, she committed suicide 13 years later. In *The Fifty Minute Hour*, psychiatrist Robert Lindner (1955) described the case of "Laura," a patient with bulimia nervosa.

These psychoanalytic case studies focus on symptoms as manifestations of intrapsychic issues such as oral impregnation fears, oral eroticism, rejection of femininity, and unconscious hatred of the mother; they ignore cultural and biologic factors. Lesser-known case studies noted bulimic behavior among young girls in boarding schools and refugee children, which suggests a connection to insecure attachment and separation fears; this theory is held today regarding the onset of eating disorders during adolescence (Johnson and Connors, 1987).

The term *compulsive overeating* was first used during the 1950s to describe binge eating among the overweight and obese population (Hamburger, 1951; Stunkard, 1959). Compulsive eating was compared with alcoholism, with its similar cravings and secret binges followed by shame and guilt. *Binge eating disorder* is a new term for this disorder.

During the mid-1970s, psychologist Marlene Boskind-Lodahl described a group of normal-weight women whom she saw at Cornell University's mental health clinic who shared the anorectic individual's fear of fat and drive for thinness. These women also regularly binged and purged. In her 1983 book, the author described her clinical experience and new research with this group, who represented the first wave of the current outbreak of eating disorders (Boskind-Lodahl and White, 1983). Russell (1979) coined the term *bulimia nervosa*, which linked bulimia with anorexia nervosa.

ETIOLOGY

Researchers have studied a variety of etiologic theories regarding eating disorders from biologic, psychologic, psychoanalytic, behavioral, and addiction viewpoints. Currently there is no clear agreement regarding what causes eating disorders. However, many opposing theories have come together to form a framework that better explains eating disorders as multidetermined syndromes. Researchers now believe that eating disorders are caused by an interaction of biologic susceptibility, including genetic markers for neurobiologic vulnerability related to premorbid temperament (Kaye, 2007), and environmental influences, including family, social, and cultural environments. A predisposed individual experiences stress, often related to the developmental tasks of adolescence, and decides to diet, which triggers the eating disorder (Box 18-2).

Biologic Factors

The many physiologic abnormalities found in patients with anorexia nervosa and bulimia nervosa suggest a biologic etiology. The homogeneity of the symptoms is striking; anorexic patients express remarkably similar thoughts and beliefs and engage in identical odd behaviors, which suggests a genetic etiology. A confounding factor is that extreme behaviors of starving, bingeing, and purging themselves cause a range of neurobiologic, metabolic, and behavioral abnormalities. Some of these effects make the patient continue the behavior. For example, starving decreases appetite and delays gastric emptying, which results in less desire to eat (Polivy and Herman, 2002). Many of these changes reverse with refeeding and the cessation of purging, but not all of them do.

Significant research into the genetics of eating disorders is currently taking place, including a study by the National Institute of Mental Health and an international multisite project sponsored by the Price Foundation. Twin and family studies suggest that up to 50% of the risk for eating disorders is possibly genetic. Relatives of anorexic patients are 12 times as likely to develop anorexia nervosa and 4 times as likely to develop bulimia nervosa. Researchers believe that a gene on chromosome 1 increases the risk for anorexia nervosa and that a gene on chromosome 10 increases the risk for bulimia nervosa (Bulik et al, 2003; Grice et al, 2002; Klump et al, 2001). It is impossible that a single gene causes eating disorders. The concept of the additive effects of several genes for high-risk personality traits and neurobiologic dysfunction is a more significant theory. New research shows significantly high basal serotonin levels and oversensitivity in the serotonin system of anorexic patients. Researchers wonder if this creates constant anxiety that is relieved by starving, which decreases serotonin. Bulimic patients show low basal serotonin levels, which are associated with depression. Serotonin levels and mood both improve with bingeing. Serotonin dysregulation is often present premorbidly and persists in many patients after recovery, which suggests a fundamental biologic dysregulation that the person tries to modulate with eating disorder behaviors (Bailer et al, 2004 and 2005; Kaye et al, 2001a). Research with recovered anorexic patients also shows overactive dopamine receptors related to excessive worry and a lack of positive response to common comforts and pleasures, such as food (Kaye et al, 1999; Kaye, 2005).

Sociocultural Factors

By adolescence, everyone has been exposed to countless advertisements by the diet and fashion industries that encourage them to strive for an idealized body and that promise that dieting and exercise will help them to achieve that goal. This "ideal" body shape is unrealistically thin for girls and equally unrealistically lean and muscular for boys. Most normal-sized adolescents feel dissatisfied with their bodies (Groesz et al, 2002). Teenagers from families that nurture and reward them with food; that equate food with pleasure, comfort, and love; or that use food as punishment by imposing dieting and food restrictions may view food as damaging or bad. The preanorexic or prebulimic person often observes their parents' struggles to balance all of society's expectations. Some have watched their mothers try to maintain a feminine image while striving to achieve in the business world. Some also observe their dieting parents and listen to their parents' self-criticism about weight and shape.

Another risk factor is participation in sports that encourage weight loss, such as cheerleading, wrestling, and running track. Participation in intensely competitive sports that encourage perfectionism and compulsive exercise also carries a high risk.

Psychologic Factors

Although the same sociocultural pressures challenge all adolescents, only a few (approximately 8%) develop eating disorders. Some teens have temperaments and coping styles that seem to protect them from eating disorders, whereas other teens have personalities and coping styles that put them at risk. Some high-risk personality traits are common to all

BOX 18-3	HIGH-RISK PERSONALITY TRAITS FOR THE DEVELOPMENT OF EATING DISORDERS

All Eating Disorders
Low self-esteem
Compliance and conflict avoidance
Sense of ineffectiveness Alexithymia (i.e., difficulty naming and expressing emotions) Interoceptive deficits (i.e., the inability to accurately identify and respond to bodily cues)
Alexithymia (i.e., difficulty naming and expressing emotions)
Interoceptive deficits (i.e., the inability to accurately identify and respond to bodily cues)

Anorexia Nervosa
Perfectionism
Rigidity
Risk and harm avoidance

Bulimia Nervosa
Impulsivity
Emotional dysregulation (i.e., oversensitivity to and difficulty with modulating emotions and behavior)

eating disorders, whereas some personality traits are more specific to anorexia nervosa or bulimia nervosa (Box 18-3).

Cognitive therapy literature describes certain distorted thinking patterns as characteristic of people who have eating disorders (Lock and Le Grange, 2005a and 2005b). These include dichotomous thinking (i.e., individuals view situations as either all good or all bad), control fallacies (i.e., individuals feel solely responsible for the happiness and failure of others), and personalization (i.e., individuals compare themselves endlessly with others and perceive others' behavior as a direct reaction to them) (see Chapter 14).

Familial Factors

Many personality traits are genetically determined, but researchers believe that the environment affects the personality as well. Families are a strong environmental influence. In 1978, Minuchin and colleagues described a stereotypic "eating disorder family" as Caucasian, upper middle class, intact, enmeshed, rigid, and hostile. Today, eating disorders occur among all socioeconomic levels, races, and cultures and are seen with a range of interactive family styles. Enmeshed families have poor boundaries, expect conformity, and discourage individuality and the direct expression of feelings. Parents are often controlling, critical, and demanding. They sometimes demonstrate poor conflict-resolution skills, which is displayed as the denial of disagreement, conflict avoidance, or constant and unproductive arguing. The result is tension and a fear of conflict.

These families often put a lot of importance on body image, social acceptance, and achievement. Research demonstrates the powerful influence of the parental encouragement of dieting and preoccupation with body image (Davis et al, 2004). Girls who do not identify with their mothers are at higher risk for low self-esteem and eating disorders (Hahn-Smith and Smith, 2001). A poor marital relationship increases the risk of eating disorders in children (Wade et al, 2001). If a child sees the drive for thinness, dieting, or other extreme behaviors in her role models, he or she is likely to try dieting as an attempt to improve her self-esteem.

In extremely dysfunctional families, the damage is often severe. Alcoholism and physical and sexual abuse have devastating effects. Emotional abuse is subtly damaging. In some cases, parents do not encourage the child to be independent, to develop self-trust, or to have pride in his or her individuality. If the child learns to avoid conflict to please others and learns to fear adult responsibilities, adolescence is a crisis. A sense of competence never fully develops, and the pressures to separate and to be an individual during adolescence are terrifying to both the child and the parents.

Confronted with this crisis, it is not surprising that the adolescent feels overwhelmed and out of control. The myth of thinness as the key to confidence, success, and control is compelling. The adolescent begins dieting, loses weight, begins to feel better, continues dieting and losing weight, and experiences a sense of control and accomplishment. Unfortunately, secondary gains such as attention and envy from peers—and often from parents—reinforce this behavior. Later, when people tell her she is getting too thin, the adolescent feels a sense of power and control that she has never felt before. By losing weight, she not only has gotten attention, but she also has frustrated those who try to make her eat normally. These secondary gains are often very rewarding, especially to a perfectionist, conflict-avoidant individual with low self-esteem. The diet has distracted her from her actual conflicts and given her a sense of mastery. Although this mastery is false, the adolescent does not want to lose it.

Sometimes the individual is unable to stick to the diet. Binge eating often begins as a reaction to the deprivation of dieting. Bingeing not only relieves hunger but also numbs pain and distracts an individual from actual conflicts. It sometimes represents an angry rebellion against the pressure to be thin. The relief of a binge is temporary, and it is quickly followed by guilt about eating and panic about the loss of control and potential weight gain. Purging reverses the binge—and the guilt. Figure 18-1 illustrates the interrelationship of all the etiologic factors in the cycle of eating disorders.

EPIDEMIOLOGY

Eight million women and 1 million men currently suffer from eating disorders. Studies using strict *Diagnostic and Statistical Manual of Mental Disorders,* fourth edition, text revision (DSM-IV-TR) criteria estimate that 3% to 10% of adolescent and college-aged women and 2% of adolescent males are bulimic. The rate of these conditions is 2% among the general population. Disturbed eating patterns, including dieting with the occasional use of diet pills, laxatives, or vomiting, occurs among 13% of young women. Binge eating without purging

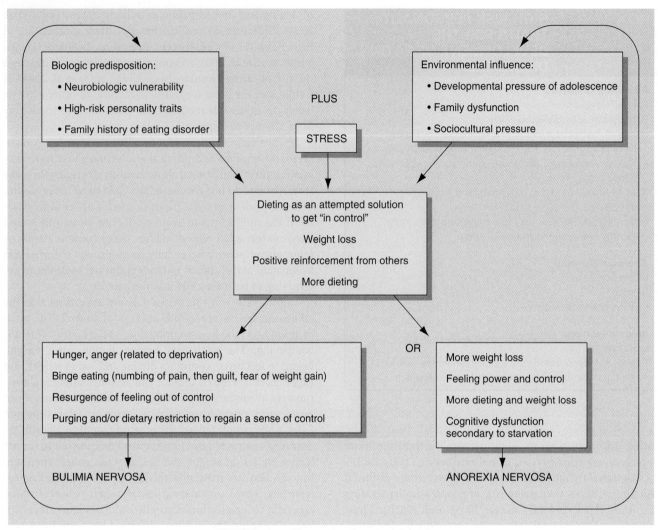

FIGURE 18-1. The cycle of eating disorders.

at least once a week occurs in approximately 5% to 20% of all women and slightly fewer men. Studies show anorexia nervosa to be consistent at a rate of 0.5% to 1% among adolescent and college-aged women. Anorexia nervosa is much less common among males. Box 18-4 summarizes the incidence and prevalence of eating disorders.

Sex Ratio

Eating disorders mostly affect females, although more cases among men are emerging. Since the early 1980s, the ratio of male-to-female cases of all three eating disorders has increased from 1:100 to 1:10. A few gender differences have emerged, and these have specifically demonstrated that men with eating disorders are more likely to have premorbid obesity and to exercise excessively (Fernandez-Aranda et al, 2004; Lewinsohn et al, 2002b).

Age of Onset

Most eating disorders begin during adolescence. About 86% of those with eating disorders report an onset before the age of 20 years. The average age of onset of bulimia nervosa is 18

years, with 80% of cases reported with an onset between the ages of 15 and 30 years. For anorexia nervosa, the peak age range of onset has decreased from 14 to 18 years to 11 to 18 years. Many cases of anorexia nervosa have occurred in children as young as 8 years old. The range of onset ages for both disorders is 8 to 70 years.

Cross-Cultural Studies

The incidence and prevalence of eating disorders around the world are similar among European countries, the United States, Canada, Mexico, Japan, Australia, and other Westernized countries that have plentiful food supplies. In the United States, there is no difference in incidence among racial, ethnic, or socioeconomic groups.

Mortality

The mortality rate with eating disorders is higher than that seen with any other psychiatric diagnoses, and it has been reported at 4% to 20% (Agras, 2001; Crow et al, 2009; Papadopoulos et al, 2009). Medical complications, substance-use–related death, and suicide are the main causes

BOX 18-4	EPIDEMIOLOGY OF EATING DISORDERS

- Approximately 7 million women and 1 million men suffer from eating disorders in the United States.
- The average age of onset is 11 to 18 years for anorexia nervosa, with cases being seen in children as young as 8 years old; the average age of onset is 17 years for bulimia nervosa.
- Approximately 5% to 8% of adolescent and college-aged women and 2% of adolescent men have bulimia nervosa.
- Approximately 2% of women and less than 1% of men in the general population have bulimia nervosa.
- Less than 1% of the general population has anorexia nervosa.
- Approximately 10% of adolescent and college-aged women have subclinical anorexia nervosa; 15% have subclinical bulimia nervosa.
- Approximately 5% to 20% of the general population (both male and female) binge regularly but do not purge.
- Approximately 90% of patients with eating disorders are female, which is a decrease from the 95% to 99% found in past studies.
- Approximately 50% of those with eating disorders recover; 77% report having had the disorder for 1 to 5 years.
- Mortality rates for bulimia nervosa are 4% to 19%; for anorexia nervosa, mortality rates are 6% to 20%. The rate increases to 20% for those who have had anorexia nervosa for 20 years.
- Similar incidence and prevalence rates are found among the Western countries, where food is abundant and dieting is common.
- Comorbidities include the following: Axis I: mood disorders (dysthymic disorders, major depressive disorder), anxiety disorders (generalized anxiety disorder, social phobia, obsessive-compulsive disorder, posttraumatic stress disorder), dissociative identity disorder, substance-related disorders. Axis II: personality disorders (borderline personality disorder, histrionic personality disorder, obsessive-compulsive personality disorder).

From the American Psychiatric Association: *Diagnostic and statistical manual of mental disorders,* ed 4, text revision, Washington, DC, 2000, American Psychiatric Association.

of death among this population. The suicide mortality ratio is significantly higher with bulimia nervosa, anorexia nervosa, and eating disorders not otherwise specified (American Psychiatric Association, 2000; Crow et al, 2009; Papadopoulos et al, 2009).

Comorbidity (Co-occurrence)

Comorbidity is the concurrent existence of two or more disorders. Depression is diagnosed in 40% to 75% of individuals with eating disorders, and it is more frequently diagnosed among patients with bulimia nervosa than with anorexia nervosa. Two thirds of eating disorder patients are diagnosed with comorbid anxiety disorders, specifically generalized anxiety disorders, obsessive-compulsive disorder, and social phobia (Kaye et al, 2004; Milos et al, 2002). With anorexia nervosa, obsessive-compulsive disorder is the most frequent co-occurring diagnosis, followed by mood disorders, posttraumatic stress disorder, social phobia, and dissociative disorder (Lewinsohn et al, 2002a; Milos et al, 2002). Substance use disorders occur in up to 17% of eating disorder patients, but they coexist more frequently with bulimia nervosa and anorexia nervosa, binge eating/purging type, than with anorexia nervosa, restricting type (Franco et al, 2005; von Ranson et al, 2002). Eating disorder symptoms predict the type of drug use, with bingeing associated more with alcohol and tranquilizer abuse, purging associated with more with the abuse of multiple drugs, and restricting associated more with amphetamine abuse (Harrop and Marlatt, 2010).

Careful diagnosis is necessary to separate the side effects of starvation and purging from the symptoms of co-occurring mood disorders.

The occurrence of comorbid personality disorders is well known to clinicians who deal with eating disorders. Three fourths of patients with eating disorders have an Axis II diagnosis. Borderline personality disorder is the Axis II diagnosis that is most commonly associated with eating disorders. Histrionic, schizotypal, and obsessive-compulsive personality disorders are also prevalent (Johnson et al, 2006). A quarter to a third of eating disorder patients report a history of childhood sexual abuse. These individuals have a higher incidence of co-occurring dissociative disorders and impulsive, self-injurious behavior (Paul et al, 2002; Wonderlich et al, 2001).

CLINICAL DESCRIPTION

Eating disorders are an easily recognizable group of psychiatric diagnoses. Refusal to eat, severe weight loss, and self-induced vomiting are unmistakable indicators of an eating disorder. However, making a precise DSM-IV-TR diagnosis and determining specific nursing diagnoses to reflect a particular patient's case are challenging and complicated tasks.

Anorexia nervosa and bulimia nervosa are the two specific eating disorder diagnoses in the DSM-IV-TR classification. The category of eating disorder not otherwise specified is provided to diagnose individuals with disordered eating who do not meet the criteria for anorexia nervosa or bulimia nervosa. The DSM-IV-TR Criteria boxes on pages 422 and 423 detail the criteria for these three diagnoses. The clinical symptoms of anorexia nervosa and bulimia nervosa are in the Clinical Symptoms boxes on pages 423 and 424.

Obesity is not included as an eating disorder in the DSM-IV-TR classification, because all cases of obesity do not involve psychiatric illness. Obesity itself is classified in the *International Statistical Classification of Diseases and Related Health Problems,* tenth edition, as a general medical condition (American Psychiatric Association, 2000).

The inclusion or exclusion of binge eating disorder (BED) in the DSM-IV-TR classification has been a controversial issue. BED is cited as an example of an eating disorder not otherwise specified, and it is included in the DSM-IV-TR as a proposed diagnosis for further study. BED is described specifically as recurrent episodes of binge eating during which the individual eats more than most people eat during a similar period and feels out of control while eating. Other criteria include distress, guilt, and disgust regarding the behavior (APA, 2000) BED will likely be included as an eating disorder diagnosis in the DSM-V.

Anorexia nervosa and bulimia nervosa are distinct diagnoses, but the conditions have many of the same features.

Many underweight patients with anorexia nervosa binge and purge, and many patients with bulimia nervosa use fasting or exercise but not purging to compensate for binges. The subtypes as well as the eating disorder not otherwise specified category assist the physician with making the most precise diagnosis. For example, if an individual meets the criteria for both bulimia nervosa and anorexia nervosa, the diagnosis of anorexia nervosa, binge eating/purging type, is made, because it is the only category that includes all of the symptoms (i.e., neither subtype of bulimia nervosa deals with weight loss). Half of individuals with eating disorders "migrate" from one diagnosis to another over time. This finding indicates that eating disorder diagnoses require further refining (Milos et al, 2005).

DSM-IV-TR CRITERIA

Anorexia Nervosa

A Refusal to maintain body weight at or above a minimally normal weight for age and height (e.g., weight loss leading to maintenance of body weight less than 85% of that expected, or failure to make expected weight gain during period of growth leading to body weight less than 85% of that expected)

B Intense fear of gaining weight or becoming fat even though underweight

C Disturbance in the way in which one's body weight or shape is experienced, undue influence of body weight or shape on self-evaluation, or denial of the seriousness of the current low body weight

D In postmenarchal females amenorrhea (i.e., the absence of at least three consecutive menstrual cycles) (A woman is considered to have amenorrhea if her periods occur only after hormone [e.g., estrogen] administration.)

Specify type:

Restricting type: During the current episode of anorexia nervosa, the person has not regularly engaged in binge eating or purging behavior (i.e., self-induced vomiting or the misuse of laxatives, diuretics, or enemas).

Binge-eating/purging type: During the current episode of anorexia nervosa, the person has regularly engaged in binge-eating or purging behavior (i.e., self-induced vomiting or the misuse of laxatives, diuretics, or enemas).

From the American Psychiatric Association: *Diagnostic and statistical manual of mental disorders,* ed 4, text revision, Washington, DC, 2000, American Psychiatric Association.

DSM-IV-TR CRITERIA

Bulimia Nervosa

A Recurrent episodes of binge eating. An episode of binge eating is characterized by both of the following:

1 Eating, in a discrete period of time (e.g., within any 2-hour period), an amount of food that is definitely larger than most people would eat during a similar period of time and under similar circumstances

2 A sense of lack of control over eating during the episode (e.g., a feeling that one cannot stop eating or control what or how much one is eating)

B Recurrent inappropriate compensatory behavior to prevent weight gain, such as self-induced vomiting; misuse of laxatives, diuretics, enemas, or other medications; fasting; or excessive exercise.

C The binge eating and inappropriate compensatory behaviors both occur, on average, at least twice a week for 3 months.

D Self-evaluation is unduly influenced by body shape and weight.

E The disturbance does not occur exclusively during episodes of anorexia nervosa.

Specify type:

Purging type: During the current episode of bulimia nervosa, the person has regularly engaged in self-induced vomiting or the misuse of laxatives, diuretics, or enemas.

Nonpurging type: During the current episode of bulimia nervosa, the person has used other inappropriate compensatory behaviors, such as fasting or excessive exercise, but has not regularly engaged in self-induced vomiting or the misuse of laxatives, diuretics, or enemas.

From the American Psychiatric Association: *Diagnostic and statistical manual of mental disorders,* ed 4, text revision, Washington, DC, 2000, American Psychiatric Association.

DSM-IV-TR CRITERIA

Eating Disorder Not Otherwise Specified

The *eating disorder not otherwise specified* category is for disorders of eating that do not meet the criteria for a specific eating disorder. Examples include the following:

1 For females, all of the criteria for anorexia nervosa are met except that the individual has regular menses.
2 All of the criteria for anorexia nervosa are met except that, despite significant weight loss, the individual's current weight is in the normal range.
3 All of the criteria for bulimia nervosa are met except that the frequency of binge eating and inappropriate compensatory mechanisms occurs less than twice a week or for less than 3 months.
4 The regular use of inappropriate compensatory behavior by an individual of normal body weight after eating small amounts of food (e.g., self-induced vomiting after the consumption of two cookies).
5 The individual repeatedly chews and spits out, but does not swallow, large amounts of food.
6 Binge-eating disorder: recurrent episodes of binge eating in the absence of the regular use of inappropriate compensatory behaviors characteristic of bulimia nervosa.

From the American Psychiatric Association: *Diagnostic and statistical manual of mental disorders,* ed 4, text revision, Washington, DC, 2000, American Psychiatric Association.

CLINICAL SYMPTOMS

Anorexia Nervosa

Behavioral Symptoms

Self-starvation (i.e., reported intake restriction and refusal to eat)
Rituals or compulsive behaviors regarding food, eating, or weight loss
Engages in self-induced vomiting, laxative or diuretic use, or excessive exercise to lose weight
Wears baggy clothes or inappropriate layers of clothing

Physical Symptoms

Weight that is 15% below ideal weight
Amenorrhea (i.e., the absence of three or more menstrual cycles when they are expected to occur; this may be primary or secondary)
Slow pulse and decreased body temperature
Cachexia (i.e., muscle wasting), sunken eyes, protruding bones, and dry skin
Growth of lanugo (i.e., fine hair) on the face and body
Constipation
Cold sensitivity
Bradycardia

Orthostatic hypotension
During adolescence, weight loss may delay puberty and retard growth

Psychologic Symptoms

Denial of the seriousness of the current low weight as well as denial of hunger
Body image disturbance (i.e., seeing the self as unrealistically fat when the person is actually at or near the ideal weight or experiencing parts of the body as unrealistically fat or out of proportion) (Figure 18-2)
Intense and irrational fear of weight gain that does not diminish as weight is lost
Constant striving for the "perfect" body
Anxiety around food and mealtimes
Self-concept that is unduly influenced by shape and weight
Preoccupation with food, cooking, nutritional information, and feeding others
Shows delayed psychosexual development or lacks age-appropriate interest in sex and relationships

PROGNOSIS

The course of the illness with eating disorders is variable. Some individuals recover fully from a single and time-limited episode of anorexia nervosa or bulimia nervosa. Many teens with anorexia nervosa who recover their normal weight later develop bulimia nervosa. Many individuals with eating disorders follow a chronic course or a pattern of relapses and remissions. Others show slow improvement after several years of treatment.

Long-term outcome studies show a more promising prognosis for those patients who continue treatment. More than 50% show improvement after 5 years (Lowe et al, 2001; Polivy and Herman, 2002). Weight restoration is necessary but not sufficient for recovery. Individuals need to resolve the core

problems related to their eating behavior as well as the underlying psychologic issues (Sysko, 2005). Outcome literature indicates that long-term cognitive-behavioral, family, or interpersonal therapy, often in combination with antidepressant medication, results in the most sustained improvement (Dare et al, 2001; Keel et al, 2002; Lowe et al, 2001).

DISCHARGE CRITERIA

The client will do the following:
• Be free from self-harm.
• Achieve the minimum (i.e., within 10%) normal weight as determined by the treatment team.
• Consume adequate calories to maintain a minimum normal weight.

CLINICAL SYMPTOMS

Bulimia Nervosa

Behavioral Symptoms

Recurrent episodes of binge eating (i.e., the consumption of a large amount of food in a discrete period of time)

Engages in **purging** behaviors to compensate for the binge, such as self-induced vomiting; the use of laxatives, diuretics, diet pills, ipecac, or enemas; excessive exercise; and periods of fasting

Physical Symptoms

May experience fluid and electrolyte imbalances from purging:

    Hypokalemia (low potassium levels)

    Alkalosis (high alkaline levels in body fluids)

    Dehydration

    Idiopathic edema (tissue swelling)

Cardiovascular

    Hypotension (low blood pressure)

    Cardiac arrhythmia/dysrhythmia (irregular heartbeat)

    Cardiomyopathy (heart muscle problem)

Endocrine

    Hypoglycemia (low blood sugar)

    May experience menstrual dysfunction

Gastrointestinal

    Constipation or diarrhea

    Gastroparesis (i.e., delayed gastric emptying)

    Esophageal reflux (i.e., the backflow of food from the stomach)

    Esophagitis (i.e., the inflammation of the esophagus)

    Mallory-Weiss syndrome (i.e., tears in esophagus)

    Dental enamel erosion

    Parotid gland enlargement (these are glands situated below and in front of each ear)

Psychologic Symptoms

Body image disturbance (see Figure 18-2)

Persistent overconcern with body weight, shape, and proportions

Mood swings and irritability

Self-concept that is unduly influenced by body weight and shape

Denial or minimization of seriousness of binge/purge behavior and risk of death

Secrecy and shame associated with binge/purge behaviors

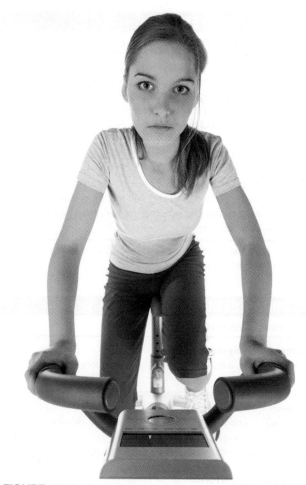

FIGURE 18-2. An individual's appearance influences self-concept. Patients with eating disorders often have a distorted view of their physical appearance and perceive themselves as unrealistically large. From Sorrentino SA: *Mosby's textbook for nursing assistants,* ed 6, St. Louis, 2004, Mosby.

- Attend group therapy sessions that encourage healthy eating patterns and a positive self-image and self-concept.
- Interact with peers who support the patient in maintaining healthy behavior.
- Keep follow-up appointments with the therapist, psychiatrist, and dietitian.

- Demonstrate the ability to follow the treatment regimen recommended to occur after discharge (i.e., compliance with medication, food plan, control of the binge/purge behavior, and plan for follow-up care).
- Verbalize awareness and understanding of the psychologic issues related to the eating disorder behavior and the maladaptive use of food and weight control to try to cope with these issues.
- Demonstrate the use of improved coping abilities to respond to stress and to manage anxiety and dysphoria.
- Exhibit developmentally appropriate boundaries within the family system and other interpersonal relationships.

THE NURSING PROCESS

ASSESSMENT

The nursing assessment of patients with eating disorders involves sensitivity, thoroughness, and sharp observation skills. The first few minutes of the interview are essential, because first impressions set the tone for the entire treatment experience. Patients with eating disorders are sensitive to others and quick to judge whether others are trustworthy. If the nurse forms a therapeutic alliance immediately, this will prevent many of the power struggles that are common (see the Case Study #1 and the Nursing Assessment Questions

CASE STUDY #1

Sienna is a 19-year-old college student who was brought to the emergency department by her boyfriend after she fainted in the shower. The boyfriend took the nurse aside and confided that Sienna was bulimic and that he was concerned that her eating disorder was related to the fainting episode. He said that Sienna was secretive and somewhat defensive about the bulimia. The initial physical examination showed no injuries from the fall, and Sienna's vital signs were normal. Her parotid glands appeared to be enlarged, and her weight appeared to be within a normal range. Her affect was tense and anxious. Sienna avoided eye contact with the nurse and mumbled that she had recently been up late studying and had not been getting enough sleep.

Critical Thinking

1 How should the nurse approach Sienna? How can the nurse bring up the subject of bulimia nervosa?
2 If Sienna responds defensively or with denial, how should the nurse respond?
3 What further physical assessments should be performed?
4 What other information is needed to complete the nursing assessment?

NURSING ASSESSMENT QUESTIONS

Eating Disorders

1 How do you feel about being here today? *To determine whether the patient is self-referred or forced into treatment and to assess the patient's willingness to participate in treatment*
2 Have you ever talked with anyone before about your eating disorder? *To assess the patient's level of self-disclosure and to reduce his or her anxiety and feelings of shame*
3 Have you been in therapy before? *To assess the patient's treatment history and to get details of previous treatment, including the name of the associated clinician, the dates of treatment, the outcomes, and the patient's experience with treatment*
4 Describe your weight throughout your life. Include the following factors when discussing weight:
 Current weight, including fluctuations during past 6 months
 Desired weight
 Lowest and highest weight (excluding pregnancy)
 Perception of childhood and adolescent size and shape
 Perception of current size and shape
 Family history of eating disorders or obesity
 Family history of dieting or preoccupation with thinness
 Childhood experiences related to weight and eating
 To determine the patient's premorbid weight and his or her perceptions of his or her body
5 How do you feel about the way your body looks? *To assess the patient's body dissatisfaction and body image distortion*
6 Assess your dieting history:
 When did you first diet?
 What started your dieting?
 What happened when you dieted?
 Did you lose or gain weight?
 Has anyone encouraged you to lose weight?
 What dieting behaviors have you used?
 To determine any use of fasting, structured diet, restriction, or diet products or programs
7 Assess your binge eating:
 Do you binge eat?
 When was the first time you binged?
 Get details about typical binge eating, including when and where it occurs, its duration and frequency, the type and amount of food ingested, and any rituals or patterns involved. Ask the patient if secrecy, hiding, stealing, or lying is involved. Assess the patient's level of control (i.e., can the patient interrupt a binge after it has begun?). *To determine the nature of the patient's bingeing to plan effective treatment; habits that are long-lasting are usually more challenging*
8 Help the patient to identify the feeling states associated with the binge: before bingeing, during the planning stages, and during and after the binge. Ask the patient to focus on past binge episodes and to answer this question: "Did you feel angry or anxious?" *To determine the patient's feelings about binge behaviors*
9 Assess the patient's food cravings (e.g., time of day, day of week, where in the menstrual cycle, any association with place [i.e., car, work, home, or store]). *To determine if the patient is able to associate his or her cravings with specific times or situations*
10 Assess the patient's purging behavior, including the following:
 Type (e.g., vomiting, diuretics, laxatives, diet pills, ipecac, thyroid pills, amphetamines, cocaine, exercise)
 Frequency (times per week)
 Amount of food purged
 Age at first purging episode
 Date of last purging episode
 To identify the patient's usual methods of purging
11 Assess the patient's menstrual history (i.e., onset of menses, regularity, premenstrual syndrome, menstrual dysfunction, and any hormone therapy). *To determine the effect of dysfunctional behaviors on menses*
12 Assess the medical side effects of the patient's eating disorder. *To identify any concomitant medical problems*
13 Assess for any comorbid (co-occurring) factors (e.g., mood disorders, anxiety, substance abuse). *To determine if there are other factors that will complicate the patient's problem*

box). Because many patients with eating disorders have one or more coexisting disorders, it is critical for the nurse to assess for the co-occurring disorders (see Box 18-4).

NURSING DIAGNOSIS

Nursing diagnoses are made from the information obtained during the assessment phase of the nursing process. The accuracy of diagnosis depends on a careful, in-depth assessment. Nursing diagnoses are prioritized according to patient needs from most urgent to least urgent.

Anorexia Nervosa

Safety or health risks of anorexia nervosa include the following:
- Risk for self-mutilation
- Risk for imbalanced body temperature
- Deficient fluid volume
- Risk for imbalanced fluid volume
- Constipation
- Perceived constipation
- Imbalanced nutrition: less than body requirements
- Delayed growth and development
  Perceptual, cognitive, and emotional disturbances include the following:
- Anxiety
- Disturbed body image
- Hopelessness
- Powerlessness
- Chronic low self-esteem
  Problems with communicating with and relating to others include the following:
- Sexual dysfunction
- Impaired social interaction
- Social isolation
  Disruptions in coping abilities are as follows:
- Ineffective coping
- Disabled family coping
- Ineffective denial
  Patient and family teaching needs may include the following:
- Deficient knowledge regarding nutrition and medical side effects of anorexic behavior
- Noncompliance with refeeding process

Bulimia Nervosa

The safety and health risks associated with bulimia nervosa include the following:
- Risk for self-mutilation
- Risk for imbalanced fluid volume
- Constipation
- Perceived constipation
- Imbalanced nutrition: less than body requirements
  Perceptual, cognitive, and emotional disturbances are as follows:
- Anxiety
- Disturbed body image

- Hopelessness
- Chronic low self-esteem
  Problems with communicating and relating to others include the following:
- Sexual dysfunction
- Impaired social interaction
- Social isolation
  Disruptions in coping abilities may manifest as follows:
- Compromised family coping
- Disabled family coping
  Patient and family teaching needs may include the following:
- Deficient knowledge regarding nutrition and side effects of bulimic behavior
- Noncompliance with treatment program

OUTCOME IDENTIFICATION

Outcome criteria come from nursing diagnoses and are the expected patient responses to be achieved (see the Case Study #2). Outcomes are prioritized according to patient needs from most urgent to least urgent.

Anorexia Nervosa

The client will do the following:
- Participate in therapeutic contact with staff.
- Consume adequate calories for his or her age, height, and metabolic needs.
- Achieve a minimum normal weight.
- Maintain normal fluid and electrolyte levels.
- Resume a normal menstrual cycle.
- Demonstrate improvement in body image with a more realistic view of body shape and size.
- Demonstrate more effective coping skills to deal with conflicts.
- Manage family conflicts more effectively.
- Verbalize awareness of underlying psychologic issues.
- Achieve ideal body weight for his or her age, height, and metabolic needs.
- Perceive body weight and shape as normal and acceptable.
- Resume sexual interest and age-appropriate sexual behavior.
- Demonstrate an absence of food rituals, preoccupation with food, or fears of food.

Bulimia Nervosa

The client will do the following:
- Participate in therapeutic contact with staff.
- Maintain normal fluid and electrolyte levels.
- Consume adequate calories for his or her age, height, and metabolic needs.
- Cease binge/purge episodes while in the inpatient setting and cease dieting.
- Demonstrate more effective coping skills to deal with conflicts.

Kayla is a 26-year-old married mother of a 2-year-old child. Kayla has been hospitalized after a suicide attempt during which she overdosed on a combination of 100 laxatives and a full bottle of her antidepressant medication. She is currently seeing a psychiatrist for depression and bulimia nervosa. The nursing assessment reveals that Kayla currently binges and purges up to three times per day. Purging consists of self-induced vomiting as well as the use of laxatives (usually 5 or 6 pills every day). At 5 feet and 9 inches tall, Kayla is within a normal weight range at 140 pounds. She is participating in unit activities willingly, although her affect is depressed. She is eating very little at meals, and she has agreed not to purge while in the hospital.

Critical Thinking

1 How will the nurse determine Kayla's therapeutic involvement with the staff and her peers?

2 What are realistic expectations of Kayla for eating regular meals? What data should be monitored to track the improvement of her nutritional status?

3 How will the nurse recognize improvements in Kayla's eating behaviors and her cessation of purging?

4 How will Kayla demonstrate an awareness of any psychologic issues underlying her bulimia?

• Demonstrate age-appropriate boundaries with his or her family.
• Verbalize an awareness of underlying psychologic issues.
• Demonstrate an improved awareness of body sensations and emotional states.
• Perceive body shape and weight as normal and acceptable.

PLANNING

The nurse's attitude toward the patient with an eating disorder is as critical to the plan of care as any specific therapeutic intervention. Patients with eating disorders appear fragile, and, although they are vulnerable, they are often quite rigid and frustrating. If the nurse does not form a good working alliance with a firm yet compassionate approach, patient care quickly turns into a series of power struggles, and the treatment will fail. The plan of care has to include consistent and collaborative efforts by the patient, the family, and the interdisciplinary staff.

IMPLEMENTATION

For the patient with an eating disorder, the nurse needs to implement a balanced plan of action that includes behavioral interventions to interrupt the cycle of eating disorder behavior as well as psychologic interventions to improve emotional regulation, interpersonal skills, and an awareness of other psychologic issues. A safe and structured environment is essential to prevent self-harm, to promote weight gain or nutritional restoration, and to help the patient to express in words what the patient is acting out with the behavior. A safe environment is necessary to teach more effective coping skills, to monitor the use of medications, and to coordinate the multidisciplinary efforts of the treatment team.

Nursing Interventions

Nursing interventions are prioritized according to patient needs, from most urgent to least urgent.

1. Provide a safe and nonthreatening environment. *This ensures safety and prevents violence.*

2. Assess the patient for any risk of suicide (i.e., suicidal ideation, gestures, or plans). *This prevents self-harm (see Chapter 22).*

3. Engage the patient in a therapeutic alliance. *This encourages the patient to express a wide range of thoughts and feelings, including any self-destructive urges.*

4. Restore the patient's minimum weight and nutritional balance through a behavioral program. For anorexia, this includes refeeding with food, food supplements, and tube feedings when necessary. For bulimia, this includes eating meals prescribed by a dietitian and avoiding purging by having the nurse remain with the patient for at least 1 hour after each meal. *This promotes health and wellness.*

5. Create a structured and supportive environment with clear, consistent, and firm limits. *This helps to establish a predictable routine and promotes internal control that the patient currently lacks.*

6. Coordinate with the dietitian to construct a behavioral plan for the patient that includes weight-gain goals of approximately 3 pounds per week, specific eating goals of eating 100% of meals, and reinforcements of increased privileges for compliance and goal achievement. *Structure helps the patient to gain self-control and reduces the anxiety generated by noncompliance and an unpredictable routine.*

7. Encourage the patient to express thoughts, feelings, and concerns about his or her body and body image. *Verbalization helps the patient to transform a sense of shame, guilt, and fear into specific areas of conflict, and it clarifies the original issues (e.g., self-esteem, intimacy, sex, adult responsibility, identity).*

8. Continue to help the patient to increase his or her understanding of body image distortion. *The goal is for the patient to recognize that preoccupation with perceived flaws is a distraction from more complex issues and that his or her attempt to alter his or her natural body size or shape will not work without resorting to life-threatening behaviors.*

9. Assist the patient with recalling positive eating experiences, such as a time when the patient was able to eat a normal portion of sweets and stop without bingeing. *This emphasizes the fact that the patient is capable of engaging in successful episodes of eating and promotes hope.*

10. Assume a caring yet matter-of-fact approach without being overly sympathetic or overly confrontational or authoritarian. *This assists the patient with maintaining clear boundaries and avoids power struggles.*

11. Normalize the patient's lack of appetite and feelings of fullness as typical of the early refeeding process. Normalize fears of obesity as part of the distorted thinking that is typical of eating disorders. *This helps the patient to accept the treatment plan and to not set up power struggles on the basis of distorted thinking and distorted body cues.*

12. Intervene with the patient's anxiety by helping the patient to increase his or her tolerance for distress and to reframe anxiety as a signal of unrecognized feelings and needs. *The patient's experience that anxiety is a tolerable emotion will bring relief and start the process of problem solving* (see Chapter 10).

13. Offer positive feedback when the patient follows the treatment plan and works to maintain the goals of the individual contract. For example, "You have eaten three new foods this week" or "You listen attentively in group." *Praise increases self-esteem, promotes compliance, and encourages the repetition of positive behaviors.*

14. Engage the patient in therapeutic interactions and groups (e.g., individual therapy, group therapy, family therapy, occupational/recreational therapy). *This will encourage the patient to express the feelings and conflicts created by eating disorder behaviors in a supportive environment and to reduce anxiety* (see Chapter 26).

15. Assist the patient with identifying issues of low self-esteem, separation and individuation, family dysfunction, and fear of maturity. *This will help the patient to reveal and process any psychologic conflicts related to the eating disorder.*

16. Discuss with the patient how an obsession with food and weight is a way to avoid more difficult life problems and challenges. *This will help the patient to increase awareness and to gain insight into the dynamics of the eating disorder.*

17. Collaborate with the dietitian to teach the patient about adequate nutrition for the patient's height and body type. Educate the patient about metabolic adaptations that are characteristic of starvation and refeeding, such as the need to increase kilocalories as energy expenditure increases. *This will counter the patient's erroneous information about ideal weight and size and help him or her to understand the nutritional requirements for restoring health.*

18. Collaborate with the social worker, the family therapist, the physician, and other members of the interdisciplinary team. *This will promote consistency when implementing the treatment plan.*

19. Teach adaptive therapeutic strategies (e.g., cognitive, communication, assertive). *This will promote realistic thoughts, feelings, and coping behaviors and help the patient to realize that it is irrational to believe that losing weight will solve his or her problems* (see Chapter 26).

20. Educate the family about healthy eating behaviors as well as the importance of normal developmental separation and individuation. *Education about these issues will promote mutually satisfying interpersonal relationships among family members* (see the Patient and Family Teaching Guidelines box on this page).

21. Collaborate with the occupational therapist to teach the patient about appropriate exercises. *This will reduce compulsive behavior and encourage the patient to exercise in moderation.*

PATIENT AND FAMILY TEACHING GUIDELINES

Eating Disorders

Teach the Family
- Stress that the cycle of eating disorder behaviors is life threatening and must be interrupted.
- Emphasize that eating disorder behaviors are hard to change and that the idea of gaining weight or stopping purging is terrifying to the patient.
- Explain that the patient experiences common underlying issues, such as low self-esteem, separation and individuation conflicts, interoceptive deficits, fear of maturity, and conflict avoidance.
- Encourage the patient to share what has been learned in group and individual therapy about psychologic issues related to the eating disorder.
- Encourage the patient to directly verbalize thoughts and feelings about family interactions.
- Promote weight gain as prescribed in the treatment plan, and describe eating disorder behaviors and signs of relapse.
- Recognize how the patient's anxiety promotes controlling behaviors that can set up a power struggle and patient rebellion; this reinforces and worsens the eating disorder.
- Direct the family to follow the meal plan without exception, and explain that fewer choices reduce anxiety for the patient.
- Understand that the family's well-intentioned attempts to be supportive will sometimes backfire, and remind them to set age-appropriate rules that the patient is expected to follow.

Teach the Patient
- Expect to not feel hungry as a result of starvation or purging. Follow the meal plan, despite feeling full.
- Expect to feel fat and uncomfortable because of the distorted thinking and interoceptive deficits that are characteristic of eating disorders.
- Increase tolerance for these distressing feelings.
- Express thoughts and feelings in therapeutic interactions.
- Transform various feelings about one's body into concrete concerns.
- Be specific about thoughts and feelings: "What exactly are you afraid will happen?" or "What does, 'I'm freaking out' specifically mean?"

Additional Treatment Modalities
Interdisciplinary Treatment Team

The interdisciplinary team consists of representatives from the fields of nursing, psychiatry, medicine, psychology, pharmacology, dietary education, social work, occupational therapy, and spiritual guidance, as needed. Interdisciplinary treatment team meetings are an opportunity to share assessment information and the development of a multidisciplinary treatment plan. Nurses often coordinate this plan and make sure that it is implemented. As managed health care has taken over more of the mental health care industry, hospital stays have become shorter, and fewer specialty units for the treatment of eating disorders exist. Patients with eating disorders are often admitted to general psychiatric units or medical units, which puts nurses in a leadership role with regard to the coordination of the treatment team. A successful treatment outcome depends on how well team members work together.

Biologic Modalities

Patients with anorexia nervosa who are more than 15% below their ideal body weight need close medical monitoring. After the initial assessment and treatment for the effects of starvation (e.g., amenorrhea, osteopenia, osteoporosis, vitamin and mineral deficiencies), nurses need to monitor the patient closely while refeeding takes place. Refeeding with meals, supplements, or a nasogastric tube normally begins with approximately 1000 to 1600 kcal/day as tolerated and increases daily to 3000 to 4000 kcal/day, depending on the patient's ideal weight. A weight-gain goal of 3 pounds per week is considered safe. Self-starvation results in energy-conserving metabolic changes, which shift quickly as refeeding progresses. Rapid increases in energy expenditure necessitate the continued increase of kilocalories to achieve weight gain. The risk of refeeding syndrome, which is a possibly life-threatening complication, is high during the early phase of treating a severely malnourished patient. Nurses are able to prevent edema, congestive heart failure, hypophosphatemia (i.e., a low phosphate level), and other serious electrolyte imbalances with slow refeeding and careful monitoring (American Psychiatric Association Work Group on Eating Disorders, 2000).

Patients with bulimia nervosa require initial assessment for acute fluid and electrolyte imbalances (particularly serum potassium) and for any of the dangerous side effects related to their individual purging behaviors. Bone mineral density screening for osteopenia and osteoporosis and assessment for amenorrhea are necessary as well. If purging is not completely stopped, electrolytes will require continual monitoring.

There are many other modalities or methods for the treatment of eating disorders. The Additional Treatment Modalities box lists these methods, and the next section discusses them in greater detail.

Pharmacologic Modalities

Data show that selective serotonin reuptake inhibitor (SSRI) medications—particularly fluoxetine (Prozac)—are effective for the treatment of bulimia nervosa, although the dose needed for the "antibulimic" effect is usually 60 mg or more. No SSRI or selective norepinephrine reuptake inhibitor

❖ CLINICAL ALERT

If the patient is compliant with the contract but does not make the expected weight gain, then the nurse will suspect that the patient is purging and report this to the treatment team, which will probably recommend that the nurse confront the patient regarding the suspected purging behavior. Increased supervision after meals and during the administration of supplements to prevent purging will follow. The nurse will remain in the room with the patient for an hour after eating or will have the patient sit at the nursing station for that period. In addition, the nurse should supervise the patient in the bathroom and stand outside the door, which should remain partially open. The contract may be amended to include these changes. If patient weight gain does not occur in a few days, the nurse will initiate tube feedings.

ADDITIONAL TREATMENT MODALITIES

Eating Disorders

- Biologic
- Pharmacologic
- Psychotherapeutic
  - Individual psychotherapy
  - Behavioral therapy
  - Cognitive therapy
  - Family therapy
  - Group therapy
  - Expressive therapies
- Adjunctive therapy
  - Occupational therapy
  - Nutrition education and counseling
  - Social work

💊 MEDICATION KEY FACTS

Eating Disorders

There is empiric evidence that selective serotonin reuptake inhibitors (SSRIs) (fluoxetine [Prozac], sertraline [Zoloft], fluvoxamine [Luvox], citalopram [Celexa]) and selective norepinephrine reuptake inhibitors (venlafaxine [Effexor]) can be effective for the treatment of binge-eating disorder and bulimia nervosa. The first-line strategy that is widely accepted for anorexia nervosa is SSRIs. Although these drugs can be helpful for treating the comorbid mood disorders, SSRIs have no direct effect on refeeding or weight restoration. Fluoxetine can be helpful after treatment to prevent relapse. The atypical antipsychotics olanzapine [Zyprexa] and risperidone [Risperdal] have shown mixed results for the treatment of the anxiety related to refeeding in a patient with anorexia nervosa, although aripiprazole [Abilify] is showing more promising outcomes.

See Chapter 12 for Medication Key Facts related to SSRIs and selective norepinephrine reuptake inhibitors.

medication directly treats anorexia nervosa, but fluoxetine (Prozac) is effective for preventing relapse in weight-restored patients (Kaye et al, 2001b; Mitchell et al, 2001; Zhu and Walsh, 2002). Atypical antipsychotic agents have shown some success for helping low-weight anorexic patients tolerate the extreme agitation related to weight gain and also for the treatment of obsessive-compulsive behaviors (Mitchell et al, 2001). A drawback of these medications is that olanzapine (Zyprexa), risperidone (Risperdal), and quetiapine (Seroquel) have significant weight gain as a common side effect. This would seem to be a benefit when treating anorexia nervosa; however, patients often refuse the medication or are noncompliant when they experience a sudden increase in appetite. A recent study of aripiprazole (Abilify) shows very promising results because it reduces the extreme anxiety without the same side effects, thereby allowing patients to tolerate their recommended refeeding plan (Trunko et al, 2010.)

SSRI medications treat co-occurring mood disorders in patients with eating disorders. This helps treatment by relieving depression and anxiety enough for the patient to do the work of psychotherapy. Bupropion (Wellbutrin) is contraindicated because of its tendency to lower the seizure threshold in patients with eating disorders. Benzodiazepine antianxiety medication is used sparingly, and it is not generally useful as a long-term treatment as a result of the potential for abuse. (see the Medication Key Facts box, pages 429).

Medical side effects of eating disorders require the use of medication. Nurses treat hypokalemia (i.e., a low potassium level) with oral or intravenous potassium supplements. Nutritional anemia is treated with iron supplements. Gastroparesis (i.e., delayed gastric emptying) is treated with metoclopramide (Reglan). Infected parotid glands are usually treated with antibiotics. Laxative dependence is often treated with a combination of stool softeners, bran, fiber, fluids, and decreasing doses of laxatives. If the patient is taking very high doses (e.g., 50 to 100 laxatives at a time), abrupt withdrawal is dangerous, and gradual withdrawal is performed under close supervision (see Chapter 25).

Psychotherapeutic Modalities

Individual Psychotherapy. Individual psychotherapy is a preferred treatment for eating disorders. Psychodynamically oriented therapists recommend long-term, insight-oriented therapy to repair early developmental failures or traumas and to teach adaptive coping skills. Most therapists recommend active therapies such as behavioral techniques for symptom management; cognitive restructuring to change distorted thinking patterns; and dialectic behavioral therapy to increase distress tolerance, to improve assertive communication, and to improve interoceptive awareness and proprioception with mindfulness techniques. Cognitive therapists are likely to recommend structured short-term therapy with more focus on changing thought patterns and less on insight. Most therapists, whatever their orientation, use hospitalization as a means for managing acute exacerbations of either the eating disorder symptoms or the associated mood disorder symptoms.

Behavioral Therapy. The self-monitoring of eating behaviors and eating disorder symptoms is an effective behavioral intervention. Behavioral contracts for weight gain, for regulating eating and exercise, and for extinguishing binge/purge behaviors are also useful. Exposure to the problem (e.g., the binge food) with response prevention (e.g., stopping the purge) is an effective behavioral intervention for bulimia nervosa. For example, a patient eats "bad" or binge foods, and the nurse prevents the purge behavior by remaining with the patient for 1 hour after the patient eats and supervising bathroom use. (see the Clinical Alert box on pages 429).

Cognitive Therapy. Most patients with eating disorders have distorted thoughts and beliefs related to food, weight, self-concept, and interpersonal relationships. Cognitive therapy techniques such as keeping track of these thoughts, identifying distortions, challenging their validity, and replacing them with rational and evidence-based experiences help change cognitive distortions. Cognitive therapy that has been modified for the young adolescent population is showing positive results (Wilson, 2006). Cognitive-behavioral therapy is a combination of challenging distorted thinking and resisting eating disorder behaviors (see Chapter 26).

Family Therapy. The primary goal of family therapy is to actively involve the entire family in stopping the patient's eating disorder behaviors. Improving family interactions is a longer-term goal. This is a new approach to family therapy that research has shown to be very effective. Adolescents with eating disorders are expected to participate in family therapy. Educating the family about eating disorders is essential, because the eating disorder behavior often becomes the focus of the family, thereby leading to power struggles that reinforce the behavior (see the Research for Evidence-Based Practice box).

Group Therapy. Group therapy is a way for patients to discuss problems with other members who share the same experiences. Patients with anorexia nervosa and bulimia nervosa often set themselves apart from others. They avoid eating with others, they secretly binge and purge, and they lie about their behaviors. This often results in feelings of isolation and shame, and, with anorexia nervosa, it reinforces the negative secondary gains related to feeling "special." Being in an eating disorder group offers patients a safe place to self-disclose and to be understood while preventing secondary gains related to being "different."

Expressive Arts Therapy. Expressive arts therapy is the use of nonverbal activities of art making, music, dance, journal writing, and poetry. Patients with eating disorders have alexithymia (i.e., difficulty naming their feelings) and interoceptive deficits (i.e., the inability to accurately identify and respond to bodily cues), and they often have difficulty finding the words needed for talk therapy. Therefore, the use of expressive arts therapy allows for nonverbal self-disclosure and the experiential exploration of the inner experience. It also bypasses intellectual defenses and helps the patient to be more present in his or her bodily experience.

Adjunctive Therapy

Occupational Therapy. Occupational therapy helps patients with eating disorders to learn how to plan meals, shop, and cook for themselves, especially if they have not eaten properly for many years. Although the dietitian will do the actual meal planning, occupational therapy will help the patient to carry out the plan. Education about healthy moderate exercise is also necessary to alter compulsive exercise patterns (see Chapter 26).

Nutrition Education and Counseling. Nutrition education and counseling includes the following: (1) calculating the patient's ideal weight range using the basal metabolic index and other methods; (2) planning a refeeding program; and (3) meal planning. Although patients with eating disorders are obsessed with food, most have distorted information about nutrition. Refeeding and maintaining recovery require 30% to 50% more caloric intake than normal, so ongoing nutritional counseling is needed (Weltzin et al, 1991). A registered dietitian conducts nutritional education and counseling with the nurse's input (see Box 18-5).

Social Work. Hospital social workers are helpful for finding community resources such as day treatment services, outpatient individual and family therapists, support and therapy groups, residential treatment facilities, and vocational rehabilitation. They also provide individual and family therapy with the nurse's input. Patients with chronic eating disorders often do not function well in society, and social workers help these patients to make the transition from the hospital to the community.

EVALUATION

The nurse evaluates the progress of the patient with an eating disorder in an organized and timely manner in accordance with the outcomes identified in the care plan. For the patient with an eating disorder, the evaluation includes physiologic, behavioral, psychologic, social, and cultural assessments. Laboratory values, vital signs, weight, and food and fluid intake provide the data that are used to evaluate physiologic responses to treatment. Observing and recording the patient's affect, level of program participation, specific eating behaviors, peer interactions, and responses to staff provide evaluative data that help the team to track the patient's behavioral responses to treatment. The use of active listening while interacting with the patient during group therapy, during activities, and during individual interactions provides additional data from which to evaluate the patient's psychologic and behavioral responses to treatment. The evaluation of outcomes also reveals the effectiveness of the interventions used by nursing and the rest of the treatment team (see the Case Study #3 on pages 433).

BOX 18-5   REFEEDING PROCEDURE

If Savannah does not eat 90% of her meals on day 1, she will receive three dietary supplements on day 2. Supplements will continue daily until she eats 100% of her meals.

If Savannah does not finish her supplements on day 2, she will be tube fed on day 3. Tube feeding will continue until she eats 100% of all meals for 1 day.

If Savannah refuses tube feeding, she will be discharged.

RESEARCH FOR EVIDENCE-BASED PRACTICE

Lock J, Le Grange D: Family-based treatment of eating disorders, *Int J Eat Disord* 37(Suppl):S64-S67, S87-S89, 2005; Lock J, Le Grange D: *Help your teenager beat an eating disorder*, New York, 2005, Guilford Press; and Eisler I et al: A randomised controlled treatment trial of two forms of family therapy in adolescent anorexia nervosa: a five year follow up, *J Child Psychol Psychiatry* 48(6):552-560, 2007.

Family therapy has always been a vital component of eating disorder treatment. Because most eating disorders begin during adolescence, including parents in treatment is the standard of care. A well-researched family-based approach was developed at the Maudsley Hospital in London during the 1980s and used at Stanford University and the University of Chicago. Family-based treatment (sometimes referred to as the *Maudsley method*) represents a very different approach from traditional family therapy for anorexia nervosa, which operated from the position that dysfunctional family systems caused eating disorders and focused on separating the patient from the family. The theory was that, by giving the patient more control over his or her eating, normal autonomous behavior would emerge; as the patient completed the developmental tasks of separation and individuation, he or she would give up the eating disorder behaviors. Family-based treatment does not hold these assumptions about the etiology or psychodynamics of eating disorders. This approach states that the causes of eating disorders are unknown and that families are not necessarily to blame, and it focuses on anorexia nervosa as a life-threatening mental illness that must be interrupted. This approach points to evidence that early and aggressive intervention leads to better outcomes and prevents the more severe and chronic form of the illness. Family-based treatment sees parents as the main agents of change in the treatment process. Parents implement the behavioral contract designed by the treatment team, especially the meal plan. The team members instruct the parents about how to get the patient to eat. They also teach the patient's siblings about how to support the patient to eat. To prevent counterproductive power struggles, the treatment team closely observes the family's efforts and coaches them. The team offers constant support to keep the family from giving up on the treatment goals. Outcome studies of this approach to anorexia show a 90% improvement rate as compared with an 18% improvement rate for those receiving individual therapy. Five-year follow-up studies show that 70% of patients remained in recovery with this type of treatment. This method also shows promising results for the treatment of bulimia. The National Institute of Mental Health is currently conducting a 5-year outcome study of this approach.

◎ NURSING CARE PLAN

Savannah is a 19-year-old college sophomore who is hospitalized for severe cachexia (i.e., she weighs 95 pounds at a height of 5 feet 7 inches) with hypokalemia (i.e., a low potassium level), nutritional anemia, and cardiac dysrhythmia. She arrived home complaining that she was too tired to concentrate on her studies. Her parents, who had not seen her in several months, were stunned at her weight loss and immediately took her to the family physician, who hospitalized her. Savannah's physician reports that she has been dieting and excessively exercising for the past 2 years but that she had always stayed within 10% of her ideal body weight. Savannah had been in individual psychotherapy during her first year of college, but she now states that she did not continue with therapy as she had promised she would. As her weight dropped, Savannah became more rigid with her exercise regime and spent many hours studying to keep up her grades. She rarely socialized, and she has no close friends at college. Savannah minimizes her weight loss, complains of feeling fat, is sullen and angry, and wants to be discharged.

DSM-IV-TR Diagnoses

Axis I   Anorexia nervosa, binge eating/purging type
Axis II   Rule out obsessive-compulsive personality disorder
Axis III Deferred
Axis IV   Moderate (3) (unable to meet college demands; lives away from family)
Axis V   GAF = 40 (current); GAF = 65 (past year)

Nursing Diagnosis *Imbalanced nutrition: less than body requirements related to self-starvation and possible purging behavior as evidenced by severe weight loss, hypokalemia, and cardiac dysrhythmia*

NOC Nutritional status: food and fluid intake; Nutritional status: biochemical measures; Weight control; Symptom control; Body image; Knowledge: diet
NIC Eating disorders management; Weight gain assistance; Nutrition management; Weight management; Teaching: prescribed diet

CLIENT OUTCOMES	NURSING INTERVENTIONS	EVALUATION
Savannah will consume adequate calories for her age, height, and metabolic needs (e.g., 100% of each meal will be consumed by the end of the hospital stay).	Initiate refeeding in collaboration with the treatment team (Box 18-5). *The patient's starving behavior is out of control, and she cannot begin eating again on her own.* Require Savannah to follow the meal plan selected by the dietitian. Savannah will feel safer and less anxious if she feels that she is following a medical refeeding treatment plan rather than choosing to eat on her own.	Savannah eats only 25% of her meals on day 1, but, on day 2, she eats 50% of her meals and drinks all three dietary supplements. After 7 days, she is eating 100% of all meals, and the supplements are discontinued. Savannah follows the meal plan recommended by the dietitian.
Savannah will achieve a minimum normal weight (within 10% of the ideal weight for a height of 5 feet 7 inches; approximately 122 pounds).	Weigh the patient daily with her back facing the scale. *Knowledge of daily weight changes will reinforce Savannah's obsession with her weight. Not knowing will help her to tolerate weight gain and help her to let go of her current overcontrol of her body.*	Savannah achieves her goal weight by discharge.
Savannah will gain an average of 4 pounds per week.	Continue to implement the refeeding plan and contract as needed *to maintain the patient's expected weight.*	Savannah maintains her expected weight.

Nursing Diagnosis *Disturbed body image related to psychologic conflicts (fear of growing up, fear of sexuality) as evidenced by complaints of body dissatisfaction, fear of weight gain, and minimizing weight loss when more than 15% below minimal normal weight (e.g., 95 pounds at a height of 5 feet 7 inches)*

NOC Body image; Identity; Sexual identity; Self-esteem
NIC Body image enhancement; Self-esteem enhancement; Anxiety reduction; Truth telling

◎ NURSING CARE PLAN—cont'd

CLIENT OUTCOMES	NURSING INTERVENTIONS	EVALUATION
Savannah will demonstrate realistic perceptions of her body shape and size.	Encourage the patient's expression of thoughts and feelings about her body. *Verbalizing specific concerns will help Savannah to uncover psychologic issues related to her body image.*	Savannah verbalizes awareness that she is underweight and that her dissatisfaction with her body has to do more with psychologic issues than with her weight.
Savannah will demonstrate increased insight into her body image distortion.	Collaborate with the dietitian to give fact-based information to counter Savannah's irrational beliefs about her body size and shape (e.g., "You are 20 pounds below the minimum healthy weight for your age and height"). *Factual information given by more than one team member reinforces the difference between Savannah's perception of her weight and her actual weight.*	Savannah verbalizes that she perceives herself as being heavier than her actual weight. She also understands that she cannot achieve and maintain an unrealistically low weight without being ill.
Savannah will demonstrate an enhanced self-concept on the basis of positive characteristics rather than totally on the basis of her body shape.	Give Savannah truthful feedback about the positive qualities that she demonstrates on the unit. *Savannah's self-concept is influenced by her body rather than who she is as a person, and she needs to view herself in terms of her true qualities.*	Savannah verbalizes positive truthful qualities about herself that are unrelated to her body, such as "I know I'm a worthwhile person because people like me" and "Many people say that I have a talent for art."

GAF, Global Assessment of Functioning; NIC, Nursing Interventions Classification; NOC, Nursing Outcomes Classification.

CASE STUDY #3

Lilly is a 17-year-old young woman admitted to the hospital for increasingly out-of-control bulimic symptoms, including binge-ing and purging up to 10 times a day and abusing laxatives. During her first week of hospitalization, the primary focus was to correct Lilly's fluid and electrolyte balance and to monitor her to prevent purging. Lilly slept for long periods of time during the first week. She participated superficially in group sessions, and she mainly complained of physical discomfort related to the cessation of her purging behavior and use of laxatives. During the second week of treatment, the team set goals to help Lilly become more involved in the psychologic issues related to her bulimia. The interventions included encouraging

Lilly to work on underlying issues of self-esteem and family dysfunction.

Critical Thinking

1 How will the nurse evaluate Lilly's progress with regard to working on underlying issues? What three specific patient outcomes would indicate such progress?
2 What specific observations should the nurse make during group sessions to evaluate Lilly's progress?
3 What verbalizations expressed by Lilly would indicate progress in her work on underlying issues?

▍CHAPTER SUMMARY

- Eating disorders are syndromes with physiologic, behavioral, and psychologic features.
- Self-starvation, binge eating, and purging behaviors have existed for many centuries, but, until recent times, eating disorders were rare.
- The reasons for the recent outbreak of eating disorders are unclear, but many believe that they are related to current cultural trends in the fashion industry, the diet industry, and the women's movement.
- Eating disorders have a multidetermined etiology that includes biologic, genetic, sociocultural, psychologic, and familial factors.
- There is a high incidence of depression among patients with eating disorders and their families.

- Personality traits that are common among individuals with eating disorders include low self-esteem, perfectionism, interoceptive deficits, harm avoidance, ineffectiveness, alexithymia, and compliance.
- Common dynamics in the families of origin of persons with eating disorders include a focus on achievement, body image, and social acceptance; enmeshment; poor conflict-resolution skills; difficulty with age-appropriate separation and individuation; emotional dysregulation; chaotic family situations; and sexual and emotional abuse.
- Most individuals with eating disorders are female, although the incidence among males is increasing. Bulimia nervosa is more common than anorexia nervosa. Eating disorders are most common among high school and college

CHAPTER SUMMARY—cont'd

students, although the incidence is growing among younger children.

- Patients with eating disorders often have other psychiatric diagnoses. Common Axis I diagnoses are mood and anxiety disorders. Common Axis II diagnoses are borderline, histrionic, and obsessive-compulsive personality disorders.
- Anorexia nervosa and bulimia nervosa are distinct diagnoses in the DSM-IV-TR classification, but they have many of the same features.
- The course of the illness is either chronic or episodic, and it requires long-term or repeated episodes of treatment.
- Interdisciplinary treatment is indicated to deal with the multifaceted nature of eating disorders.
- Medical complications of eating disorders are life threatening. Self-induced vomiting and the abuse of laxatives and diuretics cause serious electrolyte imbalances that lead to cardiac dysrhythmias and cardiac arrest.
- Nurses need to take a firm, professional, yet compassionate approach to avoid the power struggles that commonly undermine the treatment of individuals with eating disorders.
- The plan of care needs to balance behavioral interventions that interrupt the cycle of behavior with psychologic interventions that deal with fundamental issues and that promote positive coping skills.

- A safe and structured environment is necessary to prevent self-harm, to promote nutritional restoration, to help the patient to understand the meaning of his or her behavior, and to learn more effective coping skills.
- Nurses need to refeed patients in a structured manner, with clear expectations and consequences. Positive reinforcement is more effective than punishment, and consistency is essential.
- The patient needs to understand how he or she is using the eating disorder to avoid psychologic issues. The nurse assists the patient with balancing attention between restoring nutritional health and dealing with fundamental conflicts.
- SSRI antidepressants are used to treat the coexisting depression of patients with eating disorders; these drugs often help to decrease binge urges in patients with bulimia. Atypical antipsychotics are used to treat the extreme agitation and anxiety generated by the refeeding process, thereby enabling patients to tolerate eating.
- Therapists usually recommend long-term individual psychotherapy of various modalities or methods for all patients with eating disorders. Family therapy is essential for adolescents. Group psychotherapy is also a widely used treatment method.

REVIEW QUESTIONS

1. A nurse assesses an adolescent female with anorexia nervosa. Which physical findings support the diagnosis? You may select more than one answer.
   1. Temperature of 96.9°F
   2. Pulse rate of 48 bpm
   3. Sensitivity to heat
   4. Oily skin
   5. Facial lanugo
2. If a patient's ideal body weight is 124 pounds, which current weight meets the diagnostic criteria for anorexia nervosa?
   1. 105 pounds
   2. 109 pounds
   3. 112 pounds
   4. 119 pounds
3. A patient with an eating disorder has a history of taking 20 to 30 laxative products per day. Which interventions should be added to the plan of care? You may select more than one answer.
   1. Immediate discontinuation of all laxative products
   2. Daily oral stool softener medications

3. Intake of fiber and bran products
4. Liberal oral intake of fluids
5. Gradual downward titration of laxative medications

4. Prioritize the following nursing diagnoses for a patient with bulimia nervosa:
   1. Imbalanced nutrition: less than body requirements
   2. Powerlessness
   3. Social isolation
   4. Risk for imbalanced fluid volume
5. A nurse assesses the personality traits of a patient with an eating disorder. Which comment by the patient indicates bulimia nervosa rather than anorexia nervosa?
   1. "I try to do what my parents want, but I usually don't get things right."
   2. "I feel good. I feel just fine. I don't have any problems."
   3. "I don't look as good as most of my friends. That's why I don't have many dates."
   4. "If I want to do something, I just do it. I don't like to analyze things too much."

REFERENCES

Agras W: The consequences and costs of the eating disorders, *Psychiatr Clin North Am* 24:371-379, 2001.

American Psychiatric Association: *Diagnostic and statistical manual of mental disorders*, ed 4, text revision, Washington, DC, 2000, American Psychiatric Association.

American Psychiatric Association Work Group on Eating Disorders: Practice guideline for the treatment of eating disorders (revision), *Am J Psychiatry* 157(Suppl 1):1-39, 2000.

Bailer U et al: Altered 5-HT2a receptor binding after recovery from bulimia-type anorexia nervosa: relationships to harm avoidance and drive for thinness, *Neuropsychopharmacology* 29:1143-1155, 2004.

Bailer U et al: Altered brain serotonin 5-HT 1a receptor binding after recovery from anorexia nervosa measured by positron emission tomography and (carbonyl11c)way-100635, *Arch Gen Psychiatry* 62:1032-1041, 2005.

Bell R: *Holy anorexia*, Chicago, 1987, University of Chicago Press.

Binswanger L: The case of Ellen West. In May R et al, editors: *Existence*, New York, 1958, Basic Books.

Boskind-Lodahl M, White W: *Bulimarexia: the binge/purge cycle*, New York, 1983, WW Norton.

Brumberg J: *Fasting girls*, New York, 1989, New American Library.

Bulik C et al: Significant linkage on chromosome 10p in families with bulimia nervosa, *Am J Hum Genet* 72:200-207, 2003.

Crow S et al: Increased mortality in bulimia nervosa and other eating disorders, *Am J Psychiatry* AiA:1-5, 2009.(166:13 42-1346 doi: 10.1176/appi.AJP,2009.09020247 (American Psychiatric Association).

Dare C et al: Psychological therapies for adults with anorexia nervosa: randomized controlled trial of outpatient treatment, *Br J Psychiatry* 178:216-221, 2001.

Davis C et al: Looking good—family focus on appearance and the risk for eating disorders, *Int J Eat Disord* 35:136-144, 2004.

Eisler I et al: A randomized controlled treatment trial of two forms of family therapy in adolescent anorexia nervosa: a five year follow-up, *J Child Psychol Psychiatry* 48(6):552-560, 2007.

Fernandez-Aranda F et al: Personality and psychopathological traits of males with eating disorders, *Eur Eat Disord Rev* 12:367-374, 2004.

Franco D et al: How do eating disorders and alcohol use disorder influence each other? *Int J Eat Disord* 38(3):200-207, 2005.

Grice D et al: Evidence for a susceptibility gene for anorexia nervosa on chromosome 1, *Am J Hum Genet* 70:787-792, 2002.

Groesz L et al: The effect of experimental presentation of thin media images on body satisfaction: a meta analytic review, *Int J Eat Disord* 31:1-16, 2002.

Hahn-Smith A, Smith J: The positive influence of maternal identification on body image, eating attitudes and self esteem of Hispanic and Anglo girls, *Int J Eat Disord* 29: 429-440, 2001.

Hamburger W: Emotional aspects of obesity, *Med Clin North Am* 35:483-499, 1951.

Harrop E, Marlatt G: The comorbidity of substance use disorders and eating disorders in women: prevalence, etiology and treatment, *Addict Behav* 35(5):392-398, 2010.

Johnson C, Connors M: *The etiology and treatment of bulimia nervosa*, New York, 1987, Basic Books.

Johnson JG et al: Personality disorders evident by early adulthood and risk for anxiety disorders during middle adulthood, *J Anxiety Disorders* 20(4):408-426, 2006.

Kaye W: Neurobiology of anorexia and bulimia nervosa, *Physiology and Behavior* 94(1):121-135, 2007.

Kaye W et al: Altered dopamine activity after recovery from restricting-type anorexia nervosa, *Neuropsychopharmacology* 21:503-506, 1999.

Kaye W et al: Altered serotonin 2A receptor activity in women who have recovered from bulimia nervosa, *Am J Psychiatry* 158:1152-1155, 2001a.

Kaye W et al: Double-blind, placebo controlled administration of fluoxetine in restricting and restricting-purging-type anorexia nervosa, *Biol Psychiatry* 49:644-652, 2001b.

Kaye W et al: Comorbidity of anxiety disorders with anorexia nervosa and bulimia nervosa, *Am J Psychiatry* 161:2215-2221, 2004.

Kaye W et al: Comorbidity of anxiety disorders with anorexia and bulimia nervosa, *Am J Psychiatry* 161:2215-2221, 2005.

Keel P et al: Long-term impact of treatment in women diagnosed with bulimia nervosa, *Int J Eat Disord* 31:151-158, 2002.

Klump K et al: The evolving genetic foundations of eating disorders, *Psychiatr Clin North Am* 24:215-225, 2001.

Lewinsohn P et al: Epidemiology and natural course of eating disorders in young women from adolescence to young adulthood, *J Am Acad Child Adolesc Psychiatry* 31:1284-1292, 2002a.

Lewinsohn P et al: Gender differences in eating disorder symptoms in young adults, *Int J Eat Disord* 32:426-440, 2002b.

Lindner R: The case of Laura. In *The fifty minute hour*, New York, 1955, Holt, Rinehart & Winston. General Psychiatry 37:103 and 1035, York, WW Norton and Co.

Lock J, Le Grange D: Family-based treatment for eating disorders, *Intl J Eat Disord* 37(Suppl): S64-S67, S87-S89, 2005a.

Lock J, Le Grange D: *Help your teenager beat an eating disorder*, New York, 2005b, The Guilford Press.

Lowe B et al: Long-term outcome of anorexia nervosa in a prospective 21-year follow-up study, *Psychol Med* 31:881-890, 2001.

Milos G et al: Comorbidity of obsessive-compulsive disorders and duration of eating disorders, *Int J Eat Disord* 31(3):284-289, 2002.

Milos G et al: Instability of eating disorder diagnoses: prospective study, *Brit J Psychiatry* 187:573-578, 2005.

Minuchin S et al: *Psychosomatic families: anorexia nervosa in context*, Cambridge, Mass, 1978, Harvard University Press.

Mitchell J et al: Combining pharmacotherapy and psychotherapy in the treatment of patients with eating disorders, *Psychiatr Clin North Am* 24:315-323, 2001.

Papadopoulos F et al: Excess mortality, causes of death and prognostic factors in anorexia nervosa, *Br J Psychiatry* 194:10-17. 2009.

Paul T et al: Self-injurious behavior in women with eating disorders, *Am J Psychiatry* 159:408-411, 2002.

Polivy J, Herman P: Causes of eating disorders, *Annu Rev Psychol* 53:187-213, 2002.

Russell G: Bulimia nervosa: an ominous variant of anorexia nervosa, *Psychol Med* 9:429-448, 1979.

Stunkard A: Eating patterns and obesity, *Psychiatry Q* 33:284-292, 1959.

Sysko R et al: Eating behavior among women with anorexia nervosa, *Am J Clin Nutr* 82:296-301, 2005.

Trunko M et al: Aripiprazole in anorexia nervosa and low weight bulimia nervosa: case reports, *Int J Eat Disord* 2010, Wiley Periodicals, Inc. (in press). Available at: http://eatingdisorders. ucsd.edu/documents/fulltext.pdf. Accessed January 28, 2011.

von Ranson K et al: Disordered eating and substance use in an epidemiological sample. I. Associations within individuals, *Int J Eat Disord* 31:389-403, 2002.

Wade T et al: Investigation of quality of the parental relationship as a risk factor for subclinical bulimia nervosa, *Int J Eat Disord* 30:388-400, 2001.

Weltzin TE et al: Abnormal caloric requirements for weight maintenance in patients with anorexia and bulimia nervosa, *Am J Psychiatry* 148:1675-1682, 1991.

Wilson G et al: Cognitive-behavioural therapy for adolescents with bulimia nervosa, *Eur Eat Disord Rev* 14:8-16, 2006.

Wonderlich S et al: Eating disturbance and sexual trauma in childhood and adulthood, *Int J Eat Disord* 30:401-412, 2001.

Zhu A, Walsh B: Pharmacologic treatment of eating disorders, *Can J Psychiatry* 47:227-234, 2002.

Online Resources

Academy for Eating Disorders: www.aedweb.org

Anorexia Nervosa and Related Eating Disorders: www.anred.com

Mental Health America: www.nmha.org

National Alliance on Mental Illness: www.nami.org

National Association of Anorexia Nervosa and Associated Disorders: www.anad.org

National Eating Disorders Association: www.nationaleatingdisorders.org

National Institute of Mental Health: www.nimh.nih.gov

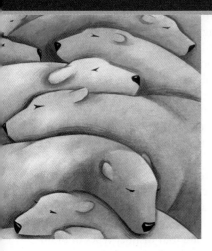

CHAPTER

19

Sleep Disorders: Dyssomnias and Parasomnias

Nancy Stark Napolitano

"Sleep is that golden chain that ties health and our bodies together."

Thomas Dekker

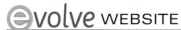 WEBSITE

http://evolve.elsevier.com/Fortinash/

OBJECTIVES

- Describe the major categories of sleep disorders.
- Discuss the factors and patients' presenting signs and symptoms of each sleep pattern disturbance.
- Develop an understanding of the assessment tools that identify sleep disorders in patients across the life span.
- Discuss how nursing and medical experts make differential diagnoses as they relate to problems of sleep pattern disturbance among their patients.
- Apply the nursing process to patients who are experiencing major alterations in their sleep–wake cycles.

- Formulate relevant nursing diagnoses for patients who demonstrate significant abnormalities in their sleep–wake patterns.
- Design comprehensive nursing care plans that reflect guiding practices for restorative sleep for patients in acute care, long-term care, and community-based settings.
- Evaluate the effectiveness of interdisciplinary interventions to promote restorative sleep in patients who are experiencing sleep pattern disturbances.

KEY TERMS

cataplexy
circadian rhythm
dyssomnias
insomnia

narcolepsy
non–rapid eye movement sleep
parasomnias
rapid eye movement sleep

sleep apnea
sleep paralysis

Sleep is a basic human need that is fundamental to human survival. Although an individual's sleep pattern typically changes as he or she progresses through the life span, adequate amounts of restorative sleep are necessary during each phase of human development to maintain the best level of physical and psychologic functioning. People are not always aware of the essential role that restorative sleep plays in their everyday lives until sleep becomes disrupted as a result of an acute or chronic sleep pattern disturbance. Psychiatric nursing practice frequently involves the management of patients with sleep pattern disruptions, because these disruptions often coexist with certain types of mental disorders. Sometimes patients experience a disruption in mental health functioning as a result of a sleep pattern disturbance.

The average nightly sleep duration for the average adult has fallen from approximately 9 hours per night to approximately 7 hours per night. This common problem results from many sleep pattern disturbances that are either self-imposed or that occur as a result of a primary or secondary sleep pattern disorder. Some common causes of sleep deprivation include insomnia, narcolepsy, breathing-related sleep disorders, circadian rhythm sleep disturbances, recurrent

437

nightmares, sleep terrors, and sleepwalking disturbances. The resulting sleep deprivation often presents significant health and safety concerns for the affected individual.

Excessive sleep loss is catastrophic and has far-reaching consequences. Current data from the National Transportation Safety Board indicate that fatigue from sleep deprivation accounts for more than 100,000 highway accidents and 1500 deaths every year (NIH, 2006a). Sleep deprivation also leads to increased risks of having both work-related accidents and substandard work performance on the job. This is especially true when a patient has a job that involves nighttime work assignments or rotating shift work.

Ongoing sleep deprivation also significantly affects the individual's overall quality of physical and psychologic health. Persistent sleep deficits are an increased risk factor for such conditions as coronary heart disease, high blood pressure, and impaired cognitive performance (NIH, 2006a). In addition, sleep pattern disturbances coexist with such mood disorders as major depression, bipolar disorder, and generalized anxiety disorder (American Psychiatric Association [APA], 2000).

THEORETIC PERSPECTIVES

Physiologic and Homeostatic Sleep Regulation

Sleep is a temporary state of unconsciousness that many think restores and repairs the body (Saladin, 2010). Although research has not identified a specific sleep neurotransmitter, several interconnected and complex biochemical and neurologic processes work together to directly or indirectly influence the sleep–wake cycle. Many researchers agree that daily patterns of neuroendocrine function act on certain areas of the brain to control sleep and wakefulness (Drake, 2010). Researchers also believe that certain neurotransmitters such as adenosine, acetylcholine, and melatonin have a sleep-promoting function, whereas serotonin, hypocretin, and norepinephrine most likely maintain arousal (Doghramji et al, 2007, Sadock and Sadock, 2008).

The regular recurrence of the sleep–wake cycle is one example of a physiologic circadian rhythm that is highly influenced by the body's internal biologic clock. Located in the hypothalamus of the brain, this biologic clock or regulator known as the *suprachiasmatic nucleus* is able to adjust sleep–wake intervals in a cyclic 24-hour pattern because of its sensitivity to the external cues of light and darkness. Researchers postulate that the presence of sunlight and other types of artificial light creates the necessary neurosensory stimulation of the photoreceptors in the retina that will eventually suppress the release of melatonin (a chemical mediator that promotes sleep) from the pineal gland. When this takes place, a state of wakefulness occurs during daylight hours. By contrast, a state of darkness promotes sleep as a result of melatonin release. Thus, during a 24-hour period, the biologic clock suppresses and then stimulates the release of melatonin to synchronize sleep and wakefulness with the use of the external cues of light and darkness (Drake, 2010; Guyton and Hall, 2010).

An individual who has a relatively normal day–night sleep pattern typically goes through a recurrent cycle of sleep and wakefulness within a defined 24-hour period because of the influence of the body's biologic clock. However, if the cues for light and darkness are disrupted in some way (e.g., as a result of night shift work or travel across several time zones), the individual will most likely experience some type of sleep disturbance because of the interruption of the sleep-regulating cues of light and darkness from the external environment (Drake, 2010).

When an individual progresses from a state of wakefulness to a stage of sleep, there are changes in his or her brain-wave activity that are evident on an electroencephalogram (EEG) recording. These changes occur in accordance with states of sleep and wakefulness. There are four distinct types of brain waves: alpha, beta, theta, and delta. Each of these categories contains brain-wave activity that has a distinct range of amplitudes and frequencies, depending on the activity of the cerebral cortex during the various stages of the sleep cycle (Saladin, 2010) (Figure 19-1).

Alpha waves occur at a frequency of 8 Hz to 13 Hz, and they occur most often in adults who are awake but resting and not attending to any particular mental task. Beta waves occur at a frequency of 14 Hz to 30 Hz, and they occur when an individual is mentally active and receptive to sensory stimulation. Theta and delta waves are low-frequency waves, and both occur in adults who are experiencing sleep states. Theta recordings are usually at frequencies of 4 Hz to 7 Hz, and they also occur in children during awake states. Delta waves involve slower wave frequencies as compared with theta recordings, and they usually occur at frequencies of less than 3.5 Hz. Delta waves occur in adults who are in deep sleep stages and in infants during states of wakefulness (Saladin, 2010).

Normally, a restorative sleep pattern has two distinct stages of sleep: non–rapid eye movement (NREM) sleep (and its associated four sleep stages: 1, 2, 3, and 4) and rapid eye movement (REM) sleep (Sadock and Sadock, 2008) (Figure 19-2). During the NREM sleep cycle, an individual initially enters the first of four stages of sleep and repeats them in a cyclic fashion throughout the sleep episode. The individual first enters into stage 1 NREM sleep after closing his or her eyes and drifting into a light sleep state (Saladin, 2010). The EEG of an individual who is in stage 1 NREM sleep demonstrates many alpha waves. The person is able to be aroused easily during this state of the sleep cycle (Saladin, 2010). If he or she is not awakened during stage 1 NREM sleep, the individual will enter stage 2 NREM sleep, during which he or she will become less easily aroused. The predominant EEG recording during this stage reflects high K complexes and spindle-like tracings at frequencies of 12 Hz to 14 Hz (Sadock and Sadock, 2008). Soon thereafter, the individual will enter stage 3 NREM sleep, and theta and delta wave activity will appear on EEG recordings (Saladin, 2010). During this stage of NREM sleep, the vital sign recordings (i.e., body temperature, pulse, respiration, and blood pressure) usually reflect a decline from baseline values, and the

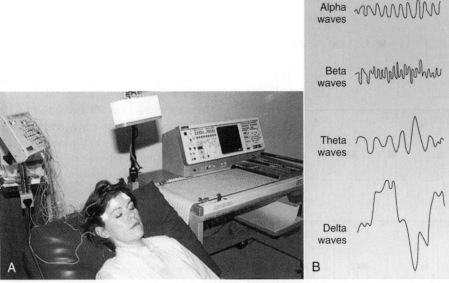

FIGURE 19-1. The electroencephalogram. **A,** Photograph showing a person undergoing an electroencephalogram test. Notice the scalp electrodes that detect voltage fluctuations within the cranium. **B,** Examples of alpha, beta, theta, and delta waves seen on an electroencephalogram. (From Lewis SM: *Medical-surgical nursing: assessment and management of clinical problems,* ed 7, St. Louis, 2007, Elsevier.)

individual is in a deeper sleep state as compared with the two previous NREM stages. The individual will then progressively enter stage 4 NREM sleep, during which arousal is difficult. Vital sign recordings are usually at their lowest level as compared with a baseline recording, the muscles are very relaxed, and the brain-wave activity shown on the EEG reflects a predominance of delta wave (i.e., slow wave) activity (Saladin, 2010).

After moving from wakefulness through stages 1 through 4 of NREM sleep, the person then goes back from stage 4 NREM to stage 2 NREM sleep. Next, the individual enters the active sleep stage known as REM sleep. The first REM period of the sleep episode takes place approximately 90 minutes after the individual first falls asleep, with subsequent REM periods occurring four to five times at 90-minute intervals throughout the sleep episode (Saladin, 2010). Each REM period usually lasts from 5 to 30 minutes, depending on the individual. For example, if the individual is extremely tired, REM sleep is shorter or does not occur at all during the sleep episode. However, when the individual becomes less fatigued, the REM periods typically increase in frequency and duration throughout the sleep cycle (Guyton and Hall, 2010).

REM sleep is an active cerebral state. During this stage of sleep, there is an increase in cerebral metabolism, with brain waves paralleling those that are seen during an awake state (Guyton and Hall, 2010). This stage of sleep is also called *paradoxic sleep* because of the seemingly contradictory findings of active brain wave activity in a difficult-to-arouse person (Saladin, 2010). The individual has decreased muscle tone and irregular muscle movements during this stage of

sleep. Active dreaming also takes place, and this is usually associated with the presence of rapid eye movements.

Normal sleep patterns and requirements vary across the life span. On average, the newborn sleeps approximately 16 hours a day, with 50% of the total sleep time spent in REM sleep. Over the course of the first 6 months of life, the infant's sleep patterns continually change so that, by the end of the first 6 months, they will closely resemble adult sleep patterns. The infant also typically develops more consolidated sleep patterns within the first few years of life, and he or she usually has uninterrupted blocks of sleep without the need for a daytime nap by the age of 4 years. As the child ages, his or her nighttime sleep requirements usually decrease so that, by the adolescent period, the sleep requirements are the similar to those of an adult. Although adolescents require approximately 9 to 10 hours of sleep per night, they sometimes experience daytime sleepiness as a result of a phase delay in their sleep–wakefulness pattern. The adolescent typically does not experience sleepiness until the early morning hours, and he or she does not wake up naturally until the late morning or early afternoon. Therefore, adolescents experience sleep disturbances as a result of activities that require them to wake early, such as school or social obligations. Sleep patterns of young adults show that they spend 25% of their total sleep time in REM sleep, whereas middle and older adults spend even less time in REM sleep than young adults. Thus, during middle and older adulthood, a person experiences more fragmented sleep, with the development of a daytime napping pattern that is especially seen in the older adult who has difficulty with uninterrupted nocturnal sleep (NIH, 2006a).

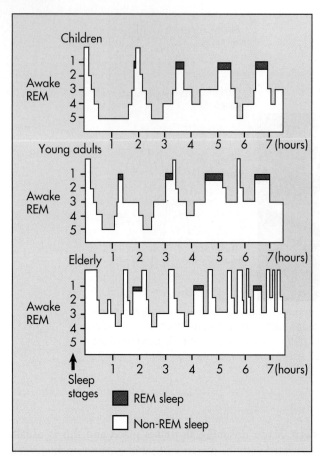

FIGURE 19-2. Normal sleep cycles. Rapid eye movement sleep occurs cyclically throughout the night at intervals of approximately 90 minutes in all age groups. Rapid eye movement sleep shows little variation in the different age groups, whereas stage 4 sleep decreases with age. In addition, elderly persons awaken frequently and show a marked increase in their total awake time. REM, rapid eye movement. (From McCance KL, Huether SE: *Pathophysiology: the biologic basis for disease in adults and children*, ed 5, St. Louis, 2006, Elsevier.)

HISTORIC PERSPECTIVES

The ancient Greeks theorized that a benevolent force known as *Hypnos,* or the god of sleep, controlled sleep. The dreams that take place during the sleep state were believed to be symbolic messages sent from the Greek gods. During the second century AD, the professional diviner Artemidorus Daldianus was responsible for interpreting the meaning of these messages, and he eventually wrote a five-volume Greek work titled *Oneirocritica,* or *The Interpretation of Dreams.* It was Daldianus' belief that, if a person's dreams were linked to his or her previous life experiences, then the dreams were insignificant and not symbolic of a message from the Greek gods. Throughout this time period, dreaming was generally thought to be an outward manifestation of the internal mental acts that took place throughout the previous day (Klosch and Ulrich, 2005).

Some 1700 years later, the Viennese physician Sigmund Freud (1856–1939) challenged Daldianus' conclusions in his

1899 publication of *The Interpretation of Dreams.* Freud postulated that dreams were in fact very significant and that they were symbolic of unconscious desires. It was Freud's belief that dreams were an outward expression of the unconscious mind and that they could be accurately analyzed with the use of free association. In essence, one could uncover the individual's unconscious desire for wish fulfillment through dream analysis (*Freud's dream theory,* 2006).

Around the same time, renowned Austrian psychiatrist Alfred Adler (1870–1937) developed a general theory of dream analysis that would later lay a foundation for other Neo-Freudian theorists who would follow. One of the basic views of Adler's theory was that dream content could be linked to individual mastery and that the dream's mood or feeling state could prepare an individual for current and future problem-solving needs. The dream content was an expression of the individual's character and his or her ongoing challenges to overcoming inferiority (*Adler's dream theory,* 2006).

Carl Gustav Jung's (1875–1961) dream theory eventually became one of the most influential theories in analytic psychology. Jung viewed dreams as being representative of the individual's mental world, and he saw them as being expressed in a symbolic language that characterized both the objective and subjective nature of the dream experience (*Jung's dream theory,* 2006).

There was no support for sleep research until the 1950s, when Nathaniel Kleitman and Eugene Aserinsky began recording the eye movements of sleep subjects. Kleitman and Aserinsky uncovered the physiologic processes associated with REM sleep. During their laboratory analysis, these researchers observed that young sleep subjects had cyclic periods of rapid movements of the eyes during certain stages of their sleep cycle. They eventually determined that these REM periods of the sleep cycle were associated with a relatively high percentage of self-reported dream states, high brainwave activity, and little or no skeletal muscle movement. This discovery was a significant breakthrough in sleep research, and it formed the basis for future theories related to sleep (Klosch and Ulrich, 2005).

Almost 10 years after this REM sleep discovery, French neurophysiologist Michael Jouver discovered an association between pontine (brainstem) stimulation in the brains of cats and the associated onset of REM phases of sleep. However, his research did not find any link between REM sleep and higher-order brain activity; the brainstem—specifically the pons varolii—appears to be responsible for stimulating REM activity, at least in cats (Klosch and Ulrich, 2005).

During the 1970s, the research of Allan Hobson and Robert W. McCarley of Harvard Medical School provided further support for a biochemical basis for sleep and dreaming. Hobson and McCarley presented two complementary theories—the reciprocal–interaction theory and the activation–synthesis theory—that attempted to explain how REM phases were activated and inhibited during the sleep cycle. During reciprocal interaction, the researchers asserted that the REM phases of the sleep cycle and the dreaming that takes place during this time are turned on and off throughout the night by neurons in the brainstem (pons). The activation–synthesis theory explains how the higher brain centers operate during the dream experience.

These researchers claimed that the chemical messenger acetylcholine was responsible for sending impulses to various brain regions (i.e., the pons, cortex, and limbic areas), which resulted in the initiation of REM activity and the associated dream state. The cessation of the REM sleep state and thus of dreaming took place through the release of the "REM off" chemical messengers: norepinephrine and serotonin. Unlike Jouver, Hobson and McCarley found higher brain centers to be participating during dreaming (Klosch and Ulrich, 2005).

Although previous theoretic and empiric data have contributed greatly to the current understanding of the nature of sleep, much is still unknown. The prevalence of sleep pattern disturbances has generated an increased public awareness of this problem. Consequently, current research continues in this area as the search for a deeper understanding of sleep becomes known.

ETIOLOGY

There are many complex and multifaceted causes of sleep disturbances. In some instances, it is difficult to find strong evidence to support some causes, because many areas of sleep research are still in their beginning stages. In addition, a sleep disorder such as insomnia sometimes begins as a result of precipitating factors (e.g., genetics, stress) and continues to become a chronic condition because of perpetuating circumstances (i.e., contextual conditioning).

According to the *Diagnostic and Statistical Manual of Mental Disorders,* fourth edition, text revision (DSM-IV-TR) (APA, 2000), sleep disorders are either primary or secondary, depending on their presumed cause (Box 19-1). Primary sleep disorders include the dyssomnias and parasomnias. The dyssomnias include sleep disorders that occur as a result of abnormalities of the physiologic mechanisms that regulate sleep and wakefulness. Alternatively, parasomnias are primary sleep disorders that occur as a result of the activation of physiologic systems at incorrect times during the sleep–wake cycle, thereby resulting in abnormal behavior or physiologic events during the sleep state. Parasomnias are often paroxysmal sleep disturbances that are more common among children. Secondary sleep disorders are most often related to psychiatric illnesses (e.g., mood disorders), the effects of substances, or general medical conditions (APA, 2000).

Biologic Factors

Biochemical alterations in neurotransmitters such as serotonin, melatonin, norepinephrine, and dopamine may play a major role in the deregulation of sleep and wakefulness (Sadock and Sadock, 2008). An inherent physiologic imbalance of these chemical mediators increases an individual's chance of a developing a sleep pattern disturbance. In addition, the development of a substance-induced sleep disorder syndrome sometimes occurs among individuals who use

---

BOX 19-1 PRIMARY SLEEP DISORDERS

Primary sleep disorders are presumed to arise from endogenous abnormalities in sleep–wake generating or timing mechanisms, and they are often complicated by conditioning factors.

Dyssomnias
Characterized by abnormalities in the amount, quality, or timing of sleep:
- Primary insomnia
- Primary hypersomnia
- Narcolepsy
- Breathing-related sleep disorder
- Circadian rhythm sleep disorder (formerly *sleep–wake schedule disorder*)
- Jet lag type
- Shift work type
- Delayed sleep phase type
- Dyssomnia not otherwise specified

Parasomnias
Characterized by abnormal behavior or physiologic events that occur in association with sleep, specific sleep stages, or sleep–wake transitions:
- Nightmare disorder (formerly *dream anxiety disorder*)
- Sleep terror disorder
- Sleepwalking disorder
- Parasomnia not otherwise specified

Data from the American Psychiatric Association: *Diagnostic and statistical manual of mental disorders,* ed 4, text revision, Washington, DC, 2000, American Psychiatric Association.

---

certain prescribed drugs and over-the-counter medications at the same time. Patients who stop taking these medications are also at risk for a substance-induced sleep disorder, because these people are often incapable of restoring healthy sleep patterns (APA, 2000). Examples of substances that influence sleep include alcohol; stimulants such as caffeine, amphetamines, and cocaine; and sedatives such as opiates, hypnotics, and antianxiety medications.

Researchers believe that narcolepsy results from a deficiency of hypocretin, a neurotransmitter that is produced by the hypothalamus. This deficiency is thought to result from an autoimmune response caused by genetic or environmental factors (Simon and Zieve, 2009a).

Genetic, Hereditary, and Familial Factors

There has been a connection between a genetic predisposition or familial association and some types of sleep disturbances. For example, there is a fairly consistent association between a familial predisposition and primary insomnia (APA, 2000), and a genetic association for narcolepsy is also supported (Simon and Zieve, 2009a). Obstructive sleep apnea also has a familial association, with current research indicating a rise in the prevalence of this disorder among younger Americans (APA, 2000; National Sleep Foundation, 2008).

Psychiatric, Cognitive, and Behavioral Factors

Some sleep pattern disturbances also occur with some mood and anxiety disorders (APA, 2000). In some instances, it is difficult to determine whether the sleep pattern disturbance is a precursor to the onset of the psychiatric illness or whether the illness, in some significant way, influenced the development of a sleep pattern disturbance. In particular, patients with insomnia usually report the onset of sleep problems after experiencing a fairly sudden onset of psychologic stressors (APA, 2000). In addition, insomnia is also a diagnostic criterion for several psychiatric disorders, including depression, dysthymia, mania, and generalized anxiety disorder (APA, 2000; Phillips et al, 2008). Lastly, substance use, abuse, and discontinuance also affect an individual's ability to obtain restorative sleep.

General Medical Condition

Sleep disturbances such as insomnia, daytime sleepiness, and sleep fragmentation may also be a result of the direct physiologic effects of a general medical condition on the sleep–wake system (APA, 2000). For example, sleep fragmentation often occurs in patients who are experiencing chronic pain (Phillips et al, 2008). Sleep pattern disturbances can also be present when a patient has a biochemical alteration that results from a medical illness such as an endocrine disorder.

Sociocultural and Environmental Factors

Self-induced sleep deprivation is the cause of sleep problems in both adolescents and adults. The delayed onset of nocturnal sleep in adolescents, demanding work and school schedules, and social demands are a few of the many factors that pose challenges to attaining and maintaining the necessary amount of restorative sleep.

EPIDEMIOLOGY

Because of the temporary nature of many sleep disturbances and the lack of formal diagnoses, some sleep disorders go unreported. Thus, the true prevalence of sleep disorders is difficult to determine, but epidemiologic surveys suggest that they are becoming more common than ever before. Approximately 47 million to 70 million people in the country do not get adequate sleep because of some type of sleep disturbance, and half of these individuals report chronic sleep pattern disturbances (NIH, 2006b). In a survey conducted by the National Sleep Foundation, 65% of respondents reported that they had experienced some type of sleep disturbance for a few nights a week or more during the preceding year (National Sleep Foundation, 2008). The data reflect a growing trend in sleep disturbances among adults in the United States.

Dyssomnias

Insomnia is one of the most common sleep disorders in the United States. Although some individuals experience brief periods of insomnia throughout their lifetime, it is estimated that 30 million adults have a persistent problem with insomnia, which can disrupt daily functioning (NIH, 2006b). The prevalence of this disorder increases with age, and it is more common among women across all age groups (Passarella and Duong, 2008). There is also a link between insomnia and psychiatric illness, most commonly major depression and dysthymia (Phillips et al, 2008).

Narcolepsy and hypersomnias are two types of primary sleep disturbances that are characterized by excessive daytime sleepiness. Narcolepsy is the most studied of all hypersomnias, and it is more prevalent than once thought (Simon and Zieve, 2009a). Between 135,000 and 250,000 people have narcolepsy, although the average time between symptom onset and formal diagnosis is approximately 10 to 15 years (NIH, 2006b). The delay in a formal diagnosis is most likely the result of this disorder being mistaken for other common causes of excessive daytime sleepiness (Simon and Zieve, 2009a).

Breathing-related sleep disorders are a group of disorders that are characterized by excessive daytime sleepiness caused by a sleep-related breathing condition such as obstructive or central sleep apnea syndrome (i.e., the temporary cessation or absence of breathing) (APA, 2000; Simon and Zieve, 2009b). Epidemiologic data indicate that 18 million Americans have obstructive sleep apnea (NIH, 2006). The estimated prevalence of this disorder is 24% among the adult male population and 9% among the adult female population (Pagel, 2008). Obstructive sleep apnea also affects approximately 2% of children. When the condition is found in children, it is usually the result of adenotonsillar hypertrophy, craniofacial abnormalities, and neuromuscular conditions, all of which result in airway obstruction during sleep (Simon and Zieve, 2009b). The development of metabolic syndrome in children is also being seen as an increasing risk factor for their subsequent development of breathing-related sleep disorders (Korner et al, 2008).

Individuals with circadian rhythm sleep disturbance rarely seek medical treatment. Therefore, the true prevalence of this sleep disturbance is difficult to estimate. The delayed sleep phase subtype of the disorder affects up to 4% of adults and up to 7% of adolescents (APA, 2000). The shift work and jet lag subtypes of the disorder often result in more severe symptoms for late-middle-aged and elderly people. Up to 60% of night shift workers have the shift work subtype of circadian rhythm sleep disorder (APA, 2000).

Parasomnias

Sleep terror disorder occurs in 1% to 6% of the child population, and it is more common among boys than girls (Kaplan and Sadock, 2004). These sleep pattern disturbances typically occur in children between the ages of 3 and 8 years, with the episodes usually taking place during NREM sleep cycles.

Nightmare disorder can happen at any age to an individual of either gender. The essential features associated with nightmare disorder are the repeated occurrences of frightening dreams that interrupt sleep and that cause the patient significant distress or major disruptions in social or occupational functioning (APA, 2000). A child who is experiencing nightmares is usually able to recall the event (this is not typical in a child with sleep terrors), and he or she usually outgrows the disorder as he or she ages. Sleepwalking disorder (somnambulism) typically occurs around the ages of 4 to 8 years, with the peak prevalence seen in children who are 12 years old. This disorder, like sleep terror disorder, is more common among boys than girls. Both sleep terror disorder and sleepwalking disorder tend to run in families (Kaplan and Sadock, 2004).

Clinical Description

According to the DSM-IV-TR, sleep disorders are best classified according to their presumed cause. The primary sleep disorders are caused by alterations in internal processes that influence sleep and wakefulness. Secondary sleep disturbances generally develop as a result of medical or mental conditions, or they occur as a result of the use of substances (APA, 2000).

Dyssomnias
Insomnia

The dyssomnia known as *insomnia* is characterized by a predominant complaint of difficulty initiating or maintaining sleep or of experiencing nonrestorative sleep for at least 1 month. This sleep disturbance typically leads to excessive daytime sleepiness and causes significant impairment in daily functioning (APA, 2000). Transient periods of insomnia can occur throughout an individual's lifetime and may be attributed to anxiety-producing situations that are self-limiting for the affected individual. The anxiety can occur either in response to an anxiety-producing situation or in anticipation of an anxiety-provoking experience (Sadock and Sadock, 2008). In this situation, after the anxiety decreases, the sleep pattern disturbance typically lessens or abates, and no treatment would be indicated. Alternatively, chronic insomnia is characterized by the inability to initiate or maintain restorative sleep for at least 1 month (Passarella and Duong, 2008). The sleep pattern disturbance often interferes with the individual's social or occupational functioning (see the Case Study #1).

Narcolepsy

Narcolepsy is the sudden onset of brief sleep attacks that last 10 to 20 minutes and that typically take place two to six times per day (Kaplan and Sadock, 2004). Thus, a person with narcolepsy will suddenly fall asleep while engaging in meaningful activities such as driving a car, eating, or interacting with people (Doghramji et al, 2007). The symptom onset for narcolepsy typically manifests during puberty or adolescence (Kaplan and Sadock, 2004). (See Clinical Alert box #1).

In addition to excessive daytime sleepiness, approximately 70% of people with narcolepsy also experience cataplexy, which is a common sign of the disorder (APA, 2000). Cataplexy is the sudden loss of muscle tone and voluntary muscle movement (Simon and Zieve, 2009a). Strong emotional experiences such as laughing or crying may cause this reaction. Persons with narcolepsy also report sleep paralysis, which means that they are not able to speak or move just

---

CASE STUDY #1

Janet is a 55-year-old woman who has insomnia. She gives a history of having frequent awakenings during the night that usually start about 1.5 to 2 hours after she goes to sleep. Janet states that she initially started having sleep problems when she was under an immense amount of stress as a result of a chronic illness. She currently has her illness under adequate control, but she continues to have problems maintaining a continuous pattern of sleep on a regular basis. She noticed her sleep disturbance continued after she returned to work after a 2-month medical leave from her job.

Critical Thinking

1. What factors support a diagnosis of insomnia?
2. Formulate two nursing diagnoses that may be relevant to Janet's plan of care.
3. What can the psychiatric nurse teach Janet about her illness? What lifestyle changes can Janet make that may improve her sleep quality and limit the progression of her problem?
4. What treatments are typically employed to treat this type of sleep disturbance?
5. How will the health care team members know if Janet's condition is improving?

❖ CLINICAL ALERT #1

Patients with narcolepsy experience excessive daytime sleepiness that results in multiple sleep attacks that typically take place at inappropriate times during the patient's normal period of wakefulness. The psychiatric nurse needs to teach the patient to manage narcolepsy by discussing the triggers that provoke it (e.g., strong emotional stimuli, sleep deprivation) and the available treatment strategies that may help to prevent it (e.g., forced daytime napping, adherence to medical treatment).

---

before the onset of or upon awakening from a brief sleep attack. In addition, some report hallucinations and experience vivid sensory perceptual experiences either upon awakening (i.e., hypnopompic hallucinations) or when entering the brief sleep episode (i.e., hypnagogic hallucinations) (APA, 2000; Doghramji et al, 2007). These four classic symptoms of narcolepsy—excessive daytime sleepiness, cataplexy, sleep paralysis, and hallucinations—are sometimes referred to as the *narcoleptic tetrad* (Doghramji et al, 2007).

Breathing-Related Sleep Disorders

Breathing-related sleep disorders are a group of disorders that result from a sleep-related breathing condition such as obstructive or central sleep apnea syndrome or central alveolar hypoventilation (APA, 2000).

Persons with obstructive sleep apnea typically have some degree of narrowing or the complete obstruction of the upper airway, which results in loud snoring episodes and regular apneic periods during sleep that last for 10 to 30 seconds. Many affected individuals have a large neck circumference and are obese (Heyworth, 2009). These individuals often wake up briefly during the night and experience excessive daytime sleepiness as a result of the periods of breathing cessation that are experienced during the night (Hirshkowitz, 2008) (see the Case Study #2 and Clinical Alert box #2).

Circadian Rhythm Sleep Disorder

Circadian rhythm sleep disorders are a group of sleep pattern disturbances with a persistent or recurrent pattern of sleep disruption that result from a difference in an imposed sleep–wake cycle and the individual's own circadian sleep–wake pattern requirements. Circadian rhythm sleep disorders result from a delayed sleep phase, jet lag, shift work, or an unspecified source (APA, 2000). Daytime sleepiness is common because of the delayed sleep onset and the mandatory early awakening related to employment or social obligations. Insomnia also occurs.

The jet lag type of the circadian rhythm sleep disorder involves periods of sleepiness and alertness that occur at an inappropriate time of day relative to local time (APA, 2000). These patterns of sleep and wakefulness occur after repeated travel across more than one time zone.

The shift work type of the circadian sleep disorder is usually the result of night shift work or frequently rotating shift work (APA, 2000). The individual with this type of sleep pattern disturbance typically experiences insomnia during the major sleep period or excessive sleepiness during the major awake period (APA, 2000). These symptoms are usually most pronounced right after the individual changes schedules, but, in some cases, the symptoms do not improve with the passage of time.

The delayed sleep phase of the circadian rhythm sleep pattern disturbance occurs when the individual has a persistent pattern of late sleep onset and late awakening times and is unable to fall asleep and wake up at the desired earlier times (APA, 2000). However, when sleep can be maintained, it may be uninterrupted until the normal awakening period.

Parasomnias

In general, parasomnias involve the presence of abnormal behavior or physiologic events that occur in association with sleep, specific sleep stages, or sleep–wake transitions (APA, 2000).

Nightmare Disorder

Nightmare disorder is one type of parasomnia that usually takes place during the REM period late in the sleep cycle. Individuals with this disorder frequently experience fragmented sleep as a result of waking up during the night with frightening dreams that threaten their survival, security, or self-esteem. Patients are usually able to recall the nightmares in vivid detail (APA, 2000).

Sleep Terror Disorder

An individual with sleep terror disorder experiences arousal during NREM sleep. This individual will typically awaken during the early part of the night, and the awakening is usually caused by manifestations of extreme anxiety or panic (Sadock and Sadock, 2008). It is not unusual for the person to scream or cry and to appear disoriented during a sleep terror episode. As with sleepwalking, the individual with sleep terror disorder is usually not able to recall the event.

Sleepwalking Disorder

Sleepwalking disorder (somnambulism) is also considered a parasomnia (APA, 2000). Individuals with a sleepwalking

---

◆ CLINICAL ALERT #3

Episodes of complex motor activity that take place during slow wave sleep characterize sleepwalking. Some examples of sleepwalking activities include waking from sleep during the first third of the night and walking around inside the home or unlocking the doors and going outside. This presents a safety risk, because the individual may also engage in dangerous activities such as operating machinery during the sleepwalking phase. The psychiatric nurse needs to teach the patient and family members about the factors that increase the likelihood of a sleepwalking episode (e.g., distended bladder, environmental noise, psychosocial stressors, alcohol and sedative-hypnotic drug use) and develop a plan to minimize its occurrence. Safety is the number one priority when planning care for this patient.

---

disorder typically will repeatedly engage in such complex behaviors as walking, dressing, toileting, and driving all while they are in a deep NREM stage of sleep (Sadock and Sadock, 2008). While sleepwalking, the individual appears to be in a trance, and arousal is difficult. At times, the individual awakens while performing complex tasks, but most frequently he or she returns to sleep and later awakens without any recall of the events that took place during the sleepwalking episode (APA, 2000) (see Clinical Alert box #3).

Parasomnia Not Otherwise Specified

A sleep disorder related to another mental disorder involves a prominent complaint of a sleep disturbance (e.g., insomnia, hypersomnia) that results from a diagnosable mental disorder (e.g., a mood disorder, an anxiety disorder) (APA, 2000).

A sleep disorder that results from a general medical condition involves a prominent complaint of sleep disturbance that results from the direct physiologic effects of a general medical condition on the sleep–wake system (APA, 2000).

A substance-induced sleep disorder involves prominent complaints of sleep disturbance that result from the use or the recent discontinuation of use of a substance (including a prescribed medication). Specific substances that may cause this condition include alcohol, amphetamines and related stimulants, caffeine, cocaine, opioids, sedative-hypnotics, and anxiolytics (APA, 2000).

PROGNOSIS

In general, the prognosis for the majority of sleep disorders is good, provided that the problem is diagnosed and accurately identified in a timely manner. The clinical courses for sleep pattern disturbances are variable, with some presenting as self-limiting occurrences and others resulting in recurring and persistent health challenges. For example, such disorders as insomnia and circadian rhythm sleep disorders have a high rate of recurrence and relapse, whereas narcolepsy and some types of breathing-related sleep disturbances are manageable with treatment. Of all types of sleep disturbances, researchers have studied insomnia and obstructive sleep apnea the most.

DISCHARGE CRITERIA

Most people with sleep pattern disturbances are not hospitalized for the sleep disorder unless the particular disorder is life threatening (e.g., a breathing-related sleep disorder with extensive periods of apnea). In these instances, the criteria for discharge relate to the particular situation under consideration. For example, a patient with a serious breathing-related sleep disorder develops a variety of problems (e.g., hypoxia, arterial hypertension, cardiac dysrhythmias) as a result of prolonged periods of apnea. Therefore, the patient needs to have these problems resolved before he or she can be safely discharged to the community or home setting. Patients with sleep disorders and coexisting psychiatric or medical conditions who are hospitalized need to meet the discharge criteria that are standard for the relevant psychiatric or medical condition.

A large percentage of primary sleep disorders also go undiagnosed, generally because the affected individuals attribute their symptoms to factors other than the sleep pattern disturbance itself and do not seek treatment for the disorder until late into the disease process. For instances in which a health care provider identifies a sleep problem during the course of the illness, the affected individual is usually treated in an outpatient setting.

The client will do the following:

- Demonstrate a satisfactory understanding of his or her illness and of the common strategies for appropriate management.
- Identify physical and psychosocial stressors that exacerbate the sleep disturbance.
- Identify signs and symptoms of the sleep pattern disturbance and focus on the initial clinical manifestations that indicate the need for early intervention.
- Identify a social support network that will be instrumental in helping the patient to achieve his or her previous or highest level of functioning.
- Verbalize adequate knowledge of the predisposing, precipitating, and perpetuating factors that are commonly associated with sleep pattern disturbances.
- Demonstrate a sufficient understanding of the treatment plan, including of any prescribed medications (e.g., intended use, action, dose, side effects, contraindications, interactions with other substances).

▌THE NURSING PROCESS

ASSESSMENT

The assessment of the individual with a sleep pattern disturbance is a complex process because of the various symptom profiles that present. For example, an individual with primary insomnia minimizes his or her symptoms of daytime fatigue, excessive sleepiness, or mental sluggishness. It is important that the nurse obtain both subjective reporting data from the affected individual and his or her bed partner as well as a comprehensive database from objective and quantifiable data

BOX 19-2	ASSESSMENT OF SLEEP PATTERNS AND ROUTINES

- Number of hours of sleep per night
- Time of day or night that the patient goes to bed or falls asleep
- Any recent changes in established sleep patterns and routines; if changes are reported, determine what factors seem to affect sleep, and assess for both inhibiting and enhancing factors
- Regularity of sleep routine (regular or irregular)
- Night time awakenings (describe)
- Presence of daytime napping (describe)
- Use of sleep aids or substances that disrupt sleep (e.g., sleep medications, stimulants, antidepressants, alcohol)
- Present stressors and those from the recent or remote past
- Objective reporting from the bed partner (e.g., snoring, apneic periods) or from parents (e.g., sleepwalking, nightmares, sleep terrors)

sources. The data obtained from the sleep history will determine if the patient has a significant problem with his or her sleep pattern and if referral to a sleep specialist is necessary.

The nurse obtains subjective data by using a sleep history questionnaire or by having the patient keep a sleep diary (Box 19-2). The observations of the bed partner or parents are also beneficial during the data-gathering process. The nurse will use rating scales such as the Epworth Sleepiness Scale to gain objective data about the patient's sleep habits (Doghramji et al, 2007). The nurse also obtains data by checking for physiologic indicators of sleep pattern disturbances while the individual sleeps. Nurses today are able to assess the quality of sleep cycles in a sleep laboratory by monitoring multiple physiologic processes while the patient sleeps. This includes observing EEG activity, electrooculographic activity (i.e., extraocular eye movements), electromyographic activity (i.e., muscle movement), heart rate and rhythm, respiratory rate, and blood pressure with the use of polysomnography testing (i.e., multiple sleep tests). Health care providers are able to do additional testing if they suspect that the individual has a problem with a particular disorder. For example, if they suspect that a patient has a breathing-related sleep disorder, then they will measure such factors as oxyhemoglobin saturation (the presence of oxygen in the blood), exhaled carbon dioxide levels (changes in carbon dioxide levels that can adversely affect breathing), breathing effort (labored breathing indicates a problem), airflow measurements, and muscular efforts during breathing.

NURSING DIAGNOSIS

Nurses formulate diagnoses on the basis of the information obtained during the patient assessment. After they are formulated, the diagnoses will direct the development of a comprehensive treatment plan that will be most effective for achieving the pre-established treatment goals for the patient with sleep disorders. Nursing diagnoses are prioritized according to patient needs, from most urgent to least urgent. The following nursing diagnoses are the most applicable for patients with sleep pattern disturbances (Carpenito-Moyet, 2009; North American Nursing Diagnoses Association International, 2009):

- Sleep deprivation
- Readiness for enhanced sleep
- Insomnia
- Ineffective breathing pattern
- Anxiety
- Fatigue
- Ineffective coping
- Ineffective role performance
- Risk for injury
- Impaired spontaneous ventilation

OUTCOME IDENTIFICATION

Nurses develop realistic patient-centered treatment plan goals on the basis of appropriate outcomes. These outcomes are the anticipated behavioral responses to expect from a patient with sleep pattern disturbances after he or she actively participates in the plan of care. Outcomes are prioritized according to patient needs, from most urgent to least urgent. Following are several examples of patient outcomes that address some of the expected behaviors of a patient who demonstrates healthy and adaptive behavioral responses to sleep pattern disturbances. The patient will do the following:

- Identify the primary causes of the sleep pattern alterations.
- Communicate appropriate interventions for a particular sleep pattern disorder and implement them.
- Demonstrate a significant reduction of sleep pattern disturbances through self-reports and objective evaluation measures.
- Participate actively in discharge planning with members of the acute care and community-based practice health care team.

PLANNING

Collaborative planning requires the active participation of the patient with the members of the multidisciplinary health care team. Treatment considerations reflect evidenced-based health care practices and include the patient. The treatment plan needs to be comprehensive and to include relevant biologic, psychosocial, and cognitive treatment modalities. This approach will be most effective for helping to restore sleep patterns in the affected patient.

IMPLEMENTATION

Nurses develop an individualized plan of care for each patient to achieve that patient's anticipated behavioral outcomes.

The plan needs to be comprehensive and appropriate to the level of care that the patient requires in the clinical setting. Most patients with sleep pattern disturbances present in the community practice setting unless the sleep disturbance is a co-occurring problem that is associated with a psychiatric condition or a medical disorder. In the latter instance, the patient often presents in the acute care setting. In either case, nurses work directly with the patient, the members of the multidisciplinary health care team, and the patient's family and significant others to design the plan of care.

Nursing Interventions

Nursing interventions are prioritized according to patient needs, from most urgent to least urgent.

1. Monitor the patient's sleep patterns and identify risks (e.g., breathing-related sleep disorder, sleepwalking, narcolepsy, daytime fatigue) *to prevent harm and injury to the patient.*

2. Teach the patient how to keep a sleep diary *so that he or she will identify patterns that promote sleep pattern disturbance.*

3. Develop a sleep hygiene plan and educate the patient about sleep hygiene practices *to promote rest and sleep in the sleep-deprived patient.*

4. Teach the patient about useful strategies for symptom management *to promote a sense of control over the problem.*

5. Help the patient to structure and maintain a quiet and comfortable environment that is conducive to sleep *to promote sleep and rest during designated periods throughout the day and night.*

6. Help the patient to identify specific stressors that affect his or her ability to obtain restorative sleep *to help the patient to avoid or reduce stressors and obtain restorative sleep.*

7. Promote the development of adaptive coping skills, such as relaxation techniques, through patient and family education *to assist the patient with managing the psychosocial stressors that negatively affect his or her ability to obtain restorative sleep.*

8. Identify the patient's social support system *to foster the use of this resource in the patient's adaptation to perceived psychosocial stressors.*

9. Promote compliance with prescribed medication plans for the treatment of a co-occurring psychiatric illness or for the short-term treatment of a primary sleep disorder. *The use of medications is an effective intervention for the treatment of primary or secondary sleep pattern disturbances.*

10. Teach the patient the importance of limiting the intake of substances that cause a substance-induced sleep disorder (e.g., alcohol, amphetamines and other stimulants, nicotine, caffeine). *The use of prescription medications such as opioids, sedative-hypnotics, and anxiolytics also affects sleep quality, and the patient should only use them when directed to by his or her health care provider. Some substances negatively affect a patient's ability to attain restorative sleep.*

11. Educate the patient about the effect that short- and long-term circadian rhythm disturbances have on restorative sleep patterns, and explore ways to establish regular sleep patterns when sleep routines are disrupted. *Knowledge will inform and empower the patient to accept help and to initiate learned strategies to restore regular sleep patterns.*

12. Refer the patient to a sleep disorder specialist as needed *to determine if advanced practice interventions are necessary. Further testing, such as polysomnography, is sometimes necessary to arrive at a differential diagnosis for the patient.*

Additional Treatment Modalities
Pharmacologic Modalities

Medications that treat primary sleep pattern disturbances are either sedative-hypnotic drugs or stimulants. The particular types of pharmacologic agents prescribed to treat sleep problems are dependent on whether the goal of therapy is to induce sleep or to stimulate wakefulness. In addition, the treatment plan sometimes includes other prescribed psychopharmacologic agents (e.g., antidepressants, anxiolytics), especially if the sleep pattern disturbance occurs with another psychiatric illness. Patients may also use over-the-counter medications in an attempt to manage symptoms of their illness. Many times, patients attempt to manage symptoms with over-the-counter medications before seeking treatment from the health care provider.

Dyssomnias

Insomnia. The benzodiazepine and nonbenzodiazepine sedative-hypnotic drugs, along with other nonpharmacologic treatments, can be used for a patient with insomnia. In general, this treatment lasts no longer than 2 weeks, because tolerance and withdrawal syndromes can result from the long-term use of some of these pharmacologic agents (Clayton et al, 2010). This is especially true for the benzodiazepine drugs because of their high addictive potential. Benzodiazepine hypnotics, such as triazolam (Halcion), temazepam (Restoril), and flurazepam (Dalmane), have the greatest potential for psychologic and physiologic dependency, and they are not commonly the first-line treatment for this disorder. They also interfere with REM sleep.

Nonbenzodiazepine hypnotics such as zolpidem (Ambien) and zaleplon (Sonata) have less abuse potential, and they cause less of a problem with rebound insomnia and REM sleep as compared with the benzodiazepine drugs. Eszopiclone (Lunesta) is a new nonbenzodiazepine hypnotic for insomnia. Lunesta has been effective for reducing sleep latency among patients with problems with insomnia, and it is also effective for helping the patient to maintain sleep. Ramelteon (Rozerem) is the first melatonin receptor stimulant that has been approved by the U.S. Food and Drug Administration (FDA), and it has shown promising results for the treatment of insomnia (Clayton et al, 2010) (Box 19-3).

Antidepressants are sometimes prescribed, especially for patients with coexisting problems with depression and

BOX 19-3   ESZOPICLONE (LUNESTA)

- Eszopiclone is categorized as a nonbenzodiazepine hypnotic drug (schedule IV controlled substance) that is indicated for the treatment of insomnia.
- The exact mechanism by which it works is unknown, but researchers believe that its effect on sleep induction and sleep maintenance is related to its effect on γ-aminobutyric acid receptor complexes.
- The results of clinical trials of eszopiclone have indicated that it is effective for decreasing sleep latency (i.e., the amount of time an individual takes to fall asleep) and for improving sleep maintenance (i.e., the amount of time an individual remains asleep once he or she enters the sleep cycle)
- Eszopiclone has central nervous system depressant effects and therefore has synergistic effects when given with other central nervous system depressant drugs (e.g., psychotropics, anticonvulsants, antihistamines, other drugs and substances that may produce central nervous system depression [e.g., alcohol]).
- Caution patients who are taking eszopiclone about performing psychomotor tasks (e.g., driving a car, operating machinery) while taking this medication.
- There are no known contraindications to the use of this drug at the present time. Side effects of this medication are similar to those associated with other hypnotics and are usually mild. These include drowsiness, dizziness, and lightheadedness. Adverse effects include unpleasant taste in the mouth, dry mouth, dizziness, viral infections, infections, and a variety of abnormal thinking and behavioral changes.
- The recommended dose (for nonelderly patients) is 2 mg by mouth taken just before bedtime; 1 mg by mouth is recommended for elderly patients. If the patient is having a problem maintaining sleep, the dose can be increased to 3 mg for nonelderly patients and 2 mg for elderly patients, if necessary.
- Eszopiclone is categorized as a pregnancy category C drug. Data from long-term clinical trials in pregnant woman are not available.

Data from Sepracor Inc: *Lunesta (eszopiclone) tablets (drug insert) 2005* (website): www.lunesta.com/PostedApprovedLabelingText.pdf. Accessed April 24, 2006.

insomnia. Most drugs in this category decrease REM sleep and are effective for the treatment of depressed patients with marked insomnia (Clayton et al, 2010).

Many patients use over-the-counter medications that contain antihistamines for symptom management. Such drugs as Sominex and Unisom contain diphenhydramine, which is an antihistamine that has both sedative and anticholinergic effects (e.g., dry mouth, blurred vision, constipation, nasal congestion, urinary retention) (Clayton et al, 2010).

Narcolepsy. The primary aim of the treatment of narcolepsy is the symptomatic management of this disorder. Central nervous system stimulants such as modafinil (Provigil), dextroamphetamine (Dexedrine, Dextrostat) and methylphenidate (Concerta, Ritalin) may be prescribed to manage excessive daytime sleepiness. In addition, antidepressants such as the selective serotonin reuptake inhibitors (Prozac) and tricyclic drugs (Tofranil) may be effective for managing the associated cataplexy (Doghramji et al, 2007; Kaplan and Sadock, 2004). Sodium oxybate (Xyrem) is the only drug that is approved by the FDA to manage the

💊 MEDICATION KEY FACTS

Sleep Disorders

Benzodiazepines (triazolam [Halcion], temazepam [Restoril], flurazepam [Dalmane]), nonbenzodiazepines (zaleplon [Sonata], zolpidem [Ambien], eszopiclone [Lunesta]) and the melatonin receptor stimulant ramelteon (Rozerem)
- These drugs are hypnotics for the treatment of insomnia.
- The abrupt or too-rapid withdrawal of benzodiazepines may result in pronounced restlessness, irritability, insomnia, and seizures.
- Long-term administration in children is associated with rickets because of the altered vitamin D metabolism that occurs with benzodiazepines.
- Paradoxic central nervous system excitation can occur when using antihistamines with benzodiazepines.
- Herbal considerations: Kava kava, chamomile, and valerian may increase central nervous system depression.
- Dietary considerations: Caffeine may counteract sedation and increase insomnia with benzodiazepines. Grapefruit may alter absorption with benzodiazepines. High-fat and heavy meals may delay the onset of sleep by approximately 2 hours in patients who are taking nonbenzodiazepines.

Other Therapies For Insomnia
Antidepressants (trazodone [Desyrel], mirtazapine [Remeron], amitriptyline [Elavil]), antihistamines (diphenhydramine [Benadryl]), and melatonin receptor agonists (Ramelteon)
- In general, these drugs have a low rate of side effects and adverse events.
- Amitriptyline is not recommended for older adults because of its anticholinergic effects.

Over-the-Counter Products
- Over-the-counter products, alternative treatments, and complementary therapies have not been systematically evaluated; efficacy data are lacking, and there are concerns about side effects.
- Herbal products (e.g., melatonin, valerian) are not regulated by the US Food and Drug Administration, and preparations may vary. Avoid taking melatonin with antidepressants, because melatonin is structurally related to serotonin. Valerian is possibly associated with hepatotoxicity.

Stimulants for Hypersomnia
- Cerebral stimulants (psychostimulants) such as methylphenidate (Ritalin, Concerta) and dextroamphetamine (Adderall) are used for narcolepsy.
- Modafinil (Provigil) is indicated for narcolepsy and other sleep disorders. Central nervous system stimulants may potentiate the action of modafinil.

excessive daytime sleepiness and cataplexy seen in narcoleptic patients (Doghramji et al, 2007). In addition, a sleep–wake schedule that includes regularly scheduled naps helps some patients with narcolepsy (Kaplan and Sadock, 2004).

Hypersomnia. The pharmacologic treatment of primary hypersomnia sometimes includes the use of central nervous system stimulant drugs such as amphetamines and modafinil (Provigil) (Kaplan and Sadock, 2004). Nonsedating antidepressants like bupropion (Wellbutrin) are also effective for symptom management for some patients with this disorder (Kaplan and Sadock, 2004).

Breathing-Related Sleep Disorders. Obstructive sleep apnea syndrome is the most common type of breathing-related sleep disorder that often results in ineffective breathing patterns. Medications such as selective serotonin reuptake inhibitors and tricyclic antidepressants can be used to treat apnea, because they decrease the time that the patient spends in REM sleep, when apnea is most likely to take place. Health care providers usually discourage patients with this disorder from using sedating substances such as alcohol, because these types of sedatives often exacerbate the problem (Kaplan and Sadock, 2004). Sedating substances relax the airway, thus increasing the risk of longer apneic episodes throughout the night. See additional treatment modalities for obstructive sleep apnea in the following sections.

Circadian Rhythm Sleep Disorders. The use of short-acting hypnotics that will induce sleep is also useful for short-term treatment.

Parasomnias

Nightmare Disorder. Pharmacologic agents that suppress REM sleep, such as the tricyclic antidepressants and benzodiazepine hypnotic drugs, treat the symptoms that are associated with nightmare disorder (Kaplan and Sadock, 2004). This disorder is frequently self-limiting in children, and it is usually manageable with short-term psychotherapy and desensitization (First and Tasman, 2004).

Sleep Terror Disorder. In the rare instance that medication management is necessary, small doses of diazepam (Valium) administered at bedtime are effective for improving this condition (Kaplan and Sadock, 2004).

Sleepwalking Disorder. Drugs that suppress stages 3 and 4 sleep, such as benzodiazepine hypnotics, have been used for the management of this disorder (First and Tasman, 2004; Kaplan and Sadock, 2004). The primary concern is to provide for the patient's safety while he or she is experiencing the sleepwalking episode. If possible, the affected individual needs to occupy the bedroom on the ground floor of the house to prevent falls. Locking windows and exterior doors and removing dangerous objects from the environment can also be beneficial. (See Chapter 25 for more information about medication for this condition.)

Psychotherapeutic Modalities

In addition to pharmacologic treatment modalities, the psychiatric nurse also participates in the planning of interventions that focus on the psychotherapeutic aspect of sleep disorder treatment. These modalities include patient

---

BOX 19-4 SLEEP HYGIENE PRACTICES

- Go to sleep and awaken at the same time each day to promote a consistent sleep–wake pattern. Try to avoid daytime napping.
- Reduce or eliminate the use of stimulants (e.g., caffeine, nicotine) and other substances (e.g., alcohol) that interfere with sleep.
- Avoid physical exercise or mental stimulation just before bedtime.
- Practice effective coping strategies to manage stress (e.g., progressive relaxation, deep breathing, listening to relaxing music).
- Create an environment that is conducive to restorative sleep (i.e., comfortable temperature, quiet environment, comfortable clothing, and low-level lighting).
- Develop a bedtime routine that will be conducive to promoting sleep (e.g., taking a warm bath, reading a book, practicing meditation).

RESEARCH FOR EVIDENCE-BASED PRACTICE

Humphries J: Sleep disruption in hospitalized adults, *Medsurg Nurs* 14(8):391-395, 2008.

The objective of this descriptive study was to identify the frequency of occurrence and the characteristics of sleep disruption among selected 18- to 55-year-old patients who were hospitalized in one of two identified acute care hospitals in the central United States. Researchers collected data regarding sleep disturbance, sleep effectiveness, and daytime sleep supplementation with the use of the Verran and Snyder-Halpern Sleep Scale from 22 research participants during their third and fourth nights of hospitalization. Study subjects consistently reported high rates of sleep disturbance, poor sleep effectiveness, and difficulty with supplemental daytime sleep during days 3 and 4 of their hospitalization. Although the application of the research findings of this study is somewhat limited because of the small sample size and the use of convenience sampling, this study does provide important information for consideration in clinical nursing practice. Additional research that examines the type and prevalence of environmental conditions that disrupt sleep during a patient's hospitalization and practice considerations that would be effective for minimizing sleep pattern disturbances is warranted.

---

education about behavioral modification and cognitive reframing. For example, patient education begins with an emphasis of sound sleep hygiene practices (Box 19-4) to promote the best possible conditions for restorative sleep. For instances in which a sleep problem such as insomnia is of a chronic nature, the patient is often conditioned to expect that he or she will have sleep problems no matter what. In this situation, the use of techniques to decondition or unlearn previous behaviors with cognitive behavioral therapy will be effective (Jacobs et al, 2004; Kaplan and Sadock, 2004) (see the Research for Evidence-Based Practice box and Chapter

24). In addition, patients with chronic insomnia are sometimes discouraged because prior treatments have been ineffective for symptom management. Thus, the nurse needs to provide the patient with psychosocial support as the patient participates in ongoing behavioral changes. This type of support helps patients who have transient problems with insomnia that results from stressful life events to know that the sleep pattern disturbance will usually improve when the underlying cause is minimized or eliminated.

Additional treatment modalities for obstructive sleep apnea often include the use of continuous positive airway pressure (CPAP). This treatment requires the patient to wear a mask during sleep. Positive pressure is applied to the airways, thus minimizing airway obstruction and improving ventilation. In some cases, patients use oral appliances to assist with clearing the airway passage. Overweight patients are also encouraged to lose weight. In addition, some patients have a surgical intervention known as *uvulopalatopharyngoplasty* to minimize airway obstruction by removing the tonsils and the excess tissue of the soft palate (Ballard, 2008).

The primary aim when managing a circadian rhythm sleep disorder is to establish some degree of regularity in the sleep–wake cycle by synchronizing sleep–wake patterns with typical daily schedules. The patient benefits by identifying external environmental cues that he or she can link to a certain phase of the sleep–wake pattern. Trying to manipulate the sleep schedule by encouraging the patient to sleep earlier than his or her previously established "late night" patterns usually helps with some circadian rhythm sleep disorders (e.g., delayed sleep phase type, jet lag type). Another strategy is progressively delaying the bedtime and awakening times over a few weeks' duration, so that the patient eventually attains a regular sleep–wake schedule that is more compatible with his or her lifestyle. The nurse then assists the patient with gradually adjusting the timing of the sleep–wake cycle by administering light therapy or encouraging the patient to spend a certain amount of time out in the sunlight. Exposure to light is effective for advancing the delayed sleep phase and thus progressively shifting the sleep–wake cycle (First and Tasman, 2004). Synchrony of sleep–wake patterns to light and dark schedules is often beneficial for these types of sleep disorders. Sleep pattern disturbances that are caused by rotating shift work or night shift work are more challenging to manage. However, anything that the patient is able to do to establish some regularity in the sleep–wake pattern will be beneficial to the overall quality of sleep (Thorpy, 2010) In addition, the patient's adherence to sound sleep hygiene practices is very important. Treatment planning that requires the participation of a sleep care specialist is sometimes necessary, especially for instances in which the patient presents with many complex problems.

EVALUATION

Ongoing evaluation is crucial for determining whether the patient is progressing toward the desired outcomes or if the nurse needs to revise the treatment plan. The psychiatric nurse and the members of the health care team—including the patient, when appropriate—need to participate in both formal and informal evaluation processes to determine the patient's progression along the health care continuum, including whether desired outcomes are occurring in a timely manner and if the modification of the plan is necessary at any point during the nursing process.

◎ NURSING CARE PLAN

Thomas is a 17-year-old moderately obese male with mild to moderate anxiety who had been experiencing excessive episodes of loud snoring, gasping, labored mouth breathing, and abnormal chest and abdominal movements during sleep that were accompanied by periods of breathing cessation (sleep apnea). His symptoms continued for approximately 6 months' duration and left him exhausted during the day. Thomas insisted that his symptoms would all disappear when he lost some weight and exercised more, but his hectic school schedule and busy social life prevented him from focusing on diet and exercise. Thomas also suffered from excessive daytime sleepiness as a result of his constant interrupted sleep patterns. His normal REM cycle was also interrupted, which compromised his biologic need for a sound and deep dream sleep. In addition, Thomas's condition seemed to exacerbate his usual mild anxiety, and he became more irritable, often without reason. He developed a habit of consuming large amounts of caffeine-containing soda and energy drinks throughout the day to stay awake at school. When Thomas stated that he would become sleepy while driving his car home from school or a social event, his parents realized that his condition was placing him in danger. One afternoon, after a close call while driving home from school, Thomas's parents finally insisted that Thomas see his pediatrician, who referred Thomas to a sleep clinic for evaluation. Tests indicated that Thomas was experiencing a breathing-related sleep disorder (obstructive sleep apnea), and CPAP was prescribed. After other physical causes were ruled out, Thomas was instructed to engage in weight reduction and exercise and activity programs that were commensurate with his age and condition.

DSM-IV-TR Diagnoses

Axis I   Breathing-related sleep disorder (obstructive sleep apnea) Anxiety traits noted
Axis II   Deferred
Axis III   Moderate obesity
Axis IV   Moderate: 4 to 5 (anxiety/irritability, resistive to treatment,)
Axis V   GAF-71 (current); GAF-81 (past year)

◎ NURSING CARE PLAN—cont'd

Nursing Diagnosis *Ineffective breathing pattern related to inadequate ventilation, obesity, obstructive sleep apnea, and mild to moderate anxiety as evidenced by loud, persistent snoring and gasping and labored mouth breathing during sleep, resulting in periods of wakefulness; unusual chest and abdominal movements; breathing cessation episodes that continue throughout the night; interrupted REM cycle (deep, dream sleep); daytime sleepiness, fatigue, and exhaustion; and increased anxiety symptoms (restless, agitated) and irritability (angers easily)*

NOC Respiratory status: ventilation; Anxiety level
NIC Airway management; Ventilation assistance; Anxiety reduction; Nutrition management; Exercise promotion; Emotional support

CLIENT OUTCOMES	NURSING INTERVENTIONS	EVALUATION
Thomas will demonstrate a regular and nonlabored breathing pattern during regular sleep hours, with normal chest movements on inspiration and expiration and an absence of snoring, gasping, mouth breathing, and sleep apnea.	Support Thomas in using the prescribed breathing treatment of CPAP every night during normal sleep hours. *CPAP is a time-tested breathing method that has been specifically designed to regulate efficient ventilation and respiratory function and to eliminate mouth breathing, snoring, gasping, and sleep apnea, thereby resulting in a regular and nonlabored breathing pattern and REM sleep during normal sleep hours.*	Thomas's breathing is regular, with normal chest movements on inspiration and expiration. Snoring, gasping, and mouth breathing are reduced or absent. No sleep apnea has been noted.
Thomas and his parents will learn about the CPAP breathing equipment (i.e., how to apply the mask, plug in the unit, turn on the machine, and clean and care for the unit components).	Instruct Thomas and his parents about the application of the CPAP unit, such as applying the mask properly and snugly over the nose, plugging in the apparatus to a regular electrical wall outlet, and cleaning and caring for the unit. *The use of a new piece of equipment, especially one that involves breathing and respiratory function and the use of a mask, is often scary and confusing the first time. The nurse's teaching skills and professional approach will often calm patient and family fears, anxieties, and confusion and result in greater compliance with treatment.*	Thomas and his parents demonstrate effective application and care of the CPAP breathing equipment.
Thomas will begin a weight-reduction program with the help of nursing and nutritional services, and he will resume a weight that is recommended for his age and physical condition.	Encourage Thomas to engage in a safe, time-tested weight-management program that is commensurate with his age, height, and physical condition. *Excess weight contributes to some forms of breathing-related sleep disorders, and it exacerbates snoring, gasping, mouth breathing, sleep apnea, and ineffective ventilation. Reaching the appropriate weight will help Thomas to eliminate or reduce symptoms and promote a healthier lifestyle.*	Thomas has enrolled in a weight-reduction program with professional recommendations.
Thomas will begin an exercise and activity program commensurate with his age, physical condition, lifestyle, and capabilities with the recommendation of an exercise physiologist.	Engage Thomas, with his parent's support, in the prescribed exercise and activity program that complements his lifestyle. *Exercise and activity often expedite weight loss when accompanied by a nutritional and weight-management program, which will reduce Thomas's breathing-related sleep disorder symptoms in a more timely manner.*	Thomas regularly participates in an exercise and activity program and a weight-management program, with his parent's support.
Thomas will continue to comply with the treatment and enjoy uninterrupted sleep throughout each night, with the cessation of his previous breathing-related sleep disorder symptoms and an absence of fatigue, exhaustion, or sleepiness during the day.	Praise and support Thomas for his continued use of the CPAP unit at night and for his adherence to his new nutritional and weight management program and his activity and exercise regimen. *Praise and support of the patient's treatment plan help the patient and family to connect the success of the patient's treatment with the need for continued compliance and offer hope and confidence in the treatment as well.*	Thomas continues to use the CPAP unit each night and to comply with the activity and exercise and weight management programs, with his parent's support. Thomas reports less fatigue, exhaustion, and daytime sleepiness.

Continued

◎ NURSING CARE PLAN—cont'd

CLIENT OUTCOMES	NURSING INTERVENTIONS	EVALUATION
Thomas or his parents will contact appropriate professional and technical support persons for any questions or concerns about CPAP procedure or apparatus.	Construct a list of support contact persons for Thomas and his parents. *Access to professional support persons to address questions and concerns or to help restore or replace faulty CPAP equipment will increase the patient's confidence and allay fears and anxieties about the treatment.*	Thomas and his parents contact CPAP professionals as appropriate and are aware that their insurance will pay for a new CPAP mask every 6 months.

Nursing Diagnosis *Anxiety related to breathing-related sleep disorder symptoms (inadequate ventilation, loud snores, gasps, labored mouth breathing, periods of breathing cessation [sleep apnea]) during normal sleep hours and fatigue, exhaustion, and sleepiness during daytime hours as evidenced by agitation (angers easily); restlessness (unable to relax during the day or during periods of nighttime wakefulness); and rapid heart rate during anxious periods*

NOC Anxiety self-control; Symptom control; Vital signs; Stress level; Acceptance: health status; Coping
NIC Anxiety reduction; Vital signs monitoring; Anger control assistance; Exercise promotion: stretching; Teaching: procedure/treatment

CLIENT OUTCOMES	NURSING INTERVENTIONS	EVALUATION
Thomas will demonstrate a reduction in anxiety to a tolerable level (i.e., decreased episodes of anger, agitation, and restlessness) and a normal heart rate after using CPAP for a period of 1 week to manage symptoms associated with his breathing-related sleep disorder.	Encourage Thomas, with his parent's help, to use his prescribed CPAP treatment every night for as long as necessary. *The patient's use of CPAP will reduce many of the physical symptoms known to exacerbate anxiety, such as ventilation problems, rapid heart rate, interrupted nighttime sleep, gasping for air, and sleep apnea.*	Thomas demonstrates reduced anxiety, anger, agitation, and restlessness since using the CPAP unit. His heart rate is within normal limits.
Thomas will demonstrate a reduction in both physical and psychosocial symptoms of anxiety, with decreased anger, agitation, and restlessness.	Teach Thomas some strategies to reduce symptoms of anxiety: simple breathing and relaxation techniques (e.g., deep breathing and tensing and relaxing the muscles), activities and exercises (e.g., simple stretching), cognitive-behavioral techniques (e.g., reframing, which involves the conversion of words like *anxious* into less threatening terms such as *eager* and *curious*; see Chapter 26). *Time-tested anxiety-reducing strategies decrease anxiety provoked by a variety of biologic and psychosocial stressors, most of which are usually unknown by the patient. In this situation, the patient's physical symptoms seemed to exacerbate his anxious nature and required both biologic and psychosocial interventions.*	Thomas is using learned anxiety-reducing strategies on a regular basis and relates a significant reduction in the physical and psychosocial symptoms of anxiety and a decrease in anger, agitation, and restlessness.

GAF, Global Assessment of Functioning; NIC, Nursing Interventions Classification; NOC, Nursing Outcomes Classification.

▍CHAPTER SUMMARY

- Sleep pattern disturbances continue to present health challenges to patients across the life span.
- The causes associated with sleep pattern disturbances are many and include familial, biochemical, psychiatric, sociocultural, and environmental considerations.

- The DSM-IV-TR categorizes sleep pattern disturbances according to their presumed etiology (i.e., dyssomnias and parasomnias).
- The detection and accurate diagnosis of sleep problems are crucial to the effective management of the disorders.

CHAPTER SUMMARY—cont'd

Diagnostic tools include a sleep questionnaire, journal, or diary; sleep rating scales; and polysomnography testing.
• Common treatment plans for sleep disturbances include psychopharmacology, cognitive behavioral therapy, contextual deconditioning, relaxation training, stimulus control, sleep restriction, surgery, and the medical management of underlying medical causes.

• Patient and family education are critical to the successful management of sleep disturbances. Education often includes topics such as sleep hygiene, symptom identification and management, and treatment effectiveness.

REVIEW QUESTIONS

1. While completing a patient history, the patient states, "I have been having problems sleeping, and I think I need medication to help me sleep. I've seen a lot of commercials on television about sleep drugs." Which of the following statements would be the most appropriate nursing response?
   1. "Medications are one type of treatment that may help some people with sleep problems. Tell me more about how you get ready for bed and your sleep history."
   2. "You should make an appointment with a psychiatrist. Sleep disturbances are usually a sign of mental illness."
   3. "All of the medications for insomnia are addictive. Are you sure you want to begin using them?"
   4. "There are many over-the-counter medications that can help you sleep better. Talk to your pharmacist."

2. A patient has a new prescription for ramelteon (Rozerem). Which instructions would the nurse give the patient with regard to taking this medication? You may select more than one answer.
   1. "Take your medication after a high-fat evening meal."
   2. "Take your medication just before you get ready for bed."
   3. "There are some dangerous side effects with this drug."
   4. "This drug will help you to fall asleep faster and stay asleep."
   5. "This drug works better if you take it with a glass of wine."

3. An adult with major depression complains of severe sleep disturbances, daytime drowsiness, and fatigability. How would the nurse classify this sleep problem?
   1. Primary sleep disorder
   2. Secondary sleep disorder
   3. Dyssomnia
   4. Parasomnia

4. Which of the following individuals would be most likely to have obstructive sleep apnea? You may select more than one answer.
   1. A 9-year-old child with moderate obesity
   2. An 18-year-old woman with an eating disorder
   3. A 26-year-old woman with inflammatory bowel disease
   4. A 35-year-old woman with a fractured femur
   5. A 45-year-old man with a body mass index of 50

5. A nurse sees amitriptyline (Elavil) 25 mg at bedtime on the medication administration record of a patient with multiple sclerosis. The nurse's drug handbook indicates that 25 mg is a low dose for this antidepressant drug. What is the nurse's correct analysis of this situation?
   1. An error on the medication administration record is likely. Recheck the physician's order.
   2. A low dose of amitriptyline (Elavil) has been prescribed to improve the patient's sleep.
   3. A lower dose is needed because of the neurologic changes associated with multiple sclerosis.
   4. Antidepressant medications are more effective when they are given during the evening.

REFERENCES

Adler's dream theory (website): www.dreamresearch.ca/enc/adler.pdf. Accessed March 15, 2006.

American Psychiatric Association: *Diagnostic and statistical manual of mental disorders*, ed 4, text revision, Washington, DC, 2000, American Psychiatric Association.

Ballard R: Management of patients with obstructive sleep apnea, *J Fam Pract* 57(Suppl 8): S24-S30, 2008.

Carpenito-Moyet LJ: *Nursing diagnosis: application to clinical practice*, Philadelphia, 2009, Lippincott.

Clayton B et al: *Basic pharmacology for nurses*, ed 15, St. Louis, 2010, Elsevier.

Doghramji P et al: Staying awake: understanding, diagnosing and successfully managing narcolepsy, *J Fam Pract* 56(Suppl 11): S17-S32, 2007.

Drake C: The characterization and pathology of circadian rhythm sleep disorders, *J Fam Pract* 59(Suppl 1):S12-S17, 2010.

First M, Tasman A: *DSM-IV-TR mental disorders: diagnosis, etiology, and treatment*, New Jersey, 2004, John Wiley & Sons.

Freud's dream theory (website): www.dreamresearch.ca/enc/freud.pdf. Accessed March 15, 2006.

Guyton A, Hall JA: *Guyton and Hall textbook of medical physiology*, ed 12, Philadelphia, 2010, Saunders/Elsevier.

Heyworth T: Obstructive sleep apnea, *Canadian Journal of Health and Nutrition* 324:64-66, 2009.

Hirshkowitz M: The clinical consequences of obstructive sleep apnea and associated excessive sleepiness, *J Fam Pract* 57(Suppl):S9-S16, 2008.

Humphries J: Sleep disruption in hospitalized adults, *Medsurg Nurs* 14(8):391-395, 2008.

Jacobs G et al: Cognitive behavior therapy and pharmacotherapy for insomnia: a randomized controlled trial and direct comparison, *Arch Intern Med* 164:1888-1896, 2004.

Jung's dream theory (website): www.dreamresearch.ca/enc/jung.pdf. Accessed March 15, 2006.

Kaplan HI, Sadock BJ: *Synopsis of psychiatry: behavioral sciences, clinical psychiatry*, Baltimore, 2004, Lippincott Williams & Wilkins.

Klosch G, Ulrich K: Sweet dreams are made of this, *Sci Am Mind* 18:39-45, 2005.

Korner A et al: Metabolic syndrome in children and adolescents—risk for sleep-disordered breathing and obstructive sleep apnea syndrome? *Arch Physiol Biochem* 114(4):237-243, 2008.

National Institutes of Health, Department of Health and Human Services: *In brief: your guide to healthy sleep*, Bethesda, Md, 2006a.

National Institutes of Health, Department of Health and Human Services: *Research on sleep and sleep disorders (reissue of PA-95-014)*, Bethesda, Md, 2006b.

National Sleep Foundation: *2008 Sleep in America Poll: summary of findings*, Washington, DC, 2008. NSF for Health Care Professionals.

North American Nursing Diagnoses Association International: *NANDA-I nursing diagnoses: definitions and classification 2009-2011*, Oxford, UK, 2009, North American Nursing Diagnoses Association International.

Pagel J: The burden of obstructive sleep apnea and associated excessive sleepiness, *J Fam Pract* 57(Suppl 8) S3-S8, 2008.

Passarella S, Duong M: Diagnosis and treatment of insomnia, *Am J Health Syst Pharm* 65:927-934, 2008.

Phillips B et al: Sleep disorders and medical conditions in women, proceedings of the Women and Sleep Workshop, National Sleep Foundation, Washington, DC, March 5-6, 2007, *J Womens Health* 17(7), 1191-1199, 2008.

Sadock BJ, Sadock A: *Kaplan & Sadock's concise textbook of clinical psychiatry*, ed 3, Philadelphia, 2008, Lippincott Williams & Wilkins.

Saladin K: *Anatomy and physiology*, ed 5, New York, 2010, McGraw-Hill.

Simon H, Zieve D: Narcolepsy, *A.D.A.M* 1-8, 2009a. University of Maryland Medical Center (website): www.umm.edu.

Simon H, Zieve D: Obstructive sleep apnea, *A.D.A.M*.1-10, 2009b. University of Maryland Medical Center (website): www.umm.edu.

Thorpy M: Managing the patient with shift-work disorder, *J Fam Pract* 59(Suppl 1):S24-S31, 2010.

Online Resources

National Sleep Foundation: www.sleepfoundation.org

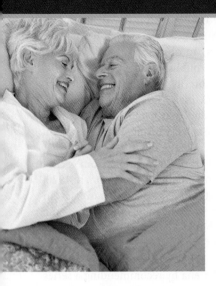

Sexual Disorders: Sexual Dysfunctions and Paraphilias

Kathryn Thomas and Shelly F. Lurie-Akman

"Life without sex might be safer, but it would be unbearably dull."

H.L. Mencken

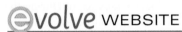 WEBSITE

http://evolve.elsevier.com/Fortinash/

OBJECTIVES

- Describe divergent etiologic theories of sexual dysfunction.
- Identify current statistics regarding the prevalence of sexual dysfunction.
- Name the categories of sexual dysfunction according to the *Diagnostic and Statistical Manual of Mental Disorders*, fourth edition, text revision, and the North American Nursing Diagnosis Association International.
- Discuss effective assessment techniques for patients who complain of a sexual dysfunction.
- Explain the recommended treatment approaches for sexual dysfunction from medical, psychologic, and relational perspectives.

- Apply the nursing process to the care of patients with sexual dysfunctions.
- Describe the different diagnoses of the sex offender (paraphilic) population.
- Discuss the focus of treatment for paraphilic disorders.
- Explain at least two types of treatment and their effects on illness symptomatology.
- Analyze the relationship between treatment and recidivism.
- Apply the nursing process to the care of patients with sexual (paraphilic) disorders.

KEY TERMS

andropause
5-dehydroepiandrosterone
Depo-Provera
   (medroxyprogesterone
   acetate)
duplex ultrasound
dyspareunia
ego dystonic pedophile
ego syntonic pedophile
EROS-CTD system

exogenous testosterone
flibanserin
hypogonadal syndrome
intracorporeal injections
Kegel exercises
lovemap
Lupron Depot (leuprolide)
MUSE
paraphilias

penile nerve function
   studies
penile–brachial index
phosphodiesterase type 5
   inhibitors
plethysmography
psychoeducation
PT-141
sensate focus
sexting

sexual recidivism
sexual response cycle
spectatoring
triggers
vaginal dilators
vaginismus
victimization
voyeurism

SEXUAL DYSFUNCTIONS

This chapter explores two categories of sexual disorders: sexual dysfunctions and paraphilias. Many people report that they are dissatisfied with their sexual lives, and they may present with a whole host of troubling complaints. These complaints best fall under a category of disorders known as *sexual dysfunctions*. Sexual dysfunctions include the lack of desire for or interest in sex, the inability to get aroused or to be orgasmic, experiencing orgasm so quickly that it leaves both the participant and the partner dissatisfied, having pain rather than pleasure with sex, and vaginal constriction that does not allow for penetration. The reported incidence of sexual dysfunction is likely extensive. Historically, Masters and Johnson (1966) estimated that 50% of individuals would experience a form of sexual dysfunction during their lifetimes. This can be a concerning discovery for both individuals and couples. The good news is that, over the past few decades, there has been enormous research interest in this area. New treatments are now available, and even more are proposed. There are fresh ideas abounding and much more help available than there ever was before. Paraphilias (sexual deviations) are discussed in the second half of this chapter.

HISTORIC AND THEORETIC PERSPECTIVES

American society has historically encouraged the belief that healthy and normal sex is heterosexual, married, monogamous, procreative, and noncommercial. Social norms regarding sexual behaviors were closely linked to medical and religious views. At the turn of the last century, many viewed sex as something to be restrained and controlled, especially for females. Women who enjoyed sex were pathologic, yet their problems with "hysteria" were treated with orgasmic release facilitated by medical doctors with the use of a variety of devices. The Reverend Sylvester Graham (of Graham Cracker fame) and Dr. John Harvey Kellogg (of Kellogg's Corn Flakes) preached that male ejaculation reduced precious, health-preserving vital fluids, and they encouraged men to abstain from masturbation and any unnecessary sexual behavior (Stearns, 2010); they also claimed that their food products facilitated this restraint. Despite these influences, American biologist Alfred Kinsey (1894–1956) and his colleagues found that record numbers of Americans were being sexual, enjoying sex, and curious to know more about it (Kinsey, 1948 and 1953).

Austrian neurologist Sigmund Freud (1856–1939) played an influential role in the modern understanding of sexuality. According to Freud, childhood experiences had a subconscious influence on sexual behavior during adulthood. Infantile feelings such as the fear of castration and penis envy, along with actual experiences, combined to create sexual dysfunctions. Freud believed that sexuality was ultimately the cause of many of the difficulties that people faced (Freud, 1977). As a result of Freud's theories, many used psychoanalysis—and its uncovering of the unconscious, which held old fears and traumas—for the treatment of sexual dysfunction for more than 50 years.

In 1966, William Masters, an obstetrician and gynecologist, and Virginia Johnson published their classic book, *Human Sexual Response*. Before its publication, the authors observed more than 10,000 male and female volunteers engaged in masturbatory and partnered sexual activity (Masters and Johnson, 1966). As a result of this research, Masters and Johnson were able to describe exactly what happens to the body during erotic stimulation, from excitement to plateau to orgasm and, finally, to resolution. In 1970, they published a second text, *Human Sexual Inadequacy*, in which they discussed their work helping others overcome sexual dysfunction. In this book, Masters and Johnson outlined the probable causes of dysfunction and gave detailed prescriptions for treatment. They shifted the emphasis of treatment to the behavioral arena by recommending a series of specifically directed exercises performed in a 13-day intensive format and guided by a dual therapy team. During the course of this work, Masters and Johnson developed many specific techniques, including sensate focus and the squeeze technique (Masters and Johnson, 1970), both of which are still used today.

Since the time of these monumental pioneers, researchers have learned much about sexual dysfunctions and about sexuality in general. Structured treatment programs such as Masters and Johnson's did not always solve every problem. Sexuality is too complex to be reduced to a sex manual solution. Helen Singer Kaplan (1974) identified the need for behavioral techniques along with psychoanalysis. Kaplan is also responsible for the development of a model of the sexual response cycle, which includes desire, arousal, and orgasm. This model is the basis for the *Diagnostic and Statistical Manual of Mental Disorders*, fourth edition, text revision (DSM-IV-TR), designations for sexual dysfunction. There were many more theorists and researchers who contributed to the modern knowledge of human sexuality, but that discussion is beyond the scope of this chapter.

During the mid-1990s, a great deal of research interest was generated regarding the origins of male erectile functioning that eventually led to the development of phosphodiesterase type 5 (PDE5) inhibitors (e.g., Viagra), which is a testosterone therapy that helps males with erectile dysfunction to achieve erections (see Clinical Alert box and discussion of these drugs later in this chapter). By 1999, more researchers were becoming interested in the field of female sexuality. Rosemary Basson proposed a new theory of the sexual response cycle that was most applicable to females (Basson et al, 2010). She suggested an intimacy-based sexual model whereby spontaneous sexual desire is not the only antecedent to sexual interaction, which explained why couples often have sex for nonsexual reasons. The model suggests that intimacy needs lead to sexual stimuli, which in turn lead to sexual arousal, desire, and finally to enhanced intimacy. Sexual desire is not only spontaneous, but it can be elicited by intimacy. Sex therapy today involves combinations of pharmacologic, physical, behavioral, educational, communication-enhancing, and psychodynamic techniques.

ETIOLOGY

There are a wide range of etiologic antecedents for sexual dysfunction. Categories include physical/biologic, psychologic/emotional, cultural, and relational. Several factors often contribute to one person or one couple's inability to have satisfying sex (Box 20-1).

Physical/Biologic Factors

Over the past several decades, there has been increasing interest in brain, neurochemical, and hormonal research and its relationship to sexual functioning. For example, researchers know that testosterone stimulates sexual desire in males and females (Lindau et al, 2007). An understanding of the role of the two divisions of the central nervous system has helped with the understanding of why stress reduces sexual arousal and interest. Vascular, neurologic, and endocrine disorders as well as a range of problems such as cancer, connective tissue and pain disorders, depression, incontinence, and sexually transmitted diseases all contribute to the development of sexual dysfunctions (Moalem, 2009). Substance abuse is epidemic in U.S. society, and it can seriously affect an individual's ability to function sexually. Medications—especially antidepressants, antihypertensives, and hormonal treatments—also affect sexual satisfaction.

Psychologic/Emotional Factors

There is a long-standing debate about the role of nature versus nurture in sexual development and functioning. Many believe that psychologic issues are more important to the etiology of sexual dysfunctions than any other factor. There is currently much literature and discussion about the effect of childhood sexual trauma on later sexual functioning (Harvey et al, 2010). Anxiety, stress, and depression also contribute to changes in sexuality. Masters and Johnson (1970) created the term spectatoring; this psychologic phenomenon involves the tendency to observe, monitor, and critique one's own sexual activity, thereby detracting from the actual experience. Positive and negative perceptions of one's body image affect sexual interest and function. Wolf explored this impact on women in her classic 1991 work entitled *The Beauty Myth*. However, lately there has been attention given to the fact that body image can affect male sexuality as well, perhaps most especially in gay men (Kraft et al, 2009).

Cultural Factors

Cultures vary distinctly with regard to the interpretations that they have for sexual behavior. Gender roles can be prescribed, and different social standards are set for men and women when it comes to how they should behave. Sexual myths influence attitudes toward sex. For example, the myth that men are always ready for sex may give women the wrong idea about men, which in turn can lead both genders to behave sexually in ways that are not natural or gratifying for either

BOX 20-1	**ETIOLOGIC FACTORS FOR SEXUAL DYSFUNCTIONS**

Physical/Biologic Factors

Vascular
Cardiac disease
Diseases of the blood vessels

Neurologic
Stroke
Head injuries
Spinal cord disorders
Epilepsy
Parkinson's disease
Peripheral nerve disorders

Endocrine
Diabetes
Altered hormonal levels (especially testosterone)

Pharmacologic
Antidepressants
Antihypertensives
Hormonal therapy
Mind- and mood-altering substances
Alcohol

Other Causes
Cancer
Connective tissue disorders, including arthritis
Pain disorders
Depression
Incontinence
Sexually transmitted diseases

Psychologic/Emotional Factors
Childhood experiences
Body image
Anxiety and stress
Learned pattern for response

Cultural Factors
Misinformation regarding sex
Lack of sex education
Different social standards for men and women
Sexual myths and attitudes
Religion

Relational Factors
Differences in sexual desire or interests
Lack of attraction
Lack of communication
Lack of trust

partner. Religiosity is an interesting cultural issue to contemplate. Many religions place restrictions on sexual behavior that is other than procreative. However, when they were polled, 70% of Catholics said that they think their church should lift its ban on birth control. Many religions advocate for a happy and vital sexual relationship, albeit generally within the context of marriage (Hollinger, 2009).

Relational Factors

Problems within relationships, including financial and family stress, often pull a couple apart and disrupt their sexual satisfaction. Couples often have poor or ineffective communication regarding their sexual likes and dislikes. Couples often do not discuss what they do or do not enjoy sexually or share their feelings about the experience. Differences in sexual drives and interests further complicate the relationship. Money (1986) used the term lovemap to describe one's idealized picture of who and what types of behaviors make up one's sexual arousal pattern. Lovemaps vary from individual to individual; therefore, a couple is sometimes not well matched with regard to their attraction to one another or the sexual activities that interest them. John Gottman, who has extensively studied relationship satisfaction, suggested that the best predictor of relationship duration and happiness is the ratio of positive-to-negative interactions (Gottman et al, 2007).

EPIDEMIOLOGY

In 1999, a major national survey of sexuality—which is still the most-quoted study of what men and women do sexually—found that American men and women between the ages of 18 and 59 years reported sexual dysfunction 31% and 43% of the time, respectively (Laumann et al, 1999). Recent studies have looked more specifically at particular groups of people, particular ages, and coexisting factors, such as the reportage of the degree of sexual distress that accompanies dysfunction. The accuracy of the data is also an issue. Overall, men do not seek care for a sexual problem, and therefore their incidence may be underreported (Newman, 2010). A recent large-scale study out of Boston included 32,000 women between the ages of 18 and 100 or more (Shifren et al, 2008) Thirty-nine percent of the women reported low levels of desire, 26% had arousal difficulties, and 21% reported problems with achieving orgasm. However, only 12% reported distress related to any of these problems. Looking at reported problems alone was not seen as sufficient criteria for a diagnosis without also evaluating the degree of distress that results from the dysfunction. When comparing previous peer-reviewed research, Derogatis and Burnett (2008) found that sexual dysfunctions are prevalent worldwide and that the occurrence of such dysfunctions increases directly with the age of men and women. Thus, gender and age need to be considered. In addition, studies report difficulty as a result of poor definitions and inadequate study design with regard to determining accurate incidence data. A July 2010 study that was performed in Norway and that involved individuals between the ages of 18 and 67 years suggested that, during the month before the study, 52% of respondents in the 60- to 67-year-old age range struggled with decreased desire. Twenty-three percent of participants in the 18- to 29-year-old age range complained of pain, and 18% of men in this younger group reported premature ejaculation. Twelve percent of men in their 60s said that they had erectile dysfunction, and 34% of women in their 60s felt that they no longer had adequate lubrication (Træeen et al, 2010).

CLINICAL DESCRIPTION

In the current clinical classification system of the DSM-IV-TR, sexual dysfunctions are divided into sexual desire disorders, sexual arousal disorders, orgasmic disorders, sexual pain disorders, sexual dysfunction caused by a general medical condition, substance-induced sexual dysfunction, and sexual dysfunction not otherwise specified (see the DSM-IV-TR Criteria box #1). The first three categories are based on Kaplan's stages of the sexual response cycle (1974). There are currently proposals being made for the DSM-V classifications. For example, it is possible that sexual aversion disorder will be deleted and other disorders combined. The proposed categories for the combined diagnoses are interest/arousal disorders and genitopelvic pain/penetration disorder.

PROGNOSIS

Nurses need to have an understanding of what types of treatment are available and how successful they are to properly guide and instruct their patients. In some cases, treatment outcomes are excellent, whereas in others they are poor. For example, hypoactive sexual desire disorders tend to have a more negative prognosis than other disorders. There are several reasons for this, with the first being a lack of known physiologic factors. Second, defining desire is an inaccurate and controversial process (see the Research for Evidence-Based Practice box #1). The last is that, among those who complain of desire disorder, relationship factors may be the actual culprits. By contrast, premature ejaculation has several relatively successful treatment strategies. Current interest in this area will eventually lead to better understanding and more effective interventions.

Masters and Johnson (1970) estimated that, 5 years after treatment, only 5.1% of patients had relapsed. However, no one has ever replicated their studies, and many have questioned their evaluation techniques. In general, many believe that sexual dysfunctions are difficult to treat. The literature lacks many long-term follow-up studies; thus, estimating prognosis is difficult. The drug companies provide statistics regarding the efficacy of such products as Viagra and Cialis. These products have been useful for men but much less so for women. Most therapy for sexual dysfunction involves the use of cognitive-behavioral techniques. The success of these techniques directly reflects the patient's willingness and persistence in implementing them.

DISCHARGE CRITERIA

After intervention, the patient will do the following:
- Develop a better understanding of the cause and symptoms of the disorder.
- Develop communication strategies with his or her partner to express desires, likes, and dislikes.

DSM-IV-TR CRITERIA #1

Sexual Dysfunctions

Desire Phase Disorders

Hypoactive sexual desire disorder: A deficiency or absence of sexual fantasy or drive for sexual activity

Sexual aversion disorder: Aversion to or avoidance of genital sexual contact with a partner

Arousal Phase Disorders

Female sexual arousal disorder: Inability to attain or maintain an adequate lubrication/swelling response of sexual excitement

Male erectile disorder: Inability to attain or maintain an adequate erection

Orgasm Phase Disorders

Female orgasmic disorder: Delay in or absence of orgasm after sexual excitement phase (must be persistent or recurrent)

Male orgasmic disorder: Delay in or absence of orgasm following sexual excitement phase (must be persistent or recurrent)

Premature ejaculation: Onset of orgasm and ejaculation with minimal sexual stimulation (must be persistent or recurrent)

Sexual Pain Disorders

Dyspareunia: Genital pain associated with sexual intercourse (not resulting from a general medical condition)

Vaginismus: Involuntary contractions of the perineal muscles with penetration (not resulting from a general medical condition)

Sexual Dysfunction Due to a General Medical Condition

Use same subtypes as above but indicate the underlying medical condition

Substance-Induced Sexual Dysfunction

Use same subtypes as above and indicate specific substance

Sexual Dysfunction Not Otherwise Specified

Does not meet criteria for the category of sexual dysfunction

Data from the American Psychiatric Association: *Diagnostic and statistical manual of mental disorders,* ed 4, text revision, Washington, DC, 2000, American Psychiatric Association.

RESEARCH FOR EVIDENCED-BASED PRACTICE #1

Carvalheira AA et al: Women's motivations for sex: exploring the *Diagnostic and Statistical Manual,* 4th edition, text revision criteria for hypoactive sexual desire and female sexual arousal disorders, *J Sex Med* 7(4 Pt 1):1454-1463, 2010.

This study involved 3687 women in Lisbon, Portugal, who completed an Internet-based survey. Outcome measures included self-reported issues regarding sexual desire, fantasy, and arousal. These questions were developed by the team performing the research. The researchers were interested in exploring a woman's motivation to be sexual; the predictors and incidence of sexual desire, fantasy, and arousal; and the woman's ability to recognize her arousal. The study is pertinent to the current discussion that is leading up to the publication of the DSM-V regarding the definition of hypoactive sexual desire disorder. For women in particular, sexual desire and fantasy do not appear to be universal experiences, and the motivation for sex may be something altogether different. The results have shown that women in long-term relationships engaged in sex with no sexual desire more often than women in shorter-term relationships. In longer-term relationships, women did not initiate sex as often, and they reported less sexual satisfaction with their partners. When identifying women who were easily aroused, the investigators found that 15.5% had sex only when they felt desire, but 30.7% typically engaged sexually without initial desire. Rather, the desire was generated after they were aroused. Sexual fantasies were reported to be sporadic in the majority of women. Religion, ease of arousal, and frequency of orgasm appeared to be factors in the degree to which women had a fantasy life. Conclusions reached by the investigators are similar to those found in other research: women's motivation to be sexual is variable, and often arousal is needed before desire is elicited. With regard to the development of diagnostic criteria, it is essential that the issues raised by this research are considered. The duration of the relationship and whether the woman is adequately stimulated are important factors. Sexuality for women is often more responsive than driven by desire. Previous definitions do women a disservice, because they presume that the sexual response cycle begins with fantasy and desire as a prerequisite.

- Develop appropriate coping strategies to deal with frustrations and setbacks.
- Demonstrate the use of appropriate intervention techniques that are designed to alleviate the specific disorder.
- Express increased satisfaction with his or her sexual functioning.

Sexuality is essential to the well-being of individuals and of couples, so nurses need to be aware that assisting their patients with the achievement of positive sexual expression is an important goal (see the Case Study #1). Facilitating this goal is a rewarding but difficult task. It demands that nurses reflect on their own attitudes and values as well as their comfort with and knowledge of sexuality. The overall goal of intervention is the achievement of sexual satisfaction, and the nurse recognizes that sexual satisfaction and the length of time that it takes to achieve varies from individual to individual and from couple to couple.

THE NURSING PROCESS

ASSESSMENT

Any discussion of sexuality can be difficult and sensitive for many people. When discussing sexuality with patients, nurses need to recognize that they are not immune to the feelings, beliefs, values, and attitudes that affect others. Therefore,

CASE STUDY #1

Ben and Christine are a couple in their mid-30s. They have been together for 5 years and cohabiting for 3 years, and they are considering marriage. However, Ben says that, before they get married, he wants to deal with their sexual issues. He says that Christine is rarely interested in sex, that he always has to initiate, and that she often turns him down. Christine admits that she has never had a strong sexual drive, possibly because she comes from a family that was religious and never discussed sex. She agrees that she often turns Ben down, but she says that she has two reasons for this: the first is that Ben often wants to engage in what she refers to as "kinky sex," which means that he likes to role-play and even tie her up at times. The second reason is that he often ejaculates quickly, which leaves her unsatisfied. Ben says that it is important for him to be creative in the bedroom; he believes that this is important for maintaining long-term sexual interest. He admits that at times he ejaculates shortly after entry and that this has been a long-standing issue. He never wanted to discuss it before because he was embarrassed. Both Ben and Christine say that there are so many good things in their relationship that they will do whatever it takes to work on these sexual issues.

Critical Thinking

1 What symptoms of sexual dysfunction or dissatisfaction does this couple exhibit?
2 What are the precursors or antecedents to the couple's sexual problems?
3 Which nursing diagnoses are appropriate for this couple?
4 How would you help Ben and Christine to achieve greater sexual satisfaction?

BOX 20-2   PRINCIPLES OF SEXUAL ASSESSMENT

- Before beginning a sexual assessment, examine your own feelings, attitudes, and level of comfort.
- Ensure a private and quiet space, ample time, and an unhurried attitude for the assessment.
- Do not ask questions about sexuality first. Begin with background information, and fit the sexual assessment into the overall assessment.
- Begin questioning about sexuality with the least sensitive areas, and then move to areas of greater sensitivity. For example, begin by asking, "Where did you first learn about sex?"
- Maintain appropriate eye contact and a relaxed and interested manner.
- Be professional and matter-of-fact about information that is asked or obtained. Avoid extreme reactions. The maintenance of an open and nonjudgmental attitude is essential.
- Use language that is professional but that will be understood by the patient being interviewed. This is a good opportunity to teach the patient about the words of sex.
- Remember, the nurse's tone of voice and manners reflect trust. If patients feel that they can trust the nurse, they will be more open.
- Sex is not something that most people are used to talking about, and this can make interviewing difficult. However, if the nurse has the right attitude, patients will generally be open, willing, and even eager to talk.

when the nurse is dealing with patient-related sexual issues, both the nurse and the patient sometimes experience discomfort. A holistic nursing assessment includes sexuality as it relates to the importance of the patient's well-being. A firm knowledge base, expert use of the nursing process, and a nonjudgmental attitude are necessary to work with this group of patients.

Assessment is always the beginning point, and it is an essential phase of working with patients with sexual dysfunction. Nurses need a clear understanding of the complexity of the symptoms and the areas of dysfunction. Sexual dysfunctions happen throughout various phases of the sexual response cycle. Some sexually based issues reflect individual functioning, but they may also be couple related. Sexual assessment includes all assessment factors, such as background, physical health, religious and cultural beliefs, education, occupation, significant relationships, and social relationships. In addition to the assessment of the specific complaint, the nurse also considers the individual's or couple's perspective of the problem and the associated desire to change.

The sexual history is an important aspect of the assessment (Box 20-2). Alfred Kinsey and his colleagues (1948) suggested beginning with the least awkward topic (e.g., sex

education) and then working toward more difficult and personal topics. The sex history includes early childhood experiences, history of masturbation, teenage experiences, the use of erotica and fantasies, contraception history, relationship history, sexual orientation, satisfaction with sexuality, and an opportunity for questions and concerns. Nurses are not usually trained in taking a sexual history; however, it is a skill that nurses can learn and implement by using their already well-developed techniques of interviewing and communication. In addition, there are tools available that can assist them (e.g., the Derogatis Sexual Functioning Inventory).

NURSING DIAGNOSIS

After assessment, the nurse is in a position to analyze the findings and arrive at diagnoses. It is best to use the DSM-IV-TR diagnoses of sexual dysfunctions with the North American Nursing Diagnosis Association International (NANDA-I)–approved nursing diagnoses to reflect specific problems. A combination of medical and nursing diagnoses helps to ensure that the nurse develops adequate plans for intervention. The nurse determines diagnoses on an individual basis and carefully selects them from the NANDA-I list (NANDA-I, 2008). Nursing diagnoses are prioritized according to patient needs, from most urgent to least urgent. Nursing diagnoses that are common for sexual dysfunctions include the following:

- Anxiety
- Fear
- Hopelessness
- Chronic pain
- Ineffective sexuality pattern
- Sexual dysfunction
- Ineffective coping
- Risk-prone health behavior
- Disturbed body image
- Social isolation
- Ineffective role performance
- Deficient knowledge (of problem and aspects of treatment)
- Impaired verbal communication (unable to express oneself)
- Situational low self-esteem
- Defensive coping

OUTCOME IDENTIFICATION

During this phase of the nursing process, expected patient outcomes derived from the nursing diagnoses are created. Outcomes are prioritized according to patient needs, from most urgent to least urgent. Outcomes common for sexual dysfunction include that the patient will do the following:

- Describe the specific sexual problem to the nurse by the second visit.
- Make an appointment for a physical examination (if appropriate) by the time of the third visit with the nurse.
- Discuss feelings associated with the identified sexual problem by the time of the third visit with the nurse.
- Participate in sex therapy sessions (if appropriate) by the time of the fourth visit with the nurse.
- Practice recommended strategies learned in sex therapy by the sixth week of therapy.
- Describe two strategies learned to enhance sexual functioning after the sixth week of therapy.
- Incorporate strategies learned during sex therapy into routine sexual activity by the end of therapy and on an as-needed basis after therapy.

PLANNING

After a thorough assessment, the establishment of the diagnoses, and the identification of outcome criteria, it is time to start the planning phase of the nursing process. Planning involves formulating an individualized plan of care that is designed to address all issues presented; the nurse and the patient then work together to define realistic treatment goals. Individuals and couples who are dealing with sexual dysfunction need to carefully consider what they are willing to do to work toward these goals. The plan of care is often different for individuals with the same problem because of each person's values, beliefs, attitudes, and perceptions of the problem. For example, a patient with a primary orgasmic dysfunction

has difficulty with masturbatory exercises as a particular treatment strategy because he believes that touching one's own genitals is unacceptable. When a patient's individual beliefs prevent the implementation of a plan of care, treatment success depends on the further exploration of the problem or an alternative plan of care.

PATIENT AND FAMILY TEACHING GUIDELINES #1
Sexual Dysfunctions

Teach Individual Patients
- Engage in breathing and relaxation techniques to reduce anxiety.
- Incorporate ways to increase comfort with and knowledge of one's body, using gradual and progressive touch. These exercises can be done in the shower or the bath or with the use of a mirror.
- Begin specific body image exercises that involve positive affirmations and mirror work.
- Practice the use of fantasy, erotica, self-stimulation, and toys to enhance sexuality.
- Provide information about human sexual response principles and current knowledge of the hormonal and biochemical control of sexual functioning.

Teach Couples
- Teach couples to schedule their sexual experiences for mutually agreed upon times.
- Help couples to develop communication skills that enhance the ability to openly discuss sexuality, including ways to express likes and dislikes.
- Suggest that couples take turns planning a favorite sexual or sensual scenario that they will then act out together.
- Create a positive sexual atmosphere through the use of sexual humor, flirtation, touch, and the enjoyment of one another. Help couples to have fun together.
- Inform couples about theories regarding the individuality and variance of sexual interest and levels of desire.
- Encourage couples to try something new, such as a full body or genital massage, sexual play at spontaneous moments, or variations in the time or location of sexual activity.

IMPLEMENTATION

Good background knowledge of the specific nature of the problem and the possible etiologies is needed to begin the implantation process. Implementation includes education, counseling, and assistance with identifying specific strategies, referrals, and support (see the Patient and Family Teaching Guidelines box #1). The nurse also needs to be aware of various treatment modalities and the prognosis for recovery with each intervention. The nurse's role is to help the patient to express concerns about sexual functioning; to express his or her feelings about the impact of these concerns; and to build his or her knowledge base, self-esteem, and communication skills. The nurse is also capable of recommending a physical examination, a treatment, and sex therapy. Nurses also monitor patient compliance and progress in treatment and help to develop appropriate discharge planning. Nurses need to stress to the patient or couple that treatment success largely depends on following through with the plan of care.

A trusting, open, and comfortable relationship is necessary to help patients with the exercises, knowledge, and interventions that are necessary to create more satisfying sexual relations. It is difficult enough to discuss sexual difficulties with others, so, without a comfortable relationship between the nurse and the patient, many sexual problems will go unrecognized and untreated. Sexual issues and problems that are associated with the maturing process are increasingly common because the population that embraced the birth control pill must now cope with the complexities of acquired immunodeficiency syndrome, menopause and inadequate production of sex hormones in males (hypogonadal syndrome). Women may experience depression and a lack of sexual desire that results from diminished hormone levels and related painful intercourse (dyspareunia) Men may feel trapped in their jobs or careers or their relationships. Sexually active adults who are not in monogamous relationships may have concerns about sexually transmitted diseases, although there are protective methods to reduce risk. It is important for the nurse to examine all of the individual's sexual issues and problems within the context of a relationship. The implementation of a plan of care most often involves both members of a couple; placing the blame on either partner may affect the couple's ability to heal.

Nursing Interventions

The following nursing interventions are prioritized according to patient needs from most urgent to least urgent.

1. Assist the patient to better understand the human sexual response. Recommend appropriate reading materials such as Masters and Johnson's *Human Sexual Response* and Helen Singer Kaplan's *The New Sex Therapy*. Other reading materials to introduce include Rosemary Basson's intimacy-based model (Basson et al, 2010). *The patient's knowledge of the human sexual response forms a foundation for his or her understanding of other aspects of sexual functioning and their relationship to sexual disorders.*

2. Teach the patient about sexual dysfunctions, including possible etiologies, symptoms, and treatment options. Include various methods of assessment, such as physical, urologic, gynecologic, and laboratory examinations as well as a psychosocial sexual assessment. *Through education, patients are able to understand why changes in sexual functioning are happening to them, and they are better able to identify symptoms that signal a sexual problem.*

3. Educate the patient about positive communication and relationship skills. Support and reinforce the patient by facilitating these skills. Provide communication and relationship-based homework assignments. Suggest bibliotherapy, such as Gottman and colleagues' *Ten Lessons to Transform Your Marriage. Problems in the relationship*

as well as the inability to communicate are often the causes of sexual dysfunctions. Positive communication and relationship skills enhance intimacy and sexuality.

4. Help the patient to explore his or her fears and anxieties related to sexuality. Do this in a private, trusting, and open atmosphere. Encourage the patient to talk about what he or she learned about sexuality and what his or her experiences were. Teach breathing and relaxation techniques to facilitate ease when dealing with these issues. *An open forum for discussing sexuality, accompanied by time-proven strategies, helps patients to overcome some of the repressed feelings that they have and to be more open to satisfying sexual experiences.*

5. Assist the patient with enhancing his or her self-esteem related to sexuality. Encourage positive self-talk, such as affirmations, cognitive therapy exercise, and body-image exercises (see Chapter 26). Discuss variations of sexual expression and treatment. *A lack of self-esteem is often a contributing factor for sexual dysfunction, and time-tested treatments and strategies will help to improve the patient's self-esteem and self-image.*

6. Refer the patient to physical treatment modalities or sex therapy, as applicable. *These therapeutic interventions will help to maximize patient success when dealing with sexual dysfunction.*

Additional Treatment Modalities

Upon completion of a careful assessment and the determination of a specific diagnosis of sexual dysfunction, the nurse must choose from several possible treatment modalities (see the Additional Treatment Modalities box). The history of sex therapy involves the use of psychodynamic and cognitive-behavioral techniques, because originally theorists believed that the reasons for sexual problems were psychologic and relational in nature. However, the current emphasis is on physiologic causation (although often causes are unknown) and on treatments that combine biologic, psychologic, and couples-related approaches.

Medically Based Evaluation and Intervention Techniques for Men

A useful measure for determining penile blood pressure is the penile–brachial index. The penile–brachial index is calculated by comparing the penile systolic blood pressure, which is determined by Doppler, with the brachial systolic blood pressure at rest and after exercise. There are other invasive and noninvasive tests for the evaluation of erectile dysfunction. A number of blood studies (e.g., thyroid function) as well as urinalysis may prove helpful. Duplex ultrasounds are performed after the injection of prostaglandins to evaluate the blood flow through the penis, to determine whether venous leakage is present, and to assess the overall status of vessel health. Penile nerve function studies can be conducted to determine if there is sufficient nerve sensation. These studies can involve simple tests such as manually squeezing the penis to elicit an anal reflex, but they can also be much more complex.

ADDITIONAL TREATMENT MODALITIES

Sexual Dysfunctions

Psychophysiologic Modalities
- Anxiolytics
- Atypical antidepressants (e.g., bupropion)
- Botox
- Cialis
- EROS-CTD
- Estrogen replacement for women
- Intracavernosal injections
- Levitra
- Lidocaine-based topical cream
- MUSE
- Penile prosthesis
- Selective serotonin reuptake inhibitors
- Exogenous testosterone therapy for men
- Viagra
- Vibrators

Possibilities on the Horizon
- 5-Dehydroepiandrosteron
- Dapoxetine
- Dopamine receptor agonists
- Flibanserin
- Pheromones
- PT-141 (a compound that treats female sexual arousal disorders)
- Viagra cream
- Exogenous testosterone replacement for women

Psychosocial Modalities
- Sex therapy
- Sexual education
- Body therapies (e.g., massage, chakra balancing, tantric yoga)
- Communication techniques
- Education
- Erotic stimuli training
- Gradual dilation of the vagina
- Masturbation training
- Semans' stop–start technique and squeeze techniques for premature ejaculation
- Sensate focus

Interest has developed in research that addresses how testosterone levels affect sexual functioning in males. Although decreasing levels of testosterone are more common in the elderly population, this condition affects people in younger age groups as well. Studies show varied declines in testosterone levels among males as they age, but there is growing evidence that these decreased levels affect men negatively. Endocrine testing is sometimes necessary. In general, researchers believe that exogenous testosterone used in males improves sexual desire and possibly sexual function in general (Bassil, 2010). A low level of the male hormone, testosterone, is called *hypogonadal syndrome* or andropause, and symptoms include abdominal weight gain and decreases in bone and lean muscle mass.

Medications used for erectile dysfunction are generally considered safe as long as the patient provides a complete medical and drug history. Combining this category of medications with nitrates is contraindicated. Sildenafil (Viagra) for the treatment of male erectile dysfunction was approved for use in the spring of 1998, and this led to immediate worldwide interest. Others have introduced similar PDE5 inhibitors, including vardenafil (Levitra), tadalafil, (Cialis) and, most recently, a daily dosing option for Cialis. PDE5 inhibitors work by blocking the enzyme that breaks down cyclic guanosine monophosphate to boost the chemical's relaxing effect on penile muscles. In combination with stimulation, these drugs have been helpful for the achievement of erection in a vast number of men (Magheli et al, 2009). Intracorporeal injections of vasodilators such as prostaglandins and other substances are given directly into the corpus cavernosum to produce erection. Intraurethral pharmacotherapy involving the introduction of vasoactive drugs through a system called MUSE (medicated urethral system for erections) is still available. In males, there is a surgery that will alter penile arterial blood flow, or surgery can be used to implant prosthetic devices. Prosthetic devices come in two different general forms, and they have been developed over time, with more satisfactory results. There is a semirigid rod that is made of silicone or metal, and there are inflatable pumps of varying degrees of sophistication.

There are a variety of selective serotonin reuptake inhibitors (SSRIs) that are useful for the treatment of premature ejaculation. Dapoxetine was an SSRI medication that was specially developed for premature ejaculation, but the U.S. Food and Drug Administration (FDA) has not yet approved its use. Topical lidocaine is also used for this disorder (see Clinical Alert box #1).

> ❖ **CLINICAL ALERT # 1**
>
> Men taking Viagra, Levitra, or Cialis need to contact their physicians immediately if they experience erections that last longer than 4 hours, painful erections, chest pain, sudden loss of vision, fainting, rash, or urinary problems. Drugs are generally considered safe for erectile dysfunction as long as the patient provides a complete medical and drug history.

Medically Based Evaluation and Intervention Techniques for Women

There is currently much less available in terms of medical testing and physiologic treatments for women. However, researchers are working diligently on this situation. Laboratory tests for estrogen and testosterone levels are valuable. Vaginal plethysmography determines blood flow to the vagina, which is an indicator of arousal; however, this procedure is inconsistent and invasive. Vaginal examinations including nerve conduction studies as well as assessments for genital pain are frequently performed.

There is growing evidence that lowered levels of testosterone lead to hypoactive sexual desire in women and that testosterone replacement improves sexual functioning. However, researchers do not fully understand the relationship between testosterone levels and sexual desire in females (Mathur and Braunstein, 2010). Lowered estrogen levels cause decreased lubrication, vaginal wall thinning, and vaginal pain. Thus, detecting levels of estradiol in the blood and estrogen replacement are sometimes necessary. Localized estrogens are available that do not appear to increase circulating estrogens. Studies in women involving the use of PDE5 inhibitors have not proven to be as successful as those in men (Romanelli and Sanson, 2010). Bupropion is sometimes prescribed to women who report low sexual desire, especially those who are taking SSRI medications; it has been shown to have moderate effect.

In 2001, the FDA cleared the EROS-CTD system for use in treating the symptoms of female sexual dysfunction. This is a device that creates a gentle suction over the clitoris with the goal of bringing increased blood flow to the genitals. The blood flow then puts pressure on the nerves and causes a reaction in the clitoris. An autonomic reflex also results in increased lubrication and an increased ability to achieve orgasm (Berman, 2008).

Anxiolytics have been successful for the treatment of vaginismus. Topical preparations of lidocaine as well as gabapentin are effective for treating genital pain disorders. Currently, a few practitioners are using Botox for the treatment of vulvodynia, which is a chronic genital pain disorder.

There is current research regarding the use of transdermal and gel-based testosterone in doses that are appropriate for women. The Intrinsa testosterone patch was turned down by the FDA several years ago, but it is making a return, and a new review may be forthcoming (Shifren et al, 2008). Recently, flibanserin, which has been dubbed "the little pink pill," came before the FDA advisory council, but its approval was recommended against. This drug is an antagonist to serotonin 2A receptors and an agonist to serotonin 1A and dopamine D4 receptors (Gever, 2010). Research found it to be an effective treatment for increasing sexual interest and satisfaction among women with hypoactive sexual desire disorder. It also appeared to relieve the distress associated with the lack of desire in women (Derogatis and Burnett, 2007).

A compound called *PT-141*, which is a melanocortin and oxytocin agonist that has central nervous system effects, is showing promise for female arousal disorders. It binds to certain sites in the hypothalamus. 5-Dehydroepiandrosterone applied locally has been initially effective in trials for vaginal atrophy, and it may be used to treat various phases of the sexual response system for women (Derogatis and Burnett, 2007).

Psychologically Based Interventions

There are a range of psychologically based techniques that are used by sex therapy practitioners and clinical sexologists. In general, homework assignments and supportive counseling form the basis of sex therapy. Sex therapy often involves weekly, bimonthly, or even monthly visits to the therapist, during which time the patients have the opportunity to discuss symptoms, progress, feelings, and observations. At times, more extensive psychotherapy is necessary, depending on the individual. Treating psychopathologic conditions (e.g., depression) may be a prerequisite to sex therapy.

Masters and Johnson (1970) developed cognitive behavioral techniques for sexual therapy. These techniques have evolved over the years into more effective and comprehensive strategies. Masters and Johnson (1970) developed the sensate focus technique, which involves focusing on body sensations while shutting out other stimuli. Sensate focus is a way of developing relaxation, learning to tune in to the body rather than the thoughts, and creating an atmosphere in which there is no demand for sexual pleasure or sexual release. The idea was that individuals often were so distracted with intellectual thoughts (e.g., "I have so much to do today"), self-deprecating thoughts (e.g., "My thighs are so huge, how can anyone think I'm sexy?"), and performance anxiety (e.g., "I wonder if I'm as good as her previous lover") that they lost touch with the actual experience.

Sensate focus techniques may include giving each other weekly massages, bathing one another, or gently caressing each other's bodies with a feather duster. The partner who is being massaged must only receive the sensations without feeling the need to reciprocate. There is no expectation of arousal or orgasmic response, just a need to enjoy the sensual pleasuring.

To develop better arousal response and better orgasmic capacity, sex therapists may teach their patients masturbatory training exercises. Often, both women and men perform Kegel exercises, which involve tightening the pubococcygeal muscle to bring blood and sensation into the genital region. The patients then begin a set of structured exercises to become familiar with the feelings associated with genital stimulation. Males with erectile dysfunction can also perform masturbatory exercises with the use of erotic focus and erotic stimuli to facilitate arousal and to decrease anxiety. Stop–start and squeeze techniques are helpful for training males with early ejaculation to be more sensitive to their genital sensations and thus delay ejaculation. Both techniques involve the male masturbating to the point of ejaculatory inevitability. With the stop–start technique, the man then simply stops stimulating; with the squeeze technique, he squeezes his penis just below the glans. Either way, he waits until the sensation dissipates and then repeats the process three to four times before allowing himself to ejaculate. The aim is to be better able to control the timing of ejaculation.

The treatment for involuntary contractions of perineal muscles during penetration (vaginismus), involves the use of vaginal dilators. The gradual introduction of larger and larger dilators, in combination with relaxation techniques, will help women to overcome the fear and pain and help to decrease involuntary spasm. Sets of dilators are available online for this purpose, but women have used their fingers or other insertion-type objects as well. A cotton-tipped applicator usually serves as the first dilator, because it is small, soft, and nonthreatening.

Two other techniques that are widely used are specific sexually focused education and cognitive restructuring.

Educational needs vary from specific ways to masturbate to theories about sexual response. Cognitive restructuring involves replacing negative or unpleasant thoughts about sexuality with more positive or realistic thoughts. An example is reframing one's sexual experiences in a more positive and pleasant light. Other helpful suggestions include using erotic materials to help train sexual focus and incorporating sexual thinking and feelings into the daily schedule. Men and women are also able to have masturbation training to help enhance their sensitivity to sexual stimulation. Masturbation training and practice facilitates and improves orgasm or orgasmic potential in both men and women. Masturbation training and the goal of becoming orgasmic also involves the use of cognitive restructuring as a method to replace old beliefs about sexuality and techniques with healthy and realistic beliefs that reduce the fear of losing control (see Chapter 26 for more information about cognitive therapy).

These sex therapy techniques have proven helpful for individuals who develop sexual dysfunctions. However, without sensitivity toward and attention paid to other factors in the patient's life, these methods do not provide satisfactory results. Some of these factors include cultural and religious values, other psychologic disorders, poor sexual learning, and body image issues.

Relationally Based Interventions

It is important but challenging for therapists to place an emphasis on the couple and their relationship, if this is the context of the sexual issue. In other words, is there a true sexual dysfunction, or does the problem really lie within the relationship? If there is a relationship problem, no amount of medically based or psychologically based therapy will be enough to facilitate success. Couple issues include role changes, the introduction of children, difficulty setting aside time for intimacy, loss of passion for the partner, anger toward the partner, a sexual desire discrepancy, or a lack of trust. A core premise of sex therapy is to get the couple sexual again. One technique for this is to ask the couple to schedule sex at a mutually agreed upon time and on a regular basis. Often couples complain that they want spontaneity, but spontaneity has not always worked, and they may have found themselves in a therapist's office because sex dwindled in their relationship. Even with scheduling, spontaneity and playfulness can be built in.

Masters and Johnson (1970) said that poor communication is at the heart of the sexual problem. To improve a couple's communication, there needs to be active listening as well as learning how to ask for what one wants and enjoys. (See Chapter 4 for more information about active listening and other therapeutic skills.) Better communication can begin in the therapist's office, where both members of the couple are encouraged to talk and to listen. These skills can then be taken out into their lives. The most significant predictors of a couple's prognosis for healing their sexual intimacy issues are the respect, regard, and genuine liking that they have for one another (Gottman et al, 2007).

EVALUATION

The final step is determining the effectiveness of interventions. This is an ongoing process, and it is not just facilitated at the end of the involvement with the individual or couple. If the nurse thoroughly and carefully defines outcome criteria, evaluation is a relatively simple process of deciding whether these outcomes were met. The nursing process is cyclic, so if the nurse determines that outcome criteria were not met, then he or she will reexamine the assessment phase or any other phase of the nursing process to determine if some key underlying factors were overlooked.

To illustrate the cyclic nature of the nursing process, consider the following steps. An important nursing diagnosis identified was sexual dysfunction resulting from a lack of knowledge, limited experience, and negative beliefs about sexuality. One of the outcome criteria that the nurse developed with the patient was that the patient would acquire and read female erotica on a daily basis. The rationale was that consciously putting sex into one's life will enhance sexuality and that the practice of reading positive erotic messages will counterbalance some of the previously learned beliefs. However, if the patient does not buy the books or has left them on the table unread, the nurse needs to go back to the assessment phase and determine if something was missed. Was the patient embarrassed and guilt-ridden about the use of erotica? Perhaps the patient's reluctance is the result of some unresolved anger at her partner for leaving her, and she is trying to disrupt her treatment as a way to get back at her partner. If the nurse finds these or additional issues during assessment, the nurse will then revise the care plan to include them. The nursing diagnoses, outcome criteria, and interventions will then change as well. If the nurse did not miss anything during assessment, perhaps the outcome criteria were unrealistic. The issue of the patient's anxiety is often complex and deep, and it may be unrealistic to assume that she will be able to relax and read erotic stories. Evaluation needs to be ongoing as well.

PARAPHILIAS
HISTORY AND THEORY

The paraphilias are a group of behaviors that are commonly accepted to fall under the clinical description of sexual deviations. Paraphilias present inappropriate sexual fantasies that involve deviant sexual acts, inappropriate sexual urges, and the acting out of these fantasies and urges.

After a psychiatric syndrome is described clinically, several steps—including laboratory studies, delimitation from other disorders, follow-up studies, and family studies—are necessary to establish diagnostic validity. It is generally acknowledged that no psychiatric syndrome has yet to be fully validated by the complete series of these steps. However, many syndromes have had a substantial body of data published during most phases of their validation. However, little is known about the data in the other areas that

◎ NURSING CARE PLAN

Michelle, a 42-year-old woman, mentions to the nurse during a routine history and examination that she has some sexual issues to discuss. She tells the nurse that her partner of 5 years recently broke off the relationship because of these sexual problems. Michelle says that she is in generally good health. She was diagnosed with depression 3 years ago, and she has been taking 20 mg of paroxetine (Paxil) daily. She is on no other medications except for a daily vitamin pill. She tells the nurse that, when she and her partner were first dating, sex seemed good in the relationship. They were affectionate to each other and had sex approximately two to three times per week. Shortly after they began living together 4 years ago, sex dropped off to monthly and then became nonexistent. She says her partner tried to initiate sex but gave up after she continually refused him. Eventually the intimacy and closeness wore away, and they fought more often. Without much discussion, her partner announced that their relationship was over and promptly moved out. Michelle said she was devastated at first but now believes that this was a wakeup call to do something about her sexual problems.

Michelle explained that she was born in Russia to a conservative Jewish family and that sexuality was never discussed. She had no formal sex education, but she recalls being interested in sex and reading books for information. She does not recall any early childhood sexual experiences, and she says that she has never masturbated. She did not date in high school, partly because of the strictness of her family. During college, she had a brief relationship with a man that she considered marrying. However, there was little attraction, and she decided to leave Russia to live in the United States. Since arriving in this country, she has had several other relationships, none of which was longer than 3 years.

According to the patient, she experiences little sexual interest. She reports that she has never put much focus on sex but that, during the past 4 years, it has become even less important to her. She says that she is concerned about this and would like to be "more normal" when it comes to sex. She says she is slow to become aroused, and sometimes she and her partner would give up after getting frustrated by her response. She rarely has orgasms. She believes that she has always had these problems to some degree but that they have gotten worse. Now that she is out of the relationship, she is not sure what to do about her sexuality, but believes that in future relationships it will again be a factor. She reports being very stressed about this, and she says that she has been avoiding social commitments out of the fear that she will meet someone.

Toward the end of the interview, Michelle shyly and reluctantly reveals that she finds sex somewhat "dirty." She also states that she in fact identifies as a lesbian and that she has had sexual relationships only with women since she was in college (and that the previously mentioned partner was actually a woman). She says that her family still lives in Russia and is unaware of her sexual orientation.

DSM-IV-TR Diagnoses

Axis I   Hypoactive sexual desire disorder
Major depression
Axis II   None noted
Axis III   None known
Axis IV   Moderate = 3 (primary relationships, socialization, anxiety)
Axis V   GAF = 55 (current); GAF = 65 (past year)

Nursing Diagnosis *Sexual dysfunction related to deficient knowledge, beliefs about sexuality, and side effects of medication as evidenced by patient's reported lack of sexual interest and arousal and questions about the source of sexual problems*

NOC Sexual functioning; Sexual identity; Role performance
NIC Teaching: sexuality; Sexual counseling; Self-awareness enhancement; Role enhancement

PATIENT OUTCOMES	NURSING INTERVENTIONS	EVALUATION
Michelle will complete one factual book about sexuality by the next session with the nurse.	Suggest that Michelle read *Real Sex for Real Women* by Laura Berman by the next session. *This will help to educate the patient about human sexuality to overcome some of her deficits.* Schedule a follow-up appointment *to ensure continuity.*	Michelle reports that she had read the book and was able to discuss what she had read.
Michelle will read women's erotica on a daily basis.	Suggest that Michelle read books of female erotica for a short time every day. *This will help to enhance her awareness of sexuality and to overcome some of the previously learned messages.*	Michelle did not buy a book on female erotica until 2 days before her appointment. She has read sexual stories since then.
By the next session with the nurse, Michelle will make an appointment with her psychiatrist to discuss her medication.	Instruct Michelle to discuss the potentially negative sexual side effects of paroxetine (Paxil). *The nurse is aware that SSRIs diminish sexual interest and affect arousal.*	Michelle reports that, after discussing the medication side effects, she and her physician decided to do a trial of bupropion (Wellbutrin) for depression.

NURSING CARE PLAN—cont'd		
PATIENT OUTCOMES	**NURSING INTERVENTIONS**	**EVALUATION**
Michelle will agree to enter sex therapy with a qualified therapist by the next session.	Encourage Michelle to receive treatment for her sexual issues. *Sex therapy is helpful for patients who want to overcome sexual difficulty and anxiety.* Educate Michelle about techniques of sexual therapy. *She will be better informed to make appropriate choices for herself.* Refer Michelle to a qualified sex therapist *for continued professional help.*	Michelle reports that she has an appointment with a sex therapist in 2 weeks.

GAF, Global Assessment of Functioning; NIC, Nursing Interventions Classification; NOC, Nursing Outcomes Classification.

establish clinical validity. For example, although there are some laboratory tests and follow-up studies of sexual deviance, there are few family studies of paraphilias.

The following question remains prominent when managing this complex and challenging group of patients: are all patients who are engaging in sexually inappropriate behaviors considered to have paraphilic disorders, or are they just bad people who act out in an inappropriate sexual manner? This chapter will present detailed concepts that will enable the reader to formulate a differential diagnosis after performing a comprehensive psychiatric assessment and psychosexual history.

LEGAL IMPLICATIONS

Forensic Psychiatry and Paraphilias

Forensic psychiatry is the application of psychiatry for legal purposes. This highly specialized area of psychiatry addresses issues related to criminal responsibility and competency to stand trial for various crimes that have been committed. Formulating a forensic opinion about the paraphilias is difficult at best. A person who has committed a sexual crime in response to psychotic processes, such as hallucinations or delusions, may be considered to not be criminally responsible (insanity plea); however, this individual may not be diagnosed with a paraphilic disorder. A person who commits a sexual crime in response to "recurrent, intense, sexually arousing fantasies, sexual urges or behaviors involving (1) nonhuman objects, (2) the suffering or humiliation of oneself or one's partner, or (3) children or other nonconsenting persons" (American Psychiatric Association, 2000) may meet the criteria of a paraphilic disorder. Such a disorder may or may not include forensic issues, as previously stated. An important aspect to explore during a forensic evaluation is the patient's ability to appreciate the criminality of the behavior (sexual crime) and the ability to conform the behavior to the requirements of the law, which is not intended to address the patient's ability to control himself or herself. This is a part of the forensic opinion, and, depending on the results of this assessment, the outcome may be a prison sentence or a sentencing to a maximum security forensic psychiatric facility until such time that the patient is assessed as no longer being a danger to society.

The Sexually Violent Predator Act

In 1990, the state of Washington's legislature enacted a bill known as the *Community Protection Act*, which provided for the civil commitment of sexually violent predators (SVPs). After a term of incarceration, an SVP may be civilly committed against his or her will to a state psychiatric facility until such time that he or she is deemed to be safe to return to the community. This was the foundation and model legislation for the development of similar laws referred to as the *Sexually Violent Predator Act*, which has been passed into legislation in 20 states, the District of Columbia, and within the federal government.

The law in Texas provides for outpatient commitment only, whereas the other states provide for inpatient commitment. Pennsylvania has a law that is just for juveniles coming from the juvenile justice system and not from the prison system. The realization of the costs of such programs may have influenced the rest of the states as far as deciding to even approach the possibility of SVP commitment laws. Although there should never be a price tag placed on promoting societal safety, the costs of SVP programs range from $40,000 (in Massachusetts) to $237,000 (in the District of Columbia) for each resident per year. California has built a 1500-bed facility just for SVPs (Fitch, 2007).

The aforementioned law established a civil commitment procedure for "any person who has been convicted or charged with a sexually violent offense and who suffers from a mental abnormality or personality disorder which makes the person likely to engage in the predatory acts of sexual violence" (Wash. Rev. Code Ann. §71.09.030, 1991). Washington state law defines a predatory act as "… an act directed toward a stranger or an individual with whom a relationship has been established or promoted for the primary purpose of victimization" (Wash. Rev. Code Ann. §71.09.030, 1991). Therefore, it is conceivable that most sexually violent predators are either pedophiles or rapists.

In 2006, a federal law for the civil commitment of "sexually dangerous persons" was enacted as part of the Adam Walsh Child Protection and Safety Act. This applied to those offenders who had completed their sentence in the federal system but who were not yet ready to be released into the community. The problem here is that there are no federal commitment facilities; hence, these offenders are committed to the custody of the United States Attorney General, who then tries to convince state officials to civilly commit these patients to one of their state facilities (Fitch, 2007).

THE ROLE OF TECHNOLOGY AND THE TREND OF "SEXTING": LEGAL IMPLICATIONS

Continuing advances in technology have made it very easy for consumers to access and transmit any kind of information via the Internet and cell phones. Currently there is a trend that is practiced primarily by young teens called sexting. Sexting occurs when someone transmits sexually explicit photos of themselves or others, other sexual images, or sexually graphic text messages via a cell phone or the Internet (Kazdin et al, 2009).

In 2008, the National Campaign to Prevent Teen and Unplanned Pregnancy and CosmoGirl.com conducted a survey of 1280 teens between the ages of 13 and 19 years. The purpose was to attempt to identify the magnitude of this potentially dangerous trend among young adolescents. It was reported 66% sent "sex messages" and that 49% sent "sexy pictures" of themselves. The survey results indicated the possibility that this behavior is more prevalent among the female population, because, as young teens, girls may want to elicit a boy's attention or be noticed more in a different light (National Campaign to Prevent Teen and Unplanned Pregnancy, 2008).

There are many negative outcomes of sexting, including potentially becoming a serious criminal offender. Nurses need to be aware that this trend does indeed exist, and they must educate adolescents and their families about the ramifications of such behavior. In addition, it would be prudent for the nurse to be aware of state laws and to educate adolescents about them.

The reader should not lose sight of the fact that it is illegal to possess and distribute sexually explicit photos, objects, and text messages that involve a minor to anyone. The literature reveals that there are several cases in which adolescents have actually received prison sentences for sending or receiving sexy photos of their 15-year-old girlfriends and then "accidentally" sending the photos to others. This may well result in a child pornography conviction, and now these teenagers will have to register themselves as sex offenders within their states (Levine, 2009).

As of February 2009, Levine identified 10 states in which minors have been arrested for sexting. The sadness of this all is the criminalization of children who are not child predators but rather who engaged in sexting (Lithwick, 2009). Teens need to know how serious this is. They should be reminded and cautioned that, after they hit "Send," the message is gone, and the damage is potentially done.

ETIOLOGY

It is unclear what may predispose an individual to develop a paraphilic disorder. Several studies have attempted to suggest causative factors and to determine the prevalence of sexual

---

BOX 20-3   ETIOLOGIC FACTORS FOR PARAPHILIAS

Biologic Factors
Chromosomal functioning
Hormonal levels

Experiential Factors
History of sexual abuse

Environmental Factors
Use of pornography during childhood and adolescence

Hereditary Predisposition

---

deviancies (see the Research for Evidence-Based Practice box #2). Research has not been able to determine the cause-and-effect etiology of the paraphilias.

Biologic Factors

It is important to acknowledge that people do not voluntarily decide what types of sexual arousal patterns that they will have. Researchers have suggested possible etiologies (Box 20-3). In the biologic domain, two areas are addressed: chromosomal functioning and hormonal levels.

In 1942, Klinefelter and colleagues described Klinefelter's syndrome as a condition that is characterized by (1) the development of gynecomastia (enlarged breasts) at the time of puberty; (2) aspermatogenesis (low sperm production); and (3) an increased secretion of follicle-stimulating hormone by the pituitary gland in the brain.

With this particular syndrome, the patient presents with 47 chromosomes instead of the normal 46; an extra X chromosome is present. The patient may be thought of as a male (XY) with an extra X chromosome or as a female (XX) with an extra Y chromosome. Patients with this syndrome look like males at birth. Hence, parents naturally raise them as males and assign them male sex roles. However, Money and colleagues (1957) described an otherwise normal 8-year-old boy with Klinefelter's syndrome who insisted that he felt more comfortable dressed in girl's clothing. Patients with Klinefelter's syndrome have very small testes, and they produce little testosterone and virtually no sperm. They also experience problems with sexual orientation and with the nature of their erotic desires.

Some theorists suggest that biologic factors may be etiologic considerations for the development of sexual disorders and that early life experiences may contribute to the development of paraphilic disorders.

Federhoff and colleagues (1994) reported the identification of patients with genetically based neuropsychiatric disorders who present with sexually deviant behaviors. Thirty-nine patients with Huntington's disease presented with paraphilias and hypoactive sexual disorders. Similarly, patients with Tourette's syndrome may have higher rates of paraphilic-like behaviors.

RESEARCH FOR EVIDENCE-BASED PRACTICE #2

Beauregard E et al: An exploration of developmental factors related to deviant sexual preferences among adult rapists, *Sex Abuse* 16:151-161, 2004.

The purpose of this study was to explore possible etiologic factors that contribute to the development of deviant sexual desires and behaviors. Researchers obtained information about the developmental factors of 118 sexually aggressive patients via the Computerized Questionnaire for Sexual Aggressors (Proulx et al, 1994). Researchers determined sexual preferences via penile plethysmography. The exploration of the relationship between developmental factors and deviant sexual arousal was performed with the use of multiple regression analyses.

The authors identified three developmental factors that related to deviant sexual preferences: (1) a sexually inappropriate family environment; (2) the use of pornography during childhood and adolescence; and (3) deviant sexual fantasies during childhood and adolescence. These results suggest that developmental factors play a part in the etiology of deviant sexual preferences. However, nurses need to be aware that these results are not all inclusive; other biologic factors play a role as well.

The authors have identified that a limitation to their study was the use of a small sample size, and they suggest that further studies are necessary in this area. Future studies also need to address other etiologic factors that contribute to the development of sexual deviance.

Hereditary/Environmental Factors

Gaffney and colleagues (1984) found evidence that suggests the familial transmission of paraphilic disorders. Groth (1979) identified children who were sexually active with adults during childhood as being environmentally influenced and therefore potentially predisposed to the development of a pedophilic disorder. This is an example of victim turned victimizer or, in this case, sex offender.

CULTURAL VIEWS OF UNTOWARD SEXUAL PRACTICES

A review of the literature revealed that some untoward sexual practices may be driven by cultural and religious beliefs or the customs of a specific country and not necessarily driven by the desire for sexual arousal. It is important for the nurse to elicit and include patient information about religious and cultural or customary beliefs during the initial evaluation before formulating a diagnosis.

Female genital mutilation (female circumcision) still occurs in 28 African countries; it is predicated upon religious and customary beliefs (Maurice, 2006) and not of a paraphilic nature. In other words, this act may be thought of as an example of sexual sadism, but this is not the case. There is no evidence that sexual arousal occurs with this religious and customary practice (Bhugra, 2008).

The same is true for countries such as Cambodia, where sex slavery and prostitution are prevalent among children and young adolescents. In Cambodia, daughters are thought of as items up for sale for the sake of the family. Because this belief exists, it is not uncommon for a mother to sell her 7-year-old daughter to a pimp for the money (Pesta, 2009). Another cultural belief that plays into this "accepted" practice is that many local men reportedly believe in the myth that having sex with a virgin will bring about good luck and good health. However, these men may be true pedophiles who want to play out their violent sexual fantasies with child sex slaves. There is no way to validate either scenario at this time (Pesta, 2009). The reader needs to keep in mind that, although prostitution and human trafficking are illegal in Cambodia, it has been reported that it is customary for officials to be paid to ignore the illegalities and to allow these practices to continue (Pesta, 2009).

EPIDEMIOLOGY

According to the DSM-IV-TR, although paraphilias are not generally diagnosed in clinical facilities, the sizeable commercial market of paraphilic pornography and paraphernalia suggests that its prevalence in the community is "likely to be higher" (American Psychiatric Association, 2000). The paraphilias that most commonly present problems are pedophilia, voyeurism, and exhibitionism. About half of patients with paraphilias who are seen clinically are married (American Psychiatric Association, 2000).

Some clinicians have addressed the presence of comorbidities (co-occurrences) in a certain percentage of the paraphilic population (Kafka and Hennen, 2002). Some of these patients may also be suffering from mental illnesses that may have gone unrecognized. Examples of co-occurring illnesses may include mood disorders, anxiety disorders, substance use disorders, and personality disorders. The presence of a co-occurring illness that goes unnoticed may have an effect on the patient's course of treatment and his or her prognosis (Seligman and Hardenburg, 2000).

It would behoove the reader to be cognizant of neuropsychiatric disorders and mental states that have been associated with hypersexual behaviors, such as frontal lobe damage and sexual deviancy. Other diagnoses to be considered are psychotic disorders, affective disorders, and cognitive disorders.

CLINICAL DESCRIPTION

The essential diagnostic features of a paraphilia are "recurrent, intense sexually arousing fantasies, sexual urges, or behaviors generally involving (1) nonhuman objects, (2) the suffering or humiliation of oneself or one's partner, or (3) children or other nonconsenting persons that occur over a period of at least 6 months" (American Psychiatric Association, 2000). Another criterion is that "the behavior, sexual urges, or fantasies cause clinically significant distress in social, occupational, or other important areas of functioning"

DSM-IV-TR CRITERIA #2
Paraphilias

Exhibitionism
The exposure of one's genitals to an unsuspecting person(s) followed by sexual arousal

Fetishism
Use of objects (e.g., panties, rubber sheeting) for the purpose of becoming sexually aroused

Frotteurism
Rubbing up against a nonconsenting person to heighten sexual arousal

Pedophilia
Fondling or other types of sexual activities with a prepubescent child (usually under age 13 years who has not yet developed secondary sex characteristics). Heterosexual pedophiles are sexually attracted to female children under age 13 years. Homosexual pedophiles are sexually attracted to male children under age 13 years. **Ego syntonic pedophiles** do not view this type of behavior as troublesome and will not voluntarily seek treatment for it. **Ego dystonic pedophiles** are concerned and troubled with this type of behavior and sometimes voluntarily seek treatment to deal with it. There are several types of pedophiles:
Homosexual
Heterosexual
Bisexual (sexual attraction to both males and females)
Limited to incest (sexual attraction to a child in one's immediate family)
Exclusive type (sexually attracted to children only)
Nonexclusive type (may also be sexually attracted to adults of either sex)

Sexual Masochism
Being the receiver of pain (either physical or emotional), humiliation, or suffering for the purpose of becoming sexually aroused

Sexual Sadism
The infliction of pain (either physical or emotional) or humiliation onto another person followed by sexual arousal

Transvestic Fetishism
The act of cross-dressing (heterosexual males wearing female clothing) for the purpose of becoming sexually aroused

Voyeurism
Observing unsuspecting persons who are naked, in the act of disrobing, or engaging in sexual activity ("peeping Tom") followed by sexual arousal

Paraphilia Not Otherwise Specified
Disorders that do not meet the criteria for the aforementioned categories:
Telephone scatologia: Obscene phone calling; "900" sex lines
Necrophilia: Sexual activity with corpses
Partialism: Exclusive focus on a particular body part for sexual arousal
Zoophilia: Sexual activity involving participation with animals (bestiality)
Coprophilia: Sexual arousal by contact with feces
Klismaphilia: Sexual arousal generated by use of enemas
Urophilia: Sexual arousal by contact with urine
Ephebophilia*: Fondling or other types of sexual activities with postpubescent children (usually between the ages of 13 to 18 years) who are developing secondary sex characteristics (e.g., pubic hair, breasts)
Paraphilic coercive disorder*: Rape; aggressive sexual assault involving an act of sexual intercourse against one's will and without consent

*Not included in the DSM-IV-TR.
Data from the American Psychiatric Association: *Diagnostic and statistical manual of mental disorders,* ed 4, text revision, Washington, DC, 2000, American Psychiatric Association.

(American Psychiatric Association, 2000). DSM-IV-TR Criteria box #2 summarizes the criteria and description of the paraphilias.

In 1994, Kafka introduced the term *paraphilia-related disorders* (PRDs). These consist of a group of sexual syndromes that are characterized by hypersexual but culturally sanctioned behaviors. Kafka (2007) defines PRDs as "recurrent, intense sexually arousing fantasies, urges or behaviors involving essentially normative aspects of sexual expression that cause distress or significant psychosocial impairment." Some examples of PRDs as listed by Kafka (2007) are compulsive masturbation, telephone and cyber sex, pornography dependence, and PRD not otherwise specified.

PROGNOSIS

Nurses should be cautioned when attempting to predict sexual recidivism, which is the chronic and repetitive inappropriate acting out of sexual behaviors that are considered to be unacceptable that have or have not resulted in criminal conviction. Patients who are currently undergoing treatment for a sexual disorder may have a lower level of sexual recidivism (Berlin et al, 1991). A study by Berlin and colleagues (1991) revealed a higher reoffense rate for those patients who do not receive (or who have never received) treatment as compared with those engaged in treatment. Treatment compliance is a therapeutic issue that nurses who are treating this population must address (see the Case Study #2).

One could surmise that, with continued treatment compliance and strict patient monitoring, these patients may present as a lesser risk to society. It is important for nurses to also acknowledge that treatment efficacy cannot be proven at this time. Further studies are warranted in this area.

DISCHARGE CRITERIA

The patient will do the following:

- State the nature of his or her specific paraphilic disorder and its impact on the self and others (e.g., if a breakdown occurs, if cognitive distortions are present).
- Identify his or her personal **triggers** (i.e., stimuli that heighten unacceptable sexual cravings and that provoke inappropriate sexual behaviors).
- Develop appropriate relapse prevention strategies.
- Communicate and problem solve effectively.
- Practice appropriate coping strategies.
- Identify support systems.

THE NURSING PROCESS
ASSESSMENT

The patient with a sexual disorder may exhibit a variety of behavioral symptoms, depending on the nature of the disorder. Some symptoms are more difficult to assess than others. The patient with a pedophilic disorder may exhibit perceptual disturbances. It is not uncommon to hear such a patient state, for example, that a child "looked older than he was." This may also be perceived as a cognitive distortion.

Cognitive distortions may be present in the patient with a sexual disorder. The two cognitive distortions that are most often present in this patient population are denial and rationalization. Denial is a defense mechanism that is used to avoid dealing with problems and responsibilities related to one's behaviors; rationalization is a defense mechanism that is used to justify upsetting behaviors by creating reasons that would allow the individual to believe that the behaviors were warranted or appropriate. These are the most critical issues that the nurse must address early during the therapeutic process. It is a good indication that such cognitive distortions are present when a patient makes a statement such as, "Well, the child didn't fight me and agreed to have sex with me."

Another symptom that requires assessment is a disturbance in feeling. Patients with paraphilic disorders commonly lack remorse for their actions. If they do experience remorse, they may be unable to acknowledge it because of cognitive distortions. Occasionally, patients with a pedophilic disorder may claim to experience feelings of "being loved" by the child with whom they have had inappropriate sexual activity.

Patients with paraphilic disorders should also be assessed for the presence of behavioral and relating disturbances. These are assessed by the patient's inability to develop age-appropriate relationships, his or her altered relationships with others, and social withdrawal that may occur as a result of embarrassment or media attention (see the Nursing Assessment Questions box).

NURSING DIAGNOSIS

After collecting patient assessment data, the nurse is ready to begin formulating diagnoses. In doing so, the nurse may find that the patient has symptoms that are indicative of more than one diagnosis, such as a paraphilic disorder, a psychoactive substance disorder, and a personality disorder. Multiple diagnoses are not addressed in this chapter. However, it is important for the nurse to be aware of this possibility.

When addressing nursing diagnoses for the patient with a paraphilic disorder, the nurse has many diagnoses from which to choose and selects those that are specific and appropriate to each individual on the basis of the analysis of comprehensive data collected during the assessment.

Nursing Diagnoses for Paraphilias

- Risk for other-directed violence
- Ineffective coping
- Ineffective denial
- Interrupted family processes
- Deficient knowledge (of the illness and aspects of treatment)
- Noncompliance (with the therapeutic regimen)
- Ineffective sexuality patterns
- Impaired social interaction

OUTCOME IDENTIFICATION

Patient-centered outcomes should relate to the patient's nursing diagnoses and be the opposite of the defining characteristics. Outcomes should be stated in clear, measurable, and behavioral terms and include a time frame, when feasible, during which the patient is expected to achieve them. Outcomes may be described as expected or anticipated, and they are viewed as specific goals to be achieved through the implementation of the plan of care. Examples of behavioral terms that the nurse may want to use when developing patient-centered outcomes include such things as "The patient will state/list/perform/participate in the following."

The patient will do the following:
- State two sexually inappropriate behaviors within 3 days of admission.
- Write a list of triggers that provoke inappropriate sexual acting out within 1 week of admission.
- Describe two appropriate coping strategies within 1 week of admission.
- List several relapse-prevention strategies that are appropriate to his or her disorder within the second week of admission.
- Actively participate in weekly group psychotherapy sessions for patients with sexual disorders.
- Verbalize two appropriate methods for meeting his or her sexual needs by the time of discharge.
- Explain the importance of medication compliance and follow-up care with outpatient group psychotherapy by the time of discharge.

PLANNING

After diagnoses have been established and patient problem identification has occurred, the nurse is ready to begin developing a plan of care that is specific to the individual patient. Patient care should be based on mutually agreed upon, realistic, patient-centered outcomes. The nurse should involve the patient in the development of an individualized plan of care, with the expectation that the patient will participate in the planning process.

In the population of patients with paraphilic disorders, it is not uncommon to find cognitive distortions. Nurses must be aware of this possibility as they obtain patient input into the development of the plan of care. For example, a patient who is in denial of a paraphilic disorder may not be able to fully cooperate with the planning of care or to view patient-centered outcomes as realistic.

IMPLEMENTATION

The nurse should work with the patient to develop an individualized plan of care that will help the patient to identify the presence of cognitive distortions (if appropriate), to prevent reoffending by identifying triggers that provoke inappropriate sexual activity, and to develop effective relapse-prevention strategies (see the Patient and Family Teaching Guidelines box #2). The nurse should also explain the significance of treatment on recidivism and stress the importance of medication compliance and follow-up care with outpatient group psychotherapy.

PATIENT AND FAMILY TEACHING GUIDELINES #2

Relapse-Prevention Strategies for Paraphilias

- Teach the patient and his or her significant others how to identify triggers that provoke inappropriate sexual thoughts and desires by listing the precursors to inappropriate sexual acting out (e.g., the patient with a pedophilic disorder who claims that he must drive by the schoolyard at 3 PM to get home [if the schoolyard is a level 5 trigger for this person]).
- Be sure that the patient understands that relapse-prevention strategies are based on the identification of triggers. Identifying triggers helps the patient to avoid reoffending behaviors.

Providing nursing care to such a patient may be difficult because of the sensitive nature of these disorders. Nurses must recognize this possibility and be aware of their own comfort level when discussing sexual issues with these patients. Identifying the presence of a paraphilic disorder may have devastating effects on patients and their significant others. It is important for nurses to include significant others in the interventions to the extent that they can participate.

Nursing Interventions

1. Help the patient to confront cognitive distortions through direct questioning methods that promote reality orientation regarding the patient's offending behavior. Open confrontation by the nurse may be needed, including an explanation of the impact of these distortions on treatment outcomes. Journaling may assist with the breakdown of cognitive distortions and help the patient to track inappropriate sexual fantasies. Patient must be aware of the presence of a problem and willing to acknowledge its existence to potentiate treatment success.

2. Educate the patient and significant others about paraphilic disorders and aspects of treatment, such as identifying triggers that provoke inappropriate sexual activity and methods that help the patient to avoid relapse. Encourage active participation in the educational process by compiling lists in a journal for review by the patient and the nurse. Copies of these lists should be placed in the patient's medical record to inform other team members about the patient's progress. This knowledge helps to provide a foundation for treatment.

3. Enhance the patient's compliance with treatment by openly discussing with him or her the effect that inappropriate sexual behaviors on others. Provide research studies regarding the effects of treatment on recidivism rates and handouts about the scope of treatment and how compliance can assist the patient with regaining control of his or her sexual behaviors. Compliance with treatment may reduce the risk of relapse.

4. Teach the patient appropriate coping strategies, assertiveness skills, and problem-solving techniques to promote relapse prevention.

5. Promote the patient's development of appropriate social skills, and provide support and encouragement to the patient for his or her efforts to control of the disorder. Peer-to-peer mentorship may be appropriate to enhance appropriate social skills and feelings of acceptance. The patient may feel guilty about his or her behavior and become socially isolated. The support and encouragement of the patient will signify that there are healthy, functional, and acceptable aspects of his or her personality. (Guay, 2009).

Additional Treatment Modalities

After careful assessment to determine the specific diagnosis of paraphilic disorder, a range of treatment modalities can be instituted (see the Additional Treatment Modalities box).

Pharmacologic

The need for medications is based on the collaborative efforts of the multidisciplinary team to assess the intensity and impulsivity of the patient's disorder and symptoms.

Antiandrogenic Medications

Depo-Provera (Medroxyprogesterone Acetate). A 500-mg dose of Depo-Provera given intramuscularly once a week has been prescribed with some success for patients with paraphilic disorders (Berlin and Meineke, 1981). This form

---

> ### ADDITIONAL TREATMENT MODALITIES
> #### *Paraphilias*
>
> - Antiandrogenic medications
> - Depo-Provera
> - Lupron Depot
> - SSRIs
> - Individual and group psychotherapy and psychoeducation
> - Insight-oriented therapy
> - Goal-directed therapy
> - Occupational and recreational therapy
> - Family therapy and couples counseling

of external control helps patients to develop their own internal controls to avoid relapse. Patients have reported that this medication lowers the frequency and intensity of inappropriate sexual thoughts and fantasies.

The nurse needs to be aware of several side effects of this drug. Because this type of medication decreases testosterone levels and sperm production, the patient who is receiving Depo-Provera may not be able to father a child. Common side effects include weight gain, increased blood pressure, and fatigue. The nurse may suggest a dietary consultation to help the patient to maintain a healthy weight and to decrease the possibility of weight gain. Blood pressure readings must be taken before each dose. In general, if the diastolic blood pressure is 100 mm Hg or greater, then the medication should be withheld. The nurse must communicate with the physician about blood pressure readings and whether or not to administer the medication.

The medication is viscous, and it should be given in doses of no more than 500 mg per muscle. The gluteal muscle may also be used for the administration of Depo-Provera. It is not necessary to administer this medication via Z-track, because there is no conclusive evidence that this method of injection increases absorption. Patients may complain of pain at the injection site, and they need to be reassured that the pain will subside within a day. If the drug is given in the deltoid muscle, the nurse may want to instruct the patient to engage in range-of-motion exercises (e.g., moving the shoulder and arm in a circular motion).

Depo-Provera should not be administered without informed consent and the patient's signature on a consent form that explains about the medication and its therapeutic and nontherapeutic effects. The nurse may review this form with the patient after a decision has been made by the physician to include this as part of the patient's individualized plan of care.

Lupron Depot (Leuprolide). Leuprolide may be a more powerful antiandrogenic drug. It acts similarly to Depo-Provera by lowering testosterone levels in the patient with a paraphilic disorder. This medication is usually prescribed as 7.5 mg given intramuscularly once a month; it is also available a dose of 1 mg per day given subcutaneously.

Side effects include a decrease in libido (the desired result), bone pain, osteoporotic changes, gynecomastia, hair growth, weight gain, high blood pressure, dizziness, headaches, mood swings, and phlebitis. The nurse must have the knowledge to assess for the presence of nontherapeutic effects.

At the outset of treatment with Lupron Depot, patients should be prescribed 250 mg of flutamide (Eulexin) given by mouth three times a day to enhance the testosterone-suppressing aspects of Lupron Depot by blocking testosterone receptors. This should be prescribed because of the increase in testosterone production that occurs within the first 2 to 4 weeks after having started treatment with Lupron Depot.

Again, it is important for the nurse to monitor the patient's blood pressure before administering Lupron Depot. The same criteria should apply for Depo-Provera. (see Clinical Alert box #2).

> ### ❖ CLINICAL ALERT #2
>
> Patients who are receiving Depo-Provera or Lupron Depot should also be monitored for bone mass density, because these powerful antiandrogenic medications may precipitate osteoporotic changes. Patients may also be prescribed bisphosphonate medications (e.g., Fosamax) to address this potentially dangerous side effect.

Selective Serotonin Reuptake Inhibitors. Current literature contains several case reports regarding the treatment of paraphilic disorders with SSRIs such as Prozac and Zoloft. These medications have fewer side effects than the antiandrogenic medications. Single case reports address the efficacy of paraphilic treatment with SSRIs by increasing serotonin activity, thereby decreasing sexual appetite. It is important to note that further research is warranted because of the absence of double-blind chart studies in this area (Kafka, 1997).

Antiepileptic or Anticonvulsant Medications. A review of the literature reflects a few documented case studies in which a relatively new pharmacologic approach to paraphilic treatment has been identified. These agents (e.g., Topiramate) have been used as treatment options for patients with compulsive and impulsive sexual behaviors (Greenfield, 2006). Some of these behaviors may be seen in the compulsive masturbator or the hypersexual patient; however, this is not to confuse the reader into believing that compulsive masturbation and hypersexuality are paraphilic disorders. Further studies are warranted in the area of paraphilic treatment with anticonvulsant medications. (see Medication Key Facts box).

Psychotherapy and Psychoeducation Groups

Nurses may lead or co-lead psychotherapy and psychoeducation groups with the physician or with another member of the treatment team if he or she has the appropriate group psychotherapy credentials.

The purposes of group psychotherapy and psychoeducation are to address cognitive distortions and to provide education to this patient population regarding the identification of triggers, relapse-prevention strategies, the importance of treatment compliance, self-esteem issues, appropriate coping strategies, and problem-solving skills.

> ### 💊 MEDICATION KEY FACTS
> #### *Sex-Drive Depressants*
>
> Sex-drive depressants are indicated for the reduction of sexual arousal and libido and for inappropriate or disruptive sexual behavior in patients with dementia.
>
> **Progestogens**
> Medroxyprogesterone (Depo-Provera)
> * This drug decreases sperm count and produces hot flashes, sweating, impotence, and insomnia.
> * Smoking while taking this drug may increase the risk for deep vein thrombosis.
>
> **Luteinizing Hormone–Releasing Hormone Agonist**
> Leuprolide (Lupron Depot) and goserelin (Zoladex Implant)
> * Leuprolide decreases sperm count and produces hot flashes, anxiety, and insomnia.
> * A serious side effect is a decrease in bone density with long-term use.
> * Severe allergic reactions include rash, pruritus, urticaria, itching, flushing, and purpuric skin lesions.
>
> **Antiandrogen and Progestogen**
> Cyproterone (Androcur)
> * This drug causes the atrophy of the seminiferous tubules and gynecomastia with chronic use.
> * Dietary considerations: The use of this drug may impair carbohydrate metabolism and fasting blood glucose levels. Hypercalcemia and changes in plasma lipids can also occur.

Recreational and occupational therapy may also be provided to assist the patient with time structuring, which may be viewed as a relapse-prevention strategy (see Chapter 26 for more information).

Family and couples therapy may also be recommended, depending on the individual patient care needs. This form of therapy is usually provided by the social worker, but it may also be provided by a masters-prepared nurse or a physician.

EVALUATION

Nurses must continually evaluate the effectiveness of their interventions on patient behavior to successfully treat this population. If identified nursing interventions are not helping the patient to achieve his or her outcomes, revisions must be made to the nursing care plan. The nurse may want to discuss the plan with the patient and obtain his or her assistance when revising it. The areas in which patient outcomes have been successfully achieved should be identified as resolved. If newly identified problems arise, these should also be addressed in the patient's plan of care.

When treating the patient with a paraphilic disorder, it is not unrealistic to expect the patient to acknowledge the presence of the paraphilic disorder, to identify triggers, to develop relapse-prevention strategies, and to state the importance of treatment compliance after discharge. If these outcomes are not met by the time of discharge, the patient would be at a greater risk for reoffending. The need to protect both the patient and society from possible relapse or recidivism is critical (see Clinical Alert box #3).

❖ CLINICAL ALERT #3

The nurse should be alert for signs of noncompliance with treatment or signs that are indicative of potential relapse as evidenced by such things as the patient's refusal to take medications or to attend therapy sessions. Patient statements such as "I don't know why I need this; I'm just here because the courts sent me"; social withdrawal; the presence of cognitive distortions; and a lack of candidness may all be viewed as risk factors for noncompliance.

The minimal expected period for outpatient treatment is 2 years, although the actual length of treatment may be considerably longer, and it is sometimes geared to align with the length of the patient's probationary sentence. These patients need to be carefully monitored for any changes in their status that could lead to relapse. Monitoring may occur through weekly outpatient group therapy or, if group treatment is not indicated, by periodic visits with the patient's therapist.

A patient is formally discharged from outpatient treatment on the basis of his or her level of progress and his or her current status regarding the paraphilic behaviors. One should not be confused into thinking that because a patient has been discharged from paraphilic treatment that this means the patient is now "cured." There is no proven cure for the paraphilic patient at this time.

After a patient has committed a sexual crime and been diagnosed with a paraphilic disorder, he or she will forever be considered a sexual offender and must register with his or her state's sex offender registry. The term *chronic sex offender* is a misnomer. These patients are similar to those patients with a chronic condition like diabetes who are asymptomatic and whose disease is controlled with diet and exercise; these patients are and will always be diabetic, but hopefully their condition will remain well controlled.

◎ NURSING CARE PLAN #2

Martin is a 50-year-old vice president of a major corporation who has been diagnosed with voyeurism. He occasionally acted out by engaging in voyeuristic activities at his country club in the ladies' locker room, where he would secretly masturbate while "peeping." Martin's wife is currently unaware of his behavior, but she suspects that something is wrong. When she confronted Martin about her suspicions, he denied the existence of any problems.

Martin voluntarily agreed to treatment, primarily out of concern that his wife will discover his disorder. He also began to recognize that he spends a great deal of time on the job fantasizing or engaging in voyeuristic and masturbatory activities. Martin has been lying to his wife about his whereabouts for approximately 10 years.

The treatment team focused on assisting Martin with the development of appropriate coping strategies. Treatment also included psychoeducation regarding trigger identification and appropriate relapse-prevention strategies. The need for couples counseling to disclose the secrets of Martin's behavior was also addressed. Martin was given medroxyprogesterone (Depo-Provera, 500 mg intramuscularly each week) to help him to control his inappropriate sexual behaviors.

DSM-IV-TR Diagnoses

Axis I Voyeurism
Axis II Deferred—compulsive traits noted
Axis III None
Axis IV Moderate = 3 (marital conflict, job stress, anxiety)
Axis V GAF = 61 (current); GAF = 61 (past year)

Nursing Diagnosis *Ineffective sexuality pattern related to the use of cognitive distortions and the presence of defense mechanisms (denial) as evidenced by engaging in socially unacceptable sexual behaviors (public masturbation) and voyeurism without regard for others*

NOC Sexual identity; Role performance; Self-esteem
NIC Sexual counseling; Behavior management: sexual; Coping enhancement

PATIENT OUTCOMES	NURSING INTERVENTIONS	EVALUATION
Martin will identify two sexual behaviors that are socially unacceptable within the first week of admission without the presence of cognitive distortions.	Monitor for the presence of cognitive distortions via a thorough sexual history. *The presence of cognitive distortions indicates whether Martin is able to identify socially unacceptable behaviors and if he requires further treatment.*	Martin readily identifies his voyeuristic and public masturbatory behaviors as inappropriate within the first week of admission.

Continued

◎ NURSING CARE PLAN #2—cont'd

PATIENT OUTCOMES	NURSING INTERVENTIONS	EVALUATION
Martin will verbalize the effects that his behavior has on others within 2 weeks of admission. (Examples: "I know my behaviors cause other people pain"; "I realize that my wife has also been a victim of my sexual behaviors.")	Educate Martin about the impact of his socially unacceptable behaviors on others through individual and group therapy sessions. *The patient's knowledge of the effects of his socially unacceptable behaviors on others is often the beginning of treatment compliance.*	Martin verbalizes an understanding of the effects of his behavior on others within 2 weeks of admission.
Martin will participate in group therapy sessions for patients with sexual disorders, and he will openly discuss his inappropriate sexual behaviors within 1 week of admission.	Encourage Martin's participation in a group for patients with sexual disorders. *These patients frequently believe that they are the only ones who engage in inappropriate sexual behaviors, which leads to feelings of hopelessness, embarrassment, and isolation. Group therapy provides confrontation, support, and hope.*	Martin actively participates in group therapy sessions within the first week of admission. He states that the group encouraged him to talk openly about his diagnosis within the second week.

Nursing Diagnosis *Ineffective coping related to the inability to trust his wife with his secret and inadequate problem-solving skills as evidenced by the use of maladaptive coping methods such as lying, denial, ineffective communication with his wife (i.e., the inability to discuss thoughts and feelings regarding his disorder), anxiety, and fear that his wife will discover his secret*

NOC Coping; Social interaction skills; Impulse self-control; Anxiety self-control
NIC Coping enhancement; Behavior management: sexual; Impulse control training

PATIENT OUTCOMES	NURSING INTERVENTIONS	EVALUATION
Martin will effectively communicate his thoughts and feelings about his disorder and behaviors with his wife and the health care staff within 1 week of admission.	Activate Martin to verbalize his thoughts and feelings about his current coping methods (e.g., lying, nondisclosure) by providing a nonjudgmental and supportive environment in which disclosure can occur. *This will help Martin to begin to understand the impact of his present coping strategies on himself and his wife.*	Martin verbalizes many thoughts and feelings about the impact that his disorder has on his marriage within 1 week of admission.
Martin will identify concerns that he has about disclosing his disorder and behaviors to his wife by the time of discharge.	Educate Martin and his wife about his disorder, its implications, and its treatment. *Educating Martin and his wife about his disorder and aspects of treatment will calm their fears and anxieties and assist them with developing trust and establishing an effective and supportive relationship.*	At the time of discharge, Martin is able to share his secret with his wife, who is very supportive and eager to learn more about how she could help her husband cope with his disorder.
Martin will formulate two achievable relapse-prevention strategies by the time of discharge.	Help Martin to formulate appropriate strategies to use at significant times during his vulnerability *to assist with avoiding relapse and to prevent him from reoffending.*	Martin discusses two relapse-prevention strategies with the staff. He will call his wife before leaving work, and he will discuss inappropriate sexual thoughts and impulses with his wife or his therapist when they occur.

Nursing Diagnosis *Deficient knowledge of illness and aspects of treatment related to cognitive distortions, anxiety, and uncertainty as evidenced by failure to seek prior treatment for the disorder and inappropriate sexual behaviors*

NOC Knowledge: sexual functioning; Knowledge: treatment procedures
NIC Teaching: sexuality; Teaching: disease process; Learning facilitation

NURSING CARE PLAN #2—cont'd

PATIENT OUTCOMES	NURSING INTERVENTIONS	EVALUATION
Martin will verbalize a basic understanding of his illness within 1 week of admission.	Evaluate Martin's current level of knowledge regarding his illness and his readiness to learn by asking direct questions. *A patient needs to demonstrate readiness to learn for learning to occur.* Create a climate that is conducive to learning (e.g., a quiet, private, and safe environment). *Learning has a better chance of occurring when there are no distractions and when the nurse has the patient's complete attention.*	Martin is beginning to learn about his illness and the triggers that provoke his sexual thoughts and feelings. He says that he is ready to learn how to deal with his inappropriate sexual impulses.
Martin will identify the triggers that tend to provoke his inappropriate thoughts and feelings within 2 weeks of admission (e.g., having too much free or unstructured time).	Educate Martin about the importance of trigger identification and the use of relapse-prevention strategies as critical steps in his treatment. *The use of effective treatment strategies will help Martin to gain more control of his inappropriate sexual behaviors.* Suggest that Martin write a list of triggers that provoke sexually inappropriate activity, and then review this list with him. *This will help the nurse to evaluate Martin's insight into his disorder and symptoms, and the exercise of writing will help to reinforce learning.*	Martin continues to recognize the elements and situations that trigger his inappropriate sexual thoughts and feelings. He states that he will take steps to obstruct them, such as filling in his free time with appropriate activities. Martin is able to write a list of triggers that provoke his inappropriate sexual behaviors.
Martin will formulate two relapse-prevention strategies: (1) construct a schedule of appropriate planned activities to fill in free or unstructured time; and (2) open the lines of communication with his wife. These strategies will be in place by the time of discharge.	Help Martin to develop at least two appropriate relapse-prevention strategies for his identified triggers. *A concrete and realistic plan will provide Martin with workable and achievable strategies to prevent relapse.*	Martin has successfully developed two relapse-prevention techniques that will help to block triggers and to prevent sexually offensive behaviors.
After discharge, Martin will join a community support group for patients with sexual disorders.	Help Martin to join a community support group for patients with sexual disorders. *An outpatient peer support group will provide Martin with the continuity of care and realistic feedback that he needs to prevent relapse.*	Martin agrees to join a community support group for patients with sexual disorders, and his wife supports this plan.

GAF, Global Assessment of Functioning; NIC, Nursing Interventions Classification; NOC, Nursing Outcomes Classification.

CHAPTER SUMMARY

- Sexual dysfunctions include a wide range of problems that affect individuals and couples and that lead to distress and dissatisfaction.
- Sexual dysfunctions are the most common of all sexual problems that come to the attention of health care practitioners. The prevalence of sexual dysfunctions is 43% among women and 31% among men.
- A history of sexual repression and incorrect information about sex contribute to the high incidence of sexual problems that are reported.

- Pioneers such as Freud, Kinsey, Masters and Johnson, Kaplan, and Basson have added to the understanding and acceptance of sexuality. Some have developed methods to help overcome the range of associated problems.
- Sexual dysfunctions are complex in nature and develop from many biologic, psychologic, cultural, and relational causes.
- The prognosis for the treatment of individuals who experience sexual dysfunction is complicated by the lack of effective outcome studies. Each disorder has its own

CHAPTER SUMMARY—cont'd

prognosis, and each situation is unique. Motivation, acceptance, commitment, and interest by the individual or the couple are necessary for treatment.

- According to Kaplan, sexual dysfunctions are categorized by the phase of the sexual response cycle. Thus, specific dysfunctions include desire, arousal, and orgasm phase disorders. Sexual pain disorders are also within the rubric.

- The nurse needs to have a sufficient understanding of human sexuality, an awareness of his or her feelings and values regarding sexuality, and a commitment to include sexuality and sexual concerns as part of patient care in a nonjudgmental manner.

- The establishment of a plan of care should include the patient's significant other. When both members of the couple are involved, blame is less likely to occur.

- Assessment is holistic and includes the patient's or couple's sexual history and interviewing as well as the necessary laboratory and medical diagnostic techniques.

- Nursing diagnoses correlate with the DSM-IV-TR diagnoses for sexual dysfunctions. The blending of both medical and nursing diagnoses will help nurses to establish accurate and individualized patient profiles that include specific sexual issues and also diagnoses such as anxiety, body image disturbances, and spiritual distress.

- Nursing interventions need to include patient education about human sexual functioning, sexual response, and sexual dysfunctions; helping patients to improve their communication; support for the patients' fears and anxieties; support for the enhancement of the patient's self-esteem; and referral for professional help.

- Many complex diagnostic and treatment modalities have been developed for sexual dysfunctions. These include medical, psychologic, and relational methods and involve neurologic, surgical, endocrine, and vascular treatments as well as specific sex therapy techniques and couples-related therapy. There are currently more therapeutic modalities for males than for females.

- Paraphilia is defined as sexual deviations or disorders that present with inappropriate sexual fantasies that involve deviant sexual acts, inappropriate sexual urges, and the acting out of these fantasies and urges.

- A family history that is positive for the presence of a paraphilic disorder or a history of victimization may predispose other family members to developing a similar or different paraphilic disorder.

- Interventions should be based on the patient's individual needs. The plan of care includes the confrontation of cognitive distortions, the exploration of the effects of inappropriate sexual behaviors on others, psychoeducational group therapy to teach the patient how to identify triggers that provoke inappropriate sexual thoughts, the development of relapse-prevention strategies and the effects of treatment on illness symptomatology, the importance of treatment compliance during and after the hospital stay, and the development of appropriate coping strategies and problem-solving skills.

- The patient with a paraphilic disorder who is compliant with treatment has a decreased risk of sexual recidivism.

- Establishing a plan of care should include the patient to the extent that he or she is able to participate, and goals should reflect mutual agreement between the nurse and the patient.

REVIEW QUESTIONS

1. A nurse assesses four newly hospitalized patients. Which patient would it be most important for the nurse to ask about sexual functioning?
   1. An 8-year-old boy receiving chemotherapy for myelogenous leukemia
   2. A 24-year-old woman having a laparoscopic appendectomy
   3. A 35-year-old woman having a laparoscopic cholecystectomy
   4. A 58-year-old man with a diabetic foot ulcer
2. A 56-year-old woman complains to the nurse, "My husband just isn't interested in sex anymore. I guess we're too old." Select the nurse's best response.
   1. "As people get older, sex is less important. Develop other aspects of your relationship."
   2. "Men experience hormonal changes, just like women. For men, it's called viropause."
   3. "Have you talked to him about his sexual fantasies? Maybe that would pique his interest."
   4. "There are other, more important things in life. Let's discuss your grandchildren."
3. A nurse counsels an adult who had an ileostomy 4 months ago. The nurse asks about sexual activity since the surgery. The patient says, "We haven't had sex. My spouse is afraid of hurting the stoma." Which comment by the nurse would be most therapeutic?
   1. "You may engage in sexual activities now. Make sure that the bag is sealed so that it doesn't leak during sex."
   2. "Try some new positions for sexual activities so you don't put any pressure on the stoma."
   3. "The stoma is healed, but sexual intimacy can be psychologically difficult after an ileostomy."
   4. "There are other ways than sex to have intimacy with your spouse. What other activities interest both of you?"

REVIEW QUESTIONS—cont'd

4. After discovering his wife masturbating, a husband tells the nurse, "I guess I just don't satisfy her anymore." Select the nurse's best response.
   1. "Masturbation is a normal part of human behavior."
   2. "How many times have you seen her masturbate?"
   3. "Did she use any foreign objects to masturbate?"
   4. "Let's refer you and your wife to a sex therapist."

5. Which statements by a patient with a paraphilia indicate that treatment was effective? You may select more than one answer.

   1. "I will come to the clinic for my leuprolide injections once a month."
   2. "I will limit my sexual activities to watching pornographic videos."
   3. "I volunteer at an elementary school, so I have supervision when I'm near children."
   4. "I have new software that prohibits me from visiting sexually oriented chat rooms."
   5. "When I get urges to have sex with children, it's best for me to stay at home."

REFERENCES

American Psychiatric Association: *Diagnostic and statistical manual of mental disorders*, ed 4, text revision, Washington, DC, 2000, American Psychiatric Association.

Bassil N, Morley JE: Late-life onset hypogonadism: a review, *Clin Geriatr Med*, 26:197-222, 2010.

Basson R et al: Summary of the recommendations on sexual dysfunction in women, *J Sex Med* 7:314-326, 2010.

Beauregard E et al: An exploration of developmental factors related to deviant sexual preferences among adult rapists, *Sex Abuse* 16(2):151-161, 2004.

Berlin FS et al: A five-year plus follow-up survey of criminal recidivism within a treated cohort of 406 pedophiles, 111 exhibitionists and 109 sexual aggressives: issues and outcomes, *Am J Forensic Psychiatry* 12:5-28, 1991.

Berlin FS, Meineke CF: Treatment of sex offenders with antiandrogen medication: conceptualization, review of treatment modalities and preliminary findings, *Am J Psychiatry* 138(5): 601-607, 1981.

Berman L: *Real sex for real women*, New York, 2008, DK Publishing.

Bhugra D: Paraphilias across cultures. In Heiner R, editor: *Deviance across cultures*, New York, 2008, Oxford University Press.

Carvalheira AA et al: Women's motivations for sex: exploring the *Diagnostic and Statistical Manual*, 4th edition, text revision criteria for hypoactive sexual desire and female sexual arousal disorders, *J Sex Med* 7(4 Pt 1):1454-1463, 2010.

Derogatis LR, Burnett AL: Key methodological issues in sexual medicine research, *J Sex Med* 4:527-537, 2007.

Derogatis, LR, Burnett, AL: The epidemiology of sexual dysfunctions, *J Sex Med* 2:289-300, 2008.

Federhoff JP et al: Sexual disorders in Huntington's disease, *J Neuropsychiatry Clin Neurosci* 6:147-153, 1994.

Fitch WL: *Laws and programs for the special civil commitment of sex offenders*, presented at the NASMHPD Commissioners Summer 2007 Meeting, Denver, Colo.

Freud S: *On sexuality*, New York, 1977, Penguin Press.

Gaffney GS et al: Is there familial transmission of pedophilia? *J Nerv Ment Dis* 172:546-548, 1984.

Gever J: *Flibanserin boosts sex life of low-libido women* (website): www.medpagetoday.com/obgyn. Accessed May 28, 2010.

Gottman JM et al: *Ten lessons to transform your marriage: America's love lab experts share their strategies for strengthening your relationship*, New York, 2007, Random House.

Greenfield DP: Organic approaches to the treatment of paraphiliacs and sex offenders, *J Psychiatry Law* 34(4):437-454, 2006.

Groth AN: *Men who rape*, New York, 1979, Plenum Press.

Guay DR: Drug treatment of paraphilic and non paraphilic sexual disorders, *Clin Therapeutics* 31(1):1-31, 2009.

Harvey ST, Taylor JE: A meta analysis of the effects of psychotherapy with sexually abused children and adolescents, *Clin Psychol Rev* 2010, Vol 30, Issue 5, July 2010, pp 517-534. E-published. doi:10.1016/j.cpr.2010.03.006

Hollinger, DP: *The meaning of sex: Christian ethics and the moral life*, Grand Rapids, Mich, 2009, Baker Academic.

Kafka MP: Paraphilia related disorders: common, neglected and misunderstood, *Harvard Rev Psychiatry* 2:39-42, 1994a.

Kafka MP: Sertraline pharmacotherapy for paraphilias and paraphilia related disorders: an open trial, *Ann Clin Psychiatry* 6:189-195, 1994b.

Kafka MP: How are drugs used in the treatment of paraphilic disorders? *Harvard Ment Health Lett* 13:8, 1997.

Kafka MP: Paraphilia-related disorders: The evaluation and treatment of nonparaphilic hypersexuality. In Leiblum SR, editor: *Principles and practices of sex therapy*, ed 4, New York, 2007, Guilford Press.

Kafka MP, Hennen J: A DSM-IV axis I comorbidity study of males (n = 120) with paraphilias and paraphilic related disorders, *Sex Abuse* 14:349-366, 2002.

Kaplan H: *The new sex therapy*, New York, 1974, Brunner/Mazel.

Kazdin C, Ibanga I: The truth about teens sexting: GMA holds a town meeting to discuss the growing teen trend, *ABC News*, New York, aired April 15, 2009.

Kinsey A et al: *Sexual behavior in the human male*, Philadelphia, 1948, Saunders.

Kinsey A et al: *Sexual behavior in the human female*, Philadelphia, 1953, Saunders.

Klinefelter HF et al: Syndrome characterized by gynecomastia, aspermatogenesis without A-Leydigism, and increased excretion of FSH, *J Clin Endocrinol Metab* 2:615-627, 1942.

Kraft C et al: Obesity, body image, and unsafe sex in men who have sex with men, *Arch Sex Behav* 35:587-595, 2009.

Laumann E et al: Sexual dysfunction in the United States: prevalence and predictors, *JAMA* 281:537-544, 1999.

Leong GB, Silva JA: Sexually violent predator II: the sequel, *J Am Acad Psychiatry Law* 29:340-343, 2001.

Levine J: What's the matter with teen sexting? *The American Prospect* 1-2, Feb 2, 2009. www.prospect.org/cs/articles?articles=whats_the_matter_with_teen_sexting

Lindau ST et al: A study of sexuality and health among older adults in the United States, *N Engl J Med* 357:2732-2733, 2007.

Lithwick D: Teens, nude photos and the law: ask yourself should the police be involved when a tipsy teen girl emails her boyfriend naughty Valentine's Day pictures? *Newsweek* 153(8), 2009. http://proquest.umi.com.catalogue.fcsl.edu/pdqweb ?index+18&sid=1&srchmode=1&inst. Accessed December 28, 2010.

Magheli A, Burnett AL: Erectile dysfunction following prostatectomy: prevention and treatment, *Nat Rev Urol* 6:415-427, 2009.

Masters W, Johnson V: *Human sexual response*, Boston, 1966, Little, Brown.

Masters W, Johnson V: *Human sexual inadequacy*, Boston, 1970, Little, Brown.

Mathur R, Braunstein GD: Androgen deficiency and therapy in men, *Curr Opin Endocrinol Diabetes Obes* 17:242-249, 2010.

Maurice J: Female genital mutilation—new knowledge spurs optimism, *Progress: World Health Organization* (72):1-8, 2006.

Moalem S: *How sex works: why we look, smell, taste, feel and act the way we do*, New York, 2009, Harper Perennial.

Money J: *Lovemaps*, Buffalo, NY, 1986, Prometheus Books.

Money J et al: Imprinting and the establishment of gender role, *Arch Neurol Psychiatry* 77:333-338, 1957.

National Campaign to Prevent Teen and Unplanned Pregnancy: *Sex and tech: results from a survey of teens and young adults*, Washington, DC, 2008, National Campaign to Prevent Teen and Unplanned Pregnancy.

Newman L: *Male sexual dysfunction* (website): www.urology.about.com/od/sexualproblems/a/malesexualdysfunction. Accessed June 15, 2010.

North American Nursing Diagnosis Association International: *NANDA-I nursing diagnoses: definitions and classification 2009-2010*, Philadelphia, 2008, North American Nursing Diagnosis Association International.

Pesta A: Diary of an escaped sex slave, *Marie Claire* 16(11):98-100, 174-178, 2009.

Proulx J et al: CQSA: computerized questionnaire for sexual aggressors, unpublished manuscript, 1994.

Romanelli F, Sanson A: Erectile dysfunction in aging men, *Acta Biomed* 1:89-94, 2010.

Seligman L, Hardenburg SA: Assessment and treatment of paraphilias, *J Counseling Dev* 78:107-116, 2000.

Shifren JL et al: Sexual problems and distress in United States women: prevalence and correlates, *Obstet Gynecol* 112(5):970-978, 2008.

Stearns P: *Sexuality in world history*, New York, 2010, Routledge.

Træeen B, Stigum H: Sexual problems in 18-67 year old Norwegians, *Scand J Public Health* 38(5):442-456, 2010.

Wolf N: *The beauty myth: how images of beauty are used against women*, New York, 1991, HarperCollins.

CLASSIC REFERENCES

Abel GG et al: Sexually aggressive behavior. In Curran WJ et al, editors: *Forensic psychiatry and psychology*, Philadelphia, 1986, FA Davis.

Abel GG et al: Self-reported sex crimes of nonincarcerated paraphiliacs, *J Interpers Violence* 2(1):3-25, 1987.

Abel GG, Osborn C: Stopping sexual violence, *Psychiatr Ann* 22(6):301-306, 1992.

Arndt WB Jr: *Gender disorders and the paraphilias*, Madison, Conn, 1991, International Universities Press.

Baker HJ, Stoller J: Can a biological force contribute to gender identity? *Am J Psychiatry* 124(12):1653-1658, 1968.

Beitchman J et al: A review of the long-term effects of child sexual abuse, *Child Abuse Negl* 16:101-118, 1992.

Bergner RM: Money's "lovemap" account of the paraphilias: a critique and reformulation, *Am J Psychother* 42(2):254-259, 1988.

Berlin FS: Special considerations in the psychiatric evaluation of sexual offenders against minors. In Rosner R, Schwartz H, editors: *Juvenile psychiatry and the law: critical issues in American psychiatry and the law*, vol 4, New York, 1989, Plenum Press.

Berlin FS: The paraphilias and Depo-Provera: some medical, ethical and legal considerations, *Bull Am Acad Psychiatry Law* 17(3):233-239, 1989.

Berlin FS et al: A five-year plus follow-up survey of criminal recidivism within a treated cohort of 406 pedophiles, 111 exhibitionists and 109 sexual aggressives: issues and outcomes, *Am J Forensic Psychiatry* 12(3):5-28, 1991.

Berlin FS, Malin HM: Media distortion of the public's perception of recidivism and psychiatric rehabilitation, *Am J Psychiatry* 148(11):1572-1576, 1991.

Berlin FS, Meineke CF: Treatment of sex offenders with antiandrogen medication: conceptualization, review of treatment modalities and preliminary findings, *Am J Psychiatry* 138:601-607, 1981.

Bradford JM, Gratzner TG: A treatment for impulse control disorders and paraphilia, *Can J Psychiatry* 40:4-5, 1995.

Gaffney GS et al: Is there familial transmission of pedophilia? *J Nerv Ment Dis* 172:546-548, 1984.

Groth AN: *Men who rape*, New York, 1979, Plenum Press.

Kansas v. Hendricks, 521 U.S. 346-398: 1997.

Kaplan HI, Sadock BJ: Paraphilias. In Kaplan HI, Sadock, BJ, editors: *Synopsis of psychiatry, behavioral sciences, clinical psychiatry*, ed 6, Baltimore, 1991, Williams & Wilkins.

Kiersch TA: Treatment of sex offenders with Depo-Provera, *Bull Am Acad Psychiatry Law* 18(2):179-187, 1990.

Kim MJ et al: *Pocket guide to nursing diagnoses*, ed 5, St. Louis, 1993, Mosby.

Klinefelter HF et al: Syndrome characterized by gynecomastia, aspermatogenesis without A-Leydigism, and increased excretion of FSH, *J Clin Endocrinol Metab* 2(2):615-627, 1942.

Meyer WJ et al: Depo-Provera treatment for sex offending behavior: an evaluation of outcome, *Bull Am Acad Psychiatry Law* 20(3):249-259, 1992.

Money J: *Lovemaps: clinical concepts of sexual/erotic health and pathology, paraphilia, and gender transposition in childhood, adolescence, and maturity*, New York, 1986, Irvington.

Money J: *Venuses penuses: sexology, sexosophy and exigency theory*, Buffalo, NY, 1986, Prometheus Books.

Money J: Treatment guidelines: antiandrogen and counseling of paraphilic sex offenders, *J Sex Marital Ther* 13(3):219-223, 1987.

Rosen R, Lieblum S: Treatment of sexual disorders in the 1990s: an integrated approach, *J Consult Clin Psychol* 63(6):877-890, 1995.

Simon WT, Schouten PG: Plethysmography in the assessment of sexual deviance: an overview, *Arch Sex Behav* 20(1):75, 1991.

Wilson GD: An ethological approach to sexual deviation. In Wilson GD, editor: *Variant sexuality: research and theory*, Baltimore, 1987, Johns Hopkins University Press.

Online Resources

Mental Health America: www.nmha.org
National Alliance on Mental Illness: www.nami.org
National Institute of Mental Health: www.nimh.nih.gov

Crisis: Theory and Intervention

Deborah Eimer King, MSN, PhD, RN

> *"Man is not imprisoned by habit. Great changes in him can be wrought by crisis—
> once that crisis can be recognized and understood."*
>
> *Norman Cousins*

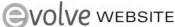

WEBSITE

http://evolve.elsevier.com/Fortinash/

OBJECTIVES

- Define the term *crisis*, and differentiate among the types of crises discussed in this chapter.
- Describe the historic context of crisis intervention, current practices, and future directions in the field.
- Identify the biopsychosocial–spiritual components of a focused crisis nursing assessment.
- Compare and contrast models of crisis intervention, and discuss how the nursing process may be used in each.
- Identify primary, secondary, and tertiary prevention strategies relevant to nursing interventions for individuals in crisis.

- Describe barriers to effective crisis intervention and resolution.
- Identify and describe self-care strategies for nurses who are working with patients in crisis.
- Identify the use of technology in crisis intervention and future trends in the field.
- Describe resilience and posttraumatic growth.
- Identify community and online resources for patients in crisis.

KEY TERMS

adventitious crisis	crisis intervention	phase-of-life (maturational crises)	resilience
coping	debriefing		risk factors
coping abilities	equilibrium	posttraumatic stress disorder	secondary prevention
crisis	external (situational crises)		tertiary prevention
crisis-focused nursing assessment	homeostasis internal (subjective crises)	primary prevention psychiatric emergency	

CRISIS

Description of Crisis

In the modern world, crises and disasters abound, and, because of modern media, people are bombarded with reminders and images of some sort of crisis on a daily basis.

Pervasive violent crimes, terrorist attacks, school shootings, the ongoing global financial crisis that came to the forefront of world media in 2008, and the massive 2010 Deepwater Horizon oil spill in the Gulf of Mexico are but a few examples. The devastation caused by natural disasters such hurricanes, earthquakes, tornados, floods, and volcanic eruptions are other striking examples. Accidents that involve motor vehicles, airplanes, trains, and buses occur daily and are linked to a multitude of tragic deaths and traumatic injuries. Each of these events ushers in any number of crises.

Human vulnerability to the life-altering impact of disasters or crises is demonstrated on international, national, local, and domestic levels. All are touched by crisis in some unique way. Nurses across all specialty areas interact with individuals, families, and communities in crisis each and every day.

On a large scale, an estimated 1.3 million women are victims of physical assault by an intimate partner each year, and one in every four women will experience the crisis of domestic violence during her lifetime (U.S. Department of Justice, 2006). Almost daily, approximately half of all humanity suffers the financial, social, and emotional crisis of poverty (Shah, 2010). The percentage of children living in poverty in the United States in 2010 will be the highest it has been in 20 years, and almost 22% of American youth will be living below the poverty line in 2010, which is the highest rate seen among America's peer nations (Foundation for Child Development, 2010).

Although a crisis may be the result of a large-scale event, it also occurs in the context of the routine, day-to-day, personal experiences that shape an individual's life.

Everyone experiences crises at some point during their lives. Millions of individuals, families, and communities are touched each day by crises that they are unable to resolve on their own. The prevalence of biologic, psychologic, social, and spiritual events that trigger crises are readily evident in daily life. A parent of four is laid off from the company that has employed family members for generations. A young woman is diagnosed with breast cancer. A drunk driver crosses a median strip and demolishes a car that is carrying a mother and her young children. Someone discovers an unplanned pregnancy. A couple divorces. An elderly couple is forced to leave their home of 40 years because they can no longer live independently. A child is diagnosed with autism. An unemployed mother and her family are evicted from their apartment. A young executive is the victim of identity theft. A teenager unintentionally overdoses on recreational substances. A young attorney loses his eyesight. A couple faces retirement after losing their pension funds. A victim of rape commits suicide. A bank forecloses on a neighbor's home.

Whether a catastrophic disaster with global impact or a crisis that occurs as part of everyday life, any of these situations can leave individuals, families, and communities struggling to adjust to situations or changes that are often unexpected, unwelcome, and overwhelming.

Opportunities that Result from Crisis

As these many examples illustrate, crises are a part of life. However, crises need not be dreaded, because they also offer potential possibilities for growth. Crises can often be positive forces, bringing with them significant opportunities for changes, life transitions, and problem resolutions. The word *crisis* is a dichotomy. It can be a stressful event with the potential to overwhelm an individual's ability to cope effectively with a challenge or threat as well as a turning point or opportunity for growth and change (Flannery, 2000). Sometimes an unplanned event will move people from complacency or apathy, thereby stretching their perspective. What appears as a negative event may resolve and produce a far better outcome. Crisis can also be defined as any situation in which a stressful life event overwhelms an individual's ability to cope effectively in the face of a perceived challenge or threat (Auerbach and Kilmann, 1997; Everly and Mitchell, 1999; James, 2008; Roberts, 2005; Wollman, 1993).

To review the evolving models of crisis intervention in disaster situations, it is important to first review relevant historic perspectives.

HISTORIC AND THEORETIC PERSPECTIVES

A variety of theorists have influenced crisis theory. Initially, Claude Bernard (1813–1878), a noted French biologist, identified the theory of physiologic equilibrium (i.e., stability of the *milieu interior*). He described equilibrium as a natural state of balance achieved by the interaction between an internal biologic feedback system and the external environment that acts to maintain the body within a normal range of functioning known as *homeostasis*. Equilibrium in both psychiatric and physiologic terms implies a steady state that resembles an optimal level of health. The term *equilibrium*, when used in psychology, refers to one's familiar state of being; crisis is a disruption of that familiar steady state. By viewing a crisis as a radical threat to what is familiar or a change from the norm, it is easy to understand why even a positive situation (e.g., the birth of a child, a promotion, winning the lottery) can trigger a stress response that is positive or good (i.e., eustress). However, an individual can interpret or perceive such positive events as negative ones, which results in a stress response that is negative (i.e., distress) (Selye, 1978). Thus, a crisis response can result from a mismatch between actual reality and what a person expects or desires (Ursin, 2002) (see Chapter 5).

Abraham Maslow's hierarchy of human needs contributes to crisis theory in that an individual has to meet physiologic or survival needs before he or she is able to concentrate on higher needs or resolve a crisis. Review Maslow's paradigm, which is diagrammed in Figure 1-1 in Chapter 1 of this book. This paradigm is an important tool for nurses who prioritize each step of the nursing process when assessing, planning, and providing patient care. Interventions begin first with a person's basic needs.

Many consider Gerald Caplan to be the father of crisis intervention techniques. He concluded that, if an individual is able to constructively resolve a crisis, that individual will gain greater personality integration and coping abilities, whereas failure to master the situation results in disorganization and ineffective coping (Caplan, 1964). Caplan identified four phases of crisis that remain foundational to current models of crisis intervention; these phases will be described in detail later in this chapter. According to Caplan, the ability to maintain or return to a state of equilibrium during a crisis depends on the individual's ability to withstand stress and anxiety, the degree of reality recognition faced when solving problems, and the range of coping abilities that the individual can use (Caplan, 1964). The individual's experience in the past with similar situations also influences his or her state of equilibrium.

Another theorist, Eric Lindemann, studied the treatment of survivors and relatives of 493 victims of the Coconut Grove fire in Boston in 1942. His studies of the psychologic symptoms of patients involved in the fire led him to believe that those individuals who were able to confront the crisis, turn to others for support, and express feelings were able to integrate the crisis into their lives in a more positive way. Those who denied the importance of the event and who did not seek assistance with the mourning process continued to have psychologic difficulties, especially depression. From his experience working with grief reactions, Lindemann proposed that grief is either "normal" or "morbid" (i.e., abnormal), depending on the individual's preexisting vulnerabilities and the ability to process loss and other stressful events. He believed that brief therapy was helpful to both the victims and their families with regard to their long-term mastery of the emotional impact of a crisis. His classic paper "Symptomatology and Management of Acute Grief" contributed significantly to early models of crisis intervention (Lindemann, 1944) (see Chapter 28).

In 1957, the Short-Doyle Act provided funds for each community to provide mental health clinics, but the emphasis was on long-term therapy. It was not until the 1970s and 1980s, when the cost of health care increased dramatically, that many began using brief therapy again because of its cost-effectiveness. Many individuals who were treated with brief therapy were in crisis, and, as brief cognitive-behavioral therapy evolved, it played a key role in the evolution of models for crisis intervention. During a crisis, maladaptive thoughts, beliefs, and perceptions of the event can often be more psychologically devastating than the event itself. By using cognitive-behavioral therapy strategies to alter the perception of the crisis, enhanced coping, problem solving, and self-efficacy often result. These are the goals of modern crisis intervention models (Flannery, 2000), and they form the foundation of current methods of crisis intervention.

A nursing framework for crisis assessment and intervention was identified by Aguilera and Mesnick (1970) about the same time that cognitive-behavioral therapy was beginning to be used increasingly in short-term therapy. This nursing model, which includes a paradigm that illustrates the effect of balancing factors during a stressful event (Aguilera, 1998), has continued to evolve since its origination, and it provides a current conceptual framework for nursing practice during crisis assessment and intervention.

When reviewing crises connected to disasters, emergency and disaster response activities were fragmented in the United States before the 1960s and the 1970s. In 1979, an executive order was signed that merged many separate disaster-related response efforts into the Federal Emergency Management Agency (FEMA). As a new agency, many unusual challenges were handled by FEMA during its first few years that demonstrated exactly how complex emergency management can be. It is apparent that handling disasters on a large scale is still a challenge.

The outgrowth of the history of crisis theory is reflected in the following sections, which describe terms, models, and strategies that can be used with the nursing process to provide care for the individual, family, or community in crisis.

DEFINITIONS OF CRISIS

Crisis has been described and defined in many ways, and several definitions are provided here. Although there is no universally accepted operational definition, crisis is generically described as a perception or experience of a situation as an intolerable difficulty that exceeds current resources and coping mechanisms (James, 2008). Crisis is a period of psychologic disequilibrium that results from the experiencing of a significant traumatic event or situation that cannot be remedied by the use of available coping strategies (Roberts, 2005). It is the subjective response to a stressful life experience that compromises an individual's stability and ability to cope or function (Roberts and Yeager, 2009). Several sources define *crisis* as any situation in which a stressful life event overwhelms an individual's ability to cope effectively in the face of a perceived challenge or threat (Auerbach and Kilmann, 1997; Everly and Mitchell, 1999; James, 2008; Roberts, 2005; Wollman, 1993).

A key element that defines crisis is the concept that the event itself is not the crisis but rather the individual's perception of the event is; the event is perceived as hazardous, threatening, or extremely upsetting to a degree at which no known coping mechanisms are effective or available (Roberts and Yeager, 2009).

CRISIS COMPONENTS

Crisis has four defining characteristics: (1) crises are specific, unexpected, and nonroutine events; (2) crises create uncertainty; (3) crises create perceptions of threat; (4) crises are processes of transformation during which the old system can no longer be maintained and the need for change is identified (Venette, 2003).

Roberts (2005) states that all crises have five common components: (1) a hazardous or traumatic event; (2) a vulnerable state; (3) a precipitating factor; (4) an active crisis state; and (5) a resolution of the crisis.

Often the crises that nurses encounter during their daily practice occur in the face of actual or perceived threats to an individual's physical/biologic, psychologic/emotional, social, or spiritual integrity, but they are time limited and without residual symptoms.

Caplan (1964) identified four distinct phases of crisis:

Phase 1: *The individual is exposed to a stressor.* This precipitant stressor triggers anxiety that leads to the use of problem-solving techniques and coping strategies in an effort to solve the problem and diminish the impact of the stressor.

Phase 2: *Previous coping and problem-solving strategies fail to relieve the stressor.* As the threat posed by the stressor persists in the context of ineffective problem solving and coping, discomfort increases. The individual is often confused, and feelings of helplessness, disorganization, and distress prevail.

Phase 3: *Resources from within and outside of the individual are mobilized to resolve the problem and to alleviate the discomfort caused by the stressor.* If all efforts at problem solving fail, anxiety may escalate to panic, and the individual may withdraw, flee the situation, and decline in function. Note that people may drop out of situations in numerous ways, including self-medication with alcohol, drugs, or other methods that have soothed them in the past. Alternatively, new problem-solving techniques may be used, and, if these are effective, a solution may be identified to lead to the resolution of the crisis.

Phase 4: *The absence of crisis resolution leads to major disorganization.* During this phase, tension escalates to a breaking point, cognitive function declines substantially, emotions become labile, and behavior may become irrational, aggressive, or self-injurious (Lowry and Lating, 2002).

Risk Factors for Crisis

Risk factors may limit an individual's ability to cope or problem solve during stressful life events or situations. These may be present across a wide range of clinical settings and include the following:

- The presence of concurrent or multiple biopsychosocial stressors
- Multiple losses, unexpected life changes, and unresolved problems
- Limitations in adaptive ability and coping skills
- Chronic physical or psychologic pain or disability
- Concurrent psychiatric disorders, substance abuse, and suicidality
- Poor social support networks
- Limited access to health care services

Nurses across many clinical settings are in unique positions to identify individuals with risk factors for crisis as a result of their daily interactions with individuals and families who are experiencing disruptions in their lives. Nurses use the risk factors assessment criteria to identify individuals and families who are at high risk for the occurrence of crises and then intervene to prevent those crises from occurring.

Types of Crises

Four major types of crises may manifest in health care practices with individuals, families, and the community: (1) external crises result from actual events or circumstances in the environment; (2) internal crises are subjectively perceived and experienced; (3) maturational crises may occur during the course of normal growth and developmental phases and milestones; and (4) adventitious crises occur as a result of extraordinary events.

External (Situational) Crises

An external crisis is precipitated by a specific external situation or event that is apparent to another observer. It usually centers on real events that threaten physical health (e.g., the inability to obtain food, clothing, or shelter) or the loss of a loved one or a valued object. Examples include the loss of a job, the death of a loved one, a change in financial status, divorce, eviction, or foreclosure. External crises may affect individuals, families, or entire communities. In addition, one external event often results in multiple crises for an individual, a family, or a community.

Internal (Subjective) Crises

An internal crisis is triggered by a subjective perception of threat to one's well-being that may not be obvious to the outside observer. Examples of internal crises are responses to aging, loss, abandonment, or a breach of loyalty that results in profound feelings of betrayal, fear, or victimization. An internal crisis may also result from a threat to a deeply held belief or value, thereby triggering spiritual distress or a loss of faith.

Any negative thought pattern or experience of emotional distress can act as an internal stressor and trigger an internal or subjective crisis. An individual or a family can view almost any situation as a crisis, depending on their own unique internal perception of the situation or event. What constitutes a crisis for one individual or family may not for another; it depends on the stressor itself and the family's internal perceptions of it. Other relevant factors include other stressors that the family is experiencing, the family's coping ability, the extent of available family resources, and prior experience with crises (Clark, 2008).

Phase-of-Life (Maturational) Crises

Humans experience normal and predictable changes throughout their lives, and these may precipitate phase-of-life or maturational crises for some individuals. Adolescence, career choices, marriage, parenthood, midlife, retirement, and aging represent some of the changes that are experienced along life's continuum. For example, a family may experience a crisis when the child leaves home for the first time for college or the military. The term *midlife crisis* describes the challenging transitions of middle adulthood. Age-related changes often bring a loss of strength, mobility, or balance; reduced memory; slower thinking; and other declining cognitive and physical abilities that may trigger crises.

Each life phase brings with it expectations from oneself and others, challenges that often increase vulnerability to crisis, and the feeling that one needs to modify coping mechanisms accordingly. Differing beliefs about life changes, what they represent, and how they are experienced by the individual or family often determine whether or not a phase-of-life crisis occurs.

Regardless of whether the crisis is internal or external, expected or unexpected, and actual or perceived, if coping abilities fail to remove the perception of threat to one's safety and restore equilibrium, a crisis will be experienced internally. It is this internal experience that becomes the focal point of crisis assessment and intervention.

Disasters (Adventitious Crises)

An adventitious crisis is precipitated by a disaster that is not part of everyday life. This type of crisis can arise from the following:

- Natural disasters (e.g., hurricanes, fires, earthquakes)
- National or global disasters (e.g., manmade disasters, including acts of terrorism, war, riots, and airplane crashes; environmental catastrophes, including oil spills and global disease outbreaks)
- Crimes of violence (e.g. rape, assault, bomb threats, homicide, violence in school settings, abuse) (see Chapter 23).

Since the 1990s, the mass media and the Internet have brought countless images of traumatic events and disasters into closer view for millions of people around the globe. The ongoing media coverage of events such as the New York terrorist attacks of September 11, 2001, and of the massive oil spill in the Gulf of Mexico in 2010 changed the landscape of awareness of the impact that multiple dimensions of adventitious crises have on people across the street as well as across the globe.

Nurses and other health care personnel must be prepared when they are called to respond to manmade disasters and to natural disasters, which appear to be occurring with greater frequency and intensity than ever before. The increasing frequency and intensity of natural disasters are the result of multiple changing global factors (Landesman, 2005; Perry, 2007; Walström, 2010).

Human Responses to Crisis

A person's response to crisis is often an ordinary response to an extraordinary event. It does not represent psychopathology but rather a struggle to find strategies and solutions that will restore the balance and equilibrium of homeostasis. During a crisis, biologic, psychologic, social, and spiritual homeostasis are disrupted, and the individual perceives a sudden loss of his or her ability to use effective problem solving and coping skills. Physical, emotional, social, and **spiritual distress** may result, and the response to such distress can be either adaptive or maladaptive.

When the response is adaptive, although the individual is temporarily unorganized, he or she is able to take action and seek a solution. When the response is maladaptive, the individual experiences prolonged or excessive periods of disorganization, tension, anxiety, hopelessness, and helplessness, and he or she is less likely to take action to find a solution. An individual's interpretation of the crisis is based on his or her perception of the event, prior learning, memory, and previous outcomes to similar situations.

Nurses use the biopsychosocial–spiritual model when assessing a patient in a crisis situation to determine if the response is adaptive or maladaptive. Intervention for patients with adaptive responses is supportive, but maladaptive responses frequently require additional intervention. In each case, the opportunity for growth and change exists.

In a crisis, an individual's coping abilities fail.

Coping is an adjustment reaction or the use of habitual patterns of behavior by an individual in response to an actual or perceived threat in an effort to maintain psychologic integrity (Aguilera, 1998). Figure 21-1 illustrates the process and outcomes of crisis.

Coping abilities emphasize various conscious and unconscious strategies that are used to deal with stress and tension.

Human coping abilities manifest as fight-or-flight reactions or freeze reactions such as anxiety, hypervigilance, sleep disturbance, emotional or physical withdrawal, denial, emotional numbing, and impaired concentration and ability to focus during normal daily functioning (Flannery and Everly, 2000). During crisis, denial is a common defense mechanism and method of coping. Denial can help people to endure and process a reality that is psychologically overwhelming for them at the time, and it can lessen the intensity of the shock that often accompanies the early phase of crisis until other coping resources can be mobilized by the individual. Coping does not imply mastery over the crisis; rather, it is the process that is used to respond to the crisis and find resolution.

During a crisis, biopsychosocial homeostasis or equilibrium is disrupted. The American Academy of Experts in Traumatic Stress (1999) identified the following immediate potential responses to crisis or trauma:

- Shock
- Numbness
- Denial
- Dissociative behavior
- Confusion
- Disorganization
- Difficulty making decisions
- Suggestibility
- Physiologic symptoms, such as nausea, vomiting, tremors, profuse sweating, and dizziness

Many individuals experience such symptoms immediately after a crisis or traumatic event, and they may continue for a limited time after the actual crisis event.

According to the *Diagnostic and Statistical Manual of Mental Disorders,* fourth edition, text revision (DSM-IV-TR), an *acute stress disorder* (ASD) may manifest when a person is in crisis (American Psychiatric Association, 2000). ASD is an anxiety disorder that is characterized by a cluster of dissociative and anxiety symptoms that occur within 1 month of a major traumatic stressor. The immediate cause of ASD is exposure to an extreme stressor that involves a threat to life, physical integrity, or the potential for serious injury or witnessing an event that involves the death or serious injury of another person and reacting to the event with marked fear, helplessness, or horror. Either during or after the experience of the traumatic event, the individual has at least three of the following dissociative symptoms:

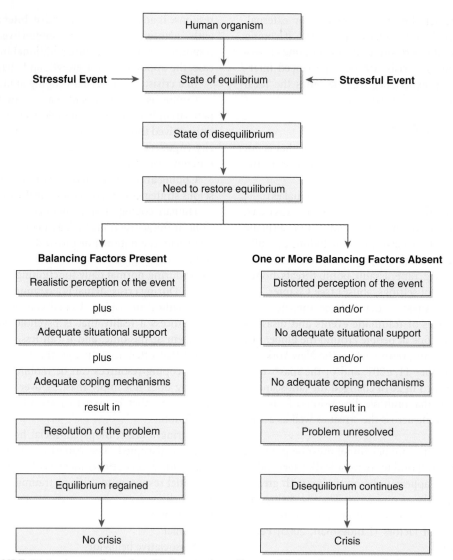

FIGURE 21-1. A paradigm that illustrates the effects of balancing factors during a stressful event. (From Aguilera DC: *Crisis intervention: theory and methodology*, ed 8, St. Louis, 1998, Mosby.)

1. A subjective sense of numbing or detachment or the absence of emotional responsiveness
2. A reduction in the awareness of his or her surroundings (e.g., "being in a daze")
3. Derealization
4. Depersonalization
5. Dissociative amnesia (i.e., the inability to recall an important aspect of the trauma)

In addition, the traumatic event is persistently reexperienced in at least one of the following ways: recurrent images, thoughts, dreams, or flashbacks; a sense of reliving the experience; or distress on exposure to reminders of the traumatic event. There is marked avoidance of stimuli that trigger recollections of the trauma (e.g., thoughts, feelings, conversations, activities, places, people) and marked anxiety symptoms or increased arousal symptoms (e.g., difficulty sleeping, irritability, poor concentration, hypervigilance, exaggerated startle response, motor restlessness). The symptoms cause clinically significant distress or impairment in social, occupational, or other important areas of functioning or impair the individual's ability to pursue goals, complete activities of daily living, or mobilize the necessary personal help and assistance. The symptoms of ASD last for a minimum of 2 days and a maximum of 4 weeks, and they occur within 4 weeks of the traumatic event (American Psychiatric Association, 2000.) These symptoms are not necessarily cause for long-term intervention; most research indicates that the immediate response to the acute event is time-limited and responsive to crisis intervention and brief therapy in the majority of cases. However, if symptoms persist for more than 1 month, additional long-term therapy is usually indicated, and assessment for other diagnoses may be also be considered, such as **posttraumatic stress disorder** (PTSD).

Several other diagnostic categories or symptom patterns are related to crisis. According to the DSM-IV-TR, crisis is not viewed as a distinct diagnostic category; rather, it is associated with several psychiatric disorders or categories of symptoms. In addition to ASD, the most common disorders include depression, anxiety, adjustment disorders, and PTSD. There has been a notable increase in the incidence of PTSD, which is due in large part to the numbers of military personnel who were diagnosed with the disorder. PTSD has been of great interest to clinicians and researchers over the past two decades, and it continues to receive attention for many reasons. PTSD is frequently associated with crises; a detailed description of the disorder appears in Chapter 10.

Nurses use the biopsychosocial–spiritual model when assessing a patient in a crisis situation to determine if the response is adaptive or maladaptive. Interventions for patients with adaptive responses are usually supportive, but maladaptive responses frequently require additional intervention. In each case, the opportunity for growth and change exists.

Psychological Stages after a Disaster. According to New York State Office of Mental Health (2006), there are predictable phases that are experienced by groups of people or communities after any type of disaster:

1. *Heroic phase.* This occurs immediately after the event, and it is a time of altruism and heroic behavior in the community.
2. *Honeymoon phase.* This occurs 1 week to 3 to 6 months after the event, when feelings of community sharing and high social attachment exist.
3. *Disillusionment phase.* This occurs 2 months to 1 to 2 years after the event, and it is characterized by feelings of disappointment, anger, resentment, and bitterness regarding the expectations of support that were not met.
4. *Reconstruction phase.* This occurs 2 months to 1 to 2 years after the event, when physical and emotional reinvestment take place.

Individuals proceed through these stages at their own pace.

Nurses who are providing care need to recognize these stages and provide appropriate interventions that are closely matched to the phase that the patient or community is experiencing. Populations that are at special risk for adverse mental health conditions after a disaster or traumatic event include children and adolescents, the elderly, refugees and migrant groups, and the developmentally or mentally disabled (Langan and James, 2005). During Hurricane Katrina, the most affected population was the poor. They were stranded on highway overpasses, roofs, and in the Superdome and Convention Center without adequate food and water, and they became quickly overwhelmed with fear and a sense of hopelessness (Rhoads, 2006).

However, even among the most vulnerable, some individuals perceive the stress associated with a disaster quite differently from others. Some individuals tend to feel empathy or survivor guilt after a disaster. It appears that a disaster often transforms behavior from isolation to increased interaction with others after the first response of shock and disbelief. Individual identities are set aside, altruism emerges, and, for a time, the focus is on the community (Dane, 2001). The literature documents that disaster experiences appear to promote personal growth and strengthen relationships in many cases (Friedman, 2005).

CRISIS INTERVENTION

An Overview

Crisis intervention involves short-term strategic therapy with action-oriented interventions that focus on solving the immediate problems related to the emotional, mental, physical, and behavioral distress that results from the crisis. Nurses help individuals to return to their precrisis level of functioning or, in some cases, to improve it. The basic goals of crisis intervention include the alleviation of the acute distress, the restoration of independent functioning, and the prevention of psychologic trauma (Langan and James, 2005). Nurses begin interventions as soon as possible after the crisis event or response, because, during a crisis, individuals are often more open to suggestions and therapeutic interventions. In addition, immediate intervention acts to stabilize psychologic disturbance and to minimize prolonged psychologic trauma.

Crisis intervention traditionally focused on individuals. However, with crises occurring on larger scales, affecting communities and geographic regions, or having a global impact, the need for group crisis intervention becomes necessary.

Global Intervention

At present, the art and science of dealing with both natural and manmade disasters is still evolving. September 11, 2001, did produce an awareness of the need for effective crisis intervention and disaster response procedures at all levels, in both the government and the private sector. The mission of FEMA is to reduce the loss of life and property and to protect communities nationwide from all hazards, including natural disasters, acts of terrorism, and other manmade disasters. FEMA leads and supports the nation in a risk-based comprehensive emergency management system of preparedness, protection, response, recovery, and mitigation (Federal Emergency Management Agency, 2009). The government now recommends and requires similar programs in a wide variety of settings, including schools, communities, and occupational settings (Everly, 2000). Since the early 21st century, the National Institute of Mental Health has funded numerous grants for large-scale research regarding the prevention and treatment of mental disorders that result from exposure to mass violence (National Institutes of Health News Release, 2002).

Crises Caused by Psychiatric Emergencies

A psychiatric emergency involves a sudden and serious psychologic disturbance that results in a behavioral state that requires intervention to prevent a life-threatening or psychologically damaging consequence. During crises that result from psychiatric emergencies, overall function is severely impaired such that the individual is unable to assume personal responsibility as a result of acute problematic behaviors. He or she is challenged to regain equilibrium without a destructive outcome for himself or herself or others.

Characteristics of a psychiatric emergency, which share features with other types of crises, include a sense of urgency or impending doom, a feeling of intolerable anxiety, and a sense of being overwhelmed and unable to cope. The individual may or may not recognize the need for assistance from others to alleviate the psychologic distress of the immediate situation. However, the primary factor that distinguishes a psychiatric emergency from other types of crises and medical emergencies is the presence or threat of danger to the self or others.

Nurses and other health care professionals encounter crises caused by psychiatric emergencies in the emergency department, the general hospital setting, the psychiatric unit, and the outpatient setting as well as in community settings such as school, residential, and occupational environments. Members of the health care team act to convert a dangerous or life-threatening crisis into problems that are addressed with intervention and target resolution. Psychiatric emergencies fall into the following three categories, which relate to many psychiatric and medical diagnoses (Lange, 2005):

1. Life-threatening behavior, including threatened or attempted suicide; individuals at high risk for suicide, assault, homicidal thoughts or actions, other violent acts toward the self or others; drug overdose (intentional or unintentional); acute psychoses caused by psychopathology, drug-induced intoxication, or psychosis; and uncontrollable anger
2. Life-disrupting behavior, including severe anxiety, loss of contact with reality, exacerbations of symptoms of mood disorders (e.g., depression, mania); the maladaptive patterns of characterologic/personality disorders; or the inability to perform activities of daily living
3. Life-impairing behavior, including intoxication, addiction, withdrawal from alcohol or drugs, toxic or idiosyncratic reactions to medication, cognitive dysfunction, illegal or high-risk behavior, or nonadherence to medical treatment regimens for medical or psychiatric diagnoses

The acute subjective distress or disturbed behavior of a psychiatric emergency is often very alarming to the patient, the family, and the community. The patient who is experiencing the psychiatric emergency is often brought to the emergency department for assessment by friends, relatives, law enforcement, or emergency responders. He or she may be referred by health care providers, agencies, or crisis hotline staff, or he or she may be in an inpatient facility already. Alternatively, there are times when a person can be brought to the hospital for emergency evaluation involuntarily, including in the following situations: 1) the person poses a *danger to himself or herself*, including sharing thoughts or threats of suicide, sharing a suicide plan, or actively using a weapon or situation to injure himself or herself; and 2) the person poses a *danger to others* as evidenced by threatening another, brandishing a weapon, or displaying erratic or unpredictable behavior. The best of all circumstances when there is a psychiatric emergency is when the patient is willing to seek emergency evaluation voluntarily. Although this does occur, patients are also frequently in a clouded mental state and have poor judgment, so many involuntary emergency evaluations are the result. Safeguarding the rights of the patient to freely choose mental health treatment and the rights of the patient and the community to remain safe are the priorities to consider when assessing the need for voluntary or involuntary emergency evaluation. Thus, emergency evaluation for an individual's dangerousness to himself, herself, or others is conducted involuntarily if the patient is unable or unwilling to do so voluntarily.

Suicide attempts and threats are among the most common psychiatric emergencies seen by the crisis nurse. Suicide ranks among the leading causes of death in the United States, and many suicides are not reported or recorded, thereby resulting in suicide statistics that are likely to be underestimated. Other crises caused by psychiatric emergencies are often the result of chronic patterns of self-destructive behavior; substance abuse or overdose; eating disorders and related medical complications; the sudden death or loss of a child, spouse, family member, or caregiver; unrelieved chronic pain; trauma; domestic violence; uncontrollable behavior; assault; abuse; sudden homelessness; or the accumulation of other biopsychosocial stressors. Populations at high risk for psychiatric emergencies include the elderly, infants, and children; individuals with weak or absent social support systems; persons who abuse substances; those without health insurance, health care, or economic resources; and those with chronic mental or medical pathologies.

Anxiety is pervasive during a crisis caused by a psychiatric emergency, and the nurse who is providing care to the patient or family experiencing this type of crisis needs to continually assess the level of anxiety being experienced by all involved persons, including the professional staff rendering care. The intense anxiety experienced by the patient who is having a psychiatric emergency can often be contagious, and a nursing priority is to remain as calm, focused, and efficient as possible when providing care and to work collaboratively to stabilize the emotional climate with all members of the crisis team.

NURSING ASSESSMENT DURING CRISIS AND DISASTER

Nursing assessment of crisis and disaster is often done both in the field (i.e., outside of a controlled, structured, and familiar care setting [e.g., hospital, clinic]) and in controlled settings (e.g., emergency department, hospital). Fieldwork includes providing mental health services in homeless shelters, encampments, temporary housing structures including tents or disaster shelters, and collaborative work with law enforcement units responding to 911 crisis calls or physical disasters (Figure 21-2). For nurses, fieldwork is an approach to crisis intervention that integrates both physical and psychiatric needs (Lerner, 2002). A summary of how to approach someone who has simultaneous physical and emotional threats to safety while the traumatic event is taking place appears in Box 21-1.

Other types of field assessments occur when a clinician is part of a law enforcement team. Many cities have made efforts to combine expertise by pairing mental health professionals

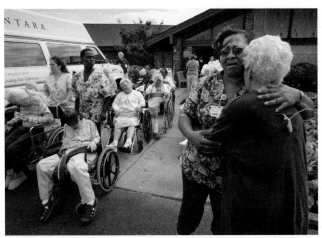

FIGURE 21-2. Crisis evokes strong emotions and the need for community action as nursing home staff and residents prepare for evacuation before a devastating hurricane. (From Win McNamee/Reuters.)

with law officers when responding to calls that involve mentally disordered patients. Both partners receive training regarding how to deescalate angry or violent persons, and the mental health partner offers additional expertise in the area of psychiatric assessment. When determining the appropriate disposition of the patient, the following components are essential and prioritized as follows:

- Ensure safety.
- Establish rapport.
- Evaluate for medical and substance-related problems.
- Use crisis intervention techniques.

Careful evaluations—whether in the field or in the hospital or a more controlled setting—reduce unnecessary violence among patients, officers, and others to bring about a peaceful resolution to the situation. Special challenges may occur when numerous community agencies are called to work together professionally in such situations. The most effective approach lies in the collaboration of providers from many disciplines and organizations and in the ability of each to put the needs of patients above individual agency or organizational politics.

A **crisis-focused nursing assessment** includes gathering comprehensive biopsychosocial–spiritual data from a variety of sources to plan interventions that will be most effective for addressing immediate problems and that will ultimately lead to crisis resolution. The more focused the assessment is in the short term, the more immediate the relief can be for the immediate problem. The assessment can then be built upon in the longer term to create a more individualized intervention or treatment plan after immediate needs are met (see Box 21-2).

After assessing the patient in crisis, the next step is the application of the comprehensive assessment data that the nurse has gathered to the variety of crisis intervention models and methods available to identify the most effective intervention techniques for the individual patient or family in crisis.

MODELS AND METHODS OF CRISIS INTERVENTION

Over the years, "psychologic first aid" and crisis intervention have proven to be effective for victims of all types of crises and disasters, especially the extreme stressors that result in psychologic trauma (Flannery, 2000). Aguilera (1998) offers five basic steps that are foundational to many of the crisis intervention models that are used in current practice and that are described in more detail later in this chapter:

1. Assessment of the individual and the problem
2. Planning of therapeutic intervention
3. Intervention
4. Resolution of the crisis
5. Anticipatory planning

In actual practice, the stages are overlapping rather than consecutive, and they link to several factors and principles that are foundational to successful crisis intervention models that target resolution and healthy outcomes.

According to Aguilera (1998), "balancing" factors that determine the effectiveness of crisis intervention strategies

BOX 21-2   CRISIS-FOCUSED NURSING ASSESSMENT

Biophysical
Chief physical or somatic complaints or stressors
Age, gender, and ethnicity
Brief health history and vital signs
Current medications and date and time of last doses
Use of herbal or homeopathic remedies
General Appearance
Brief Physical Assessment
Injury, trauma, and abnormal physical features or findings
Exposure to communicable diseases or potential toxins
Mobility status
Possibility of pregnancy, miscarriage, or active labor
Presence of others who are dependent on the person who is in crisis

Psychologic
- Chief psychologic complaints or stressors
- Perception of the event that precipitated the crisis
- Feelings and thoughts expressed by the individual
- Mental status, ability to communicate, and thought patterns
- Predominant mood
- Ability to focus and follow directions
- Predominant defense mechanisms (e.g., denial, minimization)
- Insight and judgment about the crisis and the necessary actions
- Expression of intent to injure self or others
- Suicidal or homicidal ideations
- Behavior (e.g., agitated, controlled, nonverbal, tearful)
- Appearance or report of ingestion of recreational substances, drugs of abuse, medications, or chemicals
- Report of victimization or violence
- Existing mental illness or psychiatric impairment
- Coping skills used successfully in the past
- Desired outcome or mechanism to resolve crisis
- Global Assessment of Functioning
- Indications for hospitalization or emergency evaluation

Sociocultural
- Presence of family members or social support networks
- Identification with specific community or cultural groups
- Beliefs about the crisis or disaster

- Culture-bound syndromes or symptoms
- Rituals to provide comfort, hope, or a sense of safety
- Available childcare, caregivers, or respite care providers
- Relevant legal history
- Drug and alcohol history
- Presence of community unrest, violence, or looting
- Community cohesiveness
- Community collaboration with relief agencies and resources

Environmental
Perception of safety or ongoing threats to safety
Physical safety of patient and potential threats to safety
Proximity to disaster, environmental hazards, or crime scene
Presence of food, shelter, and victimization or other environmental threats
Communication devices (e.g., cell phone, Internet, radio)
Transportation and relocation concerns
Access to emergency services, disaster relief, and supplies
Weapons or potentially injurious personal items
Access to personal belongings, valuables, hygiene, nutrition, and a safe water supply
Relevant contact with law enforcement
Weather conditions that may influence crisis recovery
Community resources and crisis hotlines
Necessary medical and life-support equipment
Access to health care or trauma facilities
Witnesses or other available historians
Extent of environmental damage and loss of life
Involvement of animals in crisis or disaster
Potential health effects

Spiritual
- Religious or spiritual affiliation
- Beliefs about the meaning or purpose of the crisis
- Presence of spiritual support (e.g., clergy, chaplain, rabbi, faith community)
- Sense of hope and overall purpose for life events
- Requests for spiritual or religious intervention
- Spiritual resources available to assist with coping
- Need for spiritual rituals (e.g., mourning or death rituals, petition rituals for assistance, gratitude rituals)

and the successful resolution of any crisis include the following: (1) the individual's perception of the event; (2) the presence of active situational supports; and (3) the person's coping mechanisms, skills, and strategies. It is critical to assess these factors when assessing the patient or family in crisis (see crisis-focused assessment). Figure 21-1 illustrates the effect of these balancing factors during a crisis. A person's perception of a crisis event may be realistic or distorted, which will either facilitate or inhibit resolution. In addition, assistance from caring and capable family, friends, and community groups often relieves the physical and psychologic burden of a crisis event. The effectiveness of a person's coping mechanisms (e.g., automatic defenses such as denial) and his or her coping

skills and strategies (e.g., learned methods) are significant determinants of the effectiveness of crisis resolution. Outcomes can also depend on the individual's previous experience with similar events, personality style, and individual response to specific crisis intervention models and strategies.

Generally agreed upon principles of intervention for cases of psychologic trauma after a crisis are as follows (Flannery, 2000):
- Intervene immediately, as close to the event as possible.
- Stabilize the victims by restoring a semblance of order and routine.
- Facilitate an understanding of the event by gathering facts, listening, and teaching.

- Focus on problem solving.
- Encourage self-reliance.

The goal of crisis intervention is to return the individual or family to their precrisis level of functioning, although, in some cases, the resolution of the crisis results in either a higher or lower level of functioning as compared with precrisis levels. During a crisis, individuals are often more receptive to intervention, and they may demonstrate greater readiness for healthy change as their distress levels increase (Velasquez et al, 1999). By focusing on the present problem and the resolution of the immediate crisis, nurses can assist individuals with seeing how adaptive changes can lead to improved health, problem solving, and solutions.

Robert's Seven-Stage Model of Crisis Intervention. Robert's seven-stage model of crisis intervention (Roberts, 1991, 2000, and 2005) has been used for intervening in acute crisis states and as a guide to proceeding with individualizing care for patients who may be in differing stages of coping. Roberts identifies seven critical stages through which patients typically pass during the process of crisis stabilization, resolution, and mastery, and he describes them as essential, sequential, and sometimes overlapping:

1. Plan and conduct a thorough biopsychosocial–spiritual assessment (see Box 21-2) that addresses the individual's dangerousness to himself or herself and others.
2. Establish rapport and rapidly establish a collaborative relationship with the individual or family in crisis.
3. Identify major problems, including those that may have triggered the crisis.
4. Encourage the expression of feelings and emotions with active listening and validation.
5. Generate and explore alternatives for coping.
6. Collaboratively develop an action plan that serves to empower the patient and that restores functioning.
7. Develop a follow-up plan to assess postcrisis status and the need for further intervention.

After the events of September 11, 2001, Roberts built on this model to develop a comprehensive and condensed framework called assessment, crisis intervention, and trauma treatment (ACT) (Roberts, 2006). The components of ACT include the following:

A: Assessment and appraisal of immediate medical needs, threats to public safety, and property damage; triage, crisis, and trauma assessment; biopsychosocial–spiritual and cultural assessment

C: Connection to support groups, disaster relief, and social services; critical incident stress debriefing (CISD) (Everly et al, 2000); crisis intervention model (Roberts, 1991, 2000, and 2005)

T: Trauma treatment plans, including treatment of traumatic stress reactions, PTSD, and trauma recovery strategies

ACT serves as a three-part conceptual framework that integrates several models of crisis assessment and intervention, to guide crisis clinicians through a sequence of planned steps in responding to all or most crisis situations, in order to pace and match interventions according to a hierarchy of needs and stages of crisis response.

Acute Traumatic Stress Management. Lerner and Shelton (2005) developed acute traumatic stress management (ATSM) to provide emergency responders with a protocol with which to respond to traumatic stress. It was designed to provide a model for first responders to address the emergent psychologic needs of persons in crisis and to offer practical strategies for helping people during a traumatic event. With the vulnerability that accompanies the experience of a traumatic event often comes a tremendous opportunity for intervention by making use of the 10 stages of the ATSM model.

Crisis Intervention with Children and Families. The U.S. Department of Health and Human Services has identified specific components and goals for crisis intervention with children and families that build on generic crisis intervention models by involving the entire family in the crisis intervention and assessment process (Gentry, 1994). An emphasis is placed on limited goals and objectives, especially with families in which disorganization and dysfunctional dynamics contribute to chaos before, during, and after a crisis. Crisis intervention with families, which is based on the pioneering work of Lydia Rapoport (1962), is guided by six primary goals that target the stabilization and strengthening of family functioning:

1. Alleviate the acute symptoms of stress that are being experienced by the family.
2. Restore the family members and the family system to optimal precrisis levels of functioning.
3. Identify the relevant events that precipitated the family crisis, and focus on an understanding of these events together with the family.
4. Identify measures that the family can take to alleviate the crisis situation, including those that are available through community resources and supports.
5. Identify and establish a connection or relationship between the family's current crisis and past experiences and patterns.
6. Assist the family with initiating new ways of perceiving, thinking, and feeling to formulate healthy and adaptive coping responses for future use.

When it respects the strengths of the family system, crisis intervention is most effective for assisting family members with identifying their own needs and the ways in which they themselves wish to proceed. Crisis can create a climate in which families have a heightened awareness of the need for change, and families may be more receptive to action plans that are directed at changes that are meaningful for them.

Any of these models can be adapted for intervention after exposure to a traumatic event, and they may be used in conjunction with brief psychodynamic psychotherapy, cognitive-behavioral therapy, and sometimes reexposure therapy or hypnotherapy. In addition, antidepressant medications frequently assist with depression, adjustment disorders, anxiety, and PTSD. Other medications (e.g., benzodiazepines, β-blockers, sedatives, hypnotics) are offered for short-term relief. The severity and type of symptoms determine whether a referral for medication is indicated. In general, when medications are indicated, the combination of medication and interactive therapy is more effective than either modality alone.

PLANNING AND EXECUTING THERAPEUTIC INTERVENTION

Nursing Approaches to Crisis Intervention

1. Express caring and consolation. Listen, observe, and encourage the expression of thoughts and feelings.
2. Assess the realities of the situation, and put tangible threats before those that are perceived and intangible to determine the degree of the crisis and the types of interventions necessary.
3. Develop and begin to use an immediate plan for intervention that is based on the comprehensive, crisis-focused nursing assessment and the crisis intervention model that best fits the patient's needs and the type of crisis situation.
4. Coordinate with other agencies. This approach is essential, particularly during large-scale disasters with tangible threats such as fires, earthquakes, wars, and acts of terror. Be familiar with resources that offer support with basic needs such as food, clothing, shelter, and financial support. Have referral information and crisis hotline telephone numbers available.
5. Anticipate future needs related to the crisis, and develop a plan with the patient for meeting these needs.

Children in Crisis

When working with children in crisis, nursing approaches should target the priorities of physical safety, psychologic safety, and reassurance (Abramovitz, 2001; Perry, 2010). In general, the goals when working with children in crisis are to prevent frightening experiences and emotions from becoming overwhelming for the child and to reinforce healthy coping to restore and reinforce feelings of control and safety rather than feelings of helplessness, threat, or danger.

Physical Safety. Consistent with Maslow's hierarchy of needs (Maslow, 1943) is the idea that basic physiologic needs (e.g., breathing, food, homeostasis) must be met before psychologic needs can be addressed. This is particularly true when children are in crisis. In addition to meeting basic physiologic needs for survival, nursing strategies target making the child's environment as safe and secure as possible, with the least amount of restrictions. Familiar and soothing objects, routines, foods, toys, and communication patterns with parents or caregivers can all help to restore a sense of structure and predictability to the physical environment and promote a sense of physical safety. Distancing children from ongoing physical threats or the "instant replay" of physical threats on the television, the Internet, and the radio is also critical to restoring a sense of physical safety so that higher-order needs can be met. A primary strategy is to find ways to facilitate communication between parents or caregivers and their children. Children seek to be in close proximity to their parents or caregivers; children often fear losing their caregivers if the caregivers are not visible to the child or if the child cannot communicate with them. Depending on the children's age groups and developmental phases, friends and members of the peer group can also help to reinforce a sense of physical safety by providing social support and tangible familiar items that serve to decrease the distress level of the child.

Psychologic Safety. When children experience a sense of psychologic safety, they have an internal sense of confidence in their ability to tolerate and manage the distress aroused by the crisis or danger that they have experienced without feeling overwhelmed or out of control. Strategies to enhance a sense of psychologic safety for children in crisis include talking with the child about the crisis or trauma in terms that he or she can understand. Avoiding the discussion of the event or not answering the child's questions only serves to increase internal distress levels rather than diffuse them. The more information that the child can be given about who, what, where, why, and how the crisis occurred, the easier it is for the child to make sense of the situation. Fear of the unknown will make a traumatized child more anxious and symptomatic. Tell the child the truth, even when it is emotionally difficult to do so. If you don't know the answer, tell the child that you don't; honesty will help with the development of trust. Just listening to the child, without necessarily having good answers to his or her questions, can be very therapeutic. Giving the child choices whenever possible can increase his or her sense of control and decrease posttraumatic distress.

Reassurance. Normalizing the child's reactions to the crisis by validating his or her feelings, thoughts, and concerns provides reassurance by explaining to the child that his or her reactions are normal and to be expected, and that others are probably experiencing similar things. This lessens the feelings of isolation and fear. Providing as consistent and predictable a pattern for daily activities as possible helps to reinforce the child's perception that caregivers are in control, which is vital to decreasing distress levels and to preventing retraumatization and relapse. Provide protection and advocacy by not hesitating to stop activities that are upsetting or retraumatizing for the child, such as setting limits with audiovisual "instant replays" of the traumatic event. The reassuring power of touch, when sought out by the child, is vital to increasing a child's sense of reassurance. Providing hugs and other forms of nonthreatening touch (e.g., holding, rocking) can be most reassuring, especially to younger children. Setting clear limits for behavior and consistently enforcing and reinforcing them reassures the child by increasing the sense of predictability in their environment. Children with special needs (e.g., developmental disabilities, other handicaps) need reassurance that is individually tailored to their cognitive abilities, communication skills, and other sensory impairments.

Adults in Crisis

A confident and caring nurse who offers both support and information and who engages the patient in rational thought or healthy diversion will minimize the negative effects of ruminating on the crisis event.

After gathering information with the use of a detailed crisis-focused assessment, the nurse explores the patient's interpretation or perception of events and, to the extent possible, identifies the patient's current and past coping skills and abilities to encourage adaptive strategies. Nurses reinforce strategies that the patient previously used and found to be successful. External stressors require physical needs to be met first, such as a place to live, safety from a perpetrator, and child care. Nurses need to target planning with regard to specific functional abilities and disabilities as well as general disturbances in mood and with the use of supportive and cognitive behavioral approaches. The discussion of a set number of sessions with the patient provides further focus for the planned interventions and emphasizes that therapy is time limited rather than open ended. This phase of intervention provides an opportunity for the patient to learn new skills and to experience growth.

Nurses review and discuss maladaptive strategies (e.g., excessive sleep, isolation, overeating, substance abuse) with the patient to explore their relative benefits and possible negative consequences. The nurse needs to support the patient with nonpunitive and noncritical approaches that assist the individual to see a cause-and-effect relationship between the stressor and the response. What is obvious to others outside of the crisis is not always obvious to the person who is experiencing the crisis. Expect ambivalence or resistance as a normal part of therapy, because therapy is an implied demand for a personal change that is upsetting, frightening, or too challenging at the time (see the Case Study).

Providing resources that will enhance the patient's ongoing recovery process is an essential component of crisis intervention. The nurse is able to offer a wide array of community resources, such as those that provide safety assessments of the home or interpersonal environment, situational supports, and assistance with activities of daily living. Online resources can be of significant assistance as well. Significant others also provide comfort by offering unconditional positive regard, and they help the affected person to preserve or regain self-esteem that was threatened or decreased as a result of the loss of control.

RESOLUTION OF THE CRISIS

The Summary

During the final stage of brief crisis therapy, the nurse helps the patient to summarize changes and to describe the increased effectiveness of coping abilities and positive outcomes. This allows the patient to reevaluate and reconfirm the progress that has been made. If the initial assessment tools measured aspects of the patient's functioning, the nurse may readminister these tools to measure progress. The nurse makes every effort to engage the patient in this process rather than merely summarizing the therapeutic events. When the patient actively participates and willingly engages in the summary procedure rather than passively listening to the nurse, the resolution process becomes more meaningful.

Open Connection

The nurse assists the patient as needed with the making of realistic plans for the future. There is a discussion of ways in which the present experience helps the patient to cope with future crises. When terminating therapy, the nurse ensures that the patient understands that, although not all of the conflicts or problems have been resolved, substantial success has led to overcoming the present crisis, and work continues when therapy ends. If additional problems that require attention are revealed during brief crisis therapy, the nurse makes any necessary referrals to address those needs.

Anticipatory Planning

Before the termination of therapy, the nurse asks the patient what the patient would do if this or a similar event occurred in the future. This is a time for the patient to reiterate what he or she has learned during the therapeutic process and to hypothetically plan and rehearse the resolving of future events. A reinforcement of primary prevention strategies, as

---

CASE STUDY

J.B. is a 37-year-old mother of two sons who are 4 and 8 years old; the younger son is autistic. Her husband has been diagnosed with cancer, and he is currently undergoing chemotherapy. He is not tolerating treatment well, and he is often physically ill. J.B. presents at the clinic requesting medication for her "nerves and insomnia." She is a new patient with no previous history of depression or anxiety. J.B. states she is having difficulty controlling her emotions and that she easily becomes tearful, frustrated, and angry with her husband and children over "small things." In addition, she reports difficulty concentrating, a 15-pound weight loss in 6 weeks, and increased distractibility. She denies the use of alcohol or drugs. Her husband is no longer able to work, the bills are accumulating, and the family is having difficulty receiving insurance reimbursement for her husband's care. Recently her autistic son had a temper tantrum in a grocery store, and a customer commented that she needed to keep the child under control. J.B.

states that she ran from the store and sat in the car crying until she was able to drive. She feels guilty that she is "unable to care for her children and make her husband's dying days pleasant." Although she states that she does not want her husband to die, she admits she will "be glad when it's over." She was having passive suicidal thoughts of running off the freeway while driving, but she said she would not really do that because of her children and her husband.

Critical Thinking

1. What are J.B.'s presenting problems, from her perception? How do they compare with her functional disabilities?
2. What survival and safety issues need to be addressed?
3. What are the priority needs for J.B. and her family? What therapeutic approaches will help?
4. What future planning needs to be addressed?

discussed previously in this chapter, is also helpful to review and reinforce at this juncture.

BARRIERS TO EFFECTIVE CRISIS INTERVENTION OR RESOLUTION

Failure to Learn from Experience

Patients often find themselves in a pattern of repeated similar crisis situations. In part, repeated mistakes result from learning to expect failure on the basis of one's prior experiences or the expectancy of no control. This is sometimes referred to as *learned helplessness,* and it is based on the seminal work of Abramson and colleagues (1978). The learning of new behaviors often takes strong motivation, an ability to think logically about the problem, tolerance for change (flexibility), willingness to change, and, most importantly, confidence or hope. More than 25 years after the publication of the original "learned helplessness" work, one of the authors, Seligman, identified the concept of "learned optimism" (Seligman, 2006), which includes strategies for helping patients to learn positive and hopeful thought patterns and behaviors, which are the ultimate determinants of successful crisis resolution.

Existing Mental Disorders

Toward the extreme end of a crisis continuum is a psychiatric emergency. This condition poses an immediate threat to safety, and it sometimes requires hospitalization, medications (antianxiety or antipsychotic), a sufficient period of time for the severe distress to subside, and crisis intervention techniques to deescalate the situation. Persons with cognitive impairments that result from major mental disorders, disability, traumatic injury, or substance intoxication often perceive reality in a distorted fashion. They frequently have greater difficulty resolving a crisis because of an impaired ability to think clearly or an inability to use executive functions (e.g., logic, reasoning, judgment) to control their behaviors. The challenge for the nurse is to maximize the patient's ability to think clearly and calmly, given the patient's limitations, before engaging in problem-solving activities.

For crisis nurses, it is important to avoid compounding an emergency by creating further trauma whenever possible. When a crisis reaches the level of requiring restrictive interventions (e.g., physical or chemical restraints, locked-door seclusion), an additional crisis exists for the patient. Some patients will perceive that the medical system has taken them hostage (Mason, 2000). The careful and adequate training of staff in the art of de-escalation and the use of the least restrictive means to maintain safety when needed reduces the potential psychologic and physical trauma to both the patient and staff and promotes the patient's sense of safety.

Secondary Gain

Secondary gain occurs when the patient uses a crisis or illness for additional personal reasons or reward, such as punishing a partner, obtaining drugs to maintain a drug habit, avoiding jail, or obtaining a letter of disability. The crisis-focused nursing assessment and a detailed history provide important clues to issues of secondary gain. For example, a dependent person or a person with histrionic or borderline traits whose partner often ignores him or her will possibly learn to gain sympathy and attention by acting out in an extreme way, such as with a suicide attempt or gesture. Patients create these types of dramatic situations or create crises, whether consciously or unconsciously, to manipulate another person or situation. In these cases, the patient responds to effective interventions in hostile or defeating ways. These competing motivations are not always immediately obvious to the therapist, but they become evident when some time has passed and when progress in therapy is unusually slow or ineffective. Typically, brief crisis therapy does not directly address these issues because of its time constraints. With adequate motivation and skilled, longer-term therapy, the nurse helps the patient to associate the crisis-seeking behavior with hidden desires or needs and then guides the patient to learn and practice more adaptive ways of meeting those needs.

Therapist-Patient Boundary Problems

Overidentification or countertransference is a reaction to the patient that originates with the therapist. Nurses who are exposed to patients' stressors that remind them of their own problems may be less effective when assessing and treating those patients with similar situations. In this event, the boundaries and roles of the patient and the nurse become unclear. The nurse is to remain realistic when working with patients who are experiencing difficult situations. The nurse maintains his or her identity while also expressing genuine concern for the patient's problem (Aguilera, 1998).

In addition to overidentification and countertransference, a nurse who is exposed to mass trauma is at risk for PTSD, depression, and other psychiatric conditions. Those who are the first to respond to disasters are among the most vulnerable to emotional dysfunction and substance use disorders, according to the Substance Abuse and Mental Health Services Administration (Goodman, 2000). Close observation is necessary to ensure safeguards for the welfare of responders to all types of crisis situations. Rest, support, peer supervision, and debriefing are essential elements for crisis workers in intervention areas, as discussed later in this chapter.

Sociocultural Considerations

A lack of economic resources, unemployment, a lack of health insurance, and limited access to health care services are all barriers to effective crisis intervention, because these conditions prevent access to primary, secondary, and tertiary prevention services. For example, in the absence of access to health promotion programs for stress reduction or crisis prevention, a crisis is more likely to occur, and it is likely to worsen without access to intervention. Unnecessary emergency department visits and hospitalizations for crises are often the result; these could often be avoided by early access to effective crisis intervention, which should occur when patients are beginning to destabilize. In addition, as a result of health care disparities in the United States, many racial and ethnic minorities and persons of lower socioeconomic status are less likely to receive screening and treatment for health problems, including mental health care and crisis intervention (U.S. Department of Health and Human Services, 1999).

Patients may also perceive barriers to needed crisis intervention services caused by language or communication difficulties, culturally held beliefs that lead to the mistrust of the formal health care system, or the perception of a crisis as a culturally familiar or "normal" occurrence. This may result in the presentation of a patient in a full-blown crisis state at a later and less treatable stage of dysfunction. A lack of culturally competent crisis intervention programs is a common barrier to the service of those in crisis. For example, clinical environments that are not compatible with or respectful of the cultures of racial and ethnic minorities often deter minorities from using crisis intervention services and from receiving effective care.

Nurses and other caregivers often have their own biases, cultural unawareness, or personal beliefs that can act as barriers to effective crisis intervention. Such barriers often distort their perceptions of the individual in crisis, influence the assessment data that they focus on, or limit their inventory of helping strategies. For example, if a nurse has been victimized by a spouse or a domestic partner, it may be difficult—at best—for that nurse to help an abuser who presents in crisis in the emergency department. If a nurse misperceives a patient with a language barrier or a certain physical appearance as not being intelligent, that nurse might unintentionally limit the information or teaching provided regarding crisis prevention and intervention strategies. To overcome their own barriers to the provision of effective crisis intervention, nurses must recognize their own biases, beliefs, and sensitivities that might distort their perceptions and limit their effectiveness as crisis helpers. Seeking counsel, training, and support to prevent those biases from influencing the care that they provide to those in crisis is critical to nurses removing their own barriers to the provision of effective crisis intervention services.

DEMANDS ON THE PSYCHIATRIC NURSE WORKING IN CRISIS

The crisis nurse needs the ability and skill to rapidly and effectively gather data about the patient in crisis, to complete a crisis-focused assessment, and to identify goals and interventions for crisis treatment. The demands on the nurse who is working with individuals and families in crisis are often emotionally challenging and potentially overwhelming.

Nurses need to continually assess their own personal feelings and internal responses when working with individuals in crisis so that they can be fully present to the patient's needs. For example, if the nurse is experiencing a heightened level of anxiety or distress in a particular patient situation, the nurse may unintentionally limit that patient's expression of his or her own anxiety or distress to reduce the anxiety or distress level of the nurse. Alternatively, if working with a particular patient triggers memories of a painful life experience that the nurse has personally experienced, an awareness

of how this might influence the nurse in establishing healthy boundaries is essential; asking a colleague to provide respite or relief or even to assume the total care of that patient may facilitate patient care and provide an opportunity for the nurse to process uncomfortable or painful personal issues.

Nurses who are working in disaster situations can experience psychologic trauma as a result of witnessing the mass destruction of homes and property, a catastrophic loss of life, traumatic injuries, horrific violence, or an overwhelming natural disaster such as a hurricane, fire, or earthquake. Debriefing is critical for both patients and health care staff to place the crisis in perspective (Everly et al, 2000). Debriefing is a process that is aimed at reducing psychologic harm, trauma, and the potential development of PTSD by helping people to process their experiences and allowing them to discuss their issues in a nonjudgmental and safe environment. Everly describes the use of both *critical incident debriefing* and *critical incident stress management* during crisis intervention.

Signs and symptoms of critical incident stress include the following:
- Physical: fatigue, sleep disturbance, headache, dizziness, elevated blood pressure, rapid heart rate, muscle tension or tremors, nausea, chest pain, shortness of breath, grinding of teeth, and changes in appetite
- Cognitive: difficulty focusing or concentrating, trouble making decisions or problem solving, negative thought patterns, flashbacks, intrusive thoughts, nightmares, and altered awareness of surroundings
- Emotional: anxiety, grief, anger, irritability, depression, panic attacks, guilt, hopelessness, psychologic numbness, decreased stress tolerance, failure of usual coping strategies, and difficulty regulating emotional responses
- Behavioral: withdrawal, restlessness, changes in social activity, changes in speech patterns, alterations in awareness of surroundings (i.e., increased or decreased awareness or distortions), suspiciousness, use of recreational substances, and engaging in high-risk behavior

The recognition of symptoms such as these is vital to helping crisis nurses to secure the help that is needed to adequately care for themselves. Accessing employee assistance program services to sort through symptoms of critical incident stress can help greatly with the identification of the need for ongoing professional assistance.

Crisis nurses can cope with the stress, fatigue, and trauma that they experience by integrating self-care strategies into their daily practice and by building healthy habits to nurture themselves. Simple strategies can go a long way in the provision of self-care for the crisis nurse. Some of these include the following:
- *Talking it out.* Find a trusted other to share your feelings with and who will allow you to get your fears and frustrations off your chest. A trusted other may be a peer, a friend, a family member, or a therapist. Employee assistance services can be very useful. Expressing your feelings will help you to diffuse symptoms and to regain focus and clarity. Remember to be mindful of healthy boundaries when

choosing with whom you share your feelings so that patient confidentiality is maintained.

- *Setting limits.* Learning to say "no" is a challenge for many professional helpers, including nurses. Having the motivation to care for others in crisis can also precipitate a crisis for the nurse who has trouble setting limits with regard to taking on more than is possible or healthy. Setting limits for our physical, cognitive, and emotional availability can prevent burnout and actually result in making us more available not only for ourselves but for our friends, our family, and our patients.

- *Nurturing relationships.* Nurses who work in crisis settings—like many other nurses—often work variable shifts, overtime, weekends, and holidays. Time away from friends, family, and one's social support system can deplete emotional resources. Strengthening relationships with coworkers and colleagues can also help to support crisis nurses in the work that they do daily, and it can build cohesive teams that can help and support each other. Maintaining meaningful relationships both at work and at home can support crisis nurses in both their personal and professional lives.

- *Developing positive stress management habits.* Nurses need to find meaningful ways to manage daily stressors so that they can "recharge," both physically and psychologically. Practicing yoga, performing relaxation techniques, listening to relaxing music, getting regular physical exercise, and obtaining adequate rest and nutrition are strategies that nurses often suggest to their patients but that they may have difficulty practicing themselves. Developing healthy conflict resolution habits, especially in the workplace, can help to diffuse cumulative work-related stress between and among coworkers. Taking breaks while at work as well as away from work—for a retreat, a mini vacation, or a more extended time away—can also be restorative, return a sense of fulfillment, and improve productivity and work satisfaction.

- *Recruiting a mentor.* Forming a developmental relationship with a more experienced crisis practitioner can help a less experienced crisis practitioner learn valuable survival skills for ongoing work in the specialty of crisis nursing. Being a mentor can help sustain and retain experienced crisis nurses who also benefit from the professional fulfillment of sharing expertise and providing support to others. A mentor helps to shape the development of the mentee by helping the mentee to build confidence through the multiple challenges of crisis nursing by providing guidance, coaching, and acceptance. Learning is encouraged as much from mistakes as from successes with the provision of constructive feedback.

- *Cultivating a sense of humor.* Humor can be one of the most adaptive and powerful strategies to help provide perspective through crisis as well as for the professional who is working with individuals in crisis. Humor has been shown consistently to relieve tension and stress, to help people bond, to provide perspective, and to foster hope and optimism. For individuals who are directly affected by crisis, the sensitive use of humor can help to lift the emotional and psychologic burden of the crisis (Sultanoff, 1995), and it can also help crisis nurses to deal with their own process of debriefing. Humor can help nurses who are working in crisis to detach from the trauma for even a few moments, give them a brief respite from emotional chaos, and role model how patients in crisis can do likewise. Humor helps all of us to bear the unbearable.

Prevention Strategies

Within the context of a public health model, the perspective of prevention emerges, and nursing strategies for crisis interventions may be viewed as prevention measures. This model also focuses on the level of population health rather than individual health, which is often relevant to a crisis that influences a community or a selected population (e.g., a disaster). Crisis intervention nursing techniques can be categorized as primary, secondary, or tertiary prevention strategies (Clark, 2008). These categories help with the refining of nursing assessment efforts, the setting of realistic goals, the identification of the most effective intervention strategies, and the evaluation and measurement of outcomes.

- *Primary prevention.* Primary prevention efforts work toward avoiding the development of a crisis. In this case, primary prevention efforts promote mental health, improve coping skills and stress management, and hopefully decrease or prevent crises from occurring. At the primary prevention level, the nurse works in partnership with the individual or family to identify potential problems, stressors, and life events that may lead to crisis so that action can be taken to prevent escalation to a crisis situation. A review of problem-solving strategies, coping skills, decision-making models, advocacy skills, mediation and conflict-resolution skills, and alternative dispute resolution strategies are some examples of primary prevention strategies that assist with the management of stressful life events before a crisis occurs. By preventing crisis from occurring, nurses can support individuals and families through life changes and transitions that produce stress by planning necessary steps ahead of time, controlling the timing and pacing of changes, mobilizing help and assistance, and modifying and reevaluating planned change as needed.

- *Secondary prevention.* Secondary prevention efforts are aimed at the early detection of a crisis, thereby increasing opportunities for interventions to prevent the progression of symptoms and the worsening of the crisis. At this level of prevention, the nurse focuses on the priority of safety for the patient and screens the patient for symptoms of crisis as well as for domestic violence, child abuse or neglect, substance abuse, legal offenses, or access to weapons. The nurse then works with the patient to identify crisis intervention strategies and goals for crisis resolution. In addition, secondary prevention during a crisis lessens the intensity of mental distress and disability during a crisis, and it can be provided across settings such as emergency departments, hospitals, mental health centers, clinics, and shelters as well as in the field.

- *Tertiary prevention.* Tertiary prevention reduces the negative impact of a crisis that has already occurred by restoring function and reducing crisis-related complications such as PTSD. The goals of this level of prevention are to facilitate optimal levels of functioning for the individual or family who has experienced crisis and to prevent further crisis-related problems from occurring. Individuals with chronic mental illness, addictions, and multiple losses or life stressors are particularly vulnerable to problems after a crisis, and they often require intense tertiary prevention strategies to regain their optimal level of functioning and to prevent the exacerbation of their often chronic symptoms.

Technology and Future Trends in Crisis Intervention

The 21st century has brought with it diverse new ways to deliver crisis intervention services, to access resources, and to communicate during crisis.

Crisis hotlines have existed in most major U.S. cities since the mid 1970s. A crisis hotline is a phone number that offers callers access to immediate telephonic emergency counseling, and it is usually staffed by trained volunteers 24 hours a day and 7 days a week. Crisis hotlines were originally started to deliver immediately accessible crisis intervention services to suicidal individuals and their friends, family, and concerned others; they have expanded in diverse ways over the years with regard to content, scope, and format. Current crisis hotlines provide crisis response services for situations that include suicide, domestic violence, rape or sexual assault, child abuse, missing and exploited children, drug and alcohol treatment, sexually transmitted disease, human immunodeficiency virus and acquired immunodeficiency syndrome, runaways, eating disorders, panic disorders, gay and lesbian issues, legal assistance, natural disaster relief, and emergency disaster services (U.S. Department of Health and Human Services, 2008). The strength of such hotlines is that they provide immediate and free personal contact with a trained counselor, with the aim of managing acute stressors and identifying coping strategies; this can be particularly helpful to a person who is in crisis. Referrals to local resources (e.g., treatment centers, shelters, counseling services) are also provided, and these include available resources for individuals without health insurance.

Online chat rooms, support groups, forums, mailing lists, message boards, blogs, newsgroups, social networking sites, and instant messaging programs now provide options for crisis intervention services 24 hours a day and 7 days a week. Such online options provide an opportunity for individuals in crisis to form supportive relationships with others in the online community who have experienced similar crises and experiences and who can share self-help strategies, resources, and community referral options (see the Online Resources at the end of this chapter).

Video calls with the use of programs such as Skype add another possible alternative for the provision of crisis intervention services and communications when a live conversation is desired, when the need to transmit visual information exists, or when individuals are in different geographic locations. Hearing impaired individuals may particularly benefit from access to low-cost or free high-quality video call options as a means of communicating with each other in sign language during a crisis. Video conferencing, which allows individuals or groups at two or more locations to communicate via live and simultaneous two-way video and audio transmissions, can help health care providers in crisis situations to collaborate regarding disaster plans, to identify needs for crisis intervention services, and to identify strategies for pooling resources across large distances. This can be especially helpful during crises such as natural disasters in rural or impoverished areas, where limited access to health care services existed even before the crisis event.

The availability of alternative vehicles for crisis counseling with experienced therapists and counselors has grown steadily during recent years. This is a growing trend that will likely shape the future of service delivery options for crisis intervention.

Other growing trends include *mobile crisis services* and in-home crisis counseling services for children and families. The goals are to assist the family with coping, to reduce crisis incidents, and to retain the child in the home, when possible. Mobile crisis services may involve in-home services, but they also include other services that are being increasingly used to improve access to crisis services. Mobile crisis services bring crisis intervention services directly to the community in the form of direct mental health services, case management, medication support, and other comprehensive services in an effort to ameliorate crisis situations, to decrease the unnecessary use of psychiatric emergency department services, or to facilitate admissions to acute psychiatric hospitals.

Resilience and Posttraumatic Growth

The capacity of human beings to cope with crisis and catastrophe in ways that are positive and that allow them to "bounce back" to homeostasis and balance is referred to as *resilience* (Masten, 2009). Resilience, which comes from the Latin *resiliens* ("to rebound or recoil"), is a dynamic process during which individuals exhibit positive coping and behavioral adaptation when faced with crisis, adversity, and trauma (Luthar et al, 2000). In science, the term *resilience* refers to the capacity of a substance to change its shape in response to a force applied to it and then recover. Through the emotional distress experienced during crises such as tragedy, loss, and trauma, resilience emerges, and it often leaves individuals stronger as a result. Some individuals have extraordinary resilience while others are not as hardy.

It is important for nurses who are working with patients in crisis to know that resilience is not a trait that people simply have or do not have; rather, it is a pattern of behaviors, thoughts, and attitudes that nurses can help patients in crisis to learn and develop. The American Psychological Association (2010) offers several strategies that can be used to help patients build resilience in the wake of crises, including the following:

1. Build social support. Helping patients to nurture relationships with friends, family, and community members that can be counted on for support and assistance during times of crisis can help them to build resilience. Those who can turn to others in the community—whether those others are family, caring community volunteers, or members of a faith-based community—build resilience to adapt to present and future crises.

2. Avoid seeing crises as insurmountable. Patients who cannot change the stressful events that they have experienced can be helped to learn that they can change how they interpret these events and how they respond to such event. Cognitive behavioral therapy techniques can be used to "reframe" a patient's negative beliefs about stressful events and to help him or her to identify areas in which he or she still has control and empowerment.

3. Accept change as part of life. Whether working with patients who have experienced an "everyday" crisis or those who have gone through a catastrophic disaster, certain life goals may no longer be attainable as a result of adverse situations. Helping patients to acknowledge their losses, to grieve them, and to accept circumstances that cannot be changed can help them to focus on circumstances that are within their power to control and change. Change—however unexpected or unwelcome—does not equal powerlessness.

4. Identify goals and take action steps toward accomplishing them. The more that patients can be helped to take action during crisis by identifying goals that are meaningful to them (followed by taking action steps toward achieving those goals), the more resilience they can build. Although outside supports—including professional help—are vital in many crisis situations, helping patients to use these resources to be actively involved in their own crisis intervention plan will build their resilience and empowerment for current and future crises.

5. Cultivate insight and self-awareness. Brief crisis intervention approaches focus on helping patients to build insight and self-awareness, including a positive view of the self. Helping patients in crisis to identify what they have learned about themselves as a result of their journey through a crisis event as well as the skills that they have developed as a result will help to foster an increased sense of self-worth, strength, and resilience. Helping patients to keep things in perspective by learning to view the crisis in a broader context can help them to maintain a hopeful outlook when it is a challenge to see the big picture. Self-care strategies, spiritual support, faith-based practices, and other practices to strengthen the individual and enhance coping can all help to build resilience.

The general belief that crisis and distress can potentially yield positive change is thousands of years old. The term *posttraumatic growth* refers to changes that surpass resilience, and it refers to movement beyond the precrisis levels of adaptation (Tedeschi and Calhoun, 1995 and 2004). Research interest in posttraumatic growth gained considerable strength during the 1990s, which resulted in the building of evidence that individuals facing a wide variety of crises, traumas, and life changes often grow substantially through the struggle with the new reality that exists in the aftermath of such events. This supports the ideas that both personal distress and personal growth can coexist and that improved psychologic health rather than psychopathology is often the result (Tedeschi and Calhoun, 1995 and 2004). The Posttraumatic Growth Inventory (Tedeschi and Calhoun, 1996) is an instrument for assessing the positive outcomes reported by persons who have experienced traumatic events; it includes a 21-item scale that measures factors such as new possibilities, relating to others, personal strength, spiritual change, and appreciation of life.

When working with individuals in crisis, nurses can instill hope by focusing on the innate human capacity to grow and flourish even under the most difficult life circumstances, and they can help patients to integrate what they have learned during the crisis into their own life story. Helping patients to simultaneously embrace both loss and growth may ultimately be the most critical and rewarding aspect of crisis nursing.

CHAPTER SUMMARY

- The challenges posed by today's crises require considerable planning, focus, and resources, especially when addressing the biopsychosocial–spiritual problems that occur after a large-scale crisis.
- Crisis intervention strategies focus on identifying an immediate precipitant, evaluating the patient's personal safety, enhancing positive coping skills to reestablish emotional equilibrium, and planning for the future. Encouraging patients to be hopeful and to build resilience is an essential aspect of effective therapy.
- Children, frail and elderly individuals, those of lower socioeconomic status, and those with preexisting mental disorders are more vulnerable to crisis and postcrisis problems. Early intervention and referral for these high-risk groups will likely lessen the amount and severity of symptoms that may be seen at a later time.
- Psychiatric mental health nurses who work in the community are especially in demand during catastrophic situations such as fires, floods, earthquakes, and acts of terrorism for those individuals who have been traumatized by the event itself and for those who have lost significant others in the tragedy. Crisis nurses and first responders are at the greatest risk for psychiatric problems themselves after these traumas, and planning for the care of caregivers is a priority for agencies that provide crisis services to the community.

REVIEW QUESTIONS

1. A category 5 tornado hits a small Midwestern town and causes the major destruction of homes and buildings. Many fatalities occur. Place in sequence the psychologic stages that the people of this community will experience.
   1. Disillusionment phase
   2. Heroic phase
   3. Honeymoon phase
   4. Reconstruction phase

2. A nurse who is on vacation comes upon a severe automobile accident. The driver emerges from the car without apparent physical injuries. Which behaviors would be expected from the driver immediately after this traumatic event? You may select more than one answer.
   1. Urinary or fecal incontinence
   2. Long-term memory loss
   3. Inability to recall the spouse's phone number
   4. Difficulty finding a driver's license
   5. Diaphoresis and trembling

3. An adult who was recently diagnosed with multiple sclerosis says, "I'm worried that I won't be able to support my family or send my children to college." This person begins drinking alcohol heavily and omitting prescribed medications. Select the correct analysis of the patient's condition.
   1. The patient is in a state of situational crisis.
   2. The patient is in a state of equilibrium.
   3. The patient is reflecting on the situational event.
   4. The patient is perceiving the event in a distorted way.

4. A parent seeks counseling after the rape and murder of a child. The parent tearfully says, "I hate the man who did this. He's being tried for the murder, but I don't know what I will do if he's not found guilty." What is the nurse's highest priority response?
   1. "Have you talked to a psychiatrist about taking some medication to help you cope?"
   2. "Do you have enough support from your family and friends?"
   3. "What resources do you need to help you cope with this situation?"
   4. "Are you thinking of killing yourself or the man who killed your child?"

5. After a major hurricane destroys a community, which statement best indicates that an individual is likely to maintain or promptly return to a state of equilibrium?
   1. "This storm wasn't so bad. It could have killed more people or destroyed the water and sewer lines."
   2. "I've been through big storms before. If we pull together, we can help each other and rebuild our community."
   3. "When my parent died 8 years ago, I got so depressed I was unable to care for my children or return to work."
   4. "I think we'll be fine. We're getting plenty of support and assistance from other communities."

6. The capacity of human beings to cope with crisis and catastrophe in ways that are positive and that allow them to "bounce back" to a balanced state after the crisis is referred to as which of the following?
   1. Resilience
   2. Homeostasis
   3. Adaptive crisis response
   4. Equilibrium

REFERENCES

Abramovitz R: *Guidelines for helping children cope with crises,* 2001 (website): www.naswnyc.org/index.html. Accessed June 1, 2010.

Abramson L et al: Learned helplessness in humans: critique and reformulation, *J Abnormal Psychol* 87(1):49-74, 1978.

Aguilera DC: *Crisis intervention: theory and methodology,* ed 8, St. Louis, 1998, Mosby.

Aguilera DC, Mesnick J: *Crisis intervention: theory and methodology,* St. Louis, 1970, 1982, Mosby.

American Psychiatric Association: *Diagnostic and statistical manual of mental disorders,* ed 4, text revision, Washington, DC, 2000, American Psychiatric Association.

American Psychological Association: *Ten ways to build resilience,* 2010 (website): http://search.apa.org/search?query=resilience. Accessed May 1, 2010.

Auerbach S, Kilmann P: Crisis intervention: a review of outcome research, *Psychol Bull* 84:1189-1217, 1997.

Caplan G: *Principles of preventive psychiatry,* New York, 1964, Basic Books.

Clark MJ: *Community health nursing: advocacy for population health,* ed 5, Upper Saddle River, NJ, 2008, Pearson Education.

Dane S, editor: Facing the unexpected: disaster preparedness and response in the United States, *Natural Hazards Observer* (26): 1-24, 2001.

Deepwater Horizon Oil Spill: NOAA assessment and restoration: http://www.gulfspillrestoration.noaa.gov/. Accessed June 12, 2010.

Everly G: Crisis management briefing(s) (CMB): large group crisis intervention in response to terrorism, disasters, and violence, *Int J Emerg Ment Health* 2:53-75, 2000.

Everly G et al: Innovations in group crisis intervention: critical incident debriefing (CISD) and critical incident stress management (CISM). In Roberts AR, editor: *Crisis interventions handbook: assessment, treatment, and research,* ed 2, pp. 77-100, New York, 2000, Oxford University Press.

Everly G, Mitchell JT: *Critical incident stress management (CISM): a new era and standard of care in crisis intervention,* ed 2, Ellicott City, Md, 1999, Chevron.

Federal Emergency Management Agency: *FEMA history*, 2009 (website): www.fema.gov/about/history.shtm. Accessed June 23, 2010.

Flannery RB, Everly GS Jr: Crisis intervention: a review, *Int J Emerg Ment Health* 2:119-125, 2000.

Foundation For Child Development: *The 2010 Child and Youth Well-Being Index (CWI). Impact of recession on children to reach new lows in 2010*, New York, 2010, Foundation for Child Development.

Friedman M: *Posttraumatic stress disorder: an overview*, A National Center for PTSD fact sheet, 2005 (website): www.ptsd.va.gov. Date Accessed: June 10, 2010.

Gentry CE: *Crisis intervention in child abuse and neglect*, 1994, U.S. Department of Health and Human Services.

Goodman D: *Responding to terrorism: recovery, resilience, readiness, and readiness, SAMHSA News*, Rockville, Md, 2000, Offices of Communication, & Public Liaison, U.S. Department of Health and Human Services.

James K: *Crisis intervention strategies*, ed 6, Florence Ky, 2008, Thompson Brooks/Cole.

Landesman LY: *Public health management of disasters: the practice guide*, ed 2, Washington, DC, 2005, American Public Health Association.

Langan J, James D: *Preparing nurses for disaster management*, Upper Saddle River, NJ, Pearson Prentice Hall, 2005.

Lange S: *Managing the psychiatric crisis*, National Center of Continuing Education, online course #3025 or #9025 2005 (website): www.nursece.com/onlinecourses/9025.html. Accessed June 20, 2010.

Lerner M: An overview of acute traumatic stress management, *Trauma Response* 8:3-5, 2002.

Lerner M, Shelton R: *Acute traumatic stress management*, 2005, The American Academy of Experts in Traumatic Stress.

Lindemann E: Symptomatology and management of acute grief, *Am J Psychiatry* 101:141-148, 1944.

Lowry JL, Lating J: Reflections on the response to mass terrorist attacks: an elaboration on Everly and Mitchell's 10 commandments, *Brief Treatment and Crisis Intervention* 2(1):95-104, 2002.

Luthar S et al: The construct of resilience: a critical evaluation and guidelines for future work, *Child Dev* 71(3):543-562, 2000.

Maslow A: A theory of human motivation, *Psychol Rev* 50(4): 370-396, 1943.

Mason T: Managing protest behavior: from coercion to compassion, *J Psychiatr Ment Health Nurs* 7:269-275, 2000.

Masten A: Ordinary magic: lessons from research on resilience in human development, *Education Canada* 49(3):28-32, 2009.

Parry ML et al, editors: *Climate change 2007: impacts, adaptation, and vulnerability: contribution of Working Group II to the fourth assessment report of the Intergovernmental Panel on Climate Change*, New York, 2007, Cambridge University Press.

Perry B: *Principles of working with traumatized children*, 2010 (website): http://teacher.scholastic.com/professional/bruceperry/working_children.htm. Accessed June 10, 2010.

Rapoport L: The state of crisis: some theoretical considerations, *Soc Serv Rev* 36(2):211-217, 1962.

Rhoades J et al: Posttraumatic stress disorder: after Hurricane Katrina, *J Nurse Pract* 2:18-26, 2006.

Roberts AR: Conceptualizing crisis theory and the crisis intervention model. In Roberts AR, editor: *Contemporary perspectives on crisis intervention and prevention*, pp. 3-17, Englewood Cliffs, NJ, 1991, Prentice-Hall.

Roberts AR: Bridging the past and present to the future of crisis intervention and crisis management. In Roberts AR, editor: *Crisis intervention handbook: assessment, treatment, and research*, ed 3, pp. 3-34, New York, 2005, Oxford University Press.

Roberts AR: Assessment, crisis intervention, and trauma treatment: the integrative act intervention model, *Brief Treat Crisis Interv* 2(1):1-22, 2006.

Roberts AR, editor: *Crisis intervention handbook: assessment, treatment, and research*, ed 2, New York, 2000, Oxford University Press.

Roberts AR, Yeager KR: *Pocket guide to crisis intervention*, New York, 2009, Oxford University Press.

Seligman M: *Learned optimism: how to change your mind and your life*, London, 2006, Random House.

Selye H: *The stress of life*, New York, 1978, McGraw-Hill.

Shah A: *Poverty facts and stats*, 2010 (website): www.globalissues.org/article/26/poverty-facts-and-stats. Accessed April 25, 2010.

Sultanoff S: Levity defies gravity: using humor in crisis situations, *Therapeutic Humor* IX(3):1-2, 1995.

Tedeschi R, Calhoun L: *Trauma and transformation: growing in the aftermath of suffering*, Thousand Oaks, Calif, 1995, Sage.

Tedeschi R, Calhoun L: The Posttraumatic Growth Inventory: measuring the positive legacy of trauma, *J Trauma Stress* 9(3), 455-471, 1996.

Tedeschi R, Calhoun L: *Posttraumatic growth: conceptual foundation and empirical evidence*, Philadelphia, 2004, Lawrence Erlbaum Associates.

U.S. Department of Health and Human Services: *Mental health: a report of the Surgeon General*. Rockville, MD, 1999, U.S. Department of Health and Human Services.

U.S. Department of Health and Human Services, Substance Abuse and Mental Health Services Administration: *SAMHSA Health Information Network (SHIN)*, 2008.

U.S. Department of Justice: *Office on Violence Against Women: working together to end the violence [annual report]*, Washington DC, 2006, U.S. Department of Justice.

Velasquez M et al: Psychiatric severity and behavior change in alcoholism: the relation of the transtheoretical model variables to psychiatric distress in dually diagnosed patients, *Addict Behav* 24(4):481-496, 1999.

Venette SJ: *Risk communication in a high reliability organization: APHIS PPQ's inclusion of risk in decision making*, Ann Arbor, Mich, 2003, UMI Proquest Information and Learning.

Walström M: *Earthquakes caused the deadliest disasters in the past decade. United Nations international strategy for disaster reduction.* 2010.

Wollman D: Critical incident stress debriefing and crisis groups: a review of the literature, *Group* 17:70-83, Geneva, Switzerland, 1993, International Strategy for Disaster Reduction.

Online Resources

American Academy of Experts in Traumatic Stress: www.aaets.org
American Nurses Association: www.nursingworld.org
American Psychological Association: www.apa.org
American Red Cross: www.redcross.org
Centers for Disease Control and Prevention: Emergency Preparedness and Response: www.bt.cdc.gov
Child Trauma Academy: www.childtrauma.org
Compassion Fatigue: www.giftfromwithin.org

Crisis Hotlines: www.allaboutcounseling.com/crisis_hotlines.htm
Crisis Intervention and Critical Incident Stress Management: www.drjeffmitchell.com
Crisis Intervention Services: www.grassrootscrisis.org
Federal Emergency Management Agency: www.fema.gov
Humor During Crisis: www.humormatters.com
International Critical Incident Stress Foundation: www.icisf.org
International Society for Traumatic Stress Studies: www.istss.org
Mental Health America: www.nmha.org
National Crisis Hotlines: www.capcsac.org/crisis-national

National Family Resiliency Center, Inc.: www.divorceabc.com
National Institute of Mental Health: www.nimh.nih.gov
Substance Abuse and Mental Health Services Administration: www.samhsa.gov
Suicide Hotlines: www.suicidehotlines.com
Trauma: www.info-trauma.org
The Survivors Club: www.thesurvivorsclub.org
U.S. Department of Energy (National Security): www.energy.gov
U.S. Department of Health and Human Services: www.hhs.gov

Suicide Prevention and Intervention

Pamela E. Marcus

"As anyone who has been close to someone that has committed suicide knows, there is no other pain like that felt after the incident."

Peter Greene

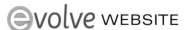 WEBSITE

http://evolve.elsevier.com/Fortinash/

OBJECTIVES

- Analyze the scope of suicide by age, gender, ethnicity, socioeconomic status, and familial factors.
- Compare and contrast biologic, psychologic, and sociologic theories regarding the etiology of suicide.
- Distinguish among suicidal ideation, gesture, threat, attempt, and completed suicide.
- Discuss key elements in the assessment of suicide risk.
- Apply the nursing process to the prevention of suicide for patients and their families.
- Construct a concept map that outlines the nursing care of a patient who has major depression and suicidal ideation.

- Describe the responsibility of mental health professionals to protect patients from self-harm.
- Discuss the use of emergency petition or involuntary inpatient hospitalization to prevent an imminent suicidal gesture.
- Discuss the roles of parents and guardians in the observation of self-destructive clues in youth and in the offering of guidance and assistance.

KEY TERMS

cognitive rigidity	imminence	suicidal ideation
conscious suicidal intention	lethality	suicidology
co-occurrence	perturbation	unconscious suicidal intention

Society has become more complex and stressful for most individuals. Some people express feelings of hopelessness, and say they do not believe that they have a future. Individuals who are unable to cope with the issues that they face often become suicidal. The National Center for Health Statistics ranks suicide as the eleventh cause of death in the United States. On average, one person dies from a suicidal act every 15.2 minutes, with 34,598 individuals completing suicide in 2007. There are approximately 25 people who have attempted suicide in the United States for every completed suicide. Teenagers and preteens have a high risk factor, with suicide ranking as the third cause of death among people in this age group. Elderly individuals who are 80 years old and older have the highest number of completed suicides; the overall number of completed suicides in this age group composed close to 50% of all of the individuals who completed suicide in 2007 in the United States. Caucasian individuals have a higher rate of completed suicide than African Americans. Firearms are the most lethal form of weapons that are used to complete suicide, with 50.2% of all individuals who completed suicide in 2007 doing so with a firearm. Women commonly die from poisoning, such as after an overdose of medication.

Individuals who are divorced, separated, or widowed have the highest rate of suicide completion (American Association of Suicidology, 2010; Conwell, 2009).

To prevent an individual from completing a suicidal act, it is essential that the nurse understand that the thoughts and behaviors that promote suicide vary for each person, and depend on the individual's response to his or her circumstances. A thorough assessment is essential to determine the appropriate intervention and level of care necessary to prevent the person from committing suicide. Interventions aimed at assisting the individual to feel less hopeless are critical during an acute crisis such as a suicidal attempt, gesture, or ideation.

Suicidal thoughts, threats, and attempts often precede a patient's search for mental health treatment. Imminent risk for suicide is one of the leading criteria for the medical care of patients who are admitted to mental health hospitals. Health professionals in all disciplines assist with assessing suicide risk and ensuring that patients receive prompt interventions to provide physical and psychologic safety. Nurses consistently contribute to these efforts because they practice in a variety of settings.

HISTORIC AND THEORETIC PERSPECTIVES

Throughout history, people have turned to suicide as a solution to their disappointments and despair. It was not until the late 1800s that pioneers such as Durkheim and Freud began to study the phenomenon from theoretic perspectives.

Sociologic Theory

In 1897, sociologist Emile Durkheim (1858-1917) first classified the social and cultural aspects of suicide into four subtypes: anomic, egoistic, altruistic, and fatalistic (Durkheim, 1951). He defined anomic suicides as acts of self-destruction by individuals who have become alienated from important relationships in their groups, especially as this relates to their standard of living (e.g., the suicides after the 1929 stock market crash). Durkheim characterized egoistic suicides as the self-inflicted deaths of individuals who turn against their own conscience (e.g., the suicide of a devout Catholic adolescent after she has had an abortion that was forbidden by her religion). Altruistic suicides are self-inflicted deaths on the basis of obedience to a group's goals rather than reflecting the person's own best interests (e.g., the deaths of the terrorist suicide bombers on September 11, 2001). Durkheim defined fatalistic suicides as self-inflicted deaths that result from excessive regulation (e.g., the suicide of a convicted prisoner who hung himself to escape a prolonged period of incarceration).

Psychoanalytic Theory

Freud viewed suicide from a psychoanalytic viewpoint. At the 1910 psychoanalytic meeting about suicide in Vienna, he described *self-destruction* as anger directed inward toward the internalized love object (Freud, 1920; Stekel, 1967). These early formulations ignored other critical feeling states, such as shame, hopelessness, helplessness, worthlessness, and fear. Later Freud incorporated many accompanying psychologic and sociologic clinical features, such as guilt, into his views about suicide (Litman, 1967).

Psychoanalysts who followed Freud had their own theories about suicide. Menninger described several sources of suicidal impulses: the wish to kill, the wish to be killed, and the wish to die. According to Jung, the suicidal person holds an unconscious wish for spiritual rebirth after feeling that life has lost its meaning. Adler identified the importance of inferiority, narcissism (self-absorption), and low self-esteem in suicidal acts. Horney believed that suicide was a solution for someone who is experiencing extreme alienation of the self as a result of a great gap between the idealized self and the perceived psychosocial self.

Interpersonal Theory

Harry Stack Sullivan (1892-1949) broadened the theoretic knowledge base of suicide by emphasizing the importance of interpersonal relationship factors. According to Sullivan, individuals are never isolated from the interactions of significant people in their lives (Sullivan, 1931). Therefore, Sullivan believed that the suicidal act needs to be viewed within the context of the perceptions of the suicidal person by his or her significant others. He viewed suicide as evidence of a failure to resolve interpersonal conflicts (Sullivan, 1956).

ETIOLOGY

Suicidology is the scientific and humane study of suicide. This research began during the early 1960s with the establishment of the Center for Studies of Suicide Prevention established at the National Institute of Mental Health in 1966. The American Association of Suicidology was then founded, in 1967. The *Bulletin of Suicidology,* which is the first professional journal devoted to the study of self-destructive phenomena, began publication in 1967. Since that time, there has been an increase in the number of suicide prevention centers, and there is a national suicide prevention hotline (1-800-273-TALK) that is accredited on the basis of clinical practice guidelines. This hotline provides counseling and crisis intervention for individuals throughout the United States who are suicidal. The American Association of Suicidology sponsors research and clinical competence and presents the findings during its yearly convention; the information is also available on the association's website at www.suicidology.org. Other websites that provide resources for suicide prevention and families who have lost a loved one to suicide are listed at the end of the chapter.

Current research is investigating the steps that a clinician needs to take to prevent an individual from committing suicide. The American Psychiatric Association has established clinical practice guidelines to outline acceptable practices that are based on this research (American Psychiatric Association, 2003). The clinical practice guidelines provide the legal standard of practice for evaluation in court if a patient completes suicide and the therapist or mental health staff is sued for negligence. The principles outlined in the clinical practice guidelines help nurses to provide safe and effective care. Along with these guidelines, one study cited six recurrent problems to consider when providing comprehensive care to patients who express suicidal thoughts (Hendin et al, 2006); these are addressed in the Research for Evidence-Based Practice box.

RESEARCH FOR EVIDENCE-BASED PRACTICE BOX #1

Hendin H et al: Problems in psychotherapy with suicidal patients, *Am J Psychiatry* 163:67–72, 2006.

This research was done to identify areas in which mental health providers can improve when providing care to individuals with imminent suicidal intent. The authors interviewed the therapists of 36 patients who had completed suicide. The therapists completed comprehensive clinical case studies, reported the medications that the patients were taking before death, and presented the patients' treatment histories in an all-day workshop. The authors identified six problem areas that were consistently evident in the therapists' clinical reports of the patients' histories before death:

1 Poor communication with treatment providers involved in the care of the patient
2 Allowing the patient or relatives to control the therapy
3 Avoidance of discussion of issues related to sexuality
4 Ineffective or coercive actions that resulted from the therapist's anxiety as opposed to the patient's clinical presentation
5 Inability to recognize the meaning of the patient's communication
6 Untreated or undertreated symptoms, such as anxiety or alcohol abuse

If the mental health providers assess their ability to address these six recurrent problem areas, there will possibly be a decrease in the completion of suicide among individuals who are receiving psychotherapy.

Biologic Factors

Researchers have studied the structure and chemistry of the brain in relation to affective or mood disorders (see Chapters 6 and 12). Research with adults has found irregularities in the serotonin systems of suicidal patients. In 1994, Nielson and colleagues studied the major metabolite of serotonin, 5-hydroxyindoleacetic acid, which is found in cerebrospinal fluid, in conjunction with the genotype tryptophan hydroxylase. This was the first report to implicate a specific gene in the predisposition to certain antisocial and suicidal behaviors regulated by serotonin (Nielson et al, 1994). Researchers have determined that there are changes in the brain's ability to manufacture and use serotonin. Postmortem studies revealed that the dorsal raphe nucleus in the brainstem sent less than the usual amounts of serotonin to the orbital prefrontal cortex (Ezzell, 2003). A research study that involved the use of a positron emission tomography study of the serotonin function in the brain of individuals who were depressed and who had a history of low-lethal (i.e., less serious) suicidal attempts and of those individuals who made high-lethal (i.e.,

more serious) suicidal attempts showed biologic differences between these two groups. Individuals who are high-lethal suicide attempters have less activity in the ventral, medial, and lateral prefrontal cortex. The individuals with a low lethality were often young and showed an increase in impulsiveness and more activity in the lateral prefrontal cortex. This research also demonstrates that there are alterations in the serotonin transporter binding that indicate serotonin hypofunction, particularly among the individuals with high-lethal suicide attempts (Joiner et al, 2005; Parsey et al, 2006). Joiner and colleagues (2005) examined the biologic aspect of suicidal behavior. They described two general categories that increase risk for suicidal completion: (1) a dysregulation in impulse control; and (2) an experience of intense psychologic pain (e.g., social isolation, hopelessness) felt by the individual with suicidal ideation and attempts. These researchers pointed out that several studies list factors such as major depression, childhood abuse, alcohol dependence, and some anxiety disorders (e.g., social phobia) that increase the risk for suicide. Twin studies demonstrated an increase in the suicide attempt rate for monozygotic twins as compared with dizygotic twins (Joiner et al, 2005). One aspect of the TORDIA study (Treatment of SSRI-Resistant Depression in Adolescents) looked at the relationship between the research participant's genetic makeup and the risk level of suicidal behavior. The researchers found that the genotypes of the individuals with a high risk for suicide had a great degree of glucocorticoid receptor subsensitivity. This result was consistent with other research studies that have linked alterations in the hypothalamic–pituitary–adrenal axis with an increased risk for suicidal thoughts and behaviors (Brent et al, 2010).

Currently there are no medications that specifically affect suicidal behavior. However, medications that regulate serotonin levels are effective for the treatment of mood disorders that often accompany suicidal ideation (see Chapters 12 and 25).

Another psychologic factor is the neurobiologic relationship between depression and suicide. Suicide most frequently occurs when and individual is depressed, and, as depression resolves, suicide risk diminishes. The biologic changes associated with depression relate to alterations in specific areas of the brain (see Chapters 6 and 12):

- *Mood.* Sadness and dysphoria are associated with limbic lesions that can be moderated with dopamine.
- *Affect.* Separate motor systems of the limbic and brainstem regions of the brain influence the control of the face and facial expressions as well as the muscular responses associated with emotional affect (e.g., crying).
- *Motivation.* Changes in the pleasure response, which is moderated by dopamine and dopamine antagonists, have an effect on motivational levels.
- *Cognitive content.* Researchers believe that frontal lobe dysfunction is related to feelings of hopelessness and worthlessness, both of which are signs of suicidal thoughts.

The explosion of knowledge in psychobiology requires that nurses integrate the psychophysiologic aspects of illness with the behavioral sciences in their own nursing practice.

Psychologic Factors

Intrapsychologic and interpersonal theories continue to dominate the psychologic view of suicidal behavior. Contemporary etiologies include the following:

- Self-directed aggression or self-destruction as an act of murder directed at the love object, which leads to states of isolation and loneliness
- Death as atonement for wrongdoings
- Death as a way to recapture the lost love object
- Suicidal death as a secondary result of the major depressive processes
- Suicidal ideation and parasuicidal behavior that result from abandonment anxiety

Most psychodynamic theorists after Freud have theorized that depression follows the loss of a significant love object and leads to feelings of helplessness, hopelessness, guilt, and diminished self-esteem. Suicide serves as a way to end those painful feeling states. This model emphasizes the functioning of the psyche and the reporting of subjective experiences.

Cognitive theory adds to the understanding of suicidal episodes by emphasizing the role of particular thought patterns, such as negativism, self-worthlessness, and a bleak view of the future Some have hypothesized that *cognitive rigidity*, which is the inability to identify problems and solutions, is a factor in suicide when it is accompanied by stress. (see Chapter 26), Edwin S. Shneidman (1918-2009) developed the term *perturbation*, which is a determination of an individual's level of distress and rated on a scale of 1 to 9. Perturbation refers to how upset, disturbed, or perturbed the individual is. Shneidman, building on his 35 years of work as a suicidologist, lectured about the common psychologic features of suicide. He defined suicide as a "response to an inner decision that the pain is unendurable, intolerable, and unacceptable. It is an unwillingness to endure that pain rather than the pain itself" (Shneidman, 1985).

It is important to understand feelings of abandonment and abandonment anxiety to prevent suicidal gestures among patients with interpersonal disturbances, especially among those individuals with borderline personality disorder (Linehan, 1993; Masterson, 1976) (see Chapter 14).

In addition, the development of behavioral approaches that are based on learning theory contributed to the understanding and treatment of mental health problems. Interventions for suicidal ideation that are based on learning theory are directed toward decreasing unpleasant events and increasing pleasant events. Tension-reducing mindfulness meditation, relaxation techniques, stress-management skills, and the rehearsal of problem-solving techniques are valuable adjuncts to the reduction of depression and suicidal behavior (Chiles and Strosahi, 2005).

Sociologic Factors

Contemporary sociologists have reinforced Durkheim's earlier work on suicide. Social scientists have supported the idea that alienation from social groups after the disruption of family, community, or social relationships leads some individuals to attempt or commit suicide.

BOX 22-1　ETIOLOGIC FACTORS RELATED TO SUICIDE

Biologic Factors

The neurotransmitters—principally serotonin, dopamine, norepinephrine, and γ-aminobutyric acid—are linked to emotional responses.

Serotonin plays a major role in the regulation of mood, and it influences the occurrence of depression and suicidality.

Genetic influences are evident; researchers believe that they have found a specific gene that predisposes a person to suicide.

Others have found that dimensions of depression (e.g., mood, affect, motivation, cognitive content) are correlated with alterations in specific brain structure.

Psychologic Factors

Self-directed aggression
Hopelessness
Unresolved interpersonal conflicts
Negativistic thinking patterns
A reduction in positive reinforcement
Difficulty with problem solving

Sociologic Factors

Isolation and alienation from social groups
Biopsychosocial influences

Suicidal thoughts and behaviors are very complex, and no single explanation is comprehensive enough to provide an adequate understanding of why they occur. A more holistic approach is to consider a biopsychosocial model that combines all of these schools of thought (Box 22-1).

EPIDEMIOLOGY

Prevalence

Suicide and suicidal behavior are present among people of all ages (including young children), among members of both sexes, and among individuals in all ethnic groups and at all socioeconomic levels (Box 22-2). In 2007, 34,598 people died as a result of suicide in the United States (Centers for Disease Control and Prevention, 2010).

Age

The two most vulnerable age groups for suicide are older adults and youths between the ages of 15 and 24 years.

Older Adults. Rates of suicide are highest among those 65 years old and older. Older adults have a suicide rate that is approximately 50% higher than all other reported suicidal statistics nationally. There were 15.9 completed suicides per 100,000 individuals in the group of adults who were older than 75 years of age. Of these, there were approximately 4 individuals who attempted suicide for each person who completed suicide among those who were 65 years old or older (Centers for Disease Control and Prevention, 2010). Caucasians have a higher rate of death by suicide than African

BOX 22-2 EPIDEMIOLOGY OF SUICIDE

Age, Gender, and Ethnicity
- Of the 34,598 completed suicides in the United States that occurred in 2007, the majority (24,725) were among white males of all ages.
- The two groups that are most at risk are youth between the ages of 15 to 24 years and white men older than the age of 65 years, with suicides increasing at the fastest rate among men who are 85 years old or older.
- Native-American adolescent males and Hispanic females are high-risk groups among the ethnic minority populations.
- Females in general attempt suicide more frequently than males.

Socioeconomic and Familial Factors
- Suicide crosses all socioeconomic levels.
- Affluent and educated overachievers are as vulnerable to suicide as people at the poverty level who are unemployed, undereducated, living in poor housing, and often the victims of crime.
- Prolonged family disruption and familial predisposition to depression and suicide (either biologically or as a learned behavior from other family members) contribute to the incidence rates.
- Family turmoil, disturbed parent–child relationships, physical and sexual abuse by family members, and hostile and rejecting parental attitudes have been found to promote suicidal behavior.

Co-occurrence with Related Health Issues
- Suicidal behavior is strongly associated with psychiatric disorders.
- Mood disorders, substance abuse, schizophrenia, borderline personality disorder, and panic disorders have a co-occurrence with high-risk suicidal behavior.
- Depression remains the single best predictor of suicide risk for all age groups.
- Suicide is the leading cause of death during the first 10 years of the course of schizophrenic illness.
- The research is mixed regarding the correlation of suicide with panic disorders, but it associated with suicide risk, especially when panic disorder coexists with depression, obsessive–compulsive disorder, or phobias.
- Independent of another specific psychiatric diagnosis, alcohol use and abuse are highly correlated with most suicidal acts, especially among youth. Suicide is underdiagnosed and underreported among older adults.
- Similarly, chronic physical illness contributes to suicidal behavior. More than half of the outpatients who committed suicide in several studies had physical health problems, such as heart disease, hypertension, obesity, and diabetes. Older adults are particularly at risk for suicide.

Americans (American Association of Suicidology, 2010). Native Americans and Alaska Native individuals have the highest rate of completed suicide; suicide is the second leading cause of death in these populations. Hispanic female high-school students are at a higher risk for completing suicide than female students who are Caucasian or African American. The Centers for Disease Control and Prevention reports that in 2007, 14.5% of high-school students of all ethnic backgrounds had reported considering a suicide attempt. Of the high-school students surveyed, 6.9% students had made a suicide attempt at least once during the year before the survey (Centers for Disease Control and Prevention, 2010).

Firearms are the most used of all methods for the completion of suicide. Of the individuals who completed suicide in 2007, 50.2% died by using a firearm. Women use poisoning to complete suicide more frequently than men do.

One of the main causes of suicide is undiagnosed or untreated depression. Many times, the person completes suicide in response to a recent loss; a physical illness with uncontrollable pain or a prolonged illness; loneliness and isolation; or a major change in roles, such as retiring or becoming a caretaker for an ill family member. Psychologic autopsy studies that provide an in-depth review of each individual who died from suicide demonstrate that more than 90% of these deaths were among individuals who had one or more psychiatric disorders. In a large aggregated study, 60% of individuals who completed suicide were diagnosed with depression. The risk of suicide increases with alcoholism, and the research shows that individuals who are dependent on

alcohol have a 50% to 70% higher risk of suicide than the general population (American Association of Suicidology, 2010).

Shneidman (1985) suggested that the high suicide rates among older adults represent a failure to adapt to significant losses, an inability to tolerate emotional pain, and negative attitudes toward the aging process related to loneliness, illness, rejection by family and society, sudden termination of meaningful work, disruption of longstanding relationships, and feelings of emptiness. As the population ages and seniors become the dominant subgroup, suicide increasingly becomes a major public health problem.

Youth. Completed suicide among the youth population is the third leading cause of death in that age group, after accidents and homicides. In 2007, there were approximately 100 to 200 youth suicide attempts for every completed suicide among these individuals (Centers for Disease Control and Prevention, 2010).

To prevent suicide among youth, it is important to understand possible causes, and to screen adolescents for psychiatric disorders, such as drug or alcohol abuse, depression, and conduct disorders. Individuals are at high risk if they are experiencing difficulty interacting with their peers. This includes bullying, the breakup of a significant relationship, a pregnancy, obesity, issues related to sexual orientation, and feelings of isolation. Adolescents are at a higher risk if there is conflict within the family or if the individual feels alienated from the family. Monitor adolescents who have experienced a peer who has been suicidal or completed suicide; this increases the possibility of a suicidal attempt (American

Association of Suicidology, 2010; Centers for Disease Control and Prevention, 2010; Goldston et al, 2008; King et al, 2009; Lenz et al, 2009).

 CLINICAL ALERT #1

Recent psychiatric sources have cited the social media networks as a possible factor in depression and suicide in teens who may be vulnerable to cyber-bullying and other negative messages (O'Keeffe et al, 2011).

Gender and Ethnicity

National suicide rates are vague with regard to the importance of gender and ethnicity when defining the scope of suicidal behavior. Suicide rates for whites are approximately twice those of nonwhites as a whole. However, it is important to note that suicide rates for African-American men have tripled since the early 1990s among those 85 years old and older.

Native-American individuals have a high degree of completed suicide. In 2007, 392 Native Americans completed suicide, which is approximately 12.1% of the Native American population (American Association of Suicidology, 2010). Assistance for Native-American youth needs to incorporate cultural aspects of the unique tribe as well as treatment for issues such as alcoholism, family conflict, and depression.

Socioeconomic Status

Suicide crosses all socioeconomic levels. Both economic well-being and poverty create circumstances that lead to the choice of suicide as a solution to stressful events.

Familial Influences

Suicidal behavior is frequently a symptom of prolonged and progressive family disruption and dysfunction. In addition, significant changes in the family (e.g., divorce, death of a loved one, social isolation) contribute to high suicide rates.

The family is most influential in the lives of children and adolescents, and it contributes to the incidence of suicidal behavior in those age groups. A suicidal adolescent often feels estranged from family members and sometimes experiences rejection and a loss of love. Actual physical or psychologic loss (e.g., death, separation, emotional distancing from the family) is one of the most significant factors to affect the high incidence of adolescent suicide (American Association of Suicidology, 2010).

There is a familial predisposition to suicide in that many suicidal adolescents often have histories of suicidal behavior among their immediate and extended families. Adolescents who completed suicide usually have mothers who had previously completed suicide. Suicidal behavior becomes a learned familial adaptation to problems and stressors (Joiner, 2005; Lenz, 2009).

Familial cultural values are also strong factors in suicidal behavior. For example, in Hispanic families, honor, centeredness, and cohesiveness are factors that can shield against suicidal behavior or contribute to it. Hispanic youth often experience conflict between traditional Hispanic values and the values of the dominant culture. Intergenerational tension, language barriers, and role conflicts also contribute to mental health problems. Adolescents who relate positively to the main culture and who still have positive relationships with their family members who have more traditional values are often at less risk for suicide (Goldston et al, 2008).

Co-occurrence with Related Health Issues

There is a relationship between suicidal behavior and the occurrence of psychiatric disorders and other health-related problems (see Box 22-2). Psychiatric illness, alcohol and other drug use and abuse, and medical illnesses are important indicators of suicidal events.

Suicidal ideation and completion often occur when individuals feel hopeless about their health problems. It is important to conduct an assessment for risk of suicidal intent with individuals with diseases of the nervous system, such as seizure disorders or multiple sclerosis; malignant neoplasms; human immunodeficiency virus or acquired immunodeficiency syndrome; chronic obstructive pulmonary disease, especially in men; chronic hemodialysis-treated renal failure, and pain syndromes (American Psychiatric Association, 2010; www.psychiatryonline.com/popup.aspx?aID=50315). Individuals with mood disorders as well as physical illness have a higher probability of suicide (Macdonald, 2010; Kjølseth et al, 2010).

Psychiatric Disorders

The presence of a diagnosable mental disorder increases the risk for suicide, regardless of age. The co-occurrence of mood disorder and substance abuse increases the probability of suicide. The risk for completed suicide secondary to a mental disorder is higher among men than women. Women attempt suicide three times more often than men do, but men complete suicide 3.6 times more often than women do (American Association of Suicidology, 2010). Approximately 90% of individuals who complete suicide have a psychiatric disorder that fits the criteria of the *Diagnostic and Statistical Manual of Mental Disorders,* fourth edition, text revision. The most commonly identified mental illnesses are mood disorders, such as depression and bipolar disorder; substance abuse; schizophrenia; and borderline personality disorder (American Association of Suicidology, 2010).

Mood Disorders. The single best predictor of suicidal thinking is the presence of a mood disorder. Two thirds of individuals who complete suicide have been clinically depressed. Although treatment is available for individuals with depression, only one in three people with depression obtain the care that is necessary to treat this illness. Untreated depression is responsible for approximately 20% of completed suicidal deaths. The possibility of suicidal risk increases with recurrent episodes of depression because of the feelings of hopelessness, worthlessness, anger, and social isolation; an inability to problem solve; and cognitive rigidity. Individuals with bipolar disorder in a hypomanic or manic state are often impulsive, thus increasing the risk for suicide. Recent studies reveal that 25% to 50% of individuals with bipolar disorder have made at least one suicidal attempt. The risk for suicidal attempts increases if the individual has had depression early in life, aggressive and impulsive behaviors, and childhood abuse. The suicidal risk increases with alcohol or substance abuse and depression (American Foundation for Suicide Prevention, 2010).

One aspect of the treatment of major depressive disorder is the use of antidepressants. In March 2004, the U.S. Food and Drug Administration had a black box warning regarding an increased risk of suicide with some of the newer atypical antidepressants. This warning indicated that antidepressants increased the risk of suicidal ideation and behavior among children and adolescents with major depressive disorder. The close observation of individuals who have been placed on antidepressants is necessary to prevent a suicide attempt (American Psychiatric Association, 2003; Brent et al, 2009; Volek et al, 2007).

Schizophrenia. Suicide is the leading cause of premature death among individuals with schizophrenia. Research shows that 20% to 40% of individuals with the diagnosis of schizophrenia attempt suicide. Approximately 4% of people who attempt suicide do so as a result of command auditory hallucinations. An estimated 10% of suicides take place during the first 10 years of schizophrenia, and the condition has an associated 15% lifetime incidence (American Foundation for Suicide Prevention, 2010). Individuals with schizophrenia have high levels of subjective stress and feelings of hopelessness, loneliness, and dissatisfaction with social relationships because of the chronic aspect of this illness. Because the onset of schizophrenia usually occurs during late adolescence or early young adulthood, the high-risk period for suicide is in between the ages of 20 and 30 years. Other risk factors associated with suicide completion in this population are active psychotic symptoms, depression, and a history of prior suicide attempts. Women have a higher completion rate after an acute exacerbation of the illness and in association with depressive symptoms and the use of alcohol. Nurses need to carefully evaluate and reevaluate this population for suicide risk, particularly during the first 10 years of a patient's illness (American Foundation for Suicide Prevention, 2010; American Psychiatric Association, 2003).

Panic Disorder. When assessing the individual for suicidal risk factors, , it is important to assess the person with a panic disorder for the possibility of suicidal ideation. There is a high co-occurrence of suicidal behavior with panic disorder, major depression, and substance abuse. Evidence supports that panic disorder in conjunction with phobias and obsessive–compulsive disorders is a risk factor for suicide and suicide attempts (American Association of Suicidology, 2010; American Psychiatric Association, 2003).

Some individuals who complete suicide have a panic disorder along with a major depressive disorder, alcohol use, and an Axis II disorder (e.g., borderline personality disorder) (American Psychiatric Association, 2003). (see Clinical Alert #2)

Borderline Personality Disorder. The criteria for borderline personality disorder in the *Diagnostic and Statistical Manual of Mental Disorders,* fourth edition, text revision,

---

❖ CLINICAL ALERT #2

Conflicting findings among researchers lead nurses and other clinicians to overlook the possible lethality of patients with panic disorders, obsessive–compulsive disorders, and phobias. A careful suicide assessment is necessary to ensure that health care providers consider this, because patients with anxiety disorders develop depression that sometimes results in suicide ideation (see Chapters 10 and 12).

---

include "recurrent suicidal behavior, gestures, or threats, or self-mutilating behavior" (American Psychiatric Association, 2000). Often the individual with this disorder experiences suicidal behavior when there is a loss or a perceived loss (Gunderson, 1984; Masterson, 1976). The trait of impulsivity is an important risk factor for suicide attempts with individuals with borderline personality disorder. Therefore, it is essential for nurses to assess the patient for impulsive behavioral patterns (Oldham, 2006) (see Chapter 14).

Alcohol and Other Drugs

There is a high occurrence of alcohol and other drug use with suicidal behavior. The practice guidelines state that alcoholism increases the rate of suicide completion by six times as compared with that seen in the general population. Alcohol is a strong risk factor for suicide, and it is present in 25% to 50% of individuals who complete suicide (American Association of Suicidology, 2010; American Psychiatric Association, 2003).

Drugs contribute to poor and impulsive decisions that lead to high-risk, self-injurious behaviors. A high percentage of alcohol- and drug-related automobile accidents among teens are suicide attempts. A study was done to explore motor vehicle collisions as a means of completing suicide; this research showed that self-harm behavior was an independent risk factor and that it resulted in multiple vehicle crashes (Martiniuk, et al, 2009).

Some factors to consider when determining the risk for suicide in individuals who abuse alcohol or drugs are co-occurring depression, the loss of a relationship or job, or a decrease in the level of functioning as a result of a medical illness. Social isolation, increased drinking, recent unemployment, and a poor social system all increase the risk of suicide. If an individual has some legal issues, he or she should be monitored for suicide risk.

Medical Illnesses

Physical health problems also play a role in persons who are at risk for suicidal behaviors because of their co-occurrence with depression. The Medical Outcomes Study, which was one of the first major national studies to link medical illnesses and depression, found that the physical and social dysfunctions associated with depression were greater than those associated with most chronic medical conditions. Researchers believe that depression causes as much physical and social impairment as chronic heart disease. In the study, depressed persons perceived their current health as poor and they

TABLE 22-1	ERRONEOUS BELIEFS AND FACTS ABOUT SUICIDE
ERRONEOUS BELIEF	**FACT**
People who talk about suicide do not commit suicide.	Most people communicate directly about their suicidal intent verbally, in writing, through artwork, and behaviorally through previous suicide attempts. These are all high-risk indicators of suicidal intent. Manipulation is not usually a factor with these individuals. Treat all messages of intent seriously.
People who are serious about committing suicide do not give clues.	Most suicidal people give warnings of their intent by giving away their possessions; wrapping up their business affairs; isolating themselves from their friends; demonstrating an increased incidence of accidents; being preoccupied with death in their writing, music, and art choices; and making self-deprecating comments related to worthlessness and hopelessness.
Young children do not commit suicide.	There were 180 suicide deaths of children between the ages of 10 and 14 years in 2007 in the United States. Consider all threats from young children seriously. Suicidal behavior is the leading cause of the psychiatric hospitalization of young children.
An improved mood means that the suicide crisis is over.	Persons who completed suicide often showed improved mood and energy before their deaths. The improved mood and energy level often mean that the person's ambivalence has ended and that he or she has made the decision to commit suicide.
Only people with the diagnosis of depression kill themselves.	Although depression is the single best indicator of suicidal risk, some people who commit suicide are not diagnosed as depressed, although they often experience depressed feelings. At risk are those with schizophrenia, substance-related disorders, panic disorder, posttraumatic stress disorder, obsessive–compulsive disorder, and the manic phase of bipolar disorder. Some people do not exhibit a specific mental disorder at all (e.g., an older man who commits suicide after learning that he has terminal cancer or after his beloved wife of 60 years dies suddenly).
Individuals who self-mutilate are really suicidal.	Self-mutilation occurs when the individual has difficulty adjusting his or her affect or is feeling numb after an emotional upheaval or trauma flashback. People who are suicidal are thinking about death; individuals who self-mutilate who are overwhelmed with unmodulated feelings.

experienced greater body pain. As compared with patients with chronic illness, the physical functioning of depressed patients was worse than that of patients with hypertension, diabetes, arthritis, and gastrointestinal and back problems. When depression and a medical condition (e.g., advanced coronary artery disease) coexisted, the patient suffered nearly twice the loss of social function that occurred when either condition existed by itself. Suicide risk also increased in the presence of such coexisting conditions (Macdonald, 2010; Kjølseth et al, 2010).

A complicating factor is that these patients tend to seek medical care for their health problems, and health care providers often miss the coexistence of a depressive disorder. It is important to assess the individual with a medical problem, particularly a chronic or potentially fatal illness, for signs and symptoms of depression.

Physical health problems often add to the emotional pain experienced by suicidal persons and sometimes contribute to their decisions to end their lives. Nurses play a critical role in assessing patients for depression and suicide risk in medical and surgical health care settings. Alerting the health care team to these findings will help to prevent suicide attempts and deaths.

Soldiers Returning From War in Iraq and Afghanistan

There have been increases in the number of suicide attempts and deaths of soldiers who have returned from the war front in Iraq and Afghanistan. The armed forces medical division, the National Institute of Mental Health, and Veteran Affairs have partnered to assist with the reduction of the rate of suicide among the soldiers and staff. The Army has implemented an ongoing study to explore the suicide potential and mental health issues among military personnel. The Army STARRS (Study to Assess Risk and Resilience in Service members) program has set the goals of rapidly identifying at-risk soldiers and providing needed services (e.g., a 24-hour crisis hotline) specifically for military personnel. The plan is meant to provide a means of encouraging resilience and decreasing suicide (National Institute of Mental Health, 2010; www.armystarrs.org, 2010).

Erroneous Beliefs about Suicide

Despite the numerous studies that have addressed suicide, the massive efforts to educate people about suicide risk, and the efforts of mental health advocacy groups, mistaken beliefs and myths still exist. Several long-standing incorrect beliefs contribute to errors in judgment when assessing individuals for suicidal intent. These beliefs are listed in Table 22-1.

CLINICAL DESCRIPTION

The assessment of suicide risk is an important skill for professional nurses in all clinical settings. However, simply voicing a concern about a patient's possible suicidality to other members of the health care team is not an adequate or safe response. The nurse needs to use interviewing skills to talk directly with the patient and his or her family about suicide during the initial nursing assessment and at points of reassessment during the treatment process. Being alert to the patient's medical history and his or her psychiatric history of suicidal behavior gives the nurse clues for identifying areas for further inquiry (see Chapter 3).

This section describes the background information that is needed to complement the assessment phase of the nursing process. Definitions of the five levels of suicidal behavior are listed in Box 22-3, along with risk factors. Often the five levels of suicidal thought or action are called *suicidal behaviors;* however, it is important to be specific when naming the types of thoughts and actions in the nursing assessment with clear descriptions or examples so that others are able to judge the patient's level of intent.

Risk Factors for Suicide

Nurses need to use their knowledge of risk factors to assist them with the assessment of intent and lethality. Risk factors that are based in part on key points from epidemiologic findings are listed in Box 22-4. Box 22-5 describes a mnemonic that is useful for remembering the warning signs of suicide.

Lethality Assessment Factors

In addition to suicide risk factors, nurses need to consider the assessment of lethality or the potential for causing death related to the level of danger associated with the suicide plan. Imminence (i.e., the likelihood that an event will occur within a specific time period), intent (i.e., the method chosen and its accessibility), and the patient's level of hopelessness often help to determine the level of lethality and the extent of interventions required for safety.

Imminence versus Nonimminence

Suicidal imminence is a subjective, clinical judgment that is made on the basis of the professional's experience, knowledge base, and intuition (see Intuitive example, Chapter 3). The determination of suicidal imminence is critical, and persons in imminent danger of killing themselves, require immediate action by the nursing staff.

Some mental health professionals define imminence as the likelihood that the person will engage in suicidal behavior within the next 24 hours. A specific suicide plan, access to lethal measures, behaviors that signal a decision to die, and an admission of wanting to die suggest imminent risk for the patient. This is especially true if these variables are combined with a sense of hopelessness, no vision of the future, or guilty thoughts. If a person has a high lethality (i.e., imminent danger to himself or herself) and refuses treatment, there is a legal consideration for safety called *involuntary hold-and-treat status.* Each jurisdiction has rules and regulations that govern involuntary psychiatric admission. However, the patient normally receives care in an inpatient setting,

---

BOX 22-3   FIVE LEVELS OF SUICIDAL BEHAVIOR

The following terms describe the five levels of suicidal thought or action:

1 *Suicidal ideation.* This involves direct or indirect thoughts or fantasies of suicide or self-injurious acts that are expressed verbally or through writing or artwork without definite intent or action expressed. Sometimes patients express this symbolically.

2 *Suicide threats.* These are direct verbal or written expressions of intent to commit suicide but without action.

3 *Suicide gestures.* These self-directed actions result in no injury or minor injury by persons who neither intended to end their lives nor expected to die as a result. However, they were done in such a way that others interpret the act as suicidal in purpose (e.g., taking eight 5-mg tablets of valium).

4 *Suicide attempts.* These are serious self-directed actions that sometimes result in minor or major injury by persons who intend to end their lives or to seriously harm themselves. Gestures and attempts that are unsuccessful and of low lethality are sometimes called *parasuicidal behavior.*

5 *Completed suicide.* The deaths of persons who end their lives by their own means with conscious intent to die are described as *completed suicide.* However, it is important to note that some suicides sometimes occur on the basis of the unconscious intent to die (e.g., engaging in high-risk activities).

---

usually for 72 hours, depending on specific state statutes. This allows clinicians to hospitalize these individuals for an evaluation of risk and to determine appropriate treatment recommendations. These patients' rights are protected to prevent abuse. Those who are judged not to be imminently in danger of hurting or killing themselves can sometimes choose less restrictive treatment options, such as partial hospitalization programs or outpatient programs. In some states, involuntary outpatient treatment assists an individual who has demonstrated a risk over time to harm himself, herself, or others. This involuntary outpatient treatment usually involves a structured outpatient program and medication administration. An advance directive is generally written that gives the individual choices in care, such as where he or she wants to be hospitalized, any specified practitioner to provide care during the crisis period, and any reactions to medications that he or she has experienced in the past. The combination of requests outlined in the advance directive and the legal statutes that mandate care provide a level of safety for the individual who is at risk. Any suicidal thoughts or behaviors—whether ideation, threat, gesture, or attempt—indicate an emergency situation and require prompt assessment and intervention. Suicide risk and imminence usually decrease after health care providers answer the cry for help and establish support systems for those who are at risk (see Chapter 9).

BOX 22-4   RISK FACTORS FOR SUICIDE

- *Age.* Persons who are most at risk for suicide are youth between the ages of 15 and 24 years and older adults who are 65 years old and older, with those 85 years old and older being the most vulnerable.
- *Sex.* Men by far have a greater incidence of completed suicides. Women have a higher rate of suicide attempts and gestures.
- *Race and ethnicity.* Suicide rates for whites are twice those of nonwhites. However, rates for African-American men who are older than 85 years of age are increasing faster than those for any other group. The group that is the second most at risk is Native-American males.
- *Physical and emotional symptoms.* High-risk indicators are serious depression, significant changes in weight, serious sleep disturbances, extreme fatigue and loss of energy, self-deprecation, anger, feelings of hopelessness, and preoccupation with themes of death and dying. Serious depression is often a sign of suicidal behavior.
- *Suicide plan.* The presence and nature of the suicide plan are the most critical factors to consider when assigning suicide risk. A plan clearly signals forethought and intent and often helps to determine the level of lethality. Plans that are more precise, detailed, and explicit about the method indicate high risk. If the method described is highly lethal (e.g., a gunshot to the head as compared with an overdose of pills) and if the method is readily available, the risk is elevated even more. Add alcohol and other drugs, poor impulse control, and limited time for rescue attempts, and the risk reaches a critical level. Plans often include giving away possessions and sometimes mention of the intent to join a deceased loved one in the

afterlife, especially if the loved one had committed suicide.
- *History of previous attempts.* The majority of persons who complete suicides have made previous suicide attempts.
- *Social supports and resources.* The availability of a support system for a suicidal person often determines the outcome of an emotional crisis. This "lifeline" of caring, support, confrontation, and limit setting—as appropriate from family, friends, and community resources—assists suicidal persons with choosing other alternatives when solving their problems. A real or perceived lack of support systems or the failure to use the support system that is available significantly increases the risk for suicide.
- *Recent losses.* One of the major emotional determinants of suicidal behavior is real or perceived losses, separations, or abandonment. Unresolved grief reactions lead to depression and suicidal behavior.
- *Medical problems.* Persons who suffer painful and debilitating acute or chronic conditions or who have terminal illness are of special concern for suicide risk.
- *Alcohol and other drugs.* These substances are often lethal companions to suicidal acts. Drugs lower inhibition, heighten depression, and quicken impulsivity. According to estimates, at least 50% of adolescents are legally drunk at the time of their death by suicide, and an even higher percentage has a history of recent alcohol or other drug abuse.
- *Cognition and problem-solving ability.* The inability to adequately identify problems and corresponding solutions greatly contributes to the choice of suicide as a solution to problems.

BOX 22-5   MNEMONIC FOR THE WARNING SIGNS OF SUICIDE:

Is Path Warm?

I	Ideation
S	Substance abuse
P	Purposelessness
A	Anxiety
T	Trapped
H	Hopelessness
W	Withdrawal
A	Anger
R	Recklessness
M	Mood change

A person with an acute risk for suicidal behavior will most often demonstrate one or more of the following warning signs:
- Threatening to hurt or kill himself or herself or talking about wanting to hurt or kill himself or herself
- Looking for ways to kill himself or herself by seeking access to firearms, pills, or other means
- Talking or writing about death, dying, or suicide when these actions are out of the ordinary

These might be remembered as expressed or communicated *ideation*.

Additional warning signs include the following:
- Increased substance (alcohol or drug) use
- Talking about having no reason for living, no future, or no sense of purpose in life
- Anxiety, agitation, inability to sleep, or sleeping all the time
- Feeling trapped and believing there is no way out
- Withdrawing from friends, family, and society
- Feeling rage and uncontrolled anger or seeking revenge
- Acting reckless or engaging in risky activities, seemingly without thinking
- Exhibiting dramatic mood changes

If any of these warning signs are observed, seek help as soon as possible by contacting a mental health professional or by calling 1-800-273-TALK (8255) for a referral.

Adapted from the American Association of Suicidology: *Home page* (website): www.suicidology.com.

BOX 22-6 **SEVERITY INDEX FOR SUICIDE RISK**

1 *Suicidal ideation.* The patient has no risk of suicide.
2 *Mild thoughts of suicide.* The individual experiences passing thoughts of suicide. For example, "This is stupid, don't think like that; you have much to do yet, like raising your child." The patient tells you that he or she is not going to make any suicide attempt. The patient has support systems in his or her life and is able to identify a purpose for living.
3 *Moderate thoughts of suicide.* The patient thinks about suicide as an option for solving his or her problems. The patient describes the feeling of wanting to go to sleep and never wake up. The patient has no plan for suicide. The patient states that he or she does not want to die so much as escape from his or her problems. The patient has support people in his or her life but does not use them because the patient feels that he or she is a burden to others. Religious beliefs help prevent the patient's suicidal tendencies.
4 *Advanced thoughts of suicide.* The patient makes a suicidal gesture that is not necessarily lethal (e.g., a small overdose, wrist cutting) or has more intrusive thoughts of suicide and tells the psychotherapist or nurse that he or

she is suicidal. The patient does not use a support system, starts to give things away, does not buy needed items, and checks insurance policies. The patient rationalizes his or her religious beliefs regarding suicide. This patient requires hospitalization to prevent a lethal suicide gesture.
5 *Severe thoughts of suicide.* The patient wants to die and cannot identify any solution other than suicide. The patient cuts off communication with others and isolates himself or herself. The patient demonstrates an increase in energy after deciding on the details of the suicide, including the means of death and the place and time that death will occur. The patient does not always tell the plan to the psychotherapist or nurse, because that person will possibly intervene and prevent the suicide attempt. If the patient is experiencing auditory hallucinations, he or she will not tell the psychotherapist or nurse about the commanding voices, because the voices are demanding that the patient not talk about the suicidal ideas. The patient has begun to question and rationalize his or her relationship with God, if any, and states that he or she is not worthy in God's eyes. The patient experiences intrusive thoughts of death and suicide throughout most of his or her thought process.

Data from Green E et al: Practice guidelines for suicide/self-harm prevention. In Green E, Katz J, editors: *Clinical practice guidelines for the adult patient*, St. Louis, 1995, Mosby.

Ideation versus Intent

Suicidal ideation, or thinking about suicide without clear intent, places a person at lower risk than a person who intends or proposes to die through a suicidal act. There are two categories of intention: conscious and unconscious.

Conscious suicidal intention involves various aspects of awareness:

- An awareness of the outcomes or anticipated results of the suicidal behavior
- An awareness of others' responses to suicide threats or attempts
- An awareness of the lethality index of the chosen method
- An awareness of rescue possibilities (i.e., part of the plan includes various avenues of rescue, or the plan is designed so that rescue is difficult or remote)

Unconscious suicidal intention is often more difficult to assess, because it requires a higher level of skill and knowledge of psychodynamic theory. Often there is a cluster of symptoms that are characteristic of the dynamics of self-destruction: depression, anxiety, guilt, hopelessness, hostility, and dependency, along with fantasies that are symbolic of death, hurting others, killing oneself, failure, and hopelessness. The motivation to hurt or kill oneself is outside of awareness, yet the patient often expresses it by extreme risk-taking behaviors. For example, a platform parachutist who jumps from low heights off of stationary objects such as buildings, towers, or cliffs has unconscious wishes to hurt himself or end his life. Others seek dangerous occupations, such as skyscraper workers, bridge builders, and high-wire artists without nets as metaphors for suicidal wishes. Some

may place themselves in dangerous and vulnerable situations that result in their deaths at the hands of others (e.g., victim-precipitated homicides). Some psychiatric patients unconsciously manipulate others through suicide threats or attempts and unconsciously arrange to be found or rescued. Unfortunately, the rescue plans sometimes fail, which results in completed suicides.

It is important to listen to the communication of intent among suicidal persons. Often individuals who were at higher risk and who have completed suicides communicated their intent in advance only to their significant others. Individuals who are at moderate risk of suicide communicate this by threatening suicide to family members or health care providers. Nurses are able to anticipate how severe the intent is by listening to the extent of the suicidal thoughts of the individual as well as to the feelings of hopelessness and the availability of a method to carry out the suicidal plan (Box 22-6).

Nurses need to carefully observe and listen for direct and indirect communication regarding the patient's suicidal intent. They need to listen not only for the words but also for the underlying themes that the words refer to or symbolize. Although a suicidal intent may seem manipulative in terms of the individual's reason for this action, nurses should never ignore it. Suicidal intent accompanied by imminence represents a high level of lethality.

Chosen Method and Accessibility

The third determining factor of lethality is perhaps the most critical. The method and its availability determine the outcome of the suicidal behavior. People are more likely to seriously injure or kill themselves if there is an easily accessible means or method.

Persons who complete suicide tend to engage in only one high-lethality act with the use of violent methods such as using firearms, piercing vital organs, hanging, jumping from high places, or using carbon monoxide poisoning. Men who complete suicides are more likely to select more violent means and to use guns or knives or hang themselves; women are more likely to jump from high places or overdose. Non-fatal attempts are done in a way that involves engaging in multiple low-lethality acts and using self-poisoning by pill ingestion (i.e., the most common method for suicide attempts), followed by wrist cutting. These methods allow time for rescue because of the slowness of their physiologic actions. Most individuals who attempt suicide use the same method for repeated suicide attempts.

Access to dangerous weapons raises an individual's suicide risk. The increase in youth suicide rates is in proportion to the increased use of firearms. The most rapid increase in firearm suicides has been in the 15- to 24-year-old age range. Because of the increasing availability of firearms and other weapons, it is important for parents to be aware of the activities and peers of their children. Parents, guardians, and teachers need to investigate any clues or signs of self-destructive behavior, symptoms of mental illness (e.g., paranoia, psychosis), and any verbalizations regarding violence toward the self or others to prevent a possible tragedy, (e.g., the shootings at Virginia Tech in which the gunman killed 32 people before he committed suicide).

Suicidal patients in psychiatric hospitals or psychiatric units in general hospitals have a high suicide risk. The most vulnerable periods for attempts are within the first 24 hours after admission and as discharge approaches. Close observation is necessary as patients move from one suicide precaution level to another. Remember that a sudden brightening of affect or a lifting of depression may signal that the patient has resolved his or her indecision or ambivalence about living or dying and made the decision to commit suicide. Some patients have attempted or completed suicide while they were not on suicide precautions at all. The observation of all patients at least every 15 to 30 minutes, whether or not they are suicidal, is vital to the detection of early clues to self-destructive behavior.

Hanging is the most prevalent suicide method that is used in hospital settings. Sharp objects are usually not available to patients as part of the safety program of the unit. However, patients have used sheets, towels, belts, cords, plastic garbage bags, shoestrings, and articles of clothing to create nooses. Other patients "cheek" their psychotropic medications and use them later in overdose attempts. Some chronically suicidal patients who sneak sharp objects into the hospital are prone to cutting attempts, usually of the wrists or the antecubital areas of the arms. Patients who have been diagnosed with borderline personality disorders or dissociative disorders are especially prone to these attempts. Searching the patient on admission and when returning from off-the-unit experiences (e.g., Alcoholics Anonymous meetings, tests or

procedures away from the behavioral health unit) is an important safety intervention to detect razors, knives, pieces of glass, and aluminum cans.

It is not possible to prevent all suicides, even in the most secure facilities (e.g., psychiatric hospitals, jails), but close observation and the continued reassessment of suicide risk minimize the chances of completed suicides. Mental health professionals have an obligation to protect patients from harming themselves, just as parents and significant adults must be responsible for youth who demonstrate signs of self-destructive behavior that requires prompt intervention. (see Clinical Alert #3)

❖ **CLINICAL ALERT #3**

Asking suicidal patients and their family members about their access to dangerous weapons must be a part of the nursing assessment. Many will verify that there are guns and other dangerous weapons in the home that are easily accessible. If the patient is experienced in firearms use (e.g., if he or she is a police officer, a member of the military, or a hunter), the risk for suicide rises sharply. Make provisions at the end of the assessment to secure the weapons, and have family and friends remove the weapons from the patient's home or from automobiles and trucks. A physician's order is usually necessary before dangerous weapons are returned to the at-risk patient.

PROGNOSIS

Suicidal behavior is a treatable mental health problem. The prognosis for many suicidal patients is related to the severity of their accompanying mental disorders. Because most suicidal behavior is connected closely with major depressive disorders, the effective treatment of depression reduces the risk of suicide. The majority of patients with depression who are treated with antidepressant medications demonstrate increased improvement or complete remission of their depressive symptoms (American Psychiatric Association, 2003). Patients with schizophrenia and panic disorder who maintain therapeutic blood levels of the prescribed psychotropic medications also have a favorable response and a positive outcome related to a reduction in suicide risk (see Chapter 25 for more information about medication).

DISCHARGE CRITERIA

Discharge criteria are necessary guidelines for both the patient and the nursing staff and lead to a completion of treatment goals. The admission assessment establishes the groundwork for discharge criteria. An accurate, thorough, and knowledgeable assessment and appropriate treatment plan promotes effective interventions and timely discharge activities. Discharge criteria help to establish time frames for the achievement of goals; to designate areas of responsibility and accountability through documentation; and to meet specific institutional, professional, certifying, legal, or funding requirements.

Discharge criteria for the suicidal patient include the following:

- Indications that the patient is no longer imminently suicidal
- Determination that the patient's living environment is safe for his or her return
- A consistent and available support system for the patient that will help to determine if the patient has self-destructive feelings
- A commitment from the patient to use psychotherapy to understand the crises that led to the suicidal ideation or attempt
- An agreement by the patient to use a suicide hotline (e.g., 1-800-273-TALK) or to call a supportive friend or family member if suicidal ideation happens again

THE NURSING PROCESS

ASSESSMENT

The nursing assessment is a critical step toward ensuring the patient's safety. Accurate assessment that continues throughout the course of care, including during hospitalization, helps the nurse to provide appropriate intervention and discharge planning. Determining an individual's risk for self-harm requires a thorough evaluation of factors that contribute to suicidality (e.g., a mental status examination, an evaluation of the patient's support resources).

The initial assessment helps to determine the presence of specific risk factors. Noting the presence of symptoms does not necessarily mean that a patient is suicidal. However, recognizing a cluster of certain symptoms within a given time frame is necessary to accurately assess suicidal intent.

When assessing the patient's risk for suicide, the nurse will observe for the following:

- *The observable behavior of the patient.* A calm patient may be highly suicidal, whereas an agitated patient is not always in danger. Although appearances are deceiving, increased irritation often signals an imminent suicide attempt as evidenced by impulsivity, restlessness, excessive motor agitation, and a brightening of the affect (Shneidman, 1985, 1996). Some individuals manifest withdrawal, apathy, irritability, and immobility that intensify with suicidality. Suicides can occur in hospitals. It is important that nurses consistently monitor a suicidal patient's behavior, affect, and interactions with others. Lethality levels increase during hospitalization, particularly as depression lifts and discharge is about to occur. (see Clinical Alert #4)
- *The history from the patient.* Careful scrutiny sometimes reveals events that contributed to current self-destructive thoughts. It is important to determine why the patient is feeling suicidal at this time. When gathering the patient's history, the nurse will identify self-defeating coping patterns and past experiences that have negatively affected the patient's self-esteem. Making a note of significant anniversary dates will help to predict a future suicide attempt.

> **❖ CLINICAL ALERT #4**
>
> A sudden change in affect for the better or a dramatic lifting of depression can be an indication that the patient has made the decision to commit suicide and is no longer ambivalent or uncertain about it. Increased energy and the ability to concentrate and plan the suicidal act facilitate suicidal actions. Be alert.

- *Information from friends or relatives.* Nurses obtain useful information about the patient's history from friends or relatives. Often it is helpful to interview the patient and family both together and separately in case the friend or relative is hesitant to speak openly in front of the patient. The nurse assesses how family members and friends feel about the patient's suicidal behavior. Family members who are angry, disgusted, or frustrated with the self-destructive patient will actually provoke the patient to complete a plan of suicide.
- *History of suicidal gestures or attempts.* The suicide attempt is often a way of coping with painful feelings. People who have used this coping style in the past are at greater risk for using it again.
- *The mental status examination.* Disturbances in concentration, orientation, and memory suggest possible organic brain syndromes or severe major depressive disorders, which reduce the patient's impulse control and increase the potential for self-harm. Disturbance in thought processing that is evidenced by command hallucinations places the patient at greater risk for acting destructively (see Chapter 3 for a discussion of mental status examination).
- *The physical examination.* Always conduct a physical examination when there are obvious signs and symptoms of substance abuse (e.g., impaired attention, irritability, euphoria, slurred speech, unsteady gait, flushed face, psychomotor agitation, needle tracks), previous suicide attempts (e.g., scars on the wrists), or debilitating medical conditions (e.g., diabetes, chronic pain).

The nurse's intuition. The nurse's own feelings of uneasiness, anxiety, or unexplained sadness are sometimes the only clues that a seemingly calm patient will act on suicidal impulses. Although these feelings seem like intuition, research suggests that "intuitive feelings" tend to be based on previous experiences in similar patient care situations. Nevertheless, if the nurse does not "feel right" about a patient, do not ignore this important source of information (see Chapter 3 for more information about intuitive reasoning). Use the questions in the Nursing Assessment Questions box to determine the patient's risk for suicide.

The following discussion refers to the Case Study. The nurse knew that the first task of assessment was to make psychologic contact with the patient. She planned to listen to how Matthew viewed his situation and then communicate her understanding of his thoughts and feelings. The nurse realized that it was important to establish rapport and trust

NURSING ASSESSMENT QUESTIONS #1

Suicide

1 Is the patient hopeless? Does the patient see no prospects for the future? Does the patient express that there are no solutions to his or her problems?

2 Has the patient made a recent suicide attempt? Are the patient's suicide attempts severe or multiple? Does the patient show impulsivity?

3 Are suicide attempts increasing in frequency or lethality? Is the patient obsessing or fantasizing about suicide or death?

4 Does the patient have insomnia with suicidal thoughts at night that continue into the early morning hours?

5 Is the patient anxious? Are there any symptoms of panic disorder or posttraumatic stress disorder?

6 Does the patient have bipolar disorder, postpartum psychosis, or psychotic depression? Is the patient experiencing pathologic grief, especially with command hallucinations, guilt, or other co-occurring conditions (e.g., chemical dependency, alcoholism, personality disorder)?

7 Is there a history of suicide by a relative or close friend? Is the patient isolated? Does the patient lack resources and available family?

8 Does the patient have detailed suicidal plans? Are lethal means available to the patient for suicide (e.g., a gun, another weapon)?

9 Did the patient leave a suicide note or give away valued possessions?

10 Is the patient becoming increasingly frustrated with his or her therapy, illness, or problems? Is the patient feeling powerless and unable to learn how to cope?

11 Has the patient been offered electroconvulsive therapy and demonstrated ambivalence about it? Has the patient interpreted the recommendation as an admission of failure and hopelessness rather than a positive solution?

A "yes" answer to any one of these questions suggests that the patient needs careful assessment by the treatment team for possible admission to a behavioral health facility, with suicide precautions instituted as per policy.

Developed by the Committee for Suicide Assessment, Sharp Mesa Vista Hospital, San Diego, Calif.

Psychologic contact does not always happen solely through verbal communication; sometimes nonverbal physical contact can be quite effective. A gentle touch on the forearm or the

CASE STUDY

Matthew, who is 26 years old, was hospitalized at the age of 19 years after overdosing on tricyclic antidepressants. At the time, Matthew's suicide attempt seemed to be linked to the end of a 3-year relationship with his girlfriend. Since the initial episode of major depression, Matthew successfully graduated from college and returned home to live with his mother after his father died. Soon, however, he began to feel frustrated and inadequate when he could not find a job that suited his education and intellectual capabilities. Matthew was eventually forced to accept a part-time position that paid minimum wage and that lacked benefits. When his steady girlfriend suddenly relocated to another state, he felt rejected and abandoned.

Matthew's mother noticed that he had become more withdrawn and isolated, and she was concerned that Matthew was possibly becoming self-destructive. After finding a loaded pistol lying on a table next to his bed, Matthew's mother phoned the local mental health crisis intervention center to discuss her concerns about her son's behavior. While talking with the intake nurse, she mentioned that Matthew had recently instructed her to donate his body organs to medical science "if anything should happen" to him. The nurse requested that Matthew come to the center immediately for an assessment to determine his risk for suicide.

Critical Thinking

1 What information did the nurse gather during the phone conversation with Matthew's mother that alerted her to Matthew's need for an immediate suicide assessment? Why is this information pertinent to suicidal ideation?

2 What other factors will the nurse consider when assessing Matthew's risk for suicide during the face-to-face evaluation?

3 Identify one factor that was noted during the assessment that will help to reduce Matthew's risk for self-harm.

with Matthew. She believed that the patient-centered approach, which was developed by Rogers (1961), facilitated open communication and in turn assisted her with more accurately assessing Matthew's risk for suicide (see Chapter 26 for more information about Carl Rogers).

The nurse used empathic listening techniques by listening for both facts and feelings (i.e., what happened and how the patient felt about it). The nurse demonstrated caring and interest by using reflective statements so that Matthew knew that the nurse truly heard what he had been saying.

When feelings were obviously present but not yet expressed, the nurse would gently comment, "I sense how upset you are by the way you are speaking. It seems like you are also angry and frustrated about what has happened."

placing of an arm around a shoulder can have an important calming effect and signify human concern as well.

The nurse demonstrated concern for Matthew by offering him a tissue when his eyes filled with tears. The nurse not only recognized and acknowledged Matthew's feelings but also responded in a calm and controlled manner; she resisted the tendency to become anxious, angry, or depressed in response to the intensity of the patient's feelings. During the assessment of Matthew, the nurse included the questions that are listed in the Nursing Assessment Questions box.

After a suicide attempt, an individual sometimes continues to be at high risk for attempting suicide again. When a patient is admitted to the hospital after a suicide attempt, ongoing assessments are necessary to determine whether the person continues to be at high risk.

1 What does Matthew understand about why his mother suggested that he come to the center for a mental health assessment? *This is asked to determine if the patient will validate his mother's concerns or deny that a problem exists.*

2 What was Matthew's intention in having a loaded gun lying next to his bed? Did he intend to kill himself or someone else? *Asking directly about a patient's intentions will decrease anxiety and feelings of humiliation and shame.*

3 Has Matthew taken antidepressants or mood-stabilizing medications in the past? Is he taking them currently? Have the medications that have been used in the past been effective for improving Matthew's mood and lowering his lethality level? Does he have access to other lethal means of suicide?

4 When was the last time that Matthew used alcohol or other drugs? When was he last intoxicated? *Patients who use alcohol and other drugs are at higher risk for completing a suicide attempt. In addition, increased impulsivity, disorientation, and confusion, which often accompany drug and alcohol use, place people at higher risk for suicide.*

5 With whom does Matthew share his feelings? *This is asked to determine if the patient has a trusted and reliable support system; if so, the lethality level is lower.*

6 What were the circumstances surrounding the death of Matthew's father? Is there a history of depression or suicide on either side of Matthew's family? *These questions determine the nature of the patient's father's death, any family history of depression, and the family's style of coping, all of which may increase the patient's risk of suicide.*

7 The nurse asks Matthew's mother, "How do you feel about Matthew's thoughts of suicide?" *This will help to determine if the patient's mother is a support resource for him.*

NURSING DIAGNOSIS

Patients who are suicidal are frequently admitted to psychiatric units, emergency departments, and intensive care units of general medical hospitals. Suicide attempts can occur before or during hospitalization. Hangings, medication overdoses, and jumping from high places are frequent methods of suicide in hospitals. An accurate nursing diagnosis that is made on the basis of a thorough and ongoing assessment is necessary when identifying and prioritizing the patient's needs for nursing interventions.

A complete nursing diagnosis is individualized and related to the patient's behaviors and nursing needs. A validation of the nursing diagnosis with the patient is necessary. However, some patients deny suicidal intent or the need for extra precautions. In the case of the diagnosis of risk for suicide or risk for self-directed violence, nurses must be cautious when determining the level of risk. It is best to err on the side of caution when diagnosing suicidality than to allow serious injury or death to occur.

The primary nursing diagnoses for these patients include the following: (NANDA-I, 2009).
• Risk for suicide
• Risk for self-directed violence
Secondary diagnoses may include the following:
• Ineffective coping
• Hopelessness
• Powerlessness
• Chronic low self-esteem
• Social isolation
• Disturbed thought processes

OUTCOME IDENTIFICATION

Outcomes come from the nursing diagnoses. They are the anticipated and expected patient behaviors or responses that are achieved as a result of nursing interventions. It is important to state outcomes in clear behavioral or measurable terms and to prioritize them according to patient needs, from most urgent to least urgent.

The patient will do the following:
• Remain safe and free from self-harm.
• Verbalize an absence of suicidal ideation, planning, or intent.
• Verbalize a desire to live and list several reasons for wanting to live.
• Agree to inform staff immediately if suicidal feelings or thoughts recur.
• Display a brightened affect with a broad range of expression, spontaneity, and speech that reflects a hopeful and optimistic attitude.
• Initiate social interactions with peers and staff, both individually and in groups.
• Use effective coping methods to counteract feelings of hopelessness.
• Express a sense of self-worth.
• Meet his or her own needs with the use of clear and direct methods of communication.
• Verbalize realistic role expectations and goals for meeting them.
• Demonstrate the absence of psychotic thinking (e.g., delusions, command hallucinations that instruct the patient to self-harm).
• Make plans for the future that include follow-up psychotherapy and adherence to the prescribed medication regimen.
• List several friends or supportive individuals (e.g., a clergy member) or use a suicide hotline (e.g., 1-800-273-TALK) to prevent a possible suicide attempt when experiencing an increase in suicidal thoughts.

PLANNING

The nurse's awareness of a patient's risk for suicide and the recurrent nature of suicide attempts necessitate a plan of care that is aimed at saving lives and restoring biopsychosocial stability. The plan of care for the suicidal individual emphasizes a reduction in the risk of self-destructive behaviors by monitoring patient behaviors and providing a safe environment; promoting the patient's feelings of self-worth and hope; improving coping skills; limiting social isolation; and building self-esteem.

IMPLEMENTATION

Primary nursing responsibilities involve the prevention of suicide. The nurse needs to recognize and effectively intervene in the potentially lethal behaviors of patients who are at risk. This process involves a continuing assessment of lethality factors to determine the patient's risk level while working with the patient to restore hope, to connect with support resources, and to develop positive alternatives to assist him or her with improved coping.

Nursing Interventions

Nurses need to implement the following interventions consistently with all hospitalized suicidal patients. Nursing interventions are prioritized according to the patient's needs for safety.

To provide safety and to prevent violence:

1. All unit precautions for preventing suicide should be strictly enforced. This includes maintaining a safe environment by doing the following:
   a. Routinely counting silverware and all other sharp objects before and after the patient's use of them
   b. Having an awareness of the patient's whereabouts at all times
   c. Providing one-to-one observation for the patient as necessary on the basis of the assessment of the patient's current lethality level
   d. Planning the staffing pattern so that the unit always has experienced staff on the floor, especially during staff mealtimes, breaks, vacations, changes of shift, or unit staff meetings (i.e., the times during which most suicides occur in hospitals)
   e. Providing a roommate for the suicidal patient
   f. Requesting that visitors clear all personal items for the patient or any gifts with staff
   g. Searching the suicidal individual for drugs, sharp objects, cords, shoelaces, and other potential weapons after a return from being off of the unit
   h. Thoroughly assessing the patient before any reason to leave the unit is granted to determine the patient's current risk level
   i. Encouraging the patient to write a no-suicide contract as a means of communication between the staff and the patient to promote self-exploration if it is within the hospital policy; encouraging the patient to try new methods of asking for assistance when feeling hopeless and isolated

These actions indicate to the patient the nurse's caring, concern, and consistent follow-through, and they offer the patient an opportunity to take charge of himself or herself when feeling hopeless and powerless. However, note that no-suicide contracts do not preclude the need for constant observation and supervision of these patients (see the Research for Evidence-Based Practice box).

2. Being mindful that most suicides occur within 90 days after hospitalization, the nurse needs to reinforce with families, guardians, social services, and legal authorities the necessity of removing any possible weapons (e.g., guns, drugs) from the person's home environment to a safe location before the patient returns home.

3. Because working with suicidal patients is emotionally draining and anxiety producing, nurses must help to create a supportive environment for themselves and for other staff, which includes clinical supervision and informal discussions regarding feelings about suicide, death, hostility, anger, depression, and other painful feelings. Developing an ongoing relationship with a suicidal patient is an intense experience during which the patient and nurse both examine their feelings about the meaning of life and death. It is an opportunity for the nurse to share a commitment to life, hope, and caring for another person. Receiving support and supervision enables the nurse to develop this kind of intense and caring relationship so that both the nurse and the patient experience less anxiety and have increased energy to work toward hope and health.

To assist with the development of improved coping skills:

1. Nurses use specific techniques that include nonjudgmental and empathic listening, encouragement, the tolerance of expressions of pain, and flexible responses to patient needs.

2. The nurse encourages the patient to focus on strengths rather than weaknesses so that the patient becomes aware of positive qualities and capabilities that have helped with coping in the past. Nurses provide learning opportunities for improved coping by introducing the patient to therapeutic modalities that assist with more positive thinking. By replacing or substituting irrational and self-deprecating thoughts, beliefs, and images, the patient becomes more capable of viewing life realistically and rationally (see the discussion of cognitive therapy in Chapter 26).

3. Nurses reduce the overwhelming effects of problems by helping patients to prioritize their concerns. Breaking the issues down into more manageable parts achieves this goal. The nurse will assist with this process by doing the following:
   a. Encouraging the patient to prioritize problems from most to least significant
   b. Supporting the patient in the finding of immediate solutions for the most urgent problems
   c. Postponing the finding of solutions to those problems that do not require immediate solutions
   d. Encouraging the patient to delegate problem solving to others when appropriate
   e. Helping the individual to acknowledge problems that are beyond his or her control

RESEARCH FOR EVIDENCE-BASED PRACTICE BOX #2

Drew BL: Self-harm behavior and no-suicide contracting in psychiatric inpatient settings, *Arch Psychiatr Nurs* 15:99-106, 2001.

No-suicide contracts have been used since the early 1970s as a means of helping the patient to take responsibility for his or her safety. This author reviewed the charts of 577 individuals with diagnoses such as major mood disorder, schizoaffective disorder, and schizophrenia to determine the effectiveness of no-suicide contracts. In the study group, 31 subjects injured themselves during the hospitalization. Each of the individuals was on high levels of observation; three patients were under constant observation, and one individual was in the seclusion room. A total of 14 out of these 31 individuals expressed suicidal intent. No-suicide contracts were used with 20 of these 31 patients. Most of the contracts were verbal.

There were two hypotheses in this study:

1 How does no-suicide contracting affect the likelihood of any self-harm behavior after controlling for the consistency of the nursing assignment, the patient's anxiety at the time of admission, the degree of environmental restriction, and the level of observation?

2 What is the likelihood of suicidal behavior (i.e., self-harm behavior with the expression of suicidal intent) for patients with no-suicide contracts as compared with patients without contracts after controlling for the consistency of the nursing assignment, the patient's anxiety at the time of admission, the degree of environmental restriction, and the level of observation?

The study demonstrated that patients with no-suicide contracts were five times more likely to harm themselves or to demonstrate suicidal gestures than were individuals without contracts. Patients with an Axis II diagnosis of borderline personality disorder (n = 10) or mental retardation (n = 2) were 10 times more likely to harm themselves than were individuals without an Axis II diagnosis. Patients who had the same registered nurse assigned during the hospitalization had a lower likelihood of self-harm.

This study demonstrated that no-suicide contracts did not prevent self-harm behaviors. If no-suicide contracts are used, it is important to attend to other risks for suicide. The consistency of assigning a nurse during the course of the hospital stay sometimes reduces the risk of self-harm.

The American Psychiatric Association clinical practice guideline states that the suicide-prevention contract (i.e., the no-harm contract) has not been rigorously researched. Without sufficient research studies, a no-harm contract cannot be endorsed as a best practice. In addition, a suicide-prevention or no-harm contract is not a legally binding document. The suicide-prevention contract may be an indication of a strong therapeutic relationship, and it represents a commitment between the clinician and the patient. It is unclear when a patient is unwilling to contract for safety whether the patient is reacting to a change in the therapeutic relationship or to a sense of reliance on the therapeutic alliance to reduce the suicidal impulses. The clinical practice guideline does not prohibit the use of the suicide-prevention contract; however, there is a cautionary statement that the clinician should evaluate the effectiveness of the no-harm contract on the basis of the therapeutic relationship. The clinical practice guideline suggests the frequent and ongoing assessment of suicidal risk. (American Psychiatric Association, 2003).

The nurse is encouraged to read the institution's policy regarding suicide-prevention contracts and to abide by this policy.

---

f. Identifying, defining, and promoting healthy adaptive behaviors in patients

g. Encouraging the continuance of healthy behaviors when improved coping strategies are demonstrated (i.e., positive reinforcement)

h. Encouraging the individual to discuss the feelings that are generated by ineffective coping (e.g., frustration, anger, inadequacy)

i. Affirming the patient's rational decisions that have been made on the basis of accurate judgment

j. Reinforcing the patient's attempts to make independent decisions

k. Acknowledging the patient's demonstrated willingness to implement improved coping behaviors (e.g., assertive communication) (see Chapter 4)

l. Responding to delusional statements by stating the reality of the situation without arguing with the patient's perceived reality

To enhance family and social support systems:

1. Enlist the family as partners in the patient's treatment. Family attendance at psychoeducation groups and family therapy is crucial to helping the patient to work through and understand complex and harmful family structures, systems, and dynamics that contribute to the individual's suicidal feelings.

2. Determine the degree of available family support that contributes to overall risk management. Inform family members about critical signs that the patient will exhibit as the depression lifts and as discharge from the hospital occurs. Encourage the removal of any lethal weapons from the patient's home environment.

3. Provide understanding and encouragement when family members express feelings (e.g., frustration, helplessness, guilt) and intense affect.

4. Contact social services to assist with any needed vocational or financial support.

5. Refer the patient to aftercare groups, support groups, and 12-step groups, as needed.

6. Refer the patient to a suicide hotline (e.g., 1-800-273-TALK) to use when the patient is feeling overwhelmed and suicidal in the future.

7. Refer the patient to sites on the Internet that provide helpful suggestions and hope (e.g., www.yellowribbon.org/).

Additional Treatment Modalities

Depending on the patient's diagnosis, pharmacologic intervention is often a primary consideration for the treatment of the suicidal patient. Antidepressants, anxiolytics, and antipsychotic medications are frequently used, depending on the individual's needs, history, and previous responses to medication intervention (see Chapter 25 for more information about medication).

Psychotherapeutic interventions vary and include insight-oriented techniques, cognitive reframing, and brief solution-focused crisis interventions (see Chapter 26).

Electroconvulsive therapy is sometimes used with adults whose response patterns reflect a lack of positive response to medication (i.e., intractable or refractory depression). These adults usually present with long-standing histories of severe depression while expressing imminent intent to die. Chapter 26 provides a detailed discussion of electroconvulsive therapy.

EVALUATION

An evaluation of the patient's response to the plan of care is crucial when working with suicidal individuals. An ongoing and all-encompassing evaluation considers the accuracy of the nursing diagnosis, the appropriateness of the intervention on the basis of the patient's response, and the timeliness with which the intervention occurred. Evaluation helps the nurse to target areas of outcomes that are critical to the patient's continued survival. A patient's lack of positive response to nursing interventions indicates the need to change the interventions, to implement other treatment modalities, or to reexamine the target dates for the completion of outcomes.

The deliberate and conscientious evaluation of a suicidal patient's response to nursing interventions helps to ensure the patient's continued safety and readiness for discharge.

◎ CONCEPT MAP CASE STUDY

Madison, a 16-year-old girl, was admitted to the adolescent psychiatric unit of a local community hospital after her nurse therapist assessed that she was imminently suicidal. Over the past year, Madison had become preoccupied with wanting to die. She reported that she had overdosed on analgesics and antibiotics three times during the last 7 months, but she never told anyone, and she did not seek medical attention. She reported that she made her first suicide attempt when she was 11 years old by self-inflicting lacerations to her wrists with a razor blade. Within the past year, she has cut her wrists five or six times. Madison complained that she felt helpless to change her relationship with her mother, who she felt misunderstood her. She often felt alienated from her mother. She reported poor school performance, increased irritability, morbid thoughts, decreased appetite, periods of insomnia, low self-esteem, and a history of sexual abuse by a babysitter's boyfriend when she was 9 years old.

During her weekly therapy session, Madison announced to her therapist: "I am no longer willing to honor our contract not to harm myself. Nothing is changing at home. My mother hates me and doesn't want me in her life. My stepdad is the only person Mom really cares about outside of herself. I hate how I look, and I hate how I am. I saved most of the pain pills my doctor gave me when I injured my leg." Laughing, she added, "I think there's enough to really put me out of my pain this time." When questioned further, Madison admitted that she was planning to kill herself. She indicated that she did not know exactly when she was going to do it, but she said, "I am not going to wait much longer." To provide for her immediate safety, the nurse therapist ordered Madison to be admitted to the hospital.

DSM-IV-TR Diagnoses

Axis I   Major depression, recurrent
Axis II   Developmental reading disorder; borderline personality traits
Axis III   Fractured left tibia, healing
Axis IV   Problem with primary support system
Axis V   GAF = 30 (current); GAF = 45 (past year)

Nursing Diagnose *Risk for suicide and risk for self-directed violence. Risk factors: dysfunctional family relationships, ineffective coping style, low self-esteem, effects of sexual abuse, verbalized intent to die, history of several previous suicide attempts, lethal suicide plan, and severely depressed mood*

NOC Suicide self-restraint; Risk control; Impulse self-control; Depression level; Aggression self-control; Abusive behavior self-restraint; Distorted thought self-control; Loneliness severity; Abuse recovery: sexual; Will to live

NIC Suicide prevention; Mood management; Behavior management: self-harm; Impulse control training; Environmental management: safety; Anger control assistance; Support group; Therapy group; Self-esteem enhancement

Continued

◎ CONCEPT MAP CASE STUDY—cont'd

Nursing Diagnosis *Ineffective coping related to negative thinking patterns, self-defeating behaviors, disturbance in self-concept, multiple stressors, and ineffective support system as evidenced by self-destructive behaviors, lack of assertive communication, impaired judgment and insight, misdirected anger, and social isolation*

NOC Coping; Suicide self-restraint; Self-mutilation restraint; Depression self-control; Stress level; Information processing; Social interaction skills; Social support; Self-esteem

NIC Coping enhancement; Anger control assistance; Anxiety reduction; Mood management; Emotional support; Support group; Support system enhancement; Teaching: individual; Therapy group

Nursing Diagnosis *Compromised family coping related to highly conflicted family relationships, enmeshed relationship with mother, hostile relationship with stepfather, and ineffective communication and parenting skills as evidenced by distancing behaviors toward patient, inability to set consistent limits, and inappropriate parent–child boundaries*

NOC Family coping; Family normalization; Family support during treatment; Family participation in professional care; Parenting performance; Caregiver–patient relationship

NIC Coping enhancement; Family support; Family mobilization; Family involvement promotion; Role enhancement; Mutual goal setting; Decision-making support

GAF, Global Assessment of Functioning; NIC, Nursing Interventions Classification; NOC, Nursing Outcomes Classification.

▌ CHAPTER SUMMARY

- Suicide is a major public health and mental health problem in the United States.
- Causes of suicide include biologic factors, psychologic factors, and sociologic factors.
- There were 34,598 suicides in 2007, which is equal to one suicide every 15.2 minutes.
- The most vulnerable groups for suicide are older adults and youths between the ages of 15 and 24 years. Caucasians and men are more likely to be at risk for suicide. Suicide crosses all socioeconomic levels.
- Suicidal behavior is strongly associated with the occurrence of psychiatric disorders and other health-related problems, such as depression, bipolar disorder, schizophrenia, panic disorders, substance abuse, some personality disorders (e.g., borderline personality disorder), and medical disorders.
- Imminence, intent, and the method chosen and its accessibility are the three determinants that indicate the level

of lethality and the levels of interventions that are necessary for safety.
- Suicidal behavior is treatable.
- Discharge criteria for the suicidal patient include indications that the patient is no longer imminently suicidal and that the patient's environment is safe for his or her return home (i.e., weapons [e.g., guns] are removed). Follow up includes outpatient psychotherapy, the possibility of antidepressant medications, and a support system in place for the patient to access.
- The plan of care emphasizes a reduction in the risk of self-destructive behaviors by monitoring the patient's behaviors, providing a safe environment, promoting feelings of self-worth and hope, improving coping skills, limiting social isolation, and building self-esteem.
- The patient is encouraged to follow the discharge plan of psychotherapy and medications, if ordered.

▌ REVIEW QUESTIONS

1. A nurse assesses five new patients who have been admitted to the psychiatric unit. Which patients would have the highest risk for suicidality? You may select more than one answer.
   1. 87-year-old white man
   2. 37-year-old African-American man
   3. 66-year-old white woman
   4. 23-year-old African-American woman
   5. 21-year-old Native-American man

2. A nurse administers medications to a patient who is on suicide observation. Which action by the nurse is most important?
   1. Inform the patient about the name, action, and side effects of the medication.
   2. Verify that the patient swallowed the entire dose of the medication.
   3. Document the patient's willingness to voluntarily take the medication.

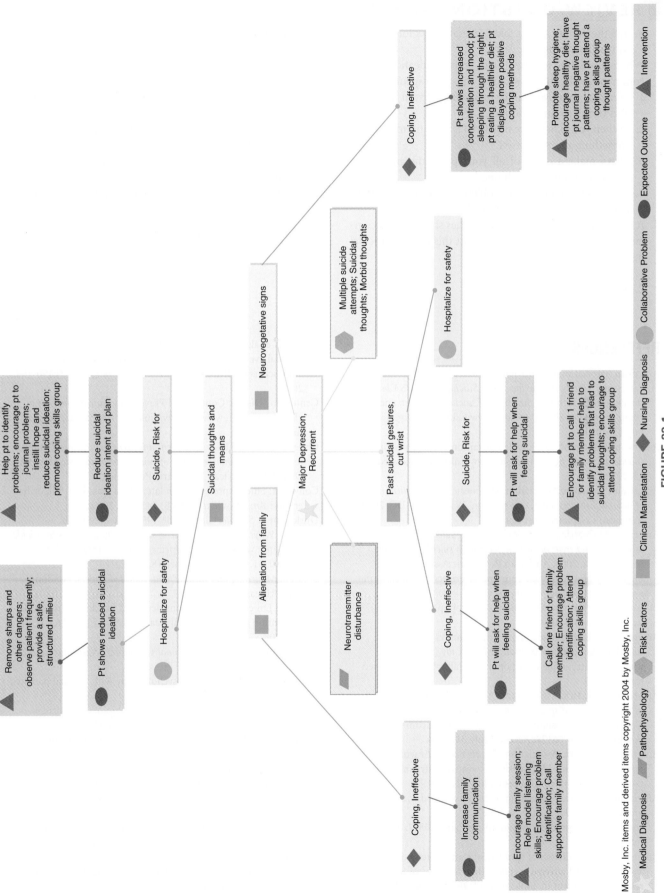

Mosby, Inc. items and derived items copyright 2004 by Mosby, Inc.

FIGURE 22-1

Medical Diagnosis Pathophysiology Risk Factors Clinical Manifestation Nursing Diagnosis Collaborative Problem Expected Outcome Intervention

4. Tell the patient that it takes several weeks for the drug to reach a therapeutic level.

3. When counseling a patient with suicidal ideation, which comment by the nurse would be most therapeutic?
   1. "I'm glad to see you taking ownership of your problems and trying to find solutions."
   2. "When you experience negative feelings, try to focus on something more positive."
   3. "Let's make a chart of all your problems and try to create solutions for each one."
   4. "Let's talk about which problems are most important and which are least important."

4. A patient draws a picture of dark skies shadowing a cemetery. How would a nurse document this level of suicidal behavior?
   1. Ideation
   2. Threat

3. Gesture
4. Attempt

5. A nurse reviews the report from a depressed patient's positron emission tomography scan. Which finding is most likely if the patient has demonstrated high-lethality suicide attempts?
   1. Increased serotonin activity in the medulla, the midbrain, and the hypothalamus
   2. Decreased serotonin activity in the ventral, medial, and lateral prefrontal cortex
   3. Decreased dopamine and glutamate receptors in the parietal and temporal lobes
   4. Increased norepinephrine and acetylcholine reserves in the thalamus and the pons

REFERENCES

American Association of Suicidology: *Facts about suicide and depression; Elderly suicide fact sheet; Suicide in the USA based on current (2007) statistics; Survivors of suicide fact sheet;* and *Youth suicide fact sheet* (websites): www.suidology.org. Accessed July 15, 2010.

American Foundation for Suicide Prevention: *Risk factors for suicide; facts and figures* (website): www.afsp.org. Accessed July 12, 2010.

American Psychiatric Association: *Diagnostic and statistical manual of mental disorders*, ed 4, text revision, Washington, DC, 2000, American Psychiatric Association.

American Psychiatric Association: *Practice guideline for the assessment and treatment of patients with suicidal behaviors*, Arlington, Va, 2003, American Psychiatric Association.

American Psychiatric Association: *Characteristics evaluated in the psychiatric assessment of patients with suicidal behavior* (website): www.psychiatryonline.com/popup.aspx?aID=56073. Accessed July 31, 2010.

American Psychiatric Association: *Circumstances in which a suicide assessment may be indicated clinically* (website): www.psychiatryonline.com/popup.aspx?aID=56140. Accessed July 31, 2010.

American Psychiatric Association: *Questions that may be helpful in inquiring about specific aspects of suicidal thoughts, plans, and behaviors* (website): www.psychiatryonline.com/popup.aspx?aID=56178. Accessed July 31, 2010.

American Psychiatric Association: *Factors associated with an increased risk of suicide* (website): www.psychiatryonline.com/popup.aspx?aID=56260. Accessed July 31, 2010.

American Psychiatric Association: *Factors associated with protective effects for suicide* (website): www.psychiatryonline.com/popup.aspx?aID=56337. Accessed July 31, 2010.

Brent DA et al: Predictors of spontaneous and systematically assessed suicidal adverse events in the treatment of SSRI-resistant depressant in adolescents (TORDIA) study, *Am J Psychiatry* 166(4):418-427, 2009.

Brent DA et al: Association of FKBP5 polymorphisms with suicidal events in the treatment of SSRI-resistant depressant in adolescents (TORDIA) study, *Am J Psychiatry* 167(2):190-198, 2010.

Centers for Disease Control and Prevention: *Suicide: facts at a glance* (website): www.cdc.gov/violenceprevention. Accessed July 30, 2010.

Chiles JA, Strosahi KD: *Assessment and treatment: clinical manual for assessment and treatment of suicidal patients*, Washington, DC, 2005, American Psychiatric Publishing.

Conwell Y: Suicide prevention in later life: a glass half full, or half empty? *Am J Psychiatry* 166(8):845-849, 2009.

Durkheim E: *Suicide*, Glencoe, Ill, 1951, The Free Press.

Ezzell C: *Why? The neuroscience of suicide: physical clues to suicide* (website): www.sciam.com/print_version.cfm?articleID=000D8D31. Accessed October 18, 2003.

Freud S: *Mourning and melancholia, collected papers*, London, 1920, Hogarth Press.

Goldston DB et al: Cultural considerations in adolescent suicide prevention and psychosocial treatment, *Am Psychol* 63(1):14-27, 2008.

Gunderson JG: *Borderline personality disorder*, Washington, DC, 1984, American Psychiatric Press.

Hendin H et al: Problems in psychotherapy with suicidal patients, *Am J Psychiatry* 163:67-72, 2006.

Joiner TE et al: The psychology and neurobiology of suicidal behavior, *Annu Rev Psychol* 56:287-315, 2005.

King CA et al: Adolescent suicide risk screening in the emergency department, *Acad Emerg Med* 16(11):1234-1241, 2009.

Kjølseth I et al: Why suicide? Elderly people who committed suicide and their experience of life in the period before their death, *International Psychogeriatrics* 22(2):209-210, 2010.

Lenz K et al: Overview of depression and its management in children and adolescents, *Formulary* 44(6):172-193, June, 2009.

Linehan MM: *Cognitive-behavioral treatment of borderline personality disorder*, New York, 1993, Guildford Press.

Litman R: Sigmund Freud on suicide, in E. Shneidman editor: *Essays in self-destruction*, pages 324-344, New York, Jason Aronson Publishers.

Macdonald P: Caring for the older person, *Practice Nurse*, 39(3): 14-17, 2010.

Martiniuk ALC et al: Self-harm and risk of motor vehicle crashes among young drivers: finding from the DRIVE study, *Canadian Medical Association Journal (CMAJ)*, 181(11):807-813, 2009.

Masterson JF: *Psychotherapy of the borderline adult: a developmental approach*, New York, 1976, Brunner/Mazel.

National Institute of Mental Health: *Army study to assess risk and resilience in service members (Army STARRS): a partnership between NIMH and the US Army* (website): www.nimh.nih.gov/health/topics/suicide-prevention/. Accessed July 11, 2010.

Nielsen D et al: Suicidality and 5-hydroxyindoleacetic acid concentraion associated with tryptophan-hydroxylase polymorphism, *Archives of General Psychiatry* 51:34-38, 1994.

North American Nursing Diagnosis Association International: *NANDA nursing diagnoses: definitions and classification 2009-2011*, Ames, Iowa, 2009, North American Nursing Diagnosis Association International.

O'Keeffe GS, Clarke-Pearson K: Clinical Report: the impact of social media on children, adolescents, and families, *Pediatrics* 2011.

Oldham JM: Borderline personality disorder and suicidality, *Am J Psychiatry* 163:20-26, 2006.

Parsey RV et al: Lower serotonin transporter binding potential in the human brain during major depressive episodes, *Am J Psychiatry* 163:52-58, 2006.

Rogers C, editor: *On becoming a person*, Boston, 1961, Houghton Mifflin.

Shneidman E: *Definition of suicide*, New York, 1985, John Wiley & Sons.

Shneidman ES: *The suicidal mind*, New York, 1996, Oxford University Press.

Stekel W: Suicide and will. In Freidman P, editor: *On suicide*, New York, 1967, International Universities Press.

Sullivan H: Socio-psychiatric research: its implications for the schizophrenia problem and mental hygiene, *Am J Psychiatry* 10:977-991, 1931.

Sullivan H: The manic-depressive psychosis. In Perry H et al, editors: *Clinical studies in psychiatry*, New York, 1956, WW Norton.

Volek JS et al: 2007, Antidepressant treatment in (Pub Med) www.ncbi.nlm.nih.gov

Online Resources

American Association of Suicidology: www.suicidology.org
American Foundation for Suicide Prevention: www.afsp.org
Army STARRS: www.armystarrs.org
Indian Health Service www.ihs.gov
National Suicide Prevention Lifeline: www.suicidepreventionlifeline.org
Suicide Prevention Resource Center: www.sprc.org
Survivors of Suicide: www.survivorsofsuicide.com
The Link Counseling Center: www.thelink.org
Training Institute for Suicide Assessment & Clinical Interviewing: www.suicideassessment.com
Yellow Ribbon Suicide Prevention Program: www.yellowribbon.org/

Violence: Anger, Abuse, and Aggression

Ann Wolbert Burgess and Dona Petrozzi

"In violence we forget who we are."

Mary McCarthy

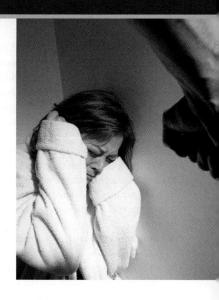

evolve WEBSITE

http://evolve.elsevier.com/Fortinash/

OBJECTIVES

- Consider violence and trauma as public health issues.
- Review various theories of family violence for application to nursing practice.
- Discuss barriers that hinder an abused woman from leaving her violent situation.
- Discuss the role of control in the etiology of domestic violence.
- Compare the child physical offender with the child sexual offender.
- Define child maltreatment in terms of emotional, psychologic, physical, and sexual abuse.

- Construct examples of how women who are raped are revictimized by society.
- Apply the nursing process to the care of victims of family violence.
- Describe the dynamics of sexual assault.
- Identify the barriers to the identification of elder abuse.
- Compare victim and offender behavior in interpersonal violence situations.

KEY TERMS

bullying
child abuse (maltreatment)
child neglect
elder abuse

enmeshed
homicide
incest
intimate partner violence

rape
stalking
violence

Few individuals in modern societies are strangers to violence, which is defined as abusive or unjust exercise of power over another. Violence may be experienced directly as victims or indirectly as observers, but in any case its impact on human lives is undeniable.

Violence may be overt or covert. The media in all its forms brings violence closer to home than most people want. Often we are witness to huge scale, real life, overt events such as the massacres on school and college campuses, the shootings on the 2009 Fort Hood military base, the senseless deaths in 2011 in an Arizona supermarket parking lot, and improvised explosive devices (IEDs) detonating before our eyes. Ravages of war and riots fill our films and the television screens as the

events are happening. Death and torture are common themes in popular video games, and even plague the very young in the form of cartoon characters. Everyday violence as an overt event is also experienced on a smaller scale that is no less devastating at the local level in homes, neighborhoods, and school and workplace settings. International, national, and local terrorism threats and events of many types are all too common.

Although actual and Internet stalking and cyberbullying activity is considered by some to be covert, it seldom misses the opportunity to directly impinge on another person's life, often with grave consequences. Much to the dismay of healthy individuals, violence in its many forms is alive and flourishing. Regardless of the threat, nurses and other skilled personnel are prepared and take the challenge to help protect, prevent, treat, and care for those in need when their lives are touched and changed by acts of violence.

The public health focus on violence has brought new experts to the field and created new collaborative partnerships among nurses, physicians, criminologists, psychologists, psychiatrists, sociologists, neuroscientists, and others. Violence began to be seen as a public health issue in 1992, when U.S. Surgeon General C. Everett Koop declared it to be a public health emergency. American society has become increasingly concerned with both the physical injuries associated with violence and the traumatic psychosocial impact that it has on its victims. It is well established that interpersonal violence can have serious deleterious effects on mental health, and these are most notably expressed as elevated levels of posttraumatic distress disorder, dissociative symptoms, and enduring personality changes (Kamphus and Emmelkamp, 2005) (see Chapters 10 and 14).

As survivors of violence continue to seek treatment in the clinical setting, nursing is expanding its professional practice and knowledge base to address the complex needs of victims of violence. Nurses are frontline responders and practice in a wide variety of settings. They need to be prepared to address the issues that relate to the assessment, care, and protection of victims of violence, whether the abuse occurs at the hands of a family member, a stranger, an acquaintance, a date, or a caregiver. Therapeutic interventions can be directed to prevent additional abuse, violence, and even death.

VIOLENCE WITHIN FAMILIES

There are daily reports of family violence in the community as well as high-profile media reports. Two examples follow.

Canadian professional wrestler Chris Benoit, 40, strangled his wife Nancy, 43, and suffocated his son Daniel, 7, before he hanged himself on a weight machine inside his home. The three bodies were found on June 24, 2007. Although no motive has been determined, speculation was that Chris Benoit suffered from repeated untreated concussions, steroid abuse, and a failing marriage. Nancy Benoit had filed for divorce in May 2005 after a domestic abuse incident, but she had withdrawn the filing in August 2005.

Mackenzie Phillips, 49, the former star of 1970s and 1980s sitcom "One Day at a Time," told Oprah Winfrey on September 23, 2009, on primetime television that she was first raped by her father—John Phillips, the lead singer of The Mamas & The Papas—in a hotel room when she was 18 years old while passed out after a drug binge. She stated that she continued to use drugs and to have consensual sex with him for years. The relationship continued long after she married Jeff Sessler when she was

19 years old, and it only ended when she became pregnant and feared that her father was the baby's father. Her father paid for an abortion.

Michelle Phillips—Mackenzie Phillips' step-mother and also a former member of The Mamas & The Papas—told The Hollywood Reporter that she believed that the allegations were false. Michelle Phillips said that Mackenzie had "a lot of mental illness" and that "she's had a needle stuck up her arm for 35 years and is jealous of her siblings, who have accomplished a lot and did not become drug addicts."

The Benoit case involves steroid drug abuse, untreated head trauma, and domestic violence. The Phillips case involves drug abuse and prolonged incest.

The problem of family violence has always existed. Women have been battered by their partners in almost every society in the world. Intimate partner violence was accepted practice. The beginning of services for battered women and children dates back to 1885, when the Chicago Protective Agency for Women, which was established to help women who were victims of physical abuse, provided legal aid, court advocacy, and personal assistance to affected women. However, by the 1940s, few shelters remained, in part as a result of the marital separations caused by World War II.

The history of childhood is replete with suffering; it has been well documented from biblical times to the present. The landmark Wilson case of 1874 pricked the American social conscience and opened America's eyes to the plight of many children. Eight-year-old Mary Ellen Wilson lived with her adoptive parents in New York City. She was held there in chains, starved, and beaten. The police responded but could do nothing because it was a "family matter," and the parents held the "rights" (Zigler and Hall, 1989). A man named Henry Berg was contacted. He had founded a protective group the preceding year, The Society for the Prevention of Cruelty to Animals. Berg was able to extricate Mary Ellen from her family's torture chamber.

This section presents definitions and current statistical trends from a developmental perspective regarding family violence. It covers bullying behavior as a precursor to abusive dating relationships and courtship abuse; partner threat and violence; domestic violence and pregnancy; batterer stalking patterns; domestic homicide; child abuse, neglect, and sexual assault; and elder abuse. It also discusses key concepts of family violence, such as socialization into violence and learned socialized violence; the psychodynamics of violent behavior, including altered attachment, jealousy, guilt, and revenge; and the biology of trauma.

BULLYING BEHAVIOR

Because of its connection to violent and aggressive behaviors that result in serious injury to the self and to others, bullying is now considered a major public health issue. Once viewed as a ritual of childhood and adolescence, bullying has now captured media headlines both nationally and internationally (Burgess et al, 2006).

Bullying is the abuse of power by one person over another through repeated aggressive behaviors. One of the first researchers on the topic, Olweus (1993), defines a bullied person as an individual who is exposed repeatedly over time to negative actions on the part of one or more persons. For bullies, power may arise from physical strength and maturity, from a higher status within a peer group, from knowing another child's weakness, or from recruiting the support of other children. As bullies age, they rely less on physical means to intimidate their victims and turn to indirect forms that entail verbal abuse and social exclusion (Olweus, 1991).

Bullying can occur in both direct and indirect ways. Males and females tend to differ with regard to the ways that they bully. Girls are less likely to bully physically and more often engage in relational aggression. This type of bullying involves a deliberate isolation and exclusion of the victim from friendship. Slander, spreading rumors, and manipulation are frequent tools of the relational bully, who also engages other students' assistance in his or her scheme with the use of threats of exclusion if they do not comply.

Victimization in particular is of great concern as a result of the potentially debilitating effects of chronic peer rejection, such as increased anger and depression, low self-esteem, and social withdrawal. Children form their interpersonal and self-schemas on the basis of their social interactions. Not all bullies graduate to having psychiatric disorders, but a persistent pattern of antisocial behavior during childhood and adolescence can be predictive of future difficulties. Olweus (1993) identifies at-risk personality traits in children as aggression toward animals or other children, a lack of empathy, and the destruction of property. Nurses are conducting research on childhood teasing and bullying. For example, the use of bibliotherapy is an innovative approach that has been recommended to school nurses as they work to promote healthy school environments (Gregory and Vessey, 2004).

DEVELOPMENTAL ASPECTS OF THE FAMILY AND ITS STRUCTURE

Just as there are developmental stages and tasks for the child who is maturing into an adult, the family may be viewed as progressing through three developmental phases. *The first phase* begins with dating, courtship, and marriage; *the middle phase* includes partnership and work, with childbearing and parenting being options; and *the third phase* continues with a work focus, optional grandparenting, and retirement. Because violence within families has only recently surfaced as a legal matter, research into the causes and consequences is limited. As a first step, definitions are provided to begin classification for the research process.

Family

Nowhere in the criminal law and its administration is the social construction of violent crime changing more rapidly than in the area of what constitutes family violence and society's response to it (Reiss and Roth, 1993). As a result of the myriad of different statutes and regulations, there is no national legal definition of a family.

Trends in family violence must be interpreted against a decline in the percentage of households that contain exclusively married couples and their biologic children. Violence between growing numbers of same-sex and opposite-sex cohabiting partners is increasingly being regarded as family violence, regardless of legal marital status. Violence between divorced or separated former couples is also considered family violence.

The National Research Council's Panel on Understanding and Preventing Violence (Reiss and Roth, 1993) considered all violent behavior within a household as family violence, specifically spouse assault, physical and sexual assault of children, sibling assault, and physical and sexual assault of other relatives who reside in the household. The panel defined physical violence as behaviors that threaten, attempt, or actually inflict physical harm and thereby expanded violence to include more than just the actual physical act (Crowell and Burgess, 1996).

The Dynamic Nature of Family Violence

There are several characteristics that distinguish family violence from stranger violence. Although there is a continuing relationship among its members that is similar to that of other relationships (e.g., teacher and student, employer and employee, child and caretaker), daily interaction in a shared domicile increases the opportunities for violent encounters. Because these individuals are bound together in a continuing relationship, it is quite likely there will be repeat violations by the offender. An unequal power relationship makes one more vulnerable to the aggression and violence of the offender. Moreover, the offender often threatens additional violence if the incidents of violence are disclosed. The victim may refrain from disclosure in anticipation of stigmatization and denigration. Finally, episodes of violence often occur in private places, are invisible to others, and are less likely to be detected or reported to police (Reiss and Roth, 1993).

Phase 1: Assault During Courtship and Marriage

The first phase of family life includes dating, courtship, and marriage. Although dating does not necessarily lead to courtship or marriage, it is instructive to review data about early relationship problems and dating aggression (Rhatigan and Street, 2005). Theories of both marital and dating aggression identify conflict as an important causal factor that leads to aggression between partners. Dating violence appears to begin as early as the age of 15 or 16 years. Typical tactics include slapping, pushing, beating, and threatening with or using weapons. Recurring and escalating episodes of violence in a relationship are quite common if the relationship is not terminated. Research has indicated that approximately 44% of acquaintance rape victims (as compared with less than 1% of stranger rape victims) are likely to be sexually assaulted more than once by the same offender (Gidycz and Layman, 1996). About 50% of the victims do terminate the

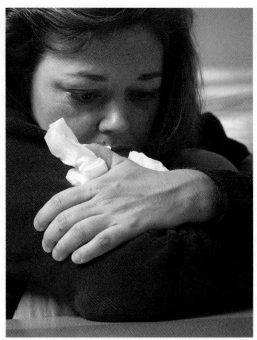

FIGURE 23-1. Physical abuse is the most common cause of injury to women in the United States. Battering occurs in all ethnic, religious, and socioeconomic groups. Although the batterer is unprovoked, the woman is made to feel that the abuse is her fault.

relationship. Victims of acquaintance rape are often in a state of denial during the aftermath of the rape, and they often present for treatment years after the assaultive incident.

Although large-scale surveys have documented the prevalence of abuse in teen dating relationships, this type of violence often escapes attention or concern. Research indicates that a large number of college students experience physical aggression in their dating relationships. Estimates of the prevalence of dating aggression among college students range from 20% to as high as 50%.

Violence can continue within marriage. Spousal assault is the single most common cause of injury for which women seek emergency medical attention. In a study of the emergency treatment of women in a metropolitan hospital, the investigators reported that battered women were 13 times more likely than other women who were receiving emergency care to be injured in the breast, chest, or abdomen, and they were three times as likely to be injured while pregnant (Stark and Flintcraft, 1982 and 1991) (Figure 23-1).

Stalking

Stalking is part of the constellation of behaviors that are associated with partner violence, especially when there is a difficult breakup with an intimate partner. Stalking takes various forms and has varying definitions across states. From a legal point of view, stalking is the willful, malicious, and repeated following and harassing of another person, with fear of violence resulting in the victim. In a pilot sample of self-reported batterers, 36 out of 120 who stalked and who were charged with domestic violence revealed three stalking groups: one in which the discrediting of the partner was the key; a second that revolved around love turning to hate; and a third that involved violent confrontation with the former partner (Burgess et al, 1997). A second study of 165 batterers suggested stalking behaviors varied from seemingly benign acts or efforts at being reasonable to hidden, threatening, and frightening behaviors. Batterers were found to contact estranged partners for two major reasons that elicit a range of contradictory and ambivalent emotions. The conscious motive, for the most part, appears to be altruistic, although the emotions range from longing to hostility, confusion, and revenge. By contrast, individuals with secret and clandestine behaviors were angry and aggressive and indicated a propensity for abusive action (Burgess et al, 2001).

Violence and Pregnancy

Prebirth violence can include sex-selective abortion or battering during pregnancy that affects birth outcome (Carretta, 2008). It has been estimated that as many as one in five teenagers are the victims of domestic violence during pregnancy (Parker et al, 1993). Recent research estimates that, in as many as two thirds of teenage pregnancies, adult males are the fathers (Males and Chew, 1996). Although domestic violence during pregnancy is often preceded by a history of abuse, pregnancy may act as a trigger that increases the frequency and severity of the violence. This increase may be related to the financial implications of the pregnancy and birth, the stress surrounding altered relational and sexual roles, and the increased attention on the growing pregnancy. In addition, pregnancy disclosure, especially in cases of questionable paternity, may also potentiate an already volatile situation.

Phase 2: Assault of Women and Children

Family violence can escalate to homicide. Several patterns are noteworthy: newborns and children between the ages of 1 and 4 years are more vulnerable to homicide than are children between the ages of 5 and 9 years (Federal Bureau of Investigation, 1990). Infants and small children are more likely to be killed by their mothers than their fathers, perhaps in part as a result of differential risk exposure; the risk of homicide for children who are younger than 5 years old is greater for male than female children, according to a case-control study (Winpisinger et al, 1991).

According to Bureau of Justice Statistics, in 2004, female murder victims were substantially more likely than male murder victims to have been killed by an intimate partner. About one third of 1159 female murder victims were killed by an intimate partner in 2004, whereas about 3% of 385 male murder victims were killed by an intimate partner that year. Of all female murder victims, the proportion killed by an intimate partner declined slightly until 1995, when the proportion began increasing, although it has stabilized recently. Of male murder victims, the proportion killed by an intimate partner has dropped (Bureau of Justice Statistics, 2004).

Case Study #1 qualifies as a catastrophic crisis because of the deaths of the mother and her infant, the disclosure of the wife as a silent battered woman during the marriage and pregnancy, and the suicide of the abuser.

CASE STUDY #1

On October 23, 1989, a frantic man called 911 and told police that he and his wife had been shot. The story that Charles Stuart told that day turned a city upside down, and it still reverberates more than two decades later (Boston Channel, 2009). The Boston police received an emergency call that a pregnant woman and her husband, driving home from a childbirth class, had been shot by an unknown assailant. Police located the couple and rushed them to a local hospital. Surgeons were unable to save the young woman. Her baby was born by caesarean section but died 10 days later. After a lengthy investigation, the police identified the prime suspect as the woman's husband, Charles Stuart. Before he could be arrested, Stuart jumped off a bridge and drowned. Stuart's brother was arrested and charged with aiding in a felony; he had disposed of two bags containing the murdered woman's jewelry as well as the murder weapon. Police divers located the evidence.

Phase 3: Assault of the Elderly

Surprisingly little is known about the occurrence of domestic violence against elders in families, for several reasons. First, most studies do not distinguish between elder abuse and elder neglect. Second, families are unlikely to report the abuse, since the responsible person may be a son or daughter. Third, many elderly people are homebound, with no one available to see what is happening.

There are presently about 39 million individuals in the United States who are more than 65 years old; the U.S. Census Bureau projects that more than 62 million Americans will be 65 years old or older in 2025 (McCoy and Hansen, 2004). Older women (67%) are far more likely than men (32%) to suffer from abuse, and slightly more than half of the alleged perpetrators of elder abuse are female (53%) (National Center on Elder Abuse Study, 2004). Because older victims usually have smaller support systems and fewer physical, psychologic, and economic reserves, the impact of abuse and neglect is magnified, and a single incident of mistreatment is more likely to trigger a downward spiral that leads to a loss of independence, a serious complicating illness, and even death (Burgess and Hanrahan, 2006).

Explanations of Family Violence

Most theories regarding the causes of family violence are only partial explanations. Either they attempt to explain a single type or a few types of family violence (e.g., partner assault), or they seek to identify a particular factor or set of factors that account for some of the observed variations in behavior between violent and nonviolent persons or acts (National Research Council, 1993). The leading explanations of family violence are derived from social, cultural, and transgenerational perspectives (Box 23-1).

The Social and Cultural Perspective

Sociologists have attempted to develop an integrated theory of several cultural and structural determinants and of social

BOX 23-1   ETIOLOGIC THEORIES RELATED TO FAMILY VIOLENCE

PSYCHIATRIC AND MENTAL ILLNESS MODEL

Social learning theory
Aggression as a learned (not instinctual) behavior
Family role modeling
Desensitization to violence as a result of repeated exposure via the media
Sociologic theory
Unemployment
Poverty
Crime
Teenage pregnancy
Isolation
Anthropologic theory
Sexual inequalities
Social organization
Cultural patterning
Feminist theory
Explanatory use of constructs of gender and power
Analysis of the family as a historically situated institution
Importance of understanding and validating women's experiences
Empowerment of women

learning. For example, feminist theory asserts that the unequal power distribution between men and women subjects women to male dominance in all spheres of life (i.e., work, family, and community life). Power extends to the sexual relationship as well as to work and social relationships. The various ways in which coercion is used depend on men's use of their physical and social power to maintain that dominant position.

Within this framework, growing up in a patriarchal society that emphasizes male dominance and aggression and female victimization, children are socialized into their respective sex roles. In addition, they learn through their experiences in the family or through exposure to the media. This learning becomes reinforced in the larger community, where male and female roles similarly rest on elements of macho culture.

Recent changes in family organization and structure may account for some family aggression. Changes that affect social and moral bonding among family members are probably most significant. One such change since the 1970s is the deinstitutionalization of children without families, the mentally ill, the homeless, and the disabled. The temporary placement of children in foster homes, via adoption, and informally with relatives exposes children to risks of violence from caretakers for whom the minimal moral constraints of the parenting role are less salient.

A second major change is the increase in the number of children who are not living with their natural parents. These numbers are substantial and growing as a result of serial cohabitation, divorce, desertion, incarceration, substance abuse, and death.

Social Isolation

Social isolation has been identified as a characteristic of some families that are at high risk for the physical and sexual abuse of a spouse or children. The isolation may be forced on the partner by the abuser. Alternatively, shame may prompt the visibly battered spouse to withdraw even further. Victims often become isolated from friends, the family of origin, neighbors, or anyone who could become acquainted with the events. Some families isolate themselves in subtle ways by using unlisted telephone numbers or cell phones. They lack a means of transportation so that they cannot visit others, and their homes may be physically shuttered from the gaze of outsiders. They often lack community ties of any kind.

Generational Transmission of Violence

The transmission of violence from one generation to the next is as much a component of subculturation as any other learned behavior. Straus and colleagues (1980) reported that, among adults who were abused as children, more than one fifth later abuse their own children. However, Widom (1989) cautions the reader that the methodologic limitations of these studies, especially their retrospective design, restrict the validity of conclusions about the long-term consequences of abuse during childhood. Regardless, most health care professionals remain concerned about the potential dangers.

Developmental Traumatology: A Neurobiologic Perspective

The growing field of developmental traumatology is providing insights regarding how the mechanisms of abuse and neglect that result from early childhood trauma can affect adult survivors (Kreidler and Kurzawa, 2009). Early sustained abuse can produce physiologic changes in the developing brain that result in difficulty with modulating emotional responses (e.g., anger, depression), with interpreting social situations, and with thinking, which can contribute to impulsivity, antisocial behavior, and sexual misconduct (Schwartz et al, 2006). Essentially, early life attachments, also called *bonding*, translate into a blueprint of how the child will perceive situations outside of the family. Positive attachment that is based on warmth, affection, caring, protective behaviors, and accountability lead to basic trust; this is at the core of the building of a social human being. Through attachment, the person gets feedback about the emerging of self. Around 18 months of age, there is a consolidation of a sense of self. The early development of the ability to self-soothe provides an inner core of calmness and the ability to avoid being overwhelmed by stimuli that results in an integrated sense of self.

Social bonding can fail or become narrow and selective. Caretakers can either ignore, rationalize, or normalize various behaviors in the developing child or, through their own problems (e.g., violent behavior), support the child's developing distortions and projections. An ineffective social environment can occur through the ignoring of aggressive or sexual behavior or by failing to intervene to correct behavior.

BOX 23-2   EPIDEMIOLOGY OF VIOLENCE

Battered Women

1.8 million wives in the United States are abused every year by their husbands

25% to 50% of all women are abused by their intimate partners at least once

20% to 25% of women who seek treatment in emergency departments are there as a result of battering injuries

2% to 8% of these women identified abuse as the cause of their injuries

7% to 17% of pregnant women experience physical abuse by their partners

Physically Abused Children

2 million children are seriously abused each year by their parents and caregivers

Of these, 1000 die as a result of their injuries

25% of the 2 million abused children are physically abused; 20% are sexually abused; and 55% are neglected

25% of the 2 million abused children are younger than 5 years old; 60% are between the ages of 5 and 14 years

Children younger than 3 years old are at a greater risk for fatal abuse than are older children

Abused and neglected children are at greater risk for later delinquency, adult criminality, and violent crimes than are nonabused or non-neglected children

Sexually Abused Children

50% of psychiatric patients have histories of physical and sexual abuse

The average age at which child incest begins is 6 years, with an average duration of 7 years

Rape

Only 10% to 20% of rapes are reported to the police

More than 90% of rape victims are women

20% of female college students are raped at some time during their college education

The most common age group for rape victims is 16 to 25 years

In 84% of rape cases, the victim is acquainted with the perpetrator

Only 5% of rapists were psychotic when they raped their victims

In 90% of rape cases, victims and perpetrators are of the same race

---

The child who lacks protection by a caretaker experiences tremendous anxiety; he or she is overwhelmed and may survive by dissociating himself or herself from the trauma. This dissociation also inhibits a sense of feeling connected to the outside world. With the earliest manifestations of this numbing, children are cruel to animals, siblings, friends, and even parents and grandparents. There is a lack of sensitivity to the pain of others, and there can be a distorted association of pain with various events. Children become isolated and disconnected from others. In a Massachusetts case, a 14-year-old youth took a 7-year-old mentally disabled boy into the woods and beat the boy to death. The youth had told people that he was going to do this, and no one intervened.

This cruel and detached behavior can be noted in date abuse that occurs in junior and senior high schools. One example from the 1990s was the gang rape of a developmentally disabled girl that happened in Glen Ridge, NJ. In that case, several high school male students inserted objects into the girl's vagina while other male high school students watched. They had no sense of their impact on the victim. The case came to light when the abusing males tried to videotape a planned second incident with the teenager.

Although attachment theory was intended as a revision of psychoanalytic theory, it has been infused with biologic principles, control-systems theory, and cognitive psychology. Although it began with an attempt to understand the disturbed functioning of individuals who had suffered early separations or traumatic losses, it is a theory of normal development that suggests explanations for some types of atypical development. Since Bowlby's preliminary formulations (1958), attachment theory has stimulated research into socioemotional development and the growth of interpersonal relationships (see Chapter 7).

Family violence has been linked to mental illness and personality disorders, although the links have been established for clinical populations rather than with the use of case-control methods or general population surveys. Studies of women's shelter populations report that depression is quite common among women who are chronic victims of domestic violence. Clinical studies have consistently found a high incidence of bipolar depression, anxiety disorders, posttraumatic stress disorder (PTSD), panic disorder, and suicide ideation among chronically abused women (Kamphuis and Emmelkamp, 2005). A large group of batterers have been diagnosed as having borderline personalities that include a constellation of behavioral shifts: anger outbursts, rage, intense jealousy, blaming, recurring moods, trauma symptoms, haunting fear of isolation and loss, binge drinking and repetitive self-destructive thoughts (Dutton, 1995).

Assaultive and Homicidal Behavior

How can interpersonal violence be explained, especially partner violence and homicide? It is difficult, because there is a transgression of a basic sense of connectedness between people, and it causes many to wonder how this kind of behavior can exist. However, it is known that early attachment disturbance and the impairment of self-regulation are major diagnostic issues among traumatized children (van der Kolk and Fisler, 1994).

With courtship violence, the aggressor may not want the relationship to end. There can be terroristic and death threats, stalking behavior, parking outside of the victim's house, and the making of harassing phone calls. The harasser cannot tolerate separation. He or she feels abandoned, angry, and depressed, and he or she may become suicidal. Rage is often behind the depression. Rejection is an attack on the ego. Frequently these individuals feel that they cannot manage on their own, and the limbic system is actually affected. These

---

BOX 23-3	**BEHAVIORS OF THE ABUSER**

Economic abuse, including the strict control of money (even when the woman earns it), food, clothing, transportation, and other resources
Sexual abuse, including marital rape and forcing the woman to participate in sexual activities against her will
Threats and intimidation, including threats of taking the children from the woman or hurting them or other family members
Threatening to injure or kill family pets
Isolating the woman from any support system, including her family, friends, and health care professionals
Constantly demeaning and insulting the woman
Intentionally breaking material objects to terrorize the woman

---

individuals may lack impulse control. Although fantasy calms these patients temporarily, the fantasies are often filled with rage at the partner. The distorted thought is this: "I killed her because I love her" (Box 23-3).

THE NURSING PROCESS

ASSESSMENT

Universal screening for domestic abuse should be performed on all women who are seen in the clinical setting, particularly pregnant women, who should be assessed at least every trimester. Because battering during pregnancy is one of the major causes of complications of pregnancy, nurses need to be attuned to the risk factors of domestic violence during pregnancy. Even older widows may have serious unresolved issues relating to abusive relationships with their deceased husbands. To obtain an accurate history of the domestic violence victim, the nurse should not question the victim in front the suspected abuser, family members, or friends. Walton-Moss and Campbell (2002) cautioned against the use of such terms as *abuse* and *battering*, because many abused women do not include these ideas in their images of themselves and their lives.

Obtaining disclosure about abuse is complicated. Carretta (2008) cautions that nurses need to be selective and creative when asking questions. For example, nurses can ask whether the woman feels safe at home instead of asking if she is abused. Nurses may also assess the partner relationship and ask, "What happens when an argument arises?"

It is important to understand that the woman may love her partner and that she desperately wants to believe him when he promises that the abuse will never happen again. Nurse responses to a positive screen should be designed to validate and support the victim's experience. Phrases such as "I believe you" and "No one deserves to be beaten" are examples of supportive responses to domestic violence victims. In addition, the nurse must provide a safe environment that is conducive to disclosure.

BOX 23-4	**GENERAL CASE HISTORY QUESTIONS FOR THE ABUSED INDIVIDUAL**

1. Have you ever been emotionally or physically abused by your partner or by someone who is important to you?
2. Within the last year, have you been hit, slapped, kicked, or otherwise physically hurt by someone? If yes, by whom, and how many times?
3. Within the last year, has anyone forced you to have sexual activities? If yes, who, and how many times?
4. Are you afraid of your partner or of anyone else that you have mentioned?

During the assessment and when taking the woman's history, it is recommended that the nurse begin with the least sensitive questions and gradually progress to the more sensitive ones. Questions should be simple and direct, and they should reflect the language and terms that the woman herself uses (see the Nursing Assessment Questions box). The Nursing Research Consortium on Violence and Abuse has developed a simple four-item questionnaire that was adapted by Campbell and Humphreys (1993) for the obtaining of a general case history (Box 23-4). These questions may be followed by additional questions.

When women do present with suspicious physical injuries, a delay in seeking treatment or an illogical explanation for the injury is a clue that may indicate abuse. Often abused women seek treatment for the indirect effects of their violent relationships. Complaints may reflect the stress of these violent relationships or residual pain from previous injuries. These women frequently appear depressed, anxious, and fatigued. Behaviors manifested by these depressed victims may include soft speech, poor visual contact, hypervigilance, decreased interest in daily activities, and suicidal ideation. The abused woman typically has more chronic, pain-related, and vague complaints than her nonabused counterpart. The health history may indicate frequent accidents and other traumatic injuries such as lacerations, bruises, and fractures. Spontaneous abortions, suicide attempts, and substance abuse may also be reported.

The assessment of the battered woman begins with the nurse's critical examination of his or her own beliefs and biases about battering autodiagnosis. For example, if the nurse believes that a woman has brought the problem on herself for not leaving the abusive relationship, then this attitude, consciously or unconsciously, will most likely be communicated to the battered woman. The nurse's attitude and resulting interactions may re-victimize the woman.

Because holistic assessments are the foundation of the nursing process, culture is an important consideration during that assessment. Culture often defines how the battered woman interprets and responds to the violence that has been perpetrated against her. Understanding the battered woman's culture is also critical for developing a treatment plan. Culture is an important determinant of whether the battered woman seeks assistance from community resources such as the police and shelters. Some ethnic women are isolated and unaware of community resources for abused individuals; they may be suspicious of caregivers outside of their own cultural group and fear being ostracized by their cultural group if they reach out to the broader community. Most battered women's shelters make a concerted effort to reach out to women of all colors and ethnic groups. When caring for a patient from a minority culture, it is the nurse's responsibility to learn about the patient's culture. Questions about the woman's culture are appropriate, but they must be presented in a sensitive and respectful way so that the woman understands that the nurse is concerned and intent on learning more about the woman's values and customs in an effort to provide effective holistic nursing care.

An understanding of culture is as important when working with the male batterer as it is when working with the battered woman. Before treatment strategies can be planned for the abuser, his cultural attitudes, values, and beliefs must be acknowledged and respected. However, no cultural beliefs and traditions can be accepted or tolerated at the expense of another person's health and well-being. Because the physical abuse of women—including rape—by their partners is common, it is critical to ask about physical, sexual, and emotional abuse in the histories of all women. The nurse must also ask if the abuser hits the children. Protective services must be notified if the children have been or are being abused (see Chapter 9).

NURSING ASSESSMENT QUESTIONS #1

For the Battered Woman

1. We often see women who have been hurt by their partners. Is your partner responsible for your injuries?
2. Has your partner ever hurt you?
3. Have you noticed any pattern to this behavior, such as an increase in frequency and severity?
4. Does he threaten to use or has he ever used a weapon to hurt you?

Box 23-5 presents the most important physical examination indicators of wife and woman abuse.

The nurse must accurately document all statements that the woman makes. Open-ended questions that reflect what the woman is disclosing should be used so that she feels in charge of the interview. Documented information must include the name of the abuser and when and how the abuse occurred. The nurse should record direct quotes from the victim and document them with quotation marks. An inquiry into the safety of other persons in the home is also the responsibility of the nurse. If it is discovered that children or disabled or elderly persons are being abused in the home, then the appropriate protective agency needs to be notified.

It is crucial to reassure the woman that the documentation is confidential and that her partner will not be allowed to have access to it without her permission. Retaliation by the batterer is always a major concern for the abused woman. However,

---

BOX 23-5   **PHYSICAL INDICATORS OF POSSIBLE ABUSE**

General Appearance
Anxious and frightened; depressed and passive; ashamed and embarrassed; poor eye contact; weight problems; looks to partner for answers and partner does all of the talking; partner exhibits smothering and extremely possessive behavior

Skin
Contusions, abrasions, minor lacerations, scars, and burns, particularly on the breasts, arms, abdomen, chest, neck, face, and genitals

Musculoskeletal
Fractures and sprains, especially of distal bones (e.g., skull, facial bones, extremities) as compared with proximal bones; dislocated shoulders; evidence of previous fractures

Genital and Rectal
Evidence of vaginal or anal rape, such as bruising, edema, and bleeding; also evidence of direct kicks or punches in this area

Abdominal
Internal bleeding or other injuries; chronic pelvic pain

Neuropsychologic
Acute stress disorder; hyperactive reflexes; chronic headaches and backaches; paresthesias from previous injuries

---

the woman should understand that she has the right to access her records and that these will be valuable to her in child custody cases or if she chooses to file charges against the abuser.

It is imperative to assess the woman's potential danger in cases of domestic violence. Information regarding the pattern of abuse and its severity and frequency is vital. Other critical signs that indicate increased danger are that the abuser has a weapon, that he has been violent outside of the house, that he is a substance abuser, that he has been stalking the woman, and that he has threatened suicide or homicide. At times, the woman may contemplate suicide. It is well documented that the battered woman is at greatest risk of harm when she tries to leave her abuser (Gelles, 1997; Walton-Moss and Campbell, 2002). Therefore, the woman must become aware of this risk, and the nurse must assist her with the development of a safety plan. Such a plan typically involves helping the victim to create an emergency exit from the home and to plan a time to escape as well as providing the phone numbers of nearby shelters, crisis lines, and community resources. The woman should also be referred to the local victim's assistance program.

NURSING DIAGNOSIS

The following nursing diagnoses are examples of those that are relevant to the case study of Nina (see Case Study #2), and

they are based on information identified in the case study. However, all nursing diagnoses are formulated from information obtained during the assessment phase of the nursing process. The accuracy of the diagnoses depends on a careful, in-depth assessment. On the basis of the information that was provided, can you identify additional nursing diagnoses?

- Pain related to injuries sustained by battering as evidenced by difficulty breathing deeply and sleeping (multiple fractures)
- Risk for injury related to present and past abuse by husband
- Anxiety and fear related to threat of further battering
- Ineffective family coping related to abuse by husband and denial by wife

OUTCOME IDENTIFICATION

The following outcome criteria are derived from the nursing diagnoses identified in the case study of Nina. These outcomes are the expected behaviors that Nina will demonstrate as a result of her plan of care. Stabilizing Nina's physical condition and securing her safety are the immediate short-term goals.

The patient will do the following:

- Report a decrease in pain resulting from abuse-related injuries.
- Demonstrate relaxed breathing pattern and verbalize feeling more relaxed.
- Demonstrate decreased fear and anxiety by being able to discuss her abuse and explore possible options for resolving it with the nurse.
- Verbalize an awareness of her increasingly dangerous situation, because her abuse has intensified over time.
- Discuss with the nurse the implications for herself, her spouse, and other family members if she remains in the present abusive situation, and explore with the nurse alternative means of family coping.
- Demonstrate an awareness of the need for safety by taking steps to protect herself in the future.
- Devise plans to secure her safety in case of future threats of abuse.
- Take advantage of community resources that increase her self-esteem and independence, and become involved with an outreach group for battered women.
- Explore potential litigation against her husband and requesting a restraining order.

PLANNING

The plan of care for any survivor of violence will focus on addressing critical physical problems, collecting appropriate evidence, securing the immediate safety of the victim, examining the implications of the abuse on the woman and other family members, and discussing future plans for safety. In the case of a battered woman such as Nina, who acknowledges the abuse only when confronted by the nurse, all possible options must be explored, because they may need to be used in the future. The nurse will develop the care plan with the

CASE STUDY #2

Nina's husband, to whom she has been married for 10 years, brought Nina to the emergency department. Her husband was very attentive to her, spoke reassuringly, and appeared to be very concerned about Nina's condition. According to her husband, a day ago Nina slipped as she was getting out of the bathtub. When she slipped, she bumped her head on the faucet and then fell on her arm. As her husband spoke, Nina sat quietly with her head down. She cradled her right arm and appeared to be in severe pain. Her right eye was red and swollen shut, and she seemed to have some difficulty breathing. Despite protests from her husband, the nurse interviewed Nina separately from her husband in a private consultation room. Although the nurse inquired directly whether Nina's husband had beaten her, Nina denied the abuse. The physician performed complete physical and neurologic examinations, and a series of radiographs were taken. When Nina returned from the radiology department, the physician told her that she had fractures of the wrist, of some of her facial bones, and of several ribs. Nina was also informed that the X-rays indicated multiple previous healed fractures of the ribs and the pelvic girdle. The nurse spent time explaining to Nina how unlikely it was for her injuries to result from a fall in the bathtub. The nurse also reassured Nina that nothing she could have done would deserve such abuse by another person. Nina finally acknowledged that her husband had abused her, but she insisted that she had no intention of leaving him because he was a good husband. According to Nina, the only time her husband is abusive is when she fails to fulfill her domestic responsibilities and therefore she provokes him into losing his temper and beating her. Nina has no children and no family nearby, except for a younger sister who is currently overwhelmed with her own family problems. Nina is psychologically and economically dependent on her husband, and she has no means of financial or psychologic support.

Critical Thinking

1 What is the first priority for the nurse who suspects abuse when assessing a woman?
2 How should the nurse respond to the shame, guilt, and self-blame of the battered woman?
3 What should a nurse do if he or she becomes angry with and rejecting of a battered woman who is in denial about being battered?
4 If you suspected that your neighbor was in an abusive situation, what signs would you look for in the relationship?

---

patient and recognize that any effort to impose personal beliefs on the battered woman is fated for failure. Instead, the patient needs reassurance that she is capable of making appropriate decisions for herself, even if her decision is to return to her abuser. It is only through empowerment—and not through threats and intimidation—that the woman is most likely to develop the strength to make independent decisions that foster growth.

IMPLEMENTATION

When the battered woman's physical condition has been stabilized, it is critical to assess her future safety and to collaboratively explore her fears, anxieties, and concerns. Despite the need to leave the abusive situation, the woman may strongly believe that she has no other option except to return to her abuser. If the woman chooses to return to the batterer, it is important to respect this decision. Making a decision to leave the batterer is usually a gradual process. However, it is critical that the woman realizes that she has options. The nurse may serve as the key factor in a beginning awareness that other options do exist.

At present, all states have laws that provide some level of protection for survivors of domestic violence. However, the reality is that there is a large gap between the actual laws and their implementation by the police and the criminal justice system. In some localities, police are mandated to arrest the abuser if there is evidence of probable violence. In many states, the police must provide the battered woman with information about local shelters, domestic violence crisis lines, and her legal rights. However, if the police do not provide the information, the nurse can advise the battered woman of her legal rights.

In recent years, some women's rights advocates and criminal justice experts have been debating mandatory reporting laws for domestic violence (Walton-Moss and Campbell, 2002). Women's rights advocates claim that mandatory domestic violence reporting laws discourage battered women from seeking treatment for their injuries, because the women fear that their situations will be reported to the police and consequently that they will be in even greater danger of abuse. Because some women are not ready to deal with the police, being forced to do so could be nontherapeutic and disempowering and even increase their risk of abuse. If no mandatory reporting laws exist, then the police should not be notified unless the woman consents. Although some professionals choose to maintain confidentiality if the battered woman requests it, the deciding factor with regard to reporting is the degree of danger that the woman faces.

Nursing Interventions

Primary prevention for woman abuse begins with making nonviolence a priority. Public health programs and campaigns against abuse help to promote public awareness and possibly social attitudinal change against woman abuse (Carretta, 2009). Education about the societal acceptance of violence against women as portrayed in films, television, magazines, and music must be exposed. Nurses can become more knowledgeable about factors that increase the risk of domestic violence, and they can work with other members of the community to establish public policy and programs to address these issues.

The secondary prevention of woman battering involves early case finding and decisive intervention. Specific nursing interventions depend on the stage that the battered woman is in, because a woman who is in denial about the abuse

TABLE 23-1　NURSING INTERVENTIONS FOR BATTERED WOMEN

INTERVENTIONS

Report abuse to police.
Provide medications to relieve pain and anxiety.
Discuss the validity of the woman's anxiety.
Encourage the woman to discuss the events that led to past and present abuse.
Point out the increasingly violent nature of the relationship, and acknowledge concern for her safety.
Insist that no person has the right to abuse another.
Explore the effectiveness of her current coping skills, and suggest additional skills.
Focus on her strengths, endurance, and abilities.
Discuss the destructive societal expectations of women.
Discuss the frequency of woman abuse.
Explore family and friends as support possibilities.
Discuss the potential for using community resources (e.g., shelters, hotlines, police).
Describe current laws regarding domestic violence.
Explore the implications of pressing charges against the batterer.
Explore the meaning of the potential relationship loss.
Explore the various options for the future.
Provide a fact sheet about domestic violence.
Provide referrals.
Develop a safety plan with critical papers, money, clothing, and other essentials to be set aside for emergency exits.
Offer to be available for further questions.

BOX 23-6　ETIOLOGIC THEORIES RELATED TO CHILD ABUSE

Biologic Theory
Parents who were abused as children are at risk for abusing their own children.

Social Learning Theory
The family teaches and accepts violent behavior.
Violence is glorified in the media.
Violence is accepted in families, schools, and churches.

Environmental Theory
Socioeconomic class
Unemployment
Stressful life events

requires a different strategy from one who is determined not to return to the relationship. For relationships in which the abuse is just beginning, it may be possible to work with the marital dyad when both partners are willing. In these cases, the man accepts all responsibility for his abusive behavior of his partner, and the counseling focuses on the prevention of any further abuse. In many situations, the advanced practice psychiatric nurse is the appropriate professional to work with the battered woman.

Tertiary prevention is required when the woman has been repeatedly abused, as in the case of Nina. In such instances, the focus is on assisting the abused woman to overcome the physical and psychologic effects of the abuse and to prevent future abuse. Because the abuser frequently threatens and harasses the woman when she attempts to leave, it may be difficult for her to follow through. Frequently, these women seek assistance from local shelters that can provide safety and counseling. Nurses are often in the position to provide support and counseling to battered women in shelters. The nursing interventions identified in Table 23-1 relate to the case study that described Nina, who requires tertiary prevention measures in an emergency department setting.

EVALUATION

Evaluation is a critical component of the nursing process. Nurses who work in settings in which battered women seek treatment must be knowledgeable about the many different responses that may occur in the battered woman. The correct evaluation of outcomes and interventions depends on this recognition. When a complete nursing care plan is developed, the evaluation is based on the achievement of patient goals.

CHILD MALTREATMENT
EMOTIONAL EFFECTS OF TRAUMA ON CHILDREN AND ADOLESCENTS

Child abuse (maltreatment) is the physical, psychologic, or sexual victimization of a minor, and it has existed across time. Although it has often been misunderstood as "new" and "more common" during the past several decades, childhood victimization has been formally categorized as a pervasive public health problem that has reached pandemic levels globally. However, this formal recognition only resulted after decades of media campaigns, increased reporting, and enhanced comprehensive and sensitive assessments of childhood victims that gave them a voice and recognized their human rights (American Public Health Association, 2007a and 2007b; World Health Organization, 2004).

Because bruises, fractures, and lacerations are easily observed and detected, physical abuse is the type that is most often reported. Sexual assault is not rare, but it is often concealed by the victim and the family. Psychologic abuse is difficult to detect and treat, and it is more long lasting than physical injury.

The various types of child neglect—nutritional, medical, emotional, and caregiver—are more subtle than abuse, but they may nevertheless cause irreparable harm to the dependent child. About 10% to 15% of children who fail to thrive are nutritionally deprived, and a high incidence of such deprivation has been found in physically abused children. For religious or other reasons, parents may deliberately deprive their children of essential medical care. Some parents are detached or disengaged and unable to provide the fundamentals for normal emotional development. In addition, some children are not adequately supervised, and they therefore suffer major and repeated injuries (Box 23-6).

PHYSICAL ABUSE

Physical abuse, which was brought to the attention of health professionals during the early 1960s by pediatrician C. Henry Kempe as the *battered child syndrome,* is the intentional physical infliction of injury by a parent or caretaker. The spectrum of injuries is broad, and it may range from a few bruises to injuries that cause death.

Bruising is observed in the form of finger and palm prints on the face or buttocks and as human teeth or bite marks. Loop and lash marks on the skin are easily identified and indicative of a doubled-over cord or belt. In most true accidents, bruising occurs on only one body surface, except when a fall occurs down a flight of stairs.

Burns are another source of physical abuse. A cigarette may cause circular areas of similar size on the soles, palms, or abdomen. Hot-water burns are noted with a clear water level on the buttocks, perineum, or legs, and they may be caused by dunking the child as a disciplinary measure for problems with toilet training. Dry contact burns to the palms and soles may result from holding the child against a hot radiator.

Fractures of the long bones, ribs, or skull are often detected in abused and neglected children. Children with neurologic injuries may present in a coma or with convulsions and be found to suffer subdural or retinal hemorrhage.

PSYCHOLOGIC ABUSE

Psychologic abuse is sustained, repetitive, and damaging behavior that substantially reduces the creative and developmental potential of crucially important mental faculties of a child. These faculties include intelligence, memory, recognition, perception, attention, imagination, and moral development. Psychologic abuse impairs children's capacity to understand and manage their environment, confuses or frightens them, and renders them vulnerable (Brassard et al, 1993). Such abuse affects education, general welfare, and social life. The consequences of psychologic abuse are determined by the nature, intensity, and duration of the abuse; the damaged mental faculties and processes; the age and stage of development of the abused child; and the quality of life, treatment, and therapy after the abuse has ended.

Often the psychologic abuse of a child is ignored until the child's formative years have been impaired by the threats and rejection that are integral parts of these families' day-to-day routines. The deprivation and misery that were parts of many neglecting parents' own childhoods may be perpetuated in their roles as parents or caregivers. They are indifferent to their children; they may not wish to harm them, but they have little capacity to help them. As a result, the children are more frequently withdrawn rather than aggressive.

Abusive language and verbal expressions of hostility are present in a high percentage of severely abusing families. Some parents state bluntly that they hate their children and never wanted them. Others threaten to kill them. Frequently the children are yelled at and called derogatory names such

> ## CASE STUDY #3
>
> Emily died on March 13, 2005, at the age of 9 months. She was the youngest in a family that had been known to the Department of Children's Services for more than 3 years. Emily suffered a broken leg with no reasonable explanation only 3 weeks before incurring the injuries that led to her death.
>
> A review of Emily's case revealed several points at which the extreme danger to children in this family might have been recognized. First, the multiple injuries to a sibling during the sibling's first year of life were never recognized as suggestive of abuse by medical staff at a local hospital during sporadic clinic appointments. When severe medical neglect of another child was reported to the Department of Children's Services, the serious consequences of that neglect were not sufficiently understood, medical information concerning the siblings was not sought (which would have revealed a pattern of possible abuse), and the case was closed. In October 2001, the police arrested the mother for Risk of Injury. The arrest record states that the officers found two children hanging out of an open third-story window. There were no adults in the unheated apartment (52°F), there was animal excrement on the beds, and no food was available. The responding police officers placed the children with a relative, arrested the mother, and did not call the Department of Children's Services until the next day. The last opportunity to avert tragedy came in February and March of 2005, when Emily presented at a local hospital emergency department with a spiral fracture of her leg. This injury was reported by the hospital to the Department of Children's Services 6 days after an emergency care physician and orthopedist initially treated the child. This referral was handled by a social worker who believed the inconsistent explanation of an accidental injury that was given by the mother. Emily remained in the home and was fatally raped and abused at the age of 9 months.

as "idiot." They are referred to as objects of ridicule, with comments such as, "You are ugly, stupid, clumsy, and hopeless, and you will never amount to anything." Hopelessness, despair, and defeat are quite obvious in these children's attention-seeking and approval-seeking overtures for love. They trust no one, and they expect little except rejection.

SEXUAL ABUSE

A person may achieve sexual contact with another person in three basic ways: (1) through consent, which involves negotiation and mutual agreement; (2) through exploitation, which involves a person capitalizing on his or her position of dominance (e.g., economic, social, vocational) to take sexual advantage of a person in a subordinate position; and (3) through assault, which involves the threat of personal injury or the use of physical force. The latter two methods constitute sexual victimization. Only through negotiation and consent can sexual relations properly be achieved. However, such consent is precluded in sexual encounters between a child and an adult by virtue of the adult being mature and occupying a position of authority and dominance with regard to the child. A child, by definition, is an immature person, and most children have not developed sufficient knowledge, wisdom, or social skills to be able to negotiate such an encounter on an equal basis with an adult. Even a physically mature child is not mature enough to emotionally cope with sexual demands from an adult. The child can easily be taken advantage of by an older person or adult, and, although the child may agree to and cooperate with the sexual activity, the child does so without an awareness or appreciation of the impact that such activity may have on his or her subsequent psychosocial development (e.g., personality formation, attitudes, values, identity issues). In general, children are not well informed about human sexuality or adequately prepared for this important area of human behavior, and the offender can exploit their innocence in self-serving ways to the physical, social, psychologic, and emotional detriment of the children.

Gaining Access to the Child

The child predator may gain access to the victim through deception or by directly approaching the child. In the majority of cases, the offender will use some type of psychologic pressure (e.g., enticement, encouragement) to persuade the child to enter into sexual activity. In some cases, the offender may resort to force, either in the form of threats and intimidation or through brute physical strength.

Pressure Situations

The most common approach used by a child predator is to initially establish a nonsexual relationship with the victim that has meaning to the child. The offender becomes a familiar and trusted figure in the child's life. Over time, sexual intimacy is introduced into the context of this involvement. The offender may deceive the child by misinterpreting social standards (e.g., "All boys and girls do this, so it's okay"); misidentifying the activity (e.g., "We're going to wrestle"); tricking the child (e.g., "I'm going to give you a bath")' or presenting the activity in the context of game (e.g., "I've hidden some money in my clothes, and, if you find it, you can have it") and then rewarding the child's cooperation with money, gifts, candy, or toys. Children will exchange the sexual activity for these other nonsexual rewards, and one of the most prized rewards is attention. The offender will capitalize on the child's need for attention to lure the child into the sexual activity by making the child feel special or important.

Forced Situations

In a lesser number of cases, the offender may directly confront the child with sexual demands in the content of verbal threats (e.g., "Do what I say and you won't get hurt"); intimidation with a weapon (e.g., brandishing a knife); or direct physical assault (e.g., grabbing the child). These tactics are directed at overcoming any resistance on the part of the victim, although the intent is not to hurt the child. Such sexual assaults constitute child rape, in which sexuality becomes the means for expressing power and anger. The offender's approach is either one of intimidation, in which he exploits the child's helplessness, naiveté, and awe of adults, or one of physical aggression, in which he attacks and overpowers his victim.

Acts of Sexual Assault

The sexual abuse of children includes a wide range of sexual acts perpetrated by persons that are 5 or more years older than the victim. These acts include exhibitionism, the fondling or manipulation of the genitals, digital penetration, penile penetration of the vagina or rectum, genital contact, the insertion of foreign objects into the genitals or rectum, and the use of children in pornography and prostitution. Sexual abuse also includes noncontact sexual activity, such as sexually explicit language directed toward a child, obscene telephone calls, the showing of pornographic materials to a child, and voyeurism. Most sexually abused children experience multiple types of sexually abusive acts. The legal definition of sexual abuse varies by state jurisdiction, and nurses need to familiarize themselves with the laws in their district.

Incest

Research on intrafamilial sexual abuse indicates that incest families are highly dysfunctional, although they may appear to be normal. Studies do not find a correlation with incest and characteristics such as socioeconomic status, culture, race, and ethnicity. Rather, incest seems to cross all boundaries.

Within incestuous families, multiple forms of abuse are likely to be present, including physical and other forms of psychologic and emotional abuse. Most incestuous families are described as enmeshed, which means that they are relatively isolated from those outside of the family and that they tend to focus most of their energies on relationships within the family. Boundaries within the family are poorly defined, and members are characterized by excessive dependency on each other for physical, social, and psychologic needs. Role reversals often occur. One example is the abused child assuming a caregiver role for the parents and other family members. However, it must be emphasized that no single pattern can accurately describe the complexity of the incestuous family.

Offenders

Characteristics of offenders are primarily based on the research of those cases that have been examined within the criminal justice system and that represent situations in which the sexual abuse was disclosed. Most cases of sexual abuse are never reported, so these criminal cases are not believed to be representative of all offenders.

At present, experts recognize that child sexual offenders make up a diverse population that is difficult to classify. The offenders vary with regard to age, occupation, income, marital status, and ethnic group. Some researchers are also beginning to study the female perpetrator, because it is believed that this group is more common than studies indicate; however, existing data show that men were perpetrators in 89% of cases compared with women perpetrators in 11% of cases. Existing research on female perpetrators indicate that they are often accomplices to males or to a general pattern of abuse among all family members (Elliot, 1993).

More juveniles are being identified as offenders, and they demonstrate more violent behavior than do typical adult offenders (Prentky et al, 2006). In addition, more of these juvenile offenders are young teenagers, and this group includes a growing number of female offenders (Schwartz et al, 2006). These juvenile offenders range in age from 5 to 19 years, and they represent all ethnic, racial, and socioeconomic classes; however, 90% are male. The majority of adult offenders report beginning their deviant sexual behavior during adolescence (see Chapter 20).

Characteristics of the Nonoffending Parent

When the abuser is the father, the mother is sometimes blamed for failing to satisfy her husband's psychologic and sexual needs or for being rejecting or dominating. In addition, when the child discloses the abuse to the mother, it has been claimed that the mother commonly denies that the abuse occurred or blames the child for initiating or encouraging it, as in the case of Mackenzie and Michelle Phillips described at the beginning of this chapter.

By contrast, many nonoffending mothers are initially shocked and unable to believe their child's claim of being sexually abused by their partner. It is especially upsetting to the woman if she loves and trusts her partner, because she must now cope with her partner's betrayal in addition to her child being violated and traumatized. It is much simpler and less painful to believe that it did not occur. Nevertheless, many mothers who are initially in shock experience a process that involves a crisis of disbelief and ambivalence that is followed by gradual acceptance and eventual dedication to healing the child's trauma as well as their own.

LONG-TERM CONSEQUENCES: TRAUMA LEARNING

Nurses realize that, when traumatized children become upset, it is hard for them to calm down, because the shifts in integrative behavior are driven by biologic dysregulation. With the use of an expanded model of information processing regarding trauma, the patterns of trauma learning are reviewed and briefly discussed. There is a progression of symptomatology and behaviors among victims of a traumatic event.

Integration of Trauma: No Posttraumatic Stress Disorder

The optimal response pattern from a traumatic event is resolution of the posttrauma symptoms, with subsequent integration of the traumatic event in to the life experience of the victim. In the integrated pattern, the patient is able to relate to the sexual abuse experience, but he or she is not compelled to dwell on it or to avoid it with the use of psychologic defenses.

Posttraumatic Stress Disorder

With a classic PTSD response, a biphasic response is noted. The victim may suffer intrusive thoughts of the abuse or display avoidant behaviors. Exposure to stimuli can induce a state of hyperarousal and numbing, which may cause the victim to experience highly emotional states.

Symptoms may include hyperactivity, headaches, stomachaches, back pain, genitourinary distress, and nightmares. Symptoms of interpersonal disruption include behaviors such as excessive fear of others and an inability to assert or protect oneself. Aggressive behaviors include agitation; aggression toward peers, family members, or pets; and potentially sexualized behavior toward others. Several patterns of PTSD symptoms are noted in traumatized children:

- The anxious pattern is characterized by generalized fears and anxious recollection of the abuse situation if probed or asked. Anxiety disorders, eating disorders, and phobic and obsessive–compulsive disorders have been linked with unresolved trauma.
- The avoidant pattern is characterized by denial or recanting that the abuse has occurred. These youths may develop a substance abuse history, depression and suicidal thoughts, phobic behavior, adjustment problems, or conduct disorders.
- The aggressive pattern is characterized by sexual or aggressive behavior. Minimal acknowledgment or frank denial of prior abuse is typical. There is the testing and breaking of rules, impulsivity, and fighting with peers. Diagnostic labels of hyperactivity, learning disabilities, conduct disorders, and impulse disorders are sometimes used.
- The disorganized pattern is characterized by fragmented and sometimes bizarre behavior. Dissociative states need to be ruled out. There may be denial or frank amnesia regarding prior sexual abuse (see Chapter 10).

Delayed Posttraumatic Stress Disorder

Some victims of trauma may not initially develop PTSD but rather progress to delayed PTSD and display no visible sequelae to the event. Avoidant behaviors include low sexual involvement, passivity, substance use to reduce tension, somatic complaints, and depression. Aggressive patterns include participating in high-risk behaviors and antisocial acts, substance use as a stimulant, and high sexual involvement.

THE NURSING PROCESS
ASSESSMENT

As with the assessment of other victims of violence, the nurse should begin with an assessment of his or her own assumptions, beliefs, and attitudes about childhood sexual abuse. Nurses who believe that the child is responsible in any way for the sexual abuse will find it difficult to be supportive of the child. The nurse must be comfortable when speaking with the child about the abuse so that an attitude of discomfort is not conveyed to the child. Children are adept at picking up nonverbal cues, and the nurse's discomfort may be interpreted by the child as a sign that he or she should not talk about the abuse with the nurse or that he or she is not believed.

As with all nursing assessments, a holistic approach is essential. Because childhood sexual abuse trauma is highly complex and affected by multiple interacting factors, it is important to gain as much information as possible without subjecting the child to unnecessary and repeated probing and questioning. Most often, the nurse encounters the sexually abused child in the emergency department or an outpatient clinic. Often the mother or another caregiver brings the child to a medical facility to determine if the child has been sexually abused. Whenever there is a suspicion of childhood abuse, a complete physical examination must be conducted.

The primary objective is to establish a trusting relationship with the child so that he or she can relate relevant events and cooperate with the physical examination. It is important to assess the relationship between the caregiver and the child to determine if the child is more comfortable with or without that person. Usually younger children do not want to be separated from their caregiver, whereas older children may be too inhibited to disclose in front of the caregiver for a variety of reasons, such as fear of being blamed by family members, disbelieved, or instrumental in the family break up. Sometimes the child may retract the disclosure in an effort to protect the abuser, with whom he or she may have an ambivalent relationship. Finally, the developmental age of the child is an important factor in his or her ability to successfully provide data about the abuse; the younger the child, the less able he or she may be to describe events and to understand the interviewer's questions.

The majority of children who have been sexually abused do not display any physical signs of abuse if the disclosure has been delayed for weeks or if there has not been any vaginal or anal penetration. The occurrence of oral copulation or mock intercourse is also difficult to physically document unless the child is examined within a short time after the activity.

In addition to the lack of physical evidence, the sexually abused child may not display any observable signs of emotional trauma, and he or she may deny, retract, and be inconsistent with regard to the description of the abuse. Caregivers often interpret this behavior to mean that the abuse did not occur and that the child is lying. The significance of absent physical or emotional signs must be clearly explained to the child's caregivers. Conversely, multiple emotional and psychologic indicators may be present; however, because many of these signs can also reflect other problems, their presence alone is not a conclusive sign that sexual abuse has occurred. The diagnosis of sexual abuse is difficult and challenging, because there is no single profile or set of symptoms that guarantees its presence. Many of the following signs and symptoms must be viewed only as potential indicators of sexual abuse, whereas others are highly probable indicators. The American Professional Society on Abused Children Task Force (2002) has developed detailed

psychosocial protocols and guidelines for health care professionals who interview and evaluate children for sexual abuse. Guidelines for the evaluation of physical signs of sexual abuse have been published by Giardino and colleagues (2002). The indicators addressed in Boxes 23-7 and 23-8 are derived from these two sets of guidelines and from clinical observation.

NURSING ASSESSMENT QUESTIONS #2

For the Sexually Abused Child

1 Do you know why you have come to see me?
2 What have you been told?
3 What kinds of games do you and (the alleged abuser's name) play when your mom isn't around?
4 Are there any games that you and (the alleged abuser's name) play that you don't like?

Clearly, the meaning of any child's acting-out behavior needs to be explored. Such behavior in abused children usually reflects the anger, confusion, and sense of betrayal that the child is experiencing and unable to discuss. Although many abused children are able to act out their feelings through rebellious and delinquent behavior, others withdraw, blame themselves, become guilt ridden, and continuously try to be a "better" or "good" child. Such children may function at a high level in school and even be praised and admired for what appears to be mature behavior, because they often assume major responsibility for adult caregiver roles in their homes. Finally, some children with abusive histories do not exhibit signs of trauma during childhood but instead go on to exhibit them later in life. As previously discussed, the presence of sexual abuse trauma depends on a wide variety of complex factors; in particular, the degree to which the child receives validation, protection, and support after disclosure is crucial to the resolution of the trauma.

The assessment of child sexual abuse should include a physical examination, interviews with the child and family members, outside information from sources such as teachers and babysitters, and psychologic tests, if needed.

In general, the interview with the child should take place in an environment in which the child feels safe and comfortable. As with all sensitive topics, questions should begin with the least sensitive and most positive topics and progress to the most sensitive and direct ones. Initial questions are meant to gain the trust of the child and to assist him or her to relax and to become more spontaneous. The developmental age of the child is a critical factor in the type and level of question that is used; therefore, all techniques must be modified according to the child's needs. Small children may have difficulty with nondirective and open-ended questions. Interviewers must be extremely cautious to not use leading questions (e.g., "Daddy likes to tickle your bottom, doesn't he?").

The nurse's role is to provide comfort and safety for the child. Thus, the immediate physical and psychologic needs of

BOX 23-7	PHYSICAL INDICATORS OF POSSIBLE CHILD ABUSE AND NEGLECT

General Appearance
Excessive fearfulness and watchfulness
Disheveled and malnourished
Failure to thrive
Multiple injuries
No history of significant trauma

Skin
Unexplained bruises, welts, and scratches in various stages of healing (i.e., different colors)
Regular patterns of bruises and welts (e.g., bite marks, marks from electrical cords)
Untreated infected wounds
Lacerations from rope burns, especially on the neck, wrists, ankles, and torso
Bruises on the buttocks, genitalia, thighs, side of the face, trunk, and upper arms

Burns
Small round cigarette burns (however, infected insect bites can resemble cigarette burns)
Immersion burns (these have even boundaries that are glove like, sock like, or symmetric; accidental burns are asymmetric with splash marks)
Patterned burn marks (e.g., from an iron or grill)

Fractures
Fractures in infants that are younger than 1 year old
Fractures of the femur, humerus, posterior ribs, skull, and long bones and any uncommon fractures

Head Injuries
Skull fractures and subdural hematomas (these are the leading cause of death among abused children)
Brain hemorrhages or contusions without external signs of injury (e.g., shaken baby syndrome)
Alopecia caused by hair pulling

Abdominal Injuries
Ruptured liver or spleen
Ruptured blood vessels
Kidney, bladder, or pancreatic injuries
Injuries to the jejunum or duodenum
Injuries to the eyes, ears, nose, and mouth
A wide variety of injuries, including missing teeth, bruising, perforation of the tympanic membrane, epistaxis, nasal fractures, retinal hemorrhage, detachment, corneal abrasions, and periorbital hematomas

Other Types of Abuse and Neglect
Munchausen's syndrome by proxy
Deprivational syndromes

BOX 23-8	PHYSICAL, BEHAVIORAL, AND PSYCHOSOCIAL INDICATORS OF POSSIBLE CHILDHOOD SEXUAL ABUSE

General Appearance
Varies from normal to anxious, fearful, and depressed

Probable Physical Examination Indicators
Bruises, lacerations, or bite marks on the breasts, neck, buttocks, extremities, and oropharynx
Presence of sexually transmitted disease, including human immunodeficiency virus
Presence of adult pubic hair and semen
Edema, abrasions, petechiae, and erythema of the genital area
Lacerations of the vagina or anus
Alterations in or enlargement of the hymenal orifice
Dysuria caused by periurethral trauma
Rectal fissures, chafing, erythema, bruising, lacerations, and perianal scarring
Semen in the oropharynx or the nasopharynx
Scar tissue of the labia minora, hymenal membrane, and anus

High-Risk Family History Indicators
Substance abuse in caregivers
History of abuse in parents
Domestic violence
Inadequate impulse control or mental illness in caregivers
Alleged offender with sexual dysfunction, poor coping skills, and poor social skills
Socially isolated family
Sexual abuse of sibling

Behavioral Indicators
Disclosure and spontaneous discussion of the abuse
Preoccupation with drawing genitals or anxious avoidance of anything to do with genitals or sex
Inappropriate sexual play behavior with dolls or other children, compulsive masturbation, inserting objects into the vagina or anus, sexualized kissing, fondling the genitals of others, and imitating intercourse
Dissociation
Avoidance of particular people
School and learning problems
Antisocial behavior, promiscuity, and substance abuse
Running away and other self-destructive behavior

Possible Psychosocial Indicators
Increased anxiety, fears, and depression; low self-esteem
Multiple somatic complaints
Signs of posttraumatic stress disorder

the child must be determined and addressed. After these needs have been addressed, it is always critical for the nurse and other health care professionals to make a determination as to whether the child will be safe if returned to his or her home.

Eventually, the child must be asked directly about the possibility of sexual abuse. In a nonemergency situation, questions such as those in the Nursing Assessment Questions box could be used with a small child whose father, stepfather, or other male caregiver is suspected of the abuse.

CASE STUDY #4

Suzy is a 5-year-old girl who was brought to the emergency department by her mother and stepfather, Mr. and Mrs. Jones, because she was bleeding from her vagina. Mrs. Jones reported that, while she was bathing Suzy in the tub, the phone rang, so she left Suzy for a few minutes to answer it. Mr. Jones claims that he went in to check on Suzy when he heard her crying and found her standing in the tub crying and bleeding from the vagina. Mr. and Mrs. Jones maintained that Suzy tried to get out of the tub but slipped and injured herself on the tub faucet. No other persons were in the home at the time of the accident. Suzy was obviously distressed, and she was unable to give a history. She clung to her mother, and she would not allow anyone—including her stepfather—to touch her. On physical examination, Suzy was found to have lacerations of the hymenal membrane and the vaginal wall, trauma to the surrounding perineal area, and old scarring.

Critical Thinking

1 What are the possible mechanisms for the injury that Suzy received?
2 How would you best prepare Suzy for her physical examination?
3 What kinds of questions and comments would be appropriate and helpful to Suzy?
4 How can the nurse structure the environment so that Suzy will feel safer?

NURSING DIAGNOSIS

The following nursing diagnoses are based on the data identified in the case study on Suzy (see the Case Study). Nursing diagnoses are formulated from the information obtained during the assessment phase of the nursing process. The accuracy of the diagnoses depends on a careful, in-depth assessment.

- Pain related to injuries sustained from sexual abuse
- Anxiety and fear related to further abuse
- Risk for injury related to sexual abuse by stepfather (possible prior incidents of sexual abuse by stepfather and increased chances of recurrence)
- Disabled family coping related to sexual abuse by stepfather and mother's possible denial as evidenced by the mother's inability to protect her daughter

OUTCOME IDENTIFICATION

The outcome criteria for Suzy are derived from the nursing diagnoses that were identified previously. These outcomes are the expected behaviors that Suzy and her mother will demonstrate as a result of the plan of care.

For Suzy, the first priority is addressing the physical trauma of the sexual abuse, which is the hymenal and vaginal laceration and the localized trauma to the perineal area. The presence of scar tissue indicates prior abuse. Depending on the extent of damage and bleeding, Suzy may require surgical

repair of her injuries. On the basis of her plan of care, the first outcome will focus on stabilizing her physical condition. The second priority will be to ensure that the abuse will not recur and that the child will be protected in the future.

Outcome Identification for Child Sexual Abuse

The child will do the following:
- Report a decrease in pain and anxiety.
- Discuss her present perceptions, distortions, and fears with the nurse.
- Verbalize an awareness that she will be protected in the future and that no one will be allowed to injure her again.

The child and parent will do the following:
- Follow through on referral sources for the child and her family. Because Suzy's abuse was ongoing and severe, she will require an individual therapist.
- Participate in individual or group therapy. Many organizations exist that conduct groups for survivors, nonoffending parents, offenders, and siblings in families in which sexual abuse has occurred. All family members need to be assessed for the level of their therapy needs.
- The mother will attend parenting classes, because she will require assistance with learning how to nurture, support, and protect her daughter in the future.

The *Diagnostic and Statistical Manual of Mental Disorders*, fourth edition, text revision (DSM-IV-TR) does recognize the sexual abuse of children. Many adult survivors have been identified as experiencing PTSD, but symptoms for both children and adult survivors of abuse vary greatly, and no single profile has been identified that would clearly describe sexual abuse survivors. However, sexual abuse can be reported under the DSM-IV-TR Axis IV, which focuses on psychosocial and environmental problems.

PLANNING

The plan of care for the abused child begins with stabilizing the child's physical needs, securing the child's safety, and addressing the child's psychologic needs (Table 23-2). Because the child depends on the parents for the continuation of these goals outside of the hospital, the family system must also be assessed (Table 23-3). In the case study of Suzy, the stepfather is the suspected abuser; therefore, it must be clearly established that the stepfather will not have access to his stepdaughter and that the mother is capable of nurturing and protecting her child in the future. Police and protective services reports must be completed by the attending staff.

IMPLEMENTATION

Education about the signs and symptoms of childhood sexual abuse is important so that nurses are able to recognize them and take swift action in all potential cases. Because the child's safety is critical, nurses should be knowledgeable about the laws in their states and about the policies and procedures of their institutions for caring for all survivors of abuse, especially children, who are the most vulnerable. In Suzy's case,

TABLE 23-2	**NURSING INTERVENTIONS FOR THE PHYSICALLY ABUSED CHILD**

NURSING INTERVENTIONS (SECONDARY PREVENTION)

Develop a trusting relationship with the parents.

Be direct and open but supportive.

Obtain a holistic history, including the stresses and problems that the family is experiencing.

Explore how the events that led to the abuse might be altered in the future.

Explore alternative strategies for childcare problems.

Discuss basic child growth and development.

Provide the parents with basic materials about child growth and development.

Have the parents apply child development principles.

Discuss the need for parenting classes.

Discuss strategies for anger control.

Discuss reporting laws regarding child abuse.

Explain the child welfare function of protective services.

Take steps to inform protective services.

Observe parent–child interactions unobtrusively.

Involve parents in childcare during the child's hospitalization, when appropriate.

Discuss the physical impact of abuse with parents.

Discuss the short- and long-term psychologic effects of child abuse.

Provide a referral to postdischarge public health child nursing.

The public health nurse will coordinate services and monitor parental progress.

The public health nurse will role model and assist the parents with applying principles learned in parenting classes to their own lives.

Have the father discuss how he will maintain his anger skills.

Teach the mother to intervene if the father exhibits negative parenting.

Assist the parents with the development of social support systems.

Explore community resources with the family.

TABLE 23-3	**NURSING INTERVENTIONS FOR THE SEXUALLY ABUSED CHILD**

NURSING INTERVENTIONS

Call the police and protective services.

Provide medication as needed; reassure the child that he or she is safe and that no one will hurt her again.

Encourage him or her to talk about her fears and concerns.

Reassure him or her that she is not to blame and that her abuser did a bad thing by hurting her.

Verify that the appropriate agencies have been notified and that they will follow through.

Document the mother's responses in terms of supporting her child and being committed to protecting her child in the future.

Provide support and education about potential resources (e.g., treatment centers, social services, criminal justice system).

Educate the mother about the signs and symptoms of abuse that the child may exhibit and how to support her child.

Assess the mother for her ability to cope with possible feelings of grief and betrayal.

the stepfather is removed from the home. Nurses are often the coordinators who ensure that protective services and law enforcement agencies are notified, that treatment referrals are made, and that plans are followed through. Usually the court mandates treatment after investigations by protective services and the criminal justice system are made.

Types of long-term treatment depend on the child's developmental level and the mother's potential for supporting and protecting the child in the future. With a younger child, play therapy is often used, because the child often has difficulty verbalizing feelings about his or her abuse. Group therapy with other young children is also useful, because common fears and misperceptions can be addressed. As the child becomes able to repeatedly address these fears and misperceptions, they will gradually be resolved. Group therapy with

other children is also a powerful modality for teaching the child self-assertive behavior and about how to self-protect in the future.

Adult survivors of this type of abuse have a multitude of treatment modalities that have recently become available, including antidepressant medications to treat depression, anxiety, and complex PTSD. Practice guidelines from the International Society for Traumatic Stress Studies (Foa et al, 2000) provide evidenced-based practice interventions for PTSD in both children and adults. These research guidelines indicate that cognitive behavioral therapy is effective for addressing the distorted guilt, blame, shame, and low self-esteem that survivors of childhood sexual abuse experience. Group therapy that incorporates cognitive behavioral interventions is also a powerful modality. Somatic techniques are helpful for treating the psychobiology of PTSD with the use of mind–body integration exercises. These modalities include hypnotherapy, eye movement desensitization, reprocessing, imagery, deep breathing, art therapy, body-focused therapy, and thought field therapy (Kamphuis and Emmelkamp, 2005) (see Chapters 26 and 27).

EVALUATION

Ongoing evaluation of patient and family outcomes reveals the efficiency of all interventions, and it is critical to ensure that the child is protected and supported during recovery. In addition, an ongoing evaluation of the caregiver is needed to determine if the family is following through with the plan of care and to address any problems that may arise. A reliable evaluation of the mother's motivation and ability to support and protect her child requires both short- and long-term assessment. Sometimes the mother may become involved with another partner who is a risk factor. Thus, the mother must be able to confront her own behavior and the decisions that she makes with regard to the safety of her children.

ELDER ABUSE

Elder abuse is frequently compared with child abuse, because, in both cases, neglect is common. However, with elder abuse, elders continue to have the rights of adults unless they are declared incompetent by a judge. Therefore, decisions cannot be legally forced on the elder as they can with children. Elders have the right to choose to remain in a particular environment, even when it is obvious that they are being abused or neglected.

TYPES OF ELDER ABUSE

The age that defines a person as an elder varies from 60 to 65 years; the definitions of the different types of elder abuse follow:

The physical abuse of an elder is defined as the use of physical force that may result in bodily injury, physical pain, or impairment. Physical abuse may include striking (with or without an object), hitting, beating, pushing, shoving, shaking, slapping, kicking, pinching, and burning. In addition, the inappropriate use of drugs and physical restraints, force feeding, and physical punishment of any kind are also examples of physical abuse. Nurses can observe for signs and symptoms of bruises, black eyes, welts, lacerations, and rope marks; bone or skull fractures; open wounds, cuts, punctures, or untreated injuries in various stages of healing; sprains, dislocations; and internal injuries or bleeding.

Sexual abuse of an elder is defined as nonconsensual sexual contact of any kind with an elderly person or sexual contact with a person who is incapable of giving consent. It includes all types of sexual assault or battery, such as rape, sodomy, coerced nudity, and sexually explicit photographing. Nurses can observe for bruises around the breasts or genital area; unexplained venereal disease or genital infections; unexplained vaginal or anal bleeding; and torn, stained, or bloody underclothing.

The emotional or psychologic abuse of an elder is defined as the infliction of anguish, pain, or distress through verbal or nonverbal acts. Emotional and psychologic abuse includes but is not limited to verbal assaults, insults, threats, intimidation, humiliation, and harassment. Other examples include treating an older person like an infant; isolating an elderly person from his or her family, friends, or regular activities; giving an older person the "silent treatment"; and enforcing social isolation. Nurses can observe for an elder who is emotionally upset or agitated; who is extremely withdrawn, noncommunicative, or nonresponsive; or who is exhibiting unusual behavior that is usually attributed to dementia (e.g., sucking, biting, rocking).

BOX 23-9 **ETIOLOGIC FACTORS RELATED TO ELDER ABUSE**

Biologic Theory
Psychopathology of the abuser

Social Learning Theory
Dependency (financial and relational)
Social isolation
Transgenerational violence

Environmental Theory
External stress

Neglect is defined as the refusal or failure to fulfill any part of a person's obligations or duties to an elder. Neglect may also include the failure of a person who has fiduciary responsibilities to provide care for an elder (e.g., failing to pay for necessary home care-services) or the failure on the part of an in-home service provider to provide necessary care. Neglect typically means the refusal or failure to provide an elderly person with such life necessities as food, water, clothing, shelter, personal hygiene, medicine, comfort, personal safety, and other essentials that are included in an implied or agreed-upon responsibility to an elder. Nurses may observe dehydration, malnutrition, untreated bedsores, poor personal hygiene, and unattended or untreated health problems.

THEORIES OF ELDER ABUSE

Although many theories seek to explain elder abuse, no single theory is completely adequate (Box 23-9). Sengstock and Barrett (1993) identify three main foci for theories on elder abuse: (1) abuser characteristics; (2) situational stress; and (3) family relationships. Pillemer (1986) identified five risk factors for elder abuse, which can be articulated within the three foci of Sengstock and Barrett: (1) the psychopathology of the abuser; (2) external stress; (3) dependency; (4) social isolation; and (5) transgenerational violence.

ELDER SEXUAL ABUSE

The incidence of elder sexual assault is difficult to estimate with any degree of confidence. The National Citizens' Coalition for Nursing Home Reform identified 1749 cases of such abuse in the institutionalized elderly during its first 3 years of keeping records starting in 1996. Furthermore, according to the National Crime Victimization Survey, 261,000 rapes and sexual assaults occurred in the United States in 2000, with collateral data from the National Crime Victimization Survey of 2000 identifying 3270 of these victims as being 65 years old or older. Of note is that serious underreporting continues to occur, with an estimate of only 30% of these cases being reported to police.

A National Institute of Justice report notes fear of the offender as the major reason for nonreporting (Tjaden and Thoenes, 2006). Such underreporting of sexual abuse continues to occur in all age groups in a significant number of cases, with the extent of nondisclosure or nonreporting estimated to be as high as 68% (Bureau of Justice, 1996). For elders, the typically inherent nature of dependence on others (e.g., family members, caretakers, agency staff) in combination with physical frailty and alterations in mental status can result in an increased risk of abuse with subsequently low rates of reporting.

From a medical standpoint, bruises may be attributed to the aging process rather than to an assault. Sometimes nursing procedures are blamed to explain genital bruising and bleeding in institutionalized elderly as either a "botched catheterization" or "rough perineal care." Bruising of the abdominal area may be attributed to tight restraints. Clearly, there are multiple reasons to believe that the known cases of elder sexual assaults underestimate the true number of such cases.

DIFFICULTIES WITH RECOGNIZING ELDER TRAUMA

Although the sexual assault of elders has likely been ongoing throughout time, it is clearly recognized as both a contemporary and emergent public health issue that requires increased awareness, comprehensive and sensitive assessment, and foundational approaches for effective intervention to promote adaptive coping and mental health (Vierthaler, 2004).

There is no prevalence data regarding PTSD among elders who have been victimized by others during a crime or as a result of other forms of elder abuse. However, the literature suggests that elderly victims may meet the diagnostic criteria for PTSD. The delayed onset of PTSD is an infrequently diagnosed variant of the disorder that is receiving attention among older combat veterans.

Another reality with older adults is comorbid disorders. There are many physical illnesses that are attributed to elders, including cardiac, respiratory, and cognitive problems; psychiatric conditions are present as well, including depression, substance misuse, and personality disorders, which many of which may mimic diagnoses on the anxiety continuum, including PTSD (Iancu et al, 1998).

Older adults who reside in nursing homes are an especially vulnerable group. They often require assistance with basic activities of daily living (e.g., bathing, dressing, feeding) as a result of physical and cognitive impairments. These disabilities make an individual dependent on others and an easy target for a sexual predator (Burgess et al, 2000).

There are approximately 17,000 nursing homes in the United States, and these house 1.5 million older adult residents (U.S. General Account Office, 2002). In a study of 5297 nursing homes in Pennsylvania, New Jersey, and New York, a quarter of these nursing homes had serious complaints that involved allegations of situations that harmed residents or that placed them at risk of death or serious injury (U.S. General Account Office, 2002). Concerns about the quality of care have mostly been focused on malnutrition, dehydration, and other forms of neglect. However, there is mounting concern about physical violence by those whom have been entrusted with their care, particularly sexual abuse (Burgess et al, 2000).

Reasons for the untimely reporting of allegations concern the following: (1) residents may fear retribution if they report the abuse; (2) family members are troubled with having to find a new place because the nursing home may ask the resident to leave; (3) staff do not report abuse promptly for fear of losing their jobs or of recrimination from coworkers and management; and (4) nursing homes want to avoid negative publicity and sanctions from the state.

ELDER ABUSE OFFENDERS

Most sexual assaults of the elderly are not witnessed. However, when the victim is infirm as a result of cognitive deficits, the lack of an eyewitness is a complicating issue during the assessment and investigation of these cases. The challenge is to reconstruct the events that surrounded the possible sexual injury. A widely held social belief regarding sexual abuse and assault is that offender motivations are sexual in nature (Safarik, 2002). More recently, the professional research suggests that sexual attacks are prompted by the offender's inherent need to dominate and oppress the victim (Safarik, 2002). In cases of rape of the elderly, it has been contended that the victims are more likely to suffer more brutality and violence during their attacks than their younger counterparts (Jeary, 2005). A theoretic explanation for this difference includes the idea that elderly victims are perceived by the offender as authoritative or even oppressive (Safarik, 2002). The use of violence helps the perpetrator to overcome this oppression by venting hostility and rage onto the victim.

In a review of 125 elder sexual abuse cases, Burgess and colleagues (2005) found that the age range of the perpetrators is between 16 and 85 years, with the average age being 37 years. Mental deficiencies or physical disabilities were noted to be sparse in this population. The use of alcohol and drugs was found in nearly half (44%) of these cases. Elder victims were more likely to have an established relationship to the offender (59%). "Almost half of the offenders were acquaintances (48%), 26% were caretakers, 19% were residents in same nursing home, and only 3% were strangers" (Burgess et al, 2005, p. 40).

THE NURSING PROCESS
ASSESSMENT

It is critical to interview the elderly patient apart from the caregiver. In a hospital setting, it is quite easy to simply assert that hospital policy mandates that patients be seen alone. If the nurse is conducting the interview at the patient's home, it may be much more difficult to gain private access to the elder. This assessment must determine whether an abuser who lives with the elder is a substance abuser or if he or she has a history of mental illness or violence, because these factors may further compromise the nurse's safety. Sometimes it is possible to identify a family member who is trusted and who is able to provide the nurse with an opportunity to

---

BOX 23-10   PHYSICAL INDICATORS OF ACTUAL OR POTENTIAL ELDER ABUSE AND NEGLECT

General Appearance
Anxious, fearful, and passive
Poor eye contact
Looks to caregiver for answers
Poor hygiene and inappropriate dress
Underweight or malnourished
Physically handicapped
No glasses, false teeth, or hearing aid, despite need

Skin
Contusions, abrasions, burns, and scars in various stages of healing
Decubitus ulcers and urine burns
Rope marks

Abdominal and Rectal
Distended abdomen
Bleeding
Fecal impactions

Musculoskeletal Fractures
Evidence of old healed fractures
Current fractures and sprains
Limited range of motion
Contractures

Genital and Urinary
Vaginal lacerations, bruises, and infections
Urinary tract infections

Neurologic
Slurred speech
Confusion

NURSING ASSESSMENT QUESTIONS #3
For the Abused Elder

1. Are you happy living with (the name of the suspected abuser)?
2. Please tell me about your financial assets and how they are managed?
3. Whom do you turn to when you are feeling down?
4. How are family disagreements handled in your household?
5. Has anyone ever hurt you or touched you when you didn't want to be touched?

In addition to possible physical signs and symptoms of elder abuse and neglect, it is also necessary to assess the older adult for signs of exploitation and abandonment. Signs of exploitation include complaints by elders or evidence of the misuse of their money, the loss of control over their finances, material goods taken without consent or approval, and unmet financial needs that are inconsistent with their actual financial status. Signs of abandonment include reports by or evidence of elders being left alone and helpless for extended periods without adequate assistance.

NURSING DIAGNOSIS

The following nursing diagnoses are based on the assessment data gathered by the nurse who interviewed and examined Marjorie (see the Case Study). These diagnoses represent a few of the possibilities that might be relevant for similar cases. Nursing diagnoses are formulated from the information obtained during the assessment phase of the nursing process see. The accuracy of the diagnoses depends on a careful and in-depth assessment.

- Decreased cardiac output and activity intolerance related to a change in health status (i.e., congestive heart failure)
- Depression related to a physical illness, a loss of role functioning, and a lack of social support
- Moderate to severe anxiety related to a change in health status and role functioning
- Ineffective family coping related to alcohol abuse by caregivers and caregiver role strain
- Disturbed personal identity related to changes in health status and role functioning

No diagnosis in the DSM-IV-TR is currently appropriate for the abused older person.

OUTCOME IDENTIFICATION

Outcome criteria for this section are based on the nursing diagnoses derived from the Case Study of Marjorie. These outcomes are the expected behaviors that someone like Marjorie will demonstrate or achieve as a result of the implementation of the plan of care and the associated interventions. Because Marjorie came to the emergency department with severe cardiac distress, the first priority is stabilizing

visit the elder as well as to ensure the safety of the nurse. Having another nurse present during a home visit is always an option, but at no time should nurses intentionally place themselves in dangerous home-visit situations.

It is not uncommon for both the abuser and the abused to maintain secrecy about the abuse. As with other types of family violence, abusers frequently threaten their victims with harm if they disclose the abuse. Even without threats of retaliation, however, a great deal of time often lapses before the abused elder is comfortable disclosing the mistreatment. Reluctance is usually a result of shame or self-blame or of fear of abandonment, institutionalization, or serious consequences for the abuser. Box 23-10 identifies physical indicators of actual or potential elder abuse. Many of these symptoms are present with normal aging. Therefore, as with other types of family violence, the nurse must perform a comprehensive assessment and consider the physical symptoms within the broader context of the patient's life history (see the Nursing Assessment Questions box).

CASE STUDY # 5

Eighty-year-old Marjorie Jones is brought to the emergency department by her daughter and son-in-law, and she is anxiously holding her chest and gasping for breath. Marjorie is currently on medication for congestive heart failure. She is underweight, dehydrated, and without her dentures, and she has poor hygiene. When asked about her missing dentures, she states that they have been lost for several months and that no one has been able to find them. After receiving medical treatment to stabilize her heart condition, Marjorie begins to feel much better and is able to give a brief history to the nurse in the privacy of her hospital room.

Marjorie appears depressed and withdrawn, and she has difficulty making eye contact. She states that, because of her inability to maintain her own apartment any longer, she moved in with her daughter and son-in-law 18 months ago. Until that time, Marjorie had a full life with her widowed friends, and she had participated in social activities. She had had a part-time housekeeper since her husband died 5 years ago, and she had been able to maintain her independence quite well until she developed congestive heart failure.

Marjorie reports that life is different for her now that she is no longer independent. She states that she is having a difficult time adjusting to being "so dependent" and that she "misses her friends." She denies ever being hurt by anyone. After gentle questioning, Marjorie gradually admits to having difficulty living with her daughter and son-in-law because of their alcohol abuse. Although neither individual has harmed Marjorie physically, they discourage her friends from visiting her, and they continually demand exorbitant room-and-board payments. Recently, she noticed that some of her jewelry disappeared. Marjorie is left alone for long periods, sometimes for entire weekends, which is frightening to her because she is physically unable to provide for her own needs and has no access to the telephone. In addition, she becomes dyspneic periodically and experiences chest pressure.

Critical Thinking

1. What is the first priority for the nurse regarding the care of an older person who may be a victim of abuse, neglect, or exploitation?
2. What is the best way to assist an older patient like Marjorie to disclose feelings, concerns, and fears?
3. What type of mistreatment has Marjorie been experiencing from her daughter and son-in-law?
4. What characteristics require assessment in Marjorie's daughter and son-in-law?

---

her congestive heart failure so that she can regain normal cardiac output as evidenced by normal vital signs, freedom from chest pain and dyspnea, and decreased anxiety and fear. The remainder of Marjorie's nursing diagnoses relate to her psychosocial needs, including her depression. Because of her change in health status and her dependency on caregivers who are exploitative and neglectful, Marjorie is feeling helpless, frightened, and depressed.

Outcome Identification for Elder Abuse

The patient will do the following:

- Explore options that may exist in relation to her home situation. Because Marjorie is an adult, she cannot be forced to leave her children's home or to press charges against them. If there are mandatory reporting laws in Marjorie's state, her children's abusive behavior will have to be reported.
- Verbalize feelings about her change in health care status, her dependency on her children, the treatment that she has received from her children, and available options for dealing with these concerns.

PLANNING

As with other victims of family violence, securing safety is a major aspect of the plan of care for abused older adults. In the case of Marjorie, stabilizing her congestive heart failure had to be achieved before her abusive home situation could be assessed and before a plan of care for this aspect of her life could be established. Because most states have mandatory elder abuse reporting laws, it is critical that nurses and other health care professionals remain open to the possibility of elder abuse whenever there are potential indicators for it. As noted previously, many times older adults will deny the existence of the abuse; therefore, it is necessary to establish a trusting relationship with older patients to facilitate disclosure. The nurse is often in the best position to assess and identify abused patients. Thus, the plan of care should include the nurse's taking time to communicate concern, compassion, and a desire to explore options and resources; this can determine whether patients disclose critical information or continue to suffer in silence.

IMPLEMENTATION

As with other cases of family violence, the nurse is often called on to function as the coordinator of care. In Marjorie's case, the nurse may need to work closely with the social worker to develop and implement the plan of care. Because the nurse has frequent opportunities to discuss Marjorie's problems with her, he or she will be a key person in assisting Marjorie to identify her feelings, recognize her strengths, realistically assess the situation, and explore all possible options before making decisions. Thus, the nurse is in a position to address the total biopsychosocial, spiritual, and cultural needs of the patient.

Nursing Interventions

As previously mentioned, nursing interventions focus on meeting the biopsychosocial, spiritual, and cultural needs of the patient. Thus, the nurse can assist Marjorie with accepting the limitations of her congestive heart failure and encourage her to optimize her self-care abilities. The highest nursing priority is to balance Marjorie's safety and autonomy. It is also

TABLE 23-4	NURSING INTERVENTIONS FOR THE ABUSED ELDERLY
NURSING INTERVENTIONS	

Monitor the patient's response to decreased cardiac output.

Monitor the patient's response to medications.

Provide reassurance and support.

Educate the patient about medications and limitations.

Monitor the patient for increased depression and suicide potential.

Explore with the patient the reasons for feelings of helplessness and grief.

Discuss the patient's capabilities and strengths.

Explore options that provide the patient with increased control.

Explore ways for the patient to increase self-care.

Explore the patient's feelings related to family abuse.

Explore the patient's options for remaining with family versus making alternate living arrangements.

Coordinate referrals.

Show respect for the patient's decisions.

Evaluate the caregiver's motivation for seeking and using assistance.

Evaluate the family's coping skills.

Evaluate possible substance abuse by the caregiver.

Evaluate the caregiver's willingness to acknowledge and work on family problems.

important to assist Marjorie with learning about the community resources that are available to her in terms of maximizing her mental and physical health. Marjorie will require assistance with dealing with how she feels about being a burden to her daughter and son-in-law as well as with the abuse that they mete out. A plan must be made with the family if Marjorie insists on remaining with them, and this plan must clearly explain the family's obligations, Marjorie's rights, and the consequences of abusive or neglectful behavior in the future. Ongoing monitoring and evaluation are necessary; this is a role that is becoming more important for nurses as they provide ever-increasing amounts of care for older patients in their homes.

The home health care nurse must be prepared to provide counseling, referrals, support, and education to older patients and their families (Table 23-4). Sometimes the caregiver may be in desperate need of stress-management techniques, general information about the aging process, basic nursing care principles, and community agencies that provide assistance for older adults. Providing such support may dramatically ease the burden of caring for the older relative and prevent the occurrence of abuse and neglect.

EVALUATION

Evaluating the effectiveness of the outcomes and nursing care plan for elders who have been abused is important, because

the abuse may continue and even escalate if older patients choose to return to the abusive environment. In a situation like Marjorie's, the potential for escalating abuse is significant, because she will probably require increasing assistance from dysfunctional caregivers who are at high risk for continuing the abuse as a result of their substance abuse. However, nurses are often not in a position to follow up with patients after the patients leave the hospital.

Sengstock and Barrett (1993) claimed that certain clues can be helpful for determining whether nursing interventions will be successful. These include the willingness of the older patient to acknowledge the abuse and the willingness of the older patient and the abusive family members to accept outside interventions or the removal of the elder from the abusive environment. Although many resources for the older patient exist in most communities, the family cannot be assisted if they deny the existence of the abuse. Like battered women, older patients may experience multiple occasions of abuse before they gradually make the decision to leave their abusive environment.

RAPE AND SEXUAL ASSAULT

Sexual violence may include attempted or completed rape, sexual coercion and harassment, sexual contact with force or threat of force, and threat of rape (World Health Organization, 2002). More than half of all victims of sexual crimes, including rape and sexual assault, are women who are younger than 25 years old. Often this violence occurs within the context of dating or acquaintance relationships, with the female partner the likely victim of violence and the male partner the likely perpetrator.

CULTURAL COMPONENTS OF RAPE AND SEXUAL ASSAULT

Cultural Values and Sexual Assault

The way a cultural or ethnic group defines gender roles and the woman's place in society affects how rape will be perceived. In the United States, multiple examples of male superiority and female subjugation exist in popular literature, media, fashion, art, and language. These cultural symbols help to form attitudes and beliefs that are then further translated into laws, court proceedings, police behavior, educational curricula, and social service programs (Dasgupta, 1998).

Myths that blame victims for rape, and broad conceptualizations of sexual assault are influenced by ethnic-specific cultural values and norms. Cultural values are the underpinnings of beliefs and attitudes, and they assist the victim, friends, family, police, and any other affected individuals with deriving meaning from the experience.

Research Related to Rape and Culture

Researchers have attempted to increase the modern understanding of the cultural definition of rape. Sexual abuse and rape by an intimate partner is not considered a crime in many countries around the globe, and women in many societies do not consider forced sex by a known partner to be rape (Leininger, 1996). Culturally sanctioned beliefs about the rights and privileges of husbands have historically legitimized a man's domination over his wife and warranted his use of violence to control her. However, women who have been forced into sex by an intimate partner may be at risk for the same results and consequences as if they had been raped by an unknown assailant (e.g., sexually transmitted diseases, physical trauma, emotional issues).

ADOLESCENT POPULATIONS

Statutory Rape

Over the last decade, there has been a growing interest in the partnering of adolescent females with older adult males, which is often referred to as *adult–teen sex.* Although most adult women do partner with slightly older males, the application of this social norm to adolescent females has been linked to an increased risk for victimization, including physical and sexual violence. Furthermore, imbalances in power and control, financial resources, levels of life experience, and even physical strength and stature may place younger females who are partnered with adult males at risk for experiencing unplanned and unprotected sex, unwanted pregnancy, and exposure to sexually transmitted infections, including human immunodeficiency virus and acquired immunodeficiency syndrome. Although partnering with an older male may be considered consensual in nature by the female, her peers, and possibly her family, sexual relationships with significantly older males may meet the legal definition of statutory rape. As such, several teen advocacy and pregnancy prevention programs have called for the increased use of existing statutory rape laws to help with the prosecution and punishment of adult men who have sex with adolescent females (Harner et al, 2001).

Developmentally, adolescents must learn to control their newly gained independence from their parents as they master developmental milestones (e.g., driving a car, dating) and learn to negotiate new relationships with peers and intimate partners. As such, youth—which is associated with limited knowledge and lack of experience in interpersonal relationships—is a significant risk factor for the experiencing of sexual victimization (World Health Organization, 2002). Adolescents are particularly vulnerable when their youth is coupled with early menarche, early dating, and early sexual activity, all of which have all been linked with an increased risk for the experiencing of victimization by an intimate partner (Harner, 2003).

Like adult victims, adolescent victims of sexual violence may experience negative physical health consequences after sexual victimization. Although physical injuries do not always occur as a result of violence, victims may suffer physical trauma to the genital tract, including vaginal bleeding, bruises, lacerations, and contusions (World Health Organization, 2002). Trauma may be more extensive among younger females, especially those who have not yet reached menarche

and who thus have less elastic and more easily damaged vaginal tissue. Virginal adolescents may also be at increased risk for physical trauma, including hymeneal and perineal tears. This trauma in turn increases the adolescent's risk of contracting sexually transmitted infections, including gonorrhea, chlamydia, herpes, and human immunodeficiency virus. According to the Centers for Disease Control and Prevention (2001), the risk of sexually transmitted infection after rape is between 3.6% and 30%.

Victims may also be at risk for experiencing an unplanned pregnancy. Among adult victims, almost 5% of pregnancies are the result of rape (Centers for Disease Control and Prevention, 2001). The incidence of rape-related pregnancies among adolescent victims is likely higher, because younger women may be unaware of or have limited access to postcoital contraceptives and may not be using any long-term contraceptive method (e.g., birth control pills) at the time of the assault (Wilson and Klein, 2002).

Several factors have been linked with an increased risk for either experiencing or perpetrating sexual victimization during adolescence, including age and developmental level, previous victimization, drug and alcohol use, and adherence to rigid social roles that dictate acceptable behaviors.

Risk Factors

Alcohol has been cited as one of the major risk factors for both experiencing and perpetrating sexual victimization. It is important to note that, although alcohol has been strongly linked to sexual assault and other violent crimes, its relationship with victimization is one of correlation and not causation. Alcohol acts as a central nervous system depressant that decreases inhibition and impairs the judgment of users. For females, intoxication—especially binge drinking, which is defined as four or more drinks in a row for women and five or more drinks in a row for men—may decrease an individual's awareness of a partner's actions and advances and make it more difficult to stop sexual advances that have gone too far. In their study of sexual victimization on college campuses, Fisher and colleagues (2000) noted that drinking enough alcohol to get drunk was significantly related to the experiencing of sexual violence.

Alcohol use and intoxication are also significantly related to the perpetration of sexual violence. Among male users, intoxication has been linked with the misinterpretation of sexual cues as well as the overestimation of a woman's sexual interest, which may ultimately result in increased aggression and forced or coerced sex. Belief in the myth that alcohol use increases sexual arousal among both parties may also serve to legitimize and excuse sexually aggressive and coercive behaviors that would not otherwise be acceptable. Furthermore, despite advances in neutralizing gender-based roles and stereotypes, the preservation of outdated beliefs that dichotomize women into categories of "good" and "bad" may lead would-be perpetrators to view women who drink alcohol as sexually available and appropriate targets as compared with their nondrinking counterparts.

CASE STUDY #6

Nancy, a college sophomore, and her roommate took the campus bus to study at the school library. After they had studied for 3 hours, two male students invited the young women back to their dorm room to play cards. The game required the loser to drink a glass of beer. Over the new few hours, the four became intoxicated, and the women missed the bus back to their dormitory. The young men said that they would sleep on the couch, and they offered their beds to the women. Nancy fell asleep immediately, but she was awakened to the presence of one of the young men, who removed her clothes and proceeded to force sex on her despite her protests. The next morning, the women returned to their dormitory and attended classes. Nancy became increasingly anxious and distressed. She could not get the thought of the rape out of her mind. She was unable to concentrate in class, to do her homework assignments, to continue her part-time job, or to attend social functions. By the end of the semester, she had failed two courses and was on academic probation. Her roommate encouraged her to report the rape to the Women's Health Center, which she did. In turn, she reported the rape to local police, but criminal charges were not filed. A civil suit was filed against the university and later settled out of court. Nancy received short-term counseling and attended group sessions at the local rape crisis center.

Drug Use

Although victims may be sexually assaulted after knowingly ingesting illegal drugs (e.g., marijuana, heroin, cocaine), they may also be unknowingly drugged by so-called "date rape drugs." Two of the more common date rape drugs, γ-hydroxybutyrate and Rohypnol, are central nervous system depressants that, when dissolved in both alcoholic and non-alcoholic beverages, become odorless and tasteless. After a person has ingested these drugs, he or she becomes disoriented and confused and may be rendered unconscious for several hours. In an effort to reduce the incidence of drug-facilitated rape, pharmaceutical companies recently included a color additive in the drug Rohypnol. In addition to similar preventative measures, the criminalization of drug-facilitated rape is also enforced under the Drug-Induced Rape Prevention and Punishment Act of 1996 and the Hillory J. Farias and Samantha Reid Date-Rape Drug Prohibition Act of 2000. However, despite these efforts, sources of date rape drugs remain plentiful in the United States, internationally, and online. As with other substances that are knowingly or unknowingly ingested by victims, memory impairment, which is a common side effect of the medication, may make it difficult for victims to remember and identify the perpetrators of the crimes (Harner, 2003).

Prior Victimization

The correlation between earlier victimization and the later perpetration of physically and sexually violent crimes cannot be ignored. It has been postulated that males who were exposed to early victimization, including experiencing child physical or sexual abuse as well as witnessing domestic violence within the family, may be more prone to adapting to these negative experiences by using externalizing behaviors. These behaviors may include the increased acceptance and use of aggression, violence, and control within future relationships as well as other maladaptive behaviors, including lying, stealing, substance use, and truancy.

Previous victimization, including experiencing or witnessing violence during childhood, has also been linked with future victimization. Sexual victimization during childhood is frequently a predictor of the experiencing of future sexual victimization. Although past victimization does not guarantee future victimization, previous victimization—including a lack of control over one's body, sexuality, and choices—may set relational norms that become acceptable in future intimate relationships. Furthermore, if childhood victimization went unrecognized or unreported—especially by someone charged with that child's care—the now adolescent victim may feel that his or her victimization is unimportant and that his or her abuse is of little consequence (Harner, 2003).

DYNAMICS OF RAPE

Rape is an interactional process that involves at least two people and a control issue. One person feels that he or she must gain control over the other person. It becomes clear when talking with rape victims that, from their point of view, rape is an act that is initiated by the assailant; it is not primarily a sexual act but rather an act of aggression, power, and violence. One factor of great importance to victims is how the assailant gained access to and control of them (i.e., the style of attack). Two main styles of attack are known as the *blitz rape* and the *confidence rape*. The assailant has two goals: the physical control of the victim and the sexual control of the victim. Some rapists gain control with a direct physical action (e.g., a sudden surprise attack), whereas others use verbal ploys in an attack that has the qualities of a confidence game. With both types of attacks, the rapist gains sexual control of the victim by force and without consent.

The blitz rape occurs out of the blue and without any prior interaction between the assailant and victim. In a split second, the attacked individual's lifestyle is shattered: he or she has become a victim. As one survivor reported, "He came from behind. There was no way to get away. It happened so fast—like a shock of lightening going through you. I was so helpless at the time."

From the victim's point of view, there is no ready explanation for the man's presence. He suddenly appears, his presence is inappropriate, he is uninvited, and he forces himself into the situation. Often he selects an anonymous victim and tries to remain anonymous himself. He may wear a mask or gloves or cover the victim's face as he attacks.

The "mark"—to use the language of the criminal world—is the person who is destined to become the victim of some form illegal exploitation. The classic example of the blitz-type rape is the woman down the street who, from the assailant's point of view, is the "right mark at the right time." He is looking for someone to capture and attack. The victim happens on the scene, and she becomes the target. Victims who have experienced a blitz attack describe being jumped on, grabbed, pushed, or shoved when the assailant approached them from behind. Children and adolescents who were victims of blitz rape were often walking home from school or a friend's house or playing with neighborhood friends when the attack occurred.

The confidence rape involves a more subtle setup than the blitz style. The confidence rape is an attack in which the assailant obtains sex under false pretenses by using deceit, betrayal, and often violence. There is interaction between the victim and the assailant before the assault. The assailant may know the victim from some other time and place and thus may already have developed some kind of relationship with her. Alternatively, he may establish a relationship as a prelude to the attack. Often there is quite a bit of conversation that occurs between the victim and the assailant. Like the confidence man, he encourages the victim to trust him, and then he betrays this trust. An analysis of rapists' talk during rape revealed a number of linguistic strategies that are used to control the victim before, during, and after the rape.

One of the linguistic strategies used by the rapists is the *confidence line*. This verbal "line" is used in various ways in terms of the rapist, such as offering or requesting assistance or the victim's company; promising information, material items, social activities, employment, or business transactions; making reference to someone that the victim knows; or trading on social pleasantries and niceties.

MOTIVATION DURING RAPE

When working with identified rapists, both convicted and not convicted, it becomes apparent that sexual desire and frustration are not their dominant motives. The majority of rapists are engaged in consensual sexual relationships. If sex is not the primary motive, then what is? Clinical work with offenders and victims reveals that rape is in fact serving non-sexual needs; it is the sexual expression of power and anger. Rape is motivated more by retaliatory and compensatory motives than sexual ones; it is a pseudosexual act that is complex and multidetermined and that addresses issues of hostility and control. The defining issue in rape is the lack of consent on the part of the victim. Sexual relations are achieved through physical force, threat, or intimidation. Therefore, rape is first and foremost an aggressive act, and, in any given instance of rape, multiple psychologic meanings may be expressed with regard to both the sexual and aggressive components of the act.

EFFECTS OF RAPE ON THE VICTIM

Victims suffer a significant degree of physical and emotional trauma during the rape, immediately after the assault, and for a considerable time period afterward. Victims consistently describe certain symptoms over and over. A cluster of symptoms has been described as the *rape trauma syndrome*, which

most victims experience; it includes physical, emotional, and behavioral stress reactions that result from the person being faced with an event that threatens his or her life or integrity (Burgess and Holmstrom, 1974).

Victims show two main styles of emotion: *expressed* and *controlled*. In the expressed style, the victim demonstrates such feelings as anger, fear, and anxiety. The victims express these feelings by being restless during the interview, becoming tense when certain questions are asked, crying or sobbing when describing specific acts of the assailant, or smiling in an anxious manner when certain issues are stated. In the controlled style, the feelings of the victim are masked or hidden, and the interviewer notes a calm, composed, or subdued affect. It is not uncommon for victims to have a flat affect, to be stoic in demeanor, or to be highly emotional. It is frequently observed that people in prison will shut down and inhibit their feelings, because they do not know whom they can trust.

Victims express other feelings in conjunction with fear. These range from humiliation, degradation, guilt, shame, and embarrassment to self-blame, anger, and revenge. Victims report feeling distressed by reminders or cues of the assault. Seeing a man who looks like the assailant will evoke a strong emotional reaction. Victims become cautious with all people; after a stranger rape, the victim expects the assailant to be everywhere.

Many symptoms develop after a rape or a sexual assault. The woman will feel numb, and she continually tries to block the thoughts of the assault from her mind; that reaction may be observed as a flat affect or indifference. She will say that she is trying to push it out of her mind, but the thought of the assault continually haunts her. There is a strong desire for the victim to try and think of how she could undo what has happened. She reports going over in her mind how she might have escaped from the assailant and how she might have handled the situation differently. However, she usually ends up believing that she would have been beaten or killed if she had not done what the assailant demanded.

Dreams and nightmares of two types are major symptoms seen among rape victims. One type is a situation in which the victim dreams of being in a similar situation and is attempting to try and get out of the situation but fails; these dreams are similar to the actual rape itself. The second type of dream occurs as time progresses. The dream material changes, and frequently the victim will report mastery in the dream. Often the victim will see herself committing acts of violence such as killing and stabbing people. The power gained in this second type of dream may represent mastery, but the victim still has to deal with this violent image of herself.

Trauma and the Limbic System

One way to explain the long-term effects of rape and sexual assault is to understand the neurobiology of trauma and its effect on the limbic system. The importance of psychologic trauma is how it affects the brain, particularly key regulatory processes that control memory, aggression, sexuality, attachment, emotion, sleep, and appetite. The affected location of the brain, the limbic system, is the alarm system that protects the individual in the face of danger. It is the beginning place where all sensory information enters the human system and is encoded. When trauma occurs, the neurohormonal system releases epinephrine, which helps to prepare an individual to act during dangerous states. However, when individuals are trapped and cannot remove themselves either through fleeing or fighting, there is a particular type of learning called *trauma learning* that occurs that does not allow for a reduction of stress through the adaptive means of the fight-or-flight response. As a result of excesses and depletion of stress hormones in the brain structures responsible for interpreting and storing incoming stimuli, alterations occur in memory systems. The individual becomes immobilized, and, as the level of autonomic arousal increases, there is a move into a numbing state as a result of the release of opiates in the brain. This numbing state accounts for the disconnection of the processing and encoding of information. In a sense, when the trauma is over, the alarm system remains somewhat stuck between the accelerated fight-or-flight response and the numbing state, which causes an alteration in the individual's adaptive capacity. This alteration is a cellular change that becomes fixed in its patterning and that is difficult to change or extinguish. Of particular importance are various theories of modulating effects in the brain. We can all appreciate this fight-or-flight response and numbing in the face of danger; what we are now understanding is that trauma can have a lasting effect on basic processes of adaptation and growth (see Chapter 7).

Because these neurosystems of arousal and numbing are intricately related to information processing and memory, there is a distinctive type of memory in which experiences are recalled as if they were happening (e.g., a flashback). Thus, when external events trigger an association with the abuse itself, the person is thrown into this panic memory and feels subjected to a hostile and exploitative environment even though nothing like that is currently present. Internal events can also trigger a trauma-specific reaction called *night terrors.* These experiences are not like typical dreams; rather, they involve a vivid and visceral response, and the individual feels as if the trauma is currently occurring.

CHAPTER SUMMARY

- Violence in general and family violence in particular are major public health concerns.
- Because nurses assume many roles in a variety of settings, they are in prime positions to advocate and intervene for those who are the victims of family violence.
- Interpersonal violence is more likely inflicted by someone that the victim knows.
- Battering is a common cause of injury to women in the United States.
- Domestic violence is generally defined as physical, psychologic, and sexual abuse that is primarily directed at women by men for the purpose of maintaining control and power.
- Emotional and psychologic abuse can be just as traumatic as direct physical abuse.
- Most child physical and sexual abuse is perpetrated by an adult that is known to the child.
- Actions that ensure protection and safety for the victim are the most important nursing interventions in abusive situations.
- Elder abuse is becoming a greater public concern as the number of older persons in the population is growing.

REVIEW QUESTIONS

1. A patient walks into the doctor's office complaining of headaches. She is accompanied by her husband, who answers the physician's questions despite the physician asking the patient the questions. The patient avoids eye contact and has a depressed affect, and her shoulders are slumped. The nurse assesses that the patient may have which of the following issues?
   a. She is suffering from major depression.
   b. She is a battered wife.
   c. She is afraid to be with people.
   d. She is experiencing migraine headaches.

2. A 24-year-old patient is admitted to the emergency department with a broken wrist, a swollen and bruised eye, and a fractured jaw. The patient agreed to tell the nurse what actually happened if she promised not to tell anyone. The patient admitted that her husband abused her and that he has abused her in the past, approximately four to five times, but only when he was drunk. Which of the following would be the most appropriate nursing intervention?
   a. Treat her physical injuries, suggest she talk to a counselor, but keep the patient's secret to maintain trust.
   b. Ask her to bring in her husband so that he can get a referral for therapy.
   c. Report the abuse to the police.
   d. Have her talk to another victim of domestic violence.

3. An 8-year-old patient is referred by his teacher for individual therapy. The patient has been aggressive at school, and he has missed many days of school. In addition, the teacher recently found bruises on his back. Which of the

REVIEW QUESTIONS—cont'd

following would be the best short-term goal for this patient?

a. The patient will develop a trusting relationship with the therapist.

b. The patient will be free from aggressive behavior.

c. The parents will attend parenting classes.

d. The patient will consistently attend school.

4. High-risk factors for childhood sexual abuse include which of the following?

a. Undereducated parents

b. Low-income families

c. Multiple siblings

d. Parents who were sexually abused as children

5. A 75-year-old female patient is admitted to the hospital for pneumonia. The nurse observes that the patient's clothes are old and dirty and that they have holes. The patient also has decubiti on her sacral area. The best question to assess for the possibility of abuse would be which of the following?

a. "How long have you lived with your son?"

b. "How much money do you have in your bank account?"

c. "Describe a typical day at home. What do you have to eat, what you do during the day, and what time you bathe?"

d. "Who buys your clothes for you?"

REFERENCES

American Public Health Association: *Policy statement database. Child abuse. Policy date: 1/1/1975. Policy number: 7512* (website): www.apha.org/advocacy/policy/policysearch/default.htm?id=790. Accessed October 5, 2007a.

American Public Health Association: *Policy statement database. Prevention of child abuse. Policy date: 1/1/1986. Policy number: 8614(PP)* (website): www.apha.org/advocacy/policy/policysearch/default.htm?id=1129. Accessed October 5, 2007b.

Barnett OL et al: *Family violence across the lifespan: an introduction*, Thousand Oaks, Calif, 1997, Sage.

Boston Channel: *The Stuart case*, 2009 (website): www.thebostonchannel.com/chronicle/21306398/detail.html. Accessed January 17, 2010.

Bowlby J: The nature of the child's tie to his mother, *Int J Psychoanal* 39:359-373, 1958.

Brassard M, Hart S: *Psychological maltreatment*, Washington DC, 1993, Violence Update, National Criminal Justice Reference Service.

Burgess A, Hanrahan N, Baker T: Forensic markers in elder female sexual abuse cases, *Clinics in Geriatric Medicine* 21(2):399-412, 2005.

Burgess A, Holmstrom L: Rape trauma syndrome, *American Journal of Psychiatry* 131:981-986, 1974.

Burgess AW et al: Sexual abuse of nursing home residents, *J Psychosoc Nurs Ment Health Serv* 38(6):10-18, 2000.

Burgess AW et al: Pathological teasing and bullying turned deadly: shooters and suicide, *Victims and Offenders* 1:1-14, 2006.

Burgess AW et al: Stalking behaviors within domestic violence, *J Fam Violence* 12(4):389-403, 1997.

Burgess AW et al: Batterers stalking patterns, *J Fam Violence* 16(4), 2001.

Burgess AW, Hanrahan N: *Identifying forensic markers in elderly sexual abuse*, Washington, DC, 2006, National Institute of Justice.

Campbell JC, Humphreys J: *Nursing care of survivors of family violence*, St. Louis, 1993, Mosby.

Caretta C: Domestic violence: a worldwide exploration, *Journal of Psychosocial Nursing and Mental Health Services* 46(42):26-35, 2008.

Carretta CM: Domestic violence, *J Psychosoc Nurs* 46(3):26-35, 2008.

Centers for Disease Control and Prevention, National Center for Injury Prevention and Control: *Intimate partner violence fact sheet*, 2001 (website): www.cdc.gov/ncipc/factsheets/ipvfacts.htm. Retried December 2, 2002.

Crowell NA, Burgess AW: *Understanding violence against women*, Washington, DC, 1996, National Academies Press.

Dasgupta SD: Women's realities: defining violence against women by immigration, race, and class. In Bergen RK, editor: *Issues in intimate violence*, Thousand Oaks, Calif, 1998, Sage.

Dutton DG: *The domestic assault of women: psychological and criminal justice perspectives*, Vancouver, British Columbia, Canada, 1995, UBC Press.

Elliot D, Briere J: Sexual abuse trauma among professional women: validatinng the Trauma Symptom Checklist-40, *Child Abuse and Neglect* 16(3):391-398, 1993.

Foa EB et al: *Effective treatments for PTSD*, New York, 2000, Guilford Press.

Gelles R: *Intimate Violence in Families* 3rd ed, Thousand Oaks, California, 1997, Sage Publishers.

Giardino A et al: *Sexual assault: victimization across the life-span*, Maryland Heights, Mo, 2002, GW Medical Publishing.

Gidycz CA, Layman MJ: The crime of acquaintance rape. In Jackson TL, editor: *Acquaintance rape: assessment, treatment and prevention*, Sarasota, Fla, 1996, Professional Resource Press.

Gregory KE, Vessey JA: Bibliotherapy: a strategy to help students with bullying, *J Sch Nurs* 20(3):127-133, 2004.

Harner H: Childhood sexual abuse teenage pregnancy, and partnering with adult men; exploring the relationship, *Journal of Psychosocial Nursing and Mental Health Services* 43(8):20-28, 2005.

Harner H et al: Caring for pregnant teenagers: medicolegal issues for nurses, *J Obstet Gynecol Neonatal Nurs* 30:139-147, 2001.

Harner H, O'Donnell S: Forensic evaluation of adolescents and adults, *GW Medical Publishing* 2003.

Iancu et al: *Information of sexual abuse in elders PTSD and the anxiety continuum, including PTSD*. 1998. Retrieved January 2009, from medscape.com: www.medscape.com.

Jeary K: Sexual abuse and sexual offending against elderly people: A focus on perpetrators and victims, *Journal of Forensic Psychiatry & Psychology* 16(2):328-343, 2005.

Kamphuis J, Emmelkamp P, Bartak A: Individual differences in post=traumatic stress following post-intimate stalking: stalking severity and pschosocial variables, *British Journal of Clinical Psychology* 42(2):145-156, 2005.

Kamphus JH, Emmelkamp PM: 20 years of research into violence and trauma, *J Interpers Violence* 20(2):167-174, 2005.

Kreidler M, Kurzawa C: Trauma Spectrum Disorders: clinical imperatives, *Journal of Psychosocial Nursing and Mental Health Services* 47(11):26-33, 2009.

Leininger M: Major directions for transcultural nursing: a journey into the 21st century, *J Transcult Nurs* 7(2):28-31, 1996.

Males M, Chew KS: The ages of fathers in California adolescent births, 1993, *Am J Public Health* 8(4):565-568, 1996.

McCoy K, Hansen B: Special report: havens for elderly may expose them to deadly risks, *USA Today*, May 25, 2004.

National Center on Elder Abuse: 2004 survey of state adult protective services: abuse of adults 60 years of age and older. 2006.

National Research Council: *Understanding child abuse and neglect*, Washington, DC, 1993, National Academies Press.

Olweus D: Bully/victim problems among school children: basic facts and effects of a school based intervention program. In Pepler D, Rubin K, editors: *The development and treatment of childhood aggression*, Hillsdale, NJ: 1991, Lawrence Erlbaum.

Olweus D: *Bullying at school: what we know and what we can do*, Oxford, UK, 1993, Blackwell.

Parker B, McFarlane J, Socken K: Physical and emotional abuse in pregnancy: A comparision of adult and teenage women, *Nursing Research* 42:173-178, 1993.

Pillemer D, Finkelhor D: The prevalence of elder abuse: A random sample survey, *The Gerontologist* 28(1):51-57, 1988.

Prentky R, Janus E, Barbaree H, et al: Sexually violent predators in the courtroom: Science on trial. *50*. William Mitchell Legal Studies Research Paper, 2006.

Reiss AJ, Roth JA: *Understanding and preventing violence*, Washington, DC, 1993, National Academies Press.

Rhatigan D, Street A: The impact of intimate partner violence on decisions to leave dating relationships: A test of investment model, *Journal of Interpersonal Violence* 20(12):1580-1597, 2005.

Safarik M, Jarvis J, Nussbaum K: Sexual homicide of elderly females: Linking offender characteristics to victim and crime scene attributes, *Journal of Interpersonal Violence* 17(5):500-525, 2002.

Schwartz A, Bradley R, Penza K, et al: Pain medication use among patients with posttraumatic stress disorder, *Psychosomatics* 47(2):136-142, 2006.

Sengstock MC, Barrett S: Abuse and neglect of the elderly in family settings. In Campbell JC, Humphreys J, editors: *Nursing care of survivors of family violence*, St. Louis, 1993, Mosby.

Stark E, Flitcraft A: Spouse Abuse. In ML R, MA F, editors: *Violence in America: A Public Health Approach* (pp. 123-157), New York, 1991, Oxford University Press.

Stark E, Flitcraft A: *Women at Risk: Domestic Violence and Women's Health*, Thousand Oaks, California, 1982, Sage Press.

Straus MA: Wife beating: how common and why? In Straus MA, Hotaling GT, editors: *The social causes of husband-wife violence* (pp. 23-36), Minneapolis, 1980, University of Minneapolis Press.

Tjaden P, Thoennes N: *Extent, nature and consequences of rape victimization: Findings from the National Against Women Survey*, Washington DC, 1998, National Criminal Justice Reference Services.

U.S. General Account Office: *Nursing homes: more can be done to protect residents from abuse (report to congressional requesters)*, Washington, DC, 2002, United States General Accounting Office.

van der Kolk B, Fisler R: Child abuse and neglect and loss of self-regulation, *Bull Menninger Clin* 58(2):145-168, 1994.

Vierthaler K: Best practices for working with rape crisis centers to address elder sexual abuse, *Journal of Elder Abuse & Neglect* 20(4):306-322, 2008.

Walton-Moss J, Campbell J: *Intimate Partner Violence: Implications for Nursing*, 2002. Retrieved January 2009, from Online Journal of Issues in Nursing: www.nursingworld.org/ MainMenuCategories/ANAMarketplace/ANAPeriodicals/OJIN/ TableofContents/Volume72002/No1Jan2002/ IntimatePartnerViolence.aspx.

Widom CS: Does violence beget violence? A critical examination of the literature, *Psychol Bull* 106(1):3-28, 1989.

Winpisinger KA et al: Risk factors for childhood homicides in Ohio: a birth certificate-based case-control study, *Am J Public Health* 81(8):1052-1054, 1991.

World Health Organization (2004). *International plan of action on aging: report on implementation* (EB115/29). Geneva.

World Health Organization: In *Abuse of the elderly*, 2002. Retrieved February 28, 2006, from World Health Organization Web Site: http://www.who.int.

World Health Organization. In *World report on violence and health: abstract*, 2002. Retrieved February 28, 2006, from World Health Organization Web Site: http://www.who.int.

Zigler E, NW H: Physical child abuse in America: past present and future. In Cicchetti D, Carlson V, editors: *Child Maltreatment and Research on the Causes and Consequences of Child Abuse and Neglect* (pp. 38-75), New York, 1989, Cambridge University Press.

Online Resources

Intimate Partner Abuse

National Coalition Against Domestic Violence: www.ncadv.org

U.S. Department of Justice Office on Violence Against Women: www.ovw.usdoj.gov

Minnesota Center Against Violence and Abuse: www.mincava.umn.edu

National Domestic Violence Hotline: www.ndvh.org

Family Violence Prevention Fund: www.fvpf.org

Child Abuse and Neglect

American Professional Society on the Abuse of Children: www.apsac.org

Child Welfare League of America: www.cwla.org

National Clearinghouse on Child Abuse and Neglect Information: www.calib.com/nccanch

Elder Abuse

American Society on Aging: www.asaging.org

Clearinghouse on Abuse and Neglect of the Elderly: www.cane.udel.edu

National Center on Elder Abuse: www.elderabusecenter.org

National Committee for the Prevention of Elder Abuse: www.preventelderabuse.org

National Fraud Information Center: www.fraud.org

Woman Abuse

The National Women's Health Information Center: Sexual Assault and Abuse: www.womenshealth.gov/violence/types/ sexual.cfm

Rape, Abuse and Incest National Network: www.rainn.org

Sexual Abuse Nurse Examination Information: www.forensic-science.com/course_description/fs207.html

Violence Against Women Online Resources: www.vaw.umn.edu

Forensic Nursing

Dona Petrozzi and Ann Wolbert Burgess

"No problem can withstand the assault of sustained thinking."

Voltaire

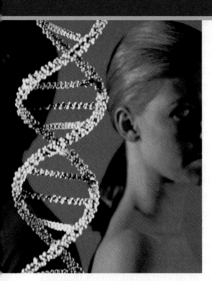

evolve WEBSITE

http://evolve.elsevier.com/Fortinash/

OBJECTIVES

- Discuss the history and development of forensic nursing.
- Describe relevant pertinent legislation and its impact on the discipline of forensic nursing.
- Define the roles and responsibilities of the sexual assault nurse.
- Discuss proper evidence collection techniques to use with the sexual assault patient.
- Identify potential complications associated with the sexual assault patient.
- Discuss the prevalence of weapon-related assaults.
- Discuss proper evidence collection techniques to use with the weapon-related assault patient.

- Identify potential physical and emotional complications associated with the weapon-related assault patient.
- Discuss the effect of violence on the family of the weapon-related assault patient.
- Identify complications associated with family members of a homicide victim.
- Define the roles and responsibilities of the correctional nurse.
- Define forensic risk and its relationship to the practice of forensic nursing.

KEY TERMS

advanced practice forensic nursing	fact witness	forensic nursing	homicide survivor
expert testimony	forensic clinical nurse	forensic psychiatric nurse	nurse death investigator
expert witness	forensic correctional nurse	forensic risk	sexual assault nurse examiner
	forensic health care system	forensics	

Although the roles have not specifically been identified, professional nurses have served a variety of roles within the forensic health care system throughout nursing's history. Qualified nurses have always assumed the care of crime-related patients and their families in hospitals, community centers, prisons, and forensic psychiatric units. However, it has been only within the past 20 years that forensic nursing has emerged as a recognized specialty within the forensic health care system. This emergence of the forensic nursing specialty highlighted existing gaps in the management of crime victims and perpetrators, particularly forensic issues in the clinical area such as the identification of risk factors, evidence collection, and the psychologic complications of violence.

Forensics pertains to public debate in courts of law; thus, the interface of law and nursing implies a legal case that may involve criminal or civil matters. Clinical forensic practice concerns itself primarily with survivors of violent crime or liability-related trauma. The statistics on violence help to substantiate the clinical need and demand for forensic nursing services. More than 1.6 million people died from violence in 2001 (World Health Report on Violence, 2002). In addition, millions of people were also injured as a result of violence, and many continue to suffer from physical, sexual, reproductive, and mental health problems, thereby making violence a leading public health issue.

Forensic nursing, which is one of the newest practices recognized by the American Nurses Association, is gaining momentum nationally and internationally, in part as a result of nursing's professional recognition in research. Forensic nursing science research highlighted the need for the integration of formalized forensic nursing expertise into the arena of forensic health care, particularly with regard to living patients. In the inaugural issue of the *Journal of Forensic Nursing*, editor Louanne Lawson (2009) noted that a professional discipline is defined, in part, by its published research and that its future depends on the research that is currently being conducted.

The professionalization of forensic nursing has served a crucial role in the development and refinement of forensic health care practice worldwide. Incorporating nursing expertise into forensic health care has offered a practical perspective in the application of knowledge and skills to the care and protection of people who are treated in the forensic health care environment. To reinforce the necessity of forensic nursing in health care settings for managing the assessment and treatment of forensic patients, formalized academic programs and professional organizations began to emerge in the United States in 1995. Furthermore, the Joint Commission now mandates that health care institutions formally detect and manage issues that pertain to potential or actual violence in their patients. It is pertinent for professional nurses to be proficient in the assessment, care, and protection of crime-related patients, because nurses are the first to identify and therapeutically intervene with individuals who have been exposed to violence.

THE HISTORY OF FORENSIC NURSING

The extant literature on forensic nursing is in general agreement that the practice of forensics has a long and accepted history in medicine and psychiatry. As noted by Lynch and Burgess (1998), the first separate discipline of forensic medicine began early during the 16th century, whereas forensic nursing's history has been traced to the 18th century, when midwives were called into court to testify on issues pertaining to virginity, pregnancy, and rape. Lynch (2009) wrote that the term *forensic* has traditionally been associated with death or murder because, until recently, forensic pathology or death investigation was the only type of forensic work that received widespread attention. According to Lynch, clinical forensic nursing practice represents an era of nursing that has developed in direct response to the increase in criminal and interpersonal violence in our society.

Lynch explained that the current theoretic model of forensic nursing evolved from the role of the police medical officer found in the United Kingdom and European countries. The clinical forensic medicine practitioner is hired by the police department and is responsible for facilitating the management of the crime victim from the scene of the incident and throughout the legal process. Goll-McGee (1999) wrote that forensic nurses deal with the population of people whose lives have been affected by societal violence. Barton (1995) pointed out that forensic nurses fill a gap where the health care system interacts with the legal system by meeting the needs of victims and perpetrators of violent crimes through enhanced quality of care and preventive services. Observation, documentation, preservation, and notification are critical for determining the legal outcomes of cases that involve violence (Malestic, 1995; Wick, 2000).

Nelson (1998) dates the official coining of the term *forensic nursing* to 1992, when approximately 70 nurses gathered in Minneapolis for the first national convention for sexual assault nurse examiners. This led to the founding of the International Association of Forensic Nurses, which is an international professional organization of registered nurses that was formed to develop, promote, and disseminate information about the science of forensic nursing. The American Nurses Association recognized forensic nursing as a subspecialty in 1995, and it defines forensic nursing as "the practice of nursing globally when health and legal systems intersect" (2009, p. 3).

LEGISLATION

Violence Against Women Act

Societal attention to violent crime against women first gained momentum during the 1970s as part of the women's rights movement. Feminists brought to light the inadequate responses of the criminal justice system in crimes against women, and, as a result, victim assistance programs began to be developed in 1972. These programs highlighted key features of the victim experience, including methods to address the psychosocial impact of trauma and interventions to gain assistance and recognition from the criminal justice system. On the basis of this foundation, the victim's movement became nationalized in 1985, when the National Victim Center was established. It was not until the 1990s that the federal government took action and developed legislation that focused on the problem of crimes against women (see Box 24-1).

The Violence Against Women Act was passed in 1994 as Title IV of the Violent Crime Control and Law Enforcement

---

BOX 24-1	SIGNIFICANT EVENTS IN FORENSIC NURSING'S HISTORY

1972: First organized victim assistance programs
1985: National Victim Center established
1992: Joint Commission on Accreditation of Healthcare Organizations mandates the assessment of violence
1994: Violence Against Women Act passed
1995: Formal academic forensic nursing programs developed

Act. This Act allocated funds for law enforcement, community prevention agendas, and victim treatment programming. Subsequent revisions of the bill in 2000 and 2005 have expanded the focus of crimes against women to include dating violence, stalking and Internet crimes, safe housing for abused families, and crimes against children and the elderly. These revisions have allowed forensic health care professionals to develop standard protocols for the victims of violent crimes and to enhance the protective mechanisms provided in the clinical setting.

EDUCATION AND CREDENTIALING OF THE FORENSIC NURSE

The five primary routes for educational preparation in forensic nursing are as follows: (1) continuing education coursework; (2) certificate programs; (3) undergraduate nursing education; (4) graduate nursing education; and (5) postdoctoral education or fellowships (Burgess et al, 2004). In addition, there are two levels of practice: basic and advanced.

Basic forensic nursing is practiced by registered nurses who have the knowledge and skills to fulfill a specific role (e.g., sexual assault nurse examiner). Basic forensic nurses achieve specialized competencies through training programs, continuing education programs, and certification programs. Most generalists are prepared at the diploma, associate's, and bachelor's degree levels (American Nurses Association, 2009).

Advanced practice forensic nursing incorporates specialized knowledge and skills. These nurses hold master's or doctoral degrees, and they are licensed, certified, and approved to practice in the roles of clinical nurse specialist, nurse practitioner, or certified nurse–midwife (American Nurses Association, 2009).

Fact and Expert Witnesses

Forensic nurses may provide both fact and expert witness testimony. A fact witness is a person with knowledge about what happened in a particular case who testifies in the case about what happened or what the facts are. Fact witness testimony consists of the recitation of facts or of a chronology of events; this is different from an expert witness, whose testimony consists of the presentation of an opinion or a diagnosis.

An expert witness is a person who—by virtue of education, training, skill, or experience—is believed to have expertise and specialized knowledge in a particular subject beyond that of the average person. This knowledge is presented in court to provide an opinion about an evidence or fact issue within the scope of the expert witness' expertise.

The following questions are generally asked to qualify a nurse for expert testimony (Shindul-Rothschild and Burgess, 2007, pp. 144-145):

- Please state for the record your formal education beyond the high-school years.
- What is your highest earned educational degree in the field of nursing?

- Was this degree earned from an accredited institution of higher education?
- Please state what practicum and internships you completed.
- Are you licensed to practice nursing? If so, in what jurisdiction?
- Is your clinical experience inpatient or outpatient or in a specialized agency?
- How many years did you spend in these practice settings?
- What medical and psychiatric diagnoses did the patients that you worked with have? What were their age ranges?
- Were you involved with assessment, treatment, or both?
- If you were involved with treatment, what types of interventions did you employ?
- Do you currently possess prescription privileges, or have you possessed these privileges in the past? If so, for what length of time and in what jurisdiction?
- Do you have admitting privileges at any facilities? If so, which ones?

Specialty Areas and Practice within Forensic Nursing
Sexual Assault Nurse Examiners

Sexual assault nurse examiners (SANEs) provide care to and collect evidence from victims of sexual assault. SANE training programs have existed in the United States since 1976. As described in the SANE Standards of Practice (ANA, 2009) the SANE is an expert in history taking and assessment; the treatment of trauma response and injury; the documentation and collection of evidence and its management; the emotional and social support required during a posttrauma evaluation; and the testimony required in court proceedings (Speck and Peters, 1999).

The International Association of Forensic Nurses (2002) has published SANE education guidelines to serve as a framework for the training and education of SANEs. The International Association of Forensic Nurses has developed a certification program that is valid for 3 years that leads to the designation of SANE-Adult and Adolescent (SANE-A). Eligibility criteria to sit for the examination include the holding of a valid U.S. registered nurse license with a minimum of 2 years of practice as a registered nurse; the successful completion of an adult and adolescent SANE education program that includes either (1) a minimum of 40 continuing-education contact hours of didactic instruction or (2) three semester hours (or the equivalent) of academic credit in an accredited school of nursing; and current SANE competency validated by an appropriate clinical authority.

The U.S. Department of Justice Office for Victims of Crimes (2001) reported that SANE programs have made a profound difference in the quality of care provided to sexual assault victims. These programs offer victims prompt, compassionate care and comprehensive forensic evidence collection. The work of these nurses has led to more effective investigations and the better prosecution of perpetrators, and it has addressed the long-standing issue of retraumatizing victims when they come to the hospital for medical care and forensic evidence collection. The report traced the establishment of the first SANE programs to the mid 1970s in Minneapolis, Minn; Memphis, Tenn; and Amarillo, Texas. By 1991, approximately 20 SANE programs existed in the United States; in 1996, there were 86 known programs; by 1997, that number rose to 116; and, by 1999, it was estimated that there were more than 300 programs in existence.

Sexual Assault Statistics. Despite the nationalization of victim programs in the United States, rape and sexual assault continues to be a significant public health issue. In 2008, the FBI Uniform Crime Report reported that there were 71,264 rapes and 5803 attempted rapes. Typically, the sexually assaulted patient will present to the emergency department after the assault.

Initial Assessment. It is the role of the forensic nurse to immediately assess the sexual assault victim for evidence of acute physical injuries, such as head or facial trauma, excessive bleeding, penetrating injuries, and fractures. Evidence of such injuries would take precedence over all other interventions, because physical injuries could be potentially life threatening. See the Research for Evidence-Based Practice box regarding examination methods as well as Box 24-2, which illustrates methods for collecting evidence. Second, the forensic nurse assesses the victim for indications of shock and stress. Common responses of the sexual assault victim during the acute phase of sexual assault include numbing, dissociation, hypervigilance, hyperarousal, and shock. See the case study of Mary, a sexual assault victim. (see Chapter 20).

BOX 24-2   COLLECTING PHYSICAL EVIDENCE FROM THE SEXUAL ASSAULT VICTIM

1 The sexual assault victim will remove his or her clothes, including undergarments.
2 Each item of clothing is placed in a separate paper bag and sealed for blood, semen, and DNA testing.
3 The sexual assault victim is assessed for bodily injury by noting specific symptoms such as bleeding and bruising.
4 The presence of such injuries is clearly documented and photographed.
5 The fingernails, the oral mucosa, and internal and external vaginal areas of female victims are swabbed and then dried.
6 Each swab is placed in a separate paper envelope and then sealed.
7 Upon the completion of evidence collection, all samples will be placed in a refrigerated area for preservation.

BOX 24-3   ASSESSMENT FOR ACUTE TRAUMATIC STRESS IN THE SEXUAL ASSAULT VICTIM

1 Is the patient alert and oriented?
2 What are the patient's vital signs?
3 Is the patient able to answer questions?
4 Does the patient remember what happened?
5 Does the patient appear frightened or agitated?
6 Does the patient startle with the slightest sound?

CASE STUDY #1

Mary, a 22-year-old woman, comes to the emergency department in the middle of the night. She appears disheveled, with torn clothing, visible bruises, and scratches; she is crying inconsolably. There is a distinct odor of alcohol on her person. She has difficulty answering questions, but she is able to report she was at a party drinking alcohol when she blacked out. She awoke to find herself lying on the street in a puddle. Mary claims that she cannot remember what happened, but she feels soreness between her legs and on her neck and breasts. Further assessment of Mary reveals that her serum blood alcohol level is twice the legal limit and that she has a history of bipolar illness. Mary is not currently taking her prescribed medications.

Critical Thinking Questions
1 What is the nurse's first priority when caring for Mary?
2 When assessing Mary, what is the nurse's primary focus?
3 What interventions help to prepare an agitated patient for a physical examination?
4 What prejudices could arise in the nurse who is unprepared for this role?
5 How do nurses overcome their biases?

To adequately address the unique needs of the sexual assault victim, a forensic nurse is required to have specific knowledge of the dynamics involved in a sexual assault as well

as of criminal offenses. The primary purpose of the sexual assault examination is to provide law enforcement with clear, concise evidence and documentation related to crimes of sexual assault. Indications of injuries in a sexual assault context would potentially be noted, primarily on the face, torso, breast, and genital areas. When this occurs, forensic photo documentation can accurately record these injuries, and it may be used later for evidentiary support of the legal charge. Throughout the sexual assault examination, the SANE would provide assurances of safety and protection to enhance the comfort of the patient as the sexual assault examination progresses to completion. Throughout the physical examination, the SANE will be attuned to the victim's mental status and monitor him or her for signs and symptoms of anxiety, panic, and grief. The interview consists of obtaining the victim's recall of the events that transpired. As SANE nurses document these interviews, they primarily record as many direct quotes as possible.

Sexual assault victims are at high risk for psychosocial complications related to the rape (Box 24-3). It is important for the SANE to provide proper education and resource materials to the victim to help ameliorate the complications associated with sexual trauma. Appropriate referrals and follow-up appointments are crucial for these patients, because they are at extreme risk for posttraumatic stress disorder (PTSD), depression, anxiety disorders, and other psychologic sequelae.

Forensic Nurses and Clinical Nurse Specialists

Forensic nurses and clinical nurse specialists work not only with crime victims and their families but with those involved in paternity disputes; those who suffer from liability-related injuries that result from vehicular or pedestrian accidents, occupational injuries, and medical malpractice injuries; and those whose injuries occurred as a result of food or drug tampering (Burgess and Lynch, 1998). Forensic clinical specialists work at the intersection of health care and the legal system, with an emphasis on a holistic approach to the delivery of patient care in medicolegal cases and the initiation of preventive education.

A major practice area for forensic nurses is a hospital's emergency department, because police frequently bring crime victims for care into such settings. Two important aspects for forensic nurses who work in this area are treating victims of weapon-related assaults and working with the families of crime victims. Both are described below.

RESEARCH FOR EVIDENCE-BASED PRACTICE #1

Somers MS: Defining patterns of genital injury from sexual assault, *Trauma Violence Abuse* 8(3):270-280, 2007.

Somers conducted a research review of the examination and detection of genital injuries in sexual assault victims. Vaginal examination with the use of a colposcope and toluidine staining provided the most accurate detection of genital injury, particularly in common areas such as the posterior fourchette, the labia minora, and the hymen. The use of digital imaging in combination with toluidine staining and the colposcopic examination will be instrumental in the development of the standardized measurement of genital injuries. Clear documentation of these types of injuries is crucial to the successful prosecution of sexual offenders.

Care of Weapon-Related Assault Victims

Weapon-related assault includes any physical injuries that are inflicted by a weapon such as a firearm, a knife, a hammer, and so on. Injuries from violent crime are a persistent public health concern; they induce considerable strain on victims, their families, and community members

Weapon Assault Statistics. According to the Federal Bureau of Investigation Uniform Crime Report published in 2006, there were 720,652 aggravated assaults that year. Violent crime victims experience physical and social disability that result in a dramatic loss of functioning and productivity (Discala and Sege, 2004). Survivors of assault-related injuries report significantly high rates of short-term and long-term disability, particularly related to the loss of mobility and chronic pain issues (Greenspan and Kellerman, 2002) as well as to psychologic symptoms of depression, anger, anxiety, and grief; this can adversely affect the physical well-being and potential survival of the patient (Mohta et al, 2003).

Violent-crime survivors require a multitude of health care services both during their hospitalizations and as they return to the community, such as medical and surgical follow-up appointments, physical therapy, and psychologic therapy. However, adequately managing these conditions can be challenging for these patients after hospitalization as a result of limited health care resources and financial constraints (Kroll, 2008).

Consequently, incidents of violent crime can be economically burdensome to health care institutions and their surrounding communities. It is estimated by the National Center for Injury Prevention and Control (2000) that the costs of direct medical expenditures and productivity losses in the United States are in excess of $20 billion each year, averaging between approximately $15,000 and $32,000 per victim (Cunningham et al, 2009). In the state of Massachusetts alone, these costs are estimated to be more than $18 million each year (Hume et al, 2007).

As a result of the high incidence of violence in urban neighborhoods, posttraumatic illness is considered to be prevalent, particularly among children and adolescents (Clark et al, 2007). In a study conducted by Rich and Grey (2005) of surviving gunshot victims, 65% reported trauma symptoms such as recurrent thoughts, nightmares, and hypervigilance. Rather than being engaged in formal treatment, 67% of this study's participants reported the use of illicit substances, mainly marijuana. The primary purpose for this substance use is to aid in numbing the victim from the effects of intrusive thoughts and to allow victims to self-medicate themselves for the treatment of insomnia and irritability.

NURSING PROCESS FOR WEAPON-RELATED ASSAULT VICTIMS

Assessment

Gunshot and stabbing victims often present to the trauma center with multiple entry wounds, thereby increasing the risk of physical complications and subsequent disability. McKinley and colleagues (1999) reported that the most common points of entry, from highest to lowest, are the spinal cord (44%), the abdomen (32%), the neck (27%), and the chest (24%). Greenspan and Kellerman (2002) report that the degree of physical disability is strongly correlated with the body area that is injured. For example, firearm injuries to the brain, the spinal cord, or the lower body resulted in higher disability in the areas of physical functioning and chronic pain, particularly as compared with injuries to the chest or the abdomen. In addition, violence-related spinal cord injuries involved higher rates of paraplegia as compared with those spinal cord injuries that resulted from nonviolent causes (e.g., motor vehicle accidents, falls) (Box 24-4).

Common comorbidities associated with severe gunshot injuries include pain, infection, hemothorax, pneumothorax, orthopedic fractures, and peripheral nerve damage (McKinley et al, 1999). These complications can have significant implications with regard to patient treatment, which can

BOX 24-4	WEAPON-RELATED TRAUMA	
COMMON AREAS OF INJURY	**COMPLICATIONS**	
Spinal cord Abdomen Neck Chest	• Chronic pain • Immobility • Self-care deficits • High risk for skin breakdown • Low self-esteem • Loss of independence • Change in familial roles • PTSD	

CASE STUDY #2

Marcus is a 19-year-old man who was the victim of a gunshot wound to the chest 1 year ago. He presents to the emergency department complaining of chest palpitations, diaphoresis, and poor sleep. In addition, Marcus reports the use of marijuana daily and the use of alcohol several times per week. His vital signs do demonstrate moderate tachycardia and hypertension. Marcus has not been to follow-up appointments in 6 months, and he has no current primary care physician. Upon further assessment, Marcus reveals that he has episodes of anxiety and depression as well as chronic nightmares, which have caused him to miss work and school.

Critical Thinking Questions

1 What nursing diagnoses will be applied to Marcus' treatment plan?
2 What are the primary interventions for Marcus?
3 In terms of follow-up care, what are Marcus' primary needs?
4 What concerns would the nurse have when discharging Marcus from the emergency department?

prolong hospitalization and delay patient recovery (Greenspan and Kellerman, 2002). In a study conducted by Discala and Sege (2004) of patient outcomes among patients who were hospitalized for nonfatal gunshot injuries, a high rate of short-term disabilities was associated with injuries to the extremities (55.9%). Long-term disability was largely associated with central nervous system injury (70%).

Nursing Diagnosis

The nursing diagnoses that are commonly applied to weapon-related trauma victims are always applied on the basis of observations and assessments that take place during the initial period after admission to the emergency department. Nursing diagnoses made at this time will also serve as a communication tool to the receiving units of the patient (e.g., operating department, intensive care unit, surgical unit).

Weapon-related trauma diagnoses include the following:
• Altered tissue perfusion related to cardiopulmonary injury
• Fluid volume deficit related to active fluid and blood loss
• Acute pain related to traumatic injuries
• Fear related to victimization by a weapon
• Powerlessness related to uncertainty of illness

See the case study about Marcus, who demonstrates mental and emotional symptoms as a result of weapon-related trauma.

Intervention

Life-saving interventions for weapon-related injuries begin with an assessment of the following: patient physical status (i.e., vital signs); the number and location of wounds to determine the degree of patient acuity; and fluid and blood loss. Initial treatment goals revolve around protecting the body's supply of blood and capitalizing on the body's physiologic response to a loss of blood. The number and location of the injuries inform the treating practitioners about the level of intervention required to sustain life, which may be intubation, chest tube placement, or surgical intervention.

Weapon-related trauma victims are often conscious upon arrival to the emergency department. Victims frequently demonstrate signs and symptoms of shock, fear, anxiety, and poor recall of the event. In this circumstance, it falls to the treating nurse to determine the mental status of the patient,

to conduct a pain assessment, and to provide education about the patient's ongoing procedures. In so doing, the nurse provides comfort and assures the patient that his or her needs will be addressed.

Evidence Collection in the Emergency Department

During the initial stages of treatment, law-enforcement officials are usually present in the emergency department. In a typical situation, a forensic nurse will provide information about the patient's identity, the number and location of the injuries, and patient acuity to the police officers. Releasing patient information in the context of a criminal act is exempt from confidentiality standards and laws, because the release of this information is for the protection of the victim; it is used to investigate the crime and potentially to apprehend the perpetrator.

All clothing is removed from the patient. Items of clothing are usually cut off as a result of the urgency of the situation. Proper forensic procedure is to cut around visible holes in the clothing. As the clothing is removed, it is immediately placed in a paper evidence-collection bag, sealed, and released directly to the police. Bullet fragments found externally on the patient are removed with a gloved hand and placed in a sealed, hard, plastic container. Personal belongings such as patient identification, cell phones, and any illegal weapons or drug paraphernalia are stored separately from clothing and again placed in paper bags, sealed, and released to the police.

Outcome Identification

Some outcomes of weapon-related trauma victims occur over the course of the hospitalization and require consistent monitoring and modification. A high priority is placed on those physical outcomes that preserve life and improve the overall condition of the patient, such as the following:

- Improved cardiopulmonary function: stable vital signs; improved oxygen saturation rates with and without thoracotomy tubes
- Fluid volume stabilization: stable vital signs; laboratory results within normal limits
- Pain will be adequately managed: decreased complaints of pain

In acute traumatic situations, the patient's physical condition requires immediate attention. However, the forensic nurse continually prioritizes all aspects of the nursing process and considers the patient's psychosocial needs and those of the family as important elements of total patient care.

Care of Trauma Victims' Families

The families of violent crime victims experience high levels of stress and anxiety that often inhibit family members' abilities to cope with and understand the current circumstances. For example, family member responses to traumatically injured patients include shock, fear, denial, suspiciousness, and anger toward caregivers, particularly during the initial phases of emergency treatment (Redley et al, 2003; Tolbert-Washington, 2001). The nurse's failure to recognize maladaptive family responses can exacerbate the risk of mental illnesses such as depression, anxiety disorders, and PTSD for both the patient and the family (Mohta et al, 2003). As a result of these findings, it is pertinent for nurses to adopt a family-centered approach that encompasses family members in caring interventions so that they are recognized as part of the patient's context or environment.

NURSING PROCESS IN TRAUMATIC VICTIMS' FAMILY CARE

Assessment

During the immediate aftermath of a traumatic event, the family must simultaneously deal with a variety of stressors. Family members must contend with the uncertainty of the traumatic injury, the unknown health care environment and personnel, the sudden injection of violence into their family, and extensive questioning from local and state law enforcement. Complications associated with a family member being shot, stabbed, or otherwise wounded during a violent crime can have long-ranging traumatic effects on the relatives of these victims and interfere with their ability to understand and cope with the experience.

PTSD is not exclusive to victims who are affected by violence. Contemporary research indicates that exposure to violence includes but is not limited to violent victimization. Witnessing a violent crime and having knowledge of a violent crime in the family or community are also considered precursors to posttraumatic illness (Brady et al, 2008). Posttraumatic symptoms have been noted to be more common among preadolescent and adolescent age groups than among school-aged children (Stein et al, 2003). In addition to demonstrating symptoms of PTSD, these adolescents may also exhibit dysfunctional behavior at school, and violent and antisocial behavior (Brady et al, 2008). Furthermore, young people who live in poor urban neighborhoods are more likely to be exposed to multiple incidents of violence during their adolescence, which can create severe social dysfunction (Brady et al, 2008). In addition, research has provided evidence that continuous exposure to violence is strongly linked to major depression and anxiety disorders, particularly among women (Clark et al, 2007) (see Chapters 10, 12, and 23).

Adult response to community violence exposure in urban neighborhoods has rarely been examined in the professional literature. However, it has been noted that adults are not exempt from posttrauma responses after exposure to violence. Clark and colleagues (2007) concluded in their study of urban women that exposure to community violence increased the possibility that women would experience depression and anxiety symptoms. At an inner city mental health clinic, 83% of the African-American participants reported the experience of a traumatic event, and 44% demonstrated posttraumatic symptoms (Schwartz et al, 2005). In addition, the presence of PTSD—particularly among those who have been exposed to violent crimes—demonstrates a heightened risk for negative health outcomes (Feldman-Hertz et al, 2005). For example, cardiac disease, intestinal problems, and chronic pain are common disorders found in patients with PTSD.

NURSING DIAGNOSIS

The nursing diagnoses that are commonly applied to family members of weapon-related trauma victims are always applied on the basis of observations of and communication with the family during the initial period after arrival to the emergency department. These diagnoses include the following:

- Interrupted family processes related to the traumatic injury of a family member
- Disabled family coping related to the sudden and violent nature of the injury to a family member
- Caregiver role strain related to the complex nature of recovery from a traumatic injury
- Homicide

Intervention

It is apparent that major injury to a person affects more than the person who is injured when a caring family is involved. Families often suffer deep emotional trauma when a loved one is involved in this type of crime. The mini care plan in Box 24-5 provides a synopsis for addressing family responses to their family member's injury as well as a list of staff interventions with rationales.

Posttraumatic Stress Disorder and Homicide Survivors

There is little empiric research regarding the presence of PTSD among the family members of victims who survived

BOX 24-5	MINI CARE PLAN FOR THE FAMILY OF A VIOLENT CRIME VICTIM	
FAMILY RESPONSE	**INTERVENTIONS**	**RATIONALES**
Shock	Provide a comfortable and private place for family members.	Allows the family to have privacy to adjust to what is happening
	Establish rapport with the family members by introducing yourself and explaining your role.	Provides the family with a contact person for questions that arise
	Assess the mental statuses of the family members.	Ensures that the family is alert, oriented, and able to understand the information provided
Fear	Offer comfort measures as needed or as requested by the family.	Decreases the fear response
	Ensure that the patient and the family are safe from further harm.	Helps the family to feel protected
Denial	Determine what the family members know about what has happened.	Ensures that the family is able to grasp what has happened and what is happening
	Allow the family to have access to the other members of the clinical team as soon as possible.	Helps with the situation becoming more of a reality
Suspiciousness	Convey factual information about the condition of the patient in layman's terms.	Tells the family that you are not hiding facts from them
	Detail the specific plan of care that is being given to the patient.	Conveys a sense of trust
	Provide accurate timelines with regard to when the family members are able to see the patient.	Conveys honesty to the family
Anger	Allow for the safe ventilation of family members' feelings.	Provides a sense of relief for the family

shootings and stabbings. According to Feldman-Hertz and colleagues (2005), the term homicide survivor applies the immediate family and friends of deceased victims of violence. Contemporary research indicates that homicide survivors are prone to psychologic distress and posttrauma symptoms beyond those that grief and bereavement models assert should be present (Murphy et al, 1999; Thompson et al, 1998). In a study of distress levels of family members of homicide victims, Thompson and colleagues found that participants experienced high levels of psychologic distress as a direct result of the homicide. Confounding the emotional effects of homicide on the family is the presence of external stressors, such as the closeness of the relationship with the victim, financial strain, and role changes within the family structure.

Survivor studies have also been conducted with parent participants to determine the presence of gender differences and PTSD. Murphy and colleagues' study revealed that 60% of mothers of homicide victims and 40% of fathers met the *Diagnostic and Statistical Manual for Mental Disorders*, fourth edition, text revision, criteria for PTSD. In terms of gender differences, fathers were more likely than mothers to report poor health and nonproductivity. Alternatively, mothers were more than two times as likely to consume alcohol regularly. Murphy and colleagues (2002) found in their study of parental coping that mothers preferred to use emotion-focused coping, whereas fathers preferred coping mechanisms that focused on restraint, acceptance, and suppression (Box 24-6).

BOX 24-6	FACTS: PARENTS OF HOMICIDE VICTIMS

- Mothers are more likely than fathers to suffer from PTSD-like symptoms.
- Mothers are more likely than fathers to use alcohol.
- Fathers are more likely than mothers to suppress their feelings about the homicide.

Nursing diagnoses that are often associated with PTSD and homicide are as follows:
- Risk for complicated grieving related to the sudden death of a family member
- Potential for posttrauma response related to exposure to violence within the family

Once again, the family members are clearly victims of an event of this magnitude.

Forensic Psychiatric Nurses

The forensic psychiatric nurse can testify about mental disorders and state-of-mind issues. They provide care to the mentally disordered in secure settings, and refine the care of cases that involve self-injurious behavior and increased risk of victimization (Mason and Mercer, 1996). Forensic nurses with established areas of expertise as a result of practice or research may testify as expert witnesses. Nurses can also testify regarding nursing diagnoses used in the care and treatment of patients (Shindul-Rothschild and Burgess, 2007). A bill passed in the Massachusetts legislature in 2002 included clinical nurse specialists among the recognized specialists that the courts may use when they require a mental health assessment for patients who need the court to appoint a guardian or a conservator. This legislation is especially useful for nurses and clinical nurse specialists who work with the mentally ill and older adults. The legislation recommended that the law be covered in nursing course curricula.

Death Investigators and Nurse Coroners

Forensic nurses also work as death investigators. O'Brien wrote that death is another point on the continuum of nursing care: "Situations exist all around us, both in the hospital setting and the community at large, with forensic implications relevant to the living and the dead. Death, all too often, is the outcome of reckless human behavior or tragic unintentional circumstances. Nurses, in all professional practice segments, must be educated and astute to acts with criminal or civil forensic implications" (2003, p. 1). O'Brien emphasized the importance of having nurse death investigators with special training to handle natural death cases, which are not law enforcement's focus; as many as 70% of the cases referred to the medical examiner's office are a result of natural causes.

The American Board of Medicolegal Death Investigators offers standardized certification for death investigators. This training includes 30 hours of classroom content and a skills check by a preceptor who is a medical examiner or a registered death investigator. Passing a 4-hour registry examination and 4000 hours of hands-on experience working with the medical examiner's office are required for certification.

Forensic Correctional Nurse

Forensic correctional nurses provide care to inmates of correctional facilities such as prisons, juvenile homes, jails, and penitentiaries. The American Nurses Association's Corrections Nursing: Scope and Standards of Practice was revised in 2006 and states that "[m]atters of nursing judgment are solely the domain of the registered nurse." A major emphasis of this work is primary health care. These services include intake screenings and evaluations, health screenings, direct patient care, the assessment and evaluation of an individual's health behavior, teaching, counseling, and helping inmates to assume responsibility for their own health. The nurse also may identify and provide community linkages for inmates after discharge.

The specialty of correctional nursing has been visible for more than 30 years. Although its early days are not well chronicled, it appears to have emerged largely in response to the forces that propelled correctional health care in general, such as the 1976 U.S. Supreme Court ruling in *Estelle v. Gamble.*

Before the 1970s, much inmate health care was provided by other inmates, correctional officers, and the occasional physician. The first documentation of correctional nursing may be a 1975 article by Rena Murtha, a director of nursing

for a large correctional system. In her account, nurses were "a tool of the warden, a slave of the physician and an unknown to the patient" (Muse, 2009).

Correctional nursing has experienced considerable growth during the past 30 years. The complex health needs of patients who are entering correctional systems require nurses with specialized knowledge and skills. Correctional nurses play a critical role in ensuring inmates' access to care and in health care delivery. It is the nurse with whom the inmate interacts most frequently and with whom the officer consults when an inmate has a health problem.

As in most health care settings, correctional nurses are the primary clinical providers of care. Registered nurses are necessary to lead care delivery and to direct the licensed nurses who work under their guidance. Correctional nurses must be clinically competent and well grounded in nursing practice. They must possess excellent skills in the areas of assessment and critical thinking. Their judgment is critical to the inmates' access to care (Muse, 2009).

Clinical Practice in Correctional Settings

Statistics. According to the Bureau of Justice Statistics (2009), there were approximately 1 million violent offenders between the ages of 18 and 39 years who were incarcerated at the end of 2008. The U.S. prison system reportedly spends in excess of $68 billion each year to house, clothe, and feed all of its incarcerated individuals. More than 250,000 incarcerated offenders are believed to have been diagnosed with major mental illnesses, which are largely untreated in the prison setting. A major reason for this is the funding restrictions of prison treatment and rehabilitative programs. The increased structure of the prison environment and the restriction of activity may exacerbate offenders' mental health symptoms (e.g., violent behavior, psychosis, self-destructive behavior, suicidal ideation) during their incarceration. Without proper treatment and intervention, these offenders are at higher risk for violence recidivism, which is the criminal behavior of an offender after being released from incarceration. The Bureau of Justice Statistics (2009) reports that 67.5% of paroled offenders will be criminal recidivists within 3 years of their release, either repeating their original offense or committing a more severe offense.

In addition to major mental illnesses, a common issue that is seen in prison and offender populations is substance addiction. According to the National Center on Addiction and Substance Abuse at Columbia University (1998), 80% of inmates have a significant history of substance abuse or addiction. Substance abuse and addiction—particularly involving alcohol—are strongly correlated with the commission of violent crime in the United States. Without proper treatment, it is expected that inmates with substance abuse issues are also at higher risk for violence recidivism.

A lack of proper attention being paid to the issues that are presented by these incarcerated offenders poses substantial challenges to urgent care centers and emergency departments. Inmates are often released from prison without access to basic needs such as housing, finances, and health care.

Consequentially, they present to community centers and emergency departments with acute psychiatric symptoms or substance-related intoxication. Unfortunately, emergency departments and urgent care centers are only able to provide short-term treatment solutions that involve little to no follow up with these patients. An added stress to these visits is the assessment and management of risk factors that pertain to violent actions, which is also known as *forensic risk*. The term forensic risk is defined as the potentiality that a forensic patient is dangerous and likely to perpetrate some form of violence on another person. Failure to address these issues of risk in these health care settings is a public health danger that can adversely affect the community.

Forensic Risk

To address issues related to a person's prospective dangerousness or risk for future violence, judicial branches of government have delegated the bulk of this responsibility to the forensic mental health community (Borum, 1996). Forensic mental health professionals are often called upon by the court system to evaluate violent offenders for the presence of acute mental illness, competency, and risk for public danger. However, this system is not without its problems. This approach has been widely criticized for being unstructured and totally reliant on subjective clinical judgment (Doyle and Dolan, 2002). As a result, professional literature in this area has now begun to investigate the adequacies of risk-assessment strategies conducted within the forensic health care setting. Unfortunately, research contributions have had little impact on health care standards, legislation, and public health policy with regard to the assessment and prevention of violence (Borum, 1996).

As the professional discipline of forensic psychiatric nursing continues to contribute to the body of knowledge related to forensic risk, it is persistently challenged to develop methods to address the complex issues of risk assessment and management as well as the associated constructs of dangerousness and recidivism in the practice environment. Risk assessment and management are central aspects of forensic nursing practice, and they serve as the basis for all clinical decision making throughout the therapeutic process; they are designed to limit and control the incidence of violence (Doyle and Dolan, 2002) (Box 24-7). Forensic psychiatric nurses are called upon to engage and participate in multidisciplinary exercises to empirically validate the concept of risk. This will not only contribute to the growing body of forensic nursing knowledge, but it will also allow the discipline to have the capacity to develop effective interventions that pertain to risk in the clinical and community settings.

A central aspect of nursing in forensic psychiatric practice is the assessment and management of the risk of violence; for more information, see the Research for Evidence-Based Practice box. Nurses are in the unique position of having frontline access to patients for monitoring and observation. Nursing interventions involve critical-thinking skills, and they are focused on determining the risk of violence in the clinical environment. Identifying precursors for violence such

BOX 24-7	INTERVENTIONS FOR THE MANAGEMENT OF FORENSIC RISK
SYMPTOMS	**INTERVENTIONS**
Irritability and agitation	Mood-stabilizing medications
	Mood journaling
	Anger-management tools
	Assisting the patient with identifying precipitants of mood changes
Psychosocial stress responses	Identifying specific sources of stress
	Identifying potential plans to manage each stressor
	Conflict-resolution skill building
	Identifying community resources that will be able to assist the patient
Behavior or attitude changes	Monitoring behavior
	Regular mental status examinations
	De-escalation techniques

as agitation and irritability, new or existing psychosocial stressors, and changes in attitude or behavior are key aspects that affect the prediction and management of violence (Doyle and Dolan, 2002). Valuable interventions such as individualized care planning, rapport building, conflict-resolution skills, self-awareness, and knowledge of the disease processes and de-escalation techniques are essential to the appropriate management of violence (Spokes et al, 2002). The use of information obtained with the use of ongoing nursing assessments and intervention planning by interdisciplinary team members will only contribute to enhancing the caring experience for the violent offender and to identifying new themes for research.

RESEARCH FOR EVIDENCE-BASED PRACTICE #2

Cloyes KG et al: Time to prison return for offenders with serious mental illness released from prison, a survival analysis, *Crim Justice Behav* 37(2):175-187, 2010.

This empiric study compared two groups: offenders with a serious mental illness and "healthy" offenders. Findings indicate that 23% of the offender population released from prison between the years of 1998 and 2002 met the criteria for severe mental illness. Of the psychiatric diagnoses that were involved, major depression was the most common, followed by bipolar illness I and II. Results of the study revealed that offenders with serious mental illness were more likely to return to prison earlier than "healthy" offenders. Higher reincarceration rates among mentally ill prisoners demonstrates the importance of psychiatric screening and treatment programs throughout the prison system.

During the past decade, forensic nursing has progressed to include all aspects of crime-related health care, including the biopsychosocial complications of exposure to violence, the risk-factor assessment of both victims and perpetrators, and the identification of community violence-prevention strategies. The practice of forensic nursing shares a common professional purpose with other forensic disciplines: to offer expert knowledge as part of the holistic care of victims and perpetrators as they navigate through the justice system. Basic to the success of forensic nursing is interdisciplinary collaboration with medical staff and law-enforcement officials as a pathway to providing comprehensive interventions and the proper management of evidence in the treatment setting.

CHAPTER SUMMARY

- Forensic nursing has emerged as a clinical specialty within the past 20 years.
- Nurses assume many responsibilities within the forensic health care delivery system as they incorporate nursing expertise into the care and protection of people who are affected by crime.
- The passage of the Violence Against Women Act fostered the development of programs that would directly address crimes against women.
- The National Victim Center, which was established in 1985, focuses its attention on community programming and women's treatment centers.
- Rape and sexual assault continue to be considerable public health issues in the United States.
- Sexual assault victims are at high risk for psychosocial complications such as anxiety, panic, and grief.

- Violent crime victims require a multitude of health care services that involve both physiologic and psychologic interventions.
- PTSD is considered to be quite prevalent among victims of weapon-related trauma and their families.
- Prisoners are commonly diagnosed with mental illness and substance addiction, which require intervention and treatment in the prison setting.
- Forensic risk assessment and management are primary functions of forensic psychiatric nurses in prisons, community programs, and hospital settings.
- Adequately addressing risk in the prison population will assist with decreasing criminal recidivism and preventing violence.

REVIEW QUESTIONS

1. The highest percentage of visible injuries related to sexual assault is found in the genital area as compared with other areas of the body.
   1. True
   2. False
2. Which of the following is the most common point of injury seen with weapon-related assault?
   1. The spinal cord
   2. The abdomen
   3. The neck
   4. The chest
3. A family in the emergency department has just been told that their family member has been killed as a result of a fatal gunshot wound. Several of the family members begin yelling until it escalates into physical fighting. Which of the following is an appropriate nursing diagnosis in this situation?
   1. Risk for posttrauma syndrome.
   2. Disabled family coping

3. Risk for complicated grieving
4. Caregiver role strain
4. A primary nurse who is responsible for caring for a prisoner who has a history of violence should pay special attention to all except which one of the following symptoms?
   1. Anger
   2. Anxiety
   3. Agitation
   4. Anhedonia
5. Fathers of homicide victims are more likely to experience PTSD than mothers of homicide victims.
   1. True
   2. False

REFERENCES

American Nurses Association: *Scope and standards of forensic nursing*, Washington, DC, 2009, American Nurses Association.

Barton S: Investigating forensic nursing, *Kansas Nurse* 70(6):3-4, 1995.

Borum R: Improving the clinical practice of violence risk assessment technology: guidelines and training, *Am Psychol* 51(9):956-968, 1996.

Brady SS et al: Adaptive coping reduces the impact of community violence exposure on violent behavior among African American and Latino male adolescents, *J Abnorm Child Psychol* 36:105-115, 2008.

Burgess AW et al: Forensic nursing: investigating the career potential in this emerging specialty, *Am J Nursing* 104(3):58-64, 2004.

Clark C et al: Witnessing community violence in residential neighborhoods: a mental hazard for urban women, *J Urban Health* 85(1):22-38, 2007.

Cunningham R et al: Before and after the trauma bay: the prevention of violent injury among youth, *Ann Emerg Med* 53(4):490-500, 2009.

Discala C, Sege R: Outcomes in children and young adults who are hospitalized for firearm related injuries, *Pediatrics* 113(5):1306-1312, 2004.

Doyle M, Dolan M: Violence risk assessment: combining actuarial and clinical information to structure clinical judgments for the formulation and management of risk, *J Psychiatric Mental Health Nursing* 9:649-657, 2002.

Feldman-Hertz M et al: Homicide survivors: research and practice implications, *Am J Prev Med* 29(5 Suppl 2):288-295, 2005.

Goll-McGee B: The role of the clinical forensic nurse in critial care, *Crit Nurs Q* 22(1), 1999.

Greenspan AI, Kellerman AL: Physical and psychological outcomes 8 months after serious gunshot injury, *J Trauma Injury Infect Crit Care* 53(4):709-716, 2002.

Hanrahan NP et al: Core data elements tracking elder sexual abuse, *Clin Geriatr Med* 21:413-427, 2005.

Hume C, Salmon J, Ball K: Associations of children's perceived neighborhood environments with walking and physical activity, *Am J Health Promot* 21:201-207, 2007.

Kroll T: Rehabilitative needs of individuals with spinal cord injury resulting from gun violence: the perspective of nursing and rehabilitation professionals, *Appl Nurs Res* 21:45-49, 2008.

Lawson L: The state of forensic nursing science, *Journal of Forensic Nursing* 1(1):5, 2005.

Lynch V: Forensic nursing defending human rights, *Journal of Clinical Forensic Medicine* 1(3):166-170, 2009.

Malestic S: Fight violence with forensic evidence, *RN* 58(1):30-32, 1995.

Mason T, Mercer D: Forensic psychiatric nursing: vision of social control, *Aust N Z J Ment Health Nurs* 5:153-162, 1996.

McKinley WO et al: Clinical presentations, medical complications, and functional outcomes of individuals with gunshot wound induced spinal cord injury, *Am J Phys Med Rehabil* 78(2):102-107, 1999.

Mohta M et al: Psychological care in trauma patients, *Injury* 34:17-25, 2003.

Murphy SA et al: PTSD among bereaved parents following the violent deaths of their 12-28 year old children: a longitudinal prospective analysis, *J Trauma Stress* 12(2):273-291, 1999.

Nelson J, Brewster A, Hymel K et al: Victim, perpetrator, family, and incident characteristics of 32 infant maltreatment deaths in the United States, *Child Abuse and Neglect* 22(2):91-101, 1998.

Redley B et al: Accompanying critically ill relatives in emergency departments, *J Adv Nurs* 44(1):88-98, 2003.

Rich JA, Grey CM: Pathways to recurrent trauma among young black men: traumatic stress, substance use and the "code of the street," *Am J Public Health* 95(5):816-824, 2005.

Schwartz AC et al: Posttraumatic stress disorder among African Americans in an inner city mental health clinic, *Psychiatr Serv* 56(2):212-215, 2005.

Shindul-Rothschild J, Burgess A: (Chapter 10) Psychiatric nursing. In Dattilip FM, Sadoff NL, editors: *What Jurists and Attorneys Need to Know About Qualifying Mental Health Professionals*, 146-156, Mechanicsburg, PA, 2007, Pennsylvania Bar.

Speck P, Peters S: Forensics in NP practice, *Advanced Nursing Practice* 7(11):18, 1999.

Spokes K et al: HOVIS-The Hertfordshire/Oxfordshire violent incident study, *J Psychiatr Ment Health Nurs* 9:199-209, 2002.

Stein BD et al: Prevalence of child and adolescent exposure to community violence, *Clin Child Fam Psychol Rev* 6(4):247-264, 2003.

Thompson MP et al: Comparative distress levels of inner city family members of homicide victims, *J Trauma Stress* 11(2):228-242, 1998.

Tolbert-Washington G: Family advocates: caring for families in crisis, *Dimensions of Critical Care Nursing* 20(1):36-40, 2001.

Wick J: Forensic nursing, *AORN Journal* 58(1):585, 2004.

Psychopharmacology

Pauline Chan

"The discovery of psychoactive drugs made an enormous difference to clinical practice."

Leon Eisenberg

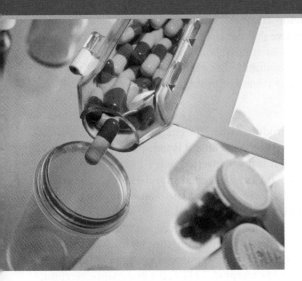

evolve WEBSITE

http://evolve.elsevier.com/Fortinash/

OBJECTIVES

- Describe and discuss the patient considerations and nursing responsibilities related to antipsychotic medication therapy.
- Describe and discuss the patient considerations and nursing responsibilities related to antidepressant medication therapy.
- Describe and discuss the patient considerations and nursing responsibilities related to mood stabilization therapy.

- Describe and discuss the patient considerations and nursing responsibilities related to anxiolytic and hypnotic medication therapy.
- Describe and discuss the patient considerations and nursing responsibilities related to stimulant medication therapy.

KEY TERMS

agranulocytosis
akathisia
atypical antipsychotics
conventional antipsychotics
extrapyramidal side effects

hypertensive crisis
metabolite
neuroleptic malignant
    syndrome
neuroleptics

photosensitivity
psychotropic
rapid cycling
refractory
serotonin syndrome

serum level monitoring
side effects
sustained release
tardive dyskinesia
titration

The National Institute of Mental Health estimates that 26.2% of Americans 18 years old and older—more than 1 in 4 adults—suffer from a diagnosable mental disorder during any given year. According to Substance Abuse and Mental Health Services Administration, about half (46.6%) of all Americans will have a mental illness during their lifetimes, and, for most, the symptoms will manifest during the teen years. About 20% of Americans will experience mood disorders, and 28.8% will experience anxiety disorders. Nearly a quarter (24.8%) will experience an impulse control disorder, and 14.6% will experience a substance abuse disorder.

Until the discovery of chlorpromazine (Thorazine) and other psychoactive medications, patients with mental illness

had few options and often were left untreated. Edward Shorter (1998), in his book *History of Psychiatry,* summarized the discovery of chlorpromazine for psychiatry as being as important as the discovery of penicillin for general medicine. The significant discovery that chlorpromazine reduces agitation, hallucinations, and psychotic symptoms marked the beginning of the era of psychopharmacology. During the years after this discovery, researchers developed additional antipsychotic medications. Initially, these included more phenothiazines, as represented by chlorpromazine, and then other structurally different chemical compounds such as the butyrophenone class, as represented by haloperidol (Haldol). During the 1960s, researchers studied these drugs to establish clinical efficacy with the use of the double-blind, placebo-controlled study method, which greatly increased the knowledge of the mechanisms of action of these drugs. The studies also provided evidence that the various antipsychotic drugs are also effective, although their potency varies. New medications continually emerge as a result of ongoing research in an effort to alleviate debilitating psychiatric symptoms and also to reduce many of the adverse side effects that occur with the use of psychopharmacotherapy.

MODE AND MECHANISM OF DRUG ACTION

The *mode of action* of a drug describes what the drug does to the body; the *mechanism of action* describes how the drug works to affect the symptoms, cure the disease, or cause side effects.

Neurotransmitters

To understand the modes of action of psychotropic medications, it is important to understand the neurotransmitter systems in the brain that are affected during psychopharmacotherapy (Kramer, 2002). The classic neurotransmitters include the following: acetylcholine, histamine, serotonin, dopamine, norepinephrine, epinephrine, aspartic acid, γ-aminobutyric acid, glutamic acid, glycine, homocysteine, and taurine. A thorough discussion of the brain's neurotransmitter systems appears in Chapter 6.

The four neurotransmitters that are the most important for the study of psychotropic medications are as follows:
1. Acetylcholine
2. Dopamine
3. Serotonin (also called *5-hydroxytryptamine* or *5-HT*)
4. Glutamate (glutamic acid)

Acetylcholine

Numerous receptors for acetylcholine exist, and the major subdivisions are the nicotinic and muscarinic cholinergic receptors. There are numerous muscarinic receptors; the M1 postsynaptic receptor is the most important because of its mediating effect in the memory function, which is linked to cholinergic neurotransmission. It is also related to the side effects of anticholinergic drugs, such as dry mouth, blurred vision, urinary retention, and constipation. Dopamine and acetylcholine have a reciprocal relationship. Dopamine suppresses cholinergic activities in the nigrostriatal dopamine pathway.

Dopamine

Dopamine is produced in dopaminergic neurons from the precursor tyrosine. Receptors for dopamine regulate dopaminergic neurotransmission. There are four dopamine receptor pathways in the brain:
1. The nigrostriatal dopamine pathway controls movements.
2. The mesolimbic dopamine pathway is involved in such things as pleasurable sensations, the euphoria that results from drugs of abuse, and delusions and hallucinations that result from psychosis.

3. The mesocortical dopamine pathway mediates positive and negative psychotic symptoms as well as the cognitive side effects of antipsychotic medications.
4. The tuberoinfundibular (endocrine) dopamine pathway controls the release of prolactin.

Serotonin

Serotonin is produced when the enzyme tryptophan hydroxylase converts tryptophan after it is transported into the serotonin neuron. It is first converted into 5-hydroxytryptophan, and it is then further converted into 5-HT by the enzyme aromatic amino acid decarboxylase. Serotonin is an inhibitory catecholamine that is stored in the vesicles until it is released by neuronal impulses. The enzyme monoamine oxidase type A destroys serotonin, thereby forming an inactive metabolite. There are numerous subtypes of serotonin receptors. The key receptor, $5-HT_{1D}$, is a presynaptic receptor, and other key postsynaptic receptors are $5-HT_{1A}$, $5-HT_{2A}$, $5-HT_3$, and $5-HT_4$. At least five serotonin pathways exist in the central nervous system (CNS). Serotonin mediates cognitive effects, emotions, panic, memory, anxiety, violence, aggression, sexual function, and sleep–wake cycles through the various pathways. Serotonin also interacts with many dopamine pathways, and it has the ability to inhibit dopamine release.

Glutamate

Glutamate or glutamic acid is an amino acid that is synthesized in the brain and that functions as a major excitatory neurotransmitter. Glutamate has been identified in an increasing number of neurologic and psychologic disorders. The psychoactive drug phencyclidine has the ability to block the N-methyl-D-aspartate receptor channel. Because glutamate is the neurotransmitter of the cortical and hippocampal pyramidal neurons, researchers hypothesize that the effects of phencyclidine reflect interference with glutamatergic neurotransmission in these brain regions.

PSYCHOTROPIC PHARMACOTHERAPY ASSESSMENT

Before starting pharmacotherapy treatment, a thorough assessment of the patient is necessary. Many drugs cause psychiatric symptoms ("Drugs That May Cause Psychiatric Symptoms," 2002), and it is important to evaluate the patient carefully. Treatment focuses on the stabilization of the illness with the goal of achieving *remission*, which is defined as a complete return to the baseline level of functioning and the absence of symptoms. After remission, the patient enters the *maintenance phase*, during which the goal is to optimize protection against the recurrence of illness. Equally important is the consideration of treatment that maximizes patient functioning and that minimizes subthreshold symptoms and the adverse effects of treatment with medications.

More recently, the term *recovery* has been used. Recovery does not mean total remission; rather, it emphasizes the individual's growth and achievement despite living with a mental

---

BOX 25-1 **VARIABLES THAT AFFECT DRUG THERAPY**

Drug-Related Variables
- Mode and mechanism of action
- Available dosage form: oral (solid, liquid, or sublingual) or parenteral
- Bioavailability of various formulations
- Onset, peak, and duration of action
- Serum half-life
- Method of elimination from the body (hepatic or renal)
- Side effects and toxicities (both predictable and idiosyncratic)
- Cost (drug price, administration, and monitoring costs)

Patient-Related Variables
- Diagnosis
- Other disease states (e.g., cardiovascular, liver, or renal disease)
- Other medications
- Age and weight
- Previous responses and history of side effects, in both the patient and his or her family
- Willingness and ability to comply
- Insight into his or her illness
- Financial issues and health insurance
- Support systems

BOX 25-2 **SYMPTOMS OF PSYCHOSIS**

Positive Symptoms
- Delusions
- Hallucinations
- Disorganized speech
- Disorganized behavior
- Catatonia
- Agitation

Negative Symptoms
- Blunted affect
- Passiveness
- Social apathy and withdrawal
- Alogia (inability to speak)
- Avolition (inability to decide)
- Anhedonia (lack of pleasure)
- Lack of attention or spontaneity

Cognitive Function Impairment
- Thought disorder
- Incoherence
- Loose association
- Difficulty with processing information

Aggressive and Hostile Symptoms
- Verbal abuse
- Assault
- Sexual acting out
- Poor impulse control

Depressive and Anxious Symptoms
- Worry
- Guilt
- Anxiety
- Irritability
- Depression

---

illness. Recovery focuses on the improvement of the patient's quality of life and self-actualization.

Variables That Affect Drug Therapy

When assessing patients before or during pharmacotherapy, it is necessary to incorporate information that addresses both drug- and patient-related variables before the initiation of therapy. Box 25-1 describes common drug- and patient-related variables.

PSYCHOSIS

In the past, the medical community thought psychosis was caused by the overactivity of dopamine neurons; this was referred to as the *dopamine hypothesis of psychosis*. Psychosis is traditionally described as having positive and negative symptoms, but research has concluded that this not an adequate description. Instead, researchers now describe psychosis with five symptom dimensions: (1) positive symptoms; (2) negative symptoms; (3) cognitive symptoms; (4) aggressive/hostile symptoms; and (5) anxious/depressed symptoms (Box 25-2).

Many think that positive symptoms occur as a result of the overactivity of the dopamine neurons in the mesolimbic dopamine pathway (increased brain activity) and that negative symptoms occur as a result of cortical dopamine deficiency in the mesocortical pathway of the brain (decreased brain activity). Antipsychotic medications are prescribed for the treatment of psychosis.

Antipsychotic Medications

Antipsychotic medications, which were previously known as *major tranquilizers* or *neuroleptics*, have been the mainstay of treatment for schizophrenia and other psychotic disorders since the introduction of chlorpromazine in 1952. These medications are effective, and they were directly and indirectly responsible for the deinstitutionalization of patients diagnosed with schizophrenia during the 1950s and 1960s. Antipsychotic medications are generally divided into two broad categories: the conventional or typical antipsychotics and the atypical or unconventional antipsychotics. The conventional antipsychotics are similar with regard to mode of action and efficacy, but they differ with regard to side effects and potency. These medications block D_2 receptors in the limbic region of the brain. The atypical antipsychotics, which are also referred to as *second-generation medications*, differ with regard to mode of action, side effects, and potency. As compared with conventional antipsychotics, the atypical antipsychotic agents generally have a lower potential for extrapyramidal effects and possibly no greater efficacy for the treatment of negative symptoms and cognitive symptoms.

TABLE 25-1   ANTIPSYCHOTIC MEDICATIONS

GENERIC NAME (TRADE NAME)	POTENCY	RECOMMENDED DOSAGE RANGE (mg/day UNLESS OTHERWISE NOTED)*	CHLORPROMAZINE EQUIVALENTS (mg/day)†
First-Generation Antipsychotics			
Phenothiazines			
Chlorpromazine (Thorazine)	Low	300–1000	100
Fluphenazine (Prolixin)	Very high	5–20	2
Fluphenazine decanoate (Prolixin Decanoate)	Very high	6.25–75 mg/3 weeks	—
Perphenazine (Trilafon)	High	16–64	10
Thioridazine (Mellaril)	Low	300–800	100
Trifluoperazine (Stelazine)	High	15–50	5
Butyrophenones			
Haloperidol (Haldol)	Very high	5–20	2
Haloperidol decanoate (Haldol Decanoate)	Very high	100–450 mg/month	—
Others			
Loxapine (Loxitane)	High	30–100	10
Molindone (Moban)	High	30–100	10
Thiothixene (Navane)	High	15–50	5
Second-Generation Antipsychotics			
Aripiprazole (Abilify)	—	10–30	—
Clozapine (Clozaril)	—	150–600	—
Olanzapine (Zyprexa)	—	10–30	—
Quetiapine (Seroquel)	—	300–800	—
Risperidone (Risperdal)	—	2–8	—
Ziprasidone (Geodon)	—	120–200	—

*Dosage range recommendations are adapted from the 2003 Schizophrenia Patient Outcome Research Team Recommendations.
†Chlorpromazine equivalents represent the approximate equivalent to 100 mg of chlorpromazine (relative potency); this applies to first-generation antipsychotics only.

Clozapine is the only atypical antipsychotic that has shown evidence of greater efficacy as compared with older typical antipsychotics for the treatment of refractory (treatment-resistant) illness.

Indications

Antipsychotics are used for the treatment of psychosis (American Psychiatric Association, 2010), which includes a wide spectrum of illnesses such as schizophrenia, schizoaffective disorders, and delusional disorders. Atypical antipsychotics are used as adjunctive or monotherapy for bipolar disorders (Schatzberg and Nemeroff, 2001). Patients with psychosis that results from secondary causes (e.g., electrolyte or hormonal imbalances, drug abuse, brain tumors, mania, depression with psychotic features) also benefit from treatment with short-term antipsychotic medications while the underlying illness is being treated. Table 25-1 lists the various types of antipsychotic medications and their dosages.

Goals of Therapy

Frequent assessment with the clear documentation of behavioral changes is needed, and patients are taught how to recognize signs and symptoms as well as side effects. Patients are encouraged to follow through with the agreed-upon treatment plan on a long-term basis, with support from the care team. It is thought that the use of a shared decision-making process will more likely influence patients to achieve recovery.

Absorption, Distribution, Metabolism, and Excretion

Sometimes the presence of food, antacids, anticholinergics, and smoking influences the absorption of drugs. Cigarette smoking tends to activate hepatic enzymes, which causes the faster metabolization of drugs; thus, smokers sometimes require higher doses. The distribution of the drug depends on the route of administration, with intramuscular injections generally having greater bioavailability than oral preparations. Many drugs are metabolized in the liver and excreted through the kidneys.

Clinical Use and Efficacy

Although antipsychotics are important and effective medications, they have many side effects. A major principle for nurses and other health care providers is to use the lowest possible effective dose for the shortest amount of time.

Target symptom response varies with time. Positive symptoms are the most responsive, and symptoms such as combativeness, hostility, psychomotor agitation, and irritability are often relieved within hours. Affective symptoms, anxiety, tension, depression, inappropriate affect, reduced attention span, and social withdrawal often take 2 to 4 weeks to respond. Cognitive and perceptual symptoms such as hallucinations, delusions, and thought broadcasting usually take 2 to 8 weeks to respond. The most negative symptoms—poor social skills, unrealistic planning, are poor judgment and insight—are psychologic processes and require a longer time to improve. Given the varied time course of different symptoms, keep in mind that increases in the medication dose will not hasten the relief of slow-responding symptoms and may result in an unnecessarily high dose of treatment.

Antipsychotic therapy usually begins with divided doses three or four times a day. This regimen is useful for determining a patient's ability to tolerate a medication and to minimize the initial impact of side effects. After an effective total daily dose is established and the patient has had time to develop tolerance to side effects, the medication is often reduced to once or twice a day. The reduced frequency of administration increases the likelihood of compliance with the regimen.

Drug Level Monitoring. In general, the gastrointestinal (GI) tract absorbs antipsychotics well, and the liver extensively metabolizes them. The half-life of a medication varies widely among individuals, but it is usually between 20 and 40 hours in adults, with the drug reaching the steady state after 4 to 7 days. Serum level monitoring (i.e., obtaining blood samples to determine drug concentration) is not routinely useful. Serum level monitoring is useful in some specific situations, including when there is a lack of response to normal doses after 6 weeks, when there are severe or unusual adverse reactions, or when patients are physically ill, elderly, or young children. The side-effect profile and specific needs of each patient largely determine the choice and dosage of medication.

Treatment Therapy for Acute Episodes. Atypical antipsychotics such as olanzapine (Zyprexa) 10 to 20 mg daily, risperidone (Risperdal) 3 to 6 mg daily, quetiapine (Seroquel) 300 to 800 mg daily in divided doses, ziprasidone (Geodon) 120 to 180 mg daily, and aripiprazole (Abilify) 10 to 30 mg daily are currently first-line treatments for acute episodes. Clozapine (Clozaril) is not a first-line treatment; it is usually reserved for refractory illness because of its risk for the serious adverse effect of agranulocytosis.

Adverse Effects of Antipsychotics: Nursing Management

Adverse effects of antipsychotics medications can be troublesome, or even painful or dangerous for patients. Nurses are continually watchful for their occurrence and intervene immediately when necessary. The conventional antipsychotics block the D_2 receptors and the extrapyramidal motor system. Therefore, although they are effective for the treatment of psychosis, these medications also induce undesirable extrapyramidal side effects (EPS) (movement disorders). In addition, antipsychotics also block noradrenergic, cholinergic, and histamine receptors to varying degrees, thereby

---

BOX 25-3 SIDE EFFECTS ASSOCIATED WITH RECEPTOR BLOCKADE

Dopamine$_2$
- Extrapyramidal side effects
- Prolactin

Histamine$_1$
- Sedation
- Weight gain

Cholinergic
- Dry mouth
- Blurred vision
- Sinus tachycardia
- Constipation
- Impaired memory and cognition

Alpha$_1$
- Orthostatic hypotension
- Reflex tachycardia

Serotonin$_2$
- Weight gain
- Gastrointestinal upset
- Sexual dysfunction

---

resulting in a unique side-effect profile for each drug. Box 25-3 lists the side effects associated with receptor blockade.

Extrapyramidal Side Effects. The use of high-potency conventional antipsychotic medications poses a higher risk for EPS. High-potency conventional antipsychotic medications include fluphenazine (Prolixin), perphenazine (Trilafon), trifluoperazine (Stelazine), and haloperidol (Haldol). Four symptoms of EPS are described next. Table 25-2 lists adjunctive medications that are used to treat EPS.

Dystonia. Dystonia reactions include spasms of the eye (oculogyric crisis), neck (torticollis), back (retrocollis), tongue (glossospasm), or other muscles, which are often frightening to the patient. Fortunately, these symptoms are readily reversed with the intramuscular injection of 50 mg of diphenhydramine (Benadryl) or of 1 or 2 mg of benztropine (Cogentin), followed by oral agents to prevent recurrence.

Dystonia reactions usually occur during the early stages of treatment, and they are common after the intramuscular injection of antipsychotics. They seldom occur after 3 months of treatment. Risk factors include the administration of high-potency agents, large doses, and parenteral injections.

Pseudoparkinsonism. Symptoms include decreased movements (bradykinesia, akinesia), muscle rigidity (cogwheel and lead pipe), resting hand tremor, drooling, masklike face, and shuffling gait. This side effect is often misdiagnosed, untreated, or unrecognized. Some patients have a behavioral form of akinesia, which is characterized by a lack of motivation, blunted affect, decreased speech, and apathy, thereby making it difficult to distinguish this symptom from negative symptoms of the illness that is being treated.

TABLE 25-2	ADJUNCTIVE MEDICATIONS USED TO TREAT EXTRAPYRAMIDAL SIDE EFFECTS			
GENERIC NAME (TRADE NAME)	**EQUIVALENT DOSE (mg)**	**DOSE RANGE (mg)**	**DOSAGE FORMS***
Anticholinergic			
Benztropine (Cogentin)	1	1–8	Injectable and capsule
Trihexyphenidyl (Artane)	2	2–15	Extended-release capsule and elixir
Antihistamine			
Diphenhydramine (Benadryl)	50	50–400	Capsules, liquid, and injectable
Dopamine Agonist			
Amantadine (Symmetrel)	n/a	100–400	Capsule and liquid only

*All of these medications are also available as tablets unless otherwise noted.

Physicians need to be on the alert for this symptom complex for proper diagnosis, and nurses are alert for the recognition of medication-related symptoms as compared with illness-generated symptoms.

Treatments include the reduction of the antipsychotic medication dose; a change to an antipsychotic medication with less potential for EPS; and the use of an oral antiparkinsonian agent such as benztropine (Cogentin), trihexyphenidyl (Artane), diphenhydramine (Benadryl), or amantadine (Symmetrel). EPS are not treated prophylactically.

Akathisia. Symptoms of akathisia include restlessness, pacing, rocking, and the inability to sit still. These symptoms are often dose related. Akathisia is sometimes confused with anxiety and agitation. To differentiate the diagnoses of akathisia and anxiety or agitation, careful observation of the patient is warranted. Akathisia improves with decreasing antipsychotic dose, whereas anxiety and agitation worsen. Akathisia is also difficult to control over a period of time, whereas anxiety and agitation are not. Propranolol (Inderal) with a daily divided dose of 30 to 90 mg is usually an effective treatment. It is advisable to monitor the patient's blood pressure when using this agent. A benzodiazepine such as lorazepam (Ativan) 1 mg orally or clonazepam 0.5 mg twice daily is often helpful.

Tardive Dyskinesia. Tardive dyskinesia manifests as the abnormal movement of any voluntary muscle group after a prolonged period of dopamine blockade. The most commonly affected muscles are those of the face, mouth, tongue, and digits, which results in grimacing, lip smacking, tongue poking, and writing movements of the fingers and toes. These movements are often severe and disabling. Risk factors include longer lengths of time of antipsychotic use and exposure, high doses, high-potency drugs, the use of conventional (typical) antipsychotics, and the patient being more than 50 years old. There is no effective treatment for tardive dyskinesia; however, the use of vitamin E has shown some benefit. Atypical antipsychotics have a much lower risk of causing tardive dyskinesia (less than 1% with risperidone and olanzapine), and clozapine carries no risk of causing tardive dyskinesia. Thus, to prevent tardive dyskinesia, conversion to atypical antipsychotics is a viable option and should be considered whenever possible. Note that clozapine carries the risk of producing agranulocytosis.

❖ **CLINICAL ALERT #1**

Tardive dyskinesia occurs as a result of the upregulation of dopamine receptors; in other words prolonged blockade results in an increase in the number of receptors. EPS, on the other hand, occurs as a result of the temporary blockade of these same receptors. Therefore, when tardive dyskinesia occurs, decreasing the dose temporarily worsens tardive dyskinesia but improves EPS; increasing the dose temporarily improves tardive dyskinesia but worsens EPS. A long-term solution is to decrease the dose and change to an atypical antipsychotic medication.

The recognition of tardive dyskinesia during its early stages is crucial. Patients need to be examined with the use of the Abnormal Involuntary Movement Scale or the Dyskinesia Identification System: Condensed User Scale. The Abnormal Involuntary Movement Scale should be performed no less than every 6 months while the patient is taking either typical or atypical antipsychotics.

Neuroleptic Malignant Syndrome. Neuroleptic malignant syndrome (NMS) is a medical emergency (Berkow, 1992). A patient with NMS has symptoms that include a decreased level of consciousness, greatly increased muscle tone (rigidity), and autonomic dysfunction (i.e., hyperpyrexia, labile hypertension, tachycardia, tachypnea, diaphoresis, and drooling). Muscle necrosis or rhabdomyolysis is sometimes so severe that it causes myoglobinuric renal failure as large amounts of myoglobin are released from the muscle tissue and excreted in the urine, thereby causing myoglobinuria.

NMS is potentially fatal, with a mortality rate of about 10%, and it occurs in approximately 1% of patients who are using antipsychotics. Major identified risk factors for the development of NMS include a history of NMS, the use of adjunctive and polypsychotropic medications, rapid dose titration, the use of high-potency antipsychotics at high doses, and the use of parenteral antipsychotics. Young male patients are more frequently affected. Most of the time NMS occurs during the early stages of treatment with antipsychotics, but it may at times occur even after years of treatment.

Laboratory findings are an important diagnostic aid with this diagnosis. Typically, laboratory abnormalities include leukocytosis (15,000 to 30,000 cells/mm^3), greatly elevated creatine phosphokinase levels (more than 3000 IU/mL), and myoglobinuria (Hermesh et al, 2002).

Initial treatment includes admission to an intensive care units as well as the following:

- Immediate discontinuation of all antipsychotic medications
- Hydration of the patient, including the intravenous infusion of fluids
- Administration of acetaminophen (Tylenol) along with cooling blankets for hyperthermia
- Consideration of an intravenous heparin infusion to reduce the risk of pulmonary emboli
- Management of arrhythmias
- Monitoring of renal function
- Intravenous infusion of dantrolene (Dantrium), a direct muscle relaxant, to reduce muscle rigidity and to treat hyperthermia that results from breakdown of muscle tissues. (The initial dose of dantrolene is 1 to 3 mg/kg daily by intravenous infusion. Dantrolene should be continued for a week after symptoms have resolved. An oral formulation can be used after the patient is discharged.)
- Consideration of use of dopaminergic drugs such as bromocriptine (Parlodel), amantadine, or anticholinergic drugs. (The initial dose of bromocriptine is 2.5 mg orally three times daily.)

Most patients recover from NMS. When the patient has recovered, it is advisable to wait for 1 to 2 weeks before restarting the antipsychotic medication. Carefully evaluate patients for the need for antipsychotics. Consider possible alternatives such as lithium, carbamazepine (Tegretol), and divalproex sodium (Depakote). If the practitioner determines that the patient should continue with an antipsychotic medication, another antipsychotic medication with a different chemical structure will be prescribed, and doses will be slowly titrated. Note any history of NMS in the patient's medical record. The patient should not receive depot antipsychotic drugs (i.e., haloperidol or fluphenazine) because of the long half-lives of these drugs.

Recently, patients with a history of NMS have been prescribed the atypical antipsychotics. It is important to note that NMS has also occurred with the use of any antipsychotic medication. The most important rule is careful monitoring for recurrence and relapse. Monitor patients for additional signs and symptoms, such as psychomotor excitement, refusal of food, anuria, and weight loss.

Drowsiness. Drowsiness is most common during the first days of treatment, and it usually disappears within 1 to 2 weeks. Sedation is particularly significant with the low-potency conventional antipsychotics such as chlorpromazine and thioridazine (Mellaril). Patients need to avoid alcohol, medications such as antihistamines (these are common in some cough and cold preparations), and sleeping aids. Some patients take the daily dose at bedtime instead of during the daytime to avoid interference with daily activities.

Anticholinergic Side Effects. The use of low-potency conventional antipsychotics such as chlorpromazine and thioridazine presents a greater risk of anticholinergic side effects. Tolerance sometimes develops over the first 4 to 8 weeks. Anticholinergic side effects are mostly annoying and usually not serious; they include dry mouth, blurred vision, constipation, urinary retention, nasal congestion, and ejaculatory inhibition. The following interventions are often useful suggestions for the patient:

- *For dry mouth*: Use ice chips, lemon swabs, and sugarless gums or candies.
- *For blurred vision*: Read in well-lighted areas for short periods, and vary the distance of the reading materials from your eyes.
- *For constipation*: Exercise regularly (this includes walking), drink plenty of fluids, eat plenty of fruits and vegetables, and use a stool softener such as docusate sodium (Colace).
- *For urinary retention*: Medical attention is often necessary. Oxybutynin (Ditropan) is successful in some cases.
- *For nasal congestion*: Use nasal decongestants to relieve symptoms.
- *For ejaculatory inhibition*: This is more prominent among men who use thioridazine. Refer the patient to a physician for further interventions or medication change.

Cardiovascular Side Effects

Postural Hypotension. Postural hypotension is dizziness associated with sudden changes in position, such as lying down and getting up. The use of low-potency antipsychotics such as chlorpromazine and thioridazine presents a greater risk for postural hypotension as a result of γ-adrenergic receptor blockade. Advise patients to rise from beds or chairs slowly to avoid the risk of falling. This is especially important with older adults.

Arrhythmias and Palpitations (Changes in Heart Rhythm). Arrhythmias and palpitations sometimes occur with higher medication doses or in patients with preexisting heart disease as well as in combination with certain drugs, such as thioridazine and ziprasidone (Geodon).

Changes in QT Intervals. Perform a baseline electrocardiogram, and repeat it at maximum dose titration. Carefully monitor for changes in electrocardiogram. Some patients will need to use an alternative medication (Taylor, 2002). Atypical antipsychotics, ziprasidone, and risperidone have been associated with a prolonged QT interval. Therefore, it is recommended to regularly monitor all patients who are taking antipsychotics.

Weight Gain. Clozapine and olanzapine have higher weight gain potential (Box 25-4). Carefully monitor the patient's blood glucose levels, and screen for adult-onset diabetes. Weight gain is especially significant when the patient is taking other drugs, such as lithium, divalproex sodium (Depakote), or mirtazapine (Remeron), which also cause weight gain.

Counsel patients about weight gain and obesity before initiating antipsychotic therapy. Record the patient's weight as a baseline, and monitor it weekly. Excessive weight gain will possibly indicate the need for a change of antipsychotics. Preventive education includes dietary counseling, including calorie counts, portion sizes, the choosing of low-fat and

---

BOX 25-4	ANTIPSYCHOTIC MEDICATIONS ASSOCIATED WITH WEIGHT GAIN*

- Clozapine
- Olanzapine
- Low-potency conventional antipsychotics (e.g., chlorpromazine)
- Quetiapine
- Risperidone
- High-potency conventional antipsychotics (e.g., haloperidol)
- Ziprasidone and molindone

*Ranked from greatest to least potential.

low-calorie foods, and exercise. Excessive weight gain—along with a high blood glucose level, high blood pressure, and high cholesterol and triglycerides levels—increases the risk factors that contribute to the development of metabolic syndrome, which can lead to diabetes and other chronic illnesses.

❖ **CLINICAL ALERT #2**

Neuroleptic malignant syndrome (NMS) is a medical emergency that may be fatal if left untreated. Nurses will observe excessive muscle rigidity, fever, rapid heartbeat, diaphoreses, and drooling. The immediate discontinuation of antipsychotic medications is necessary, and this should be followed by the treatment of other adverse symptoms.

Photosensitivity and Skin Changes. Phenothiazines such as chlorpromazine induce photosensitivity reactions. Haloperidol sometimes causes photosensitivity, but this is rare. The word *photosensitivity* is a general term that is used to describe either the common phototoxic response or the uncommon photoallergic reaction. The phototoxic response is a nonimmunologic reaction that resembles sunburn and that occurs immediately after exposure to sunlight, usually within hours. Clinical signs and symptoms include erythema, pain, and edema. Photoallergic reactions are immunologic and require previous exposure to the photosensitizing agent, and they are commonly delayed (i.e., they usually occur 1 day to 2 weeks after exposure to sunlight). Clinical signs and symptoms include papulovesicular eruption, pruritus, and eczematous dermatitis. The treatment of sunburn includes topical burn cream and antihistamines, whereas steroids are often indicated for photoallergic reactions. Advise patients to wear protective clothing and to use a good sunscreen during outdoor activities. Titanium dioxide is the least likely sunscreen product to cause photosensitivity disorders (Reid, 1996). Skin discoloration (e.g., grayish-blue skin is associated with antipsychotic use. Low-potency conventional antipsychotics such as chlorpromazine and thioridazine are associated with skin pigmentation. The

management of these side effects requires switching the patient to another antipsychotic.

Poikilothermia. The loss of the ability to regulate internal body temperature with environmental temperature change occurs and is often problematic for older adults. Closely monitor older patients who are using antipsychotics when they are in the outdoors during hot weather.

Galactorrhea and Gynecomastia. Galactorrhea and gynecomastia are the result of dopamine blockade, which results in hyperprolactinemia. The management of these side effects includes patient counseling and may require medication change.

Short-acting Typical (Conventional) Antipsychotics

Antipsychotics are often prescribed in the hospital on an as-needed basis for agitation and for the acute symptoms of psychosis. An injection of haloperidol lactate can be administered intramuscularly or intravenously for acute agitation. The starting dose is 1 to 2 mg given intramuscularly or intravenously, and this may be repeated every hour until the patient responds. Haloperidol lactate given every 4 to 6 hours is usually adequate. For patients with delirium, haloperidol lactate is most frequently administered intravenously. Caution should be used when administering this drug to elderly patients; they are usually given a much lower dose, starting with 0.25 mg every 4 hours as needed.

Long-Acting Injectable Typical (Conventional) Antipsychotics

Long-acting antipsychotics may be prescribed for patients whose symptoms interfere with their ability to take daily doses of any medication or who do not have reliable persons to help them monitor their lives. Instead of taking oral doses, their medications are administered by injection once every 3-4 weeks.

Fluphenazine Decanoate Injection. Fluphenazine decanoate is administered intramuscularly or subcutaneously. The onset of action is about 24 to 72 hours. Normally, the patient will see the effects of the drug within 48 to 96 hours. The patient receives subsequent dosages in intervals according to his or her response. A maintenance therapy dosage is usually established after 4 weeks.

Haloperidol Decanoate Injection. Haloperidol decanoate can be given only as a deep intramuscular injection. The maximum dose should not exceed 100 mg. If an additional dose is necessary, the initial injection does not exceed 100 mg, with the balance of the dose given in 3 to 7 days as a separate injection. Patients receive haloperidol decanoate usually every 4 weeks or monthly.

Table 25-3 compares haloperidol decanoate and fluphenazine decanoate with regard to onset, peak time, half-life, and therapeutic range. The pharmacokinetic response after intramuscular injections varies among patients.

Atypical Antipsychotics

EPS occurs much less frequently with use of atypical medications, and there is much less risk for the development of

TABLE 25-3	PHARMACOKINETICS COMPARISON OF DEPOT ANTIPSYCHOTICS	
	HALOPERIDOL DECANOATE	**FLUPHENAZINE DECANOATE**
Onset	Slow onset	1–3 days
Time to peak	6 days	2–4 days
Half-life	21 days (3 weeks)	14–26 days (2–3 weeks)
Therapeutic range	100–450 mg/month	12.5–75 mg/3 weeks

tardive dyskinesia as compared with high doses of high-potency typical antipsychotics. Clozapine is the first atypical antipsychotic that demonstrated efficacy for the treatment of both the positive and negative symptoms of schizophrenia. Subsequently, risperidone, olanzapine, quetiapine, ziprasidone, and aripiprazole were approved for use in the United States. Olanzapine, risperidone, quetiapine, and aripiprazole are the first-line treatment for schizophrenia because of their effectiveness and their favorable side-effect profiles. Ziprasidone is also considered first-line treatment, but it has a greater capacity to prolong the QT/QTc interval in the heart as compared with other antipsychotics; it should be used with caution. Clozapine is not a first-line therapy because of the risk of agranulocytosis; it is used for the treatment of refractory illness. The most recent study (CATIE I and II, 2005 and 2006) advocates the use of low to moderate doses of mild-potency first-generation antipsychotics for first-line therapy, along with the atypical antipsychotics. In the CATIE III study (2006), clozapine's effectiveness was further demonstrated with a longer time to discontinuation for any reason (i.e., a patient stays on clozapine therapy longer) than quetiapine and risperidone.

Both CATIE, and other important government-funded studies that do not include funding from pharmaceutical manufacturers avoid potential funding source bias.

The newer atypical antipsychotics (i.e., asenapine, iloperidone, and paliperidone) are effective for the treatment of schizophrenia. Because they are new on the market, they are not considered first-line therapy.

A complete list of atypical antipsychotics and their U.S. Food and Drug Administration (FDA)–approved indications are listed below:

Clozapine. Clozapine is a dibenzodiazepine. It was the first atypical antipsychotic that was introduced for use in the United States.

Mechanism of Action. Researchers believe that the high receptor affinity for D_4 and $5-HT_2$ is responsible for the many advantages of clozapine as compared with the typical antipsychotics. Positron emission tomography scanning techniques have demonstrated the dramatic difference between the atypical antipsychotic clozapine and the conventional antipsychotic haloperidol (Figure 25-1).

Clinical Use. Clozapine is used for refractory illness. The dose is usually titrated slowly to avoid side effects such as sedation and orthostatic hypotension. The initial dose is 12.5 mg daily on the first day, which is then quickly titrated to 12.5 mg twice a day. The dose may be increased in 25-mg increments every other day until an optimal dosage of 300 to 500 mg/day is reached. To avoid oversedation, patients take the larger dose in the evening.

Risks. Agranulocytosis is the decrease or lack of agranulocytic white blood cells (WBCs), which places a patient at risk for acquiring infections. It occurs in 1% to 3% of patients. In the United States, patients who are taking clozapine (Clozaril) are required to register with the Clozaril National Registry. The patient is monitored very closely by the physician and pharmacy and clozapine is discontinued

Clozapine is discontinued permanently if the total WBC count falls below 2000/mm^3 or if the absolute neutrophil count falls below 1000 mm^3. Patients who are at risk for agranulocytosis, such as immunocompromised patients (e.g., patients with acquired immunodeficiency syndrome or active tuberculosis), are not good candidates for clozapine therapy. In addition, the patient should not receive other medications (e.g., carbamazepine) that carry the risk of agranulocytosis.

Side Effects. For clozapine include those that are similar for many antipsychotics: sedation, anticholinergic effects, orthostatic hypotension, weight gain, hypersalivation (drooling), some risk for seizures. EPS is rare (although akathisia occurs) and NMS is uncommon with clozapine use.

Risperidone. Risperidone is a benzisoxazole derivative; it blocks dopamine (D_2) receptors and 5-HT receptors. Risperidone also blocks D_1, D_4, α-1, α-2 and H_1 histamine receptors, and it is effective for treating both the positive and negative symptoms of psychosis.

Clinical Use. The usual dosage range for risperidone is 4 to 8 mg/day in two divided doses. Higher doses increase the chance of EPS and other side effects. Titrate it slowly, starting with 1 mg daily in divided doses. In the older adult, the dose is generally lower, usually starting at 25% to 50% of the usual adult dose. When titration is complete, administer a once-a-day dose at bedtime. For older patients, the bedtime dose is not always appropriate because of the risk for falls. Bedtime doses are also not appropriate for patients who experience agitation and insomnia. As compared with other atypical antipsychotics, risperidone has fewer anticholinergic side effects, and it is often preferred for older patients (Ranier et al, 2001). A long-acting injection of risperidone (Risperdal Consta) is available. The initial dose is 25 mg given by deep intramuscular injection every 3 weeks. The dose is sometimes increased to 37.5 mg every 2 weeks up to a maximum dose of 50 mg every 2 weeks. Before administering long-acting injections, give patients risperidone orally to ensure that there are no serious adverse side effects.

Side Effects. Common side effects are insomnia, hypotension, agitation, and headache. Hyperthermia sometimes occurs, especially among older patients. Additional side effects

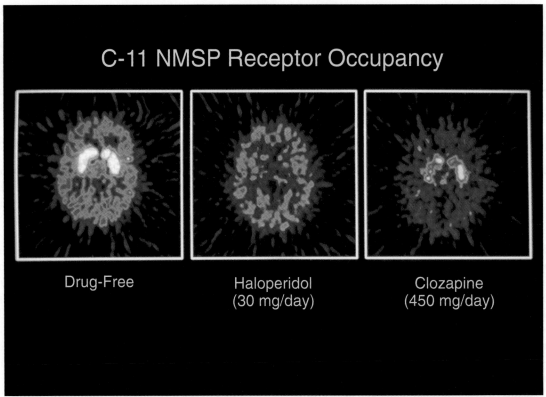

FIGURE 25-1. A transaxial positron emission tomography scan image at the level of the basal ganglia. Carbon-11 *N*-methylspiperone (NMSP) is a radioactive tag that binds and thus highlights dopamine type 2 (D_2) receptors. The three panels are from the same 36-year-old man with schizophrenia. In the first panel, the man is drug free, and the D_2-rich basal ganglia are highlighted by the NMSP. Note the absence of NMSP in the next panel, 6 weeks later, when the patient was taking haloperidol, 30 mg/day, with 85% of his basal ganglia D_2 receptors occupied with haloperidol. Finally, with the man taking clozapine, 450 mg/day, only 37% of the D_2 receptors are occupied by drug. Although the psychosis was responsive to both medications, motor side effects were considerable with haloperidol and absent with clozapine. (Data from Tamminga CA et al: Unpublished research. Maryland Psychiatric Research Center, University of Maryland at Baltimore.)

include the following: Low incidence of EPS and tardive dyskinesia, hypotension, weight gain, hyperprolactinemia.

Olanzapine. Olanzapine is a thienobenzodiazepine. It is an atypical antipsychotic with greater D_2 blockade and weaker D_4 and α-adrenergic blockade. Structurally, olanzapine is similar to clozapine, but it does not involve the risk of agranulocytosis. Olanzapine is effective for the treatment of the positive and negative symptoms of schizophrenia. It is also approved for use as monotherapy for bipolar disorder in manic episodes. It is effective for the treatment of schizoaffective disorders.

Clinical Use. The recommended starting dose is 5 to 10 mg daily at bedtime, and it is often titrated to 20 mg/day. The rapidly disintegrating olanzapine tablet is particularly useful for patients who prefer a rapidly disintegrating tablet without the need to swallow the entire tablet. Olanzapine is available as an intramuscular injection, and it treats agitation (i.e., overexcited, hostile, or threatening behavior) in patients with schizophrenia or bipolar disorder. Elderly patients with

dementia-related psychosis who are treated with atypical antipsychotic drugs like olanzapine are at an increased risk for death as compared with placebo.

Side Effects. Side effects related to use of olanzapine include the following:

- *Sedation and anticholinergic side effects*, weight gain, adult onset diabetes may occur, risk for seizures, hyperprolactinemia.

Quetiapine. Quetiapine is a dibenzothiazepine derivative with weak affinity for serotonin 5-HT$_{1A}$, 5-HT, dopamine D_1, D_2, histamine H_1, adrenergic α-1, and α-2 receptors. Quetiapine has no appreciable affinity for cholinergic muscarinic and benzodiazepine receptors.

Clinical Use. The recommended initial dose of quetiapine is 25 mg twice a day, with increases in increments of 25 to 50 mg twice or three times a day on the second or third day, as tolerated, to a target range of 300 to 400 mg daily on the third or fourth day. Subsequent titration generally occurs in no less than 2 days with 50-mg increments. The usual dosage range for the treatment of schizophrenia is 150 to 750 mg/day. Doses of more than 800 mg/day are not recommended. The FDA has recently approved a new once-a-day dosing formulation, which directly helps to improve patient adherence to the medication regimen.

Side Effects. There are side effects involved with the use of olanzapine. Nurses will monitor cholesterol and triglycerides because levels may be elevated with quetiapine.

Ziprasidone. Ziprasidone is a benzisothiazol piperazine derivative and a 5-HT$_{2A}$ and D$_2$ antagonist. It is also a 5-HT$_{1A}$ agonist and therefore has greater protection against adverse EPS. Ziprasidone also inhibits norepinephrine reuptake.

Clinical Use. The recommended starting dose of ziprasidone oral capsule is 20 mg twice a day to be taken with food. It is usually titrated with increments of 20 mg every 2 days up to 80 mg twice a day. An increase in dose to more than 80 mg twice a day is not recommended.

Ziprasidone for injection is indicated for the treatment of acute agitation among patients with schizophrenia when the use of ziprasidone is appropriate and when a rapid control of agitation is necessary. Patients with a diagnosis of schizophrenia who experience agitation frequently manifest behaviors that interfere with their care (e.g., threatening behavior, escalating or urgently distressing behavior, self-exhausting behavior). Be aware that elderly patients with dementia-related psychosis who are treated with atypical antipsychotic drugs like ziprasidone are at an increased risk of death as compared with placebo.

Risks and Contraindications. Because of ziprasidone's dose-related prolongation of the QT interval and the known association with fatal heart arrhythmias with QT prolongation by some other drugs, it is contraindicated among patients with a known history of heart problems (Glassman and Thomas Bigger, 2001).

Ziprasidone should be avoided in combination with other drugs that prolong the QT interval. (see the Research for Evidence-Based Practice box).

Side Effects. The most common side effects of ziprasidone use are GI discomfort, including nausea, dyspepsia, constipation, diarrhea, and dry mouth. CNS side effects include drowsiness, akathisia, dizziness, EPS, dystonia, and hypertonia. Cardiovascular side effects include tachycardia and postural hypotension. Dermatologic side effects include rash and fungal dermatitis. Other side effects include abnormal vision and upper respiratory infections. Side effects associated with intramuscular injections include pain at the injection site, headache, postural hypotension, bradycardia, nausea, constipation, dizziness, drowsiness, and sweating.

Summary

In general, providers should initially administer antipsychotic medications in divided doses to minimize side effects and to determine the patient's ability to tolerate the medication. After an effective dose has been established, simplify the dosage regimen to once-a-day dosing. Studies have shown that patient medication adherence and compliance improve with daily dosing or less-frequent dosing. Nurses continually observe for major side effects that may occur. This is especially important with patients whose psychosis may prevent them from telling the nurse when they experience certain side effects.

RESEARCH FOR EVIDENCE-BASED PRACTICE

FDA Alert: *Increased mortality in patients with dementia-related psychosis*, April 11, 2005.

This alert reported that patients with dementia-related psychosis who were treated with atypical (second-generation) antipsychotic medications were at an increased risk of death as compared with patient taking a placebo. On the basis of available data, the FDA requested that the package inserts of all atypical antipsychotics include a *black-box warning* that described this risk and that noted that the drug is not approved for the treatment of this condition. The decision was made after the FDA reviewed reports of analyses of 17 placebo-controlled trials that enrolled 5106 elderly patients with dementia-related behavioral disorders that revealed a risk of death among the drug-treated patients of between 1.6 to 1.7 times that seen in the placebo-treated patients. Researchers performed clinical trials with Zyprexa (olanzapine), Abilify (aripiprazole), Risperdal (risperidone), and Seroquel (quetiapine). Over the course of these trials, which averaged about 10 weeks in duration, the rate of death in drug-treated patients was about 4.5% as compared with a rate of about 2.6% in the placebo group. Although the causes of death varied, most of the deaths appeared to be either cardiovascular (e.g., heart failure, sudden death) or infectious (e.g., pneumonia) in nature.

The GI tract generally absorbs antipsychotic medications well. To improve medication adherence and compliance, liquid doses are available. Most atypical antipsychotics are available in an oral rapidly disintegrating tablet form, which readily dissolves on the tongue. Olanzapine and ziprasidone injections are available for the treatment of acute agitation among people with schizophrenia or bipolar disorder. In addition, risperidone is available in depot long-acting intramuscular injection that can be administered every 2 weeks for added convenience.

MAJOR DEPRESSION

Antidepressants

The first modern antidepressant medication, imipramine, was marketed in 1958. This tricyclic compound is a modification of the structure of the antipsychotic chlorpromazine. The reason imipramine and similar drugs are called *tricyclics* (TCAs) is because of the compounds' three-ring chemical structure. Dr. Roland Kuhn, a Swiss psychiatrist, originally administered imipramine to patients with schizophrenia and found no clinical efficacy. Astute observation and the persistence of Dr. Kuhn, who studied the use of imipramine in patients with depression, quickly led to proving imipramine's efficacy for the treatment of depression. This success served as the catalyst in the search for additional antidepressant medications that exhibited improved efficacy and that reduced side effects. At the same time, advances in the understanding of the role of serotonin in depression pointed toward a new class of antidepressants, the selective serotonin reuptake inhibitors (SSRIs).

Indications

The antidepressants have many therapeutic uses, but the primary approved use is to treat major depression as defined by the DSM-IV-TR (Katon and Sullivan, 1990). Antidepressants are also effective for the treatment of a number of other conditions, including the following:

- Anxiety
- Obsessive-compulsive disorders
- Panic disorders
- Bulimia
- Anorexia nervosa
- Posttraumatic stress disorder
- Bipolar depression
- Social phobia
- Irritable bowel syndrome
- Enuresis
- Neuropathic pain
- Migraine headache
- Attention-deficit/hyperactivity disorder
- Smoking cessation
- Autism

Biologic Theory

The biologic theory states that depression occurs because of a decreased amount of or the inadequate function of the catecholamine neurotransmitters norepinephrine or serotonin. Antidepressant drugs affect the responses of these neurotransmitters. Presynaptic neurons synthesize these neurotransmitters, which are incorporated into vesicles. The action of the various antidepressants causes the vesicles to release their contents into the synapse. After they are released, neurotransmitters cross the synapse and affect receptors on the postsynaptic neuron. Most of the neurotransmitters are taken back into the presynaptic neuron to conserve this valuable resource; then they reenter the synthesis process and are incorporated into the vesicles for future use. The cyclic antidepressants partially block the reuptake of norepinephrine and serotonin. Initially, this results in increased amounts of neurotransmitter in the synapse, which reduces the number of receptors on the postsynaptic membrane. This change in receptor density, called *downregulation*, takes several weeks to occur, and it is temporarily associated with the antidepressant response (Figure 25-2).

According to the biologic theory, a patient who fails to respond therapeutically to one antidepressant will respond more favorably to a different antidepressant. It makes sense to switch to an antidepressant that more specifically affects the neurotransmitter that is associated with that individual patient's depressed state. Even with the strength of the biologic hypothesis, a single theory does not fully explain the etiology of depression. The efficacy of medications and the ability to measure the complex effects of neurons offer important clues for a better understanding of the causes of depression.

Major Classes of Antidepressants

Selective Serotonin Reuptake Inhibitors (SSRIs). SSRIs remain first-line drug therapy for the treatment of depression (Celexa, 2000) because of their safety and favorable adverse effect profile. Unlike the TCAs, there have been no fatalities associated with the overdose of an SSRI. Escitalopram oxalate (Lexapro) is one of the newest SSRI to be approved by the FDA (Lexapro, 2002).

SSRIs work by inhibiting the reuptake of 5-HT, which results in an increase of 5-HT concentrations in the synapse. There are six SSRIs currently approved by the FDA, and more are being studied. Except for fluvoxamine, which is approved for use to treat anxiety, all of the SSRIs are approved for the treatment of major depression disorder. All SSRIs are effective for the treatment of panic disorders, obsessive-compulsive disorders, bulimia nervosa, social phobia, and posttraumatic stress disorder.

Efficacy. The efficacy among SSRIs is similar. Choosing a particular antidepressant depends on the patient's acceptance and tolerance of the adverse effects and, to a lesser extent, the cost. Adverse effects differ among the SSRIs, mainly because of their differing affinities for the 5-HT receptor subtypes. Some patients tolerate one antidepressant better than another, so it is important to assess the patient thoroughly before choosing a particular drug. To maximize patient acceptance and compliance with these medications, monitoring side effects is important and needs to continue for the duration of therapy.

Half-lives. The half-lives of SSRIs differ; this difference must be considered when choosing a particular dosing schedule. For example, fluoxetine has the longest half-life and an active metabolite, norfluoxetine, prolongs the drug effect. This enabled the development of a sustained-release fluoxetine formulation that allows the patient to take the drug once a week (Claxton et al, 2000). This is a convenient dosing schedule that normally improves patient compliance.

Cost. The cost of SSRIs is taken into consideration. Fluoxetine is now available in a generic formulation, although Prozac is the only fluoxetine that is available in a sustained-release formulation that is suitable to be taken once a week. Paroxetine is available in a sustained-release formulation as Paxil CR, but it still requires a once-a-day dose. There is a slight advantage to using Paxil CR, because the slow-release formulation helps to reduce GI upset. There appears to be no advantage as compared with the regular Paxil formulation in the clinical setting, because Paxil CR cannot be cut or split in half to save cost. Pill splitting or cutting reduces the overall cost of some of the SSRIs. For example, paroxetine 20-, 40-, or 60-mg tablets are priced comparably regardless of the dose.

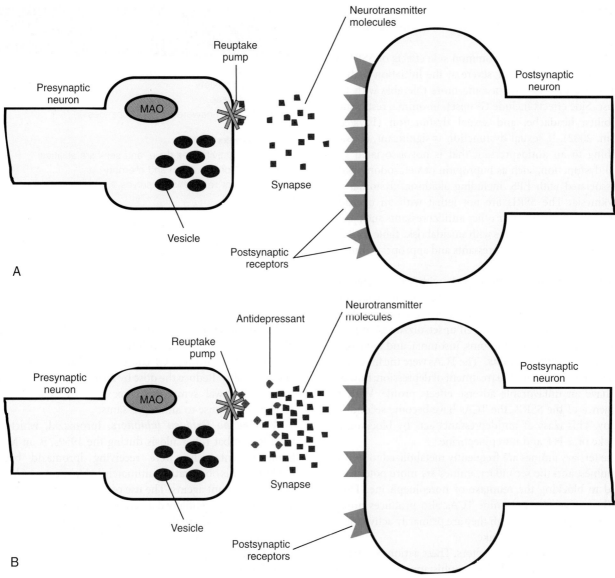

FIGURE 25-2. Neurotransmitter responses to antidepressant therapy. A, In the depressed state, sparse amounts of neurotransmitter are available in the synapse of a depressed person. B, With treatment, the reuptake of neurotransmitter is blocked by the antidepressant drug *(in red)*. The result is increased amounts of neurotransmitter in the synapse. After several weeks, the post-synaptic receptors have decreased (i.e., downregulated), which is associated with resolving depression. For the sake of clarity, this drawing omits numerous receptors and postsynaptic intracellular mechanisms that may ultimately prove to be important components of the patho-physiologic substrate of depression and the antidepressant response.

By splitting or cutting in half a higher-dose tablet (e.g., using half of a 40-mg tablet for a 20-mg dose), the patient is able to substantially reduce the cost of the medication.

Serotonin Syndrome. SSRIs are subject to a variety of drug interactions, some very serious, as a result of associated complex metabolism process. The potential drug interactions of SSRIs with other drugs that also affect serotonin lead to the serotonin syndrome, which is life threatening. Interacting drugs include monoamine oxidase inhibitors (MAOIs), dextromethorphan, meperidine, and sympathomimetics. The

clinical signs of serotonin syndrome include confusion, hypo-mania, restlessness, myoclonus, hyperreflexia, diaphoresis, shivering, tremor, and diarrhea.

Serotonin syndrome is treated in an acute care hospital setting in the following ways:
- Discontinuation of the medications that are causing the increase in serotonin
- Supportive measures, such as cooling blanket for hyper-thermia; benzodiazepines (e.g., clonazepam) for myoc-lonus (i.e., the sudden twitching of muscle or muscle

parts without any rhythm or pattern); anticonvulsants for seizures; and antihypertensives for increased blood pressure

Side Effects. The most common side effects of SSRIs are mild. They are often more severe at the initiation of treatment, but they lessen or become more tolerable with time and use. Side effects include GI upset, insomnia, restlessness, irritability, headache, and sexual dysfunction (Fava and Rankin, 2002). If sexual dysfunction is significant, consider switching to an antidepressant that is not associated with sexual dysfunction, such as bupropion or nefazodone. SSRIs are associated with EPS, including akathisia, dystonia, and bradykinesia. The SSRIs are not lethal with an overdose, which is an advantage over other antidepressants such as the TCAs, especially for patients with suicidal risk. Table 25-4 lists the side effects of all antidepressants and appropriate nursing interventions.

Discontinuation of Therapy. A withdrawal syndrome can occur, thereby making it important to gradually taper the SSRIs over 2 to 4 weeks. Symptoms of the withdrawal syndrome include severe headache, GI upset, dizziness, impaired concentration, flu-like symptoms, insomnia, and anxiety.

Tricyclic Antidepressants. The TCAs were the first widely used antidepressants for the treatment of depression; however, they have an unfavorable adverse effects profile. With the emergence of the SSRIs, the TCAs have become second-line therapy. This class of antidepressants acts by blocking the reuptake of 5-HT and norepinephrine.

The tertiary amines are frequently metabolized to secondary amines, and the secondary amines are more potent with regard to blocking the reuptake of norepinephrine. This is why the use of tertiary amine TCAs also produces norepinephrine response, although they are primarily active for the blocking of serotonin reuptake.

TCAs also act on other receptors. These actions contribute to the adverse effects, including antihistaminic effects, anticholinergic effects, and effects on cardiac conduction.

Anticholinergic Side Effects. All TCAs have substantial anticholinergic side effects, such as dry mouth, blurred vision, GI upset, constipation, urinary retention, and confusion. Among the TCAs, desipramine and nortriptyline have the least intense anticholinergic side effects. All of the TCAs are very sedating, and patients usually take them at bedtime. Because they cause cardiotoxicity, an electrocardiogram is recommended before the initiation of therapy and should be repeated periodically. TCAs cause orthostatic hypotension. Instruct patients, especially the elderly, to rise slowly to prevent falls. Another disadvantage of TCAs is the risk of fatality with an overdose, particularly among patients with suicidal risk.

Monitoring Parameters. Therapeutic blood level monitoring is useful to confirm that the administered dose is maintaining a serum drug concentration within the effective range and to prevent toxicity and serious adverse effects. Avoid TCAs in elderly patients because of anticholinergic side effects, orthostatic hypotension, sedation, and cardiac arrhythmias. SSRIs are preferred for elderly patients.

BOX 25-5	TIME COURSE OF RESPONSE TO ANTIDEPRESSANTS

First Week
Decreased anxiety
Improved sleep
Patient often unaware of these changes

1 to 3 Weeks
Increased activity, sex drive, and self-care abilities
Improved concentration and memory
Psychomotor retardation resolves

2 to 4 Weeks
Relief of depressed mood
Less hopelessness
Suicidal ideation subsides

Discontinuation of Therapy. TCAs should be tapered for discontinuation. Abrupt withdrawal leads to a withdrawal syndrome that involves GI complaints, dizziness, insomnia, and irritability. Reduce the dose by 25 to 50 mg/week to minimize withdrawal symptoms. Box 25-5 explains the time course of response to antidepressants.

Monoamine Oxidase Inhibitors. Iproniazid, which was used to combat tuberculosis during the 1950s, is an MAOI. Some patients who were receiving iproniazid became euphoric. This observation ultimately led to the use of MAOIs as antidepressant agents. The use of MAOIs is now limited as a result of the potentially dangerous side effects and the strict dietary modifications that are necessary with its use, which will be described later in this section. Thus, the search for new antidepressant agents continued.

Mode of Action. The neurotransmitters norepinephrine, serotonin, and dopamine are monoamines. In the CNS, these molecules are synthesized inside of the presynaptic neuron. The maintenance of cellular homeostasis requires a mechanism to degrade monoamines. Monoamine oxidase is an enzyme that is found in the mitochondria of cells that participate in the normal process of degradation of these amines; MAOIs inhibit this enzyme initially, which results in the increased availability of these neurotransmitters. As with other antidepressants, these initial neurotransmitter increases result in postsynaptic receptor *downregulation* that is temporally related to the antidepressant response, as described earlier.

Clinical Use and Efficacy. MAOIs are used for the treatment of atypical (novel) depression, major depression without melancholia, or depressive disorders that are resistant to TCAs. Hypersomnia, hyperphagia, anxiety, and the absence of vegetative symptoms characterize atypical depression. In addition, MAOIs have been used with variable success for the treatment of other disorders, such as certain anxiety disorders, eating disorders, and some pain syndromes (e.g., migraines).

TABLE 25-4   SIDE EFFECTS OF ANTIDEPRESSANTS WITH NURSING INTERVENTIONS

SIDE EFFECTS	NURSING INTERVENTIONS
Anticholinergic Effects	
Dry mouth	Offer sugarless gum and candy or artificial saliva; for persistent problems, treat with pilocarpine 1% rinse and spit (4 drops of 4% pilocarpine and 12 drops water) or bethanechol (Duvoid, Urecholine) 5 mg sublingual or 10–30 mg once or twice daily
Blurred vision: disturbance of near vision; far vision usually preserved	Ask if the vision prescription is current; try pilocarpine 1% eyedrops or bethanechol 10–30 mg three times daily
Urinary retention	When not caused by benign prostatic hypertrophy, may be treated with bethanechol 10–30 mg three times daily
Constipation	Prevent by encouraging fluids (medication givers may offer), fruits and vegetables, and mild physical exercise (walks) Treat with bulk-forming laxatives (e.g., Metamucil 1–2 tablespoons every morning or docusate 100 mg daily or twice daily); avoid stimulant laxatives when possible; if needed, limit duration to avoid laxative dependence or treat with bethanechol 10–30 mg once or twice daily
Anticholinergic delirium (also known as *atropine psychosis*)	Monitor for agitation restlessness, psychotic signs and symptoms, and myoclonic jerking; sometimes occurs with or without peripheral anticholinergic signs; hold anticholinergic drugs; physostigmine 5 mg given intravenously rapidly reverses the condition but requires life-support backup and cardiac monitoring
α-Blockade	
Orthostatic hypotension	Consider other contributing factors, such as low-salt diets, restricted fluid intake, and dehydration; antihypertensive medications exacerbate this condition; advise the patient to change positions slowly, to dangle his or her feet for 1 minute in a sitting position when rising from prone, and to sit immediately when lightheaded; offer support hose and exercises to strengthen the calf muscles to improve venous return
Sexual Dysfunction*	
Decreased libido	Neostigmine 7.5–15 mg 30 minutes before anticipated intercourse
Impaired erection	Often an anticholinergic problem; change to less anticholinergic drug or try bethanechol
Priapism	Rare disorder associated with trazodone; prolonged painful and nonsexual erection; medical urgency treated with epinephrine injections to the OPS Corpora cavernosa; may require surgical intervention that leads to permanent impotence
Impaired ejaculation	Requires switching drugs; try neostigmine 7.5–15 mg 30 minutes before anticipated intercourse
Inhibition of orgasm	Less serotonergic drug; try cyproheptadine 4 mg daily; note that cyproheptadine, a serotonin antagonist, has caused a loss of antidepressant efficacy in some patients; the addition of bupropion has been successful
Hematologic	
Agranulocytosis	Exceedingly rare allergic reaction that usually occurs in the first 3 months of treatment; monitor for fever, sore throat, mucosal ulceration, and weakness; discontinue drug; change to different chemical class
Petechiae, ecchymosis, easy bruising, bleeding	Associated with selective serotonin reuptake inhibitor effect on platelets; often occurs with normal or decreased platelet counts; discontinue drug; monitor complete blood cell count and for dizziness and lightheadedness
Other	
Weight gain	Associated with cyclic antidepressants and monoamine oxidase inhibitors; recommend diet and exercise; treat with diuretics (e.g., hydrochlorothiazide for edema)
Weight loss	Associated with selective serotonin reuptake inhibitor; rarely clinically significant
Tremor	Caffeine exacerbates tremors; determine degree of interference with daily activities; propranolol 10–20 mg three to four times daily is often useful
Antidepressant withdrawal	Anticholinergic rebound results in gastrointestinal upset, cramps, and diarrhea; educate the patient about potential withdrawal symptoms; when discontinuing, taper slowly over several weeks; selective serotonin reuptake inhibitor withdrawal symptoms include nausea, lightheadedness, dizziness, faintness, fatigue, paresthesias, and flu-like syndrome

*Obtain a clear history from the patient to determine that the complaint does not predate the depression or medication use.

From Andrews JM, Nemeroff CB: Contemporary management of depression, *Am J Med* 97:24S, 1994; modified from Pollack MH, Rosenbaum JF: Management of antidepressant-induced side effects: a practical guide for the clinician, *J Clin Psychiatry* 48:3, 1987.

MAOIs are rapidly absorbed. They are metabolized in the liver, and they have average half-lives of approximately 24 hours. A majority of individuals metabolize MAOIs relatively slowly. This metabolic difference among individuals results in wide variations with respect to required doses for efficacy and sensitivity to side effects at a given dose. There is no clinically available test for this metabolic rate. Thus, many clinicians begin MAOI therapy with a 10- or 15-mg test dose. The vital signs are monitored and complaints of side effects are studied closely before beginning titration.

Contraindications to the use of MAOIs include cerebrovascular defects, major cardiovascular disease, and pheochromocytoma (a tumor of the adrenal medulla). Older patients do not tolerate MAOIs well, so their use is uncommon among individuals who are more than 65 years old. MAOIs sometimes worsen symptoms of Parkinson's disease, induce manic states in bipolar patients, and exacerbate psychotic symptoms in patients with schizophrenia. Patients with diabetes require the adjustment of their hypoglycemic medication. MAOIs are contraindicated during pregnancy.

Nurses know it is critical that patients taking MAOIs need to comply with a tyramine-restricted diet (Box 25-6) and avoid stimulant medications to prevent the risk of a potentially fatal hypertensive crisis. Thus, the patient's ability to comply with dietary and medication restrictions is an important consideration before the initiation of therapy. It is the nurses responsibility to teach the patient and the family about MAOIs. Response to therapy takes 3 to 6 weeks. Except in emergencies, discontinuations should be tapered.

Drug–Drug and Drug–Food Interactions. Dietary tyramine is a precursor in the synthesis of norepinephrine. In the presence of an MAOI, foods high in tyramine (an amino acid byproduct that is formed by the bacterial breakdown of tyrosine in fermented foods) lead to a sharp increase in available norepinephrine and a potentially fatal hypertensive crisis. Tyramine is not the only factor in food that interacts with MAOIs. For instance, fava beans contain dopamine, which affects blood pressure in the presence of MAOIs. Previously, dietary restrictions for MAOIs were extensive and made compliance unlikely. Estimates of compliance with an MAOI diet have been as low as 40%. However, for several reasons, there are not an overwhelming number of MAOI hypertensive reactions. Foods, different brands of prepared foods, and a patient's susceptibility to this interaction all vary widely. For instance, although a cup of coffee elevates blood pressure and causes headaches, some patients who take MAOIs benefit from a cup of coffee as an adjunct to treat hypotension on awakening. Thus, patient education consists of simple, clear, written and verbal instructions to absolutely avoid certain foods. Nurses need to review warnings about other foods that cause problems in some patients or when consumed in large quantities. Patients need to maintain dietary restrictions for 2 weeks after discontinuing MAOIs. All patients need to know the warning signs of hypertensive crisis, which include headache, stiff neck, sweating, nausea, and vomiting. Patients with such symptoms need to seek medical attention immediately.

BOX 25-6 **DIETARY RESTRICTIONS FOR PATIENTS WHO ARE TAKING MONOAMINE OXIDASE INHIBITORS**

Prohibited
- Aged cheeses
- Ripe avocados
- Ripe figs
- Anchovies
- Bean curd and fermented beans
- Broad beans (e.g., fava, Italian)
- Yeast extracts and yeast-derived vitamin supplements
- Liver
- Delicatessen meats (especially sausage)
- Pickled herring
- Meat extracts (e.g., Marmite, Bovril)
- Fermented foods
- Chianti and sherry

Allowed in Moderation
- Beer and ale (tyramine content varies with brand and can be especially high in imported beers and some nonalcoholic beers)
- White wine and distilled spirits
- Cottage cheese and cream cheese
- Coffee (2 cups/day)
- Chocolate
- Soy sauce (tyramine content varies with brand)
- Yogurt and sour cream
- Spinach, raisins, tomatoes, eggplant, and plums

❖ CLINICAL ALERT #3

It is extremely important for nurses to teach patients to avoid certain foods and other drugs when taking MAOIs to avoid a hypertensive crisis. Nurses teach patients about these facts and discuss them with patients and their families; give their patients lists of potentially dangerous foods and drugs as reminders; and document the nursing actions that occur during nurse–patient interactions.

Many drugs also interact with MAOIs and lead to hypertensive crisis or dangerous hypotension (Box 25-7). Many over-the-counter medications are dangerous when taken with MAOIs, including diet pills, nasal decongestants, asthma medications (including inhalers), and cough suppressants (dextromethorphan). Literally hundreds of over-the-counter and prescription combination products under many different brand names contain sympathomimetics that are unsafe to use with MAOIs. Therefore, nurses need to educate every patient who is taking an MAOI to consult a physician, dentist, nurse, or pharmacist before taking any additional medication. Although hypertensive events are generally more dangerous and more common, the response to a sympathomimetic medication or dietary indiscretion is sometimes hypotension rather than hypertension. Whether a hypotensive or hypertensive reaction (described below under Other Side Effects) ensues is a function of the overall adrenergic tone of the patient and is not predictable.

The *treatment of hypertensive crisis* usually begins with nifedipine (Procardia, Adalat) 10 mg. Absorption from oral administration is extremely rapid, and the patient's blood pressure often lowers in a matter of minutes. Monitor the patient's vital signs every 10 to 15 minutes until the patient is stable. Other therapies include the γ-adrenergic blockers phentolamine (Regitine) 5 mg given intravenously and chlorpromazine 50 mg given by mouth.

Patients who fail to respond to a non-MAOI antidepressant usually wait at least 2 weeks before starting an MAOI. An important exception to this is fluoxetine. Because of the long half-life of fluoxetine and its active metabolite norfluoxetine (approximately 7 to 10 days), patients who are discontinuing fluoxetine need to wait at least 5 weeks before starting an MAOI. In general, this class of medication is not suitable for patients with suicidal risk or with the cognitive inability or unwillingness to follow the rigid regimen of dietary and drug restrictions.

Other Side Effects. Orthostatic hypotension is a common initial and sometimes persistent side effect of MAOIs. Dangling the feet when rising from a prone position, changing positions slowly, wearing support stockings, and increasing fluid and salt intake are often effective treatments. A caffeinated drink in the morning is useful as long as the nurse has monitored the patient's vital signs initially. Edema, sexual dysfunction, and weight gain are also common and often lead to drug discontinuation. Complaints of insomnia occur with all MAOIs. Moving the last dose of the day to an earlier time is helpful. Complaints of confusion or feeling drunk indicate an excessive dose. Although these drugs do not have direct effects on cholinergic receptors, anticholinergic-type side effects (e.g., dry mouth, urinary hesitancy, constipation) are common. Sometimes MAOI-induced pyridoxine (vitamin B6) deficiency causes paresthesias (numbness, prickling, tingling feelings). This is treated with oral pyridoxine.

The abrupt discontinuation of MAOIs may produce a withdrawal syndrome and so should be avoided. Symptoms include nausea, sweating, palpitation, nightmares, hallucinations, delirium, and paranoid psychosis.

Other Antidepressants

Duloxetine. Duloxetine is a selective serotonin and norepinephrine reuptake inhibitor. The FDA has approved it for the treatment of major depression in adults and for diabetic neuropathy as well. Venlafaxine and desvenlafaxine are the only other selective serotonin and norepinephrine reuptake inhibitors that have been approved for use in United States. Duloxetine inhibits serotonin and norepinephrine, and it weakly inhibits dopamine reuptake in the neuronal synapse. Duloxetine is available in 20-, 30- and 60-mg enteric-coated delayed-release capsules.

It is well absorbed orally. To avoid toxicity, careful consideration is given by prescribers when adding other medications.

Venlafaxine. Venlafaxine is a selective serotonin and norepinephrine reuptake inhibitor. Unlike TCAs, it does not affect other receptors that cause the undesirable adverse effects such as anticholinergic and antihistaminic side effects.

Because venlafaxine affects both serotonin and norepinephrine, patients with a less-than-optimal response to an SSRI use it (Thase et al, 2001). It is also used to treat anxiety disorders (Gelenberg et al, 2000).

Formulations and Dosage. Venlafaxine is available in regular and sustained-release formulations. Patients take regular tablets two or three times a day. Patients take Venlafaxine XR, the sustained-release formulation, once a day. If the patient cannot tolerate a single sustained-release dose, then the dose is divided to reduce side effects such as GI upset. The initial dose of regular-release venlafaxine is 50 to 75 mg/day, which is administered in two or three divided doses with food. The dose is increased by 75-mg increments every 4 days. Doses beyond 225 mg do not usually demonstrate increased efficacy; however, severely depressed patients often need up to 350 mg/day. The maximum recommended dose is 375 mg/day.

Side Effects. The most common adverse effect is GI upset, which is more significant among older patients. Venlafaxine causes increases in blood pressure, and patients with uncontrolled hypertension need to use it with caution. The increase in blood pressure is dose related. Other side effects are similar to those that are associated with the SSRIs, including insomnia, restlessness, headache, and irritability.

Trazodone. Trazodone is an SSRI, and it also blocks 5-HT$_{2A}$ receptors. Because of its sedative effects, trazodone is used as an agent to counteract insomnia.

Formulations and Dosage. The therapeutic dosage range is 50 to 600 mg/day. Patients should take the lowest effective dose.

Side Effects. Sedation is a frequent and often intense side effect. Therefore, trazodone is currently used as a hypnotic and an antidepressant adjunctive therapy to SSRI to counteract insomnia. The most frequent cardiovascular side effect during therapy is postural hypotension, which is often accompanied by syncope, especially among patients who are taking concomitant antihypertensive therapy (Spivak et al, 1987). The adjustment of antihypertensive medication is necessary if it is administered concurrently.

A rare but serious side effect is priapism. Priapism is painful, persistent, abnormal penile erection that is unaccompanied by sexual stimulation. This is an emergency, and it requires prompt medical attention.

Patient Education. Discuss sedation, the risk of falls, and orthostatic hypotension with the patient. Warn male patients of the potential serious side effect of priapism.

The trazodone long-acting tablet (Oleptro) is a once-a-day formulation. Available dosages are 150- and 300-mg tablets. It is indicated for treatment of depression. The long-acting formulation is not FDA approved for use in children.

Bupropion. Bupropion has inhibitory effects on dopamine and norepinephrine reuptake, and it has a lesser effect on serotonin reuptake (i.e., it is commonly referred to as a *norepinephrine and dopamine reuptake inhibitor*). The exact mechanism is unknown.

Half-life and Dosing Schedule. Bupropion has a short half-life, and patients take doses three times a day. An extended-release product is available for twice-daily dosing. The recommended initial dose of bupropion is 200 mg/day, which is administered as 100-mg doses once in the morning and once in the evening. To prevent the risk of seizure and adverse effects such as dystonia, the maximum single dose of bupropion SR is limited to 150 mg/dose and 450 mg/day, and the non–sustained-release dose is 100 mg/dose.

Side Effects. Common side effects include nervousness, headache, and insomnia. Seizure is a significant risk; titrate the dose and follow the dosing schedule closely. Another common side effect is dystonia.

Bupropion is available as a 24-hour extended-release formulations (XL) and as a 12-hour extended-release formulations (ER) that is administered twice a day.

Other Therapeutic Uses. Bupropion is helpful for the reduction of cigarette, alcohol, and drug cravings (Chengappa et al, 2001). Zyban is the brand name of bupropion as labeled for use as an adjunct therapy for cigarette smoking cessation (Bupropion, 1997). Bupropion is an antidepressant that is often used in association with alcohol and drug detoxification and rehabilitation.

Mirtazapine. Mirtazapine increases both norepinephrine and serotonin in the synapse. It also blocks serotonin receptors (Davis and Wilde, 1996).

Dosage. The recommended starting dose is 15 mg/day as a single dose. It is preferable to give the dose in the evening, before sleep. The effective dose range appears to be 15 to 45 mg/day.

Side Effects. The major side effects are sedation and weight gain (Gorman, 1999). Interestingly, sedation is more prominent with a lower dose. Weight gain is significant, and it is sometimes desirable for older patients. Other side effects

include constipation. Serious but rare side effects include neutropenia, agranulocytosis, and hepatotoxicity. Regular monitoring parameters include complete blood cell counts and liver function tests.

Other Therapeutic Uses. Mirtazapine, 15 mg orally, is often administered the night before surgery to reduce insomnia and to minimize presurgical anxiety.

> ❖ **CLINICAL ALERT #4**
>
> Antidepressants sometimes increase the risk of suicidal thinking and behavior in adults as well as in children and adolescents with depression and other psychiatric disorders. Families and caregivers will closely watch children and symptoms.

Methylphenidate and dextroamphetamine may be used occasionally as antidepressants; both have been effective for treating depression in some older patients. The dose range is 5 to 40 mg/day for methylphenidate and 10 to 30 mg/day for dextroamphetamine.

Not all patients are suitable for treatment with these drugs, and patients with the potential for drug abuse should be especially closely watched. Avoid these drugs for patients who are already anxious, or psychotic.

Lithium

Lithium is sometimes prescribed for refractory (treatment-resistant) depression. Therapeutic blood-level monitoring is an imperative requirement. Use lithium with caution in older patients and in patients with renal impairment.

Thyroid Therapy

Patients with low thyroid function often exhibit symptoms of depression. Levothyroxine (T_4) is used, and some patients require combination therapy that includes antidepressants. Patients require monitoring and periodic thyroid function tests.

Herbal Supplements

Saint John's wort is a mild herbal antidepressant that is commonly used in Europe and that has gained considerable popularity in the United States. Caution patients that Saint John's wort should be avoided in combination with other antidepressants (see Chapter 27).

BIPOLAR DISORDERS

Mood Stabilizers

The role of mood stabilizers in the treatment of bipolar disorders is significant; these include role of mood stabilizers, the treatment of bipolar disorder, and include lithium, valproate, carbamazepine, and other anticonvulsant mood stabilizers. Many of the anticonvulsant mood stabilizers have risks of adverse drug reactions and drug interactions (Frances et al, 1996). Atypical (second-generation) antipsychotic drugs have received FDA approval for the treatment of acute mania or mixed episodes of mania and depression. In addition, the FDA has approved olanzapine and aripiprazole for the maintenance treatment of bipolar disorder. The FDA has also approved the fixed-dose combination of olanzapine and fluoxetine (Symbyax) for the treatment of the depressive phase of bipolar disorder. Many patients prefer taking the combination once daily in the evening, because olanzapine is sedating.

Lithium. Lithium, which is a single ion, was medicinally used for more than a century for several ailments, but its use for mania was discovered by accident. Physicians have used lithium for the treatment of bipolar mania for more than 50 years. It has antimanic, antipsychotic, and antidepressant activity; however, it is most effective for the treatment of pure mania and less effective for the treatment of a mixed-state mood disorder (Bipolar Disorder, 1999).

Therapeutic Dosage Regimen. Close monitoring by the nurse of the patient's laboratory reports of blood serum lithium levels is imperative. The therapeutic index or the range between the therapeutic and toxic levels of lithium is narrow. The diligent nurse is therefore instrumental in helping patients to avoid potentially severe adverse reactions to this medication. The therapeutic index varies slightly among facilities, and the nurse's responsibility is to follow current procedures.

Patients usually begin lithium in low divided doses to minimize side effects. The dose is titrated according to the patient's response and the appearance of side effects until the serum lithium concentration is within the range of 0.5 to 1.2 mEq/L (Tohen and Grundy, 1999). A typical starting dose is 300 to 400 mg three times a day, depending on the patient's age and weight.

With a given dose regimen, lithium levels achieve a steady state after 5 days. Because of its narrow therapeutic index, lithium levels must be checked periodically at steady state and after each dose increase. It is appropriate to check lithium levels more frequently when rapid titration is necessary, such as for the treatment of acute mania or when the nurse suspects toxicity. As levels reach the upper limits of the therapeutic range, they should be checked more frequently to minimize the risk of toxicity. Older patients are more at risk for lithium toxicity, and they may need the dose adjusted, with the upper end of the therapeutic range being approximately 0.6 mEq/L.

In addition to the monitoring of serum lithium levels, other baseline and periodic monitoring includes the following: renal function, thyroid function, urinalysis, complete blood cell count with differentials, serum electrolytes, electrocardiogram, and weight. It is advisable to perform a pregnancy test for women of childbearing age before initiating lithium therapy. Order renal function and thyroid function tests periodically, and carefully monitor them.

Clinical Use

Acute Treatment. Lithium is effective for the acute and prophylactic treatment of both manic and depressive episodes in patients with bipolar disorders. The first-line treatment is to combine lithium or valproate with an antipsychotic.

For less ill patients, monotherapy with lithium and valproate or an atypical antipsychotic such as olanzapine or risperidone is used. Benzodiazepines are often helpful as a short-term adjunctive treatment.

For patients who have rapid cycling bipolar disorder, which involves four or more mood disorder episodes within 12 months, valproate plus an antipsychotic is sometimes preferred over lithium. Carbamazepine or oxcarbazepine may be used instead of lithium or valproate. Antidepressants should be tapered or discontinued. Psychosocial therapy is used in combination with pharmacotherapy.

Other Uses of Lithium. Lithium is also prescribed for the acute treatment of major depressive disorder, for the prevention of recurrent major depression, and for the treatment of cluster headaches.

Side Effects and Toxicity. As many as 75% of patients treated with lithium experience some side effects. Lithium toxicity is closely related to serum lithium levels, but it also occurs when levels approach the upper end of the therapeutic range. Some side effects are minor, and lowering the dose can reduce them. Side effects that are correlated with peak serum levels (e.g., tremors) may be reduced by changing to a slow-release formulation or by changing to a single bedtime dose. Box 25-8 shows the potential side effects of lithium therapy in relation to blood serum concentration levels.

Mild to Moderate Effects. Some of the strategies that are used to manage persistent side effects include β-blockers to treat tremor; diuretics for polydipsia, polyuria, or edema; and topical antibiotics or other preparations for acne. Manage GI upset by changing the dose to a slow-release or controlled-release formulation or by giving the drug with meals. If the patient uses a diuretic, reduce the lithium dose (sometimes up to 50%) because of increased intrarenal reabsorption induced by diuretics. In addition, it is advisable to monitor the patient's electrolyte balance, particularly sodium and potassium. A starting dose of 5 mg twice a day of amiloride, a potassium-sparing diuretic that does not alter the lithium level, is recommended. Lithium sometimes induces hypothyroidism. Perform thyroid function tests, and prescribe levothyroxine for these patients as appropriate. Treat any exacerbation of psoriasis with dermatologic preparations. However, in some cases, the discontinuation of lithium is necessary.

Severe Toxicity and Lithium Overdose. As the serum level increases to greater than 2.5 mEq/L, the risk of permanent neurologic impairment is significant. In these cases, it is important to reduce the serum level rapidly. Hemodialysis is the only reliable method to rapidly reduce the serum level, especially in the presence of acute poisoning or when a patient deteriorates rapidly and is showing clinical signs of intoxication, such as coma, convulsions, cardiovascular collapse, or respiratory failure. Nurses continuously monitor patients, especially in the case of an overdose of sustained-release lithium, because the manifestation of symptoms may be delayed.

Patient Education. During patient education, nurses address the potential side effects of lithium as well as

BOX 25-8   LITHIUM SIDE EFFECTS

Transient Effects and Mild Toxicity
- Fine tremor
- Gastrointestinal upset
- Mild polyuria and polydipsia
- Muscle weakness and lethargy

Persistent Effects
- Fine tremor
- Mild polyuria and polydipsia
- Increased white blood cell count
- Nontoxic goiter and hypothyroidism
- Exacerbation of psoriasis
- Acne
- Alopecia
- Weight gain
- *Effective acute treatment and prophylaxis: 0.5–1.2 mEq/L*

Moderate Toxicity
- *Lithium level: 1.5 mEq/L*
- Coarsening of tremor
- Reappearance of gastrointestinal symptoms
- Confusion
- Sedation and lethargy
- *As levels increase:*
- Ataxia
- Dysarthria
- Mental status deterioration

Severe Toxicity
- *Lithium level: 2.5 mEq/L*
- Seizures
- Coma
- Cardiovascular collapse
- Death

potential drug interactions. Counsel patients to monitor their fluid intake according to activity and exercise levels and to avoid a salt-restricting diet. In addition, advise patients about potential drug interactions with thiazide diuretics, angiotensin-converting enzyme inhibitors, nonsteroidal anti-inflammatory drugs, and cyclooxygenase-2 inhibitors. Women of childbearing age need to discuss the use of lithium and other psychotropic medication if they should become pregnant. Follow-up appointments and monitoring are important for all patients.

Valproate. Valproate is an anticonvulsant medication that is effective for the treatment of manic episodes, and it is the first-line treatment for rapid-cycling bipolar disorder. It is more effective than lithium for the treatment of bipolar disorder with prominent depressive symptoms. It is also effective for the adjunctive treatment of schizoaffective disorder (Bogan et al, 2000).

Absorption, Distribution, Metabolism, and Excretion. The body rapidly absorbs valproate orally, with peak serum concentrations occurring within 4 hours. Valproate is metabolized extensively in the liver and excreted in the urine.

Dosage and Titration Regimen. It is generally advisable to start with a dose of 20 to 30 mg/kg per day in hospitalized patients. This usually occurs with the use of a divided dose regimen until the desired serum level is reached.

In the outpatient setting or in older patients, doses are titrated until the serum level is stabilized. When the patient is stable, it is advisable to simplify the dose to once or twice a day to enhance patient compliance. Extended-release divalproex (Depakote ER) is available for once-a-day dosing.

Side Effects. The main reasons for using valproate for bipolar disorders are its relative safety and the more rapid abatement of symptoms as compared with lithium. Minor side effects include sedation and GI distress. These occur early during the course of treatment, and they typically resolve with continued treatment or dose adjustment. Divalproex has a wider therapeutic range than lithium. Inadvertent overdose is uncommon, and accidental or intentional poisoning is less likely to be lethal than with lithium, thereby making it a preferred choice over lithium for older patients. In rare incidences, however, valproate causes serious adverse effects.

Common dose-related side effects include the following: (1) sedation; (2) GI distress, nausea, vomiting, diarrhea, dyspepsia, and anorexia; (3) benign transaminase elevation; (4) osteoporosis; and (5) tremor. These side effects are often transient. Other side effects that are persistent include hair loss, increased appetite, and weight gain. Mild asymptomatic leukopenia and thrombocytopenia sometimes occur, but the associated levels usually return to normal when the patient discontinues therapy.

Hepatotoxicity. Patients with a history of hepatic disease are at higher risk for hepatotoxicity. Hepatic failure has occurred mostly in children 2 years old or younger who are receiving multidrug therapy. Life-threatening pancreatitis has occurred in both children and adults shortly after initial use as well as after several years of use. Baseline liver function tests are necessary before the initiation of valproate therapy. Monitor for clinical signs of hepatotoxicity as well as laboratory levels of liver enzymes.

Persistent Gastrointestinal Distress. Indigestion, heartburn, and nausea are common side effects of valproate therapy. Taking the dose with food, using enteric-coated tablets, or changing of formulation to divalproex instead of using valproic acid is generally helpful. The administration of a histamine-2 antagonist such as famotidine (Pepcid) is sometimes helpful. If the patient vomits and has severe abdominal pain, monitor his or her serum amylase level and carefully evaluate for pancreatitis.

Tremor. Essential tremor is a common side effect of valproate. Dose reduction or the administration of a β-blocker such as propranolol (40 to 160 mg in divided doses) reduces this effect.

Sedation. This is a common side effect, and it is more prominent at the initiation of therapy. A more gradual titration is often necessary. The once-a-day bedtime dose with the use of an extended-release formulation of valproate is also useful.

Hematologic Effects. Mild leukopenia (i.e., a total WBC count of more than 3000/mm^3) is usually reversible with dose reduction or discontinuation. Discontinuation reverses mild cases of thrombocytopenia, but more serious cases have occurred. For patients who are receiving anticoagulation therapy, monitor an appropriate test of clotting function closely.

Serious Adverse Effects. Rare and idiosyncratic but potentially fatal adverse effects with divalproex include fatal hepatic failure, pancreatitis, and thrombocytopenia. Monitoring parameters include hepatic function and a complete blood cell count on a regular basis (usually every 6 months).

Potential Drug–Drug Interactions. Valproate displaces highly protein-bound drugs from their binding sites, thereby resulting in the increased blood levels of the drugs that have been displaced. An example is the drug interaction of valproate with lamotrigine; the use of valproate increases the lamotrigine blood level twofold.

Patient Education. Patient education includes the management of minor side effects as well as of the signs and symptoms of hepatic and hematologic side effects. Advise patients to report these potentially serious side effects promptly.

Other Uses. Valproate is an anticonvulsant, and it is effective for the treatment of grand mal, petit mal, myoclonic, and temporal lobe seizures. The drug is much less effective for focal or complex partial seizures. It is also indicated for prophylaxis for migraine headache and as an adjunctive therapy for pain management.

Carbamazepine. Carbamazepine and oxcarbazepine (Trileptal) are also anticonvulsants, and they are alternative treatments for acute bipolar mania in place of lithium or divalproex.

Mechanism of Action. Carbamazepine is structurally related to imipramine, which is a TCA. Carbamazepine has psychotropic effects, and it is less sedating than most anticonvulsants. The drug elevates mood in some depressed patients, and it is a second-line treatment for bipolar disorder. Although carbamazepine is effective for the treatment of psychiatric disorders, it does not have a neurochemical profile that resembles that of classic antipsychotics. However, data suggest that carbamazepine decreases dopamine turnover without directly blocking dopamine receptors.

Absorption, Distribution, Metabolism, and Excretion. Carbamazepine has a unique pharmacokinetic profile. Metabolism occurs via the cytochrome P4503A4 enzyme. Initially, it has a half-life of approximately 36 hours. However, carbamazepine induces its own metabolism during treatment; this is complete within 3 to 5 weeks. After this period, the half-life is about 24 hours. For this reason, the patient does not reach the steady state until about 4 weeks after initial therapy. In addition, with increasing carbamazepine doses in children, a dose-dependent autoinduction process occurs.

Extended-release capsules taken every 12 hours provide steady-state plasma levels that are comparable to those obtained with immediate-release tablets taken every 6 hours at the same milligram dose. Food increases bioavailability; therefore, providers recommend giving carbamazepine with food.

Dosage Regimen and Monitoring Parameters. Carbamazepine doses range from 200 to 800 mg/day. The dose is usually started at the lower end of the range and titrated upward in accordance with response and side effect tolerance. For patients who are more than 12 years old, carbamazepine is usually initiated at 200 to 600 mg/day in divided doses. The usual manner of titration increases the dose by 200 mg/day. For hospitalized patients with acute mania, the dose is initially titrated faster. Rapid titration causes an increase in side effects such as drowsiness, dizziness, ataxia, and diplopia.

Side Effects and Toxicity. Overdoses or the undetected excessive accumulation of carbamazepine can be fatal. Signs of carbamazepine toxicity include dizziness, ataxia, sedation, and diplopia. Acute toxicity results in stupor or coma. Treatment includes gastric lavage and the management of symptoms.

Rare and idiosyncratic but potentially fatal side effects include agranulocytosis, aplastic anemia, thrombocytopenia, hepatic failure, exfoliative dermatitis (e.g., Stevens-Johnson syndrome), and pancreatitis. Other serious side effects include cardiac conduction disturbances.

A complete blood cell count with differential and platelet count as well as liver function tests are recommended every 2 weeks during the first 2 months of therapy. If the results of the tests are normal, then the tests can be done every 3 months thereafter. However, whenever there are signs or symptoms of hepatic, hematologic, or dermatologic reactions, the patient should have laboratory tests performed more frequently.

The patient can manage minor side effects (e.g., nausea) by taking carbamazepine immediately before or after meals, by dividing the doses throughout the day, by changing to a sustained-release form, or by using a histamine-2 antagonist such as famotidine. Cimetidine (Tagamet) is not recommended because of potential drug–drug interactions. Manage sedation and dizziness by decreasing the dose or shifting the dose to bedtime.

Patient Education. It is important for nurses to counsel patients to monitor for signs and symptoms of hematologic and hepatic abnormalities so that the patients can report them promptly. Instruct the patient to notify the physician immediately if a rash occurs.

Potential Drug–Drug. Erythromycin, calcium channel blockers, and SSRIs increase carbamazepine levels, whereas carbamazepine decreases the levels of many other drugs, including antipsychotics, some steroids, oral contraceptives, thyroid hormones, benzodiazepines, TCAs, and anticonvulsants.

The concomitant use of clozapine increases the risk of aplastic anemia, and patients need to avoid this. The concomitant use of lithium sometimes causes an acute state of confusion.

Oxcarbazepine. Oxcarbazepine is as effective as carbamazepine for the treatment of bipolar disorder, and patients usually tolerate it better. This is often an alternative for patients who are unable to tolerate carbamazepine.

Risks. Hyponatremia is a major concern with oxcarbazepine therapy, and some limit its use as an anticonvulsant and antineuralgic. The mechanism is thought to be the result of an antidiuretic-hormone–like action on the kidney. Most cases of hyponatremia are asymptomatic, although confusion and an increase in seizure frequency have occurred in some patients. Hyponatremia with oxcarbazepine occurs most commonly among older patients and during the administration of high doses of the drug (Houtkooper et al, 1987; Johannessen and Nielsen, 1987; Kloster et al, 1999; Nielson et al, 1988; Pendlebury et al, 1989; Steinhoff et al, 1992; Van Amelsvoort et al, 1994; Zakrzewska and Patsalos, 1989).

Side Effects. Headache, drowsiness, dizziness, ataxia, tremor, abnormal gait, fatigue, sedation, encephalopathy, and oculogyric crises have occurred with the administration of oxcarbazepine. Sedation, difficulty with concentration, and memory impairment are also associated with its use.

Hyperlipidemia, antidiuretic hormone effects, altered reproductive hormones, weight gain, and effects on thyroid function have also occurred with the administration of oxcarbazepine. The use of oxcarbazepine is associated with decreases in the T_4 hormone but not in the T_3 or thyroid-stimulating hormone (Micromedex, 2003).

Lamotrigine. Researchers have studied lamotrigine in bipolar depression and in rapid-cycling bipolar disorders; it has been effective for the treatment of both conditions (Botts and Raskind, 1999).

Dosage Titration and Risk. The initial dose of lamotrigine is 25 mg once a day, and it is increased in 25-mg increments every other week. When the patient is taking valproate in addition to lamotrigine, reduce the dose of lamotrigine by half because of potential drug interactions. Lamotrigine requires a slow titration; the titration schedule must be followed to minimize the risk of skin rash. Approximately 5% of patients develop a maculopapular rash, and approximately 0.1% of patients develop Stevens-Johnson syndrome, which is often fatal.

Side Effects. Common side effects include headache, dizziness, GI distress, and blurred or double vision.

Drug Interactions. Significant drug interactions occur with valproate.

Topiramate. Topiramate is a sulfamate-substituted monosaccharide that is used for the treatment of epilepsy. Topiramate is an anticonvulsant that is an adjunctive therapy for partial seizures and generalized tonic–clonic seizures. It is not used as monotherapy for bipolar disorder, but it is sometimes useful as an adjunctive therapy. Topiramate is also used for the treatment of binge eating, bulimia, cluster headache, trigeminal neuralgia, and Tourette's syndrome.

Dosage. Titrate topiramate dosage slowly, with an initial dose of 50 mg/day for the first week that is then increased in 50-mg increments per week until the patient reaches a dose of 400 mg/day in two divided doses. Slower titration is necessary to minimize side effects, primarily impaired cognitive

function (Martin et al, 1999). Slow titration also minimizes other side effects such as dizziness and drowsiness.

The dosage of topiramate is 11 to 35 mg/kg/day for children 5 years old or younger and 5.5 to 16.5 mg/kg/day for children 6 to 12 years old. The clearance of topiramate is 50% greater in children, which results in a shorter half-life. In children, topiramate has a faster elimination rate, which results in a 30% lower plasma concentration as compared with adults. Topiramate has significant drug interactions with enzyme-inducing anticonvulsants. These result in an increased clearance rate and shorter half-life.

Risks. Use topiramate with caution in patients with renal impairment, and adjust the dose (Bialer, 1993). Topiramate may cause acute myopia and secondary close-angle glaucoma; it should be avoided by patients with glaucoma. Slowly taper topiramate to avoid the risk of precipitating seizures.

Side Effects. Anemia has occurred with topiramate use. Cardiovascular effects include hypertension, postural hypotension, vasodilation, arrhythmias, palpitations, atrioventricular block, and bundle block.

The most common side effects of topiramate include drowsiness, dizziness, ataxia, speech disorders and related speech problems, psychomotor slowing, nystagmus, fatigue, confusion, language problems, anxiety, and cognitive problems. Auditory hallucinations have occurred as well.

Newer Anticonvulsants

Several newer anticonvulsants are only indicated and approved by the FDA for the treatment of seizures. These include tiagabine, zonisamide, and levetiracetam. The newer anticonvulsants listed are not FDA approved for the treatment of bipolar disorders at this time.

Treatment of Mania

The first step in the treatment of mania includes the use of a mood stabilizer such as lithium or valproate. The FDA has approved atypical antipsychotics for the treatment of mania, and these drugs have been effective.

For patients with agitation associated with mania, a benzodiazepine is often added to the initial treatment regimen until the patient stabilizes. High-potency benzodiazepines such as lorazepam and clonazepam are sometimes used. Alprazolam is not used, because its antidepressant effect precipitates mania.

Atypical Antipsychotics for Mania

The atypical antipsychotics have been effective for treating mania, and they include aripiprazole, olanzapine, clozapine, quetiapine, risperidone, and ziprasidone. The atypical antipsychotics are replacing haloperidol and conventional or typical antipsychotics. When patients receive haloperidol, a mid-range dose is often adequate for treatment. A typical dose of haloperidol is 10 to 15 mg/day.

Combination of Mood Stabilizers

Lithium is sometimes combined with valproate for the effective treatment of bipolar disorder during the manic phase.

The use of valproate in combination with carbamazepine is generally best avoided because of potential drug interactions. If there are no other alternatives and the patient is using a combination of valproate and carbamazepine, the dose of valproate needs be increased and the dose of carbamazepine needs to be lowered because of their mutual drug interactions.

Treatment of Bipolar Depression

The treatment of bipolar depression is different from the treatment of unipolar or major depression. The first attempt is the optimization of the mood stabilizer. Monitor the patient's thyroid function tests. Clinical signs of hypothyroidism include depression, which is usually treated with thyroid hormone replacement therapy. If the patient will be using an antidepressant, carefully monitor the patient, because this predisposes the patient to mania. In general, SSRIs and bupropion are safer; avoid TCAs.

Maintenance Therapy and Lifelong Intervention

Because patients with bipolar disorder face the prospect of requiring lifelong medication therapy, the noncompliance rate is high, which results in multiple recurrent episodes of mood disorders. Patients frequently discontinue their medications when symptoms subside. The goal of maintenance therapy is to prevent recurrence, and there is a fine balance between optimal therapy and patient acceptance. The risk of relapse is high with the discontinuation of a mood stabilizer, and patients often become refractory to treatment, even when they resume the use of the same drug. Therefore, it is important to educate patients to avoid stopping their medication when they feel better and to emphasize the need for prophylactic treatment despite the lack of symptoms. In addition, to avoid noncompliance with medication, patients need to know that they must tolerate an acceptable level of side effects. For example, a lithium dose between 0.8 and 1.0 mEq/L is an optimal level for maintenance therapy, but it usually causes side effects. There are attempts to maintain a level of 0.4 to 0.6 mEq/L to reduce the side effects, and this correspondingly improves patient compliance.

ANXIETY DISORDERS

Twenty million people in the United States suffer from anxiety disorders. They are the most prevalent of all psychiatric conditions, and they are among the leading causes of disability in the United States and worldwide, costing billions of dollars in lost wages and for treatment. There is also a strong association between alcohol and drug abuse and anxiety disorders worldwide (Kushner et al, 1990).

Generalized Anxiety Disorder

Excessive worry, poor concentration, insomnia, and an unidentifiable cause characterize anxiety disorder. Symptoms last more than 6 months, and the patient is not always able to function in his or her daily life. Treatment options include antidepressants, benzodiazepines, and buspirone.

Treatment Medications

Antidepressants. Several antidepressants have proven to be effective for the treatment of anxiety disorders, particularly the second-generation antidepressants. Venlafaxine is an FDA-approved antidepressant drug for the treatment of generalized anxiety disorder. Patients commonly use the sustained-release formulation (Venlafaxine XR) because of better compliance with the less-frequent dosing schedule. This drug has a somewhat more rapid onset than other antidepressants.

The advantage of antidepressants over benzodiazepines is that these drugs are also effective for patients with co-occurring disorders such as major depression or other anxiety disorders. Other advantages include a lower potential for drug dependence and abuse that occurs with many antianxiety medications. The disadvantage as compared with benzodiazepines includes a longer onset of peak action (i.e., 4 weeks versus 1 week or less) and less efficacy for the treatment of the physical or somatic symptoms of anxiety.

Antidepressant doses for generalized anxiety disorder are similar to those for major depression. Gradual titration minimizes side effects and increases patient compliance. Adverse effects of SSRIs and venlafaxine include GI upset, insomnia, irritability, headache, and sexual dysfunction. Imipramine has the side effect profile of the TCAs, including anticholinergic effects, drowsiness, and dizziness. Nefazodone causes drowsiness and liver toxicity.

Benzodiazepines. Clonazepam, lorazepam, and alprazolam are all FDA approved for the treatment of generalized anxiety disorder. The longer-acting benzodiazepine clonazepam is desirable because of its ease of dosing; patients usually take it only once or twice a day. The advantage of benzodiazepine is its rapid onset (i.e., 1 week or less). Disadvantages include cognitive impairment, decreased coordination, potential drug abuse, and withdrawal symptoms. In general, shorter-acting benzodiazepines are more difficult to taper and potentially cause more problems with withdrawal.

Buspirone. Buspirone is a 5-HT$_{1A}$ receptor partial agonist that requires a dosing schedule of two or three times a day. It is effective for the treatment of generalized anxiety disorder, but it does not appear to be effective for panic disorder.

The major disadvantage of buspirone is its longer onset, which is usually 2 to 4 weeks. Initial therapy includes the addition of benzodiazepines until the patient sees the effect of buspirone. Table 25-5 describes the therapeutic indications of hypnotic and anxiolytic agents.

Obsessive-Compulsive Disorder

Obsessive-compulsive disorder (OCD) is characterized by persistent and recurrent thoughts, images, impulses, and behaviors that are distressing to the individual and that impair daily function.

Treatment Medications

Antidepressants. SSRIs and clomipramine are effective for the treatment of OCD. Physicians prefer SSRIs because of

TABLE 25-5   HYPNOTIC AND ANXIOLYTIC AGENTS

GENERIC NAME (TRADE NAME)	APPROVED INDICATIONS	APPROXIMATE BENZODIAZEPINE EQUIVALENCY (mg)	ACTIVE METABOLITE	USUAL DOSAGE RANGE (mg/day)	HALF-LIFE (hours)
Benzodiazepines					
Alprazolam (Xanax)	A, AD, P	0.5	No	0.75–4 (A) 4–10 (P)	12–15
Chlordiazepoxide (Librium)	A, AW, PS	10	Yes	25–200	5–30
Clonazepam (Klonopin)	LGS	2.5	No	1–6*	20–50
Clorazepate (Tranxene)	A	7.5	Yes	7.5–90	20–80
Diazepam (Valium)	A, PS, SE	5	Yes	2–40	20–80
Estazolam (ProSom)	Hypnotic	2	No	1–2	10–15
Flurazepam (Dalmane)	Hypnotic	15	Yes	15–30	8–40
Halazepam (Paxipam)	A	20	Yes	20–160	10–20
Lorazepam (Lorazepam)	A, PS	1	No	0.5–10	10–20
Oxazepam (Serax)	A, AD, AW	15	No	30–120	5–20
Prazepam (Centrax)	A	10	Yes	20–60	20–80
Quazepam (Doral)	Hypnotic	2	Yes	30–50	30–50
Temazepam (Restoril)	Hypnotic	15	No	15–30	10–20
Triazolam (Halcion)	Hypnotic	0.25	No	0.125–0.25	1.5–5
Nonbarbiturate, Nonbenzodiazepine					
Buspirone (BuSpar)	A	—	—	10–60	2–4
Chloral hydrate (Noctec)	Hypnotic	—	—	500–2000	8–11
Diphenhydramine (Benadryl)	Hypnotic	—	—	25–100	3–9
Diphenhydramine (Unisom)	Hypnotic	—	—	25–100	8–12
Ethchlorvynol (Placidyl)	Hypnotic	—	—	500–1000	18–20
Eszopiclone (Lunesta)	Hypnotic	—	—	2–3	3.8–6
Rozerem (Ramelteon)	Hypnotic	—	—	8	2–5
Zaleplon (Sonata)	Hypnotic	—	—	10–20	1.1
Zolpidem (Ambien)	Hypnotic	—	—	5–10	1.5–4
Zolpidem CR (Ambien CR)	Hypnotic	—	—	6.25–12.5	2.9

A, Anxiety; *AD*, anxiety associated with depression; *AW*, alcohol withdrawal; *LGS*, Lennox-Gastaut syndrome (seizures); *P*, panic disorders; *PS*, psychotic disorders; *SE*, status epilepticus.
*Up to 20 mg/day given for seizure.

their more advantageous adverse effect profile and better patient compliance. Fluvoxamine, fluoxetine, paroxetine, and sertraline are all effective. The choice of a particular SSRI depends on side effects, patient tolerance, and potential drug interactions.

Drug Interactions. Significant drug interactions occur with clozapine, TCAs, and theophylline; a reduction in the dose of these drugs is recommended. Fluvoxamine inhibits important enzymes resulting in necessary dose adjustments for other drugs, including alprazolam.

Tricyclic Antidepressants. Clomipramine is effective for the treatment for OCD, whereas other TCAs, such as desipramine and imipramine, are not. Clomipramine has the usual side-effect profile of the TCAs including sedation, anticholinergic side effects, orthostatic hypotension, sexual dysfunction, and seizure risk. TCAs are second-line therapy.

Augmentation Therapy

Cognitive behavioral therapy is an important nonpharmacologic intervention for OCD. Other augmentation therapies include the use of the following: (1) dopamine-blocking agents; (2) buspirone; (3) lithium; and (4) clonazepam.

Dopamine-Blocking Agents. Haloperidol has been effective as an adjunct to fluvoxamine for OCD that is associated with tics. Researchers are currently studying olanzapine for use in the treatment of patients with OCD.

Posttraumatic Stress Disorder

Posttraumatic stress disorder (PTSD) involves recurrent anxiety symptoms that occur in response to very serious life events (i.e., war combat, child abuse, rape). Symptoms interfere with daily function and relationships.

Treatment Medications

Antidepressants. SSRIs are effective treatment as a class for PTSD (Foa et al, 1999b). Drug selection is based on patient preference, side-effect profile, and patient tolerance. Nefazodone and bupropion are also effective. TCAs and MAOIs are effective, but they are generally not used because of their side-effect profile and potential drug and food interactions. The use of a combination of different drug classes is often necessary.

Benzodiazepines. Benzodiazepines are an effective treatment for PTSD. Clonazepam is effective to reduce flashbacks and nightmares. The major problems with the use of benzodiazepines are *tolerance* and *dependence*. There is also risk for the patient with alcohol abuse because of additive depressant effects.

Mood Stabilizers. Lithium, divalproex, and carbamazepine are adjunct therapies for explosiveness, irritability, and other symptoms that are associated with PTSD.

Social Phobia

Social phobia is the most common anxiety disorder. Strong and persistent anxiety that results from a fear of scrutiny by others, embarrassment, or humiliation characterize this disorder. The patient's response is disproportionate and unrealistic for the situation. A high incidence of alcohol abuse and depression is associated with social phobia, because patients are often isolated as a result of their avoidance.

Treatment Medications

Antidepressants. The SSRIs, including paroxetine, fluoxetine, fluvoxamine, sertraline, and citalopram, are the first-line treatments for social phobia. Dosing is similar to that used for major depressive disorder. Slow titration increases patient compliance and tolerability. The onset of therapeutic effect is about 4 weeks, with optimal effects seen after 8 to 12 weeks.

Nefazodone is an option if sexual dysfunction is a significant side effect. Nefazodone is contraindicated for patients with hepatic impairment.

Benzodiazepines. Clonazepam and alprazolam are effective.

Gabapentin. The effective dose is 900 to 3600 mg/day. Side effects include sedation, dizziness, and dry mouth.

Herbal Therapy for Anxiety
Kava Kava

Kava kava (*Piper methysticum*) is an herb that has anxiolytic and sedative properties. It is available as a root extract in capsule form. The recommended dose for the treatment of anxiety is 100 to 125 mg dried kava kava root extract taken three times a day. It is also available in tablet form as a purified kavalactone, and the dose is 50 to 70 mg three times a day. As a tincture, the usual dose is 30 drops with water three times a day.

Side Effects. Kava kava was thought to be relatively mild and safe. Recently, the literature has warned of kava-kava–associated hepatitis, cirrhosis, and liver failure. Other side effects include altered judgment, altered motor reflexes, GI upset, skin rash, and visual disturbances.

Herb–Drug Interactions. Kava kava is associated with interactions with several drugs, including barbiturates, benzodiazepines, dopamine agonists, alcohol, and MAOIs. There is added risk with combinations of other hepatotoxic drugs.

Valerian

Valerian (*Valeriana officinalis*) has anxiolytic and hypnotic properties. It is used for the treatment of mild to moderate insomnia as well as for restlessness and tension. Valerian is available as a capsule, extract, tincture, and tea. The dose for anxiety relief is 220 mg of valerian extract three times a day.

Side Effects. Some patients have had hepatotoxicity with the long-term use of valerian. Side effects include sedation and withdrawal symptoms that are similar to those associated with the benzodiazepines.

Patient Education

Important teaching points for patients with anxiety disorders and their families include the following:
- Educate the patient that an anxiety disorder is a treatable illness and that is does not represent a personal weakness or failure.
- Educate the patient about the different types of medications that are effective for the treatment of this condition as well as their side-effect profiles, precautions, and contraindications.
- Encourage patients to participate in the decision-making process when choosing therapy.
- Medications generally take several weeks to achieve maximal effects. Encourage the patients to continue the medications although they may not see an immediate effect.
- Encourage nonpharmacologic interventions, when appropriate.
- Advise the patient regarding potential drug–drug and drug–herb interactions. Tell patients to report any medications that they are taking to their physician or health care professional. This includes herbal remedies, prescription drugs, and over-the-counter drugs.
- As with all herbal preparations, caution patients to use only those products that have the unit clearly defined on the label.
- Counsel the patient regarding the risk of mixing alcohol with these medications, especially benzodiazepines.
- Counsel the patient to avoid driving or operating machinery, because many of these drugs cause drowsiness and sedation.

Summary

Pharmacotherapy for anxiety disorders is moving away from benzodiazepines and toward the serotonergic antidepressants, particularly the SSRIs and venlafaxine. The SSRIs and venlafaxine have better safety profiles and do not involve the risk of substance abuse, tolerance, and dependence that are associated with the benzodiazepines. The disadvantage is their slow onset of action. Benzodiazepines are still widely prescribed because of their rapid onset of action and the lack of associated sexual dysfunction.

INSOMNIA

Hypnotics
Benzodiazepines

Triazolam. Triazolam (Halcion) has a short half-life and a fast onset of action. It is used to treat the patient who has difficulty falling asleep.

Temazepam. Temazepam (Restoril) has an intermediate half-life with a slow onset of action. It is for the patient who awakens early and cannot stay asleep.

Flurazepam. Flurazepam (Dalmane) has a long half-life with a fast onset of action. It is good for patients who have difficulty both falling asleep and staying asleep. The disadvantage is rebound insomnia.

Nonbenzodiazepine Hypnotics

Zolpidem (Ambien), zaleplon (Sonata), eszopiclone (Lunesta), and ramelteon (Rozerem) are the nonbenzodiazepine receptor agonists. They are structurally unrelated to benzodiazepines, and they do not appear to have abuse potential. They possess minimal muscle relaxant, anticonvulsant, or anxiolytic properties. Advantages over benzodiazepines include a lack of rebound insomnia, a lack of the development of dependence, and a lack of adverse withdrawal effects. The main disadvantage of zolpidem and zaleplon is their high cost as compared with the benzodiazepine hypnotics.

Zolpidem. Zolpidem is an oral imidazopyridine sedative–hypnotic agent.

Pharmacokinetics. Onset is within 30 minutes, and the duration is 3 to 5 hours. It is rapidly absorbed. The half-life of the drug is 2.5 to 5 hours. It is metabolized into inactive compounds (Greenblatt et al, 1998).

Dose. The usual dose is 10 mg immediately before bedtime; the dose for older adults is 5 mg. Repeating the dose is not recommended. Limit the therapy to 7 to 10 days, and reevaluate the patient if a longer duration is necessary.

Ambien CR is a dual-layer tablet that works in two distinct ways:

- The first layer dissolves quickly to help patients get to sleep fast.
- The second layer dissolves slowly to help patients stay asleep.

Ambien CR is available in 6.25- and 12.5-mg tablets. It is a controlled-release formulation, but there are no comparative sleep studies between the regular formulation and the sustained-release formulation.

Side Effects. Patients have reported dizziness, headache, GI upset, nausea, and mild anterograde amnesia. With doses of more than 10 mg/day, there is a risk of hallucinations.

Drug Interactions. Zolpidem is highly protein bound. Food decreases absorption. Avoid the use of other CNS depressants, including alcohol.

Zaleplon. Zaleplon is a nonbenzodiazepine hypnotic agent.

Pharmacokinetics. Zaleplon is a short-acting hypnotic with a rapid onset of action. The onset is within 30 minutes, and the duration is 2 hours. The half-life is 1.1 hours. Because of its short onset and short half-life, zaleplon is useful for the treatment of insomnia that occurs during the middle of the night and the early morning (Elie et al, 1999).

Dose. The recommended dose for the treatment of insomnia is 10 mg before bedtime. A 5-mg dose is sufficient for a small or low-weight patient or for an older adult. The dose may be repeated once.

Side Effects. Dizziness and headache are common.

Eszopiclone. Eszopiclone is the newest of the three nonbenzodiazepine benzodiazepine receptor agonists that are available in the United States, and it also has the longest half-life. It has a rapid onset of action (15 to 30 minutes), and it is available in 1-, 2-, and 3-mg tablets. The usual dose is 2 to 3 mg for adults. Older adult patients need to receive lower doses (i.e., usually 50% of the regular adult dose).

Rozerem. Rozerem (Ramelteon) is short acting and has a half-life of 2 to 5 hours, which is similar to triazolam. The usual dose is 8 mg; 16 to 32 mg have been administered with no apparent additional side effects, but these higher doses did not provide added benefits.

New Drugs Pending Approval

Gaboxadol and indiplon are hypnotics that are currently in development and that have not yet been approved by the FDA. Gaboxadol may have advantages over current hypnotics that are available on the market. Indiplon is an indirect γ-aminobutyric acid agonist.

Other Agents Used for Sleep

Trazodone. **Mechanism of Action.** Trazodone is a serotonin reuptake inhibitor that blocks serotonin receptors. The dose as a hypnotic is 50 to 200 mg at bedtime.

Pharmacokinetics. There is delayed onset, with a long half-life of 6 hours that may be longer for older adults and obese patients. Side effects are sedation and orthostatic hypotension. Priapism, which is a rare but serious adverse effect, sometimes occurs. Trazodone is preferred over benzodiazepines for patients who are in drug or alcohol detoxification programs or when patients need to avoid benzodiazepines.

Chloral Hydrate

Mechanism of Action. The mechanism of action of chloral hydrate (Noctec) is unknown. The active metabolite is trichloroethanol, which possesses an hypnotic effect and which is responsible for cross-tolerance.

Pharmacokinetics. The drug has a rapid onset of 30 minutes. The half-life is 8 to 11 hours. The duration of effect is 4 to 8 hours.

Dose. The recommended dose is 500 to 1000 mg at bedtime, with a maximum dose of 2 g.

Side Effects. Side effects include GI upset, nausea, vomiting, ataxia, confusion, headache, hallucinations, and rash. All patients who are using this drug need to avoid alcohol. This is recommended for the short-term treatment of transient insomnia (i.e., a few nights). It is not for initial treatment, because doses of more than 4 g can be fatal, and there are many safer drugs available (e.g., nonbenzodiazepine hypnotics).

Diphenhydramine. Diphenhydramine is widely available over the counter. Many over-the-counter sleep remedies contain diphenhydramine, including Nytol, Sominex, and Unisom. It is an antihistamine and an H_1-receptor antagonist.

Pharmacokinetics. Diphenhydramine is metabolized in the liver.

Dose. The recommended dose is 25 to 50 mg at bedtime. The maximum dosage is 300 mg/day.

Side Effects. Tolerance sometimes develops after 2 weeks. Avoid this drug in older adults because of its anticholinergic side effects.

Barbiturates. The use of barbiturates has dramatically decreased because of the many safer and better hypnotics that are now available. Table 25-5 lists their dosages and half-lives.

Melatonin. Melatonin (Micromedex, 2003) is an *N*-acetyl-5-methoxytryptamine. It is a naturally occurring hormone that is secreted by the pineal gland, and it is a byproduct of serotonin metabolism. The dose is 0.3 to 5 mg at bedtime. It is often used to counteract jetlag.

Melatonin is not an herbal product; however, it is commercially available in combination with other herbal remedies. Side effects include drowsiness and daytime fatigue. Avoid other CNS drugs when taking melatonin.

Herbal Products for Sleep

Kava Kava. The dose of kava kava for use as a hypnotic is 60 to 120 mg of dried extract (Micromedex, 2003).

Valerian. The dose of valerian for use as a hypnotic is 400 to 900 mg at bedtime. Because of its slower onset, patients need to take valerian 1 hour before bedtime (Micromedex, 2003).

AGGRESSIVE AND VIOLENT BEHAVIORS

Aggressive and violent behaviors are frequent among patients with a wide spectrum of underlying disorders. Brain injury, brain trauma, dementia, mental retardation, and seizure disorders are some of the underlying disorders that lead to aggressive and violent behaviors. CNS infections and drug abuse may also lead to aggressive behaviors. Patients with schizophrenia, mania, and personality disorders often display these behaviors.

Careful diagnosis always precedes treatment to avoid the overuse and misuse of medications. Although the FDA has not approved any medications specifically for aggression, many medications are being used, primarily for the following two purposes:

- To sedate and calm the patient and to prevent patient self-harm or harm to others
- To treat chronic aggressive behaviors

The factors that are most important during the selection of an initial emergency medication include the availability of an intramuscular injection or liquid formulation, the speed of onset, and the previous history of the patient's responses (Allen et al, 2001b).

Acute Agitation and Aggression

Sedating medications are commonly used to treat a patient during an acutely aggressive or violent situation. It is important to select a sedating medication that is limited in duration to avoid oversedation and potential adverse effects.

Antipsychotics or benzodiazepines are commonly used. Treatment does not exceed 4 weeks. When a patient requires more than 4 weeks of treatment, change the approach to address chronic treatment.

Antipsychotics

Antipsychotics are commonly used to treat acute aggressive and violent behaviors. Often it is the sedating property of the antipsychotics that produces the calming effect for the patient. An important point to remember is that antipsychotics cause side effects such as akathisia (increased psychomotor restlessness), which inexperienced nurses often mistake for increased irritability and agitation. It is an error to administer an extra as-needed dose of the antipsychotic medication in this instance, because it may worsen the patient's symptoms.

The atypical antipsychotics are becoming more commonplace for the treatment of aggressive behavior, and they have fewer side effects (see Table 25-6). The disadvantage of using atypical antipsychotics is that only ziprasidone is available as an intramuscular injection, and it is expensive. All of the atypical antipsychotics are effective, and the choice depends on the patient's condition and the side-effects profile of each drug. For example, patients with diabetes and weight gain need to avoid the use of olanzapine. Instead, quetiapine is preferred for patients with a history of EPS, and risperidone is preferred for older patients and patients who are delirious, because this drug produces fewer anticholinergic side effects (Allen et al, 2001a).

Haloperidol. In patients with brain injury and acute aggression, low-dose haloperidol is preferred. The recommended dose is 1 mg orally or 0.5 mg intramuscularly, with repeated injections every hour until aggression is controlled. After a patient shows no aggression for 48 hours, the dose of haloperidol is gradually tapered, with a decreasing daily dose schedule of 25% until the achievement of the goal of discontinuation.

For patients with dementia and schizophrenia, risperidone is often used (Ranier et al, 2001). Low-dose risperidone of 0.5 to 1 mg is preferred, and the doses should be smaller for older adults with dementia. Trazodone, which is a sedating antidepressant, has been used to treat older adult patients with sundowning syndrome and aggressive behaviors. Some providers prescribe a low dose of 50 to 100 mg.

Benzodiazepines

The sedating properties of benzodiazepines are helpful for the management of acute agitation and aggressive and violent behavior. Another advantage of the benzodiazepines is their rapid onset of action. There have been reports of paradoxic reactions in which benzodiazepines cause violent and aggressive behaviors, but these are rare.

Lorazepam is the most common benzodiazepine in use. Nurses administer it orally or by injection. It is commonly used in combination with antipsychotic medication such as haloperidol. Other nonbenzodiazepine sedating agents used include valproate, chloral hydrate, and diphenhydramine.

TABLE 25-6 ATYPICAL ANTIPSYCHOTICS: INDICATIONS APPROVED BY THE U.S. FOOD AND DRUG ADMINISTRATION

INDICATION	ARIPIPRAZOLE (ABILIFY)	ASENAPINE (SAPHRIS)	CLOZAPINE (GENERIC)	ILOPERIDONE (FANAPT)	OLANZAPINE (ZYPREXA)	PALIPERIDONE (INVEGA)	QUETIAPINE (SEROQUEL)	RISPERIDONE (GENERIC)	ZIPRASIDONE (GEODON)
Acute treatment of schizophrenia in adults	X	X	X	X	X	X	X	X	X
Maintenance treatment of schizophrenia in adults	X				X	X	X	X	X
Acute treatment of schizophrenia in adolescents (13–17 years old)	X				X		X	X	
Acute treatment of bipolar mania in adults	X	X			X		X	X	X
Acute treatment of bipolar mania in adults; adjunct to lithium/valproate	X				X		X	X	
Acute treatment of bipolar mania in pediatric patients (10–17 years old)	X								
Acute treatment of bipolar mania in pediatric patients (10–17 years old); adjunct to lithium/valproate	X								
Maintenance treatment of bipolar mania in adults	X				X				X
Maintenance treatment of bipolar mania in adults; adjunct to lithium/valproate							X		X
Acute treatment of agitation associated with schizophrenia in adults	X				X				X
Irritability associated with autistic disorder in children and adolescents (5–16 years old)	X							X	

Indication						
Acute treatment of depressive episodes associated with bipolar disorder in combination with fluoxetine			X			
Acute treatment of treatment-resistant depression in adults in combination with fluoxetine			X		X	
Adjunctive therapy to antidepressants for acute treatment of major depressive disorder in adults	X					
Acute treatment of schizoaffective disorder as monotherapy		X				
Acute treatment of schizoaffective disorder as adjunct to mood stabilizers, antidepressants, or both		X				
As monotherapy for treatment-resistant schizophrenia				X		
For a reduction in the risk of recurrent suicidal behavior in patients with schizophrenia or schizoaffective disorder				X		

Chronic Aggression

When a patient continues to exhibit aggressive behavior for more than several weeks, the choice of medication to counteract aggression is guided by the patient's underlying condition. For example, when aggression is related to schizophrenia, antipsychotic medications are sometimes used. When aggression is related to mania, lithium or valproate is used. When aggression is related to seizure disorder, carbamazepine or valproate is used.

Antipsychotics

Do not use antipsychotics solely for the treatment of aggressive behavior but rather to treat the underlying condition.

Buspirone

Buspirone, which is an antianxiety agent, has been effective for the treatment of aggressive behavior. The initial dose is 5 mg twice a day, which is increased by 5-mg increments every 3 to 5 days. The patient usually does not see the full effect for several weeks, and the effective dose may be as high as 45 to 60 mg/day.

Anticonvulsants

Carbamazepine and valproate are used to treat bipolar disorders and associated aggressive behaviors because of their important anti-kindling properties (see Chapter 12). Carbamazepine has been effective for reducing the aggressive behavior associated with dementia. Lithium is also useful for treating aggression associated with mania.

Antidepressants

Trazodone has been prescribed for the treatment of aggression associated with organic mental disorders. Other antidepressants such as the SSRIs have also been used. The dose range of the antidepressants used to treat aggression is the same as that used for the treatment of depression.

Antihypertensive Medications

The β-blocker propranolol has been effective for the treatment of aggression related to organic brain syndrome. Major side effects of propranolol include the lowering of blood pressure and of the heart rate. Remember that β-blockers may cause depression.

Special Considerations for Children

If antipsychotic medication is necessary for the treatment of aggression in children, a low-dose atypical antipsychotic such as olanzapine or risperidone is preferred (Allen et al, 2001c).

CHAPTER SUMMARY

- Although previously atypical antipsychotic medications were thought to have improved efficacy as compared with conventional antipsychotics for the treatment of negative symptoms, with the results of CATIE studies, the current thinking is that both conventional and atypical antipsychotics are equally effective for the treatment of psychosis. With atypical antipsychotics, patients have much less risk for the development of tardive dyskinesia.
- The response to antipsychotic medication is heterogeneous and varies among patients.
- In general, the sequence of symptom response is as follows: positive symptoms, affective symptoms, cognitive and perceptual symptoms, and negative symptoms.
- NMS may be a fatal response to any antipsychotic medication. Although it is most frequently associated with conventional antipsychotics, it is also associated with atypical antipsychotics. It is important to recognize NMS and to treat it early. Careful diagnosis is necessary.
- A great majority of patients respond favorably to pharmacologic treatment. Failure rates are often caused by inadequate dosing or length of trial, particularly with antidepressants.
- Antidepressants usually cause changes in energy levels; increased energy may result in a patient's suicide attempt.

- Suicidal ideation often persists, so patients are at the highest risk to act on suicidal impulses during the early stage of treatment. Protect patients, and counsel them about the delay of desired effects with the use of antidepressants.
- Pharmacotherapy for depression has risk. Therefore, knowledge of toxicity and efficacy is important for optimal therapeutic response.
- Adjunctive therapy (e.g., with antipsychotics) is often used with lithium for bipolar disorder.
- Antianxiety medications such as benzodiazepines are an adjunct to therapy for short-term use. They are often an additive in long-term therapy as well.
- SSRIs are the first-line treatment for depression and for many anxiety disorders.
- Anticonvulsants are useful for the treatment of bipolar disorders and as adjunctive therapy for pain and other conditions.
- Herbal therapy is common. Caution patients about drug–drug and drug–herb interactions, and instruct them to consult a physician regarding any symptoms that they may experience. Patients should only use products with specifically labeled unit doses.

REVIEW QUESTIONS

1. A patient has been taking citalopram (Celexa) for 2 years for depression. The patient's outcomes have been achieved, and the patient wants to discontinue the medication. Which information should the nurse provide?
   1. "It's important for you to gradually stop taking this drug over 2 to 4 weeks."
   2. "Citalopram is an antidepressant medication that is usually taken for life."
   3. "Because your depression is alleviated, you may discontinue the medication."
   4. "Stopping this medication all of a sudden can cause serotonin syndrome."

2. A patient with schizophrenia was changed to a new antipsychotic medication 3 weeks ago. The patient calls the clinic nurse complaining of sore throat, fever, and malaise. Which laboratory test would be most helpful for determining the cause of these findings?
   1. Serum lithium level
   2. Complete blood cell count
   3. Liver panel
   4. Urinalysis

3. A patient who has been hospitalized for major depression has been taking sertraline (Zoloft) for the past week and has verbalized increased energy and improved sleep. What is the highest priority question that the nurse should ask?
   1. "Have you experienced any side effects from this drug?"
   2. "How has your appetite changed since starting this drug?"
   3. "Do you think your depression is less severe?"
   4. "Are you having any thoughts of harming yourself?"

4. A patient with bipolar disorder takes lithium. After playing soccer on a hot summer day, the patient complains of nausea, vomiting, diarrhea, and thirst. The patient's hands begin to tremble, and her gait becomes unsteady. Select the priority nursing interventions. You may select more than one answer.
   1. Complete an Abnormal Involuntary Movement Scale evaluation on this patient immediately.
   2. Instruct the patient to not take any more lithium until directed to do so by the physician.
   3. Collaborate with the physician about drawing a serum lithium level immediately.
   4. Administer an antiemetic medication to the patient.
   5. Collaborate with the physician regarding increasing the patient's daily lithium dose.

5. Quetiapine (Seroquel) is prescribed for a patient who smokes two packs of cigarettes per day. Which effect would be expected?
   1. Quetiapine will have a longer half-life for the patient, so fewer doses per day are needed.
   2. The doses of quetiapine will be lower than usual because of a slowed metabolism.
   3. This patient has a higher risk for the development of tardive dyskinesia.
   4. Higher doses of quetiapine will likely be needed to achieve therapeutic effects.

REFERENCES

Allen MH et al: Guidelines 10: initial medication strategies for a violent and unmanageable child: treatment of behavioral emergencies, Expert Consensus Guideline Series: a postgraduate medicine special report, White Plains, NY, 2001a, Expert Knowledge System.

Allen MH et al: Guidelines 12: Choice of oral atypical antipsychotic for an agitated, aggressive patient with a complicating medical condition: treatment of behavioral emergencies, Expert Consensus Guideline Series: a postgraduate medicine special report, White Plains, NY, 2001b, Expert Knowledge System.

Allen MH et al: Treatment of behavioral emergencies, Expert Consensus Guideline Series: a postgraduate medicine special report, White Plains, NY, 2001c, Expert Knowledge System.

American Psychiatric Association: Diagnostic and statistical manual of mental disorders, ed 4, text revision, Washington, DC, 2000, American Psychiatric Association.

Berkow R, editor: The Merck manual of diagnosis and therapy, ed 16, Whitehouse Station, NJ, 1992, Merck & Co, Inc.

Bialer M: Comparative pharmacokinetics of the newer antiepileptic drugs, Clin Pharmacokinet 24:441-452, 1993.

Bipolar disorder: management of acute mania in adults. In Manolakis PG: Guide to drug treatment protocols: a resource for creating and using disease-specific pathways, Washington, DC, 1999, American Pharmaceutical Association.

Bogan AM et al: Efficacy of divalproex therapy for schizoaffective disorder, J Clin Psychopharmacol 20:520-522, 2000.

Botts SR, Raskind J: Gabapentin and lamotrigine in bipolar disorder, Am J Health Syst Pharm 56:1939-1944, 1999.

Bupropion (Zyban) for smoking cessation, Med Lett Drugs Ther 39:77-78, 1997.

Celexa: citalopram product information, St. Louis, 2000, Forest Pharmaceuticals.

Chengappa KN et al: Bupropion sustained release as a smoking cessation treatment in remitted depressed patients maintained on treatment with selective serotonin reuptake inhibitor antidepressants, J Clin Psychiatry 62:503-508, 2001.

Claxton A et al: Patient compliance to a new enteric-coated weekly formulation of fluoxetine during continuation treatment of major depressive disorder, J Clin Psychiatry 61: 928-932, 2000.

Davis R, Wilde MI: Mirtazapine: a review of its pharmacology and therapeutic potential in the management of major depression, CNS Drugs 5:389-402, 1996.

Anonymous: Drugs that may cause psychiatric symptoms, Med Lett 44:59-62, 2002.

Elie R et al: Sleep latency is shortened during 4 weeks of treatment with zaleplon, a novel nonbenzodiazepine hypnotic, J Clin Psychiatry 60:536-544, 1999.

Fava M, Rankin MA: Sexual functioning and SSRIs, J Clin Psychiatry 63(Suppl 5):13-16, 2002.

Foa EB et al: *Treatment of posttraumatic stress disorder, Preferred medications for guideline 3: selecting a specific medication strategy, Expert Consensus Guideline Series*, White Plains, NY, 1999, Expert Knowledge System.

Frances A et al, editors: The expert consensus guideline series: treatment of bipolar disorder, *J Clin Psychiatry* 57(Suppl 12A):1-88, 1996.

Gelenberg AJ et al: Efficacy of venlafaxine extended release capsules in nondepressed outpatients with generalized anxiety disorder: a 6-month randomized controlled trial, *JAMA* 283:3082-3088, 2000.

Glassman AH, Thomas Bigger JT: Antipsychotic drugs: prolonged QTc interval, torsades de pointes, and sudden death, *Am J Psychiatry* 158:1774-1782, 2001.

Gorman JM: Mirtazapine: clinical overview, *J Clin Psychiatry* 60(Suppl 17):9-13, 1999.

Greenblatt D et al: Comparative kinetics and dynamics of zaleplon, zolpidem and placebo, *Clin Pharmacol Ther* 64:553-561, 1998.

Hermesh H et al: High serum creatinine kinase level: possible risk factor for neuroleptic malignant syndrome, *J Clin Psychopharmacol* 22:252-256, 2002.

Houtkooper MA et al: Oxcarbazepine (GP 47.680): a possible alternative to carbamazepine? *Epilepsia* 28(6):693-698, 1987.

Johannessen AC, Nielsen OA: Hyponatremia induced by oxcarbazepine, *Epilepsy Res* 1(2):155-156, 1987.

Katon W, Sullivan MD: Depression and chronic medical illness, *J Clin Psychiatry* 51(Suppl):3-11, 1990.

Kloster B et al: *Sudden death in two patients with epilepsy and the syndrome of inappropriate antidiuretic hormone secretion (SIADH)*, Sandvika, Norway, 1999, The National Center for Epilepsy.

Kramer TA: Dopamine system stabilizers, *Medscape Psychiatry Mental Health eJournal* 7, 2002.

Kushner MG et al: The relation between alcohol problems and the anxiety disorders, *Am J Psychiatry* 147:685-695, 1990.

Lexapro: *(Escitalopram) product information*, St. Louis, 2002, Forest Pharmaceuticals.

Martin R et al: Cognitive effects of topiramate, gabapentin, and lamotrigine in healthy young adults, *Neurology* 52:321-327, 1999.

Masand P et al: Psychostimulants in post-stroke depression, *J Neuropsychiatry Clin Neurosci* 3:23-27, 1991.

Micromedex: *Micromedex healthcare series*, vol 115, Greenwood Village, Colo, 1974-2003, Thomson Micromedex.

Neurontin: *gabapentin product information*, Morris Plains, NJ, 1999, Parke-Davis.

Nielson CP et al: Polymorphonuclear leukocyte inhibition by therapeutic concentrations of theophylline is mediated by cyclic-3,5-adenosine monophosphate, *Am Rev Respir Dis* 137:25-30, 1988.

Pendlebury SC et al: Hyponatremia during oxcarbazepine therapy, *Hum Toxicol* 8:337-344, 1989.

Ranier MK et al: Effect of risperidone on behavioral and psychological symptoms and cognitive function in dementia, *J Clin Psychiatry* 62:894-900, 2001.

Rawls WN: Trazodone B, *Drug Intell Clin Pharm* 16:7-13, 1982.

Reid CD: Chemical photosensitivity: another reason to be careful in the sun, *FDA Consumer Magazine* 1996.

Schatzberg AF, Nemeroff CB: *The American Psychiatric Press textbook of psychopharmacology*, ed 2, Washington, DC, 2001, American Psychiatric Publishing.

Shorter E: *A history of psychiatry: from the era of the asylum to the age of Prozac*, Hoboken, NJ, 1998, John Wiley & Sons.

Spivak B et al: Postural hypotension with syncope possibly precipitated by trazodone, *Am J Psychiatry* 144:11, 1987.

Steinhoff BJ et al: Hyponatremic coma under oxcarbazepine therapy, *Epilepsy Res* 11:67-70, 1992.

Taylor DM: Prolongation of QTc interval and antipsychotics, *Am J Psychiatry* 159:1062, discussion 1064, 2002.

Thase ME et al: Remission rates during treatment with venlafaxine or selective serotonin reuptake inhibitors, *Br J Psychiatry* 178:234-241, 2001.

Tohen M, Grundy S: Management of acute mania, *J Clin Psychiatry* 60(Suppl 5):31-34, 1999.

Van Amelsvoort TH et al: Hyponatremia associated with carbamazepine and oxcarbazepine therapy: a review, *Epilepsia* 35:181-188, 1994.

Wagner GJ et al: Dextroamphetamine as a treatment for depression and low energy in AIDS patients: a pilot study, *J Psychosom Res* 42:407-411, 1997.

Zakrzewska JM, Patsalos PN: Oxcarbazepine: a new drug in the management of intractable trigeminal neuralgia, *J Neurol Neurosurg Psychiatry* 52:472-476, 1989.

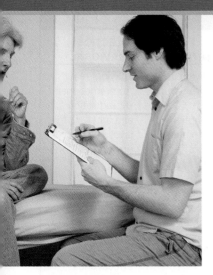

Therapies: Theory and Clinical Practice

Nancy A. Coffin-Romig

"You must be the change you wish to see in the world."

Mohandas K. Gandhi

evolve WEBSITE

http://evolve.elsevier.com/Fortinash/

OBJECTIVES

- Discuss the underlying theories of the humanistic, behavioral, cognitive behavioral, psychoanalytic/psychodynamic, supportive, and emotion-focused therapies.
- Describe the principles of individual, group, and family therapies and the role of the nurse.
- Describe the role of the nurse in maintaining a therapeutic community in the psychiatric mental health setting.

- Compare and contrast the stages and tasks of the family life cycle.
- Distinguish between occupational, recreational, art, music, psychodrama, and movement/dance therapies.
- Describe the historic evolution of electroconvulsive therapy as a biologic therapy and the role of the nurse.

KEY TERMS

activity therapies	continuous reinforcement	emotional triangle	recreational therapy
attachment	countertransference	genogram	role modeling
boundaries	curative factors	intermittent reinforcement	therapeutic milieu
classical conditioning	defense mechanisms	modeling	transference
cognitive appraisal	ego function	occupational therapy	
community meeting	electroconvulsive therapy	operant conditioning	

This chapter discusses the most common clinical therapies and their underlying theories in the field of psychiatry and mental health, (Table 26-1), and how nurses use their principles to provide nursing care to patients who are diagnosed with a mental illness. The knowledge and research that addresses the efficacy of clinical therapies are steadily growing.

Hildegard Peplau (1952 and 1992), a pioneer and educator in psychiatric nursing, regarded the nurse–patient relationship as the central framework for the implementation of therapeutic interventions. During the working phase of the nurse–patient relationship, the nurse helps the patient to identify difficulties, express feelings and thoughts, explore options and possibilities, and reinforce healthy coping. The

nurse helps the patient to change ineffective coping by providing alternative strategies for identifying and expressing underlying needs, acquiring new strategies in symptom management, adhering to medication, and role-playing interpersonal skills. (See Chapter 4 for more information about Peplau.)

THEORETIC PERSPECTIVES

Humanistic Approach

The humanistic approach emphasizes the human potential and the inherent worth of human beings as unique, self-actualizing, and self-determined with the capacity to develop

TABLE 26-1	**THEORETIC COMPONENTS OF THERAPIES**					
	PSYCHOANALYTIC	**HUMANISTIC**	**BEHAVIORAL**	**EMOTION FOCUSED**	**COGNITIVE**	**DIALECTIC BEHAVIORAL**
Basic orientation	All behavior is meaningful; unconscious impulses and conflicts influence behavior	Human beings move toward constructive change and integration	Behavior is learned	Emotion informs a person that an important need, value, or goal may be advanced or harmed in a situation	An individual's organization of thoughts and assumptions determines his or her affect and behavior	Behaviors result from emotional dysregulation and an invalidating environment
Concepts	Id, ego, and superego; unconscious and preconscious	Interpersonal relationships are the basis for health and neurosis	Conditioning; separation of the patient from the problem	Emotion schemes	Core beliefs; automatic thoughts; dysfunctional thinking	Emotional regulation; distress tolerance; interpersonal effectiveness; core mindfulness
Goal	Uncover the unconscious conflict and increase ego consciousness	Bring aspects of the self into awareness and acceptance	Modify observable behavior	Identify maladaptive emotions to make them amenable to change	Restructure cognitive appraisal, thereby changing mood and behavior	Accurately labeling emotions, monitoring behaviors, and developing a here-and-now awareness
Techniques	Dream analysis; free association	Person centered: genuineness, unconditional positive regard, and empathetic understanding	Systemic desensitization; relaxation training	Expressive enactment of the emotion; accessing needs and goals; emotional regulation	Cognitive: questioning and reattribution Behavioral: activity schedule and cognitive rehearsal	Chain analysis; telephone support; meditation skills

self-awareness. This self-awareness allows an individual to make choices that more fully enhance his or her quality of life in the full range of human experiences. Numerous therapies have developed since the movement began during the 1950s.

Abraham Maslow (1908-1970), who is considered the father of humanistic psychology, viewed human beings as being motivated by basic needs. He ordered basic needs in a hierarchy that started with survival needs, such as physiologic and safety needs, and that progressed toward more self-transcendent needs, such as love and belonging, esteem, and, ultimately, self-actualization (see Figure 1-1). Maslow theorized that an individual's coping behaviors determine that individual's ability to meet his or her basic needs and his or her satisfaction with meeting those needs. The blocking of or inability to meet basic needs leads to ineffective coping or, more seriously, to the development of psychopathology (Maslow, 1943). The nurse assists patients with identifying their current needs, how those needs are met, and the effectiveness of their coping behaviors.

Carl Rogers (1902-1987) was a renowned humanistic psychologist who developed the person-centered approach to therapy and identified *genuineness, unconditional positive*

regard, and *empathetic understanding* as the three essential elements in a therapeutic relationship. The nurse uses these elements to build trust and form a therapeutic alliance with the patient, with the goal of fostering constructive personality changes in the patients as they progress though the phases of the nurse-patient relationship (Rogers, 1957 and 1980).

Behavioral Approach

Behavioral therapies maintain that behavior is a learned response to a stimulus in the environment. The behavioral approach—in combination with cognitive and pharmacologic therapies—has proven to be effective for the treatment of attention-deficit/hyperactivity disorder, anxiety disorders, and eating disorders. The purpose of behavioral therapy is to decrease or increase the probability of an identified behavior.

Classical Conditioning

Ivan Pavlov (1849-1936) was a Russian physiologist who won the Nobel Prize for his work on the digestive system, which he studied through his famous experiments with dogs. Pavlov observed that dogs salivated whenever they anticipated that food was forthcoming, and he labeled this phenomenon *psychic secretion.* He theorized that the dogs learned to associate certain events with the presence of food and therefore salivated before tasting the food (i.e., learned association). Pavlov developed his theory of classical conditioning (1928) when he paired a neutral stimulus (a bell) with another stimulus (a food that triggered salivation). Eventually, the sound of the bell alone triggered salivation in the dogs. Extinction of this response occurred when the dogs were no longer offered food, and they therefore stopped salivating at the sound of the bell (Pavlov, 1928).

Behaviorism

John B. Watson (1878-1958) was an American psychologist who developed the behaviorism school of thought. He was influenced by Pavlov's principles and stressed the importance of the social environment with the shaping of behavior. Watson is well known for his work with a child named Albert in which the therapist made a loud noise each time Albert reached for a white rat. Eventually, Albert became frightened of the rat and later all furry animals, even without the noise. Some have questioned Watson's ethics in conducting such an experiment with a child; however, he was able to show that controlling the stimulus could change or shape behavior.

Operant Conditioning

B.F. Skinner (1904-1990) was an American behavioral psychologist who coined the term *operant conditioning* as a method for modifying behavior in animals, which he then applied to people. In operant conditioning, changing a behavior involves identifying three elements: the stimulus, the response, and the reinforcer (Figure 26-1). The stimulus is the environmental event that immediately precedes a behavior. The response is the action or overt behavior that occurs immediately after the stimulus. The reinforcer or the consequence/feedback strengthens the behavior by either raising or lowering the probability of the behavior occurring again (Skinner, 1987).

Reinforcement. There are two categories of consequences that are used in operant conditioning that are designed to increase or decrease the probability of a behavior occurring in the future by changing the type of consequences over a set time interval. The reinforcement of a behavior by rewarding each behavior on the same time interval or when a correct response occurs is known as *continuous reinforcement.* *Intermittent reinforcement* occurs when the reinforcer is delivered on a slightly different time interval or after a set number of correct responses called a *schedule* (Table 26-2). Table 26-3 describes four types of reinforcement.

Underlying Principles of Behavioral Therapy

Modeling. The principle of modeling maintains that behavioral change occurs through the observation of behaviors in others that bring positive or negative consequences (Bandura, 1969). For example, children often imitate the behavior patterns of parents, teachers, and peers. Role-playing is another form of modeling in which patients have the opportunity to observe the modeling of new behavior and then practice the new behavior and receive feedback. An example is a nurse conducting a psychoeducational group on assertive behavior. One of the roles of the nurse is to model healthy behavior and then provide guidance and feedback to patients who exhibit difficulties with verbalizing needs, speaking to the physician about medications, and managing and expressing feelings such as anxiety, anger, fear, and interpersonal conflict. The nurse provides positive reinforcement with verbal praise when the patient exhibits behavior that is adaptive for everyday social encounters.

Premack Principle. The Premack principle states that a frequently occurring positive behavioral response serves as a positive reinforcer for less frequent desired responses

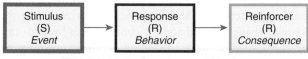

FIGURE 26-1. Operant conditioning.

TABLE 26-2	INTERMITTENT SCHEDULES	
CLASS	**METHOD**	**EXAMPLE**
Fixed interval	The first correct response or consequence is given within a set amount of time.	A child is rewarded with a star on a chart for sitting in his or her seat quietly within 1 minute after the bell rings for class to begin.
Variable interval	The first correct response or consequence is given after a set amount of time passes, but, after the consequence is given, a new time period (either shorter or longer) is set. Behavior that is reinforced by a variable interval schedule is more difficult to change or extinguish.	This is often seen with the inconsistent enforcement of rules and rewards for children by parents and teachers.
Fixed ratio	After a specified amount of a correct behavior or response occurs, a reinforcer or consequence is given.	A child is given a token at the end of the day for washing his or her hands before every meal.
Variable ratio	A reinforcer or consequence is given with a varying correct number of responses or desired behaviors. This type of variable–ratio schedule is most effective for the maintenance of behavior.	Children on the inpatient psychiatric unit receive a reward of praise by staff when they use the verbal expression of feelings instead of acting out their feelings of frustration or anger.

TABLE 26-3	TYPES OF REINFORCEMENT	
TYPE	**DEFINITION**	**EXAMPLE**
Positive	A pleasant or desirable behavior occurs and a positive reinforcer or consequence is added to increase the frequency of the response.	A teacher smiling at a student during class when the student gives a correct response to a question
Negative	A behavior is used to stop or avoid a stimulus or condition that is undesirable.	Testing the temperature of the water before stepping into the shower so as to not be burned
Punishment	A negative consequence is given in response to an undesirable behavior to weaken the frequency.	Giving a child a time out or removing points for hitting another child
Extinction	The connection between a behavior and a response is broken by removing the reinforcer.	Ignoring or walking away when a child engages in a temper tantrum

(Premack, 1959). For example, parents require their children to pick up their toys before going out to play or going online to chat with friends after their homework is completed. This principle is best used with children and adolescents when facilitating behavioral changes to increase tolerance for delayed gratification.

Shaping. Shaping is a principle that requires the use of reinforcements in a step sequence that leads to a change in a target behavior. The nurse schedules reinforcements or consequences in close approximation to the desired behavioral response. For example, a child with attention-deficit/hyperactivity disorder disrupts class by interrupting the teacher's lesson. First, the nurse designs a behavioral token system to reward the child for not speaking out during class each hour of the school day. The following week, the nurse adds the accompanying behavior of raising the hand to the first behavior and gives the child a reward. The following week, the nurse adds waiting to be called on to the two previous behaviors and gives a reward when the child performs all three behaviors in the correct sequence.

Counterconditioning. The goal of counterconditioning is to replace a negative response to a stimulus with a positive response. This method of behavior modification was developed by Joseph Wolpe (1958), an American psychiatrist who was born in South Africa (1915-1997). Wolpe's method, called *reciprocal inhibition*, aims to assist the patient with learning an alternative response to disturbing stimuli such as phobias, anxiety disorders, and pain. The most common technique of counterconditioning is systematic desensitization, which assists individuals with overcoming a fear of a particular stimulus (e.g., an animal, heights, riding in an elevator, public speaking, flying). The therapist and the patient form a systematic hierarchy of progressive encounters with the feared stimulus. A number between 1 and 10 is assigned to each encounter and leads to the final direct encounter with the feared stimulus. The therapist pairs relaxation techniques with each stage of exposure, and the patient progresses through each stage to a direct encounter with the feared stimulus until symptoms are extinguished. Recent advances in computer technology and software development have led to the development of virtual reality exposure therapy for the treatment of the phobias of flying, heights, animals, claustrophobia, and posttraumatic stress disorder

(Botella et al, 2004; Coelho et al, 2009; Krihn et al, 2004; Parsons and Rizzo, 2008; Rothbaum, 2009; Wolitzky-Taylor et al, 2008). Aversion therapy is another type of treatment that pairs a noxious response or unpleasant consequences with a stimulus. The most common form is the use of the drug disulfiram (Antabuse), which induces severe nausea, vomiting, and headache when an individual ingests alcohol. The purpose is to remove the positive effect and replace it with a negative response, thereby creating an aversion to the drinking of alcohol. (see Chapter 10).

The Role of the Nurse

The primary role of the nurse who is using behavioral therapy is to assess and identify the patient's problem behaviors in collaboration with the multidisciplinary team. Next, the nurse determines the schedule of reinforcement and the reinforcers to use. The two types of behavior management programs that are most frequently used in mental health settings are the contingency contract and token economy. The contingency contract is a written agreement between the mental health providers and the patient and family regarding the behavior change desired and the consequences for performing the desired behavior; including negative consequences. All parties sign the contract, and the nurse places it in the patient's chart with a timetable for evaluation. A token economy is a system of behavior reinforcements in which patients earn tokens by performing predetermined desired behaviors. Tokens carry a value and can be exchanged for items that have different point values.

Cognitive Behavioral Therapy

Aaron T. Beck, an American psychiatrist who was born in 1921, developed cognitive therapy at the University of Pennsylvania in the early 1960s. Cognitive therapy is based on the premise that distorted or dysfunctional thinking causes psychologic disturbances in mood and behavior. A large body of research exists to prove the efficacy of cognitive therapy for bipolar disorder (Beynon et al, 2009); depression (Beck, 1995; Jonsson and Hougaard, 2008); anxiety disorders (Beck, 1995; Hofmann et al, 2008); and the prevention and treatment of traumatic stress (Roberts et al, 2009). The therapist works with the patient to identify and correct dysfunctional thinking patterns, which in turn alleviate symptoms of depression, anxiety, and traumatic stress and help to prevent relapse in bipolar disorders.

The cognitive model proposes that perceptions and the interpretation of events through a process called *cognitive appraisal* influence emotions and behaviors. How the person thinks about a situation or event governs that individual's emotional responses and behaviors. During childhood, individuals begin to develop certain core beliefs about themselves that tend to be global, rigid, and overgeneralized.

Core beliefs for individuals who are depressed usually involve self-worth or self-esteem and are often statements such as "I am worthless," "I am incompetent," "I will never amount to anything," "I am a terrible person," and so on. These core beliefs lead to attitudes, rules, and assumptions that influence how an individual perceives a situation or event. Intermediate beliefs or attitudes, rules, and assumptions become a way to manage or deal with core beliefs. The core belief of "I am not smart" involves an intermediate belief such as, "I must get an A" or "No matter how much I study, I will never get an A." These intermediate beliefs generate automatic thoughts when a situation occurs that involves studying. In this instance, the individual says, "I don't understand the reading material." The person feels anxious and frustrated (emotion) and closes the book (behavior) (Figure 26-2).

The goal of cognitive therapy is to assist the patient with identifying automatic thoughts and connecting these thoughts to feelings. Patients have homework such as keeping a diary or log for tracking feelings, thoughts, and behaviors; reading assignments; and completing exercises. During sessions with the therapist, the patient and the therapist review logs and explore situations that generate problems. The therapist explores with the patient, the situation or event that generated distress or difficulty and then asks questions such as: "What was going through your mind at that time?" "What did you think when he told you the news?" "How did you feel after hearing your grade?" "What did you do then?" Through the process of questioning the validity of automatic thoughts, the therapist challenges intermediate and core beliefs and helps the patient to generate alternative responses.

Beck and colleagues (1979) listed the most common types of automatic thoughts or cognitive errors among depressed patients, which are as follows:

- *Overgeneralization.* The patient reaches general conclusions on the basis of a single event and excludes any other facts; these beliefs are often negative, and they lead to feelings of helplessness or hopelessness.
- *Mental filtering.* The patient filters out certain facts that are often positive to fit a core belief or an assumption about an event.
- *Catastrophizing.* The patient focuses on the negative aspects of a situation or event and predicts an outcome of failure to the exclusion of other possible outcomes.
- *Minimization.* The patient discounts the positive results of his or her accomplishments, which reinforces a negative self-appraisal; this often leads to an overemphasis on and reinforcement of negative outcomes from the past.
- *Magnification.* The patient focuses only on the negative facts of a situation and excludes other facts.
- *Dichotomization.* The patient sorts or divides events into judgment categories of good or bad and all or nothing, which leads to narrow definitions of success and failure.
- *Arbitrary inference or fortune telling.* The patient draws automatic conclusions about the outcome of a situation without considering the actual facts in the situation and alternative solutions that are available.
- *Personalization.* The patient interprets the outcome of an event as reflective only of one's actions and excluding the responsibility of others or other facts that have influenced the situation.

Dialectic Behavioral Therapy

Traditional treatment with cognitive behavioral therapy focuses on changing thoughts, feelings, and behaviors. Marsha M. Linehan, an American psychologist (born 1943), initially developed dialectic behavioral therapy (DBT) in 1993 for patients who are diagnosed with borderline personality disorder, and who often exhibit self-harm behaviors. This disorder often involves self-cutting or burning, chronic pattern of suicide attempts, impulsivity, and intense emotional displays that alternate with episodes of anxiety, shame, and depression. Several studies of DBT have found that the therapeutic techniques developed by Linehan were successful for patients suffering from borderline personality disorder (Bohus et al, 2004; Linehan et al, 1991 and 2006; Turner, 2000) and more recently for patients with other disorders, such as eating disorders (Tech et al, 2001), and for chronically depressed older adults (Lynch et al, 2003).

Linehan (1993) maintains that emotional dysregulation or difficulties are the result of an inborn temperament that leads to an inability to regulate emotions or to an emotional vulnerability, which includes high sensitivity to emotional stimuli, emotional intensity, and difficulty with returning to a more neutral emotional baseline. The other central factor is the presence of an invalidating environment that includes dismissing an individual's interpretation of feelings, thoughts, or behaviors; informing the individual that his or her description and analysis of his or her own experience is "wrong"; and telling the individual that his or her experiences are socially unacceptable or that they represent

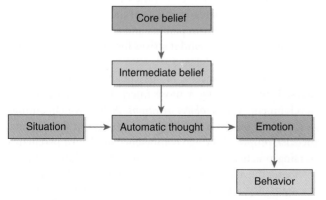

FIGURE 26-2. The cognitive behavioral model.

undesirable personality traits. In addition, an invalidating environment does not permit or ignores attempts at communicating private inner experiences of thoughts and feelings, experiences of others, and resulting self-appraisal and interpretation of the social environment. Patients who have experienced physical, emotional, and sexual abuse; patients with borderline personality disorder or eating disorders such as bulimia, anorexia, and obesity; and patients with depression and substance abuse often describe experiencing an invalidating environment. The consequences of an invalidating environment and emotional vulnerability lead to an inability to accurately describe or label inner experiences and emotional states, difficulty with tolerating distressing states, difficulty with forming realistic goals and expectations, and the inability to trust one's own thoughts, emotions, and interpretations of outer events and individuals (Linehan, 1993). Changes in patients with borderline personality disorder occur by helping the patients to build skills that involve mindfulness meditation, to reduce emotional dysregulation, and to increase validating and dialectic strategies. (Lynch et al, 2006).

Patients who are engaged in DBT receive three treatment modalities: (1) individual therapy; (2) group therapy; and (3) telephone support. The goal of treatment is to assist patients with increasing their tolerance; regulating their emotions; and learning to adopt more effective behavioral responses in a validating therapeutic environment.

Individual Therapy

Therapists identify behavioral targets and rank them as life-threatening, therapy-interfering, and quality-of-life–interfering behaviors. The patient self-monitors the behaviors via weekly diary cards, and the therapist highlights the highest-priority behaviors. Sessions focus on the analysis of events that led to the problem, and exploring the emotional responses that led to the problematic or target behavior. During this process, the therapist validates the patient's responses and offers alternative behavioral responses to the emotions that are being experienced. Telephone consultation is available between sessions to help reinforce new behavioral responses.

Group Skills Training

This second phase of treatment consists of four modules:
1. *Core mindfulness skills.* The therapist teaches meditation skills to assist the patient with developing a here-and-now awareness through observing, describing, and participating fully in one's actions and experiences, without judgment.
2. *Interpersonal effectiveness skills.* The therapist teaches effective ways of achieving objectives with other people by learning and practicing assertiveness skills, managing conflict, and maintaining relationships and self-esteem.
3. *Emotion modulation skills.* The therapist helps the patient to evaluate and manage emotional responses through exposure, the blocking of ineffective behavioral responses, and the substituting of effective responses.

4. *Distress tolerance skills.* The therapist teaches learning techniques for tolerating emotional distress and unmet needs through finding meaning and acceptance.

In a controlled study, Bohus and colleagues (2004) found that patients who participated in a 3-month inpatient DBT treatment program demonstrated statistically significant improvement in a variety of symptoms.

DBT provides nurses with opportunities for assisting patients with developing skills for managing emotional dysregulation and ineffective behavioral responses (e.g., self-harm, chronic suicide attempts).

Psychoanalytic Psychodynamic Approach

Gallop and O'Brien (2003) maintain that the psychoanalytic psychodynamic theory in psychiatric mental health nursing practice, provides a deeper understanding of how early childhood relationships and experiences heavily influence the patient's symptoms and interpersonal difficulties. Principles from the newly emerged supportive psychotherapy model discussed later in this section offer general guidelines for psychosocial interventions for nurses who are working in a variety of health care settings.

Sigmund Freud (1856-1939), an Austrian physician, is the founder of psychoanalytic theory. A variety of schools of thought regarding personality structure and development have evolved over the past century from Freud's original theory in an attempt to more fully explore the relationship between the ego and the unconscious (Jung, 1966); ego formation or object relations (Mahler et al, 1975; Winnicott, 1965) and self-psychology (Kohut, 1977; Stern, 1985); and attachment theory. The initial focus of psychoanalytic psychotherapy was on the psychic or psychologic structure of the personality. Freud (1960) proposed the structure of id, ego, and superego:

- The id is the primitive undifferentiated level of the personality that consists of drives, instincts, needs, and reflexes. It is irrational by nature and operates on the pleasure principle.
- The ego develops or emerges during the first 6 months of life and develops with the purpose of mediating between the outside world and the irrational id impulses. The ego operates on the reality principle.
- The superego is the last stage of personality structure development and represents the moral aspect of the personality. The superego consists of the internalized rules of conduct learned from parents and other authority figures regarding morality, and it strives for the ideal in personality development.

Subsequent followers of psychoanalytic theory have focused on expanding a more interpersonal model of ego development, called *object relations theory*, which outlines descriptions of ego function. Norine J. Kerr (1990), a nurse theorist, proposed the ego competency model for psychiatric nursing practice on the basis of the object relations theory involving the assessment of ego functioning in terms of ego strengths and deficits. Kerr contends that patients receive mental health treatment because of deficits or weaknesses in

BOX 26-1	EGO COMPETENCY MODEL

- **Impulse control:** Effectiveness with which impulses are adaptively controlled
- **Mood:** Ability to sustain a normal range of moods that vary appropriately with external occurrences
- **Judgment:** Ability to anticipate the consequences of one's behaviors
- **Reality testing:** Accuracy of the perception of external events
- **Self-perception:** Ability to regulate appropriate feelings of self-esteem
- **Object relations:** Degree and quality of relatedness to others
- **Thought processes:** Characteristic mode of thinking and language expression
- **Activities of daily living:** Ability to use existing ego strengths to achieve self-maintenance
- **Stimulus barrier:** Degree to which sensory stimuli are adaptively screened

From Kerr NJ: The ego competency model of psychiatric nursing: theoretical overview and clinical application, *Perspect Psychiatr Care* 26:13-24, 1990. (onlinelibrary.wiley.com/doi/10.1111/j.1744-6163.1990.tb00323.x). Published online January 2009.

ego functioning when coping with common stressors of everyday living, difficulties with social and personal relationships, and impairments in self-identity. The number of ego functions affected and the severity of deficits govern the patient's level of overall functioning and treatment goals. An assessment of ego functioning (Box 26-1) provides the nurse with important data for developing a care plan that is designed to help patients to increase their ego functioning and enhance their quality of life.

The contemporary psychoanalytic and psychodynamic approach to therapy is the existence of the unconscious as a component of the individual's personality structure. The unconscious is the location of repressed memories from childhood; particularly traumatic memories, which are seen as the source of psychopathology. Present-day difficulties with relationships or overwhelming feelings of depression or anxiety originate during early childhood relationships and traumatic experiences. Unconscious repressed unmet childhood needs or traumas influence conscious behavior. The goal of psychoanalytic/psychodynamic therapy is to bring repressed memories into conscious awareness. The psychodynamic therapist helps the patient to develop a conscious awareness of the defenses employed by the ego to ward off intrapsychic conflict.

Defense Mechanisms

Anna Freud (1895-1982), in *The Ego and the Mechanisms of Defense* (1937), developed the concept of the ego as the mediator between the id and the superego and the use of defense mechanisms when conflicts occur between the ego and the id or the superego. The defense mechanisms protect the ego by channeling the overwhelming anxiety that is generated by the conflict. Defense mechanisms operate unconsciously or

consciously, and they are sometimes adaptive or become unhealthy when they prevent an individual from confronting reality or when they impair psychologic growth (see Chapter 10 for more information about defense mechanisms). Symptoms of psychopathology are largely reflective of an ineffective use of defense mechanisms.

Transference and Countertransference

Sigmund Freud (1959) is credited with the discovery of the phenomenon of transference. The term *transference* refers to the unconscious projection of feelings, thoughts, or unsatisfied or repressed wishes, which are transferred onto the therapist or nurse in the therapeutic relationship. Transference is marked by strong feelings from the patient toward the therapist or nurse, and it can be positive or negative. For example, a patient sends letters to a nurse requesting additional contact after discharge from the hospital. The phenomenon of transference can occur in any relationship. Psychoanalytic and psychodynamic therapists assist patients with working through the projected or transferred feelings from earlier relationships as they arise in the therapist–patient relationship. The patient's reactions or feelings often evoke a response in the therapist or nurse of empathy, nurturing, approval, sexual attraction, self-importance, anger, irritability, rejection, or caretaking. These feelings or thoughts toward a patient from the therapist or nurse are called *countertransference*. An example of countertransference is a strong dislike or attraction to a patient that affects the ability of the nurse to provide care. These are conscious or unconscious feelings, and they are signaled by an overly strong emotional reaction to the patient that can be either positive or negative. As the patient does during transference, the therapist or nurse projects or displaces his or her feelings toward people in the past onto the patient, which is representative of unsatisfied or repressed needs. The recognition of transference and countertransference reactions by the therapist or nurse remains vital to maintaining the boundaries of the therapeutic relationship. A lack of awareness or consciousness leads to boundary violations and prevents progress with regard to assisting the patient with meeting treatment goals (Peternelj-Taylor and Yonge, 2003; Stiles, 2004).

Therapeutic Techniques

Psychoanalytic and psychodynamic-oriented psychotherapists primarily integrate the transference and countertransference within the therapeutic relationship as a source of unconscious material. By developing trust with the patient, the therapist forms a therapeutic alliance, which helps to promote the transference that leads to the exploration of projected wishes and needs. Together, the patient and the therapist identify defense mechanisms and carefully challenge them, thereby allowing for a gradual release of repressed memories. The psychotherapist helps the patient to explore emerging memories and associated feelings and thoughts and to integrate them into consciousness by gaining a deeper understanding of the effect of childhood memories on present symptoms. By contrast, psychoanalysts primarily use the techniques of word association (Jung, 1966) and dream analysis (Freud, 1961; Jung, 1969) when working with patients. For this technique, dreams are an objective source of material that symbolically reflects the intrapsychic conflict that causes the patient's symptoms. Patients record dreams and interpret them with the therapist. Through personal associations with symbols, images, or individuals that appear in the dreams, unconscious feelings and memories emerge. The analyst helps the patient to integrate repressed material, which eventually leads to a reduction or absence of symptoms.

Supportive Psychotherapy

A revised model of psychodynamic psychotherapy has emerged in recent years called *supportive psychotherapy* (Misch, 2000; Viederman, 2008; Winston et al, 2004). The aim of this treatment model is for the therapist to establish an authentic and meaningful dialogue or "being with the patient" to help the patient to resolve an internal conflict or crisis (Viederman, 2008). A strong therapeutic alliance through active participation by the therapist is used versus the more passive role employed by the therapist in traditional psychoanalytic and insight-oriented psychotherapy. The primary focus is on the "here and now" to gain insight into earlier experiences as they relate to the current situation. The effectiveness of supportive psychotherapy and psychodynamic psychotherapy for a wide variety of psychiatric disorders (Chrits-Christoph, 2008; Leichsenring, 2007) including quality of life among patients with breast cancer (Boutin, 2007) is widely supported by research.

Emotion-Focused Therapy

Emotion-focused therapy is based on the premise that emotion is a universal language and a fundamental experience of being human. Current research reveals that emotions serve as a primary meaning system that informs people about the significance of events to their well-being (Greenberg, 2004). Emotion-focused therapy has been effective for the treatment of adult survivors of child abuse; for sexual assault survivors; for patients with depression, anxiety disorders, and anorexia nervosa; and for couples therapy (Anderson et al, 2010; Ellison et al, 2009; Greenberg, 2004; Greenberg et al, 2010; Macintosh and Johnson, 2008; Palvio and Nieuwenhuis, 2001; Rasoli et al, 2008). Emotional schemes underlie the experiences of trauma, anxiety, depression, and other psychologic disorders. The three principles of emotion-focused therapy are: (1) increasing the awareness of emotions by attending to bodily sensations; (2) enhancing emotion regulation; and (3) transforming emotion. The aim of emotion-focused therapy is to access primary adaptive emotions (e.g., anger, fear, sadness, disgust, surprise, joy) and maladaptive secondary emotions (e.g., shame, guilt, hopelessness, helplessness, abandonment, loneliness, worthlessness). Unhealthy thoughts associated with unhealthy secondary emotions are challenged by forming a new inner voice that is based on the patient's healthy primary emotions and needs and that improves his or her emotional regulation (Greenberg, 2004). The outcome is the enhancement of emotion-focused coping skills by helping patients to come to terms with their emotional experiences.

THERAPEUTIC MILIEU

Historic Development

Maxwell Jones (1907-1990), a social psychiatrist, developed the concept of the therapeutic community during the 1950s. His goal was to develop a structure in psychiatric settings that builds a therapeutic environment (Jones, 1968). He believed that the therapeutic community was a critical factor for determining successful treatment outcomes. He based his writings mainly on his experiences and observations of long-term state psychiatric hospitals. His writings were an effort to establish hospital or community mental health treatment environments that optimize treatment outcomes for patients with psychiatric disorders. Jones (1968) identified three factors that determine the therapeutic effectiveness of the social environment:

1. The presence of two-way communication between the patients and the members of the multidisciplinary team
2. An effective decision-making process during all levels of treatment and between staff members and patients
3. Opportunities for social learning to address interpersonal problem areas

Jones (1968) saw the psychiatric setting as a living laboratory for experimenting or learning new ways of problem solving for conflicts and crises. The psychiatric setting in essence becomes a microcosm of the larger society. The roles of the nurse in promoting a therapeutic milieu include the following:

- Observing behaviors and providing opportunities for the patient to receive feedback and to develop new skills for coping with everyday interpersonal relationships
- Helping the patient with problem solving to meet basic needs
- Identifying feelings, thoughts, and behaviors in response to stressors
- Managing psychiatric symptoms and improving communication skills

The **therapeutic milieu** is an environment that is created and maintained to restore and promote optimal psychologic health and wellness. The nursing profession has always recognized the importance of the therapeutic milieu to healing. Florence Nightingale (1820-1910), a British nurse who is considered the founder of modern nursing, defined her work as organizing the environment to allow the mind and body to heal. The same principle is true for psychiatric mental health nursing.

The psychiatric unit is a social system in its own right, with patients at various points in their lengths of stay. Each patient has his or her own agenda and interacts within the milieu to meet his or her unique personal and social needs. The milieu is both a large work group with the task of healing and a community with all the tasks of communal living. The psychiatric mental health nurse is the manager of the milieu as set forth by the American Nurses Association in the standards of psychiatric and mental health nursing practice (see the inside back cover). The nursing staff manage the unit 24 hours a day, and lead the interdisciplinary team with planning and implementing patient treatment goals, performing nursing care, and overseeing unit program activities. The overall goal is the promotion and the maintenance of an optimal healing environment. The seven major elements of an optimal healing environment framework are as follows: (1) building healing spaces; (2) creating healing places; (3) developing awareness and intention; (4) experiencing personal wholeness; (5) cultivating healing relationships; (6) practicing healthy lifestyles; and (7) applying collaborative medicine. with interdisciplinary teams that employ traditional and complementary therapies (Jonas and Chez, 2004).

Functions of the Therapeutic Milieu

Walker (1994) outlines Gunderson's (1983) five functions of structure, involvement, containment, support, and validation to create a positive treatment environment or therapeutic milieu.

- Structure: organizing time; scheduling activities; providing physical space, and the physical environment; unit activities, policies, and rules; medication administration; etc.
- Involvement: patients are expected to be active and collaborative participants in the formulation of treatment goals, to participate in selected unit activities, to accept feedback, to interact with other patients, and to provide constructive feedback to others.
- Containment: those functions that are helpful for the safety of the patient, the nurse, and other patients. It includes the use of locked areas, seclusion, restraints, and frequent monitoring (i.e., one to one or close observation) that assist patients with managing aggressive behaviors, decreasing environmental stimuli, and managing personal boundaries.
- Support: the staff efforts to promote patient self-esteem and well-being by demonstrating respect, individualizing treatment and care, and fostering social support and collaboration among peers.
- Validation: acknowledging a patient's individual needs when appropriate, considering a patient's unique personal history, and accepting the patient's experience and potential.

Goals of Milieu Therapy

The goals of maintaining and supporting the therapeutic milieu are the primary responsibilities of nursing in collaboration with the patients and the multidisciplinary team. The most common goals of the therapeutic milieu are as follows:

- Providing a physically and psychologically safe environment
- Maximizing the highest level of psychologic functioning
- Identifying acute or chronic physical illnesses that are affecting psychiatric symptoms
- Promoting healthy coping behavioral strategies and symptom management

- Helping to promote independent activities of daily living
- Educating patients and their families about medications and other therapeutic modalities
- Establishing collaborative discharge planning with the patient or family and the multidisciplinary team

Structure in the Psychiatric Milieu

The goals of the therapeutic milieu are structured by the boundaries, roles, and functions of the patients and members of the multidisciplinary team. Patients are responsible for being active participants in the treatment plan by doing the following:

- Attending scheduled activities
- Participating in treatment planning and goal setting
- Meeting regularly with members of the interdisciplinary team
- Acquiring effective problem-solving skills and emotional coping strategies
- Performing self-care activities
- Adhering to the medication regimen

Nurses are primarily responsible for managing the structure of the psychiatric unit by maintaining the unit schedule of patient activities, which include the following:

- Completing hygiene and grooming
- Participating in mealtimes
- Taking medications at the prescribed times
- Participating in unit assignments (e.g., watering plants, keeping the dayroom organized, running community meetings, attending planned activity therapies)
- Meeting with multidisciplinary team members

Patients have free time for patio breaks, social interactions, and individual meetings with staff.

Boundaries

The nurse maintains boundaries in the psychiatric setting by clearly outlining the roles of the staff and the patient, meeting responsibilities for the achievement of treatment goals, and maintaining the integrity of the therapeutic milieu.

Safety

The nurse enforces the following basic rules in order to promote and maintain a safe environment for patients, staff, and visitors.

- Patients will not have access to harmful items such as sharps, belts, and shoelaces.
- Patients will not have the means to harm themselves or others on the unit.
- Approved methods for managing patients who are at high risk for aggressive behavior are available to staff.
- Therapeutic communication skills, staff training, and collaborative relationships among staff are essential for ensuring a safe environment.

Therapeutic Interactions

The responsibility of the nurse is to maintain a therapeutic relationship that is built on trust, rapport, mutual respect, and interactions that focus on the patient and his or her treatment goals (see the Research for Evidence-Based Practice box later in this chapter).

Communication

Open communication by the nurse and other team members regarding observations of patient behaviors, interactions with peers, adherence to unit activities, and individual interactions between staff and patient, helps to develop flexible boundaries for communication among the treatment team members. Evaluating the patient's treatment plan and goals is an ongoing process that requires periodic modification. Nurses provide 24-hour care and play a key role in the evaluation process (see Chapters 3 and 4).

Role-Modeling

The nurse who role-models effective interpersonal skills (e.g., respect, caring, genuineness, assertiveness, conflict resolution) promotes an environment of trust and emotional safety for patients in the therapeutic milieu. The nurse is responsible for modeling nurse–patient interactions that demonstrate and reinforce healthy boundaries between the nursing staff and patients or between patients and their peers. Role-modeling provides significant opportunities for patients to learn how to have mature and effective interpersonal interactions with staff and with each other (see Chapter 4).

Yurkovich (1989) described three phases through which patients progress during their hospitalization as they adapt to the therapeutic milieu. The role of the nurse changes to accommodate the patient's length of stay and the degree of familiarity that the patient has with the treatment setting. The nurse's function is to respond in ways that consistently promote the stated goals. The three phases and the different roles of the nurse during each phase are presented in Table 26-4.

Structure of the Mental Health Unit

Community Meeting

Most mental health units conduct some type of group meeting that is designed to review staff and patient roles and responsibilities in the milieu and to address issues that inevitably occur as part of communal living. The mental health community meeting is made up of staff and patients, and it generally occurs during the morning shift, with a brief review sometimes held in the afternoon. The goals of the meeting include the following:

- Introduce new patients to the staff, the milieu, and the other patients.
- Orient all patients to scheduled unit activities and groups, and explain the functions of the activities and groups.
- Introduce patients to their primary contact person for each shift and to the medication nurse.
- Ask each patient to state at least one goal that he or she has for the day. A goal may be as simple as taking a shower, or be as complex as preparing for discharge. All goals are accepted, because they reflect the patient's place on the health–illness continuum.

TABLE 26-4	PATIENT AND NURSE ROLES IN THE THERAPEUTIC COMMUNITY	
PHASES	**PATIENT ROLES**	**NURSE ROLES**
Newcomer	Follower	Gives information
	Seeks information	Provides introductions
	Observes group	Supports socialization
Member	Gives information	Encourages risk taking
	Gives opinions	Provides opportunities
	Encourager	for contributions
	Activator	Plans for behavioral
	Compromiser	change
Leader	Initiator/contributor	Gives feedback to
	Coordinator	patient from
	Orientor	therapeutic community
	Evaluator/critic	Provides positive
	Standard setter	feedback
	Gatekeeper	Shares an evaluation of
		patient roles in the
		therapeutic community
		with the patient

From Yurkovich E: Patient and nurse roles in the therapeutic community, *Perspect Psychiatr Care* 25:18-22, 1989.

- Review old business that patients want to bring up (e.g., "The smoking rules are way too strict." "My shower still has cold water." "What did we decide about telephone use?").
- Discuss any new business that patients have (e.g., "I suggest that we get some new videos. How do other people feel?" "I don't think the patient assignments are fair.").
- Assign each patient (with the patient's consent) to a unit activity in accordance with the patient's capability and the length of time that he or she has spent on the unit. Typical assignments include kitchen and dayroom organization, taking meeting minutes, and presenting unit rules for smoking, laundry, telephone use, visiting hours, and so on.

In summary, a community meeting provides an opportunity for patients to be oriented to the unit, to meet other patients and their primary contact persons, to voice concerns, to ask questions, to state their goals of the day, to discuss old and new business, and to problem solve regarding issues related to communal living. Because appropriate task completion is essential to mental health, the nurse carefully explains the functions and tasks of the various groups and activities offered on the unit. This promotes the opportunity for each group or activity to be used as effectively as possible for each patient.

Table 26-5 illustrates an example of an effective therapeutic community meeting. The nurse leader in this community meeting facilitated movement toward the stated goals of introductions, orientation, and organization. The nurse took the opportunity to assess the general tone of the milieu and to make observations regarding individual patients. For example, Patty seemed somewhat bewildered, and Lynette

TABLE 26-5   THERAPEUTIC COMMUNITY MEETING

PURPOSE	DIALOGUE
The leader defines the purpose of the meeting.	**Leader:** Good morning. It's Wednesday, July 28, and this is our community meeting. This is the meeting where we get ourselves organized for the day and take care of any business that comes up. This is important, because there are many people living in this community.
The leader provides structure for the task.	**Leader:** Let's do first things first and introduce ourselves and discuss what we all do here.
The leader defines tasks and explains how patients can use her in this role.	**Leader:** I'm Kerry, and I'm one of the nurses. I'll be passing out the medications today, so if any of you have questions about your medications, please see me. I'll also be leading the process group, and I'll tell you more about that later.
The leader provides structure.	**Leader:** [To each patient] Would you please introduce yourself to everybody and say something about yourself?
	Patient: Well, I think everybody knows me. I'm Cara. I've been here since Friday. I'll probably go home Wednesday or Thursday.
	Patient: I'm Kyle. I don't know if I'll ever go home.
	Patient: I'm Josh. I'm Kyle's roommate, and he snores! So loud!
The leader focuses on the task.	**Leader:** Josh, please say something about yourself.
	Patient: I'm tired. I'm not sleeping well.
	Leader: Thanks.
	Patient: I'm Paula. I just came in yesterday, and I've met a few of you. This is a real nice place.
	Patient: I'm Kirsten. I've got nothing to say.
	Patient: I'm Emily. Uh, I don't like to talk in front of people.
The leader models acceptance.	**Leader:** I appreciate your effort.
	Staff: I'm Jenna. I'm the occupational therapist. I'll be leading the 9 AM and 2 PM groups today in the activity room. I also want to meet with you, Paula, to get to know you and to make some plans with you about how you can best use occupational therapy. Could you meet with me after the meeting to set up a time?
	Paula: Sure.
The leader acknowledges effort.	**Leader:** Thanks for your introductions.
The leader defines the role of the contact person and addresses how patients can use the contact person to promote task accomplishment.	**Leader:** Each one of the staff acts as a contact person for each of you. Your contact is the person who is working with you for the day. You can talk to your contact about anything that concerns you. I'll be the contact person for Cara, Josh, and Emily. Jenna will be the contact person for Kyle, Paula, and Kirsten. Any questions so far?
The leader promotes self-responsibility by telling patients how to meet their own needs.	**Leader:** Let me introduce today's schedule to you. It's posted on the bulletin board if you forget the times. We mostly want to tell you about the activities and groups.
	Jenna: From 9 AM to 10 AM is Roles Group. This group helps you to look at the different parts you play in your various relationships. It's a good place to look for patterns that recur in your life. I will be the group leader.
The leader defines the purpose and structure of groups and activities.	**Leader:** You then have free time until 10:30 AM. From 10:30 AM to 11:30 AM is Process Group. In this group, we pay attention to how we communicate with each other. It's a good place to look at any problems that you may be having communicating with other people. I will be group leader. Lunch is at 11:45 AM, and at 1 PM you have a choice of taking a walk if you have privilege to do so or playing a game like bingo here on the unit. From 2 PM to 3 PM is the Activity Group that Jenna leads. This is where you can make something. It's a good opportunity to look at how you approach performing a task. At 3:30 PM, we go home, and the evening staff will meet with you to go over the evening schedule and staffing. Any questions?
The patient uses information and responds to the cooperative style modeled by the leader.	**Josh:** Do we have to play bingo? I hate that game.
	Leader: No, that was just what came to mind. Actually, as a group, you can choose any game that you'd like at that time.
The leader supports the patient's initiative, clarifies the situation, and models the acceptance of question asking.	**Leader:** Thanks for asking. It helps us to make ourselves clear and to share an understanding of what happens here on the unit.
The leader reiterates ways that patients can be responsible for themselves.	**Leader:** Any other questions about the schedule? [Pause] It's a lot to remember. If any questions come up during the day, check the schedule on the bulletin board or see your contact person.

Continued

TABLE 26-5	THERAPEUTIC COMMUNITY MEETING—cont'd
PURPOSE	**DIALOGUE**
The leader continues to provide structure.	**Leader:** I think we can move to the last piece of business for this meeting, and that's to deal with any issues that come up whenever so many people are living together. Is there anything that you want to talk about? **Kirsten:** I still don't have any hot water.
The leader promotes interaction.	**Leader:** I heard about that from the night staff again. It's been a while, hasn't it? **Kirsten:** Three days, and nothing has happened yet.
The leader clarifies information.	**Leader:** Well, actually, something is happening. Engineering found that the valve is broken, and they're waiting for a replacement.
The group follows up on problem solving that is probably based on the leader's earlier modeled acceptance and encouragement to be self-responsible.	**Kirsten:** [Sarcastically] Great! They're waiting, and I still don't have any hot water. **Cara:** No hot water at all? **Kirsten:** Well, my shower works, but I don't have any hot water in my sink to wash up. I don't want to take a whole shower just to wash my face. **Josh:** Why don't you just wet your washcloth in the shower? **Kirsten:** That's what I've been doing, but I get soaked and my clothes get soaked. **Cara:** Well, I don't mind if you want to use my sink for washing up, as long as you give me notice.
The patients have clarified their actions as appropriate to their roles.	**Kirsten:** Really? Thanks. I'll do that.

appeared angry. The nurse will share this information with staff and provide the context to the situation, which will be extremely useful as staff interact with the patients throughout the day. The structured meeting assists the nurse with becoming oriented to the tone of the unit and the status of the patients. This information will also help the nurse to organize the day while considering patient needs, which could change as the day goes on. Thus, the therapeutic milieu is structured to provide nursing interventions that clearly define expectations of the patient "through a mutually collaborative process in order to augment and enhance ego functions and to promote a positive sense of self" (Sebastian et al, 1990, p. 26).

GROUP THERAPY

Human beings are social by nature, and Maslow identified belonging as one of the basic needs. The meeting of needs occurs primarily in groups, beginning with the family, where physical and psychologic needs are met; this is essential for healthy growth and for the development of family members. The need for belonging and social development progresses through the life span and moves to larger social groups, such as school, church, recreation, work, local community, society, and the cultural or international community. A basic understanding of how groups function and the therapeutic role of groups helps the nurse to more effectively participate as a member and leader in professional and clinical settings. Northouse and Northouse (1998) defined a group as a "set of three or more individuals whose relationships make them in some way interdependent" (p. 196). Groups in the health care settings fall somewhere in the range between content oriented and process oriented (Figure 26-3), and the designation depends on the purpose of the group. *Content* refers to the tasks or activities needed to accomplish the goals of the group. *Process* refers to the interpersonal relationships among members of the group and the leader. All groups contain both elements and vary in accordance with the goal of the group (Northouse and Northouse, 1998). A therapeutic group is a specific type of group in which the goal is psychologic change and growth. Therapeutic groups generally fall closer to the process-oriented end of the continuum, and they are largely dependent on the level of change that members are seeking. Therapeutic groups range from having a behavior focus to a psychoanalytic approach that involves personality change.

Types of Groups

Task groups focus primarily on tasks, activities, and procedures and the quality of work that is necessary to meet the goal. There is generally some processing going on among members. Examples of task groups are committees that are formed to develop or revise a policy or procedure, to monitor quality improvement, or to plan a patient outing or unit activity. Task groups can be made up of nurses, therapists, and patients working together, or they may only be made up of members of one of these groups.

Midrange groups are groups that combine the functions of task and process. Support and self-help groups are examples of groups that provide an opportunity for individuals and families to come together to process experiences by sharing feelings and thoughts with others who have found ways to cope with similar experiences over time. Members who are further along in the process of coping (sharing information) with loss, disability, sobriety, addiction, illness, rehabilitation, and other challenges help other members by giving (altruism) their knowledge to newer members. Some self-help or support groups are led by a mental health professional or by an experienced member volunteer who is elected by other group members. Another type of midrange group is the psychoeducational group, which is the most common type of group that is facilitated by nurses in inpatient, outpatient, and

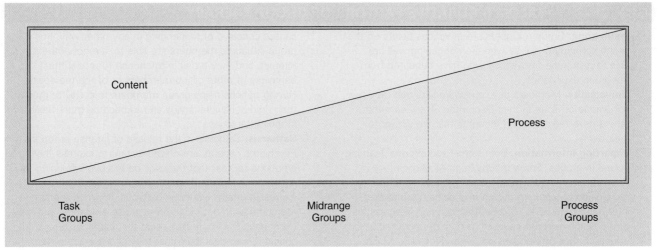

FIGURE 26-3. The emphasis on content and process in different types of groups. Psychiatric mental health nurses are most involved with process group therapy. (Modified from Loomis M: *Group process for nurses*, St. Louis, 1979, Mosby.)

community settings. This type of group has a more formal structure and more clearly stated goals. These goals generally include gaining new knowledge for the understanding and management of a psychiatric disorder, learning activities for increasing self-awareness, and developing strategies that promote effective coping skills.

Process groups focus on interpersonal relationships among members and their communication styles or patterns. A type of process group is psychodynamic group therapy. A key assumption of this type of therapeutic group is that psychopathology has its source in disordered relationships (Yalom, 2005). The goal of group psychotherapy is to help individuals to develop more functional and satisfying relationships. Because the dysfunction in each group member will eventually manifest in the group, the task of the group therapist is to monitor and support the development of the curative factors (Box 26-2) that facilitate change by assisting members with understanding their patterns of interaction within the group. Therapists hope that this greater understanding will help members to transfer their new insights to the larger society outside of the confines of the group. Irvin Yalom (2005), an American psychiatrist and an innovator in the area of group inpatient therapy, advocated the following steps to help group members to accomplish this task:

- Get feedback about how they present themselves to others.
- Assess whether their fixed patterns are realistic or effective for the current situation.
- Discover previously unknown parts of themselves (e.g., strengths, skills, abilities, desires).
- Gradually try new behaviors within the safety of the group.
- Accept ultimate responsibility for the way that they live their lives.

Group Dynamics

After the nurse establishes the goal and formation of a group, a number of factors or dynamics influence the success of the group with regard to meeting its goal. It is essential for the nurse to understand the importance of leadership, norms, cohesiveness, and roles when developing the necessary skills to practice successful nursing interventions in a group format.

Leadership

The leader's role and leadership style are determined by the goals of the group. The leader plays an important role in guiding the group to meet its goals, developing group norms, and facilitating communication among members. Leadership is the "process in which one person attempts to influence others in order to attain some mutually agreed-upon goal" (Northouse and Northouse, 1998, p. 202). The leader's ability to influence the group depends on communication skills that are positive, open, assertive, flexible, tactfully honest, and receptive while acknowledging members' issues as the group moves forward to meet the stated goal. According to Lieberman and colleagues (1973), the characteristics of an effective therapeutic group leader are as follows:

- *Emotional stimulation.* This occurs when a leader actively encourages members to express their feelings, helps them confront and reflect ideas and values in a safe setting, and role-models effective communication strategies that move the group closer to its stated goal.
- *Caring.* This is demonstrated when a leader expresses sincerity, openness, warmth, and kindness to the group members.
- *Meaning attribution.* This refers to a leader who helps members to develop insight into the underlying meaning of their behavior and who helps to provide a deeper understanding and acceptance of feelings that emerge from everyone involved in the group process.
- *Executive functioning.* This refers to the leader's ability to monitor group norms, set limits, and attend to group rules and procedures.

BOX 26-2 YALOM'S CURATIVE FACTORS OF GROUP THERAPY

1 **Instill hope.** Group members are at various points on the health continuum. Those who are not coping well are able to gain hope from those who have benefited from the group experience.

2 **Universality.** Members develop awareness that they are not unique or alone in their discomfort. They learn that others have reactions and thoughts that are similar to their own.

3 **Imparting information.** Both formal and informal learning occurs in groups. Some groups (e.g., Alcoholics Anonymous, medication-education groups, symptom-recognition groups) are designed specifically to give information. However, groups that focus on interpersonal relationships help members to gain insight about the effects of their interactions on group dynamics, which they can then generalize to the larger society.

4 **Altruism.** By and large, members of groups give credit to other group members for their support and insight. Members view their improvement as related to the work done by all group members. The knowledge that they are useful to others helps members to experience an improved sense of self-value.

5 **Corrective recapitulation of the family group.** People act as they were taught to act in their families. With psychiatric patients, these patterns are often dysfunctional, and the patient continues to repeat these dysfunctional patterns in all interactions. Group therapy provides the opportunity for patients to identify, evaluate, and change these patterns.

6 **Development of social techniques.** By interacting with others, members are able to improve their social skills. Members will often give other members feedback regarding their reactions to each other's interpersonal style. This enriches member recognition of the various effects of their style on others, and it gives them opportunities to choose and practice styles that are more in keeping with their goals.

7 **Imitative behavior.** Group members are often "caught" or trapped in a specific style of interacting because they cannot conceive of responding in any other way. In a group situation, members are able to see how others interact, and they are able to choose to model the behaviors of other group members or of the therapist. Having options helps group members to curtail or modify their rigid behavioral styles and to become more flexible in their interactions.

8 **Catharsis.** Catharsis is the release of intense emotions. Psychiatric patients are often hesitant to express these emotions for fear that they will be too overwhelming for anyone to handle and that the consequences of expressing them would be grievous. In group therapy, members learn how to express these emotions, and they experience the immediate relief that catharsis brings. In addition, members learn that they and the group have survived the expression of emotions without calamity.

9 **Existential factors.** Human beings must inevitably deal with the fact that we all exist alone in the universe, despite the presence of others. Psychiatric patients (as well as others) tend to be unrealistic with regard to their expectations of human relationships; they may think that, with the perfect mate, friend, or family, all feelings of aloneness would vanish. In group therapy, members learn that human companionship can decrease feelings of loneliness but that it does not ever completely eliminate those feelings. By not reaching for what is unattainable, members are able to enjoy what is attainable.

10 **Cohesiveness.** This is one of the most powerful benefits of an effective group. Many members experience extreme isolation during their daily lives, and they consequently feel disconnected from others, even when they are not alone. Being part of a cohesive group that achieves its stated goals allows members to experience a sense of belonging and a feeling of being part of a whole that is greater than any one individual.

11 **Interpersonal learning.** In groups that are designed to examine interpersonal relationships, the members learn to identify, clarify, and modify maladaptive behaviors.

From Yalom ID: *The theory and practice of group psychotherapy,* ed 3, New York, 2005, Basic Books.

Norms

Norms are the rules of behavior that are established by the leader and group members. They represent shared expectations regarding appropriate behaviors (Sampson and Marthas, 1990), and they serve to maintain the function and work of the group. The norms emerge out of interactions among members and the leader, and they ultimately have an effect on the development of cohesion and other curative factors. Norms are either enabling (i.e., those that assist the group with the accomplishment of its work) or restrictive (i.e., those that hinder movement toward the accomplishment of the group's goal).

Norms are either overt or covert (Northouse and Northouse, 1998). Overt norms are the rules that are explicitly known and agreed upon by all members. For example, an overt norm is the timing of group sessions (i.e., when they begin and end). The group usually agrees upon this norm during the formation phase of the group. If the normal times of the group change, the leader and the group members discuss the effects that these changes will have on the group and the group's goal. Covert norms are the unspoken or implied rules among group members. For example, actively listening without interruption when another member is talking is a covert norm. Nonverbal glances of disapproval or the stopping of dialogue usually signal the violation of this norm.

Norms tend to develop early in groups, and they are difficult to change later during the course of the group's development. The leader or group therapist and the members are all responsible for monitoring the norms and their effectiveness for meeting individual and group goals. Nurses on the

TABLE 26-6	FACTORS THAT INFLUENCE GROUP COHESIVENESS
CHARACTERISTIC	**CONSIDERATIONS**
Group goals	Clear goals that are based on similar member values and interests motivate members to seek and maintain group membership.
Similarity among members	Members are frequently attracted to other members who share similar values and beliefs. However, there are some instances in which people are attracted to those who are dissimilar from them with regard to values and attitudes.
Type of interdependence among members	Groups that function in a cooperative rather than a competitive manner tend to have higher cohesion among members.
Leader behavior	For the most part, democratic styles of leadership are associated with higher group cohesiveness than are other styles of leadership (e.g., autocratic).
Communication structures	Decentralized communication structures, which are characterized by increased member interaction, are associated with higher morale and increased satisfaction among members.
Group activities	Members who are asked to perform group activities that they believe are beyond their capabilities will feel less attracted toward the group, whereas members who believe that group activities are within their capabilities will feel more attracted toward the group.
Group atmosphere	Members are frequently attracted to groups that help them feel valued and accepted.
Group size	Group size should match the number of members needed to complete the task. Larger groups can compromise group cohesiveness if there are too many members for the task.

From Cartwright D: The nature of group cohesiveness. In Cartwright D, Zander A, editors: *Group dynamics: research and theory*, ed 3, New York, 1968, Harper and Row.

inpatient psychiatric unit are responsible for promoting norms that meet the goal of a therapeutic environment or milieu when conducting community meetings and leading psychoeducational groups.

Cohesiveness

Cohesion or cohesiveness is the extent to which group members work together to accomplish stated goals. This is the sense of "we-ness" that a group experiences. Cohesion acts as a bond among group members, and it has been associated with positive group outcomes such as increased interactions, norm conformity, goal-directed behaviors, and member satisfaction (Northouse and Northouse, 1998). Table 26-6 summarizes factors that influence group cohesiveness.

Roles

The behavior of individual members toward each other has a significant impact on the functioning of the group and the group's ability to accomplish its goal. Member behavior is categorized by the roles that are assumed by group members. These roles often reflect the characteristics and roles adopted during early family life. Three broad categories of roles assumed by group members are group task roles, group building and maintenance roles, and individual roles. Members of a group often have more than one role.

Task roles are members' behaviors that contribute to the group's ability to perform its function to meet the group's goals. The primary concern of task roles is to obtain and share information to solve problems. Group building and maintenance roles enhance the development of member relationships by supporting the ability of the group to work together and to build group cohesiveness. Individual roles are the roles that a member adopts to meet individual needs; sometimes these adversely affect group cohesion, function,

and tasks when the leader or group does not confront them. Examples of the three categories of member roles are presented in Box 26-3.

Phases of Group Development

All groups progress through the phases of development that are governed by the group dynamics that have been previously outlined. Northouse and Northouse (1998) developed a model that is based on small group research findings. The model consists of five phases: (1) orientation; (2) conflict; (3) cohesion; (4) working; and (5) termination. Understanding the phases of group development and the common characteristics of group behavior during each phase gives the nurse a framework for recognizing and assisting the group with each phase.

Orientation Phase

Individuals in this beginning phase of group development are evaluating the leader and other members with regard to trustworthiness; compatibility between individual goals and group goals; types of requirements (e.g., time, tasks, roles); level of self-disclosure required; and the establishment of norms. The role of the leader is to help group members to feel like part of the group and to achieve a sense of privacy, trust, and independence. The establishment of structure, group guidelines, and group norms is the primary responsibility of the leader.

Conflict Phase

Conflicts occur when group members compete with each other and the leader for control, influence, and authority regarding group decisions. The conflict over control is common in groups and possibly comes from resistance to the formation of a new group out of fear of entering into a new

BOX 26-3   ROLE FUNCTIONS WITHIN A GROUP

Task Functions

Initiator: Proposes new ideas, directions, tasks, and methods

Elaborator: Expands on existing suggestions and further develops the group's plans

Evaluator: Critically evaluates ideas, proposals, plans, and procedures and examines their practicality and effectiveness

Coordinator: Helps pull together ideas and themes to clarify members' suggestions and assists various subgroups with working more effectively toward their common goal

Group Maintenance Functions

Encourager: Offers praise to members, when warranted; communicates the acceptance of others and their ideas; is open to differences within the group

Harmonizer: Mediates conflicts and disagreements that emerge in an effort to relieve or reduce tension within the group

Compromiser: Assumes a position between contending sides and seeks a compromise that all parties can accept

Individual Functions

Aggressor: Acts hostile and negative toward other members; criticizes others' contributions; attacks the group and its members

Recognition-seeker: Calls attention to own activities; boasts; redirects things toward self

Help-seeker or *confessor:* Uses the group as a vehicle to either gain sympathy or achieve personal insight and self-satisfaction, without consideration for others or for the group as a whole

Dominator: Asserts authority and seeks to manipulate others in an effort to be in control of everything that happens

---

set of interpersonal relationships. It is the leader's responsibility to guide members through the conflict by helping them to negotiate issues of influence and control while accepting the conflict as a normal phase of group dynamics.

Cohesion Phase

Cohesion begins when group members have worked through conflicts and are more aware of their individual differences. A greater understanding and acceptance of differences is evident, and members begin to feel more positive toward each other. Trust begins to build, self-disclosure increases, and a greater expression of feelings, thoughts, and behaviors begins to emerge. As members continue to work as a cohesive group, the leader's role is one of minimal guidance and direction.

Working Phase

The hallmark of the working phase is the group's greater depth of self-disclosure and expression of both positive and negative emotions and thoughts. It sometimes takes up to 2

months for the working phase to fully develop, depending on such factors as group size, whether it is a short- or long-term group, and member commitment. Members of short-term task groups generally exhibit positive feelings toward each other in the form of praise, joking, a high spirit of camaraderie, and work productivity. The leader's role is minimal in task-oriented groups during this phase, unless otherwise indicated. The role of the leader in any therapeutic group varies in accordance with the issues being addressed in the group.

Termination Phase

A group disbands when the goals of the group are fulfilled or when the allotted time is up. The termination phase in long-term therapeutic groups is sometimes a time of grief and loss for group members as well as for the therapist. Feelings of abandonment, guilt, fear, anger, gratitude, positive affection, or frustration sometimes emerge during this phase. Members recognize that the uniqueness of their group can never be recreated or duplicated. Each individual member will confront this phase in accordance with previous personal experiences of loss and separation. The leader during this phase summarizes the group accomplishments and helps members to confront their feelings about individual group members, the leader, and the ending of the group as a whole.

FAMILY THERAPY

A family is a primary social group of individuals who are related by biologic lines, legal bonds of marriage, or adoption and who are emotionally related or interdependent. The developmental stage of each family member and the family's phase in the family life cycle influence the function or tasks of the family. Carter and McGoldrick (2005) outlined six stages of the family life cycle (Table 26-7). The authors defined the key emotional processes that are necessary at each stage for successful transition to the next stage of the family life cycle. As the family moves through the life cycle stages, there is an ongoing redefinition of roles, the entry and exit of members, changes in emotional and attachment needs, and the realignment of boundaries. The hallmarks of healthy family functioning include the following:

- Open communication patterns among family members for the negotiation of individual needs and tasks
- Secure attachment or emotional bonds among family members
- Flexibility and adaptability to change
- Ability to express and distinguish emotions and thoughts
- Ability to effectively manage social and economic stressors

Several schools of family therapy have emerged from the treatment models of individual and group therapies since the 1960s (Table 26-8).

Family Systems Theory

The family systems theory is the foundation for all forms of family therapy, and views the family as the primary

TABLE 26-7 STAGES OF THE FAMILY LIFE CYCLE		
FAMILY LIFE CYCLE STAGE	EMOTIONAL PROCESS OF TRANSITION: KEY PRINCIPLES	SECOND-ORDER CHANGES IN FAMILY STATUS REQUIRED FOR DEVELOPMENTAL PROGRESS
Leaving home: single young adults	Accepting emotional and financial responsibility for self	Differentiating self in relation to family of origin Developing intimate peer relationships Establishing self with respect to work and financial independence
The joining of families through marriage: the new couple	Commitment to a new system	Forming a marital system Realigning relationships with extended families to include spouse
Families with young children	Accepting new members into the system	Adjusting marital system to make space for children Joining in child-rearing, financial, and household tasks Realigning relationships with extended family to include parenting and grandparenting roles
Families with adolescents	Increasing the flexibility of family boundaries to permit children's independence and grandparents' frailties	Shifting of parent–child relationships to permit the adolescent to move into and out of the system Refocusing on midlife marital and career issues Beginning to shift toward caring for the older generation
Launching children and moving on	Accepting a multitude of exits from and entries into the family system	Renegotiating the marital system as a dyad between grown children and their parents Developing adult-to-adult relationships between grown children and their parents Realigning relationships to include in-laws and grandchildren Dealing with the disabilities and deaths of parents/grandparents
Families in later life	Accepting the shifting generational roles	Maintaining own or couple functioning and interests in the face of physiologic decline Exploring new familial and social role options Supporting the more central role of the middle generation Making room in the system for the wisdom and experience of the elderly Supporting the older generation without overfunctioning for them Dealing with the loss of a spouse, siblings, and other peers and preparing for death

From Carter B, McGoldrick M: Overview: the expanded family life cycle: individual, family and social perspectives. In Carter B, McGoldrick M, editors: *The expanded life cycle: individual, family and social perspectives*, ed 3, Boston, 2005, Allyn & Bacon.

emotional system that shapes and determines the outcome and course of one's life. A healthy emotional and psychologic environment is created by family interactions and relationships that help individual members to meet developmental tasks while allowing the family as a whole to move through the stages of the family life cycle. Relationships and functioning among family members "are interdependent, and a change in one part of the system is followed by compensatory changes in other parts of the system" (Carter and McGoldrick, 2005, p. 436). The family system strives to maintain a psychologic homeostasis or balance through emotional interactions or relationships among family members. The couple or marital dyad, siblings, and the parent–child pair are the common subsystems or relationships within the family. A relationship between two or more individuals constitutes a subsystem. Extended family members also interact to form other subsystems that affect overall family functioning. Some of the following key concepts of family systems therapy are assessed by the family therapist and the data collected are used to identify areas in need of intervention.

Attachment

Attachment refers to the emotional bonds between couples, parents, and children. Seeking and maintaining an emotional bond with significant others is an innate, primary, and motivating need in human beings across the life span (Johnson, 2003). Positive attachment is built on a strong sense of trust that someone is available to provide a sense of safety and security, and it serves as a buffer against the effects of stress, thus allowing psychologic development to proceed. A secure positive emotional attachment for a child to a parent provides a safe psychologic environment for the child through the stages of individual development and maturity, and it leads to psychologic autonomy within a network of emotional bonds between immediate and extended family members. Some forms of attachment, such as avoidant and insecure attachment, result from traumas such as physical or sexual abuse, emotional abuse, loss of a parent, mental illness in a parent (e.g., depression leading to emotional abandonment), severe illness, or trauma by war, famine, or catastrophe that affects one or more members of a family. The developmental stage of the infant, child,

TABLE 26-8	A COMPARISON OF FAMILY THERAPY MODELS	
MODEL	**DESCRIPTIONS**	**GOALS**
Psychodynamic	Regards family pathology as resulting from internal intrapsychic forces that are manifested in intimate interactions; symptoms result from family projection processes that stem from unresolved conflicts and losses in the family of origin (Boszormenyi-Nagy and Spark, 1973)	To bring about reconstructive personality change that is achieved by a working through of unconscious transference distortions among family members and with the therapist; over an extended period, patients explore the connection between past relationships and current problems (Bentovin and Kinston, 1991)
Bowen	Regards family pathology as resulting from a lack of differentiation and high anxiety; those who lack differentiation are emotionally reactive, anxious, and dysfunctional (Bowen, 1976a)	To promote differentiation and less reactivity; therapy focuses on the family of origin within a multigenerational context; the therapist coaches family members to resolve undifferentiated relationships with the family of origin (Kerr and Bowen, 1988)
Structural	Regards family pathology as resulting from stressors on a family that cannot nurture its members as a result of faulty social organization and structure as well as dysfunctional interactions among members (Minuchin, 1974)	To transform family structural patterns by challenging the family's idea of where the problem lies and how to solve it; the therapist joins the family to challenge the system from within, thereby transforming structure, patterns, and behavior (Colapinto, 1991)
Strategic	Focuses on the social context of human dilemmas and habits and avoids the use of psychiatric labels; instead, problems are seen as solvable with the use of directives to change how family members relate to one another (Lankton and Lankton, 1983)	To organize family members to take charge of problems, to facilitate the ability of family members to love and be loved, to promote the family's ability to reframe the distribution of power and responsibility, to promote shifts between hierarchy and equality, and to address personal gain and altruism that contribute to the maintenance or resolving of family problems (Madanes, 1991)
Behavioral	Problems are overt behavioral acts rather than emotional states or cognitions; combines training strategies with individual and conjoint problem solving among members (Falloon, 1991)	To change reinforcements so that family members receive rewards for desired behaviors instead of maladaptive behaviors; this occurs with the use of education, training, conditioning, and management strategies (Patterson, 1975)
Feminist	Problems result from the unique issues that women face as a result of socialization; enacts a political, institutional, and gender-sensitive viewpoint that is aimed at gender equality for defining and changing family structure and function (Goodrich, 1991)	To equalize access to influence, control, choices, resources, opportunities, and status; makes use of role-modeling, education, rebalancing of relationship power and authority, reframing of authority, and reinforcing of new beliefs (Avis, 1991)

From Haber J: Family therapy. In Lego S, editor: *Psychiatric nursing: a comprehensive reference*, ed 3, Philadelphia, 1966, Lippincott-Raven, p. 62.

or adolescent governs the extent of attachment impairment. An extensive body of research has shown that how a caregiver responds to a child's needs and expectations and how a child's needs are met lead to three distinct attachment patterns: (1) secure attachment; (2) avoidant attachment; or (3) anxious–ambivalent attachment. After observing attachment styles in children, researchers concur that being responsive, attentive, and approving leads to a securely attached child who exhibits less inhibited and more explorative behavior. Being inconsistent when responding and when giving attention leads to an anxiously and ambivalently attached child who tends to try to reestablish contact, who clings to the caregiver, and who constantly checks to see that the caregiver is nearby. Constantly ignoring or deflecting the needs and the attention of the child leads to an avoidant attachment style in which the child attempts to maintain proximity but avoids close contact with the caregiver (Siegel, 1999). Adults who have a secure attachment style have reported positive early family relationships and trusting attitudes toward others. These individuals have also been shown to have higher levels of self-esteem as compared with individuals with insecure attachment styles. Adults with an avoidant attachment style tend to view relationships as less satisfying and intimate as compared with securely attached individuals. They are also less trusting of others, and they tend to avoid getting close to others. Adults with an anxious–ambivalent attachment style view others in a relationship as unreliable and are unable to commit themselves. They also see their relationships as having less interdependence, trust, and satisfaction as compared with securely attached individuals. Parents or adults with avoidant or insecure attachment styles have difficulty with forming healthy or secure attachment with their infants and children, thereby leading to difficulties with meeting the developmental needs of infants and children as they mature into adolescence and young adulthood.

Symptom Development

The development of symptoms in a family depends on the amount of anxiety and stress that are being generated in the family and how much these disrupt the family system. The degree of symptoms in one or more family members and the level of anxiety present in relationships reflect the level of psychologic development and coping skills available for the management of internal and external stressors. For example, few symptoms appear in families with strong emotional bonds and healthy coping skills under high levels of stress, whereas other families under similar conditions exhibit symptoms that indicate high levels of anxiety that result from ineffective family coping skills that are caused by poor communication patterns and high levels of interpersonal conflict. Symptom development is generally based on the emergence of various types of stressors as the family moves through time and available psychologic and social support resources (Carter and McGoldrick, 2005). (See examples of stressor types in the Role of the Family Therapist section of this chapter.)

Emotional Triangles

An **emotional triangle** is a situation that occurs in a family that tends to redirect anxiety and to avoid actual or potential conflict between two people by introducing a third person or third issue into the mix. Although triangles decrease anxiety, they also keep the two individuals from addressing the source of the conflict that has produced the anxiety. A triangle temporarily diffuses a problem relationship, but if it becomes fixed and the original conflict is not resolved, then symptoms begin to appear in one of the members of the triangle. Identifying triangles in the family and their role in the psychologic symptoms of the family members is essential when planning interventions that help families to more effectively manage anxiety-producing stressors both within and outside of the family.

Boundaries

Boundaries are rules in the family that regulate interpersonal emotional contact between individual family members and subsystems within the family. Boundaries or rules that become rigid and that do not allow contact with outside subsystems result in isolation, limited emotional support, and disengagement. An extreme amount of stress needs to occur before an individual family member or the family as a whole seeks assistance. By contrast, enmeshment involves limitless contact and support among family members that intrude on the development of independent emotional competence. The development of boundaries for interactions between subsystems to allow for emotional independence is necessary (Nichols and Schwartz, 2001).

Genogram

A **genogram** is a two- to three-generational diagram that is designed to track family processes over time. These processes include conflicts, types of boundaries, enmeshment, disengagement, and family triangles (Figure 26-4).

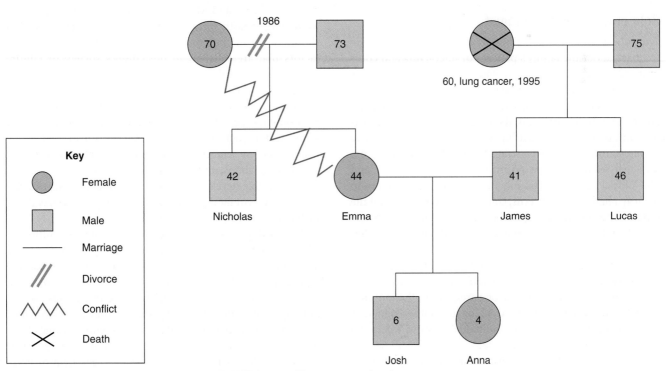

FIGURE 26-4. Three-generational genogram.

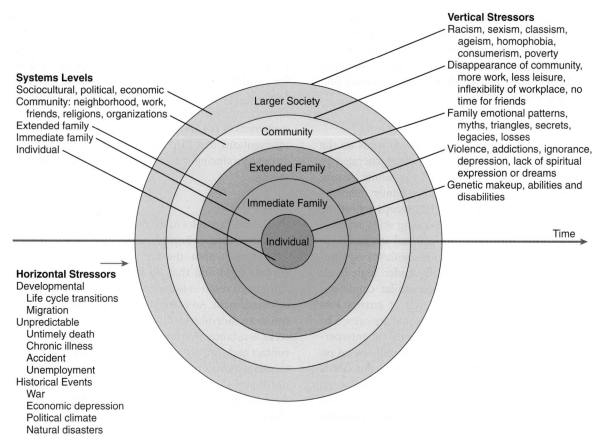

Vertical Stressors
- Racism, sexism, classism, ageism, homophobia, consumerism, poverty
- Disappearance of community, more work, less leisure, inflexibility of workplace, no time for friends
- Family emotional patterns, myths, triangles, secrets, legacies, losses
- Violence, addictions, ignorance, depression, lack of spiritual expression or dreams
- Genetic makeup, abilities and disabilities

Systems Levels
Sociocultural, political, economic
Community: neighborhood, work, friends, religions, organizations
Extended family
Immediate family
Individual

Larger Society
Community
Extended Family
Immediate Family
Individual

Time

Horizontal Stressors
Developmental
    Life cycle transitions
    Migration
Unpredictable
    Untimely death
    Chronic illness
    Accident
    Unemployment
Historical Events
    War
    Economic depression
    Political climate
    Natural disasters

FIGURE 26-5. Flow of stress through the family. (From Carter B, McGoldrick M: Overview: the expanded family life cycle: individual, family and social perspectives. In Carter B, McGoldrick M, editors: *The expanded life cycle: individual, family and social perspectives*, ed 3, Boston, 2005, Allyn & Bacon, p. 6.)

Role of the Family Therapist

The role of the family therapist is to observe and provide feedback about the family's patterns of interacting and communicating with each other, and evaluating the family's responses, strengths and weaknesses. The goal of therapy using the systems approach is to effect change by helping family members work out their differences and concerns by communicating and relating directly with each other. The therapist introduces new strategies for the family to use that will result in more positive interactions (Carter and McGoldrick, 2005). The family therapist uses a genogram to identify relationship patterns, communication styles, and the level of communication skills between the couple dyad, the parent–child dyad, the child–child dyad, and any other extended family relationships.

Family therapists view symptoms in relation to the overall family system that is exhibiting difficulty in one or more subsystems, such as the couple or parent dyad, the mother–son dyad, the father–daughter dyad, or the mother–daughter dyad. This is in contrast with individual therapy, where the focus is on a single individual.

Symptoms of psychologic distress in one family member affect other family members and also create secondary

stressors. Carter and McGoldrick (2005) identified stressors as flowing in both vertical and horizontal directions within the life cycle of the family over time (Figure 26-5). Social factors that are inherent in the family's society or culture progress downward into the community, the extended family, the immediate family, and, finally, to the individual.

Vertical stressors include societal attitudes and values regarding race, gender, work, and leisure time and individual family factors such as the generational transmission of family history, family emotional patterns and attitudes, family secrets and taboos, and cultural beliefs. Horizontal stressors are predictable developmental stressors that arise during the normal stages of family development, such as marriage, childbirth, and entering college.

Family difficulties most often arise during a transition or when moving to the next stage of the family life cycle. Carter and McGoldrick (2005) cited research that indicates that the highest points of stress occur during times of loss or when there is an addition to the family. These transitions require families to redefine their relationships as they form new emotional attachments and lose other attachments. Families enter into crisis when they do not have the psychologic resources to manage these stressors. Some families seek help or enter the mental health care system during a developmental crisis or a situational crisis. Referral to a family therapist occurs when the parents, the school system, or the juvenile court identifies a child or adolescent as not exhibiting or adhering to age-appropriate behaviors set by social or cultural standards. Examples of inappropriate behaviors include aggression, difficulty concentrating, a significant change in school performance (e.g., poor grades), an unusual or abrupt change in behavior (e.g., withdrawal in a normally outgoing child or adolescent), difficulties with peer relationships, substance use or abuse, extreme difficulty with separation, inappropriate fears, fire setting, or cruelty to animals. Some families also require additional support with the onset of an acute physical or psychiatric illness in a family member (see Chapter 17).

Role of the Nurse

The nurse plays a vital role in assessing symptoms of distress in family members and in helping the family to identify and mobilize available resources that facilitate emotional support and functioning in the family as a whole. Tapp (2000) emphasized the nurse's responsibility to acknowledge the reciprocal influence between illness in a patient and other family members. The nurse is able to employ a brief 15-minute assessment with the use of a genogram by asking the following three important assessment questions:

- *Which family members are most involved with the patient?* This involves making a genogram to illustrate the family's structure (see Figure 26-4).
- *How does the illness affect the family?* The nurse explores, with family members, the amount of distress and anxiety that are being experienced and acknowledges the family's concerns and fears.
- *How does the family affect the illness?* The nurse engages in therapeutic conversations to help the family to reveal its method of managing the demands of caregiving, to provide feedback for effective coping methods, and to suggest additional community resources and support groups for the family to use while negotiating the crisis. The goal is to help family members learn how to cope and manage family stressors, such as the loss of a child, parenting concerns, a chronic psychiatric illness, developmental disabilities, addictions, a chronic physical illness, widowhood, single parenting, and divorce.

ACTIVITY THERAPIES

Health care providers have practiced activity therapies—also known as *therapeutic activities, expressive therapies, experimental therapies,* and *adjunct therapies*—in psychiatric mental health settings since the 1980s. With the onset of managed care and cost containment, the use of these activities has diminished. In many instances, nurses pair up with recreational therapists to conduct these activities in inpatient, outpatient, and community settings.

Types of therapeutic activities include recreational, occupational, art, music, movement/dance, and psychodrama. which provide service to children, adolescents, adults, and older adults of all functional levels and diagnoses. The

RESEARCH FOR EVIDENCE-BASED PRACTICE BOX

Thomas SP et al: What's therapeutic about the therapeutic milieu? *Arch Psychiatr Nurs* 16:99-107, 2002

Nurse researchers conducted a phenomenologic study of patients in an acute psychiatric unit regarding the meaning of their inpatient experience. Three interrelated themes of "refuge from self-destructiveness"—"like me/not like me," "possibilities/no possibilities," and "connection/disconnection"—emerged in relation to the hospital experience. Patients described the hospital as a "safe house" or sanctuary that provided respite and protection from their daily struggle against self-destructive impulses. The environment was experienced as being accepting and involving a kinship with other patients that led to feeling of decreased isolation. Staff met the patient's needs for structure, food, and shelter. Being with others afforded the patients with the opportunity to talk, listen, and compare their stories, thereby finding similarities and differences that led to a decrease in the isolation that they felt as a result of their symptoms and experiences. Participants described hospitalization as opening possibilities for a future with treatment, but they also described their dread of discharge and of having to face anxieties and fears. Socialization and being with other patients was described as being highly valued. Expectations for more one-to-one time and group and activity therapies to facilitate change and less games, classes, and idle time were also expressed. Staff members who were perceived as helpful were those who "displayed an attitude of willingness to give (attention, time, information, services) and to be flexible about unit rules" (p. 104). Close monitoring by staff was not viewed as intrusive or aversive; rather, it was experienced as staff being "on top of things" and "keeping a close eye on you." The researchers concluded from the findings that nurses need to provide more one-to-one counseling and opportunities for group activities, to revise unit program activities, and to be more attentive regarding barriers to interaction (e.g., closed windows or doors at the nurses' station).

primary intent of these activities is to increase the patient's awareness of feelings, behaviors, thoughts, and sensations through the medium of art, music, or dance and to use that medium to minimize pathology and to promote mental and emotional health. Activities also allow patients to express themselves on multiple levels, to be creative, and to demonstrate conflicts, strengths, and limitations in a safe and nonthreatening environment, which will help to prepare them for life outside of the hospital. Activity therapists and nurses generally collaborate to recommend activity therapies to the patient's primary physician.

Historic Perspectives

Activity therapies date back to 2000 BC, when exercise and the arts were found to be healing, especially for melancholia, which is known today as *depression.* During the 18th and 19th centuries, the moral treatment of persons with mental illness increased, and nurses were among the first to recognize the therapeutic value of these activities. Two nurses, Susan E. Tracy and Florence Nightingale, contributed greatly to the birth of recreational therapy and occupational therapy. As the activities evolved and became more complex in theory and practice, activity therapy eventually became recognized as its own specialty, with professional, ethical, and educational standards.

Role of the Nurse

The nurse's role in activity therapies is extremely valuable for the following reasons:

- The involvement of nurses provides more availability for patient activities.
- The nurse is an additional trained professional observer who represents safety and comfort, which reduces the patient's anxiety and inhibitions.
- The collaboration of the nurse, the therapist, and the physician allows multiple disciplines to view patient problems from different perspectives, which increases the opportunity for more effective outcomes.

Occupational Therapy

Occupational therapy focuses on the assessment of the patient's task performance, cognitive functioning, psychosocial development, the recognition of strengths, and weaknesses, and adaptation to change. The nurse's role in occupational therapy includes daily contact with patients to provide encouragement, support, role-modeling, teaching, discussion, and reality testing of prescribed tasks. The nurse's assessment of overall patient functioning provides valuable information for occupational therapists. For example, during a mental status assessment, the nurse observes that a patient is experiencing cognitive decline and exhibits frustration and inability to solve problems. The nurse concludes that this patient will benefit from the occupational therapist's evaluation of cognitive functioning and problem solving skills.

Recreational Therapy

Recreational therapy, which is also known as *therapeutic recreation,* is sometimes considered the art of work, love, and play. The nurse's role in recreational therapy includes promoting activities and interactions that foster independence, responsibility, problem-solving skills, leisure activities, and interactive skills. Table 26-9 describes the various types of recreational therapy and the nurse's role in each type.

ELECTROCONVULSIVE THERAPY

Electroconvulsive therapy (ECT), is a biologic treatment that involves a brief, controlled, electrical stimulus applied to the brain which produces a change in brain chemistry that results in an improved mood state (ECT is fully described in the following paragraphs).

Historic Perspectives

ECT, which is sometimes known as *electroshock therapy,* was first used as a treatment in 1934 to "cure" psychotic disorders by inducing convulsions. Paracelsus, a 16th-century Swiss physician, gave camphor to induce convulsions as a method of treating "lunacy"; in 1764, Von Auenbrugger used the same intervention to treat symptoms of mania. In 1934, Meduna administered an injection of camphor oil to a patient with schizophrenia who had been in a catatonic stupor for 4 years. After a series of these treatments, the patient made a remarkable recovery. Meduna administered this same treatment to 26 patients, 13 of whom showed significant improvement. Reports of the success of this new form of therapy spread, and others soon explored additional methods to induce convulsions. By 1938, two Italian scientists, Cerletti and Bini, administered 11 separate transcerebral treatments with the use of an electrical stimulus to induce a seizure in a patient with schizophrenia. The patient fully recovered from his illness, and Cerletti and Bini received worldwide acclaim for their efforts (Gomez, 2004; Kavanaugh and McLoughlin, 2010). It is doubtful that this patient would be diagnosed with schizophrenia by today's standards, but the relative safety and efficacy of this procedure opened up a whole new treatment technique for psychiatry.

Modern Electroconvulsive Therapy

ECT is currently considered a safe and effective treatment for major depression. Despite advances in the pharmacologic treatment of major depression, approximately 15% of depressed people do not respond to medications and continue to experience depression. However, of this 15%, approximately 90% find relief from depression with the use of ECT, thus making it an effective treatment for patients who are resistant to pharmacotherapy.

ECT involves sending an electrical current through the brain of an anesthetized patient to induce a grand mal seizure. The exact mechanism of action is not known. Because of this lack of understanding and issues surrounding patients' rights, ECT has had a poor reputation in the public mind on the basis of media portrayal of the treatment. The most appropriate candidates for ECT are those who are experiencing a major mood disorder. Patients with melancholic, delusional, and psychotic depression also tend to respond well to ECT.

Other candidates for ECT include patients who have had prior positive outcomes with ECT, cannot tolerate the side effects of antidepressants, experience acute suicidal thoughts and behaviors, and have fluid and electrolyte imbalance because of an inability to eat or drink due to severe depression. ECT has also been used to treat mania, severe catatonia, and schizophrenia that is unresponsive to antipsychotic medications.

ECT is used for patients with mental disorders who are in the first trimester of pregnancy when pharmacotherapy is contraindicated. It is also an effective treatment for older adult patients who are experiencing mental illness and who cannot tolerate the effects of pharmacotherapy.

TABLE 26-9   RECREATIONAL THERAPY AND THE NURSE'S ROLE

THERAPY	DESCRIPTION	NURSE'S ROLE
Art therapy	The use of art to help resolve conflicts and promote self-awareness through nonverbal media	Observing the patient's use of art, encouraging verbal responses to artwork, and noting the content of the patient's artwork and how it relates to the patient's specific issues. (NOTE: Do not comment on the quality of the artwork or the patient's artistic talents. This is not an art contest but simply each patient's means of self-expression.)
Music therapy	The use of music in a defined structure to bring about change and to promote self-organization, social connection, and expression	Observing whether the patient is active or passive during the experience and noting any verbal and nonverbal feelings that are expressed by the patient. (NOTE: The patient's taste in music is not the focus of this activity.)
Movement/dance therapy	The use of movement (kinesics) to express emotions, work out tensions, develop an improved body image, and achieve body awareness and social interactions through rhythmic exercises and responses to music	Participating in the activity, observing and encouraging all patients to participate, and promoting discussion, when possible. (NOTE: The patient's dancing talents are not the focus of this activity.)
Psychodrama/sociodrama	The use of spontaneous expression and dramatic technique to act out emotional problems to promote health through the development of new perceptions, behaviors, and connection with others; a method of group psychotherapy developed by Jacob Moreno (1889-1974), a Viennese physician	Observing the patient's reactions and encouraging the patient to relate these reactions to his or her own issues. (NOTE: The patient's acting talent is not the focus of this activity.) Psychodrama is not a mainstream activity in most psychiatric mental health facilities. However, it is sometimes used in a simpler form (e.g., role-playing) in which individuals act out conflicts with significant others in a safe setting. Role-playing is often used to help children and adolescents reenact conflicts with a trusted nurse or therapist.

Contraindications to ECT include patients with space-occupying lesions in the brain that cause increased intracranial pressure. Risk factors are recent myocardial infarction, aneurysms, acute respiratory infection, cardiac arrhythmias, organic syndromes, thrombophlebitis, and narrow-angle glaucoma.

ECT is not used for patients with the following diagnoses: drug dependence, personality disorders, reactive depression, and paranoid schizophrenia. Physicians generally administer ECT treatments three times a week, with an average series including 8 to 12 treatments.

Informed Consent

Informed consent authorizes the physician to perform ECT. The health provider obtains patient consent before treatment, after thoroughly educating the patient about the procedure and preparing the patient for any possible effects. The nurse is often a witness to informed consent (see Chapter 9). In some states, two psychiatrists are required to independently document that all pharmacologic treatments have been unsuccessful.

Preparation

Basic preliminary tests before ECT include a complete blood cell count, a comprehensive metabolic profile, a urine analysis, an electrocardiogram, and a physical examination. ECT is currently performed on an inpatient or outpatient basis, depending on the physician's assessment of the patient's condition and support system. Patients scheduled for ECT must fast overnight, and they are prepared as if they were undergoing a routine operative procedure (i.e., they empty their bladders and remove any jewelry, dental appliances, and nail polish).

Approximately 30 minutes before ECT, the patient receives an intramuscular injection of atropine, typically 0.5 mg. This drug reduces secretions and protects against vagal bradycardia, which can occur with the application of the electrical stimulus.

Procedure

In the ECT treatment room, blood pressure, cardiac, and electroencephalogram monitors assess the patient's vital functions. Emergency equipment such as oxygen, suction, and a cardiac arrest cart (crash cart) is also available. The minimum staff in attendance includes the treating psychiatrist, an anesthesiologist, and a nurse.

The anesthesiologist gives a short-acting anesthetic and a muscle relaxant intravenously; muscle paralysis prevents increased movement, which reduces the risk of fracture or injury. A mouth guard is placed, and 100% oxygen is administered. After the patient has obtained anesthesia and paralysis, the ECT electrodes are placed. For bilateral ECT, electrodes are placed on the right and left anterior portion of the patient's temples. For unilateral ECT, the electrode is placed on the anterior side of the patient's nondominant temple. For example, if the patient is right-handed, the electrode is placed on the right temple.

After the electrodes are placed, a brief electrical stimulus (generally no more than 2 seconds in total duration) is applied. The body does not move because of the paralyzing agent, and the seizure is confirmed by electroencephalographic monitoring. The patient awakens after a few minutes, and oxygen is discontinued accordingly. The patient is monitored for any respiratory distress or excess secretions that may need to be suctioned.

Postprocedure

After ECT, the patient remains in the recovery room for about 1 to 3 hours until his or her vital signs are stable and he or she is alert, oriented, and able to walk without assistance. The patient is now able to eat and resume normal activity. Some patients feel sleepy and return to bed for a while. The side effects that are most frequently associated with ECT are headache and memory loss.

Patients who are experiencing headaches sometimes receive a mild analgesia and are instructed to rest. Memory impairment tends to be more pronounced with bilateral ECT. It can be quite severe during the course of treatment, but it generally improves significantly after the completion of a series of treatments.

Role of the Nurse

Nurses need to fully understand the indications, contraindications, and side effects of ECT so that they can appropriately educate, and support the patient and the family.

The nurse also ensures that the patient's rights regarding treatment are understood by the patient and accurately documented. Before and after the procedure, the nurse calms the patient's fears, and concerns; dispels myths about ECT use; obtains the vital signs; and performs other necessary nursing interventions. The nurse also comforts and reassures patients who are experiencing headache or memory loss and recognizes the need for the repetitive teaching of patients with memory loss throughout the course of treatment. This is often challenging, because the depression itself sometimes impairs the patient's memory and concentration. Nurses need to be aware that there is still some controversy about whether mild cognitive deficits remain after ECT (Blazer and Cassel, 1994). Nurses work closely with the patient, the family, the physician, and the anesthesiologist to provide a safe and effective ECT procedure and follow-up. (Kavanaugh and McLoughlin, 2010; Uko-Ekpenyong, 2007).

CHAPTER SUMMARY

- The humanistic approach emphasizes the human potential and inherent worth of human beings as unique, self-actualizing, and self-determined individuals with the capacity to develop self-awareness.
- Behavioral therapies are based on the premise that behavior is a learned response to a stimulus in the environment.
- Cognitive therapy is based on the theory that distorted or dysfunctional thinking causes psychologic disturbances in mood and behavior.
- Group therapy allows the patient to define himself or herself through human interaction and task accomplishment.
- Family therapy promotes the health and functioning of the entire family system, because it helps to define the member's roles and tasks during times of stress and transition.
- The goal of activity therapy is to increase the patient's awareness of sensations, feelings, perceptions, thoughts, and behaviors.
- Activity therapy includes occupational and recreational (art, music, movement/dance, and psychodrama/sociodrama) therapies.
- Occupational therapy focuses on the assessment of task performance, cognitive functioning, and psychosocial development.
- Recreational therapy focuses on assessing the individual's capacity to incorporate the curative elements of play and leisure into his or her lifestyle.
- The nurse's role in therapeutic activities is that of a professional observer and participant who works with the therapist to enhance the patient's capabilities and functioning within the parameters of the assigned activity.
- ECT is a safe and effective biologic treatment for major depression and other select diagnoses, despite residual negative public perceptions.
- Nurses play an integral role in preparing and educating patients and families with regard to ECT.

REVIEW QUESTIONS

1. A nurse interacts with a woman who was recently widowed when her husband was killed in a plane crash. While supporting and comforting this patient, the nurse experiences distressing personal feelings associated with the death of a parent 5 years earlier. What is the nurse's best action?
   1. Acknowledge the transference that is evident in this relationship, and discuss the phenomenon with the patient.
   2. Carefully select the words that he or she uses during interactions with this patient to avoid influencing the patient.
   3. Disregard his or her personal feelings and proceed with helping this patient to resolve her grief.
   4. Recognize the development of countertransference, and introspectively explore ways to cope with it.

2. A patient says to the nurse, "The treatment team wants me to attend individual therapy sessions to help me with my problems, but I'm not going. I've seen psychotherapy in movies, and it's not for me." Select the nurse's most therapeutic response.
   1. "Psychoanalysis is an effective short-term approach to the solving of problems. You should follow the recommendation."
   2. "Psychotherapy is just one type of individual therapy. You and your therapist can decide which type is best for you."
   3. "It is your right to decide whether or not to participate in any type of therapy, regardless of the team's recommendation."
   4. "It doesn't sound like you like this plan. Perhaps you should consider changing to a new psychiatrist."

3. A nurse talks with a patient who is engaged in an arts and crafts activity. The patient says, "I've never been artistic. I shouldn't even come to these silly groups." The patient also attends cognitive behavioral therapy sessions two times a week. Which comment by the nurse would be supportive of the cognitive behavioral therapy?
   1. "I noticed that you made interesting color combinations and encouraged others."
   2. "What activities do you think you would enjoy more than arts and crafts?"
   3. "You should try harder to finish projects that you start. You give up too easily."
   4. "These are simply recreational activities. Talk to your therapist about your reactions."

4. The following comments are made by members of a group. Which comment best contributes to the group's cohesiveness?
   1. "I need to talk about how my problems developed and get some ideas for solving them."
   2. "We aren't making progress, because our group leader has as many problems as we do."
   3. "No one in this group wants to hear anything else about failed romantic relationships."
   4. "We started out talking about losses, but we have strayed from that subject."

5. The leader opens the discussion during the first meeting of a new group. Which of the following comments would be appropriate for this phase?
   1. "Let's start by asking each person here to define his or her problems."
   2. "Let's begin by establishing the ground rules for our group."
   3. "I would like each person to explain why you are attending this group."
   4. "Bringing family members to our group will help us achieve our goals."

REFERENCES

Anderson T et al: Effects of clinician assisted emotional disclosure for sexual assault survivors: a pilot study, *J Interpers Violence* 25:1113-1131, 2010.

Avis JM: Power and politics in therapy with women. In Goodrich TJ, editor: *Women and power: perspectives for family therapy*, New York, 1991, W.W. Norton & Co.

Bandura A: *Principles of behavior modification*, New York, 1969, Holt, Rinehart and Winston.

Beck AT et al: *Cognitive therapy of personality disorders*, New York, 1979, Plenum.

Beck JS: *Cognitive therapy: basics and beyond*, New York, 1995, Guilford Press.

Bentovin A, Kinston W: Focal family therapy: joining systems theory with psychodynamic understanding. In Gurman AS, Kiskern DP, editors: *Handbook of family therapy*, vol 2, New York, 1991, Brunner/Mazel.

Beynon S et al: Psychosocial interventions for the prevention of relapse in bipolar disorder: systematic review of controlled trials, *J Psychopharmacology* 23:574-591, 2009.

Blazer DG, Cassel CE: Depression in the elderly, *Hosp Pract* 29: 37-41, 1994.

Bohus M et al: Effectiveness of inpatient dialectical behavior therapy for borderline personality disorder: a controlled trial, *Behav Res Ther* 42:487-499, 2004.

Boszormeyni-Nagy I, Spark G: *Invisible loyalties: reciprocity in intergenerational family therapy*, New York, 1973, Harper & Row.

Botella C et al: Treatment of flying phobia using virtual reality: data from a 1 year follow-up using a multiple baseline design, *Clin Psychol Psychother* 11:311-323, 2004.

Boutin DL: Effectiveness of cognitive behavior and supportive-expressive group therapy for women diagnosed with breast cancer: a review of the literature, *Journal for Specialists in Group Work* 32:267-284, 2007.

Bowen M: Theory in the practice of psychotherapy. In Guerin P, editor: *Family therapy: theory and practice*, New York, 1976, Gardner Press.

Carter B, McGoldrick M: Overview: the expanded family life cycle: individual, family and social perspectives. In Carter B, McGoldrick M, editors: *The expanded life cycle: individual, family and social perspectives*, ed 3, vols 1-26, Boston, 2005, Allyn & Bacon.

Coelho CM et al: The use of virtual reality in acrophobia: research and treatment, *J Anxiety Disord* 23:563-574, 2009.

Colapinto J: Structural family therapy. In Gurman AS, Kniskem DP, editors: *Handbook of family therapy*, vol 2, New York, 1991, Brunner/Mazel.

Chrits-Christoph P: Changes in positive quality of life over the course of psychotherapy, *Psychotherapy Theory, Research, Practice, Training* 45:419-430, 2008.

Ellison JA et al: Maintenance of gains following experiential therapies for depression, *Journal of Counseling and Clinical Psychology* 77:103-112, 2009.

Falloon IRH: Behavioral family therapy. In Gurman AS, Kniskem DP: *Handbook of family therapy*, vol 2, New York, 1991, Brunner/Mazel.

Frederickson BL: The role of positive emotions in positive psychology: The broaden-and-build theory of positive emotions, *Review of General Psychology* 2:300-318, 2001. Website is: generallythinking.com/research

Freud S: The dynamics of transference. In *Collected papers*, vol 2, New York, 1959, Basic Books.

Freud S: *The ego and the id*, New York, 1960, W.W. Norton & Co. (edited and translated by J Strachey).

Freud S: *The interpretation of dreams*, New York, 1961, Scientific Editions (edited and translated by J Strachey).

Gallop R, O'Brien L: Re-establishing psychodynamic theory as foundational knowledge for psychiatric/mental health nursing, *Issues Ment Health Nurs* 24:213-227, 2003.

Gomez GE: Electroconvulsive therapy: present and future, *Issues Ment Health Nurs* 25:473-486, 2004.

Goodrich TJ: Women, power, and family therapy: what's wrong with this picture? In Goodrich TJ, editor: *Women and power: perspectives for family therapy*, New York, 1991, W.W. Norton & Co.

Greenberg LS: Emotion-focused therapy, *Clin Psychol Psychother* 11:3-16, 2004.

Greenberg LS et al: Emotion-focused couples therapy and the facilitation of forgiveness, *J Marital Fam Ther* 36:28-42, 2010.

Gunderson J: *Principles and practices of milieu therapy*, New Jersey, 1983, Jason Aronson Inc.

Hofmann SG et al: Cognitive-behavioral therapy for adult anxiety disorders: a meta-analysis of randomized placebo-controlled trials, *J Clin Psychiatry* 69:621-632, 2008.

Johnson SM: Introduction to attachment: a therapist's guide to primary relationships and their renewal. In Johnson SM, Whiffen VE, editors: *Attachment processes in couple and family therapy*, New York, 2003, Guilford Press.

Jonas WB, Chez RA: Toward optimal healing environments in health care, *J Altern Complement Med* 10(Suppl 1):S-1-S-6, 2004.

Jones M: *Beyond the therapeutic community*, New York, 1968, Basic Books.

Jonsson H, Hougaard E: Group cognitive behavioral therapy for obsessive-compulsive disorder: a systematic review and meta-analysis, *Acta Psychiatr Scand* 119:98-106, 2009.

Jung CG: *Two essays on analytical psychology*, ed 2, vol 7, collected works, New York, 1966, Princeton University Press.

Jung CG: *The structure and dynamics of the psyche*, ed 2, vol 8, collected works, New York, 1969, Princeton University Press.

Kavanagh A, McLoughlin DM: Electroconvulsive therapy and nursing care, *Br J Nurs* 18:1370, 1372, 1374-1377, 2010.

Kerr ME, Bowen M: *Family evaluation: an approach based on Bowen theory*, New York, 1988, W.W. Norton & Co.

Kerr NJ: The ego competency model of psychiatric nursing: theoretical overview and clinical application, *Perspect Psychiatr Care* 26:13-24, 1990.

Kohut H: *The restoration of the self*, New York, 1977, International Universities Press.

Krihn M et al: Virtual reality exposure therapy of anxiety disorders: a review, *Clin Psychol Rev* 24:259-281, 2004.

Lankton SR, Lankton CH: *The answer within: a clinical framework of Ericksonian hypnotherapy*, New York, 1983, Brunner/Mazel.

Leichsenring F, Leibing E: Psychodynamic psychotherapy: a systematic review of techniques, indication and empirical evidence, *Psychol Psychother* 80:217-228, 2007.

Lieberman MA et al: *Encounter groups: first facts*, New York, 1973, Basic Books.

Linehan MM: *Cognitive-behavioral treatment of borderline personality disorder*, New York, 1993, Guilford Press.

Linehan MM et al: Cognitive-behavioral treatment of chronically parasuicidal borderline patients, *Arch Gen Psychiatr* 48:1060-1064, 1991.

Linehan MM et al: Two year randomized controlled trial and follow-up of dialectical behavior therapy vs therapy by experts for suicidal behaviors and borderline personality disorder, *Arch Gen Psychiatry* 63:757-766, 2006.

Lynch TR et al: Dialectical behavior therapy for depressed older adults: a randomized pilot study, *Am J Geriatr Psychiatry* 11:33-45, 2003.

Lynch TR et al: Mechanisms of change in dialectical behavior therapy: theoretical and empirical observations, *J Clinical Psychol* 62:459-480, 2006.

Macintosh HB, Johnson S: Emotionally focused therapy for couples and childhood sexual abuse survivors, *J Marital Family Ther* 34:298-315, 2008.

Madanes C: Strategic family therapy. In Gurman AS, Kniskem DP, editors: *Handbook of family therapy*, vol 2, New York, 1991, Brunner/Mazel.

Mahler MS et al: *The psychological birth of the human infant: symbiosis and individuation*, New York, 1975, Basic Books.

Maslow AH: A theory of human motivation, *Psychol Rev* 50:370-396, 1943.

Minuchin S: *Families and family therapy*, Cambridge, 1974, Harvard University Press.

Misch DA: Basic strategies of dynamic supportive therapy, *J Psychother Pract Res* 9:173-189, 2000.

Nichols MP, Schwartz RC: *The essentials of family therapy*, Boston, 2001, Allyn & Bacon.

Northouse P, Northouse L: *Health communication: strategies for health professionals*, Norwalk, Conn, 1998, Appleton and Lange.

Palvio SC, Nieuwenhuis JA: Efficacy of emotion focused therapy for adult survivors of child abuse: a preliminary study, *J Trauma Stress* 14:115-133, 2001.

Parsons TD, Rizzo AA: Affective outcomes of virtual reality exposure therapy for anxiety and specific phobias: a meta-analysis, *J Behav Ther Exp Psychiatry* 39:250-261, 2008.

Patterson G: *Families: applications of social learning to family life*, Champaign, Ill, 1975, Research Press.

Pavlov I: *Lectures on conditioned reflexes*, New York, 1928, International Publishers (edited and translated by WH Grant).

Peplau HE: *Interpersonal relations in nursing*, New York, 1952, GP Putnam's Sons.

Peplau HE: Interpersonal relations: a theoretical framework for application in nursing practice, *Nurs Sci Q* 5:13-18, 1992.

Peternelj-Taylor CA, Young O: Exploring boundaries in the nurse-patient relationship: professional roles and responsibilities, *Perspect Psychiatr Care* 39:55-66, 2003.

Premack D: Toward empirical behavioral laws: I. Positive reinforcement, *Psychol Rev* 66:219-233, 1959.

Rasoli R et al: Comparing effectiveness of individual and marital emotionally focused intervention based on decreasing relationship distress of couples with chronically ill children, *Journal of Family Research* 3:683-696, 2008.

Roberts NP et al: Systematic review and meta-analysis of multiple-session early interventions following traumatic events, *Am J Psychiatry* 166:293-301, 2009.

Rogers CP: The necessary and sufficient conditions of therapeutic personality change, *J Consult Psychol* 21:95-103, 1957.

Rogers CP: *A way of being*, Boston, 1980, Houghton-Mifflin.

Rothbaum BO: Using virtual reality to help our patients in the real world, *Depress Anxiety* 26:209-211, 2009.

Sampson E, Marthas M: *Group process for the health professions*, New York, 1990, Delmar.

Sebastian L et al: Whose structure is it anyway? *Perspect Psychiatr Care* 26:25-27, 1990.

Siegel DJ: *The developing mind: how relationships and the brain interact to shape who we are*, New York, 1999, Guilford Press.

Skinner BF: Whatever happened to psychology as the science of behavior? *Am Psychol* 42:780-786, 1987.

Stern DN: *The interpersonal world of the infant*, New York, 1985, Basic Books.

Stiles AS: Personal versus relational boundaries: concept clarification and therapeutic interventions, *J Theory Constr Test* 8:72-78, 2004.

Tapp DM: Therapeutic conversations that count, *Can Nurse* 96:29-32, 2000.

Tech CF et al: Dialectical behavior therapy for binge eating disorder, *J Consult Clin Psychol* 69:1061-1065, 2001.

Turner R: Naturalistic evaluation of dialectical behavior therapy-oriented treatment for borderline personality disorder, *Cogn Behav Pract* 7:413-419, 2000.

Uko-Ekpenyong G: What you should know about electroconvulsive therapy, *Nursing*, 37:56hn1-56hn2, 56hn4, 2007.

Viederman M: A model for interpretative supportive dynamic psychotherapy, *Psychiatry* 71:349-358, 2008.

Walker M: Principles of a therapeutic milieu: an overview, *Perspect Psychiatr Care* 30:5-8, 1994.

Winnicott DW: *The maturational processes and the facilitating environment: studies in the theory of emotional development*, New York, 1965, International Universities Press.

Winston A, Rosenthal RN, Pinsker H: *Supportive Psychotherapy*, 2004, American Psychiatric Association Publishers, (168 pages).

Wolitzky-Taylor KB et al: Psychological approaches in the treatment of specific phobias: a meta-analysis, *Clin Psychol Rev* 28:1021-1037, 2008.

Wolpe J: *Psychotherapy by reciprocal inhibition*, Stanford, Calif, 1958, Stanford University Press.

Yalom ID: *The theory and practice of group psychotherapy*, ed 3, New York, 2005, Basic Books.

Yurkovich E: Patient and nurse roles in the therapeutic community, *Perspect Psychiatr Care* 25:18-22, 1989.

Online Resources

American Art Therapy Association: www.arttherapy.org

American Dance Therapy Association: www.adta.org

American Music Therapy Association: www.musictherapy.org

American Occupational Therapy Association: www.aota.org

American Society of Group Psychotherapy and Psychodrama: www.asgpp.org

American Therapeutic Recreation Association: www.atra-online.com

Association of Convulsive Therapy: www.act-ect.org

Beck Institute for Cognitive Therapy and Research: www.beckinstitute.org

Behavioral Tech: Dialectical Behavior Therapy: www.behavioraltech.com

International Centre for Excellence in Emotionally Focused Therapy: www.iceeft.com

27

Complementary and Alternative Therapies

Ruth N. Grendell

"Imagine a future world where [we] believed in the natural healing capacity of human beings and emphasized prevention above treatment."

Andrew Weil

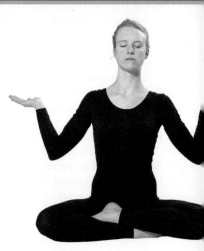

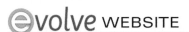 WEBSITE
http://evolve.elsevier.com/Fortinash/

OBJECTIVES

- Describe the philosophic differences between complementary and alternative medicine and traditional (allopathic) therapies.
- Discuss the use of various complementary and alternative medicine therapies, including mind–body interventions, pharmacologic and biologic treatments, herbal medications, diets and dietary supplements, and alternative systems of medical practice.

- Describe the nurse's role in providing holistic nursing care.
- Discuss the impact of integrating complementary and alternative therapies into nursing practice, education, and research.
- Outline a patient education program that focuses on the concurrent use of alternative therapies and traditional (allopathic) therapies.

KEY TERMS

allopathic (traditional/conventional) medicine
complementary and alternative medicine

concierge medicine
disease
health
holistic

illness
stress response

Hippocrates, the renowned father of medicine, followed four major principles: (1) to observe all; (2) to study the patient rather than the disease; (3) to evaluate honestly; and (4) to assist nature (Lyons, 1978). Florence Nightingale (1859) said that the nurse's major role was to provide an environment that supported the patient's healing processes. However, the traditional, or conventional, biomedical model, also referred to as allopathic medicine, appears to have a major focus on the disease rather than on perceiving the patient as a whole person.

Nevertheless, people all over the world have continued using their "tried-and-true" home remedies that have been passed down from one generation to the next. Many of these self-treatment alternatives and foods are readily available to consumers today. Many people also continue to use some of

the alternative therapies along with the prescribed therapies without informing their health care providers. In some instances, combining herbal and over-the-counter (OTC) medications with prescribed medications is potentially very harmful. Therefore, it is important that health care professionals are knowledgeable about the numerous alternative therapies that are available to the public (Cosentino, 2004).

The biomedical model is based primarily on the following assumptions: (1) the scientific method identifies the cause of a disease (i.e., a pathologic condition), and providers implement curative treatments to correct abnormal physiology; (2) the germ theory defines infections; (3) the prevention of disease is based on proper hygiene, public sanitation, and personal lifestyle choices; (4) disease is usually tangible and measurable. The terms *disease* and *illness* are often used simultaneously; however, illness is a highly individual and personal response that is exhibited as pain, suffering, or distress (Venes, 2005).

By contrast, the focus of the holistic or alternative care model is on strengthening one's inner resistance to disease and healing from within or enhancing the body's innate healing powers (Domrose, 2010). Although biomedical practices have strongly influenced the nursing discipline, nursing also has deep roots in the holistic or patient-centered perspective that considers the impact of all intrapersonal, interpersonal, and environmental interactions as contributing factors to a person's well-being or illness (American Holistic Nursing Association, 2006).

These therapies have been primarily used for pain management; for the treatment of chronic illness, anxiety, and depression; and for disease prevention. This chapter describes the contrast in philosophies and treatment modalities between biomedical and holistic models of care and discusses selected alternative therapies and their significance to the practice of nursing.

ALTERNATIVE THERAPY FIELDS

Complementary and alternative medicine (CAM) encompasses a broad range of healing philosophies, approaches, and therapies and their accompanying theories and beliefs. There are more than 1800 approaches to healing in this field. Some therapies are based on physiologic principles of modern medicine, whereas others come from concepts that are in contrast with accepted medical practices. In 1992, Congress established the Office of Alternative Medicine under the direction of the National Institutes of Health to evaluate the effectiveness of alternative therapies. In 1998, the Office of Alternative Medicine became the National Center for Complementary and Alternative Medicine (NCCAM). There are regional centers for objective, evidenced-based research on alternative therapies throughout the nation (NCCAM, 2009a). The NCCAM has classified complementary and alternative therapies into seven broad categories: (1) alternative medicine systems; (2) mind–body interventions; (3) pharmacologic and biologic-based therapies; (4) herbal medications; (5) diet, nutrition, supplements, and lifestyle changes; (6) manipulative and body-based methods; and (7) energy therapies. More than 600 CAM therapies are contained within this continually evolving NCCAM taxonomy. The 600 are formal taxonomy; more than 1800 exist less formally. The list of CAM practices is constantly revised as a result of the gradual acceptance of some CAM modalities that are based on research findings (Cosentino, 2004). Box 27-1 lists selected CAM therapies.

BOX 27-1	COMPLEMENTARY AND ALTERNATIVE THERAPY FIELDS AND SELECTED EXAMPLES

Alternative Systems of Medical Practice
Traditional Chinese medicine, including acupuncture
Ayurvedic medicine
Homeopathic medicine
Naturopathy
Environmental medicine
Culture-based community medicine (folk medicine)

Mind–Body Interventions
Meditation
Mindfulness-based therapy
Prayer
Yoga
The arts: music, dance, drama, art, and literature
Humor
Exercise
Animal-assisted therapy
Psychotherapy
Hypnosis

Pharmacologic and Biologic Treatments
Vaccines and medicines not yet approved by mainstream medicine (e.g., animal cartilage, chelating chemicals)

Herbal Medicine
Chinese herbals
European herbals
American herbals

Diet, Nutrition, Supplements, and Lifestyle Changes
Vitamins, minerals, and supplements
Designer diets (e.g., macrobiotic, cancer, weight reduction)
Food-elimination diets (e.g., for allergy detection)
Vegetarian diets
Ethnic-based diets

Manual Healing Methods
Osteopathy
Chiropractic
Massage
Acupressure
Foot and hand reflexology
Therapeutic touch

Energy Therapies
Biofeedback
Bioelectromagnetics
Light therapy
Bone-growth stimulation
Magnet therapy

HISTORIC OVERVIEW

Ancient Cultural Beliefs

In ancient times, many believed that illness was a punishment for sin or a whim of the gods—in other words, a matter of fate. Healing came through purification of the body with the use of herbs, fasting, purgatives, incantations, and ceremonies. Individuals believed that evil spirits caused diseases and adverse events; good spirits intervened on the behalf of an individual or group. People made animal sacrifices to appease the gods, and calling on spirits became part of healing rituals. However, some countries passed laws to regulate the practices of hygiene, sanitation, and the preservation of food to protect people from disease.

Hippocrates (400-377 BC) introduced beliefs that the gods did not control health, which is the state when all functions of the body and mind are normally active. Instead, health was dependent on the harmony or balance of the body, the mind, and the environment. He used a patient-centered approach to treat the whole person. The dominant beliefs in most Asian countries considered that individuals attained this balance between human beings and nature by finding inner peace and spiritual contentment and by understanding and practicing the interactive powers of the mind, body, and spirit. In many cultures, healers were priest–physicians who were referred to as *holy men* or *shamans,* and the care that they provided was shamanistic medicine (Ellis and Hartley, 2007; Topham, 2010).

BIOMEDICINE MODEL CONCEPTS

Western biomedicine (allopathic medicine) is based on a worldview that is strongly influenced by Cartesian dualism (i.e., the separation of the mind and the body) and by the Newtonian physics of the 17th and 18th centuries. In other words, "[d]isease occurs when the parts break down" (KPBS, 2006). Science and technology revolutionized the practice of medicine and facilitated a greater understanding of human biology and methods of intervention in disease and illness. In Western biomedicine, practitioners have standardized treatments and evidence-based care regimens that match the patient with a disease category of defined signs and symptoms. These technically oriented interventions aim for rapid results to reverse the deteriorative physiologic disease process and to prolong life (Topham, 2010).

HOLISTIC MODEL CONCEPTS

By contrast, the holistic perspective focuses on the healing of the total person rather than the cure of a specific disease. Each person is uniquely separate from another human being and is considered to be more than the sum of his or her individual parts—in other words, what affects one aspect of the person in fact affects all aspect (Topham, 2010). In addition to examining physical symptoms, the clinician considers the influence of cultural and genetic factors, past and current experiences, family structure, and role functions on the person's perception of health and illness and the use of coping mechanisms. Many of these therapies are preventive measures rather than treatments for disease symptoms. Research indicates that many of the CAM therapies (e.g., diet, exercise, psychologic stress-reduction therapies) are effective for preventing and managing chronic disease processes (Pelletier, 2007). CAM therapies encourage individuals to take responsibility for their own health and to participate in the recovery process when diseases do occur. A change in attitude and lifestyle, a sense of control and peace, and decreased anxiety indicate healing, although the particular disease may not be cured. Multiple methods are sometimes incorporated into the individualized plan of care. Many alternative therapies are based on Oriental and Far Eastern beliefs and practices. Unifying themes among the several alternative therapies include a person's inherent recuperative ability, the importance of self-esteem, and the influence of spiritual and emotional beliefs on health. Treatment methods are based on maintaining or restoring a balance within all aspects of the individual. Box 27-2 presents a detailed listing of themes.

Rise in Dominance of the Biomedical Model

Before the 1800s, biomedicine and alternative medicine coexisted and competed on a somewhat equal basis. During the latter part of that century, however, the biomedical model was considered superior because of the scientific discovery of microbes as the cause of many infectious diseases and the methods that were developed to eliminate those causes. Disease cure rates rose, and favorable surgical outcomes soon followed with the use of proper aseptic techniques and new anesthesia discoveries. Another significant event that legitimized biomedicine was a research report by Abraham Flexner in 1910, which indicated the need for standards for the education and licensing of physicians. The philanthropic funding of medical education institutions quickly stopped any financial assistance to schools with nonmedical and nonscientific curricula.

BOX 27-2   **COMMON THEMES OF INTEGRATIVE THERAPIES**

- Humans have recuperative powers.
- Religious and spiritual values are important to the state of one's health.
- Self-esteem and the purpose of life are positive influences in the healing process.
- Thoughts, feelings, emotions, values, and perceived meanings affect physical function.
- Most therapies rely on diet, exercise, relaxation techniques, lifestyle, and attitude changes.
- The focus is on the total person and includes one's physical, emotional, mental, and psychosocial health.
- Illness is an imbalance; interventions are directed toward the restoring of balance.
- Energy is the force that is needed to achieve balance and harmony.

As a result of the rising dominance of the biomedical model, many questioned the credibility of alternative therapies. These practices were soon relegated to the fringes of health care, and they were often referred to as quackery. Although chiropractic and osteopathic practices continued, others such as homeopathy and naturopathy were almost forgotten (White, 2009). However, today more than 40% of Americans report using alternative therapies; worldwide, more than 90% of people use them (Cosentino, 2004). Although Europe and other countries have largely accepted CAM therapies, most U.S. health care professionals ignore the fact that people use many alternative methods to manage their diseases and chronic illnesses.

Merging Philosophies

Renewed interest in mind–body interactions grew during the mid-20th century. The discovery that some people who were exposed to pathogens did not become ill led researchers to challenge the existing biologic theory and to explore other possible influencing causes. Subsequent epidemiologic studies revealed that diet, smoking, and environmental pollution were strongly associated with increased incidences of lung cancer. They also found that widowed persons had higher death rates than married persons in the same age group; that socioeconomic factors had an effect on disease; and that certain religious groups had fewer reports of illness and death from specific diseases. The technologies of modern biomedicine did not provide explanations. The strong possibility of a cause-and-effect relationship between the environment and the mind, spirit, and body in health and illness encouraged further investigation. These findings indicated that many chronic conditions are the result of common lifestyle risks (e.g., smoking, diet, sedentary lifestyle, stress). However, these factors are not treatable by means of the one-dimensional solutions prescribed by conventional (allopathic) medicine.

Psychoneuroimmunology or psychoendocrine neuroimmunology is a relatively new field that involves the study of a person's psychobiologic factors and their interaction with the stress response and its influence on health outcomes. The arousal of the hypothalamic–pituitary–adrenal axis affects the nervous, endocrine, and immune systems. Prolonged exposure to stress and high anxiety levels are linked with lowered immunity, whereas a greater resistance to illness is associated with lower stress and anxiety levels. The psychoneuroimmunology model provides a framework for screening risk factors for health problems, including stress stimuli, sociodemographic factors, lifestyle behaviors, and health history (Anderson, 2004a). Psychoneuroimmunology is also possibly the framework for the conducting of future studies of the efficacy of mind–body therapies because of its emphasis on the relationships among stress, increased cortisol levels, and the impairment of the immune system (See Chapter 5).

Scientists have explored the age-old mind–body healing modalities of other societies, particularly Oriental medicine. As a result, mainstream health care has integrated acupuncture, meditation, relaxation techniques, massage, and other related interventions into care plans. Some medical and nursing schools have included courses in CAM in their curricula. Additional researchers are conducting studies in this area, and several practitioners have published articles (Anderson, 2004b; Pelletier, 2007). However, progress in integrating CAM into mainstream medicine will be slowed because of regulatory and reimbursement measures, values, and misconceptions still held by many allopathic (biomedicine) practitioners and the lack of large-scale clinical trials to demonstrate the effectiveness of CAM (Box 27-3).

BOX 27-3 EXAMPLES OF COMPLETED AND ONGOING RESEARCH FUNDED BY THE NATIONAL CENTER OF COMPLEMENTARY AND ALTERNATIVE MEDICINE AND SAFETY WARNINGS

NOTE: Many of these studies are longitudinal and require several months or years to produce results. Large-scale, long-term, randomized clinical trials are the gold standard of biomedical research (NCCAM, 2006). Preliminary findings have been reported for some of the studies. After the performance of evidence-based studies, the Agency for Healthcare Research and Quality has issued several safety alerts. Some herbals are harmful for persons with certain health problems and because of their interactive effects with other herbals and medications. Consider the following examples:

- *Kavakava (Piper methysticum)* is a member of the pepper family that is used to treat insomnia, stress, and anxiety. It is linked with hepatitis and cirrhosis.
- *Garlic* is popular for the reduction of cholesterol levels. However, it is harmful when combined with drugs that are used for the treatment of acquired immunodeficiency syndrome. For example, it reduces the effectiveness of saquinavir by 50%.
- *St. John's wort* should not be used with protease inhibitors such as indinavir.
- *Bioterrorism protection herbals* have been advocated by some as protection against virulent infections that can be spread by biologic weapons. However, the Centers for Disease Control and Prevention state that there is no scientific basis for this practice. Anthrax and smallpox progress too rapidly for the immune system to counteract them via the use of any CAM dietary supplement.

Modified from the National Center for Complementary and Alternative Medicine: *Home page* (website): www.nccam.nih.gov. Accessed December 20, 2010.

CURRENT ISSUES

The Changing Complexion of Health Care

Modern medicine has become so expensive that it is straining the economy of the United States and of many other developed nations and putting itself beyond the reach of much of the world's population, particularly for long-term regimens. Chronic and degenerative illnesses, including cardiovascular disease, cancer, diabetes, arthritis, and depression, are reaching epidemic proportions (Bodenheimer and Fernandez, 2005; Pelletier, 2007). Nearly 70% of the U.S. health care budget is spent on the treatment of persons with chronic diseases, and costs will escalate as the baby-boomer generation grows older. The United States spent more than $1.7 trillion—or 15.3% of the U.S. gross domestic product—on health care in 2003. Researchers predict that this will increase to $4 trillion by 2015, which will be approximately 20% of the gross domestic product. These costs are straining all of the systems that finance health care (Gutierrez and Ranji, 2005).

Concierge medicine, which is also known as *boutique medicine* or *platinum medicine,* is a relatively new practice method for physicians who choose to limit their practice to patients who are able to privately pay an annual fee for extra and special services from that physician. There are a wide range of services offered that depend on the individual physician's imagination and choices. Annual fees may include e-mail communication, priority access to services, and coordination of care with a focus on illness prevention (Majette, 2009). This type of practice is obviously in the minority in the United States, but the American Medical Association and other legal governing organizations consider it to be legal and ethical. The obvious disadvantage is that it eliminates those who are not privileged and wealthy from participating.

Unfortunately, biomedical treatments and advanced technology also have negative consequences. Some microbes have become resistant to medications. Some chronic diseases that still defy scientific interventions have replaced infectious diseases as the major cripplers and killers. Side effects of many of the new "wonder drugs" sometimes involve dangerous psychologic and physiologic effects.

Consumer confidence in conventional treatment methods has deteriorated, and citizens are turning to legislators to change the health care system. Reasons for the growing dissatisfaction include the increasing costs and restrictions imposed by managed care and health maintenance organizations. Consumers also want to have more control of their health care decisions. Convenience and fewer side effects from natural substances, less invasive techniques, and the ability to choose are appealing alternatives to traditional medicine (Topham, 2010).

In December 2008, NCCAM released the most comprehensive findings regarding the use of CAM by Americans. The report was based on data from the 2007 National Health Interview Survey of 23,394 Americans 18 years old or older who answered questions about their health practices and status and their use of 27 types of CAM. Approximately 36% (4 out of every 10 people) had used some form of alternative therapy during the previous year, which represented an increase from the 34% reported in 2002. The therapies included acupuncture, hypnosis, and chiropractic care in addition to self-administered therapies such as meditation, exercise, diet-based therapies, and herbal supplements.

Barriers to the Acceptance of Alternative Therapies

Although alternative practices have been popular for centuries in Europe, Asia, and the Far East, therapeutic results were primarily reported through anecdotal reports, so the Western medical community questioned the validity of the research methods. The Western medical world continues to call for clinical studies that are to be conducted within strict, controlled limits. The U.S. Food and Drug Administration (FDA) also expressed great concern about the lack of guidelines to ensure the purity and dosage accuracy of herbal remedies and supplements (NCCAM, 2008). These substances are currently exempt from FDA approval. There is also a concern regarding claims that a certain substance is a cure-all for many health problems. The FDA continues to argue for the right to regulate these products. Another great concern is the validity of media reports, the credentials of the report writers, and the fact that no effective control exists for the more than 15,000 health care information sites on the Internet.

Many advocates of alternative therapies cannot afford the tremendous costs of FDA investigation; thus, many methods will not be tested. Additional barriers are society's heavy reliance on high-technology treatments, the dependence on pharmaceuticals, and state laws that limit the practice of medicine or the healing arts to those with professional medical licensure. Political lobbying and the advertising influence of drug manufacturers are other major barriers, although most pharmaceutical companies produce OTC compounds that are attractive substitutes to costly prescription medications.

The many barriers are typical for innovative proposals that challenge any current traditional practices. Additional concerns focus on the dangers of self-diagnosis, potential and critical delays in the seeking of appropriate medical care, potential interactions that may occur with the concurrent use of herbal treatments and other drugs with prescribed medications, and the detrimental effects of not informing health care providers about the use of CAM products. The scientific research projects at NCCAM have produced a notable shift in thinking by mainstream medical practitioners. Because the use of CAM is continuing to increase, the medical community and consumers deserve to know which therapies have demonstrated effectiveness and which have not. CAM does have limitations, and it can be harmful if it is not used properly. Biomedical medicine also includes some practices that research has not yet validated. The same stringent standards of evidence-based medicine must be employed for all therapeutic interventions, thereby helping to prevent double standards.

IMPACT OF THE *HEALTHY PEOPLE 2010* REPORT

As early as the 1970s, the rising costs of medical care led several physicians and educators to see the need for integrating technical sophistication with humanistic values. The debate surrounding quality-of-life issues required a focus on changes in educating the public and the profession. Alternative strategies evolved, such as permitting family members to assist with patient care in intensive care units, creating a homelike atmosphere during labor and delivery, presenting health education programs, and establishing self-help support groups. Health care agencies made health appraisal questionnaires available in health care facilities, and illnesses because creative opportunities for instruction on self-care. Some practitioners introduced a limited number of alternative therapies, including acupuncture and stress-reduction measures, into the system.

Health care reform became a major issue during the 1980s, and, as a result, researchers conducted several nationwide studies. The Healthy People Initiative established specific national goals and objectives that would be evaluated every 10 years. The 2000 report indicated that some progress had been made toward increasing protective and preventive measures that require the active participation of both individuals and health care providers. Specific needs of several high-risk groups were targeted, including infants, children, ethnic and low-income groups, and older adults. The two major goals for 2010 were as follows: (1) to increase the quality and years of a healthy life; and (2) to eliminate health disparities. These goals were similar to those of the 2000 report. Plans are in progress for establishing the goals for the 2020 report. The proposed shift in emphasis will be on age-group populations with high risk factors rather than on specific diseases, and an effort will be made to determine how the definition of health changes over the course of a person's lifespan (Healthy People, 2010; Centers for Disease Control and Prevention, 2008). Ongoing research will monitor the incidence of health and illness. *Statistical indicators of a healthy population* include eight aspects: (1) evidence of physical activity, (2) a reduction in obesity, (3) a decline in tobacco and substance abuse, (4) responsible sexual behavior, (5) improved mental health, (6) a decrease in injury and violence, (7) enhanced environmental quality, and (8) a more widespread application of immunizations. The nurse plays a primary role in health promotion and education. Consider these indicators as you learn about human responses to health and illness.

EXPLORING THE EFFECTIVENESS OF ALTERNATIVE THERAPIES

The Informed Patient

Physicians have less control over disease information as consumers become more active in making decisions about their methods of treatment and turn to therapies that address them as whole beings. Individuals, self-help, and discussion groups often make use of the Internet for the exchange of information. Broadcasts of documentary films and programs in health education and fitness have also enhanced public awareness of developments in health care, alternative therapies, and self-care options.

The Nurse's Role

The health of individuals, families, and communities is a major focus of nursing, with consideration for the effect of the individual's health status, health beliefs, and interactions with others and the environment. Several practice models help to guide the nurse to carry out these practices. All of the new integrative therapy (CAM) models are designed around a holistic view of the patient, which includes the individual's ability to adapt and cope with life events; the impact of social and cultural values on health and illness beliefs; and personal responsibility for healthy outcomes (KPBS, 2006; Topham, 2010).

People from every culture have different perspectives of the Western health care model and will respond in different ways. They often view the system as cold and abrupt or even rude, and they often turn away unless health care providers understand them. Knowing this, it is important to keep people of all cultures connected to the system, particularly with regard to public health concerns. It is important for the nurse to respect people's dignity, integrity, and belief systems; to negotiate a situation that allows for as much independence in the care process as possible; and to create an environment that promotes partnership with patients during all phases of the nursing process. The Joint Commission also requires documentation of the ways in which nurses meet patients' cultural needs (Frisch, 2001a; Williams, 2006).

The American Holistic Nursing Association has published standards for holistic practice (Box 27-4), and resources are available from the several nursing specialty groups (Frisch, 2001b). Nurses often integrate CAM techniques with traditional medical practices, such as teaching breathing and visualization strategies for the management of pain and the reduction of stress and anxiety. The nurse, serving as a teacher and a facilitator, empowers the patient.

APPLICATION OF SELECTED ALTERNATIVE THERAPIES

Since the mid-1970s, there has been a major effort to identify strategies that assist individuals cope with acute diagnoses and chronic psychologic and physiologic health problems as well as with managing sudden and long-term life changes. The greatest benefits of CAM therapies lie in promoting healthy lifestyles and managing chronic illnesses and diseases (Kreitzer and Disch, 2003; Pelletier, 2007; Topham, 2010).

Mind–Body Interventions
Meditation

The relaxation response to meditation consists of a wide range of beneficial physiologic and psychologic effects, including lowered heart and blood pressure rates, decreased serum levels of adrenal corticosteroids, increased immunity to disease, and a sense of calmness, peace, and mental alertness. Meditation therapies include biofeedback, visual imagery, and other stress-reduction measures, including yoga and progressive relaxation techniques. Originally, meditation was a religious practice (e.g., saying prayers, reciting scripture, saying the rosary, concentrating on a religious symbol). Nurses can teach meditative techniques, and there are a number of audiotapes that facilitate the mastery of concentration. Guidelines for meditating include a routine of selecting a special time and place, assuming a comfortable position, using deep breathing and progressive relaxation exercises, and focusing attention on a chosen mental image (Topham, 2010).

Prayer

Prayer differs from meditation in that it involves communication with God or a superior being. Prayer for healing purposes is an individual or group action or an intercessory prayer (distant prayer) conducted by other people with or without the knowledge of the individual for whom the prayers are said. Ancient forms of intercessory prayer include the laying on of hands and anointing the ill person with oil.

Prayer is silent or spoken and conversational or formal, or it may involve the recitation of a favorite form of prayer. Illness sometimes interferes with an individual's ability to

pray because of feelings of isolation, guilt, grief, or anxiety (Maier-Lorentz, 2004). Prayer is one of the therapeutic tools that nurses may use when providing spiritual care to calm a patient's worried feelings. Many hospitals have chaplains to support patients and their families of all faiths. Numerous studies—some with a strong scientific base and others that have been poorly constructed—have demonstrated significant positive associations between religion (faith) and health; therefore, nurses do not ignore the role that beliefs play in a person's ability to cope (Koenig, 2006).

Mindfulness-Based Therapy

Jon Kabat-Zinn is the founder of the Mindfulness-Based Stress Reduction (MBSR) Clinic at the University of Massachusetts Medical School. The program is based on Zen consciousness, which involves paying attention to one's own inner experience by quieting the mind and investigating the mind through personal experiences and asking questions such as "Who am I?" Individuals learn how to balance physical, mental, and spiritual health by using all of the senses. Many use MBSR to address a variety of health problems, including anxiety, eating disorders, and addictions. In an interview, Kabat-Zinn stated, "Humans are miraculous beings, and we have infinitely more capacity and dimensions associated with our brains and our nervous system and with our deep intelligences, *and I emphasize the plural*, that we usually simply ignore" (Gazella, 2005, p. 59). MBSR therapy has been proved effective for persons with prostate cancer, for those receiving bone marrow transplants, for prison inmates and staff, and for persons in multicultural settings as well as those in corporate and work environments.

The goal of the meditation process is not to change the thoughts but to allow an awareness to emerge by paying attention only to the present moment and being nonjudgmental about all thoughts that pass through the mind. Although this type of meditation is based on Buddhist beliefs, the spiritual aspects are deemphasized for a Western audience. Hatha yoga and controlled breathing eliminate distractions and permit the participant to be more objective about his or her inner thoughts. The person also learns to scan the body systematically as part of a desensitization process to inhibit the automatic learned responses to unhealthy thoughts (Telner, 2005; Laidlaw and Dwivedi, 2004; Telner, 2005). Kabat-Zinn's book *Catastrophe Living: Using the Wisdom of Your Body and Mind to Face Stress, Pain and Illness* (1990), which outlines the practices of the MBSR clinic, is a major resource for mindfulness-based cognitive therapy (MBCT) programs.

MBCT is a promising new approach for the prevention of recurring episodes of depression. The therapy uses the decentering or disengagement concept to help the individual to visualize passing events in the mind that are neither necessarily valid reflections of reality nor central aspects of the self. Culture and upbringing strongly influence the meaning of an event and an individual's response. Reframing or cognitive restructuring (cognitive optimizing) is also used (See Chapter 25).

MBCT is particularly helpful for persons who have had three or more depression episodes and who experienced depression early in life (Kabat-Zinn, 2002) (see the Research for Evidence-Based Practice box).

RESEARCH FOR EVIDENCE-BASED PRACTICE

Foley E et al: Mindfulness-based cognitive therapy (MBCT) for individuals whose lives have been affected by cancer: a randomized controlled trial, *J Consult Clin Psychol* 78(1):72-79, 2010.

The diagnosis of cancer brings its own set of anxiety and depression responses. Several clinical trials have supported the positive effects of MBCT for a variety of stressful and depressive situations. This study was conducted with 116 adult participants with mixed cancer diagnoses. The psychologic challenges after the cancer diagnosis include adjustment to the diagnosis and treatments, the disruption of life events, the reevaluation and one's life direction, and the tolerance of an uncertain outcome. The resulting negative thoughts and brooding without action to disengage from the thoughts increase anxiety and depression. Pretests and posttests for depression, anxiety, and quality of life were administered. Participants were assigned to either an immediate treatment group or a wait-listed treatment group. Treatment consisted of 8 weekly sessions, a 1-day guided meditation workshop, assigned readings, and home exercises. There were significant changes for both groups; however, improvements in anxiety, depression status, and quality of life scores were greater for the immediate treatment group. These findings may be the result of participants in the wait-listed group being in later stages of the disease by the time of treatment. Scores obtained from a 3-month posttest continued to indicate improvement for both groups. The greatest satisfaction with the MBCT program was in the gaining of a sense of control over the illness.

Johrei Meditation

Psychotherapists are also looking at Johrei, a Japanese strategy that involves a nontouch method of sending subtle energy toward another person and that includes not only paying close attention to the recipient but also being open hearted and feeling goodwill toward the recipient. The Johrei method also makes use of Zen meditation principles. In Asian languages, the term *mindfulness* means that a person is affectionate and has kind-hearted characteristics when attending to the here and now. Some have used this method in conjunction with hypnosis. A pilot study of Johrei therapy that involved persons in substance-abuse rehabilitation revealed significant decreases in depression, stress, and physical pain and improved emotional and spiritual states as compared with persons receiving only the standard therapy (Brooks et al, 2006).

Yoga

Living a balanced life is central to yoga principles. The individual achieves specific body postures (*asanas*), gentle movements, stretches, and breath control. He or she minimizes the stimulation of the senses, leads a simple life, and performs directed meditation through daily practices. Concentration on the purity of body and mind, self-restraint and contentment with life, studying relevant literature, and daily dedication to a higher being are the means to attain this balance. Originally practiced in India, yoga has become a popular practice as a part of health enhancement and as a therapy for stress reduction and for people with chronic diseases. Hatha yoga, which is also called *Hatha vidya*, is the most familiar form of yoga. Outside of India, Hatha yoga is mainly practiced for mental and physical health (Saper et al, 2009).

Use of the Arts

The use of music, dance, drama, literature, humor, and art is part of environmental therapy for patients and health care providers. Quiet background music provides a soothing atmosphere, and it is distracting medium during times of stress and pain. Music is often used in intensive care units, in birthing rooms, during dental procedures, and even as a stimulus for people with lowered levels of consciousness. Mood music allows the listener to express emotions and feelings through dancing, singing, and creative thinking. Music is also beneficial for reducing agitation among persons with dementia (Gaskill, 2004; Goodal and Etters, 2005).

Dance is an expression of joy and celebration throughout the world. Many have used it as a means to increase self-esteem and body image; to lessen depression, fear, and isolation; and to express emotions (Khazzoom, 2009). Art has often been used to help children and adults express their feelings about stressful situations and their unconscious concerns about their illnesses. Art expression has been a psychotherapy tool in geriatric centers, with children and adolescents, in hospices, in alcohol treatment programs, and in prisons. Books, poetry, and religious writings are often inspirational, and they can cause a person to become immersed in reading for long periods of time. Writing in a journal or diary is also a form of expressing one's emotions; this is called *process meditation,* and it involves a conversation with the self. Many age-specific therapies are also recommended, including storytelling, poetry, crafts, puzzles, and games.

Humor

Humor and laughter are also helpful for expressing emotions, relieving tensions and anxiety, and coping with painful or unpleasant situations. Laughter often has a positive effect on cognitive ability, respiratory and heart rates, blood pressure, and muscle tension. In some places, humor rooms supplied with videocassettes, audiotapes, books, cartoons, and artwork are available for patients, families, and agency staff; all are encouraged to use humorous artwork on bulletin boards in patient rooms and staff work areas. In his classic book, *Anatomy of an Illness as Perceived by the Patient* (1979), the famous journalist Norman Cousins wrote about the value of humor for relieving the severe pain that he experienced as a result of ankylosing spondylitis by stating that a good belly laugh when watching *Candid Camera* episodes or Marx Brothers films allowed him to be pain free for at least 2 hours at a time. Cousins wrote that humor healed him (Anderson, 2004a).

Exercise

The benefits of physical exercise are well known. Exercise brings a general sense of health and vitality, increases respiratory and cardiovascular efficiency, and promotes a longer life. People who exercise often sleep better and have improved appetites; society now considers exercise a major factor in self-care (Pelletier, 2007). People with disabilities are able to perform even simple exercises. Special Olympics events for wheelchair athletes are excellent examples of the use of exercise to enhance an individual's self-image and general health. (A discussion of tai chi exercises is included in the section about traditional Chinese medicine later in this chapter.)

Animal-Assisted Therapy

This discussion of mind–body interventions is not complete without mentioning the use of companion animals to induce the relaxation response and to enhance emotional and physiologic well-being. Animal-assisted therapy is a goal-directed intervention that has been designed to improve human physical, social, emotional, and cognitive function in a variety of settings. Animal-assisted therapy is frequently used in conjunction with occupational and physical therapies for refining fine motor skills, assisting with maintaining balance and walking tolerance, and increasing attention and self-esteem. Studies show a reduction in a person's hypertension, heart rate, and social isolation when pets are a treatment modality. Studies have also shown the benefits of this therapy to the morale of staff and caregivers. Individuals who are blind, deaf, or paralyzed use companion animals to assist them with accomplishing activities of daily living. Some acute and long-term health care agency policies now allow pets into intensive care units, pediatric wards, hospices, rehabilitation units, and geriatric and other areas. Nurses are active supporters of animal-assisted therapy (Delta Society, 2006; Topham, 2010).

Hypnosis

Hypnosis has been in use since the 18th century as a deep relaxation technique, and it is a useful tool for the treatment of substance addiction, smoking cessation, pain control, fears, and phobias. It is also successful before anesthesia induction, as a means for reducing hypertension, for relieving pain and muscle spasms in persons with cerebral palsy, for relaxing children during invasive procedures, and for dietary management. Hypnosis involves the use of mental images, concentration, the use of repetitive words and sounds, and total relaxation. Hypnosis produces an altered state of consciousness that permits the person to concentrate with minimal distraction. Self-therapy at home consists of education in self-hypnosis with the aid of guiding audiotapes that have been designed to address the individual's specific problem. Hypnosis relies heavily on the person's

openness to suggestion (KPBS, 2006). There is a concern that selective serotonin-reuptake inhibitor medications are a contributing factor to the increase in the suicide rate among people with depression. A systematic meta-analysis of several clinical studies indicated that minimal benefits come from selective serotonin-reuptake inhibitor medications as compared with placebo effects. The research recommended that the use of hypnosis in psychotherapy was a better choice (Kirsch, 2005).

Energy Therapies
Biofeedback

Biofeedback is a technique that initially involves the use of electrical equipment to assist individuals with gaining conscious control over body processes that are normally beyond voluntary command. Biofeedback training is often combined with controlled breathing techniques or meditation to provide individuals with increased awareness of their bodies. Electrodes that are attached to the affected area send information to a monitoring device that emits a signal to alert the person to changes in a particular body function (e.g., an increase or decrease in muscle tension). Transcutaneous electrical nerve stimulation is one example of this technique, and it is most often used for patients with chronic pain and muscle spasms (Topham, 2010).

Several other electrical biofeedback devices have been used to assist patients with gaining self-control of certain body functions. By watching their responses on the device, patients learn to use mental processes to control that particular body action. A therapist instructs the patient in the mental exercises during a series of sessions. Eventually the patient is able to practice the exercises without the aid of the machine. Biofeedback has been used for the treatment of multiple physical, cognitive, and behavioral symptoms. Among these are hypertension, temperature control, gastrointestinal activity, substance abuse, stress, sleep disorders, migraine headaches, and other vascular disorders (Saito and Saito, 2004).

Bioelectromagnetics

Concepts of magnetic field therapy relate to the electrical currents that exist within and external to the body, the influence of external currents on the body, and the result of physical and behavioral changes. Examples are the electromagnetic energies produced by x-rays, televisions, microwaves, and light rays. Prolonged exposure to such fields produces hazardous effects. However, scientists also discovered that lower-level energy frequencies are beneficial in the design of diagnostic and treatment tools.

Health care providers use nonthermal electromagnetic fields—which do not cause the heating of tissues—for bone repair, nerve stimulation, and wound healing; as electrostimulation via acupuncture needles for the stimulation of the immune system; and for neuroendocrine modulations. Copper bracelets as well as static or permanent magnets for arthritis pain relief have been used for many years. Magnets are taped to various areas of the body, inserted inside shoes, and placed in mattress covers. An NCCAM survey in 1999 revealed that more than $500 million in the United States and $5 billion worldwide were spent on magnet products each year. Many individuals purchase these products without consulting their health care providers. Magnets are safe except for persons with pacemakers or defibrillators. Although anecdotal accounts yield favorable responses for the use of magnets, clinical trials by NCCAM (2009) have revealed mixed results; there is no firm support for their use.

Alternative Systems of Medical Practice

Alternative systems of medical practice include traditional Chinese medicine (TCM); acupuncture; ayurvedic, homeopathic, naturopathic, and environmental medicines; and anthroposophically extended medicine, which builds on naturopathy, homeopathy, and modern scientific medicine.

Traditional Chinese Medicine

TCM involves the use of a variety of therapies, including acupuncture, acupressure, massage, herbal medicine, qigong, and tai chi. Tai chi, which is a Chinese exercise program with roots in the ancient martial arts, has gained popular appeal for people of all ages in the West. It consists of slow and gentle rhythmic movements, controlled breathing, and the creation of an "inner stillness." Individuals have used tai chi to prevent and remedy a variety of muscular and joint problems and to reduce stress, and it is an excellent exercise for persons with osteoarthritis. Other benefits include pain relief, a reduction of joint soreness and stiffness, and balance maintenance. There are many different styles of tai chi exercises, and choosing an instructor is important, because some of the movements may need to be modified. Individuals need to consult their health care providers before beginning any exercise program (Topham, 2010).

Variations of TCM are practiced in Japan, Korea, and Vietnam. Oriental medicine is centered on the diagnosis of disturbances of qi (pronounced "chee"), which is the vital energy, and the balance between the forces of yin and yang (i.e., female and male, cold and hot, dark and light). TCM diagnostic procedures consist of observing facial expressions and body movements, careful listening and questioning, and palpating body pulses. The relationship of physical and emotional behaviors is used to plan a range of traditional therapies. The most frequent TCM methods used in the United States are acupuncture and massage.

Acupuncture. Acupuncture is a process during which the practitioner inserts small needles at selected energy points of the body that correspond with energy pathways or meridians that traverse from the body surface to the inner organs. Its purpose is to activate the qi and to achieve a balance when imbalance exists. The needles are sometimes heated and attached to a mild electrical current, or they may be twirled by hand to cause vibrations. Numerous studies have revealed the positive effects of acupuncture on a wide range of disorders, including gynecologic, mental, and neurologic problems and substance dependence. Its effectiveness for pain control and anesthesia is attributed to the release of endogenous opioids (endorphins) that are produced within the central nervous system. Acupuncture is one of the most thoroughly researched and documented alternative medical practices (Eshkevari and Heath, 2005).

Ayurveda/Ayurvedic Medicine

Ayurvedic (science of life) medicine originated in India and dates back thousands of years. This method involves the use of a combination of therapies, including meditation, yoga, massage, herbs, aromatherapy, and biofeedback. In ayurvedic medicine, the body is a pharmacy that can make its own natural drugs to heal itself.

The human body is also a microcosm of the universe, with principles or *doshas* that interact to maintain balance. The basic nature (*prakriti*) or the genetic code and the relationship among the doshas remain unaltered throughout a person's life. Each dosha has a principal location in the body, with emphasis on the interdependence of health and the quality of the person's sociocultural life. When any imbalance occurs, the individual achieves a restoration of balance of the internal environment through proper diet and lifestyle (NCCAM, 2009).

Homeopathic Medicine

Homeopathic medicine is based on the belief that substances that produce certain disease symptoms in a healthy person provide a cure for a sick person who is experiencing the same symptoms. Diluted substances are used to elicit a cure (e.g., a very dilute solution that contains a poison ivy compound is used for a skin rash). The medication has to be shaken vigorously or "potentized" for its greatest effectiveness as the solution picks up energy from the dissolved substance. These products are often used for acute and chronic health problems as well as for health promotion.

The homeopathic drug market has become a multimillion-dollar industry; the FDA currently regulates these remedies, and drugs manufactured by reputable pharmaceutical companies are in the *Homeopathic Pharmacopoeia of the United States*. Some are sold as OTC drugs, but products that are used for serious conditions must be dispensed by a licensed practitioner. These medications are not tested for safety and efficacy as required for prescription and new OTC drugs, because they contain little or no active ingredients (NCCAM, 2009).

Naturopathy

A small group of physicians practice naturopathy. These physicians have been educated in the sciences, and they have received specialized training in the disciplines of alternative medicine. They use an eclectic selection of herbs, homeopathy, nutrition, TCM, hydrotherapy, and manipulative therapy in conjunction with modern scientific medical diagnostic methods and standards. Naturopathy focuses on self-healing, and practitioners individualize health care to meet the individual's needs. The basic principles include the following (Barrett, 2006; NCCAM, 2007):

- The use of therapies that do no harm
- The physician's primary role as teacher

- The establishment and maintenance of optimal health and balance
- The treatment of the whole person
- The prevention of disease via the maintenance of a healthy lifestyle
- The therapeutic use of nutrition

Many of these therapies occur in treatment spas, where practitioners use sunlight, fresh air, and water therapies. Fasting, natural food diets, colonic enemas, acupuncture, massage, and TCM are also used. Allopathic practitioners view naturopathy with skepticism (Barrett, 2006).

Environmental Medicine

Allergy treatment was the original impetus for the development of environmental medicine during the 1940s. Scientists noted that the sensitivity and allergy symptoms of some individuals improved after the elimination of certain foods, chemicals, molds, dust, pollens, or other substances. Emotional stress was also a source of immune system dysfunction. The person's environmental history became an important component of the diagnostic process by providing a chronologic account of etiologic circumstances that led to the health problem. The elimination of health hazards from the environment has become a major health issue. Examples include the removal of asbestos building insulation materials, the instillation of devices that recapture gasoline fumes and smog emissions from automobiles, the removal of certain pesticides from the market, and the elimination of preservatives and color additives from foods, medicines, and nutrition supplements.

Culture-Based Community Medicines

Many culture-based or folk medicine practices follow naturalistic methods, and a spiritual healer or shaman usually provides religious rituals, which are a major component. Symbols such as prayer wheels, sand paintings, meditation, amulets, group singing, chanting, and dancing ceremonies are part of these healing rituals. On the Navajo reservation, modern hospitals and the shaman's healing room are under the same roof. Some people believe that spells cast by the witch doctor have sometimes proved to be more powerful than Western medicines (Grendell, personal observation).

Manual Healing Methods

Included in manual healing methods are osteopathic and chiropractic medicines, massage, reflexology, and techniques that make use of pressure points and other various touch therapies.

Osteopathy and Chiropractic Medicines

Osteopathy and chiropractic medicine both involve the manipulation of soft tissues and joints, and both require specialized education and licensure to practice. Much of the public considers osteopathic practices to be mainstream medicine, and the practitioner is often the patient's primary health care provider. Chiropractic practitioners study the relationship between pressure, strain, and tension on the spinal cord and the ability of the neuromusculoskeletal system to act efficiently. Manual adjustments of the spine to correct alignment are a mainstay of treatment. Some insurance carriers have approved chiropractic medicine, and NCCAM has recently established a center to study its effects (NCCAM, 2009).

Massage

Touch, which is the basic medium of massage therapy, is a form of communication and caring. There are more than 80 different forms of massage therapy that vary from gentle stroking to deep kneading, rubbing, and percussion. Most massage is done with the hands; however, the forearms, elbows, and feet are sometimes used. The primary purposes of massage therapy are to produce muscle and total body relaxation and to increase circulation. In the past, massage techniques were in fundamental nursing courses. Massage should not be used for persons who are taking anticoagulant therapy; for patients after surgery; or for areas that involve circulatory abnormalities, open wounds, sciatica, varicose veins, thrombi, or joint or bone injuries (Topham, 2010).

Acupressure

The same meridian points that are used in acupuncture are manipulated in pressure-point therapies. These therapists use their fingertips to apply pressure to more than 600 designated points in the soft tissues. Acupressure is both a diagnostic tool and a treatment. The sessions sometimes last up to an hour, with the recipient spending equal time lying in the prone and dorsal positions for a total body treatment. The therapist also places a strong emphasis on mind, spirit, and body balance when counseling the patient. Shiatsu, which is a Japanese form that is similar to acupressure, involves the therapist applying pressure with the palm of the hand as well as the fingers.

Hand and Foot Reflexology

Reflexology, which originated in Egypt, is also referred to as *zone therapy*. This technique is based on the premise that the feet and hands are mirrors of the body, with reflex points that correspond to glands, organs, and other structures in the body. The feet are more responsive to massage than the hands. The massage of a reflex point without the use of oil, cream, or lotion stimulates the corresponding organ in that zone. The main goal is to provide relaxation by removing tension in a zone area (Allen, 2009).

Therapeutic Touch

Healing through touch can be traced back to early civilizations, and nurses have practiced various forms of therapeutic touch for many years. Benefits of contact touch such as massage have been recently identified as providing a sense of spiritual balance, relieving mental and emotional tension and anxiety, improving blood flow, easing pain, and stimulating the immune system.

Therapeutic touch also refers to a noncontact technique that has evolved from the laying on of hands associated with

Far Eastern, European, and religious philosophies. This method is based on a theory that the release of excess energy from the healer assists the ill person with the healing process. Individuals can learn the basic principles, and workshops are available throughout the country and the world. Healing touch is a similar technique, and the American Holistic Nurses Association developed a certificate program to teach it in 1993 (Zerwekh, 2008).

Pharmacologic and Biologic Treatments

Pharmacologic and biologic alternative therapies consist of a variety of drugs and vaccines that are not yet included in mainstream medicine. Some stimulate the immune system to ward off diseases and consist of older herbal remedies; all are considered nontoxic. One example is shark and other animal cartilage that is used to treat acquired immunodeficiency syndrome (AIDS), cancer, and arthritis. Cartilage possibly inhibits tumor growth by cutting off the blood supply to the tumor, suppressing autoimmune reactions, and promoting wound healing. Ethylenediaminetetraacetic acid is a chemical that binds with metallic ions and that is used as a chelation treatment for poisoning from lead and other toxic metals. It is now being proposed as treatment for ridding the body of free radicals and thus removing fat deposits from artery walls and improving cardiovascular circulation. A total of 70 studies yielded positive results. However, the American Heart Association and other organizations do not endorse its use (American Heart Association, 2006).

Herbal Medicine

The use of herbal and plant medicine is an ancient practice worldwide. Tree barks, plant roots, berries, leaves, resins, seeds, and flowers have all been ground into powders, mixed with solutions, brewed in teas, and used singly or in combination for the treatment of different ailments. One third of adult Americans—an estimated 60 million people—use herbal remedies. In all, 64% of the world's population relies on herbal remedies. More than 1500 herbs are marketed in the United States. Lists of herbs and their uses are readily available on line and in reputable health food stores to name a few.

Records of herbal medicines appeared in the Bible; in Egyptian texts extending back to 2000 BC; in Greece and Rome at the time of Aristotle; in the Muslim world; in India; and in the Orient. Each culture compiled a *materia medica* (i.e., a listing of drugs and their uses). The American Indians contributed a vast array of herbals to the colonial American medicine formulary, and herbals continued to be a mainstay of medical practices for many years. Today herbal products are marketed only as food supplements, and the FDA and other regulatory agencies consider some of these to be potentially dangerous. There are not any safety guidelines for these products. Nevertheless, the public is purchasing alternative medicines at a greater rate than ever before and adopting many remedies from other cultures.

The formulas of TCM are based on the correct ratio or balance of a variety of food herbs that are harvested and

❖ CLINICAL ALERT #1

It is important to inquire and document whether the patient is taking any herbal preparations or using any food supplements. Natural substances may cause toxic adverse effects, severe allergic reactions, and adverse drug reactions, and they may also interfere with laboratory test results (see Boxes 27-5 and 27-6).

BOX 27-5   POTENTIAL INTERACTIONS BETWEEN MEDICATIONS AND HERBALS, FOOD SUPPLEMENTS, AND ALLOPATHIC MEDICATIONS

- Ginkgo biloba may intensify the anticlotting effects of warfarin (Coumadin) and other anticoagulant drugs, including aspirin; garlic and ginseng also have similar effects when used with anticoagulant drugs.
- Many fortified foods (e.g., calcium-fortified orange juice, breakfast cereals) have high concentrations of calcium and other minerals that bind with antibiotics (e.g., ciprofloxacin, gatifloxacin, levofloxacin, tetracycline) and prevent drugs from being absorbed. Tetracycline also binds with aluminum, magnesium, and other minerals.
- Calcium carbonate antacid preparations interfere with the absorption of levothyroxine (thyroid hormone).
- Echinacea interferes with the efficacy of birth-control pills.
- Alfalfa, which is used for hot flashes, interferes with the effects of immunosuppressant drugs.
- Grapefruit juice increases the bioavailability of many drugs, such as antihypertensive drugs, cholesterol-lowering drugs, benzodiazepine and nonbenzodiazepine sedatives, carbamazepine (an anticonvulsant), sertraline (an antidepressant), cyclosporine (an antirejection drug), and amiodarone (an antiarrhythmic).
- St. John's wort reduces the blood concentrations of indinavir (a protease-inhibitor used to treat human immunodeficiency virus infection) and cyclosporine.
- Caffeine (e.g., coffee, tea, cocoa, guarana) increases blood levels of theophylline. When these substances are used together, caffeine side effects are increased, including nervousness, tremor, and sleeplessness.
- Fiber delays the absorption of drugs and nutrients, including vitamins and minerals. Patients need to take bulk-forming laxatives at least 2 hours before or after taking their medications to prevent these problems. Persons who are taking digoxin need to avoid taking their medications with bran fiber, bulk-forming laxatives, and foods that contain pectin (e.g., apples, pears).
- Foods that acidify urine include cheese, eggs, and meat, thereby extending acidity; foods that alkalinize urine include citrus and vegetables that decrease acidity. A high-salt diet increases the urinary excretion of lithium and limits drug effects (i.e., treatment for bipolar disorder).

Modified from Eberhardie C: Food supplements and herbal medications, *Nurs Stand* 20:52-56, 2005; Sparreboom A et al: Herbal remedies in the United States: potential adverse interactions with anticancer drugs, *J Clin Oncol* 22:2489-2503, 2004.

BOX 27-6 **POTENTIAL NUTRIENT AND DRUG INTERACTIONS**

- Fish oils are commonly used for rheumatoid arthritis, psoriasis, and inflammatory bowel disease and to improve immunity; however, they increase the anticoagulant action of aspirin and dipyridamole, and they produce increased bleeding if they are taken with vitamin E.
- Iron compounds reduce the absorption of carbidopa-levodopa (Sinemet) and levodopa. Antacids reduce the uptake of iron and the absorption of methyldopa.
- Broccoli, Brussels sprouts, kale, parsley, spinach, coffee, green tea, and liver are rich in vitamin K; these foods neutralize the effects of anticoagulant drugs.
- A hypertensive crisis may occur with the combination of foods that are rich in tyramine (e.g., aged cheese, fava beans, salami, pepperoni, pickled fish, red wines, some beers) and monoamine oxidase inhibitor drugs (antidepressants). The newer selective serotonin-reuptake inhibitor drugs have mostly replaced the older monoamine oxidase inhibitor drugs; however, monoamine oxidase inhibitors are still available.
- Certain foods alter the rate of drug excretion. Acidic foods (e.g., eggs, cheese, meat) lengthen the half-life of drugs; alkaline foods (e.g., citrus, vegetables) decrease the half-life of drugs. A high-salt diet hastens the urinary output of lithium, which is a common drug used to treat bipolar disorder.
- Many drugs need to be taken with food to prevent drug-related gastrointestinal irritation; however, some drugs need to be taken on an empty stomach, such as erythromycin, levodopa, most penicillins, and tetracycline. Drug absorption is often delayed or enhanced as a result of the presence of food. Fatty foods delay gastric emptying, thereby delaying the time for a drug to reach the desired peak level. High-carbohydrate meals enhance the absorption of some drugs.

Modified from Leigh E: Nutrient-drug interactions, *Nutr Sci News* 42-44, February 1, 2008.

prepared at an appropriate time to enhance their effects. Food herbs are composed of plants (85%), animals (12%), and minerals (3%). The various herbal ingredients are mixed in accordance with the disease's imbalance of yin and yang rather than with regard to the chemical makeup of the herbs. Yin and yang characteristics and their related properties of cold and heat are used to categorize diseases and medicines. These mixtures are supplements to a well-balanced diet, and they are often prescribed along with daily exercise and positive thinking in the belief that a balanced body is the result of a balanced life. Many Chinese herbal stores have captured a large share of the U.S. alternative medicine market.

Examples of commonly used herbs worldwide are ginkgo biloba, echinacea, saw palmetto, *Prunus africana*, ginseng, and St. John's wort. Both European and Oriental varieties of ginkgo biloba are used to increase circulation, to bring oxygen to the brain, and to retard the effects of aging. European studies have shown its effectiveness for improving mental

alertness, increasing circulation to the extremities, lowering cholesterol, and improving blood flow to the retina. Echinacea or purple coneflower is prized for its antiseptic properties and its ability to stimulate the immune system, and it is frequently used for the treatment of influenza, the common cold, and wounds. Saw palmetto berries and *Prunus africana* have become popular treatments for benign prostatic hypertrophy. Ginseng root has been used as a tonic in China for more than 3000 years; many have used it as an antistress agent and to alter the circadian rhythms and the amounts of circulating corticosterone. *Hypericum,* which is the principal ingredient of St. John's wort, has been called "nature's Prozac" because of its popular use as an antidepressant (Eberhardie, 2005). Examples of natural herbal remedies new to the U.S. market include black cohosh for menopausal symptoms; a mental acuity formula that is a combination of vitamins and herbs for mild memory problems; probiotic pearls, which are a dietary supplement with acidophilus and *Bifidobacterium longum* to promote healthy intestinal flora; and pantetheine plus, a triple-action combination formula that is used to enhance the breakdown of fat and cholesterol. Box 27-5 describes potential interactions among herbal medicines, food supplements, and allopathic medicines.

❖ **CLINICAL ALERT #2**

Concerns about the safety of herbal medications include the following (Eberhardie, 2005):
- Some herbal medications have been mixed with synthetic chemicals, including heavy metals.
- Safe dosages of food supplements and herbal medications may not have been established.
- The concentrations of an active ingredient are not always consistent in the liquid or pill.
- Chemical and microbiologic contamination may occur.
- Packages, labeling, and advertising policies need to be more rigorous with regard to ingredients, purposes, and effectiveness.
- Some dangers are associated with self-medication and with mixing different medicinal approaches for a certain health problem. This is particularly important to consider when interacting with patients from multicultural backgrounds.

Aromatherapy

Aromatherapy was initially used in Egypt to relieve pain, but today many individuals use it for relaxation or as an adjunct to stress-reduction measures. More than 300 essential plant oils are currently in use as inhalants, for massage and compresses, as additions to bathwater, and for use in candles. In ancient times, people used the burning of aromatic woods to purify the air. Some still use incense as part of healing ceremonies. Other examples include the use of birch oil as an anti-inflammatory agent, lavender for its calming effects and for headache relief, rosemary added to vaporizers for the relief of congestion, citrus as an energizing agent, and peppermint for nausea relief and as an antipyretic and respiratory stimulant. Aromatherapy is also included as part of Ayurvedic therapy (Topham, 2010).

Diet and Nutrition

Diet and nutritional needs are integral to both traditional and alternative therapies. Today's affluent diet, which is high in animal fats, refined carbohydrates, and partially hydrogenated vegetable oils, contributes to obesity and to many of the current health problems in the United States. Educational information provides alternative healthy diets and lifestyle changes to prevent or correct obesity, cardiovascular disease, diabetes, and other chronic health problems. Vitamins and other food supplements are frequently added to the health maintenance plan. Studies include research regarding the value of the antioxidant vitamins A and E; of β-carotene for the prevention of cataracts and cancer; and of the effects of vitamin C and nicotinic acid as replacement therapy for psychiatric patients who are receiving electroconvulsive and tranquilizer therapy. Megadoses of niacin have helped to reduce serum cholesterol. Some providers have given nutritional supplements to offset the effects of medicines prescribed for people with AIDS (Pelletier, 2007). Health food stores and the Internet are promoting popular new foods and juices. Pomegranate juice and blueberries are being promoted because of their antioxidant properties, and juice from the acai, which is a native berry from Brazil, is a "superfood" that is rich in antioxidants and omega fatty acids. Noni juice, from a plant that is found mainly in the South Pacific, is supposedly a cure for a range of health problems from high blood pressure to poor digestion. Guarana, which is a South American berry that has chemical properties similar to those of caffeine, is an ingredient that is added to "energy" food bars and drinks. Mangosteen, a Southeast Asia fruit, has been used as an antioxidant and for a variety of health problems as well.

Several diets have been developed for the treatment of specific diseases. Macrobiotic cancer diets are based on Oriental beliefs of creating a balance of yin and yang. Research by environmental medicine scientists has helped to identify potential food antigens such as chemical additives and natural food substances. Food-elimination diets reduce sensitivity to certain substances and hasten recovery from allergic responses; these diets have also been used to treat children with attention-deficit/hyperactivity disorder (Pelletier, 2007). Health care providers need to be sensitive to ethnic and cultural diets when planning health care activities. Some of these diets pose health risks because of a lack of essential ingredients or because they interact with prescribed medications (see Box 27-6). Incorporating familiar foods into the diet also facilitates a person's recovery, and substances in the diet may actually facilitate healing.

CHAPTER SUMMARY

- An historic overview reveals that contrasting perspectives exist regarding the nature of human beings. Some view individuals as whole persons composed of balanced mind, body, and spirit. Others adopt a dualistic view that separates the functions of the body from mind and spirit functions.
- Allopathic medicine has traditionally been a dualistic model with an emphasis on curative methods of biologic diseases on the basis of empiric evidence outcome criteria. By contrast, the focus of the holistic or alternative care model is on strengthening one's inner resistance to disease and "healing from within" or enhancing the body's innate healing powers.
- There is a stigma attached to alternative methods. The scientific community often labels alternative methods as hoaxes, witchcraft, or magico-religious practices and attributes results to placebo effects. Nevertheless, nurses need to become knowledgeable regarding the many CAM methods used by patients from diverse cultural and ethnic backgrounds to manage their lives. Nurses must be nonjudgmental about these practices.
- The public must become educated regarding the potential harmful effects of the concurrent use of alternative and prescription medicines. Informing health care providers when taking alternative medicines is essential. People also need to understand the consequences of self-diagnosis, self-treatment, and delays when seeking help.
- Several factors have influenced the use of CAM interventions, including the escalating costs of modern health care, restrictions imposed by third-party payers, the influence of media coverage, the introduction of ancient cultural therapies, and an increase in consumer interest in self-control, especially for promoting health and for managing chronic health problems.
- The traditional allopathic system has included some CAM interventions, especially stress-reduction therapies; however, barriers still exist for herbal medicines, dietary supplements (because of the lack of significant empiric evidence of their effectiveness), and safety control issues.
- The American Holistic Nurses Association suggests that alternative and traditional therapies complement each other in the provision of holistic care, and it recommends that nurses become familiar with alternative methods and incorporate them into the plan of care whenever possible. Use of the term integrative therapies has become a common practice.
- Nurses educate patients about the potential harmful effects of the concurrent use of alternative and prescription medicines and emphasize to patients the need to inform their health care providers about what therapies they are using.
- The concepts of caring and healing as well as commitment to global health are integral components of nursing.
- The nurse attends to a wide range of human experiences and responses to health and disease. During the provision

CHAPTER SUMMARY—cont'd

of a caring relationship, the nurse promotes healing and health maintenance.

- The goal of holistic nursing is to enhance the healing of all aspects of the whole person. The nursing profession performs independent and interdependent actions that are largely technical, such as teaching, administration, and research. Nursing is dynamic, evolutionary, and humanistic, and it is a discipline that is fundamentally based on scientific and theoretic knowledge and founded on moral, ethical, and spiritual values.

- Concepts of health, illness, and disease are deeply embedded. Cultural competency requires an awareness of one's own values and of those of the health care system. Nurses frequently have to support decisions that differ from their own cultural norms and values. Culturally incompetent care challenges the belief system of patients and their families, causes undue stress, and inhibits the healing process. Efficient and effective clinical care in cross-cultural circumstances is a new competency for all nurses to attain.

REVIEW QUESTIONS

1. A nurse assesses a newly admitted patient. The patient says, "I've been taking feverfew for my migraine headaches. It has really helped a lot." The nurse knows that there are no hazardous interactions between feverfew and the patient's current medications. Select the nurse's best response.
   1. "I'm glad feverfew helps your headaches. I'll make a note in your chart that you take it."
   2. "You should never take any medications unless you have a physician's prescription."
   3. "I also take feverfew for my own migraine headaches. It has really helped me, too."
   4. "Feverfew is not backed by reliable research for the treatment of migraine headaches."

2. A patient with chronic psoriasis takes various fish oils and vitamin E to improve his immunity and his skin condition. This physician instructs the patient to take aspirin daily to reduce the risk of heart disease and stroke. When the nurse assesses this patient 3 weeks later, which observation indicates a dangerous drug interaction?
   1. The patient's psoriatic skin lesions are dry and crusty.
   2. There are numerous bruises on the patient's extremities.
   3. The patient reports that movement occurs with less pain.
   4. Scales are being shed from the patient's psoriatic skin lesions.

3. When used in combination with an anticoagulant medication, the ingestion of large quantities of which foods would be likely to reduce medication effectiveness? You may select more than one answer.

   1. Broccoli
   2. Green tea
   3. Pickled herring
   4. Aged cheese
   5. Scrambled eggs

4. A nurse interviews for new employment at four facilities. This nurse values holism, including the healing powers of CAM. Which observations would suggest to this nurse that the facility has similar values? You may select more than one answer.
   1. The facility advertises the purchase of a new single photon emission computed tomography diagnostic device.
   2. The facility sponsors weekly articles in a local newspaper about new cures for disease.
   3. The interview includes a tour of the facility's high-tech biomedical laboratory.
   4. The interview concludes with a tour of the facility's massage therapy suites.
   5. Each patient at the facility has input into his or her plan of care and then signs the plan.

5. The nurse cares for a patient who uses alternative vitamin therapies to manage a chronic disease. The nurse believes that the vitamins are not therapeutic. Select the nurse's best initial action.
   1. Report the situation to the ethics committee.
   2. Ask the patient to discontinue taking the vitamins.
   3. Determine whether the vitamins pose any danger.
   4. Teach the patient about more effective strategies.

REFERENCES

Allen M: The rainbow room, *Reiki News* 8(4):28-29, 2009.

American Heart Association: *Questions and answers about chelation therapy* (website): www.americanheart.org/presenter.jhtml?identifer=4493. Accessed April 24, 2006.

American Holistic Nursing Association: *Mission statement, vision, and purpose* (website): www.ahna.org. Accessed January 15, 2011.

Anderson RA: The immune system and mind function, *Townsend Letter for Doctors and Patients* 265-266:102-106, 2004a.

Anderson RA: Psychoneuroimmunoendocrinology review and commentary, *Townsend Letter for Doctors and Patients* 269:126-129, 2004b.

Barrett S: *Naturopathy* (website): www.quackwatch.org/01QuackeryRelatedTopics/Naturopathy/naturopathy.htm. Accessed April 4, 2006.

Bodenheimer T, Fernandez A: High and rising health care costs: Can costs be controlled while preserving quality? *Ann Inter Med* 143:26-32, 2005.

Brooks AJ et al: The effect of Johrei healing on substance abuse recovery: a pilot study, *J Altern Complement Med* 12(7):625-631, 2006.

Centers for Disease Control and Prevention: *CDC helps launch healthy people 2020 collaboration* (website): www.cdc.gov/news/2008/03/Healthypeople2020.html. Accessed December 23, 2010.

Cosentino, B. W: Complementary and alternative medicine in the mainstream. *Nursing Spectrum Nurseweek*, December 13, 2004 (website): www2.nursingspectrum.com/articles/print.html?AID=13355. Accessed January 23, 2011.

Delta Society: *Animal-assisted therapy/activities 101* (website), 2006: http://www.deltasociety.org/Page.aspx?pid=317 Accessed January 21, 2011.

Domrose, C: Meditation offers benefits for patients and nurses, February 22, 2010 (website): http://news.nure.com/article/20100222/NATIONAL01/10222 accessed: January 22 2011.

Eberhardie C: Food supplements and herbal medicines, *Nurs Stand* 20:52-56, 2005.

Ellis K, Hartley C: *Nursing in today's world: challenges, issues and trends*, Philadelphia, 2007, Lippincott.

Eshkevari L, Heath J: Use of acupuncture for chronic pain: optimizing clinical practice, *Holistic Nursing Practice* 19(5):217-221, 2005.

Gaskill M: Forces of nature (complementary/alternative therapies), *Nurseweek* July 26:11-13 2004.

Gazella K: Bringing mindfulness to medicine: an interview with Jon Kabat-Zinn, *Altern Ther* 11:56-64, 2005.

Goodall D, Etters L: The therapeutic use of music on agitated behavior in those with dementia, *Holist Nurs Pract* 19:258-262, 2005.

Gutierrez C, Ranji U: *U.S. health care costs, Kaiser Family Foundation, 2005* (website): www.kaiseredu.org/topics.im.asp?=1andparentID=61andid=358. Accessed April 3, 2006.

Healthy People 2010: *Topics and objectives* (website): www.cdc.gov/nchs/healthy_people.htm Accessed January 24, 2011.

Kabat-Zinn J: Commentary on Majumdar et al: mindfulness meditation for health, *J Altern Complement Med* 8:731-735, 2002.

Kirsch I: Medication and suggestion in the treatment of depression, *Contemp Hypn* 22:59-66, 2005.

Khazzoom L: Drug-free remedies for chronic pain, *AARP* 2009.

Koenig H: *Separating fact from fiction* (website): www.stnews.org/Commentary-2758.htm. Accessed April 3, 2006.

KPBS: *The new medicine (video)*, San Diego, Calif, 2006, San Diego State University.

Kreitzer M, Disch J: Leading the way: the Gillette nursing summit on integrated health and healing, *Altern Ther Health Med* 9:3A-10A, 2003.

Laidlaw T, Dwivedi P: Combining cognitive, emotional, behavioral, and dare we say it, the spiritual: review of mindfulness-based cognitive therapy for depression: a new approach to preventing relapse. *Contemp Hypn* 21:205-209, 2004.

Lyons AS: Hippocrates. In Lyons AS, Petrucelli RJ, editors: *Medicine: an illustrated history*, New York, 1978, Harry N. Abrams, Inc.

Maier-Lorentz, M: The importance of prayer for mind/body, spirit, *Oncology Nurse Society News* 16:51-59, 2004.

Majette GR: From concierge medicine to patient-centered medicine homes: international lessons and the search for a better way to deliver health care in the U.S., *J Law Med* 305(4):585-619, 2009.

National Association of Cognitive-Behavioral Therapists: *What is cognitive-behavioral therapy?* (website): www.nacbt.org/whatiscbt.htm. Accessed March 28, 2006.

National Center for Complementary and Alternative Medicine. *Examples of completed and ongoing research related to use of complementary alternative medicine* (website): http://nccam.nih.gov/research/clinicaltrials/factsheet/. Accessed March 4, 2011.

National Center for Complementary and Alternative Medicine: *Comprehensive findings of complementary and alternative medicine* (website): www.altmed.od.nih.gov/nccam. Accessed March 4, 2011.

National Center for Complementary and Alternative Medicine: *NCCAM overview* (website): www.altmed.od.nih.gov/nccam. Accessed March 4, 2011.

National Center for Complementary and Alternative Medicine: *Institute of Medicine summit on integrating complementary and alternative medicine* (website): www.altmed.od.nih.gov/nccam. Accessed March 4, 2011.

National Center for Complementary and Alternative Medicine: *Magnet therapy: an overview* (website): www.altmed.od.nih.gov/nccam. Accessed March 4, 2011.

National Center for Complementary and Alternative Medicine: *Ayurvedic and homeopathic medicine* (website): www.altmed.od.nih.gov/nccam. Accessed March 4, 2011.

National Center for Complementary and Alternative Medicine: *Naturopathy: an overview* (website): www.altmed.od.nih.gov/nccam. Accessed March 4, 2011.

National Center for Complementary and Alternative Medicine: *Osteopathy and chiropractic medicine: an overview* (website): www.altmed.od.nih.gov/nccam. Accessed March 4, 2011.

Nightingale F: *Notes on nursing: what it is and what it is not*, London, 1859, Harrison, 59, Pall Mall.

Pelletier K: *The best alternative medicine*, New York, 2007, Simon and Schuster.

Saito I, Saito Y: Biofeedback training in clinical settings, *Biogenic Amines* 18:463-476, 2004.

Saper RB et al: Yoga for low back pain in a predominantly minority population: a pilot random controlled study, *Altern Ther Health Medicine* 15(6):18-27, 2009.

Telner, J: Review of Mindfulness-based cognitive therapy for depression: A new approach to prevent depression, Segal AV et al. New York, The Guilford Press, 2002. *In Can J Psychiatry*, 50:432, 2005.

Topham D: Alternative and complementary therapies. In Daniels R et al, editors: *Nursing fundamentals: caring and clinical decision making*, New York, 2010, Delmar Learning.

Venes D (editor): *Taber's cyclopedic medical dictionary*, Philadelphia, 2005, FA Davis.

White KP: What psychologists should know about homeopathy, nutrition and botanical medicines, *Prof Psychol Res Pr* 40(6):633-640, 2009.

Williams, S: Beyond belief: Transcultural nurses provide culturally competent care, *Nurseweek.* pp. 54-55, 58, May 8, 2006.

Zerwekh J: Contemporary health care delivery: trends and economics. In Zerwekh J, Claborn J, editors: *Nursing today: transitions and trends*, ed 3, Philadelphia, 2008, Saunders.

Online Resources

American Association of Oriental Medicine: www.aaomonline.org

American Holistic Nurses Association: www.ahna.org

National Center for Complementary and Alternative Medicine: www.nccam.nih.gov

Grief: In Loss and Death

Katherine M. Fortinash

"In the depth of winter, I finally learned that within me there lay an invincible summer."

Albert Camus

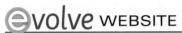 WEBSITE

http://evolve.elsevier.com/Fortinash/

OBJECTIVES

- Define *grief, bereavement,* and *mourning.*
- Describe three common responses that are seen with normal grief.
- Discuss the four major categories of grief.
- Differentiate the symptoms of grief from those of depression.
- Analyze the potential for complicated grief in high-risk patients, including children.
- Describe effective interventions for different stages of grief.

- Explain how grief can trigger other losses in various ways.
- Define *chronic sorrow,* and identify persons who are at risk.
- Explain how posttraumatic stress disorder may resemble complicated or traumatic grief.
- Discuss the profound effects of grief and loss on individuals across the life span.
- Describe grief's lifelong effects on parents who lose a child.
- Apply the nursing process to the management of patients who are experiencing grief and loss.

KEY TERMS

acute grief	childhood grief	grief work	social support
anger	chronic sorrow	guilt	tasks of grief
anticipatory grief	complicated grief	mourning	
attachment objects	delayed grief	parental grief	
bereavement	grief	postvention	

Grief is a natural and normal reaction to loss, and it is part of the human experience; however, many of us are unprepared for its daunting journey. The death of a loved one is one of the most painful experiences of a lifetime, and the grief that follows is often lonely, debilitating, and frightening. Nevertheless, studies show that most people are remarkably resilient with regard to coming to terms with death, regaining their interests, and moving forward in life (Shear and Mulhare, 2008). Although each loss is unique, experts agree that the grief response is generally multifaceted and that it involves painful psychologic, physiologic, cognitive, and behavioral changes that vary among individuals. Therefore, support throughout the grief process depends on the resilience and

diverse needs of each person and family affected (Agnew et al, 2010). Although it is most commonly associated with the death of a loved one, grief occurs when there is any significant loss, including the loss of a beloved pet or a valued object; a treasured role or identity; or a certain degree of power, control, self-esteem, dignity, or sense of worth. Grief descends on everyone, regardless of age, status, or circumstance. The following individuals are vulnerable to grief:

- The husband whose wife dies after a long marriage
- The parents who lose a child
- The parents of an infant with birth defects
- The wife who is caring for her husband with Alzheimer's disease

- The young husband whose wife has inoperable cancer
- The family of a patient in the intensive care unit
- The victim of violence (e.g., abuse, rape, war, natural disaster, terrorism)
- The young husband and father whose wife is killed in battle
- The homeless mother who is living in a shelter with her children
- The parents whose son was incarcerated for a serious crime
- The patient who is newly admitted to a psychiatric hospital
- The family of a teenager whose drug addiction is out of control
- The elderly widow who loses a beloved pet
- The family who loses their home through foreclosure
- The young husband and father who loses his job and cannot support his family
- The person who retires from a lifetime of work
- The child who loses a parent through death or divorce

In grief, we yearn and long for the person who died, and we become engulfed in sadness and disbelief as we struggle to understand the finality of the loss (Shear and Mulhare, 2008). We may think, say, and do things that are normally uncharacteristic as we attempt to battle the anguish and confusion that are a part of grief. There seems to be no relief and no end to the intense feelings that we experience, and there is no right way of coping with death. Grief has been categorized as the emotional equivalent of a raw, open wound. With great care, it will eventually heal, but there will always be a scar. Most nurses are in daily contact with grief, both other people's and their own (National Institutes of Health, 2006). Therefore, grief should be addressed to varying degrees in all schools of nursing. Nurse researchers White and Ferszt (2009, p. 239), recommend that "theoretical models of grief, and research related to care of grieving clients, should be included in nurse practitioner curriculum and continuing education programs" (see Research for Evidence-Based Practice #1 later in this chapter). The terms *grief*, *bereavement*, and *mourning*, are often used interchangeably. Their definitions may overlap somewhat, but they do have different meanings (Agnew et al, 2010):

- Grief and its associated pain were identified by Sigmund Freud (1917), the founder of psychoanalysis, as "normal and inevitable life experiences." In his landmark work, John Bowlby (1980), a psychoanalyst and psychiatrist, wrote about the attachment theory in which grief is viewed as a "natural response to loss of an attachment figure." He believed that attachment begins during early childhood, with parents, caregivers, and siblings being primary attachment objects. During adolescence, peers and romantic partners are added to this group of attachment figures, and adult attachment objects change during the remainder of one's lifetime (Bowlby, 1980). In their classic social readjustment rating scale, psychiatrists Holmes and Rahe (1967) identified the death of a spouse as the most stressful life event, ranking it at 100 on a scale of 1 to 100. Many experts cite the death of a spouse as a high risk for suicide in the elderly. These findings indicate the importance of spousal attachment during all stages of adulthood. Spouses who cannot manage the complex tasks of running a home without their partner may be vulnerable. Many sources cite the death of a child as being equally risky and disruptive. Nurse researchers Arnold and Buschman Gemma (2008, p. 658) state that "[t]he death of a child is an incomprehensible and devastating loss" (see the Research for Evidence-Based Practice #2 later in this chapter).

Each type of loss means that something meaningful has been taken away, whether it is physical, psychologic, social, or symbolic. Many sources in the literature concur that, to varying degrees, grief often triggers other losses. The complex and tumultuous effects of grief are noted in the following example:

A young husband who is grieving for his wife, who is in the last stages of cancer, also grieves for the loss of his role as husband, lover, and partner. These additional losses compound the grief that he feels for his wife. If children are involved, his grief is exacerbated as he deals with their grief and considers how these major life changes will affect all of their lives. His anticipated role as a single parent intensifies his grief (see Anticipatory Grief later in this chapter).

Each family member experiences grief in a personal way, and grief is influenced by many factors (e.g., developmental, cultural, religious, spiritual) as well as by the individual's resilience, perception of loss, available support systems, and attachment to the individual. Anthony Love (2007, p. 73), a psychologist and educator, notes that "Grief occurs with loss of symbolically important connections and involves intense emotional reactions and changes to our experiences of self, the world, and the future. Individual responses reflect factors such as personality and life history, social context and cultural practices, and the symbolic magnitude of the loss."

- Bereavement is the period after a loss, when one is experiencing the state of having lost a loved one. Bereavement typically evokes an intensely emotional response that is often experienced as acute grief (Shear and Mulhare, 2008) (see the section about Acute Grief later in this chapter). The tasks of mourning (i.e., adaptation to grief) generally begin during bereavement. The time and intensity spent in bereavement largely depend on how attached or bonded the survivor was to the deceased and how much time was spent anticipating the loss (Bowlby, 1980). Many bereaved individuals experience common grief reactions during which normal life functioning is interrupted by depressive symptoms (e.g., sadness, crying episodes, sleeplessness). Distress may be present for several months, and it gradually lessens over time as survivors use their inner personal strengths and support systems to move forward in life even as they continue to mourn (Agnew et al, 2010).

- *Mourning* is the process by which people adapt to a loss. Cultural customs, rituals, and society's rules for coping with loss influence the way that different cultural groups mourn and respond to grief, in addition to other factors listed previously (National Institutes of Health, 2006). In Western culture, mourning generally lasts for a period of weeks to months, during which time the loss and grief are gradually absorbed into the ongoing life of the individual. Although there is still longing and sadness for the deceased person, the bereaved individual eventually regains the capacity for joy for the continuity of life (Shear and Mulhare, 2008).

RESPONSES TO GRIEF AND BEREAVEMENT

Responses to grief and bereavement may be examined as a range of physical, cognitive, relating, and affective symptoms of pain. The intensity of the pain is often a surprise to the mourner. Lindemann's classic study of grief (1944) and other more current studies (Agnew et al, 2010; Anderson et al, 2008; Love, 2007; Shear and Mulhare, 2008) have identified many of the manifestations of grief, including physical distress, preoccupation with the image of the deceased, guilt, anger, hostile reactions, and disruptions in normal patterns of conduct. These and other physical and psychologic manifestations of grief are summarized in the following sections.

Physical Manifestations

Physical manifestations of grief include weakness, numbness, anorexia, feelings of choking, shortness of breath, tightness in the chest, dry mouth, and gastrointestinal disturbances. Fatigue, exhaustion, insomnia, and episodes of sobbing are common. Bereaved persons frequently seek medical attention for vague symptoms such as chest discomfort or gastrointestinal problems, some of which seem to have no physiologic basis. In addition, there is a clear link between grief and increased vulnerability to mental and physical illness, although grief is seldom a direct cause of illness or death (except for suicide). The grieving person is especially prone to myocardial infarction, hypertension, rheumatoid arthritis, depression, alcohol and other drug abuse, and malnutrition (Tomita and Kitamura, 2002.) Although rare, problems that persist or worsen may put the grieving person at risk for physical or emotional harm.

Cognitive Manifestations

Cognitive manifestations center on the patient's preoccupation with the deceased person. The involuntary nature and intensity of the preoccupation are surprising and distressing to some. It is common for the preoccupation to take the form of conversations with the deceased; with normal grief, the person recognizes that the deceased person is not actually present. In older adults especially, these conversations sometimes continue for the rest of the survivor's life. It is typical for a recently bereaved person to be preoccupied with

thoughts and memories of the departed loved one and to be uninterested in ongoing life. This preoccupation usually diminishes over time, although some individuals maintain links with the deceased for many years, and, for some people, this continues until death. These links are sometimes in the form of remembrances such as treasured things or renegotiated relationships with the deceased. Many authorities now recognize the drive to maintain links between the living and the dead as normal behavior (Shear and Mulhare, 2008). In some cultures (e.g., Chinese, Vietnamese), the failure to maintain formal links with deceased ancestors is considered to be pathologic (Kemp and Chang, 2002). Another common symptom is difficulty concentrating, which may manifest as a lapse of focus or orientation to time and place. Seeking and longing for the lost person, object, or status are universally experienced, and some grieving persons experience hallucinations. Individuals most often describe these as momentary glimpses of the person who died or brief auditory messages of two or three words that are perceived to have been spoken by the deceased individual. Some relate experiences such as smelling familiar scents (e.g., perfume or cologne connected to the deceased). In most cases, hallucinations diminish within a month or two after the loss, and they are considered part of the normal grieving process. With complicated grief, which is also known as *traumatic* or *prolonged grief,* hallucinations persist, increase in number or intensity, or become derogatory or threatening (e.g., the deceased person beckoning the survivor to join him or her). When this occurs, the hallucinations are then considered to be negative hallucinations (pathologic), and therapeutic interventions including hospitalization and antipsychotic medications are indicated (American Psychiatric Association, 2000). Complicated grief symptoms also include preoccupation with the deceased, repetitive thoughts, rumination, isolation, and excessive guilt. Complicated grief may resemble major depression or posttraumatic stress disorder (PTSD), and it often co-occurs with these disorders (Shear and Mulhare, 2008). Complicated grief is discussed in more detail later in this chapter, and Chapters 10 and 12 contain more information about anxiety and depression.

Behavioral and Relating Manifestations

Behavioral and relating problems figure prominently in the Axis IV category of the *Diagnostic and Statistical Manual of Mental Disorders,* fourth edition, text revision (see Appendix on Evolve). These conditions are listed in the form of psychosocial and environmental stressors (American Psychiatric Association, 2000). Some Axis IV problems that are directly or indirectly related to grief and bereavement include the following:

- Death of a family member
- Health problems in a family
- Inadequate social support
- Adjustment to life-cycle transition
- Inadequate finances
- Marital difficulties
- Work or career problems

Behavioral and relating manifestations of grief include disruptions in patterns of conduct that range from an inability to perform even basic activities of daily living to dragging oneself through daily activities to a restless and disorganized behavior that includes searching for that which is lost, obsessive reflection and reminiscence, and an intense sense of isolation (Hentz, 2002; Lindemann, 1944; Shear and Mulhare, 2008). The former life and patterns lose meaning and satisfaction without the lost person or object, and there does not seem to be a new life or routine to which the bereaved individual can turn to find comfort. This loss of relating and meaning is a major cause of despair or hopelessness. With complicated grief, survivors tend to avoid all efforts to come to terms with the inevitability of death and the consequences of loss (Shear and Mulhare, 2008).

Affective Manifestations

Affective manifestations of grief are often overwhelming, with sadness, guilt, loneliness, hopelessness, and anger being the most common. Symptoms that increase in intensity may meet the criteria for the diagnosis of a mood disorder (e.g., major depression, dysthymic disorder). The most common differences between symptoms of bereavement and major depression or dysthymic disorder are that psychomotor retardation, morbid guilt, and suicidal ideation are less common with bereavement and that mood disorders are of longer duration than bereavement (Hentz, 2002; American Psychiatric Association, 2000). Complicated grief may resemble significant mental health problems such as suicidality, major depression, and PTSD, or it may coexist with these disorders. Children can also experience complicated grief (Shear and Mulhare, 2008). Love (2007) categorized normal or uncomplicated grief reactions as follows:

- Emotional—sadness, anger, guilt, and anxiety
- Cognitive—preoccupied, ruminating, fantasizing, and confused
- Physical—somatic complaints and lowered immune function
- Behavioral—crying, agitated, withdrawn, searching, and avoidant
- Existential—the disruption of life's certainties and the questioning of beliefs

Guilt

Guilt is a pervasive theme in patients who are grieving, even among children as young as 2 years old. Many survivors search for their failures or omissions in the relationship, and, when they do not find significant errors, some proceed to magnify whatever small mistakes they may have made (Lindemann, 1944). Many people are tortured by these "if onlies" and "what ifs" (e.g., "If only I had called," "If only we hadn't let her take the car that night," "If only I had taken time to listen and visit more often"). Shear and Mulhare (2008) state that guilt often stems from regrets of not being able to prevent the death or suffering of the deceased or the idea that it isn't right for the bereaved person to enjoy life when the loved one is gone. Many sources indicate that some survivors believe that they should have died instead of their loved ones. This is especially true of parents whose children precede them in death (see Research for Evidence-Based Practice #2). Many researchers identify survivor guilt as a common theme among people who go through intense experiences (e.g., war, prisoner of war status, concentration camp) and survive when others do not. This has serious implications for those who survive the current wars in the Middle East. The film *Sophie's Choice*, which starred Meryl Streep as a woman who was forced to give up one of her children to the Nazis to save herself and her other child, illustrated how the character of Sophie could not resolve her guilt and ultimately committed suicide. The continued emotional abuse that she suffered at the hands of a mentally ill "rescuer" who professed to love her may have been a contributing factor to her suicide. Guilt is especially troublesome for those whose relationships with the deceased were ambivalent and characterized by unresolved or unexpressed feelings other than what the survivor did or did not do during the loved one's life. Grief that is accompanied by a sustained loss of self-esteem, and ambivalence about living is an indication that an individual is at increased risk for suicide and needs help. All that we can do with the guilt is to learn from it for the sake of other people in our lives. When a loved one dies by suicide, it is especially important to remember that we cannot control the behavior of another person, even as we search for answers (Hsu, 2002). See Clinical Alert #2 later in this chapter and Chapter 22 for more information about suicide.

Anger

Anger is common during grief, and it is sometimes directed toward the person who died, toward family members, toward the health care staff, or toward God or a higher power. Some turn anger inward toward the self. Many theorists agree that anger is generally a response to the anxiety that comes from the powerlessness and vulnerability that results from the death of a loved one and from other losses. For example, some express anger toward the deceased in statements such as, "How could she do this to me? It's not fair!" or "How does he expect me to take care of things alone?" Many survivors believe that it is wrong to feel anger toward a deceased loved one, so they turn the anger inward. Anger turned inward also reflects a survivor's inability to release the lost person or object. To those who have spent a lifetime suppressing anger, these overwhelming and "wrong" or ego-dystonic feelings (i.e., unnatural or uncomfortable feelings) are distressing and indicate to some individuals that they are "going crazy." Some need permission to express their anger. For others, if the death itself is not enough to create anger, tending to the business after a death (e.g., funeral preparations, legal matters) results in anger. The professional, cool, and detached attitude of some of the funeral directors and lawyers involved can easily evoke anger and hostility among survivors who need more warmth and understanding during this vulnerable time. Talking about anger also helps survivors to define, understand, and learn how to handle it. Suppressing anger can lead to deeper-than-normal depression or bitterness. The impulse to use drugs, including prescription drugs and alcohol, occurs for some. Bereaved persons with a history of any sort of drug misuse or mental illness are at risk for the recurrence or exacerbation of these problems.

THE STAGES AND PROCESS OF GRIEF

Stages

Grief is often described in terms of stages. Although there is variation among the different conceptions, many stage-oriented theories involve three basic levels: (1) avoidance (numbing and blunting); (2) confrontation (disorganization and despair); and (3) reestablishment (reorganization and recovery) (Kemp, 2006). Avoidance includes both the initial denial and subsequent brief periods of time when the survivor "forgets"—and then "remembers," with shock and pain—the losses and the grief. Confrontation is the often-lengthy period of active mourning and includes the most acute physical, cognitive, behavioral, relating, and affective manifestations of grief, as discussed previously. Reestablishment does not suddenly occur as a distinct stage; it happens with a gradual decrease of symptoms and ultimately in an adjustment to life without the lost person or object. The problem with stages is that they tend to be neater in theory than they are in reality. This can mislead some individuals into thinking that grief progresses in an orderly manner through definitive stages and that then, almost magically, grief is over, and the survivor establishes a new life. In reality, "[g]rieving can be a relatively slow and uneven process, so applying prescriptive stages or goals to individuals' experiences can be unhelpful" (Love, 2007, p. 73). No two people grieve the same way, even in the same family. Like a snowflake or a fingerprint, each person's grief has unique characteristics and a timetable all its own.

Process
Characteristics

It is more helpful to think in terms of a process of common and dynamic responses to grief than to think of grief as occurring in well-defined stages. Some adhere to the stages of grief defined in the literature: they initially respond to the death of a loved one with shock and disbelief that is followed by protest and despair. However, others might take a less common path. They may experience a period of emotionless cognitive activity (e.g., planning the funeral, managing the household affairs) that is mixed with waves of yearning, despair, and disorganization (e.g., sobbing, confusion, wandering). Whichever path is followed, most people gradually begin the long, painful, and varied process of rebuilding a life without the person who died. An essential feature of this process is its dynamic and changing nature (Kemp, 2006). For example, some experience periods of normal functioning that are interspersed with periods of psychologic distress or symptoms that are almost indistinguishable from those of major depression. Countless people say, "It seems like I'm doing fine, and then, for no reason at all, I start crying" (as if some external or practical reason were needed). The grief process sometimes includes all of the previously mentioned responses, phases, or symptoms, or it may include only some of them. There is not always a "stage of avoidance" or a period of organized cognitive activity; alternatively, there may be very little in the way of resolution, reorganization, or adjustment to the environment in the absence of the deceased. Moreover, when death is expected, the grief process begins before the person dies. Grief that occurs before a death or another type of loss is called *anticipatory grief,* which is discussed later in this chapter. Box 28-1 summarizes several theories of grief.

Grief Work

Grief work has been an important concept for most of the twentieth century (Hendry, 2009). Named first by Lindemann (1944), *grief work* is the means by which people move through the stages and processes of grief. Worden (1982) in Hendry (2009) identified "tasks of mourning," which suggest that work needs to be done before mourning can be completed. Grief work is both a struggle to not give in to despair and a willingness to confront the reality of the despair. Within the grief process, the bereaved person must continue to move forward with the business of life. This includes paying the bills, making decisions, and, at the same time, being able to separate him or herself from the person who died and to readjust to a world without the deceased. During grief work, the mourner begins the difficult task of turning to others for emotional satisfaction and redirecting energy that was once given to the person who died. The survivor continues to express the deep and painful emotions of grieving, which includes grieving for the self as well as the deceased and for all of the plans and dreams that will never be fulfilled. The process is exhausting, because it requires both physical and mental energy; however, it is a necessary journey both for closure and new beginnings (National Institutes of Health, 2006).

Tasks of Grief

Accomplishing the tasks of grief helps to resolve issues that may otherwise obstruct the grief process (Carpenito, 2002; Kemp, 2006). Most grief theorists agree that bereavement is a very complex issue and that people express their grief in various ways. What appears to be consistent is that mourning is necessary and that people must have the opportunity to grieve to establish equilibrium. The following is a theoretic framework of grief that describes Worden's tasks of grieving (Worden 1982 in Hendry 2009):

- *Accepting the reality of the loss.* Persons who are unable to complete this initial task may have trouble with the remaining tasks
- *Working through the pain of grief.* Although this is difficult, pain that is not completely experienced or worked through can emerge at some point as illness or depression. Grief can become complicated if there is no social system to support mourning.
- *Adjusting to an environment without the presence of the deceased.* Grieving individuals must learn to cope without the loved one in their lives.

BOX 28-1   SUMMARY OF GRIEF THEORIES

Lindemann

Grief is manifested by predictable psychologic and somatic symptomatology. Somatic distress, a preoccupation with the deceased person's image, guilt, hostile reactions, and a loss of patterns of conduct all characterize acute mourning. Dysfunctional or morbid grief reactions are distortions of some aspect of normal grief. The duration of grief and the development of dysfunctional grief are largely dependent on the success with which the mourner works through the grief.

Kübler-Ross

Elisabeth Kübler-Ross's stages of dying—denial, anger, bargaining, depression, and acceptance—are often applied to grief. The initial response to loss often includes denial, anger, and bargaining. Denial is characterized by the refusal to accept the loss. Individuals initially direct anger at the health care staff and then, later in the process, at the person who died. Bargaining and denial are often mixed in a futile attempt to reverse reality. Depression tends to be the lengthiest phase; with dysfunctional grief, it becomes chronic and meets the *Diagnostic and Statistical Manual of Mental Disorders,* fourth edition, text revision, criteria for major depression. The acceptance of the loss is a gradual process that includes aspects of previous stages. As the grief work progresses, acceptance increases.

Bowlby

Grief and loss are characterized first by numbness during which the loss is recognized but not necessarily felt as real. Numbness is followed by yearning and searching, during which time the loss is still not fully realized. During the third phase, disorganization and despair occur, the loss is understood as real, and intense emotional pain and cognitive disorganization occur. Reorganization is the final phase, and it is characterized by a gradual adjustment to life without the deceased.

Engel

The initial response to loss is shock and disbelief. Awareness of the loss and the meaning of the loss develop during the first year of mourning. Eventually, the relationship is resolved and put into perspective.

Shneidman

Conceptualizing less structure or fewer stages than other theorists with regard to grief, Shneidman views the expression of grief as being dependent primarily on an individual's personality or style of living. An individual who goes through life feeling depressed and guilty is likely to grieve similarly. One who avoids emotional investments with others will also tend to try to avoid grief.

Theory Synthesis

Grief tends to occur in several phases. The initial response to loss is shock, numbness, denial, or other means of defense against the reality and pain of loss. This initial phase is followed by painful psychologic and physical disequilibrium, which—in the case of chronic grief—lasts indefinitely. The third phase of resolution or recovery is a gradual process during which the good days begin to outnumber the bad. Ultimately, although the deceased individual is not forgotten, the individual's relationship with the deceased is resolved and placed into perspective.

- *Relocating the deceased emotionally and moving forward with life.* The mourner who accomplishes this task recognizes that the loss can be integrated into the here and now. This person can learn to find ways to maintain the memories of the deceased and still develop relationships with the living.

Kemp (2006) and Carpenito (2002) describe the following tasks of grief:

- Telling the "death story" or describing in detail the events surrounding the death or loss
- Expressing and accepting the sadness of grief
- Expressing and accepting guilt, anger, and other feelings that may be perceived as negative
- Reviewing the relationship with the deceased with significant others
- Exploring possibilities in life after the loss (e.g., new relationships, activities, sources of support)
- Understanding common processes and problems that can occur during grief
- Being understood and accepted by others

Complicating Factors

Several factors complicate grief work. First, it is extremely painful. Many people are surprised at the intensity and depth of the pain, and they often make an attempt to avoid the distress by throwing themselves back into a busy schedule or by taking a vacation. Second, the work is inherently contradictory. The pain demands expression, but many often fear that they will lose control over their feelings if they express the pain, saying "I know that if I start crying, I will never stop." Third, individuals need both emotion-based coping (e.g., expressing deep, powerful feelings) and problem-solving coping (e.g., developing strategies for going on with life) to successfully complete the work. Finally, in most of the Western world, cultural values support the avoidance of the expression of grief. For example, Western cultures value self-control highly, especially among men. There is a tendency to try to rush through grief and to get back to work or get on with one's life—as is said ad nauseam, "Let the healing begin." Rituals that formerly helped with individual and community expressions of grief are now often brief "celebrations" of the deceased's life or other upbeat and usually brief events. Memorial services have replaced the ritual of the funeral mass. The viewing of the body, which is a customary ritual by some ethnic groups, has been reduced to 1 or 2 days instead of 4 or 5 days. If the body is cremated, there is no need to visit the cemetery, which is a ritual that is growing less and less common with each generation. Cemetery visits brought peace to many survivors, who enjoyed planting flowers at the gravesite and whispering words of remembrance to their loved ones. Today's grief rituals are limited to what the public considers appropriate or what is convenient for today's busy lifestyle. After the burial or cremation, the survivors are left alone with their pain and with a long journey of healing ahead.

TYPES OF GRIEF

Types of grief include anticipatory, acute, and complicated (also known as *traumatic grief* or *prolonged grief disorder*) as well as chronic sorrow (Shear and Mulhare, 2008). Different sources indicate some disagreement about definitions (the terms *dysfunctional grief* and *pathologic grief* were often used to describe complicated grief). There is also disagreement about the time required for the resolution of a particular form of grief (see the Acute Grief section later in this chapter for a discussion of grief timelines).

Anticipatory Grief

Anticipatory grief, which is also known as *premourning,* is grief that is associated with the anticipation of a predicted death or a developing loss (Ackley, 2002; Heffner and Byock, 2002; Shneidman, 1980). Lindemann (1944) identified this type of grief as "preparatory grief," which is the grief that terminally ill patients experience to prepare for their final separation from the world. Lindemann believed that the threat of death or separation could in itself provoke a bereavement response. Prominent researcher Dr. Elizabeth Kübler-Ross (1981) identified a five-stage model of anticipatory grief that is experienced by individuals who are confronting death:

1. Denial—shock and disbelief
2. Anger—struggling with fate (i.e., "Why me?" or "It's not fair!")
3. Bargaining—making deals with a higher power in the hope of a cure
4. Depression and despair—realizing that death is inevitable
5. Acceptance—succumbing to fate with relative calmness

Although the Kübler-Ross grief model is instructive for identifying the general patterns of the grief experience, it has its limitations, as described by Maciejewski and colleagues (2007):

- It was developed for people with terminal illness and not to describe the grief responses of the survivors.
- It offers a linear process of grieving, and people do not always uniformly progress through these stages.
- It leads to typical aspects of grieving, such as regression or early acceptance, being misconstrued as evidence of complicated grief reactions (see the summary of grief theories).

Anticipatory grief sometimes begins with a catastrophic diagnosis, and it is characterized by a keen sense of vulnerability. The old and comfortable illusion of immortality that we all have when life is good suddenly disappears, and grief

for that idea begins at the time of diagnosis. In this situation, the grief is often complex. For example, in a family in which a loved one develops dementia, grief is acute (related to the current condition), ongoing (as the family gradually loses aspects of the loved one), and anticipatory (as the long-term reality of the disorder becomes clearer).

Early during the development of the anticipatory grief model, anticipatory grief was viewed as an adaptive process that helped to resolve relationships and prepare survivors for the anticipated loss. Ideally, the realization that loss was approaching gave the people involved an opportunity to work on interpersonal and spiritual reconciliation and to provide support for one another (Parkes, 1998). More recently, some clinicians and researchers have seen an association between anticipatory grief and a high incidence of depression or family withdrawal from the patient. A recent study showed that hopelessness strongly influenced preparatory grief, possibly as a result of the strong relationship between depression, hopelessness, and anxiety (Mystakidou et al, 2007). There is general agreement about the following: (1) that grief begins when a serious physical or mental illness occurs; (2) that this grief is sometimes anticipatory and involves pain, as do other forms of grief; and (3) that a lack of emotional response to serious illness or other loss is an indication that complicated grief is likely (Ackley, 2002; Carpenito, 2002). The nurse therefore needs to view anticipatory grief as normative and to understand that persons who are experiencing it will possibly benefit from intervention. It is important to emphasize that these experiences are not necessarily prescribed stages that people should pass through even though they are still often viewed this way (Maciejewski et al, 2007).

Acute Grief

Acute grief, which is usually simply referred to as *grief,* is the prototype of a painful experience after a loss. Its symptoms and process are described earlier in this chapter. Although there is agreement that acute grief is time limited, there is no agreement on how long acute (or normal) grief lasts. An early theory is that acute grief lasts approximately 1 year (Shneidman, 1980). Shear and Mulhare (2008, p. 663), say that "acute grief lasts most of the day, every day, for up to 6 months." Some researchers integrate the time span for acute grief with the severity of symptoms, the severity of the trauma or loss, the nature of the relationship, and cultural values (American Psychiatric Association, 2000; Kemp, 2006; Stroebe et al, 2000). Acute grief does not have a clear ending; gradually the sadness lessens, the pain diminishes, and eventually the mourner moves forward with his or her life, although complete recovery may never occur (Hentz, 2002). Love (2007, p. 76), states that the typical grief course includes fluctuations between anger and acceptance and that "prescriptive timelines and set stages for resolving grief cannot be imposed." In some traditional cultures (e.g., East Indian) and among some individuals of certain religions (e.g., Jewish, Hindu), grief is ongoing and not limited by time (Kemp, 2006). Within the process of healing and moving on, there are times of acute exacerbation whenever some situation or event brings back

TABLE 28-1	SIMILARITIES AND DIFFERENCES BETWEEN COMPLICATED GRIEF AND USUAL ACUTE GRIEF

Complicated Grief Similar to Usual Acute Grief
- Yearning and longing
- Sense of disbelief and difficulty accepting the death
- A mix of emotions with painful emotions usually dominant
- Preoccupation with thoughts and memories of the deceased
- Interest and engagement in ongoing life is attenuated and focused on bereavement-related activities

Complicated Grief Differs from Usual Acute Grief
- Grief is unresolved after 6 months
- Accompanied by ruminations about the death, the person who died, the bereaved person themselves, or about grief
- Repetitive images of the person who died
- Ruminations about self-blaming thoughts
- Excessive avoidance and isolation

the pain, and the mourner again feels overwhelmed with grief. Holidays, birthdays, and other significant milestones are obvious events that may revive the grief. Other precipitants are less obvious, and thus the mourner is unable to prepare for them. For example, a song, an image, or a smell that is present in an unguarded moment may invoke sadness as powerful as it was in the beginning. These moments of exacerbation also decrease over time.

Complicated Grief

"Complicated grief is the result of mourning that has been derailed and fails to reach resolution" (Shear and Mulhare, 2008, p. 666). Although there is considerable debate about what precisely constitutes complicated grief, all sources agree that it lasts longer than other types of grief and that is characterized by greater disability or other more dysfunctional patterns than usual as defined by cultural values. Love (2007) states that persons who are experiencing significant functional impairment for more than 6 months are likely experiencing a complicated grief reaction and may suffer comorbid disorders such as anxiety, depression, or PTSD. Early theorists have described complicated grief in multiple ways, and many of these definitions are still true today. Lindemann (1944) and many writers and researchers who came after him (e.g., Stroebe et al, 2000; American Psychiatric Association, 2000; Parkes, 1998; Cowles and Rodgers, 1991; Bowlby, 1980) have all distinguished normal and complicated aspects of grief. More recent researchers (e.g., Shear and Mulhare, 2008; Kristjanson et al, 2006; Love, 2007) agree that, up to some point, grief is normal and that, beyond that point, grief is considered pathologic or complicated. Table 28-1 compares the responses of complicated grief with those of usual acute grief is used with permission from Shear and Mulhare (2008):

PTSD is sometimes a feature of complicated grief in which individuals re-experience past traumatic events with extreme symptoms of anxiety (Fortinash and Holoday Worret, 2007; Love 2007; Melhem et al, 2001; Shear and Mulhare 2008). Persons who are prone to the development of PTSD include the following:
- Military personnel who fought on the battlefield
- Victims of natural disasters such as Hurricane Katrina in 2005 and the catastrophic 2010 earthquake in Haiti
- Those who experienced violent acts of terrorism such as 1999 Columbine High School shootings, the 2007 Virginia Tech massacre, the 9/11 terrorist attack, and the 2011 shooting in Tucson, Arizona
- Individuals affected by widespread devastation such as the 2010 Deepwater Horizon oil well explosion in the Gulf of Mexico
- Prisoners of war or concentration camps

A recent study showed that family members whose intensive care unit experience resulted in the discharge or death of a loved one were at risk for developing PTSD, anxiety, depression, or complicated grief (Anderson et al, 2008). If depression is the predominant feature of bereavement and if it is incapacitating 2 months after the loss, the patient may be diagnosed as having a major depressive disorder (American Psychiatric Association, 2000). Ray and Prigerson (2006) state that, when grief does not resolve within a reasonable period of time or when individuals have extreme experiences, the grieving process is most likely no longer adaptive.

Types of complicated grief include the following (American Psychiatric Association, 2000; Anderson et al, 2008; Kemp, 2006; Shear and Mulhare 2008):
- *Traumatic grief.* This occurs when there is traumatic loss, such as when a spouse is murdered, when a child dies suddenly and unexpectedly, or when rape or multiple deaths occur. PTSD is often a concurrent or complicating factor that is sometimes characterized by psychic numbing, intrusive thoughts, avoidance of stimuli, increased arousal, and other aspects of PTSD (Fortinash and Holoday Worret, 2007; Melhem et al, 2001). For some patients, there is a distortion or exaggeration of one or more normative components of grief, with anger and guilt being the most common.
- *Absent or inhibited grief.* This is characterized by the minimal emotional expression of grief, and it is sometimes related to trauma, as noted previously. Absent grief sometimes converts to delayed grief, and the individual may experience it years after the loss. Precipitating factors for the conversion to delayed grief often are powerful experiences, such as psychotherapy or religious conversion.
- *Conflicted grief.* This occurs when the relationship with the deceased individual or the lost object is characterized by ambivalence or conflict. Initial responses to the loss are often minimal, and they then intensify rather than diminish over time; the survivor feels "haunted" by the deceased. An adult survivor of childhood sexual abuse whose abusing parent dies is an example of a person who is at risk for conflicted grief.

- *Chronic grief.* This is unending grief that occurs after a loss. Chronic grief is sometimes related to the survivor and the deceased having a highly codependent relationship. In other cases, chronic grief is a result of a severe loss and a lack of resources or support to deal with the loss. Chronic grief is especially common in some cultural groups (e.g., Cambodian refugees, Native Americans).

Complicated grief is generally associated with one or more of the following (Ackley, 2002; Parkes, 2001):

- Unresolved issues in the relationship with the person who died
- Inhibited expression of grief
- Lack of social support
- The "deritualization" of Western culture (e.g., reduced mourning periods of 1 or 2 days)
- Uncertain loss (e.g., prisoners of war, kidnapping)
- Traumatic loss (e.g., by murder, in an accident)
- Multiple losses (e.g., war, natural disaster, mass murders)
- Loss that is seldom discussed (e.g., rape, abortion)
- Undervalued loss, such as that felt by some who experience miscarriages or other losses that may not be recognized by others as significant
- The accumulated effects of current grief on past unresolved grief

Chronic Sorrow

Chronic sorrow is a form of grief that often includes characteristics of other forms of grief but that differs with regard to several essential aspects. First, chronic sorrow is a response to ongoing loss, such as the chronic illness of a loved one. Second, persons who are experiencing chronic sorrow seldom experience disability (e.g., major depression), and they typically function at a higher level in activities of daily living as compared with those who are experiencing other forms of grief (Burke et al, 1992). Persons who are at risk for chronic sorrow include parents with children who have mental disabilities, schizophrenia, or other chronic illness; spouses of persons with long-term chronic illnesses, such as multiple sclerosis, alcoholism, or Alzheimer's disease; and persons with similar disorders (Lichtenstein et al, 2002; Pejlert, 2001). There is no documentation of the effects on the grief process when the cause of the chronic sorrow is removed (i.e., when the disabled person dies) see Case Study #2.

Children and Adolescents in Grief

In a recent study of 132 bereaved children and adolescents who had experienced childhood traumatic grief (CTG), Brown and colleagues (2008, p. 900) found that "CTG severity was significantly associated with the degree to which the death was viewed as traumatic." The study reported that CTG was also associated with the emotional response and degree of sadness exhibited by the child's caretakers. Although many sources agree that most children cope well even after a sudden death, some research has shown that bereaved children experienced increased incidents of psychiatric problems during the first 2 years after a parent's death (Brown et al, 2008; Cerel et al, 2006). It is important

❖ CLINICAL ALERT #1

The following increase a patient's risk for the development of complicated grief:

- Premorbid psychiatric history or history of psychosocial trauma
- Social isolation
- Relationship with the deceased that was characterized by unresolved conflict or ambivalence (e.g., a "love–hate" relationship, conflicting feelings about the deceased)
- Relationship with the deceased that was characterized by enmeshment and a high level of introjection, hence difficulty with letting go
- Tendency to suppress grief
- Young age (e.g., traumatic death of parents during childhood; see the Children and Adolescents in Grief section of this chapter)

to consider the age and development of the child; young children are strongly dependent on their parents, and the early loss of a parent can be devastating and traumatic. Many theorists agree that this is because the child lacks the emotions and mature coping skills to maintain a sense of self while grieving (Brown et al, 2008). It was also noted that more violent causes of death tended to exacerbate the grieving process in children and that "closer relationships with the deceased are associated with higher rates of suicidality, PTSD, substance abuse, agoraphobia, and other severe mental health symptoms" (Brown et al, 2008, p. 903). Melhem and colleagues (2007) wrote that young people who believed that others were responsible for their parents' deaths or who felt that others blamed them for the death had a significantly higher incidence of CTG. For many children, death represents a loss of safety, and a sense of uncertainty about the world and their own existence. The emotional support of parents and significant others is critical to the child's response to loss. As children get older and realize the permanency of death, they are more aware of its threat, and they need the protection of caring adults during this vulnerable time (Brown et al, 2008). Implications for further research in this critical area is suggested. See the interventions for childhood grief later in this chapter.

Grief and Depression

Grief and depression are often compared with one another. Grief—especially complicated grief—also shares characteristics with PTSD, particularly in that both invariably involve loss (Table 28-2).

BEREAVEMENT CARE

Before Loss

Grief is a universal experience that comes with or without warning and that occurs many times and with varying intensity throughout life. The major psychosocial determinants of

TABLE 28-2	COMPARISON OF GRIEF, DEPRESSION, AND POSTTRAUMATIC STRESS DISORDER		
ASPECT	**GRIEF**	**DEPRESSION**	**POSTTRAUMATIC STRESS DISORDER**
Process	Related to loss	Relatively static or cyclic affective disorder that is not necessarily related to loss	Relatively static anxiety disorder related to trauma; precipitating event is outside of the range of usual human experience
Manifestation of symptoms	Usually appear shortly after the loss	Sometimes associated with an identified loss	Often appear years after the trauma
Depressive symptoms	Dysphoric mood of sadness, hopelessness, and despair; anger and periods of agitation are common	Similar to but more intense than grief, except that the individual seldom expresses anger; psychomotor retardation, morbid guilt, and suicidal ideation are more common	Common; other symptoms include persistent reexperiencing of the trauma (rather than preoccupation with the image of the deceased, as with grief); increased arousal is common
Physical symptoms	Cover a wide spectrum; sometimes include heart disease and other chronic illnesses	Primarily neurovegetative	Sleep disturbances often resemble those of grief or depression; hypervigilance is common
Spiritual beliefs	Sometimes provide meaning or context	Seldom provide context or meaning	Seldom any relation

the pathology of grief are a psychiatric history before the loss and inadequate social support (Silverman et al, 2001). It makes sense then that the first and primary promotion of mental health (e.g., family involvement in community and faith activities, improved parenting, other such efforts to promote mental and spiritual health) is the best way to address grief.

When Loss Is Impending

A second point for the nurse to consider when addressing health promotion or disability prevention is in the case of terminal illness or other anticipated loss. Interventions in these situations include assisting individuals and families with working toward personal, interpersonal, and spiritual reconciliation so that they can effectively deal with anticipatory grief. Even in the best of relationships, there are sometimes unresolved issues or areas in which growth is possible. Promoting health during this stage of life includes promoting the participation of both the patient and the family in care. Clearly effective participation in care has a positive effect on the grief process after death, although long-term effects are not known for caregivers of patients with Alzheimer's disease, schizophrenia, and other similar chronic illnesses. A variety of means exist for intervention at this point, including individual informal or formal counseling in acute care settings, family support groups, hospice care, and spiritual support. Nurses and other health care professionals need to address the health needs of family members as well as those of patients (see Research for Evidence-Based Practice #1).

Health care providers offer preventive grief therapy to survivors in several circumstances. For example, hospice and palliative care programs typically offer bereavement calls or visits at specified intervals to survivors. Many hospice programs also periodically hold seminars and other events or activities for bereaved adults and children. Churches and synagogues hold grief workshops for members and others in the community. These are generally weekend or time-limited groups that are similar to self-help groups such as I Can Cope and others. Religiously oriented grief activities are also held in some cases in association with significant religious holidays related to death or remembrance.

After the Loss

The third intervention point takes place after the loss occurs (i.e., postvention). Intervention at this point is often preventive and directed toward addressing existing problems that are interpersonal in nature or related to normative or complicated grief. The tasks of grief, as discussed previously, provide a framework for intervention after loss.

SPIRITUALITY AND GRIEF

Love (2007) writes that disruptions such as the death of a loved one can result in the survivor searching for meaning in death and questioning spiritual values and beliefs. The grief experience can threaten all basic spiritual needs or issues. Meaning, hope, relatedness, forgiveness, and transcendence sometimes fall away and leave the mourner in a spiritual vacuum. The nature of God and previously held beliefs, including any easy answers to life's problems (e.g., that faith protects one from pain), are called into question and do not always support the reality of the current feelings. Grief is then interpreted as a test of faith, and the awareness or acknowledgement of anger or other negative feelings is taken as a personal spiritual failure (i.e., a source of more guilt).

Although dreams and visions are significant spiritual events in some cultures, in the context of Western cultures, they are discounted as either immaterial or pathologic. There is often reluctance by the grieving individual to discuss dream experiences and feelings about them with family, friends, or clergy. As mourners struggle to find a context for the doubt and confusion that accompanies these experiences, it is important for the nurse to listen with openness and to determine how these experiences either confirm or challenge the mourner's spiritual and religious beliefs. Some individuals are confirmed in their traditional beliefs; others see the dissolution of their faith occurring; and still others find or rediscover a deeper faith (see Chapter 8).

Grief has the potential to transform those who experience it, for better or worse (White and Ferszt, 2009). Carse (1980) says that grief can invite the survivor to a new life in which he or she can take the discontinuity of death, loss, and grief to a higher level of continuity. For others, grief is a context for retreat into an impoverished life. Interventions in grief are most effective when they are used to promote health, to offer comfort and hope, and to prevent dysfunction. Interventions are less effective during the postvention period, and they are least effective for the treatment of complicated grief.

THE NURSING PROCESS
ASSESSMENT

The nursing assessment of a person who is bereaved is based on knowledge of the normative and pathologic aspects of the grief process, the influences on the grief process, and the person's resources. Assessment encompasses the following: (1) the grief experience of the mourner; (2) the factors that inhibit or promote working through the grief process, including cultural and religious norms; and (3) the mourner's ability to mobilize cognitive, behavioral, and emotion-based coping strategies. The nurse assesses the patient's current level of functioning with the understanding that, up to a point,

---

NURSING ASSESSMENT QUESTIONS

Grief

1. Describe how it has been for you since (the person being grieved for) died.
2. How have you reacted to other major losses in your life?
3. Whom do you depend on when you are having a hard time, like now? Talk about what it's like when you ask for help.
4. Let's go over all the prescription drugs and other medicines and vitamins that you are taking.
5. How often do you have alcoholic drinks or other drugs? When you drink or take drugs, how much do you take, and how does it make you feel?

   A question not to ask is, "How are you doing?" Cultural norms are to respond to such questions with "Pretty good," "Okay," or "Fine." These answers are essentially meaningless.

---

impaired functioning is to be expected (see the Nursing Assessment Questions box).

Physical Disturbances

Physical disturbances during acute grief include weakness, anorexia, shortness of breath, tightness of the chest, dry mouth, and gastrointestinal disturbances (e.g., constipation, diarrhea, abdominal pain, gas, nausea, vomiting). Cardiovascular and gastrointestinal problems predominate among patients with chronic grief. Vague physical complaints such as unfocused abdominal pain or shortness of breath are especially common with all stages and types of grief.

Cognitive Disturbances

Cognitive disturbances are often focused on a preoccupation with images and thoughts of the deceased. This preoccupation is sometimes so pervasive that the bereaved person is unable to carry on with some activities of daily living. The inability to control thoughts is distressing to many mourners. During acute grief, these obsessive thoughts are normal; they are simply part of the process. Preoccupation that results in a significant disturbance of daily life (e.g., work) is widely considered pathologic after about 1 year after the date of death when the person who died was an adult and 2 or more years after the date of death when the deceased was a child (see Research for Evidence-Based Practice #2).

Behavioral and Relating Disturbances

Behavioral and relating disturbances often result from the depressive aspects of grief. Some people who are bereaved describe themselves as "stopped" and thus unable to participate in relationships. There is a tendency among survivors to reflect on the death and on the relationship with the deceased. During at least the earlier phases of the process, talk of the deceased tends to focus only on his or her positive qualities and to ignore the multifaceted nature of the individual. Many people who are bereaved cry with little apparent provocation, which often results in discomfort for the mourner and others. During chronic grief, the talk of the death and the relationship tends to be repetitive and superficial rather than progressive and insightful (see Case Study #1).

Affective Disturbances

Affective disturbances are primarily those of sadness or depression, anger, and guilt. Cultural norms of continuing on with everyday life and getting back to normal inhibit the expression of these feelings. People who are bereaved soon begin to feel that nobody wants to hear about their loss. Sadness and even feelings of depression are not considered pathologic unless they persist for 1 to 2 years after the death or include suicidal ideation (see Clinical Alert #2 later in this chapter).

NURSING DIAGNOSIS

When diagnosing grief or problems that occur with grief, nurses need to be mindful that the typical approach is to

Mrs. Gray is 75 years old and lives alone in the apartment that she shared with her husband for the past 21 years, since their retirement. Her husband died the previous month, after a 2-year struggle with prostate cancer. Since her husband's death, Mrs. Gray has felt sad and depressed. She wants to spend time with others, but she says, "They're happy, and I'm sad, and it's no good for anyone." For the past week, except for "forcing" herself to take her daily walk around the block, Mrs. Gray has spent most of her time alone in her apartment. She has a poor appetite, difficulty sleeping, and feels guilty about all of the things that she feels she could have done to help her husband. Most of the other residents in the apartment complex are similar in age to Mrs. Gray, and she is close to several of them. Her only child, a son, lives in another state, and he has invited his mother to move into his home with him and his wife.

Critical Thinking

1. According to your assessment, what type of grief is Mrs. Gray experiencing?
2. From your knowledge of the grieving process, what are Mrs. Gray's three most important needs?
3. What personal resources are likely to be most helpful to Mrs. Gray at the present time?
4. What questions would you ask Mrs. Gray during this stage of her grief?

identify problems of a physical or psychologic nature and then to try to alleviate the discomfort. Because grief normally includes discomfort, attempts to avoid or eliminate the discomfort—no matter how well intentioned—will impede the grieving process. Alternatively, extreme discomfort will possibly require pharmacologic intervention. The point at which discomfort is classified as extreme or abnormal rather than normal has not been defined. Therefore, an insightful diagnosis focuses on the expression of normal feelings (e.g., anger, guilt, sadness) as much as on what feelings actually exist. Nursing diagnoses are prioritized according to patient needs and safety issues.

Acute Grief

- Disturbed personal identity related to changes in roles and relationships as evidenced by the inability to establish new patterns of relating to others and the environment after the death of a spouse or loved one
- Situational low self-esteem related to pervasive feelings of guilt and cognitive distortions caused by guilt as evidenced by thinking about inadequacies in the relationship with the deceased and blaming the self for all problems in the relationship
- Impaired social interaction related to altered role performance and disruptions in usual patterns of conduct and interactions as evidenced by difficulty with adapting to life changes and with developing relationships in accordance with the current situation

Complicated Grief

- Risk for self-directed violence; risk factors include feelings of hopelessness and anger and reports and observed incidents of rage resulting from the perceived inability to live without the deceased
- Complicated grieving (unexpressed) related to fear of catastrophe if grief is expressed as evidenced by absence of expression of feelings related to the grief process
- Complicated grieving related to unresolved guilt as evidenced by frequent references to personal failings in the relationship with the deceased

Chronic Sorrow

- Chronic sorrow related to effects of the death of a loved one or experiences of chronic physical or mental illness or disability (e.g., Alzheimer's disease, schizophrenia, mental retardation, cancer) as evidenced by recurring feelings of sadness and grief that vary in intensity over time and that interfere with the person's ability to reach the highest level of personal and social well-being
- Caregiver role strain related to chronic sorrow as evidenced by caregiver withdrawal from community life to care for a loved one with a chronic condition

Other Nursing Diagnoses

- Risk for other-directed violence
- Risk-prone health behavior
- Disabled family coping
- Ineffective coping
- Ineffective denial
- Interrupted family processes
- Fatigue
- Grieving
- Hopelessness
- Posttrauma syndrome
- Powerlessness
- Insomnia
- Social isolation
- Disturbed thought processes
- Spiritual distress
- Ineffective sexuality pattern

OUTCOME IDENTIFICATION

Outcome criteria focus on the enhancement of emotional coping skills or methods (e.g., greater expression of feelings of grief) and cognitive and behavioral coping abilities (e.g., strategies to develop more functional patterns of living that are appropriate to changed life circumstances). Outcomes are prioritized according to patient needs and safety issues.

The patient will do the following:
- Verbalize the absence of suicidal ideation.
- Express grief and guilty or angry feelings related to the death rather than suppressing grief.
- Express both positive and negative feelings about the deceased rather than idealizing the qualities of the deceased.

- Explore the relationship with the deceased in a multifaceted way that includes both positive and negative aspects.
- Formulate and implement reasonable plans for adapting life and the identified role to present circumstances.
- Participate in at least one social or community activity each week.

PLANNING

The plan of care for a person with acute grief consists primarily of the following: (1) supporting the mobilization of the person's personal and community resources; (2) providing normative data about the grief process; and (3) supporting the person in her or his grief work (see Case Study #1). The next section of this chapter discusses each of these steps. Assistance is sometimes necessary to mobilize resources (e.g., family, friends, spiritual supports), because individuals are often reluctant to ask for help, and resource individuals often do not know how to provide help. In addition, some of the symptoms of grief (e.g., fatigue, sadness, anger) promote isolation rather than relationship with others. Frequently, if either the bereaved person or a support person is able to initiate contact, the other will respond appropriately. However, too often mourners and their resources exist in isolation, each wishing that they knew how to make contact with the other. Nurses can provide normative data about grief (i.e., an explanation of physical, emotional, social, and spiritual difficulties inherent in the grief process) to both the bereaved and his or her support systems. In a culture that is in many ways lacking in ritual and tradition, grief sometimes seems mysterious or pathologic, even to those who one might expect to be helpful (e.g., clergy). The nurse teaches survivors and others (e.g., family members) what they might experience during the grieving process. Bereavement and survivor groups are excellent forums for such teaching. Supporting the mourner in his or her grief work includes facilitating the telling of how the deceased died and exploring both positive and negative aspects of the relationship with the deceased, positive and negative aspects of the deceased, and cognitive and behavioral coping strategies. Assistance with mobilizing resources and providing normative data is also part of this type of support.

The plan of care for a person with complicated grieving focuses on the specific pathologic condition of the patient. The nurse also addresses normative aspects of grief, and he or she can direct plans toward the community. With community-focused planning, the nurse helps churches, synagogues, community centers, hospitals, and other organizations to develop self-help groups for bereaved persons. Nurses also serve as facilitators for such groups (see Case Study #2).

IMPLEMENTATION

The first priority when planning care for a person with complicated grief is to assess the risk for the patient becoming violent toward himself or herself or others. The patient's physical health is also a major concern. The plan should include efforts to work toward resolving the grief through

---

CASE STUDY #2

Mr. and Mrs. Black have a 25-year-old son, Kevin, who has chronic undifferentiated schizophrenia. Kevin lives at home most of the year, except for when he is admitted to the county hospital, which occurs two or three times a year. Kevin has never worked. He has no friends, he is withdrawn most of the time, he has violent episodes about once a month, and he is noncompliant with medications. The Blacks tried different hospitals until they ran out of insurance coverage for Kevin. Kevin has experienced a variety of antipsychotic medications, different therapists, alternative therapies, and spiritual counseling, but nothing has changed the course of his illness. Mr. Black works long hours at an auto parts store, and Mrs. Black stays home with Kevin. Mr. and Mrs. Black have begun seeing the clinical nurse specialist from the county hospital community outreach program. Their chief complaints as a couple and individually are overwhelming feelings of hopelessness and physical and mental exhaustion. The clinical nurse specialist has diagnosed their problem as caregiver role strain related to chronic sorrow as evidenced by the caregivers' withdrawal from community life to care for their son with chronic schizophrenia. The nurse has implemented a plan of care that includes the following: (1) weekly couples' counseling; (2) joining a regular family support group in a community facility; and (3) biweekly home visits by an outreach staff member to assist Kevin with medication compliance, which is an ongoing challenge.

Critical Thinking

1. What is your opinion about whether Kevin will experience significant improvement with regard to his disorder?
2. Part of the care plan is directed toward the parents. Why are they also receiving care instead of Kevin alone, if he is the one who is mentally ill? What might happen to Kevin if his parents are no longer able to cope with Kevin's mental illness and its challenges?
3. Discuss potential success in relation to this plan. Are the Blacks likely to achieve happiness or even contentment as a result of receiving the care described?
4. Discuss each of the following feelings that family members with relatives with chronic mental illness sometimes experience: anger, sorrow, guilt, love, and despair (See Chapter 13).

---

emotional, cognitive, and behavioral means. Chemical dependency presents a major barrier to the individual's goal attainment, and the nurse needs to address it. Dependence on antianxiety medications is common. In many cases, the approach can be growth oriented rather than directed only toward the treatment of symptoms.

Nursing Interventions

Bereavement care ideally takes place in the community before the patient deteriorates to the extent that hospitalization is required. Nursing interventions are prioritized according to patient needs and safety issues.

1. Evaluate the patient for his or her intent to kill himself or herself or to harm or kill others *to ensure safety and prevent violence.*

2. Promote a therapeutic alliance between the patient and the nurse. *Developing a working relationship is sometimes difficult because of the patient's suppressed feelings. Death and other major losses are often experienced as complete destruction of the certainty and order around which people structure their lives. It is therefore necessary for the nurse to be consistent and orderly with respect to following through on all obligations, such as schedules and appointments.*

3. Facilitate the patient's expression of feelings related to the loss, and validate the feelings already expressed by the patient. In addition, begin to introduce the possibility of other feelings related to the loss, such as ambivalence. Help the patient to take an increasingly active role in exploring and understanding the full response to the grief. *Ambivalent feelings are especially difficult for many patients to acknowledge. Many patients are prone to merely repeating feelings and thoughts rather than exploring, expanding on, and understanding them. Although some repetition of feelings, concerns, and experiences is unavoidable and somewhat helpful, it is important for the patient to understand the full grief response to begin the healing process.*

4. Help the patient to understand the relationship between himself or herself and the lost person or object and to express and understand the grief and its attendant feelings. Facilitate a review of the patient's relationship with the deceased, and help the patient to discuss and understand meanings within the relationship, including hopes fulfilled, disappointments, and strengths and weaknesses of the relationship. *It is essential for the patient to move beyond the grief that is related to the death or loss and to begin to understand the full meaning of the relationship, both good and bad.*

5. Facilitate the full expression of grief by assisting the patient with linking together the full spectrum of feelings, both positive and negative, regarding the loss and the relationship with the deceased. *It is necessary for the patient to remember the deceased as a real human being with both positive and negative qualities, to let go of the idealistic image of the person, and to begin to move forward without guilt and remorse. Some survivors are more successful at this than others.*

6. Promote interactions with others and offer limited and specific options for the patient to increase social support, both individually and in the community. Encourage the patient to continue engaging in social relationships, even when—as some mourners say—it feels as if he or she is "just going through the motions." *It is important for the patient to begin to move forward and "join the living," even if it means "going through the motions" at first. With encouragement from family and friends, the patient will eventually develop a healthy social life while experiencing (in a healthy sense) both good and bad memories of the deceased.*

Therapeutic responses to grieving persons:
- "This must be a difficult time for you. I would like to sit here with you for a while."
- "It's OK to feel anger or any other emotion at this time."
- "Most people experience these feelings during a loss."
- "Guilt is a common response when a loved one dies. Are you having any other feelings?"
- "If you want to talk about your thoughts and feelings, I am here to listen."
- "Do you have someone who can stay with you at home for awhile?"

Nontherapeutic responses to grieving persons:
- "Please don't cry; you'll upset yourself and the children."
- "You shouldn't be angry at your husband for dying."
- "Don't tell people you can't go on; you will scare them."
- "I know you feel bad now, but I promise that you'll get over it."
- "You're lucky your husband lived so long; I lost mine years ago."
- "Other people have been through much worse and survived."

Collaborative Interventions

A multidisciplinary approach by a team that consists of nurse, a psychiatrist, a psychologist, a social worker, an occupational therapist, and other health care providers is not usually necessary, although community resources are an important part of care. Because of the frequency and vagueness of physical complaints, the most important individual to be involved is the patient's nurse practitioner, physician, or other source of primary care (see Research for Evidence-Based Practice #1).

Problem-Oriented Grief Therapy

Health care providers offer grief therapy when a problem that is not necessarily complicated grief exists or is anticipated. Like other of life's unavoidable processes, the difficult and painful transitions of normative grief usually respond to understanding and support. Grief therapy often focuses on emotional responses to the loss; problem solving related to moving forward in life (i.e., undoing the bonds of attachment) (Bowlby, 1980; Parkes, 2001; Worden, 1982); or finding or reconstructing meaning in the loss or relationship (Neimeyer, 2006).

Emotional issues center around the telling and retelling of the details of the story of the death and its surrounding issues as well as the history of the relationship, with emphasis on the experience and the expression of related feelings, particularly sadness, anger, guilt, and other troubling feelings (Carpenito, 2002). During earlier phases of the process, the bereaved person recalls only the positive qualities of the deceased. As the mourner progresses through the grief work and the wound begins to heal, both the positive and negative qualities of the deceased and the relationship emerge. Problem-focused strategies address questions of developing support, relationships, and other issues inherent in "the new life" after a loved one dies. Family-oriented therapy focuses on improving communication, increasing cohesiveness, and enhancing problem solving. The death of a spouse is especially important. Researchers such as Holmes and Rahe (1967) have rated it highest among all losses, although experts cite the loss of a child as being the most risky (see Research for Evidence-Based Practice #2). The death of a spouse presents the surviving mate with a host of new responsibilities that were previously performed by the deceased (e.g., paying the bills, doing the weekly shopping, using the computer, cooking meals, mowing the lawn, driving). Widowhood is difficult at any age. For older adults who are unable to manage their home alone, the results of the loss can be as overwhelming as the grief itself. If the surviving spouse is forced to leave his or her home and move into an assisted living or other facility, the loss of home and community compounds the grief. For parents with young children, the trauma of being a single parent can be a daunting task. In addition, the loneliness experienced in suddenly living without the emotional support of a partner is profound at any age (Fortinash and Holoday Worret, 2007; Mabry, 2006).

Grief Intervention During Childhood and Adolescence

Loss that occurs during childhood predisposes a child to many physical, emotional, and behavioral problems. There is an increased risk for suicide during the adolescent period, because preteen and teenage children have a more mature understanding of death as being permanent rather than transitory (Brown et al, 2008). Interventions include listening to children and adolescents express their thoughts about death and dying and responding according to the child's understanding and developmental stage (Fortinash and Holoday Worret, 2008). A young child's questions about death should be centered on the child's own feelings and interpretation. If the child believes that Mommy or Daddy is in heaven with the angels and God and that is the family's belief, then there is no need to contradict the child, because this may be a source of comfort and peace. Some children may identify pets that died and that they were assured by their parents went to heaven; these children may assume that their parents are now happily reunited with the lost pets. Adolescents, who are more aware of the permanence of death, may feel more out of control, depending on their own coping mechanisms and sense of self; therefore, they may not be as easily comforted. Adolescents who are given some control over their lives may feel more empowered and less helpless when dealing with grief (Cerel et al, 2006; Fortinash and Holoday Worret, 2008). It is important to not shut children out of the grieving process and to include them in decisions that involve the memorial services and other necessary tasks and activities that follow. There is little known about factors that protect children and adolescents from complicated grief after the death of a parent. Melhem and colleagues (2007) noted that complicated grief scores did not increase among children who were involved in attending the funeral of the loved one and who assisted with the removal of the personal effects of the deceased. Most researchers agree about the importance of emotional support from parents and others during this vulnerable time. Adults

need to have the coping mechanisms that are necessary to contain their own emotions, because their ability to provide support is directly correlated with the success or failure of the child's adjustment after the traumatic event (Brown et al, 2008).

Medications During Grief

In response to the frequent overuse of medications to mask grief, some practitioners discourage the use of antianxiety or antidepressant medications for bereaved persons. However, even with cases of normal grief, some mourners require the short-term use of these medications during certain stages of the grief process. Selective serotonin reuptake inhibitors are the mainstay of therapy in most settings and for most problems of grief, including complicated or traumatic grief (Fortinash and Holoday Worret, 2007) (see Chapter 25).

Reassurance is an essential component of grief therapy. The absence of cultural norms for expressing or otherwise dealing with grief results in some people feeling as if their grief is the beginning of insanity. They say things like, "I'm going crazy" or "I think I'm losing my mind." Although some will not initially believe it, they need to hear from the nurse that their experience is grief, that it is normal, and that it is not mental illness. The tasks of grief, as described previously, provide a framework for therapy.

Interventions for Complicated Grief

With complicated grief, there is often unresolved grief from the past or a preexisting psychologic condition that the nurse needs to address as part of the grief therapy. Therapy thus includes the issues noted previously in addition to other interpersonal issues. Often a central issue in complicated grief is the promotion of the patient's ability to express the pain of the grief rather than only the anger or guilt (Ackley, 2002; Carpenito, 2002). It is common for bereaved persons to have ill-defined fantasies of catastrophe if their pain is expressed (e.g., "If I ever start crying, I will never stop"). Patients with complicated grief are at an increased risk for suicide and, to a lesser extent, for hurting others. Some also experience physical and mental disorders, as previously discussed.

Intervention studies are looking at the validity of the constructs of complicated grief (Bonanno, 2006). New research offers a cognitive behavioral model that suggests that patients use narrative strategies that have special meaning for them to cope with devastating loss. The cognitive behavioral model focuses on the patient's struggle to integrate the loss into his or her autobiographic memory (Boelen et al, 2006; Neimeyer, 2006). Shear and Mulhare (2008) concluded that a target psychotherapeutic approach was needed to confront complicated grief. They modified interpersonal psychotherapy on the basis of Bowlby's attachment theory of grief and loss (Bowlby, 1980). Their treatment focused on revisiting the loss and helping patients to re-imagine their ongoing relationship with the deceased, and re-envision their own future lives. The crux of this therapy is to use strategies and techniques that were used successfully in the past, to treat similar traumatic events. The researchers were guided by Bowlby's ideas about the dilemma of surrendering hope for the return of the lost loved one. Complicated grief treatment is short term, and it consists of motivational interviews and confrontive approaches, with respite periods. The goal of treatment is to "acknowledge the death and its consequences, revising the mental representation of the deceased, and redefining life goals" (Shear and Mulhare, 2008, p. 664).

The patient's primary physician, nurse practitioner, or other source of primary health care needs to be involved in or kept aware of grief treatment for several specific reasons. First, it is common for grieving patients to frequently seek medical care, often for vague or difficult-to-evaluate complaints that are actually somatic expressions of grief. An awareness of the presence of complicated grief and ongoing therapy will help health care providers to avoid unnecessary tests and treatment. Second, there is significant risk of suicide with complicated grief, and an informed health care provider needs to be alert to suicidal hints, gestures, and attempts to obtain lethal amounts of medications. According to Caico (2007) and White and Ferszt (2009), nurse practitioners are exposed to death across the lifespan, and they provide care to patients of all age groups in primary care settings (see Research for Evidence-Based Practice #1). All health care professionals who are involved in the care of a person with complicated grief need to be alert to the possibility of the patient's seeking help from multiple sources and thus the potential for lethal amounts of medication.

RESEARCH FOR EVIDENCE-BASED PRACTICE #1

White P, Ferszt G: Exploration of nurse practitioner practice with clients who are grieving, *J Am Acad Nurse Pract* 21.231-240, 2009. Copied with permission from the authors.

This qualitative, descriptive study using audio-taped interviews, explored the role of nine NPs in assessing patients in primary care settings who were grieving the death of a significant person. Requirements were that NP's were certified by the American Nurses Credentialing Center with a minimum of 5 years experience of primary care clinical practice. The purpose of the study was to describe what nurse practitioners actually do in day-to-day practice to manage their patients' grief, since little has been written about their practice with this population. Research questions were, 1. What signs and symptoms do NPs assess in patients who are grieving? 2. What strategies do NPs incorporate in their plan of care? 3. What health outcomes do NP's evaluate in the primary care setting? The nursing process was applied and assessment data were categorized as physical complaints, overall functioning, and emotional well-being or coping. Interventions included validating the patients' grief, prescriptions, and teaching. Grief that was considered ongoing or complicated was referred for further assessment and evaluation. Outcomes included relief of physical complaints, stabilized chronic illness, improved overall functioning, and improvements in patients' emotional well-being and coping abilities. The NP's were offered suggestions by other grief experts, such as expanding their roles to include counseling parents who lose a child through sudden infant death syndrome or other causes, and educating parents about children's grief responses. Implications for practice show that more research in understanding theoretical models and current research related to grief is warranted.

RESEARCH FOR EVIDENCE BASED PRACTICE #2

Arnold J, Buschman Gemma P: The continuing process of parental grief, *Death Stud* 32:658-673, 2008. Copyright Taylor & Francis Group, LLC. Copied with permission from the authors.

A study covering a span of 20 years examined the grief experiences of parents who lost a living child. Seventy-four mostly female nurses responded to a survey tool designed to examine the lifelong effects of parental grief. Causes of child death were varied and ages ranged from infancy to adulthood. Quantitative findings reported that parental grief is complex and ongoing vs. linear, and that grieving is associated with emotions that are both painful (e.g., regret, guilt, anger), and transformative. Of the 11 qualitative items, 5 dealt with specific images of grief, and 6 allowed respondents to describe the ways their lives were changed. Examples of images describing grief were "an erupting volcano, a well into which one descends, and a hollow or empty space." The last image was experienced by 75% of respondents (multiple expressions of emptiness were reported in various ways by 45 respondents). Forty-one parents responded with a whole range of their own images, which were consoling to them. Some images had religious or spiritual meanings, an example being a beautiful child happy in heaven and waiting to be reunited. Twenty-nine parents replied with a continuum of responses, such as difficulty loving their remaining children, being anxious and cautious in their relationship, having a heightened sense of love, attachment, and protection. Thirty-four respondents reported a wide range of life changes, including strain in their marriages, less communication with spouses, and distancing leading to divorce and remarriage. Some reported feeling less competent, while others felt stronger with renewed faith. Some changed roles, opting to work in labor and delivery to "help make a difference." Acceptance was a complicated process, and viewed in light of the lifelong nature of the grief. Some said acceptance was necessary because the event could not be changed. Others found it impossible as noted in the statement "I will never accept the death, rather I have found a way to live next to it". Authors suggest that support varies and is beneficial when grieving parents help each other share stories of their child's life and death.

The likelihood of suicide attempts and completion increases with grief, especially with complicated grief. The loss of psychosocial support systems is especially significant for men. A sustained loss of self-esteem, blaming of the self for the death, and ambivalence about living indicate that suicide risk is markedly increased.

EVALUATION

The nurse evaluates the patient's increasing ability to express his or her feelings and to develop effective coping strategies (e.g., increasing social interaction). It is important for the patient to express the full spectrum of feelings that are associated with the loss and that are related to the relationship with the deceased. Expressing feelings only about the loss itself is not sufficient for successful progress in grief work (see the Patient and Family Teaching Guidelines box). Remember that grief is a normal response to loss and that the feelings associated with grief are necessarily painful. The key to successful grief work depends on the individual's understanding of his or her relationship with the deceased. When that occurs, the patient is able to continue the work of investing in new relationships.

PATIENT AND FAMILY TEACHING GUIDELINES

Grief

There is little tradition related to grief in this contemporary technologic society. Therefore, it can be extremely helpful to provide persons who are bereaved with normative data about grief. This includes common physical, cognitive, behavioral, and affective responses to grief. It is helpful to write a list of grief reactions in layperson's terms and to review the list with the person who is bereaved. The power or intensity of feelings in response to loss is especially important to discuss with the bereaved person.

◎ **NURSING CARE PLAN**

Mr. Meek and his wife had been married for 45 years when she suddenly died 15 months ago from a myocardial infarction. Since his wife's death, Mr. Meek has become increasingly reclusive. He expresses extreme anger toward the doctors and nurses who were in the emergency department when his wife died. Mr. Meek keeps his home exactly as it was when his wife was alive. He has refused to dispose of any of her belongings, and he has renewed subscriptions to magazines that only Mrs. Meek read. Both Mr. and Mrs. Meek drank heavily but denied alcoholism. They had no children, and their relationship was characterized by frequent verbal abuse and occasional physical abuse. Mr. Meek continues to drink daily. He complains of heart problems, and he is angry with his physician, who insists that Mr. Meek has only mild hypertension that should respond to dietary changes and a cessation of alcohol consumption. Mr. Meek has begun keeping his curtains drawn and ignoring his neighbors and friends, and he denies the need for interpersonal relationships.

DSM-IV-TR Diagnoses

Axis I   Major depression; alcoholism
Axis II   None known
Axis III   Hypertension
Axis IV   Loss of primary support person (death of spouse)
           Problem related to the social environment (living alone, isolating self)
Axis V   GAF = 40 (current); GAF = 45 (past year)

Nursing Diagnosis *Complicated grieving (chronic distorted) related to the inability to appropriately express the full spectrum of feelings associated with his wife's death as evidenced by social isolation, projected anger, daily alcohol use, and somatic complaints*

NOC Coping; Motivation; Psychosocial adjustment: life change; Personal health status; Role performance; Depression self-control; Communication; Grief resolution
NIC Grief work facilitation; Coping enhancement; Anger control assistance; Guilt work facilitation; Support system enhancement; Emotional support; Counseling

PATIENT OUTCOMES	NURSING INTERVENTIONS	EVALUATION
Mr. Meek will engage in a therapeutic alliance with the home health nurse.	Visit Mr. Meek's home at a regular time on the same day once each week. *Constancy and dependability are essential to the development of productive relationships.*	Mr. Meek reluctantly agrees to visits from the nurse.

NURSING CARE PLAN—cont'd

PATIENT OUTCOMES	NURSING INTERVENTIONS	EVALUATION
Mr. Meek will cease the intake of alcohol at least 4 hours before and during visits with nurse.	Develop a contract with Mr. Meek in which he agrees to sobriety during visits. *Sobriety is essential to therapeutic relationships and personal growth.* Institute a chemical dependency care plan (see Chapter 15).	Mr. Meek maintains sobriety during visits. Mr. Meek enters and continues in a 12-step program or another program intended to promote sobriety.
Mr. Meek will express anger, sadness, and other feelings that are appropriately related to his wife's death.	Gradually present Mr. Meek with aspects of his grief experience that will help him to uncover his sadness and ambivalence. *Feelings of sadness and ambivalence are threatening to Mr. Meek. Do not introduce these too rapidly during the interventions.*	Mr. Meek is able to appropriately express sadness, confusion, ambivalence, and other feelings in addition to anger.
Mr. Meek will identify a variety of feelings that are expressed through anger, such as sadness, loneliness, fear, and confusion, related to the loss of his wife and partner.	Recognize the legitimacy of Mr. Meek's anger. Demonstrate the acceptance and understanding of ambivalence and other feelings such as sadness and confusion. *Anger is the means by which Mr. Meek is expressing other feelings that are not yet in his awareness. Facilitating other feelings helps to better manage anger and to promote the resolution of grief.*	Mr. Meek begins to accept the validity of anger and of feelings other than anger that are hidden behind his expressions of anger and rage.
Mr. Meek will discuss his hopes (both fulfilled and unfulfilled) and the disappointments related to his relationship with his wife.	Assist Mr. Meek with reviewing his relationship with his wife and the hopes that he and his wife held, including those that were fulfilled and those that led to his disappointments. *Although Mr. Meek's problems are attributed to his wife's death, they are also to a great extent attributable to his relationship with his wife and his difficulty with coping with losing her.*	Mr. Meek discusses his relationship with his wife in realistic terms (i.e., neither idealized nor all negative), and he expresses both positive and negative feelings about their relationship.
Mr. Meek will grieve in a functional manner for his wife, and begin to engage in social situations for the sake of their relationship, and for himself.	Facilitate Mr. Meek linking together all of his feelings and responses related to his relationship with his wife, to his life, and to his current dysfunctional behavior. Encourage his gradual return to social situations and events. *This is the full expression of grief and moving forward.*	Mr. Meek fully expresses his grief and attempts to move forward by contacting friends and family

GAF, Global Assessment of Functioning; NIC, Nursing Interventions Classification; NOC, Nursing Outcomes Classification.

CHAPTER SUMMARY

- Grief encompasses all spheres of being. Symptoms include physical, cognitive, behavioral, and affective reactions.
- Although grief is commonly presented in stages, it is more effective to conceptualize grief in terms of a dynamic process during which certain tasks are usually accomplished.
- Grief is classified as acute, anticipatory, or complicated and as chronic sorrow. Types of complicated grief include traumatic grief, absent or inhibited grief, conflicted grief, and chronic grief.
- Despite grief's inherent pain, most people do not require special interventions, and they may not benefit from grief therapy or the attending of a bereavement group (Stroebe et al, 2005).
- The potential for complicated grief decreases when patients have a healthy family life, when they provide care

for the person who is dying, when they participate in community-oriented bereavement programs, and when they receive therapy if they are at risk. Grieving children at risk for complicated or traumatic grief need to feel safe and protected by caring adults.

- Therapy for persons who are experiencing complicated grief includes facilitating the expression of suppressed feelings, mobilizing cognitive and behavioral coping skills, dealing with unresolved aspects of the relationship, releasing bonds of attachment, and encouraging reentry into socialization and into activities that give meaning to life.
- Young children need to express their own thoughts and feelings about death and dying, including the religious and spiritual aspects. Adolescents need to be given tasks that make them feel empowered and in control of their lives. Adolescents should be monitored during the grieving

■ CHAPTER SUMMARY—cont'd

process, because they can be at risk for suicide. A healthy sense of self and strong coping skills are positive qualities that may prevent complicated or traumatic grief.

- In a recent study of 74 respondents, parental grief was described as a devastating and lifelong process that involved transformative life changes. The study showed that acceptance has more than one meaning and that it is viewed in the light of the lifelong nature of this type of grief (see Research for Evidence-Based Practice #2).

- Some researchers suggest a cognitive behavioral model that focuses on the struggles of those who are experiencing complicated grief to integrate loss into their autobiographic memory. Shear and Mulhare (2008) are using a modified interpersonal psychotherapeutic approach that is based on Bowlby's (1980) attachment model of grief and loss as a way of targeting complicated grief.

■ REVIEW QUESTIONS

1. A patient who continues to be tearful and who has difficulty verbalizing feelings of sadness regarding a parent who died 11 years ago is experiencing which type of grief?
   1. Traumatic grief
   2. Conflicted grief
   3. Inhibited grief
   4. Chronic grief
2. A patient with a new diagnosis of metastatic breast cancer says, "I can't believe that this is happening to me. My mother died of breast cancer. I can't go through that." Select the nursing diagnosis with the highest priority.
   1. Grieving
   2. Ineffective coping
   3. Ineffective denial
   4. Risk for self-directed violence
3. A child dies after being struck by a car. The physician tells the parents, "Your child's injuries were so severe that there was nothing we could do." What is the initial nursing intervention?
   1. Bring the parents to a room to be alone.
   2. Explain all of the medical interventions that were attempted.
   3. Stay with the parents until a support person arrives.
   4. Give the parents a referral for a grief counseling group.

4. A man was killed during a robbery attempt 10 days ago. His widow, who has a long history of major depression, cries spontaneously when talking to the nurse about her loss. Select the nurse's best response.
   1. "The sudden death of your husband is hard to accept. I'm glad that you're able to tell me how you're feeling."
   2. "This loss is harder to accept because you have a severe mental illness. Try to focus on other activities."
   3. "Your tears let me know that you are not coping appropriately with your loss. Let's make an appointment with your physician."
   4. "I'm concerned that you're crying so much. Your grief over your husband's death has gone on too long."
5. Four teenagers are killed in an automobile accident. Three days later, which behavior indicates that one of the teenagers' parents is coping effectively with his or her loss?
   1. He or she returns immediately to his or her employment.
   2. He or she forbids other teens in the household from driving a car.
   3. He or she isolates himself or herself at home and refuses visitors.
   4. He or she marks the site of the accident with flowers.

REFERENCES

Ackley BJ: Anticipatory grieving. In Ackley BJ, Ladwig GB, editors: *Nursing diagnosis handbook*, ed 5, St. Louis, 2002, Mosby.

Agnew A et al: Bereavement needs assessment in specialist palliative care: a review of the literature, *Palliat Med* 26(1):46-59, 2010.

American Psychiatric Association: *Diagnostic and statistical manual of mental disorders*, ed 4, text revision, Washington, DC, 2000, American Psychiatric Association.

Anderson W et al: Posttraumatic stress and complicated grief in family members of patients in the intensive care unit, *J Gen Intern Med* 23(11):1871-1876, 2008.

Arnold J, Buschman Gemma P: The continuing process of parental grief, *Death Stud* 32:658-673, 2008.

Boelen PA et al: A cognitive behavioral conceptualization of complicated grief, *Clin Psychol* 13(2):109-128, 2006.

Bonanno GA: Is complicated grief a valid construct? *Clin Psychol* 13(2):129-134, 2006.

Bowlby J: Loss: sadness and depression, vol 3. In *Attachment and loss*, New York, 1980, Basic Books.

Brown EJ et al: Childhood traumatic grief: a multi-site empirical examination of the construct and its correlates, *Death Stud* 32:899-923, 2008.

Burke ML et al: Current knowledge and research on chronic sorrow: a foundation for inquiry, *Death Stud* 16:231-245, 1992.

Caico C: Educating women's healthcare professionals about the prenatal grief process, *Women's Health Care: A Practical Journal for Nurse Practitioners* 6(3):19-26, 2007.

Carpenito LJ: *Nursing diagnosis: application to clinical practice,* Philadelphia, 2002, Lippincott.

Carse JB: *Death and existence,* New York, 1980, John Wiley & Sons.

Cerel J et al: Childhood bereavement: psychopathology in the 2 years post-prenatal death, *J Am Acad Child Adolesc Psychiatry* 45:681-690, 2006.

Cowles KV, Rodgers BL: The concept of grief: a foundation for nursing research and practice, *Res Nurs Health* 14(2):119-127, 1991.

Fortinash KM, Holoday Worret PA: *Psychiatric nursing care plans,* ed 5, St. Louis, 2007, Mosby.

Fortinash KM, Holoday Worret PA: *Psychiatric mental health nursing,* ed 4, St. Louis, 2008, Elsevier.

Freud S: Mourning and melancholia. In Strachey J, editor: *The standard edition of the complete psychological works of Sigmund Freud,* vol 14, London, 1917, Hogarth Press.

Heffner JE, Byock IR: *Palliative and end-of-life pearls,* Philadelphia, 2002, Hanley & Belfus.

Hendry C: Incarceration and the tasks of grief: a narrative review, *J Adv Nurs* 65(2):270-278, 2009.

Hentz P: The body remembers: grieving and a circle of time, *Qual Health Res* 12(2):161-172, 2002.

Holmes TH, Rahe RH: The social readjustment rating scale, *J Psychosom Res* 11(2):213-218, 1967.

Hsu AY: *Grieving a suicide: a loved one's search for comfort, answers and hope,* Downers Grove, Ill, 2002, Intervarsity Press.

Kemp C: Spiritual care in terminal illness. In Ferrel B, Coyle N, editors: *Oxford textbook of palliative nursing,* ed 2, Oxford, 2006, Oxford University Press.

Kemp C, Chang B-J: Culture and the end of life: Chinese, *J Hosp Palliat Nurs* 3:173-178, 2002.

Kristjanson L et al: *A systematic review of the literature on complicated grief,* Canberra, Australia, 2006, Department of Health and Aging.

Kübler-Ross E: *Living with death and dying,* New York, 1981, Macmillan.

Lichtenstein B et al: Chronic sorrow in the HIV-positive patient: issues of race, gender, and social support, *AIDS Patient Care STDS* 18:8, 141-148, 2002.

Lindemann E: Symptomatology and management of acute grief, *Am J Psychiatry* 101(2):141-148, 1944.

Love A: Progress in understanding grief, complicated grief, and caring for the bereaved, *Contemp Nurse* 27(1):73-83, 2007.

Mabry R: *The tender scar: life after the death of a spouse,* Grand Rapids, Mich, 2006, Kregel.

Maciejewski PK et al: An empirical examination of the stage theory of grief, *JAMA* 297:716-723, 2007.

Melhem NM et al: Comorbidity of Axis I disorders in patients with traumatic grief, *J Clin Psychiatry* 62:884, 2001.

Melhem NM et al: Phenomenology and correlates of complicated grief in children and adolescents, *J Am Acad Child Adolesc Psychiatry* 46:493-499, 2007.

Mystakidou K et al: Preparatory grief, psychological distress and hopelessness in advanced cancer patients, *Eur J Cancer Care (Engl)* 17:145-151, 2007.

National Institutes of Health: *Loss, grief and bereavement (PDQ),* update June 19, 2006 (website): www.cancer.gov.

Neimeyer R: Making meaning in the midst of loss, *Grief Matters: The Australian Journal of Grief and Bereavement* 9:62-65, 2006.

Parkes CM: Bereavement. In Doyle D et al, editors: *Oxford textbook of palliative medicine,* ed 2, Oxford, 1998, Oxford University Press.

Parkes CM: Bereavement dissected: a re-examination of the basic components influencing the reaction to loss, *Isr J Psychiatry Relat Sci* 38(3–4):150-156, 2001.

Pejlert A: Being a parent of an adult son or daughter with severe mental illness receiving professional care: parents' narratives, *Health Soc Care Community* 9:194-204, 2001.

Ray A, Prigerson H: Complicated grief: an attachment disorder worthy of inclusion in DSM-V, *Grief Matters: The Australian Journal of Grief and Bereavement* 9:33-38, 2006.

Shear MK, Mulhare E, Complicated grief, *Psychiatr Ann* 38(10):662-667, 2008.

Shneidman ES, *Voices of death,* New York, 1980, Harper & Row.

Silverman GK et al: Preliminary effects of prior trauma and loss on risk for psychiatric disorders in recently widowed people, *Isr J Psychiatry Relat Sci* 38(3–4):202-215, 2001.

Stroebe M et al: On the classification and diagnosis of pathological grief, *Clin Psychol Rev* 20(1):57-75, 2000.

Stroebe W et al: Grief work, disclosure and counseling: do they help the bereaved? *Clin Psychol Rev* 25:395-414, 2005.

Tomita T, Kitamura T: Clinical and research measures of grief: a reconsideration, *Compr Psychiatry* 43(2):95-102, 2002.

White P, Ferszt G: Exploration of nurse practitioner practice with clients who are grieving, *Journal of the Academy of Nurse Practitioners* 21:231-240, 2009.

Worden J: *Grief counseling and grief therapy: a handbook for the mental health practitioner,* New York, 1982, Springer.

29

Mental and Emotional Responses to Medical Illness

Ruth N. Grendell

"In a disordered mind, as in a disordered body, soundness of health is impossible."

Cicero

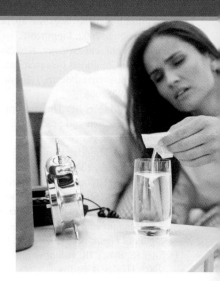

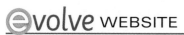 **WEBSITE**

http://evolve.elsevier.com/Fortinash/

OBJECTIVES

- Discuss the historic and theoretic perspectives related to stress.
- Define the major physiologic and psychosocial stressors and their impact on health status.
- Describe the potential negative impact that stress has on multiple body systems.
- Summarize the biologic and psychologic responses to stress.
- Discuss the adaptation to stress (i.e., cognitive appraisal, autonomic nervous system responses, and use of coping mechanisms).
- Discuss the prevalence of human immunodeficiency virus (HIV) and acquired immunodeficiency syndrome (AIDS), particularly in vulnerable populations.
- Distinguish between adjustment disorders and Axis I mood disorders in patients with HIV/AIDS with the use

- of the criteria of severity of symptoms, treatment, and prognosis.
- Examine potential interactions between the behavioral characteristics of individuals coping with HIV/AIDS and treatment adherence management.
- Discuss the benefits of providing holistic health care to vulnerable groups.
- Describe the independent and collaborative interventions that nurses and other health care professionals use for patients who are experiencing stress-related health problems.
- Apply the nursing process for patients with HIV/AIDS.
- Explain the concepts of empowerment and self-care.
- Identify factors that influence current and future trends in self-care.

KEY TERMS

acquired immunodeficiency syndrome
acute illness
acute stress disorder
AIDS dementia complex
CD4 count

cognitive appraisal
coping
daily hassles
distress
eustress
general adaptation syndrome

general inhibition syndrome
homeostasis
human immunodeficiency virus
patient empowerment
psychologic stress

psychoneuroimmunoendo-crinology
secondary appraisal
stress
viral load

The holistic health care model that is gaining prominence addresses the person's total physical, psychologic, and spiritual health and illness needs. It is patient-centered, it includes supportive services, and it provides education to address the ultimate goal of self-care management. The family and significant others are included in patient decision making, and they are active partners in the plan of care. A renewed interest in the multiple contributing factors to health and illness has prompted scientists to explore the relationship of internal and external stressors and human responses. Study findings indicate a strong communication network between the mind, the body, the spirit, and human responses. However, the conventional health care model has continued to focus primarily on the physiologic conditions of health and illness (see Chapter 27). A blended or holistic model is slowly emerging and may become the health care model of the future.

The effects of environmental factors, personal experiences, and effective or ineffective coping mechanisms on psychologic and physiologic outcomes are significant. The American Holistic Nurses Association defines each person's environment as everything that surrounds the individual—in other words, the physical, emotional, and spiritual elements of his or her surroundings (Zborowsky and Kreitzer, 2009).

As you progress through this chapter, consider the total human responses of the young woman who is diagnosed with breast cancer, to all of the subsequent events. Consider the responses of the 50-year-old man who experiences a heart attack, and the responses of an older person who loses a spouse. The total responses of a child who is subjected to abuse can have lifelong consequences. Finally, consider the responses of a survivor of an earthquake, a tsunami, or another stressful life event.

Specific nursing skills and knowledge are required to provide competent care to patients who are experiencing psychologic distress related to various types of illnesses. Human immunodeficiency virus infection and acquired immunodeficiency syndrome (HIV/AIDS) are major health care issues throughout the world; therefore, these conditions will serve as a representative example for the discussion of acute, chronic, and life-threatening illnesses and diseases and the subsequent mental and emotional responses.

MENTAL ASPECTS OF PHYSIOLOGIC ILLNESS

In ancient times, people believed that magical beings or evil spirits caused mental illness by possessing a person and interfering with the functions of the mind. Some attributed mental illness to being born under certain astrologic signs or during the phase of a full moon. Trephining, which is the drilling of holes into the skull, was often performed to allow evil spirits to leave the body. In many societies, mental illness was thought to be caused by a hex, a curse, or a head injury, and this is still the belief in some cultures today. A number of factors delayed progress in the study of mental disorders and the discovery of effective treatment modalities until well into the 20th century. Some factors included misconceptions about the cause of mental disorders and the stigma imposed

by many societies. This often resulted in the isolation of the mentally ill, who were secretly cared for by the family or institutionalized to prevent them from harming others or themselves. However, some societies honored the mentally ill and considered them to have special healing or magical gifts. From the 17th to 19th centuries, the mentally ill suffered physical and mental abuses in institutions. They were placed in chains or other physical restraints, put in ice baths, and given insulin and electric shock therapy. Some patients even had to suffer surgical frontal lobotomies, which the medical community and society now consider to be a barbaric method of diminishing higher-level cognitive functions (Beers, 1935; Dully and Fleming, 2007).

Theories of Illness or Disease: Biologic, Multicausal, and Psychosocial

The biologic model views physiologic disease as a result of malfunctions of the body's organs and cells. The signs and symptoms of diseases are observable and quantifiable. However, the model does not explain the causes of all diseases. Multicausal theories focus on the capability of every living organism to maintain its internal environment or homeostasis, which is a dynamic state that is created by the feedback and regulation processes. The three intricately connected master feedback systems in the body are the *neurologic*, *endocrine*, and *immune* systems. These systems are normally capable of managing and responding to multiple incoming stimuli from the internal and external environments. Psychosocial theories emphasize the impact of stressful stimuli and the interaction of psychologic, physiologic, and social factors as supportive factors in the adaptation process and as causative factors in the development of illness or disease (Porth and Matfin, 2008). The following discussion of the major psychosocial theories provides the framework for studying the mental, spiritual, and emotional responses to physiologic illness and disease.

General Adaptation Syndrome

Stress is an inevitable aspect of life, especially in societies in which rapid and accelerating challenges and changes exist. Hans Selye (1907-1982), an endocrinologist, was a pioneer in stress research during the 1940s and 1950s. He defined stress both as a response to noxious or stressful stimuli and as a stimulus that produces biologic, emotional, and psychologic responses. Selye based his research on the study of posttraumatic stress disorder (PTSD) that he observed in returning veterans returning from World War II. At that time PTSD was called "combat fatigue." The syndrome was experienced and identified in all wars prior to World War II and was named "soldier's heart," "battle fatigue," and others. Regardless of the names, the debilitating symptoms were the same.

Selye (1956) explained that stress as a stimulus sometimes involves a variety of events, including negative and positive situations. He noted that culture, age, developmental phase, past experiences, lifestyle, and other factors, including health status, influenced the person's response to stress. Therefore, no single factor is responsible for the cause of a person's stress response. Selye also stated that a certain amount of stress, whether negative (distress) or positive (eustress), produces mental and physiologic changes that are necessary for growth and survival.

Distress is a subjective response to internal or external stimuli that are threatening or perceived as threatening to the self. This includes fatigue, pain, fear, and acute or chronic disease.

Eustress is a nonspecific stress response that is associated with desirable events, such as one's wedding, a job promotion, or the birth of an infant. Selye found that all living things, including plant life, respond to any type of stress with predictable adaptive patterns.

Psychologic stress is all processes, whether originating in the external environment or within the internal environment of the person, that demand a cognitive appraisal of the event before a response or the activation of any other system (Marcus, 2008).

Selye labeled the three stages of the individual's innate behavioral responses to any stress stimulus as the biologic stress syndrome or the general adaptation syndrome. The three stages consist of the following: (1) a brief alarm reaction stage or the fight-or-flight stage, which alerts the individual to the presence of stressful stimuli; (2) the stage of resistance; and (3) the exhaustion stage. Selye hypothesized that the normal survival response involves a reciprocal reaction between the autonomic nervous system, the endocrine system, and the immune system. The release of the hormone epinephrine from the sympathetic branch of the autonomic nervous system places the person "on alert," and the activation of the hypothalamic–pituitary–adrenal axis results in the release of cortisol from the adrenal glands. Responses during this stage include the elevation of blood pressure; tachycardia; the constriction of blood vessels and the diversion of blood from nonessential organs to the heart, brain, and skeletal muscles; increased muscle tone; increased blood sugar levels; dilated pupils; increased alertness; and "free-floating anxiety" (Marcus, 2008; Neyland, 1998; Porth and Matfin, 2008).

During the prolonged *stage of resistance*, the neuroendocrine and adrenal systems mobilize energy resources to enhance the vasoconstrictive effects of epinephrine to maintain the elevated blood pressure and to activate the immune system. Persistent stimulation of the sympathetic nervous system results in elevated levels of cortisol and catecholamines. This affects multiple organ systems of the body, including the brain, the immune system, and the cardiovascular system (Porth and Matfin, 2008).

The *exhaustion stage* occurs when all of the individual's resources are used and the individual is unable to adapt to the stressor. Some become ill or die if they do not replenish their resources. However, if the stressor is removed or if the body is able to adapt, the exhaustion stage is reversed and has only a limited effect. In some cases, the individual "freezes" or shuts down and is unable to respond in any manner. Neurnberger (1981) labeled this reaction as the *general inhibition syndrome* or the *possum response*. This response is the result of overstimulation of the parasympathetic nervous system, and it is activated automatically as a means of survival that has a "paralyzing or numbing" effect when an individual is facing a life-threatening event (Phillips, 2010). Neurnberger believed that Selye had ignored the powerful role of the parasympathetic inhibition mechanisms, and he cited the effects of stress imposed by depression on the behavioral responses of fatigue, apathy, and other signs of psychomotor "slow down" or retardation.

Other researchers were also investigating the effects of the chemicals secreted by the autonomic nervous system for regulating cardiovascular, gastrointestinal, and motor responses. Like Selye, they too found that homeostasis was often disrupted in response to stress, and they noted that the sympathetic nervous system was particularly responsive to environmental stimuli and involved emotional reactions. Recently, technology such as positron emission tomography has helped health care providers to actually observe the living brain and the role of stress on brain function, particularly with regard to the long-term effects of PTSD. Certain portions of the brain (primarily the frontal cortex) are sometimes suppressed because of a flood of events that involve many integrated levels of control between the neuroendocrine and immune systems and multiple body systems. Prolonged exposure to stress causes atrophic changes in the hippocampus, decreases short-term memory storage, and increases the risk for depression and the poor regulation of endocrine responses to stress (Marcus, 2008; Porth and Matfin, 2008).

Appraisal–Transaction Theory

Lazarus and Folkman (1987) stated that stress is a transaction process rather than an event. This process occurs as the person makes a cognitive appraisal of each stress encounter and assesses its intensity as either harmful, a threat of harm, or a challenge to overcome. A secondary appraisal determines what the response will be, such as selecting the coping method to use to reduce the effect of the stress. The response process depends on the individual's current and past experiences with stressors. The timing of the event and the person's use of coping skills also influence the response process. Problem-focused skills are strategies that help to resolve the stressful situation. Emotion-focused coping responses related to fear and anxiety frequently manifest as ego-defense mechanisms, such as denial or repression. Lazarus also stated that the individual's methods for coping with stress and general life experiences greatly affect his or her degree of resistance to infectious microbes.

Lazarus believed that most of life's stressful events consist of the accumulation of seemingly minor daily annoyances; therefore, health care providers need to view stress within the total context and not in isolation.

Daily hassles are annoying or troublesome concerns, states of confusion or turmoil, and events that the person cannot control. The individual's perception of available social support and its effectiveness also influence the impact of an event. According to Lazarus and colleagues' research, self-generated hassles and poor coping skills are more damaging to a person's health than hassles that occur by chance. The researchers also investigated daily uplifts as buffering measures against the effect of daily hassles. Uplifts, such as a support system, meeting with friends, being satisfied by completing a task, healthy self-care, meditation, and prayer helped to maintain or restore a balance (Lavee and Ben-Ari, 2008; Lazarus, 1990). The inappropriate social behavior of children with special needs caused embarrassment (hassles) for their siblings; however, uplifts for these siblings included hugs and kisses that they received from those same brothers and sisters with special needs (Orfus and Howe, 2008).

Life Changes and Illness Theory

The research by Holmes and Rahe (1967) focused on responses to stress related to the universal life developmental phases (i.e., infancy to old age) and the universal maturational stages (e.g., marriage, death of a loved one, changing careers) as transaction processes. Their findings revealed that adaptation to many significant changes over a short period of time reduces a person's energy sources. They found that managing difficult situations and the control of one's destiny depend on effective coping, positive self-esteem, and perceived self-efficacy or internal locus of control. Ineffective coping is associated with an external locus of control, which is in place when a person feels a loss of control over his or her life events or destiny (Hellman, 2004; Witek-Janusek, 2004).

Numerous studies have used Holmes and Rahe's Social Readjustment Rating Scale. Examples of significant life changes that require a greater level of adaptation include the death of a spouse or child, marriage, divorce, personal injury, and retirement. Examples of lower significant events include holidays, vacations, a change in eating habits, and a change in residence or job. The research by Holmes and Rahe has had a tremendous impact on the practice of mind–body medicine. However, further research is necessary, because the scale does not include significant stressors such as chronic life changes, monotony, anticipated stress, or unexpected events (see Chapter 5).

Stress, Organ Maladaptation, and Disease Theory

Harold Wolff, a professor at Cornell University, studied human responses to chronic stressors from 1930 to 1962. His research indicated that, even when coping strategies are appropriate, repeated use of a response sometimes causes pathologic changes and tissue damage in a particular body system, organ, or mucous membranes throughout the body. Stewart Wolf's research in 1979 also demonstrated that chronic high levels of adrenalin, serum glucose, cortisol, and other hormones are harmful to body tissues (Hellman, 2004).

Psychoneuroimmunoendocrinology

Psychoneuroimmunoendocrinology, which was formerly called *psychoneuroimmunology,* is a relatively new multidisciplinary approach to the study of the intricate mind–body interactions among the neurologic system, the endocrine system, and the immune system. Psychoneuroimmunoendocrinology studies examine the effect of perceived psychosocial stressors and the biopsychologic stress response on the development of disease (Venes, 2009). The psychoneuroimmunoendocrinology model provides a holistic framework for research and screening risk factors of health problems, lifestyle, and sociologic factors (Anderson, 2009).

The holistic health care model includes a greater emphasis on health promotion across the life span, self-care management, and a holistic approach to the management of acute and chronic psychosocial and physiologic health problems (Colin-Thome, 2009). The nurse has a pivotal role in helping patients to recognize the impact of stress and to assist them with selecting appropriate coping mechanisms and promoting the best possible quality of life.

A forum entitled *Treating the Whole Patient: The Mind–Body Connection* was very well received during the 2009 U.S. Psychiatric and Mental Health Conference. An Internet community forum was created to continue discussions, to allow individuals to view short informational videos, and to pose questions that are responded to by the leaders of the forum. Many of the questions relate to the relationship of physical and psychologic disorders, especially depression, and the reactions that patients may have to psychotropic drugs and drugs used for the treatment of physical conditions. Additional live forums will be conducted at the next annual conference. The website for this project is included in the reference list for this chapter (Continuing Medical Education, 2010).

Coping Mechanisms

Coping is the use of resourcefulness and the ability to manage the stress of daily circumstances, such as the challenges posed by pain, disability, or acute or chronic disease. Coping mechanisms may be conscious or unconscious and adaptive or maladaptive. Conscious methods are sometimes learned; unconscious mechanisms are often referred to as *protective ego defenses.* Adaptive conscious mechanisms include distractions such as reading, praying, meditating, using relaxation techniques, and seeking social support. Examples of maladaptive conscious mechanisms are withdrawing from social contacts, changes in dietary habits, smoking, drug and alcohol abuse, or participating in other unhealthy behaviors and sudden outbursts of anger. Unconscious ego defense mechanisms include repression, denial, rationalization, and regression. Unconscious mechanisms often prevent the individual from realistically appraising himself or herself, other people, and situations (Carpenito, 2003). These examples of conscious and unconscious defense mechanisms are not all inclusive, because many people often make use of other ego defense mechanisms. The goal is to use strategies that minimize unnecessary sources of stress and to promote effective adaptive responses.

It is important to recognize that people use these responses to protect their integrity. A response is often a temporary measure until the immediate crisis is resolved or until the person is able to control the situation. A variety of problem-solving coping options are available during the appraisal process, such as wondering how to change the situation, to accept it, to seek more information, or to resist impulsive actions. The ability to regulate emotions, behavior, and the environment are critical to successful adjustment. Heightened emotions interfere with a person's ability to effectively relate to stressors. The careful and cautious assessment of the person's behavior is sometimes necessary to determine whether the nurse needs to support or change the coping mechanism. The ultimate goal of quality nursing care is to promote a healthy outcome (Lee, 2010; Phillips, 2010).

Acute Illness or Disease Responses

An acute illness or disease is a sudden interruption of a person's normal activities. In general, the duration of acute illnesses is a few weeks to 6 months. Examples of common responses are fear, anxiety, spiritual distress, feelings of powerlessness and helplessness, hostility, and anger. However, a rapid uncomplicated recovery and a return to normal activities often erase these emotions quickly (Millsbaugh, 2005 and 2008; Stuart, 2008). Responses to the diagnosis of a life-threatening disease or illness are usually intense. In some cases, the individual will shut down and withdraw or deny that anything is wrong.

The term *acute stress disorder* refers to the mental, emotional, and physiologic responses to a trauma or crisis. This phenomenon has received greater attention in the United States after incidents such as the bombing of the Alfred P. Murrah Federal Building in Oklahoma City in 1995, the terrorist attack in New York City on September 11, 2001, the failed airline bombing plot in December 2009, and shootings at schools across the country. When they are involved in such events, individuals commonly experience symptoms of dissociation (i.e., a sense of detachment or a decreased awareness of the surrounding environment), amnesia, or feelings of unreality. Some are unable to effectively cope with the situation. Symptoms occur either immediately or shortly after the traumatic event occurs, and they usually last up to a month. Immediate psychologic or spiritual counseling that allows the individual to freely express stressful feelings of fear and anxiety will help the individual to gain a clearer appraisal of the impact of the situation and assist with problem solving and with a return to a level of functioning that the person perceives as normal. The learning of stress management techniques and debriefing skills is strongly recommended for nurses who interact with individuals in these traumatic situations.

During the current wars in Iraq and Afghanistan, psychiatrists, chaplains, and other therapists provide counsel to men and women who are continually exposed to severely stressful situations. Anxiety is common, particularly for the military personnel who have had multiple deployments, which often rekindle vivid memories of previous stressful events. Many of these personnel also have anticipatory stress related to the fear of an unpredictable outcome, such as injury or death. Therapists are available day and night to help prevent the long-term progression to PTSD that occurred for so many

people after previous wars. Other stress-reducing strategies include scheduled rest periods away from the battle line, entertainment, air-conditioned tents, freshly prepared food, and access to the Internet for communicating with family and friends at home (Lenz, 2006). A few military rehabilitation centers (e.g., Walter Reed Army Medical Center in Washington, DC; Brooke Army Medical Center at Fort Sam Houston, San Antonio, Texas) are available in the United States. The military also created a new family-centered facility at the U.S. Naval Hospital in San Diego, California, to ease the transition closer to home and to manage stress-related outcomes. A rehabilitation clinic is helpful for adjustment to life with prosthetics and preparations for a new life and new career choices. Additional strategies involving telehealth and virtual reality graded exposure have been introduced for patients with PTSD (Nieves et al, 2009; Wood et al, 2009) (see Chapter 10).

Chronic Illness or Disease Responses

Chronic diseases or illnesses require continued management over a period of years or decades. Examples include diseases such as the following:

- Cardiovascular, stroke, respiratory, and renal disorders
- Cancer
- Persistent chronic diseases such as diabetes, HIV/AIDS, rheumatoid arthritis, and multiple sclerosis
- Certain long-term mental disorders, such as schizophrenia and bipolar disorder
- Ongoing impairments, such as amputations, paralysis, and blindness, which affect all age groups

Chronic diseases represent 60% of global deaths and approximately one third of the burden of global disease. The residual disability of these diseases is irreversible, and it requires education and rehabilitation for individuals and their informal caregivers. There is often a need for supervision and observation over an extended period of time.

Chronic health problems place a tremendous psychosocial, emotional, and financial burden on the individual, the family, and society. The unpredictability of a chronic disease is a challenge to the person's self-esteem, body image, and sexuality. It is also disruptive to social relationships and the role functions within the family, the workplace, and the community. Chronic health problems often take away a person's sense of autonomy and independence (Cumbie et al, 2004; World Health Organization, 2006).

Exacerbations of symptoms such as pain, fatigue, nausea, anorexia, sleep disturbances, and the steady decline in functioning ability challenge coping skills. The progression in severity of symptoms may be either rapid or slow, and it is sometimes caused by the side effects of medications, treatment failure, or complications associated with the comorbidity of another disease. Adaptation is a complex and a continuous process of restructuring life around the chronic condition, particularly with regard to accepting a loss of independence and valued roles. The uncertainty of the progress of chronic diseases often leads to depression, anger, and feelings of hopelessness and helplessness. Some feel trapped or imprisoned by their diseases (Lee, 2010). Assisting the person with reframing negative thoughts and responses to stressful situations is a cognitive strategy for strengthening the patient's and family's ability to adapt to the chronic condition and to shape its course rather than being overwhelmed by it.

HIV AND AIDS

Human immunodeficiency virus (HIV) infection and acquired immunodeficiency syndrome (AIDS) are global epidemics. The availability of new pharmacologic therapies has prolonged the progress of the disease, which is now considered a chronic disease in many developed countries. However, these therapies are not available for persons who need them in many parts of the world, so these diseases continue to be life threatening for millions of men, women, and children.

Like all viruses, HIV cannot reproduce itself unless it enters a living cell. Once it is inside a cell, this retrovirus is able to reverse itself into a single strand of DNA (deoxyribonucleic acid) that is capable of entering the cell's nucleus and that becomes a permanent part of the genetic structure of the cell. When the cell divides, the viral strand also infects the daughter cells. The rapid duplication of infected cells in the blood and lymph systems damages and destroys the body's protective cells, particularly the T-helper or CD4$^+$ lymph cells. This process results in a defect in the individual's natural immunity against disease, especially against certain opportunistic infections and AIDS-related cancers. One of the diagnostic criteria is a drop in CD4$^+$ blood. Although individuals in the symptomatic state are identifiable by a specific set of signs and symptoms, those who are infected but asymptomatic often go undiagnosed for long periods of time. Neither health care providers nor patients themselves suspect HIV infection. Infected asymptomatic individuals are capable of transmitting the disease to others, even when they remain asymptomatic. The average time between an undetected HIV infection to an AIDS diagnosis is approximately 10 years (Springer, 2004).

Both clinical and research evidence indicate that HIV infects the brain and results in central nervous system impairment in some individuals. In addition to the troublesome physical and neurologic consequences of HIV/AIDS, many individuals experience significant psychologic distress related to the awareness of their diagnosis and their subsequent adaptation to the consequences of this chronic life-threatening illness. Families and significant others are also affected by the diagnosis and experience psychologic distress of their own. Information and counseling services are available to all individuals who are struggling with an actual or potential HIV/AIDS diagnosis (Mitchell and Knowlton, 2009).

Sexual transmission and infection as a result of needle exchange among drug abusers are the primary modes of transmission. Efforts to change these high-risk behaviors are not always successful, because making these changes is exceedingly complex and involves changing behaviors that are not easy for patients to discuss with the nurse. Because impoverished African-American and Latino subgroups are disproportionately represented in the AIDS community, a focus on culturally held beliefs and needs is critical to successful interventions to prevent and treat HIV.

There are many reasons why psychologic distress—particularly feelings of anxiety and depression—among persons living with HIV or AIDS is of concern to clinicians who are caring for these individuals. These negative affective states are reflective of subjective distress and maladaptive coping. Negative affect, irritability, decreased energy, lethargy, altered performance, restlessness, and interrupted sleep strongly influence the individual's ability to endure the course of this chronic condition and its demanding treatment plan. Feelings of helplessness, negative self-image, and persistent fear and worry contribute to this as well, and these sometimes lead to suicide ideation or attempts. These conditions further tax the patient's resources and affect the person's feelings of hopefulness and quality of life. Although suicidal responses among patients with HIV/AIDS are sometimes understandable, nurses always have a responsibility to prevent any potential risk for suicide and to include it in the nursing assessments of these patients.

With HIV/AIDS, as with other life-threatening illnesses, health status carries both primary and secondary implications for quality of life and functional performance. Individuals who are symptomatic are aware of their disease and its potential to affect their lives. Both physical and psychologic symptoms have a direct impact on quality of life, but they also have an indirect impact as a result of the process of secondary appraisal of each new stressor. Individuals perceive HIV-related symptoms or the occurrence of opportunistic diseases and infections as threatening because of their meaning to the individuals. For some, these symptoms are a reminder of their vulnerability. In addition, the real or anticipated consequences of these symptoms (e.g., declining role performance, functional deficits, altered social activities) are also considered threatening. Adaptation during symptomatic HIV disease requires the rearrangement of goal-related activities to achieve a positive emotional state. When they are perceived as being outside of the individual's control, physical and psychologic symptoms are overwhelming, and this feeling sometimes leads to depression and anxiety. Some individuals perceive stable or recurring symptoms as having a global effect on many outcomes that are important to him or her. Each new symptom episode represents additional losses and less control over one's life and thus produces psychologic distress.

Highly active antiretroviral therapy (HAART) that must be taken for a lifetime has prolonged the interval between the diagnosis of HIV infection and the development of full-blown AIDS. This fact has diminished the capacity of AIDS surveillance data to monitor the underlying impact of HIV in the United States. Although there has been a decline in cases of HIV infection, patterns and characteristics of these trends raise concern. For example, research estimates that 25% of those persons with HIV infection are not aware of their diagnosis.

Cultural Considerations

There has been a rapid rise in the number of newly diagnosed HIV/AIDS cases in rural areas, where it is difficult to provide prevention and treatment interventions. One reason for this rise is that individuals who migrated from rural to urban areas are moving back to rural communities after they have been diagnosed with HIV. This backward migration has raised concern about the adequacy of health care and supportive services in regions where many do not understand HIV/AIDS and where specialists are typically not available. Poverty, isolation, stigmatization, discrimination, and lack of transportation also contribute to minimal access to care. States that have reported more than 150 AIDS cases in rural communities include Texas, Mississippi, Florida, Georgia, New York, North Carolina, and South Carolina. The thirty-eighth meeting of the Presidential Advisory Council on HIV/AIDS in February 2010 recommended several strategies to assist with the achievement of an HIV-free generation. Strategies and policies include early screening; case management; medication adherence; addressing risks for women, adolescents, and incarcerated populations; and recognizing mental problems as associated comorbidities (US Department of Health and Human Services, 2010).

A second population of concern with regard to HIV/AIDS that has also been difficult to reach is women and adolescent girls. Currently, more women are infected worldwide than men; the rates have increased 10% in Asia since 2004, and, in Africa, young girls between 15 and 24 years old represent half of all new HIV infections. Most of these women and girls are infected through heterosexual contact. Women are more biologically vulnerable than men because of the larger surface area of the female genital tract that can be exposed to infected secretions. Additional factors, particularly in patriarchal societies, include women's low social status, fear of physical abuse by a sexual partner if they request the use of condoms, poverty, and illiteracy. Many women in underdeveloped countries have at least one sexually transmitted disease, thereby making them more susceptible to HIV infection. Their HIV-positive status is often undetected, and approximately half a million newborn infants have acquired HIV. Studies estimate that 4 million women and girls were bought, sold, and forced into prostitution, marriage, or slavery in the Asian Pacific and African countries (World Health Organization, 2006). In the United States, the greatest increase in numbers of women diagnosed with HIV/AIDS is seen among African-American and Hispanic women.

Women with HIV/AIDS face the day-to-day issues of dealing with this profoundly life-threatening illness in themselves and, for many, in their young children and spouses or partners. They are both the infected and the affected, coping with their own disease courses and the challenges of caring for children who are infected. Clearly, one of the most critical psychosocial concerns is the shock of learning about one's HIV-positive status. Individuals (including older adults) who do not perceive themselves to be at risk are less likely to suspect infection and are more likely to delay testing. Once tested, they often have significantly greater difficulty coming to terms with their infection. In some instances, their partners were also unaware of their HIV serostatus or did not inform them about it. The stigma and shame attached to the diagnosis is overwhelming. Addressing the shock and disbelief surrounding the awareness of their diagnosis and their perceived fantasies related to their prognosis is critical to the care of these populations.

Patients with HIV/AIDS who have emigrated from other countries to the United States do not always trust the traditional medical care establishment. For socioeconomically vulnerable individuals, a lack of compliance with treatment is often the result of limited resources or competing needs that interfere with the ability to access and use services. Many have a cultural worldview and perspective about health and illness that medical providers do not easily understand or accept. To effectively care for these individuals, it is important for the nurse to develop trust with the patient and an understanding of the individual's perspective on health and his or her attitudes toward conventional treatment. Specifically, it is critical that the nurse understand the patient's beliefs, fears, and life goals. The initial acceptance of treatment depends on the trust that patients feel toward the provider. Black churches across the nation are involved in an education campaign to address the stigma attached to HIV/AIDS and to offer free screening services; included are the use of prayer, scriptures, and counseling (Sanchez, 2010) (see the Research for Evidence-Based Practice box).

In summary, specific characteristics of individuals and populations—including cultural and regional differences in predisposing factors and adaptive behaviors—influence all aspects of health care, from the prevention of infection to the treatment of late-stage AIDS. Culturally sensitive interventions take into account subtle as well as more obvious regional and ethnic characteristics of these populations.

ETIOLOGY OF PSYCHOLOGIC DISTRESS IN PATIENTS WITH HIV/AIDS

When establishing the basis for psychologic distress in patients with HIV disease, it is important to understand various etiologic foundations. Psychoneurologic and psychosocial theories explain the etiology of impairment and distress in persons (primarily adults) with HIV disease. The first important consideration, however, is whether the mental disorder and psychologic symptoms predate HIV infection; in other words, does the individual have a history of moderate to severe and persistent mental illness that was present before the HIV infection? Some individuals, such as those with major depression, bipolar disorder, injection and noninjection drug use, and alcohol abuse, have engaged in high-risk behaviors that resulted in their becoming infected with HIV. Because early testing and therapy are extremely effective, nurses need to closely assess and monitor these individuals for their ability to access and use existing HIV treatment services.

The following discussion focuses on mood or cognitive disorders related to an HIV/AIDS diagnosis, with or without

RESEARCH FOR EVIDENCE-BASED PRACTICE

Parks FM: Working with narratives: coping strategies in African American folk beliefs and traditional healing practices, *J Hum Behav Soc Environ* 15(1):135-150, 2007.

Narratives were provided by individuals to describe the meanings of their traumatic and illness experiences and their coping strategies. Four themes were revealed: (1) spirituality; (2) rituals; (3) the power of words; and (4) dreams. Spirituality meant gaining a feeling of self-worth and assuming one's place in the world. Relationships with family and the community were very important. Rituals included "laying on of hands," anointing with oil, and praying done for oneself or by others. Prayer was a powerful communication with a higher being or ancestor. Special life rituals included baptism, shared communal experiences, chanting, and services of a spiritual healing advisor. Words are felt to have power, and the tone of voice used increased their negative or positive power. Words also provide images that explain events that occur or will occur in the future. Dreams were related to a belief in a coexisting spiritual world as well as visions and omens of the future that are frequently interpreted by the person and others.

An interview guide was developed from the findings of the study to assist with the providing of patient-centered care. Questions included asking the person to describe coping strategies that are most helpful; what role spirituality had in life; what routine rituals were used; what folk beliefs and healing practices were most helpful; whether discovering the meaning of dreams was important; and whether the person has a "church mother" or a spiritual healing adviser.

a prior psychiatric illness. The primary *Diagnostic and Statistical Manual of Mental Disorders,* fourth edition, text revision (DSM-IV-TR), diagnoses for review are adjustment disorders with anxiety, depression, or disturbance of conduct.

BIOLOGIC/NEUROPSYCHIATRIC FACTORS

Nervous system diseases associated with HIV take a variety of forms. HIV affects the brain in the form of AIDS dementia complex, the spinal cord as vacuolar myelopathy, and the nerve endings as peripheral neuropathy. Soon after the discovery of AIDS, the frequency and severity of cognitive impairment among hospitalized patients puzzled health care providers.

Now providers know that HIV has a direct effect on the central nervous system and that it causes a subacute encephalopathy. Research suggests that important parts of the brain—the frontal cortex, the basal ganglia, and the hippocampus—are involved. Cortical atrophy and ventricular dilation have been shown on computed tomography scans, and these indicate possible permanent and significant damage to the central nervous system. The profound dementia noted in some patients with AIDS seemed disproportionate to the clinical condition, laboratory values, and gross neuropathologic findings present in these patients. Making this discovery even

more difficult was that the histories of many of these patients often revealed psychologic and cognitive problems that predated signs of immune deficiency. The understanding of all of the details of the viral effects is still incomplete. Providers know the following for certain: (1) HIV easily crosses the blood-brain barrier; (2) it is present in the brains of almost all infected persons; and (3) it directly or indirectly destroys cells in the nervous system (Cook and Tyor, 2006).

With this knowledge of histopathology, nurses are able to make accurate diagnoses of cognitive and affective changes in patients. Changes in mood may be evidence of clinical depression or represent signs of AIDS-related dementia. Even with organically based changes, the signs and symptoms are often subtle, and laboratory findings do not immediately point to irregularities. The emotional problems tend to mimic functional disorders. In addition, initially the neurologic examination, laboratory values, electroencephalogram, cerebrospinal fluid, and computed tomography scan of the brain appear normal. Also confusing is the fact that many of these high-risk and sometimes socially impaired individuals have psychosocial stresses that help to explain the emotional distress that they exhibit. Seropositivity, the absence of a premorbid or family history of psychiatric illness (including substance abuse), positive signs on neuropsychologic testing, and signs of organicity (e.g., imbalance, tremor, avoidance of complex tasks, sensitivity to drugs and alcohol) help with the differential diagnosis. Although AIDS dementias vary, there are generally two primary types: (1) dementia that is characterized by moderate signs of depression and (2) dementia with a more acute psychotic presentation. Apathy, withdrawal, fatigue, hypersomnia, weight loss, anorexia, psychomotor retardation, and subtle cognitive deficits are evidence of the first type of dementia. The acute psychotic presentation includes delusions, hallucinations, psychomotor agitation, mania with grandiosity, and profound cognitive impairment.

AIDS-related cases of moderate to severe dementia occur in approximately 7% of patients who have been newly diagnosed with HIV/AIDS and in up to 30% of those with more advanced HIV disease. Reports of the effects of HAART have indicated that the prevalence of AIDS dementia is far less of a concern. Specifically, since the onset of HAART, there has been a significant reduction in the risk for the development of HIV dementia. Not only have there been fewer cases of dementia, but there also appears to be longer life expectancy after the onset of HIV dementia. However, HAART does not destroy the virus in the brain, and the brain is possibly a reservoir for the virus. However, this partially depends on the viral load in the central nervous system and the viral strain. Despite the effectiveness of HAART, disease progression occurs, and sometimes the treatment is not effective for some individuals. Some side effects and drug interactions are difficult to live with, and there is a risk of developing drug resistance. Some individuals decide to stop treatment, thereby allowing the disease to progress and to ultimately kill them. This is devastating for the patient's families and friends (Cook and Tyor, 2006; Springer, 2004).

When a patient's impairment is determined to be primarily organically based, the influence of psychosocial phenomena is sometimes present, but this is not the initial target for intervention. Rather, health care providers treat patients with AIDS-related dementia like patients with other organically based dementias. In summary, nervous system disease is associated with HIV infection. Primary HIV disease carries the potential for neuropsychiatric complications. Behavioral and cognitive symptoms of AIDS dementia are as follows:

- Poor concentration
- Difficulties with problem solving
- Apathy
- Social withdrawal
- Forgetfulness
- Slowness of thought
- Motor deficits (e.g., tremor, impaired rapid repetitive movements, imbalance, ataxia)

Sometimes these symptoms are accompanied by delirium, delusions, and hallucinations. Many often misinterpret symptoms of depression, which include apathy, motor slowing (bradyphrenia), and attention deficits, as early signs of dementia. Some patients also abuse alcohol or cocaine and other drugs, which adds to the complexity of understanding the neurologic manifestations of advanced HIV disease. For example, cocaine psychosis closely resembles the psychosis caused by HIV (Springer, 2004).

Psychosocial Factors

With HIV disease, there is a spectrum of disorders in which psychosocial—particularly stress-related—disorders are important. Essentially four categories of individuals need intervention.

First, there are those who believe they are at risk for HIV infection but who have not gone for testing. These individuals are "the worried well," some of whom experience ongoing stress because they assume that they are indeed seropositive. They tend to exaggerate their risk rather than deny it. They display low self-esteem, anxiety, uncertainty, and, at times, irrationality. They appear to be somewhat histrionic and indecisive, and they sometimes offer clues to their concern, which indicates a desire for help. Still, their fear of being seropositive prevents them from taking care of themselves and from confronting their irrationally based concerns.

The second category of individuals who need attention is made up of those individuals who are HIV positive but asymptomatic. Although some tend to think of HIV as an acute fatal illness, most patients are either asymptomatic or even symptomatic but do not meet the criteria for full-blown AIDS. Even those who have been symptomatic often remain highly functional between symptomatic episodes. After a prolonged incubation period of months or years, most patients will go on to develop AIDS-related symptoms and AIDS. The uncertainty that these individuals have to face on a day-to-day basis becomes their primary concern.

The third category consists of individuals who are symptomatic but who have not yet developed an AIDS-defining condition. Early during the epidemic's history, these patients were diagnosed with AIDS-related complex. Symptomatic individuals are not acutely ill but tend to suffer from various AIDS-related conditions and from the side effects of the antiretroviral medications that they are taking.

In studies of symptomatic disease as compared with asymptomatic HIV disease, persons with symptoms exhibited more distress. Research suggests that the prevalence of depressive disorders increases at later stages of HIV infection before and after AIDS develops. A drop in CD4 count (i.e., the number of cells that have a protein on the surface that helps the immune system to fight disease), or a diagnosable opportunistic infection sometimes triggers further fears of impending decline in health or death. However, only AIDS-related signs and symptoms (rather than CD4 count) are associated with an increasing risk of clinical depression.

The fourth and final category of individuals who are suffering directly from HIV disease is composed of patients with full-blown AIDS. The clinical course of many AIDS-related conditions varies. For example, Kaposi's sarcoma, which is a malignant tumor of the connective tissue, sometimes presents in immunocompromised patients with AIDS as a slowly progressive disease over the course of many years. In other cases, it presents with a sudden and rapid progression that occurs over weeks to months. Both Kaposi's sarcoma and *Pneumocystis jiroveci* (formerly *Pneumocystis carinii*) pneumonia occur less frequently today than they did before HAART. With the refinement of medications to fight opportunistic diseases and infections and to lower HIV viral load or viral burden (i.e., the number of viral particles in a sample of blood), the median survival rate has markedly increased, even for those with advanced HIV disease. Available data regarding the patient's disease course, immune status (i.e., current CD4 count and viral load), and general health status can offer a clearer prognosis. The depression that these patients experience is not always simply a normal grief response to having a fatal illness. For some individuals, a pathologic process that is characterized by alienation, irrational guilt, diminished self-esteem, and pronounced suicidal ideation is sometimes present. Still, the impact of a recent AIDS diagnosis on depression and depressive symptoms required further study to determine the likelihood that an HIV-specific mood disorder exists (Springer, 2004).

Data about suicidal ideation and the numbers of suicide attempts in patients with HIV/AIDS are limited. Previous studies have suggested that suicidal ideation is common (Cooperman and Simoni, 2005). However, HAART has restored hopefulness to many who felt powerless over HIV/AIDS. Thus, although declining physical health status worsens depression and increases suicide risk, new therapies work to counteract this process. With the limited decline in physical health status as a result of new therapies, hopefulness is possible, and this can counteract feelings of despair related to the disease. Hopelessness is seen as an important risk factor for suicide. When it occurs in either the presence or absence of physical decline, nurses need to address it aggressively.

CLINICAL DESCRIPTION

The primary DSM-IV-TR diagnostic condition addressed here is adjustment disorder. Adjustment disorders among patients with HIV/AIDS are also called *severe demoralization syndromes*. These syndromes are different from a diagnosis of major depression. Major depression presents with a syndrome of low mood, in which patients complain of persistent sadness or flatness of emotional tone, and anhedonia, which is an inability to experience pleasure or satisfaction in things that ordinarily produce such responses. Patients who are experiencing adjustment disorders with depressed mood experience the same sadness as someone with major depression does, but they usually report feeling fairly normal when they are distracted from thinking about the circumstances that cause them distress. When reminded, they experience a welling up of sadness and overwhelming grief. Thus, adjustment disorders are closely linked to the overwhelming feelings that are provoked by the circumstances of living with HIV. Adjustment disorders are coded according to the subtype that best characterizes the predominant symptoms (American Psychiatric Association, 2000) (see Chapter 12).

Note that although patients may also display other psychiatric disorders (e.g., a major depressive episode, psychoactive substance abuse), adjustment disorders (e.g., acute distress disorder) with anxious or depressed mood are more common among patients who are seeking HIV treatment in community-based primary care clinics. As previously stated, this diagnosis relates to their reaction to having a serious life-threatening illness. A differentiating and defining feature of adjustment disorder is that the disorder begins within 3 months of the onset of a stressor and lasts no longer than 6 months after the stressor or its consequences have decreased. Other recurring disorders (e.g., bipolar illness, recurrent major depression) are also common, but these usually predate the patient's seroconversion or the onset of an HIV-related stressor. No one fully knows the incidence of previous psychiatric illness or substance abuse disorders among HIV-infected individuals, but many believe that it is higher for some community samples, partly on the basis of the fact that HIV is transmitted through exposure to infected needles in substance-abusing populations (Berger-Greenstein and Terrence, 2007; Irtaelski et al, 2007).

In addition to ruling out the presence of another Axis I disorder (e.g., a major depressive episode), nurses give consideration to other diagnostic categories when conducting a differential diagnosis assessment of these patients. These include bereavement reaction, psychologic factors related to a medical condition, PTSD, stress disorder, and personality disorders. Although diagnostic assessments vary, substance abuse and bereavement reactions are frequently comorbid conditions in patients whose Axis I diagnoses are either major depressive episodes or adjustment disorders with emotional features. Specific HIV-related problems that have been observed during psychiatric hospital admissions are as follows:

- Anxiety and depression related to deteriorating physical health status
- Social rejection related to HIV-seropositive status
- Increased drug use as a response to HIV seropositivity
- Shame or guilt regarding stigmatized sexual practices or drug use
- Guilt or fear about having put others at risk, including fear of retribution
- Homicidal ideation toward the person who infected the patient

PROGNOSIS

Although the prognosis for the resolution of anxiety and depression among patients with adjustment disorders is generally good, the case for resolution in persons with HIV/AIDS is not well documented, primarily because the stresses associated with HIV/AIDS persist and thus suspend the resolution of this condition. Researchers who study the psychologic and neuropsychiatric effects of HIV attempt to isolate crisis points at which psychosocial stressors or other factors lead to more serious levels of depression, anxiety, and other psychiatric problems. Because HIV infection is a chronic stressful life event that is depicted by a series of physical, functional, and psychosocial losses, anxiety and depression are likely to occur intermittently and relate to the psychologic pain that accompanies different phases of the disease process. Some experiences are severe enough to accelerate a dysphoric mood or a crisis. Although the concept of crisis points seems applicable to this population, several considerations are important.

The experience of HIV/AIDS as a crisis is highly variable. Some patients struggle with the disease, and this struggle is evident. Other patients seem to cope well and even seem to find new courage to take on healthier lifestyles. Thus, assuming that all patients experience the same level of distress denies individual differences in the ways that people cope with life stress. It is important that nurses use caution when generalizing about the inevitability of psychologic distress and what will result in a crisis for a patient.

THE NURSING PROCESS
ASSESSMENT

The psychosocial assessment of a patient with HIV/AIDS with a diagnosis of adjustment disorder, anxiety, or depression requires a thorough appraisal of primary and secondary nursing diagnoses. The clinical assessment that enables nurses to obtain relevant nursing diagnoses needs to be all-inclusive. Nurses have to address the identifying data, the current symptoms, and the history of the present problem (i.e., anxiety, depression, or conduct). Specific data about sleep patterns, appetite, and changes in weight are important when assessing the severity of the mood disturbance. Details about previous psychiatric contacts (both outpatient and hospitalizations), including precipitating events, will establish any preexisting psychiatric disorders that place the patient at risk for current or future episodes of clinical depression or anxiety. A priority area of assessment is the patient's previous and current tendency to inflict personal harm or to harm others. As previously noted, nurses need to seriously evaluate and monitor the patient's risk for suicide over time as the course of illness advances. Anger and rage are also manifested through violent behaviors, homicidal threats or gestures directed at those believed to be the source of infection, and occasionally toward society at large.

CASE STUDY

Rocio is a 29-year-old Hispanic woman married to José, who is HIV positive. Two months ago, Rocio was diagnosed as HIV positive with symptomatic HIV disease. She is positive for AIDS-related fatigue, fevers, nausea, diarrhea, dyspnea, and wasting syndrome. A thorough gynecologic examination reveals that Rocio is in the early stages of cervical dysplasia. The nurse practitioner in the women's clinic asked the psychiatric team to evaluate Rocio. She has been pregnant for 5 months, and she has three additional children who are younger than 5 years old. Rocio and José are undocumented residents who have lived in the United States for 6 months. Their primary language is Spanish. When questioned about her pregnancy and her personal health, Rocio sobbed uncontrollably. She explained that she is really worried about her children and what will happen to them. She cannot eat or sleep, and she has not told any friends or family that she is HIV positive, because she is ashamed and worried that they will not be kind to her children if they knew her diagnosis. When she is distracted from thinking or talking about her diagnosis, Rocio appears to be optimistic and grateful for the care that she is receiving at the clinic.

Critical Thinking
1 What are the patient's most immediate problems or needs related to her HIV diagnosis?
2 What assessment data reflect the patient's sensitivity to her diagnosis?
3 Why might the patient be reluctant to seek the social support she needs?
4 What stressors could contribute to the patient's fear, anxiety, sense of helplessness, and depression?

Data about the patient's family unit and current social network are particularly relevant. A description of the family unit of origin, including the family's history of traumatic events, migration, and cultural factors, help to sensitize providers to the contextual nature of the patient's responses to his or her illness and the potential for the co-occurrence of PTSD. These same data regarding current relationships are also critical, because they influence the ways that patients cope with HIV/AIDS and the availability of existing resources (see the Case Study).

Social history information is of general importance, but certain data hold special significance. The nature of the patient's social network and his or her previous and current sexual practices are important. In many cases, patients are not

only living with the personal threat of HIV, but they are also dealing with the possibility of placing others at risk. A diagnosis of HIV brings with it a variety of responsibilities to the patient's previous sexual partners.

Finally, when assessing the basis for psychologic distress, nurses conduct a thorough mental status examination on all patients. Periodic assessments occur as the disease progresses, and these allow for careful attention to and the monitoring of any undesirable findings.

NURSING DIAGNOSIS

Nurses formulate diagnoses from the data that are gathered during the assessment phase of the nursing process. The accuracy of nursing diagnoses depends on the careful and comprehensive assessment of the patient's history, presenting symptoms, behavior, and responses to actual and potential life stressors. The reliability of all informants—whether the sources are the patients themselves, their significant others, or previous data from charts—is extremely important. Multiple sources of data will confirm information and ensure appropriate assessment and diagnoses.

Nursing diagnoses for persons with AIDS who experience adjustment disorders with depressed or anxious mood are prioritized according to individual patient needs (North American Nursing Diagnosis Association International, 2008) and may include the following:
- Risk for suicide
- Anxiety
- Compromised family coping
- Ineffective coping
- Hopelessness
- Ineffective denial
- Noncompliance
- Powerlessness or risk for powerlessness
- Chronic or situational low self-esteem
- Social isolation

OUTCOME IDENTIFICATION

Outcome criteria come from the nursing diagnoses and address the responses that the patient is expected to achieve. The patient will do the following:
- Verbalize the absence of suicidal ideation and plans.
- State reduced frequency and intensity of feelings of hopelessness and powerlessness.
- Reduce ineffective denial and engage in a therapeutic alliance with staff to evaluate coping options.
- Initiate social interactions with others with HIV/AIDS (both individually and in groups) to gain information and support about coping effectively with HIV/AIDS.
- Identify barriers or problems that accelerate the exacerbation of anxiety and depression (e.g., perception of inadequate social support, perception of powerlessness over physical symptoms).
- Verbalize clear, goal-directed, short-term plans that are achievable and that focus on problem solving.

- Express improved self-esteem and self-confidence with regard to managing his or her illness and treatment and demonstrate intentions and behaviors to improve antiretroviral treatment adherence.

PLANNING

The nurse's awareness of the complexities of living with HIV disease is extremely critical to the development of an appropriate plan of care for the patient, the patient's family, and his or her friends, partners, and significant others. For patients who are diagnosed with adjustment disorders, the nurse considers a plan of action that will achieve the following results:

- Prevent self-directed violence.
- Address concerns in a clear, goal-directed, problem-solving manner.
- Increase social networking that will provide needed information and comfort.
- Monitor unfavorable effects of stressors on the patient's current level of adaptation.
- Interact with staff in an effective therapeutic alliance during therapy and when social supports diminish or when social networks cannot provide the technical expertise that the patient requires.

IMPLEMENTATION

The challenges of working and intervening with patients with HIV/AIDS are considerable and multiple. Both the patient's diagnosis and the responses to his or her disease greatly affect and often devastate families and caregivers. Therefore, it is important to consider and include families and significant others in interventions when it is appropriate and with the consent of the patient.

For example, significant others who engage in problem-solving coping methods (as compared with emotion-focused coping) are more helpful to patients who are trying to minimize the psychologic burden of adapting to their disease. Nurses need to teach significant others about the disease, its course, and what to expect over time. Trained professionals need to address any lack of knowledge. Support groups for caregivers of persons with HIV/AIDS are available, and these are particularly helpful for family members and significant others. These groups provide support and comfort for dealing with anticipated bereavement, fear of contagion, and the stress of caregiving. Support networks of a less formal design also exist to provide assistance for patients and their loved ones through newsletters and drop-in centers.

Nursing Interventions

Patients with HIV/AIDS often have numerous symptoms that require multiple interventions to address various aspects of their physical, psychosocial, and spiritual well-being. The patient's safety is paramount, and the nurse's first priority is to prevent potential or actual threats of self-harm or suicide. Subsequently, an integrated multidisciplinary approach to treatment is important. The interventions discussed here mainly focus on the patient's psychosocial needs. They are directed toward changing ineffective individual coping skills and treating impaired social interactions. Many nursing interventions for HIV parallel interventions that are used with other illnesses, particularly life-threatening cancers. However, people with HIV have unique experiences that are not similar to those of people with other life-threatening illnesses (e.g., dealing with disease contagion, the stigma and shame associated with their diagnosis, feelings of betrayal by those who have given them HIV). These features of the disease cause strong feelings that negatively affect individuals and may even affect their health status and approach to treatment. Successfully coping with HIV/AIDS is a priority for maintaining their quality of life over the course of their illness.

The primary category of intervention in the psychosocial domain is ensuring the safety of the patient and others. The nurse then focuses on facilitating adaptive coping to the multiple stressors that the patient will confront. Interventions to improve effective or adaptive coping include the following:

- Assist patients with maintaining or improving their quality of life.
- Prevent a state of hopelessness and powerlessness.
- Assist patients with managing or containing their feelings of fear, anxiety, grief, guilt, depression, and helplessness.
- Enhance patients' sense of self-worth and positive self-esteem.
- Assist patients with satisfactorily adapting their relationships as they are confronted with various stages of dependency on family, significant others, and health care providers.
- Assist patients with maintaining the highest level of functioning possible.
- Assist patients with developing a long-range plan for treatment adherence management.

Nurses also intervene to help patients cope adaptively to each phase of their HIV disease. With respect to maintaining or improving patients' quality of life, nurses are able to intervene to change the physical discomfort and psychosocial isolation that patients often experience. They teach patients to handle the pain and fatigue caused by their illness and by the side effects of HAART. In so doing, they are also helping the patient to exert control and to minimize feelings of helplessness.

There is a growing trend toward patient involvement in decision making regarding the course of treatment; this is called patient empowerment. Health care providers and their patients need to be adequately prepared to work in a partner relationship. Social support networks are important to patients with HIV/AIDS. Without them, social isolation and loneliness occur and significantly influence quality of life. In addition, disengagement is a normal process when adjusting to physical decline. The nurse needs to help the patient preserve those relationships with friends and family who are capable of meeting the patient's dependency needs. Loss of role functioning is usually painful to a patient, but it is even more painful when supportive relationships, for whatever reasons, are not available to the patient.

Managing anxiety, helplessness, grief, guilt, depression, and fear is also important to help the patient to maintain his or her quality of life. Informing the patient about HIV disease and treatment options lessens the anxiety that many patients experience, because it reduces uncertainty surrounding the disease and the likely prognosis. The nurse also needs to be aware that information does not comfort all patients. Sometimes patients do not understand or hear the instructions that the nurse provides. Nurses must individualize teaching plans according to the patient's level of written and verbal comprehension and always validate what the patient has retained by asking him or her to repeat what he or she has learned.

Supporting patients when they are confronting the multiple losses associated with their disease is comforting and helpful for reducing their negative feelings of grief and depression. These anticipated or actual losses include physical decline and the loss of social role, income, and supportive relationships. A loss of dignity related to declines in health and functional status also occurs. Anticipating losses and preparing patients to cope with these circumstances reduces the patient's psychologic distress. Nurses are also able to supplement patients' resources by providing them with knowledge of social and financial services and counseling assistance.

Helping the patient to maintain or enhance a sense of self-worth and to avoid a state of powerlessness and hopelessness in the face of this serious disease requires thoughtful consideration about the ways that the disease affects the patients. Sometimes the nurse teaches the patient how to respond to the curiosity of others. Hiding one's illness and minimizing its effects is sometimes adaptive, because it helps patients to live as normally as possible despite their symptoms and the effects of treatment. A study of HIV-positive men in Namibia revealed that many of the men felt responsible for being infected and believed that they deserved the consequences. Most had turned to religious beliefs, which became an important part of their lives and gave them a sense of control. The infection took on a new meaning for them and brought a new purpose to their lives as well as hope for a good outcome (Plattner and Meiring, 2006).

Assisting the patient with preserving relationships requires both direct and indirect intervention. Nurses help patients to understand the reasons for the reactions of their family members and friends. Less directly, they assist informal caregivers by teaching them how to respond to the patient's reactions to his or her illness and treatment. The informal caregivers of patients with AIDS are usually concerned about the contagiousness of the disease. Providing factual information to these caregivers will decrease any tendency that they may have to withdraw out of fear of becoming infected with HIV. For cases in which patients are sexually active with partners, nurses need to teach them about and encourage them to follow safe sexual practices.

A final important category of intervention is related to the treatment of acute and subacute syndromes that are associated with cognitive impairment. Dementia associated with AIDS includes cognitive, motor, and behavioral manifestations. Initial symptoms are usually memory impairment and concentration difficulties, but these symptoms are often overlooked and frequently confused with symptoms associated with depression. However, some patients complain of forgetfulness, "slowed thinking," and difficulty concentrating when engaged in conversations, watching television programs, or reading. In some cases, poor balance and coordination occur early on. As this syndrome progresses with no chance of reversal, patients become dependent on others for the completion of activities of daily living. Many patients and their caregivers fear the development of dementia. Some have observed friends whose lives were significantly compromised by AIDS dementia in all areas (i.e., cognitive, motor, and behavior). In addition, AIDS dementia is not easy to identify, and symptoms increase and decline, thereby causing a great deal of uncertainty and anxiety. For this reason, conducting an early, thorough assessment and instructing patients and caregivers about signs and symptoms are extremely important interventions.

With the arrival of new therapies, researchers are hopeful that AIDS dementia will decline and that some patients with dementia will regain their lost abilities. Whether these symptoms are reversible and what level of cognitive improvement will result are the subjects of ongoing study.

Nurses who work with patients with AIDS with associated dementia participate in the neuropsychiatric assessment of their patients by recording problems related to memory, attention span, concentration, and motor deficits. They provide support to the patient as well as to the patient's family members and friends who are assuming patient care. Caregivers or partners sometimes welcome respite care or home care, depending on the patient's functional status and needs. It is important to help patients and their families to remember treatment and medication schedules; this includes the use of checklists, bulletin boards, pill boxes, alarms, and other strategies to promote self-care management and to ease the burden of care for significant others.

Additional Treatment Modalities

Nursing interventions contribute significantly to the patient's ability to cope effectively with HIV disease. However, it is important to keep in mind that other disciplines and therapies also play a critical role in the patient's ability to deal with the psychologic distress related to HIV. Currently accepted treatments of adjustment problems in patients with HIV/AIDS parallel those for other populations with adjustment disorders, but this section addresses key differences related to the following: pharmacologic intervention, the preferred format for individual counseling, psychosocial support networks specific to persons living with HIV/AIDS and their significant others, and the use of other methods to decrease stress and to promote patients' highest level of functioning.

PHARMACOLOGIC INTERVENTION

Medical

Previously the first line of treatment for HIV was the prescription of a reverse transcriptase inhibitor (e.g., AZT). This was called *monotherapy,* because only one agent was involved. More complex courses of therapy have replaced monotherapy approaches. Combination antiretroviral therapies include HAART and mega-HAART. These treatment plans include reverse transcriptase inhibitors and protease inhibitors, which work together to interrupt the production of new viruses. Combination therapies are the most effective treatment available, but some cause disabling side effects.

Psychopharmacology

Psychotropic medications are useful for the treatment of patients with HIV disease, and there are no medical reasons to avoid their use. The most common psychotropic medications with which HIV/AIDS patients experience moderate to severe distress are antidepressants and anxiolytics. The best outcome results from the use of medications combined with cognitive behavioral counseling approaches. Counseling and psychotherapy are generally the standard of care for patients with significant and persistent depression or anxiety. Still, in the case of demoralization syndromes (i.e., adjustment disorders), some patients respond well to unstructured support with a caring provider who is not technically trained.

Antidepressant medication is sometimes prescribed if the patient manifests a significant depressed or anxious condition. Sometimes an antidepressant is given as a preventative measure in anticipation of new uncontrollable stressors. Anxiolytics are prescribed in daily dosages or as needed to reduce the patient's anxiety. The choice of antidepressant or anxiolytic and the dose of medication often depends on the patient's neurovegetative symptoms and underlying physical illness. For example, for an agitated patient with gastroenteritis who is also having difficulties with diarrhea as a result of the disease or complications of treatment, an antidepressant medication with more anticholinergic action is sometimes the best choice. This medication reduces diarrhea and provides mild sedation, thus working to the patient's advantage. In addition to the individual's overall health status and specific emotional distress, the age of the patient is important. For example, older adults and adolescents are generally treated with lower doses of psychotropic medications. The first step in antidepressant treatment is to assist the patient with consistently taking the medication and using an adequate therapeutic dose. Physicians generally begin with low doses of the chosen medication and slowly increase the level to minimize medication side effects. Remember that, in addition to the potential side effects that patients experience while taking antidepressants, they are also experiencing varying degrees of side effects from their antiretroviral medications. An antidepressant drug may interfere with the efficacy of the antiretroviral drug; however, the antidepressant may assist the patient with coping with the side effects of the antiretroviral drug and improve his or her adherence to the medication regimen. The patient should be evaluated after a 2-week period to determine whether there are improvements in mood, adverse reactions, and medication self-management.

Integrative Therapies

In the absence of a definitive cure, many patients with HIV have chosen to supplement their treatment programs with complementary and integrative therapies or treatments. Ordinarily, medical physicians do not provide these complementary therapies, but these therapies can be combined with the patient's medical treatment. Complementary therapies for patients with HIV/AIDS include mind–body remedies and herbal supplements that are aimed at reducing the individuals' symptoms or treatment side effects, enhancing their immune status, or improving their sense of well-being. Examples of these therapies include acupuncture, massage, herbs, vitamins, meditation, and stress reduction. With few exceptions, these approaches are helpful and not harmful. Exceptions are the use of St. John's wort, which reduces the blood plasma concentration of indinavir (a protease inhibitor), and garlic supplements, which interact with saquinavir (another protease inhibitor). Caution patients to discuss the use of any herbal or dietary supplements with their health care providers to prevent any adverse effects that may result from the interactions of these substances with their antiviral treatment therapy (see Chapter 27).

The stress of HIV infection is chronic and usually continues for long periods, with acute exacerbations. Nurses need to recommended alternative methods of managing stress. Along these lines, there are well-documented techniques (e.g., stress reduction, meditation, relaxation techniques) that are extremely useful to many persons at various stages of HIV/AIDS. For example, nurses are able to teach stress management strategies and progressive relaxation exercises to patients. Stress management manuals and self-help books as well as brief workshops in the community are available to help patients learn these techniques. Some of these instructional aids are also available on DVDs.

Nurses also need to recognize, discuss, and support the individual's desire to control psychologic distress through alternative methods, including spiritual practices. Spirituality as treatment is receiving increased attention, because a growing body of literature suggests that there is an important connection between how a person interprets the meaning of his or her illness and his or her ability to cope with illness and loss. Taking spirituality and prayer into account when assessing an individual's needs and resources and developing intervention strategies requires a shift in perspective.

Nurses monitor patients' self-management strategies for other reasons as well. Nurses must caution patients that bodies infected with HIV are different from disease-free systems. Weight loss generated by diet changes and physical exercise is usually more of a problem than a desired goal. Unnecessary dieting and strenuous exercise that result in a reduction of calories need to be minimized. The recommendation for exercise focuses on moderation, with the major goal of exercise being strength building and resistance training. Adding muscle mass is a good thing for these patients; burning calories is not.

EVALUATION

When nursing interventions are successful, the patient will usually show significant signs of improvement in his or her coping abilities. If these coping abilities improve, changes in patient mood, behavior, and functional abilities will also improve. Increases in patients' understanding of their illness and treatment will also be evident. A large part of the treatment of persons with HIV/AIDS is individualized teaching to help them to regain and maintain a sense of control over their lives, their symptoms, and their disease.

Effective coping is evident in the outcome criteria that are addressed in the treatment plan; in other words, patients will demonstrate an ability to manage and contain uncomfortable feelings of fear, anxiety, guilt, grief, and depression. As their ability to manage symptoms improves, the patient's self-esteem and perception of self-worth will also improve. Relationships with others, especially those in caregiver roles, will be stronger because of the added instruction and support from the nurse. The patient will demonstrate a realistic level of hope as a result of the nurse's efforts to help him or her to find meaning in life and to set small but realistic goals. Although patients do not consistently experience a strong sense of well-being, they should experience an improved quality of life on the basis of increased feelings of cognitive, behavioral, and decisional control. Helping patients to achieve control minimizes their fear, anxiety, and depression associated with HIV/AIDS while maximizing their ability to cope with their illness and multiple losses. They will be more likely to follow their antiretroviral therapy regimen when they can make choices.

CHAPTER SUMMARY

- Historically, the scientific community considered the body, mind, and spirit as separate entities. Physical health and illness were major concerns, and few paid attention to the individual's mental and emotional responses to physiologic problems.
- Multicausal and psychologic theories provide a framework for understanding the person's response to stress and its relationship to physiologic and psychologic interactions.
- Common psychosocial responses to stress and illness are fear, anxiety, feelings of powerlessness and helplessness, hostility, and anger. Depression often prohibits effective coping and adaptation.
- Coping involves the use of resourcefulness and the ability to manage the stress of daily circumstances such as the challenges posed by pain and disability or by acute or chronic disease. Coping mechanisms are conscious or unconscious, and they may be adaptive or maladaptive.
- Adaptation is a complex, continuous, and demanding process, particularly with regard to accepting a loss of independence and valued roles.
- HIV disease is a major public health problem worldwide. Some persons who are infected with HIV are asymptomatic for long periods of time. AIDS is the advanced stage of HIV disease.
- HIV/AIDS is a chronic disease that affects multiple body systems, including the brain and the central nervous system. Many individuals experience significant psychologic stress related to the awareness of their diagnosis and the subsequent need for adaptation to the consequences of this life-threatening chronic illness.
- Dramatic shifts in the numbers of persons living with AIDS have occurred as a result of the development of effective antiretroviral medication therapy. Consequently, more people are living longer with HIV, and they will ideally learn to cope effectively with the ongoing impact of their disease and its treatment.
- Certain disadvantaged minorities have a disproportionate number of AIDS cases. These populations traditionally have experienced problems with accessing health care services. Shifts in rates of HIV infection suggest that adolescent girls and women are increasingly vulnerable to HIV/AIDS.
- One principal DSM-IV-TR diagnosis among persons with HIV/AIDS is adjustment disorder. This diagnosis is differentiated from other mood disorders (e.g., major depression).
- Nurses conduct assessments and interventions in collaboration with the patient and, in some cases, with family members and significant others.
- Psychotropic medications are helpful for some patients who are experiencing more severe depression or anxiety, especially when such medications are coupled with structured or unstructured supportive counseling.
- The psychosocial needs of those who are infected with and affected by HIV are numerous and present significant challenges to quality of life and the management of treatment adherence in these individuals and their family members or significant others.
- Complementary therapies such as stress reduction, relaxation, and spirituality or prayer are useful to many patients in various stages of HIV disease.
- The current Western health care model includes a greater emphasis on health promotion across the life span, self-care management, and a holistic approach to the management of acute and chronic psychosocial and physiologic health problems.
- The nurse has an essential role in helping patients to recognize the impact of stress and assisting them with selecting appropriate coping mechanisms and promoting the best possible quality of life.

REVIEW QUESTIONS

1. During the past 2 years, the patient has had a parent die, been diagnosed with rheumatoid arthritis, lost employment, and begun divorce proceedings. Which complaints should the nurse expect? You may select more than one answer.
   1. "I'm having trouble remembering to pay my bills every month."
   2. "All this stress has helped me to focus on what I really need to accomplish."
   3. "It seems like I catch every little virus that goes through our community."
   4. "I'm beginning to feel like I am losing control of my life."
   5. "My energy levels have increased in response to these stressful events."
2. A nurse wants to research interactions between the neurologic, endocrine, and immune systems in response to psychosocial stressors. Which search term would yield the desired information?
   1. Multicausal theories of disease
   2. Psychoneuroimmunoendocrinology
   3. General adaptation syndrome
   4. Epidemiology
3. An adult is hospitalized with pneumonia and dehydration as a result of advanced AIDS. The patient is confused and delusional. Which nursing diagnosis should be included in the plan of care?
   1. Disturbed thought processes
   2. Hopelessness
   3. Powerlessness
   4. Risk-prone health behavior
4. A young adult is informed of a positive laboratory test for HIV. The patient tells the nurse, "Well, I know what I need to do now." What is the nurse's next action?
   1. Give the patient information about local support groups.
   2. Assess the patient's suicidality.
   3. Discuss the results of the newest medication research.
   4. Arrange a consultation with the social worker.
5. Which individual would have the highest risk for clinical depression?
   1. An individual with AIDS whose CD4$^+$ count has decreased over the past week
   2. An individual who believes that she has a risk for HIV infection but who has not been tested
   3. An individual with AIDS and a recent sudden onset of Kaposi's sarcoma
   4. An individual with AIDS whose viral load increased over the past month

REFERENCES

American Psychiatric Association: *Diagnostic and statistical manual of mental disorders*, ed 4, text revision, Washington, DC, 2000, American Psychiatric Association.

Anderson RA: Psychoneuroimmunoendocrinology: review and commentary, *Townsend Letter* 309:102-104, 2009.

Beers CW: *A mind that found itself*, New York, 1935, Doubleday, Doran and Co.

Berger-Greenstein JA, Terence M: Major depression in patients with HIV/AIDS and substance abuse, *AIDS Patient Care STDS* 21(12):942-955, 2007.

Carpenito L: *Nursing diagnosis: application to clinical practice*, ed 10, Philadelphia, 2003, Lippincott.

Centers for Disease Control and Prevention: *Surveillance report, 2007* (website): www.cdc.gov/hiv/topics/surveillances/reports/2007report/default.htm. Accessed March 6, 2007.

Colin-Thome D: Supporting self-care in the 21st century—a long-term conditions view, *Journal of Holistic Healthcare* 6(2):6-8, 2009.

Continuing Medical Education: *Treating whole patient: the mind-body connection forum* (website): www.cmellc.com. Accessed March 12, 2010.

Cook J, Tyor W: The pathogenesis of HIV-associated dementia: recent advances using a SCID mouse model of HIV encephalitis, *Einstein Q J Biol Med* 22:32-40, 2006.

Cooperman N, Simoni J: Suicidal ideation and attempted suicide among women living with HIV/AIDS, *J Behav Med* 28:149-156, 2005.

Cumbie S et al: Advanced practice nursing model for comprehensive care with chronic illness: model for promoting process engagement, *Adv Nurs Sci* 27:70-80, 2004.

Dully H, Fleming C: *My lobotomy*, New York, 2007, Three Rivers/Crown Publishing.

Hellman E: Theories of health promotion and illness management. In Black J et al, editors: *Medical-surgical nursing: clinical management for positive outcomes*, ed 6, Philadelphia, 2004, Saunders.

Holmes T, Rahe R: The social readjustment rating scale, *J Psychosom Med* 11:213-218, 1967.

Irtaelski DM et al: Psychiatric co-morbidity in vulnerable populations receiving primary care for HIV/AIDS, *AIDS Care* 19(2):220-225, 2007.

Lavee Y, Ben-Ari A: The association of daily hassles and uplifts with family and life satisfaction: does cultural orientation make a difference? *Am J Community Psychol* 41(1-2):89-98, 2008.

Lazarus R: Theory-based stress management, *Psychol Inq* 1:3-13, 1990.

Lazarus R, Folkman S: *Stress, appraisal and coping*, New York, 1987, Springer.

Lee G: Contributing factors of depression for persons with musculoskeletal pain in workman's compensation settings: an ecological conceptualization in rehabilitation counseling intervention, *J Rehabilitation* 76(i):3-12, 2010.

Lenz R: Army changes tack in treating combat stress, *San Diego Union-Tribune* A-21, June 4, 2006.

Marcus P: Anxiety and anxiety disorders. In Fortinash K, Holoday Worret P, editors: *Psychiatric mental health nursing*, ed 4, St. Louis, 2008, Mosby.

Millsbaugh D: Assessment and response to spiritual pain: part I, *J Palliat Med* 8(5):919-923, 2005.

Millsbaugh D: Assessment and response to spiritual pain: part II, *J Palliat Med* 8(6):1110-1117, 2008.

Mitchell M, Knowlton M: Stigma and depression symptoms among informal caregivers of people living with HIV/AIDS, *AIDS Patient Care STDS* 23(8):611-617, 2009.

National Institutes of Health: *AIDS virus hides out in bone marrow cells* (website): www.nlm.nih.gov/medlineplus/news/fullstory-96115.html. Accessed March 7, 2010.

Neurnberger P: *Freedom from stress: a holistic approach*, Honesdale, Pa, 1981, Himalayan International Institute of Yoga Science and Philosophy.

Neyland T: Hans Selye and the field of stress research, *J Neuropsychiatry Clin Neurosci* 10:230, 1988.

Nieves JE et al: Telemental health for our soldiers: a brief review and a new pilot program, *Mil Med* 174(12):1241, 2009.

North American Nursing Diagnosis Association International: *NANDA-I nursing diagnoses: definitions and classification 2009-2011*, Philadelphia, 2008, North American Nursing Diagnosis Association International.

Orfus M, Howe N: Stress appraisal and coping in siblings of children with special needs, *Exceptionality Education Canada* 18(3):166-181, 2008.

Phillips S: *Stress and coping* (course at Florida International University) (website): www.fiu.edu/faculty/phillips/NUR3055/TransStress.htm. Accessed March 5, 2010.

Plattner IE, Meiring N: Living with HIV: the psychological relevance of meaning making, *AIDS Care* 18(3):241-245, 2006.

Porth C, Matfin G: *Pathophysiology: concepts of altered health status*, ed 8, Philadelphia, 2008, Lippincott.

Sanchez L: Black churches mounting AIDS campaign, *San Diego Union-Tribune* B-1, March 11, 2010.

Selye H: *The stress of life*, New York, 1956, McGraw-Hill.

Springer L: Human immunodeficiency virus infection. In Lewis S et al, editors: *Medical-surgical nursing: assessment and management of clinical problems*, St. Louis, 2004, Mosby.

Stuart G: *Principles and practice of psychiatric nursing*, ed 9, St. Louis, 2008, Mosby.

United Nations: *UNAIDS outlook—2010: fresh perspectives and response* (website): www.unaids.org. Accessed November 24, 2010.

U.S. Department of Health and Human Services: *President's Advisory Council on HIV/AIDS 38th meeting* (website): www.aids.gov/federal-resources/policies/pachel/meeting/February-2010-minutes.pdf. Accessed February 2, 2010.

Venes D: *Taber's Cyclopedic Medical Dictionary*, ed 21, Philadelphia, 2009, FA Davis.

Witek-Janusek L: Stress. In Lewis M et al, editors: *Medical-surgical nursing: assessment and management of clinical problems*, ed 6, St. Louis, 2004, Mosby.

Wood DP et al: Combat related post-traumatic stress disorder: a case report using virtual reality graded exposure therapy with physiological monitoring with a female Seabee, *Mil Med* 174(11):1215-1222, 2009.

World Health Organization: *Chronic disease* (website): www.who.int/health_topics/chronic_disease/en. Accessed June 17, 2006.

Zborowsky T, Kreitzer MJ: People, place, and process: the role of place in creating optimal healing environments, *Creat Nurs* 15(3):186-190, 2009.

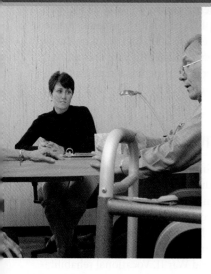

Community Mental Health Nursing for Patients with Severe and Persistent Mental Illness

Alwilda Scholler-Jaquish

"If there is any great secret of success in life, it lies in the ability to put yourself in the other person's place and to see things from his point of view as well as your own."

Henry Ford

evolve WEBSITE

http://evolve.elsevier.com/Fortinash/

OBJECTIVES

- Describe the components of community mental health nursing.
- Identify outpatient treatment options that are commonly available in community settings.
- Discuss the legal influences that affect the health care of persons in the community with severe and persistent mental illness.
- Describe ways in which nurses play an integral role in symptom management and medication compliance for persons in the home and the community.
- Analyze the impact of obesity and substance abuse, on persons with severe and persistent mental illness.

- Explain the impact of managed care on community psychiatric rehabilitation.
- Describe the cultural needs of community residents with severe and persistent mental illness.
- Explore the factors that contribute to the incarceration of persons with mental illness.
- Identify the predictors of violence in persons with mental illness.
- Apply the nursing process to patients in the community and in the home.

KEY TERMS

adult family home
adult residential treatment program
case management
clubhouse model
community mental health center

congregate care facility
deinstitutionalization
least restrictive
programs for assertive community
    treatment

psychosocial rehabilitation and skills
    training program
severe and persistent mental illness

The current emphasis in psychiatric treatment for patients with mental and emotional illness is on outpatient and community-based programs. Care in the community occurs in various places that include community hospitals, partial hospitalization programs, evaluation and treatment facilities, psychiatric rehabilitation programs, respite care, and many independent and semi-independent living arrangements. Community psychiatric mental health nursing includes a variety of treatments, methods, and activities that address the needs of psychiatric patients, especially those with severe and persistent mental illness, who are trying to maintain a stable position in the community.

ROLE OF THE NURSE

The role of the community mental health nurse is to help the patient to maintain his or her highest level of functioning and independence within the community. It is a challenging role that requires a comprehensive understanding of human behavior and development, psychiatric disorders, and prevailing treatments. Sharp assessment skills and keen insight based on experience, good judgment, and knowledge of group processes and family dynamics are also essential qualities for the community mental health nurse. In addition, it is critical for the nurse to be familiar with the available community resources and community networks, so he or she can work with the multidisciplinary treatment team to help patients and their families adjust to the community and enhance their quality of life.

Changes in the financing of psychiatric treatment have caused many variations in health care settings and in the delivery of nursing care. Medicaid and Medicare reimbursement guidelines and private insurance carriers limit the amount and types of care that are available for individuals with severe and persistent mental illness. It is not uncommon for mentally ill persons who are being discharged from acute psychiatric care facilities to have home-care visits for 1 to 2 weeks or once a month for a limited period of time. Most psychiatric nursing care takes place through home health care agencies, with federal and state orders to control spending. The psychiatric nurse's visit is often limited to 30 minutes, and it needs to include psychiatric evaluation, medication compliance, health teaching, crisis intervention, and documentation. Newer approaches to community mental health nursing include telephone contacts and communicating with patients through the Internet (Balon, 2002; Shore and Manson, 2005; Zauszniewski and Suresky, 2004).

Nurses also serve as case managers, home health care providers, and members of psychiatric teams that provide comprehensive care to persons with severe and persistent mental illness. Nurses with advanced practice or clinical specialist credentials can work as managers of a community mental health center or program and consult with staff in residential treatment centers (Laskowski, 2001; Yamashita, 2005).

Responsibilities include intake interviews, managing a caseload of patients in a community mental health setting, and providing psychiatric home health care, including the administration of psychotropic medications. Community mental health nurses are often responsible for establishing and supervising the competencies of mental health workers (Coursey et al, 2000; Edwards et al, 2005), and caring for special populations, such as severely and persistently mentally ill persons with alcohol or drug addictions, those with human immunodeficiency virus (HIV) or acquired immunodeficiency syndrome (AIDS), troubled adolescents, and diverse ethnic groups.

Advanced practice nurses typically see patients with mental illnesses in community mental health centers, in private practice, or in nurse-managed mental health clinics. The advanced practice nurse monitors behavioral changes and medication management, conducts psychoeducation, and examines patients for physical health problems. Nurse-managed mental health centers are often located in medically underserved areas where they consistently have contact with patients with severe and persistent mental illness and their families (Puskar and Bernardo, 2002; Wheeler and Greiner, 2002).

HISTORIC PERSPECTIVES

State hospitals have been in existence since the late 18th century, when the care of the mentally ill was shifted from jails and poorhouses to a more humane setting. The Great Depression significantly affected the quality of care available in psychiatric institutions. Many servicemen and servicewomen developed psychiatric conditions associated with their experiences during World War II. Vocational rehabilitation and group therapy were instituted with the passing of the Barden-LaFollete Act in 1943. Psychiatrists became interested in outpatient and group therapy, and they left the state mental hospitals. By 1955, almost 80% of psychiatrists were practicing in community settings (Accordino et al, 2001).

In 1955, state hospitals reached a peak census of 559,000 patients. During the early 1960s, a number of social, political, and economic issues brought attention to the apparent warehousing of chronically mentally ill people in state institutions. A 6-year study was conducted to evaluate the quality of care that was available in the existing mental health facilities. Because of the terrible conditions that mentally ill patients lived in, activists initiated the Mental Retardation Facilities and Community Mental Health Centers Construction Act of 1963. The intent of this act was to provide psychiatric health care in community settings.

In 1964, health insurance provided mental health coverage for individuals. The following year, Medicare began to provide health care for older adults. Medicaid, which was designed to provide health care for the poor, was passed in 1965. President Carter was instrumental in passing The national Mental Health Systems Act in 1980. This was designed to provide services for the chronically mentally ill, but funding was withheld during President Reagan's administration (1981-1989). Collectively, these events combined to create deinstitutionalization as costs increased and benefits diminished. Over the next 10 years, there was a rapid emptying of mental institutions across the country. This move to empty hospitals occurred throughout the developing world; thus, mentally ill people in many countries were displaced and on their own. Managed care was the primary focus of care during the 1990s, which was followed by increased financial limitations (Cutler et al, 2003).

Deinstitutionalization

During deinstitutionalization, federal dollars were designated for community mental health facilities; however, the enacted legislation was never funded. The goal was to provide community mental health centers to meet the needs of the community, which included a follow-up care system that would decrease the need for psychiatric hospitalization. Care for severely mentally ill persons shifted from large state hospitals to communities. Patients with identifiable family members were discharged to homes after a 20-year absence or more. Family members were wary about the sudden arrival of mentally ill individuals in their homes. Those without family were transferred to halfway houses that were supposed to provide supervision for the residents. These facilities were poorly managed, however, and many failed to meet their goal during the first few years. Persons who were discharged to their family homes or to halfway houses soon wandered off and became homeless. More than 100,000 mentally ill homeless were left to roam the streets without food, shelter, medication, or protection of any kind. In addition to the homeless, tens of thousands of older mentally ill and mentally retarded persons of all ages were transferred to nursing homes. These drastic changes in the care setting resulted in the decline of quality of care. The state hospital population decreased by 75%: it went from 504,000 to 138,000 between 1963 and 1986.

Deinstitutionalization was both a historic fact and a set of legal mandates that governed the treatment of mentally ill persons. The people who were directly affected by deinstitutionalization more than 40 years ago no longer exist; yet, the components of the process are still in place, as in the following examples: (1) Most managed care plans require patients to be discharged as soon as their psychotic episodes cease; (2) The least restrictive methods are used to control persons during psychotic episodes; (3) Most facilities only use physical or behavioral restraints for short time periods, and check the patients every 15 minutes; and (4) Patients are closely supervised in a seclusion room and released as soon as their behavior is under control.

PERSONS WITH SEVERE AND PERSISTENT MENTAL ILLNESS

The person with severe and persistent mental illness has numerous emotional, cognitive, and behavioral symptoms that are associated with specific disorders, such as schizophrenia and mood disorders. The manifestations of these disorders are also associated with the person's life history and may be obvious to the family for a long time before treatment is sought and the diagnosis is made. The family may describe the person's behavior as "odd" or "eccentric," or "different" and "unique," or even "special" and "introspective" without realizing or being willing to admit that the family member has a psychiatric illness that needs professional help. The family generally seeks treatment for the ill member when the behavior becomes irrational, threatening, assaultive, or self-destructive, or when they can no longer sustain the emotional or financial burden of caring for a person with severe psychiatric symptoms. If the individual resists help, he or she may end up as a homeless person, without the benefit of psychiatric care or hope of a better life (see Chapters 12 and 13).

Mentally ill persons who are disturbed or actively psychotic are not required to obtain psychiatric treatment unless they are a threat to themselves or others. A homeless person who is hallucinating or is a public nuisance cannot receive treatment if the behavior is non-threatening. These individuals have the right to determine their own treatment, and have the right to refuse medication. In a psychiatric setting, a physician will order certain medications on a limited basis. In some settings, a registered nurse will administer medication on an emergency basis, provided that he or she can obtain the physician's order either before or immediately after giving the medication; this occurs only if the patient poses an immediate danger to himself or herself or others. Health care providers are only able to give the drugs as a **least restrictive** intervention, which means that interventions such as talking to or distracting the patient were tried first and were unsuccessful or unsafe. Each emergency administration of medication thereafter requires a physician order as well (see Chapter 9).

Psychotropic Medications

In addition to community care, another factor that influenced deinstitutionalization was the introduction of the phenothiazine chlorpromazine (Thorazine) and lithium carbonate during the late 1950s for the treatment of mental illnesses. These drugs made it possible to discharge patients who previously experienced refractory psychosis (i.e., psychosis that did not readily respond to treatment). Today, the further development of antipsychotic medications continues to greatly influence the prognosis of psychiatric treatment, thereby leading to the rapid and often premature discharge of patients from hospitals.

The community mental health nurse faces a number of issues related to the use and misuse of psychotropic medications. It is important to monitor the dosage of medications, changes in prescriptions, and potential complications. The onset of type 2 diabetes is one of the less known side effects of commonly used antipsychotic medications. Diabetes associated with psychotropic medications has been demonstrated to be more frequent with risperidone (Risperdal) (Koller et al, 2003). Compliance with antipsychotic medications is associated with decreased hospitalization. Persons who are compliant spend more money on medications (Gilmer et al, 2004). The new Medicare drug benefit (Plan D) can negatively affect compliance, because some uncommon antipsychotics are not covered by Plan D. Aligning oneself with a medication provider requires a significant amount of skill, which can be difficult for certain populations, such as the elderly or infirm. Community mental health nurses sometimes need to assist individuals with obtaining medication coverage.

Nonadherence is a complex problem that means that a patient is not following the prescribed plan of care. Factors that affect nonadherence include the patient's attitude toward his or her illness, financial considerations, the side effects of psychotropic medications, and the patient's mental illness. It is important to assess the patient's response to medications, medication adherence, and potential side effects. Side effects include sleep disorders, night terrors, nervousness, and more serious complications, such as cardiovascular, peripheral, and anticholinergic effects (e.g., dry mouth, blurred vision, urinary retention) (see Chapter 19). Nurses need to be aware that the most troublesome side effects for patients are sexual dysfunction and weight gain. Researchers have associated weight gain with diabetes, coronary artery disease, and sleep apnea (Balon, 2002; Kohen, 2004; Reutsch et al, 2005). There is evidence that sibutramine (Meridia), an over-the-counter weight loss drug, may help the patients to control weight gain (Barclay and Vega, 2005), but it is not without side effects. Some persons with severe mental illness have sexual dysfunctions, and the psychotropic medications make these dysfunctions worse (see Chapter 20).

Educating patients and family members about psychotropic medications in a clear and concise manner, is a major responsibility of the community mental health nurse. It is essential that the person understand the importance of a regular medication regimen, and the potential seriousness of certain side effects. Teaching medication adherence and safety and assessing the patient's knowledge and needs regarding medication is an ongoing process (O'Connell, 2006). All side effects need to be documented and reported to the patient's physician (see Chapter 25).

Legal Influences

A civil rights movement also influenced deinstitutionalization in that it emphasized the rights of people with mental illness to make decisions for themselves. During this time, it was difficult to commit people to mental institutions against their will as laws supported more treatment and less restrictive alternatives in the care of persons with mental illness. Treatment rather than custodial care became the focus of institutional settings. The U.S. Court of Appeals mandated the "least restrictive alternative to hospitalization" as the guide for the placement of patients to discourage unnecessary hospitalization (Applebaum, 1999) (see Chapter 9).

There are approximately 200 mental health courts in the United States. Canada, England, France, India, Australia, and New Zealand also have mental health courts, although some countries only have one. These courts serve to divert persons with severe and persistent mental illness away from the criminal justice system (Mental Health America, 2009).

Mental health courts are multijurisdictional and community-based programs that provide court supervision and services to mentally ill offenders through the cooperation of state, county, and local nonprofit agencies, to promote their treatment, to improve their quality of life, to decrease recidivism, and to increase community safety and awareness (Breen and Breen, 2008). These programs provide comprehensive services; however, the number of people served by these courts is minimal as compared with the number of mentally ill patients that are committed to jails or prisons.

Legal and ethical issues continually challenge community mental health nurses. A signed consent is required for every treatment. Careful documentation of the care provided and the patient's response are essential. Nurses are sometimes legally responsible to warn potential victims when they become aware of a patient's potential for self-destructive behavior or actions that are harmful to others. It is important to recognize that the patient may also be at risk for physical, sexual, or emotional abuse from members of his or her own household. Nurses need to be aware of state laws that mandate patient confidentiality while sharing necessary information about a patient. For example, a nurse who learns of illegal behavior on the part of a patient (e.g., stealing clothes in response to a delusion of grandeur) or engaging in high-risk sexual behavior that results in the patient contracting HIV or hepatitis C infection needs to report such findings to the appropriate professionals. A nurse needs to develop trusting relationships with patients, but the nurse should never agree to keep patients' unsafe or illegal behaviors secret. State laws sometimes require nurses to report persons who are at risk to transmit HIV disease. In these more complex situations, the community mental health nurse needs to communicate with both the patient and the agency to find the appropriate course of action to protect the patient and the community (see Chapter 9).

CURRENT COMMUNITY MENTAL HEALTH TREATMENT SYSTEMS

Community Mental Health Centers

Community mental health centers provide outpatient services for children, the elderly, individuals who are chronically mentally ill, and those who have been discharged from an inpatient psychiatric facility. Special populations include mentally ill persons who are homeless, who are in jail, who engage in substance abuse, or who have AIDS. The services must include 24-hour emergency service as well as day treatment that may include partial hospitalization or psychosocial services. Programs are specifically designed to manage the special needs of each group. Services also provide screening for persons to determine whether they are appropriate for admission to a state mental hospital.

Funding

Community mental health centers are eligible to receive a number of federal grants through the Substance Abuse and Mental Health Services Administration. State and private grants are also available and provide for a variety of patient care needs.

Many states are now contracting with private health maintenance organizations to finance mental health services for Medicaid and Medicare patients. Nurse-managed clinics also provide mental health services, which are reimbursed by Medicaid for individuals who qualify. Documentation is the key to obtaining financial reimbursement for care. A program that does not receive reimbursements cannot continue to provide care to the neediest people.

Philosophy

Two separate philosophies that currently dominate the mental health care provider systems for persons with severe and persistent mental illness are freedom of choice versus continuity of care.

Freedom of Choice

Freedom-of-choice advocates argue that all people, regardless of their disabilities, should be able to choose from a variety of treatments. With this method, patients select from different treatments and treatment providers and receive care at a variety of agencies. With the current trend of managed care, these systems operate on the basis of managed competition, whereas, agencies compete to develop services that will best serve persons with mental disorders. Freedom-of-choice systems have experienced some common problems with patient care: (1) Individuals often have symptoms that affect their behavior, sometimes making them unpleasant or uncooperative and predisposing them to reject treatment; and (2) many agencies do not choose to develop treatment options for severe mental disorders because they disagree with the premise of freedom of choice. Both the provider and the patient have the freedom to make decisions; however, treatment providers in these systems have the right to refuse to treat anyone whose symptoms make that person resistant to accepting treatment. This leaves a patient who is difficult to treat without services. Also, some patients with severe mental disorders will withdraw from treatment as a result of impaired judgment that is caused by worsening illness when in fact the treatment actually needs to increase. Patients with severe and persistent mental illness who are in prison also have the right to refuse treatment. In this system, patients have many treatment options, but there is no central contact. This means that, if a patient stops treatment, it is less noticeable because the care comes from many places instead of through a central contact.

Continuity of Care

Continuity-of-care advocates argue that persons with severe and persistent mental illness need to have one stable treatment provider throughout all phases of their illness (Adair et al, 2005). The assumption is that some symptoms of mental illness disrupt a person's care, so the symptoms also need to be treated. In this type of system, a central care provider or case manager is responsible for assessment, securing treatment, and referral to appropriate services. A central care coordinator does not usually provide the majority of the services, but the coordinator has the primary relationship with the patient. The disadvantages of this system are that the coordinator's evaluation of the patient's condition, the situation, or the system can limit the patient's care options and that when a case manager leaves, the patient experiences a major disruption in a primary relationship and often has difficulty continuing treatment or starting a new relationship. The advantages of this type of system are that the treatment is continuous and that the patient has someone to contact who will take action to coordinate care.

Many systems—whether they offer freedom of choice or continuity of care—operate on the concept of *episodes of care*, which follows the medical model in which, the patient uses the system only when his or her symptoms require care. The advantage of this model is that it has the potential to serve increased numbers of patients, because not all patients will require services at the same time. The disadvantage is that it does not make use of primary prevention. Patients often do not see a provider until they require acute intervention. Acute and inpatient intervention is more costly, both to the system and to the patient. Generally, the more severe the episode of illness, the longer and more difficult the recovery period, which results in more disruption to the patient's life.

CULTURAL CONSIDERATIONS IN COMMUNITY MENTAL HEALTH NURSING

People in every culture throughout the world can develop mental illness. Community mental health nurses have the challenge of identifying the diverse cultural populations within their community service areas and adapting or developing programs to meet the needs of these populations. A primary goal of hospitals, community health nurses, and nurse educators is to demonstrate approaches to care that are culturally sensitive and competent for persons of all cultures and ethnic groups. Community involvement, the development of trust, and cultural sensitivity training are all necessary components to accomplish this goal (Huggins, 2003), and are essential for patient and family compliance with treatment and medication regimens.

There are many cities with large populations of Filipino Americans, Japanese Americans, Latinos, and Asians, such as Vietnamese and Chinese citizens (Hampton, White and Chafetz, 2007; Sanchez and Gaw, 2007). There are also groups of Alaskan Natives and Native Americans with special needs who do not live on reservations or in rural areas (Substance Abuse and Mental Health Services Administration, 2009). An Urban Indian Health Program was established in San Diego to provide culturally sensitive care to these individuals with physical and mental health problems (Wilkie, 2008).

Every cultural group has traditions and beliefs about the acceptance of mental illness and the ability and willingness to trust health care providers. In addition, there are problems accessing care for migrant workers, refugees, and asylum seekers (Basok et al, 2009). Some members of the Jewish community view severe mental illness as a stigma. Recently, the impact of mental health has been included as a topic to be addressed as part of the Jewish Family Services program in regions across the country. Some Jewish service centers have taken a larger role than others, including the development of a website by the Jewish Family Service of MetroWest New Jersey called GotBlue.org. It has been noted that the focus on achievements among this population has frequently resulted in the unwillingness to address mental illness (Jampel, 2009).

African Americans represent 12% of the U.S. population; however, cultural biases, misunderstanding, and stigma regarding the mental health professions can result in inadequate treatment for this group. Socioeconomic status may also limit access to health services. African Americans are more likely to rely on family and religious groups (National

Alliance on Mental Illness, 2004). The rate of mental health issues is the same in all cultural groups, but African Americans have faced inequities with regard to access to health care (American Psychiatric Association, 2009).

Stigma is an issue for all cultural groups. In some groups, there is a sense of shame or failure, whereas others fear discrimination from health care providers. It is important for the community mental health nurse to understand that such a stigma will have a negative effect on the patient's ability to accept and comply with treatment (Pinto-Foltz and Logsdon, 2009).

Persons who live in rural communities are often unwilling to seek help for severe and persistent mental illness and often have limited access to psychiatric and mental health services.

Some cultures have a negative view toward mental illness, which causes some families to hide the existence of a mentally ill family member or refuse to allow the member to live with the family (Chou et al, 2004). Native Americans who live on tribal reservations often do not have contact with mental health providers and are unable or unwilling to travel to the nearest treatment center. In Japan, there is a social stigma related to schizophrenia that prompted the Japanese people to rename the disorder *togu schitcho sho (integration disorder)*. As a result of this name change, the number of individuals receiving treatment increased by more than 50% in 3 years (Sato, 2006). In some situations, Native Americans have benefited from telepsychiatry, where professionals maintain contact through the Internet (Shore and Manson, 2005). The Arab-American and Chaldean cultural sensitivity program in Detroit have bicultural and trilingual staff that serve these diverse populations in the mental health centers and in the community (Arab-American Chaldean Council, 2002). Understanding the cultural beliefs about mental illness and being sensitive to diverse ethnic and cultural groups is a critical goal for community mental health nurses.

Language can be a barrier for many people who need care. Often the meaning behind the spoken words or those that were not spoken is more important than what is said. Understanding what the symptoms mean to the individual is very different from knowing the symptoms without understanding how they affect the patient and his or her life (Gilmer et al, 2007). It is essential to have access to individuals who speak the common languages of their community (see Chapter 8).

COMPONENTS OF COMMUNITY MENTAL HEALTH CARE

Community Mental Health Programs

Community mental health programs, such as day-treatment programs, are outpatient programs that are staffed by interdisciplinary teams. They are available during the work week, allowing patients' families to go to work or complete other household tasks. Day-treatment programs provide services in 3- to 6-hour time blocks and include at least one of the basic

treatment components of group therapy (e.g., psychoeducational classes, skills training, environment therapy, activities). Most patients attend these programs voluntarily, although some individuals are ordered to attend the program as an alternative to inpatient treatment. Research shows that the combination of these treatment programs and medication therapy is more effective for preventing relapse than the use of medication alone.

In the field of psychiatric programming, there is a philosophic difference between therapy and rehabilitation. Although both are vital to the overall treatment of mentally ill patients and share the goals of preventing relapse and further deterioration, the difference is in the focus of treatment. Therapy focuses on reducing the patient's discomfort, symptoms, and illness to promote his or her adjustment in the community. Rehabilitation focuses on the development of a person's strengths and assets and the improvement of health by restoring or increasing the person's functioning in the community. There are four main models of community psychiatric programming: (1) partial hospitalization programs; (2) psychosocial rehabilitation and skills training programs; (3) assertive community treatment programs; and (4) the clubhouse model of psychosocial rehabilitation programs.

Partial Hospitalization Programs

Partial hospitalization programs provide the most intensive treatment of the therapeutic models. They offer short-term care that is similar to that provided in an inpatient setting, except the patient is able to return home each day. Patients enter partial hospitalization programs when they are discharged from the hospital but still require specific treatment on a partial basis. Partial hospitalization programs provide less than 24 hours of daily care and also meet the needs of individuals who are living in the community and who require a higher level of care (Murer, 2007).

Treatment goals are to reduce symptoms and increase the patient's functioning to a level that the patient is able to maintain outside of the hospital and as a member of the community. A nurse who is working in a partial hospitalization program monitors the patient's symptoms and mental status, facilitates groups, teaches psychoeducation classes, plans and implements activities, and works with a psychiatrist to monitor the therapeutic effects and the side effects of medications. Careful assessment is necessary to diagnose and intervene with patients who express suicidal thoughts or plans (see Chapter 22).

A recent study supported the implementation of evidence-based approaches that were designed to enhance recovery and the need for more flexible treatment options, such as patient-centered care instead of prescribed treatment programs (Yanos et al, 2009).

Psychosocial Rehabilitation and Skills Training Programs

Community-based psychosocial rehabilitation has been provided for persons with severe mental illness for more than 40 years. Patients who struggle with disturbed thoughts (delusions) or disturbed sensory perceptions (hallucinations) are often unable to think clearly, solve basic problems, or cope effectively with activities of daily living. They are often confused and disoriented, and may develop a sense of hopelessness and low-self esteem as they become more and more helpless to deal with life's challenges. They often lack skills in communicating their thoughts and emotions to others in order to get their basic needs met. **Psychosocial rehabilitation and skills training programs** are for patients who need skills training because of neurocognitive and neuropsychiatric deficits due to their mental disorders. The primary criterion for rehabilitation training is that the patient has a deficit in skill performance or lacks the skills that are necessary for living, learning, or working.

These programs are designed for patients who have the potential for growth and who are capable of developing the skills necessary to make personal choices and to manage their illness. The mental health workers assist patients with normalizing their relationships with themselves and others to help them to successfully integrate into the community. Patients receive training and education in managing the here-and-now problems of daily living.

Mental health professionals in these programs maintain an informal relationship with the patients and their families and everyone calls each other by their first names. This type of comfortable environment encourages the patient to learn the basic skills that are needed to relate to others. The staff addresses patients' rights and assists each patient with developing a sense of empowerment. Staff members also work with the patient's family or significant persons to achieve positive outcomes for everyone involved in the patient's life.

A nurse who is working in this environment assists the patient with developing a realistic plan of care designed to achieve effective outcomes based on the patient's identified needs or problems. The nurse also develops and teaches psychosocial education and skill-building classes that address the neurocognitive needs of the patients. Neurocognitive improvement has been shown to be strongly related to rates of psychosocial improvement (Brekke et al, 2009) (see Case Study #1 on this page, Chapter 13, and Self-care deficit nursing care plan in Chapter 16).

Programs for Assertive Community Treatment

Programs for Assertive Community Treatment (PACT) also known as Assertive Community Treatment (ACT) help people with severe and persistent mental illness to stay out of the hospital. The primary goal of these programs is to assist patients with the development of community living skills. A team of mental health practitioners is available 24 hours a day and 7 days a week and each professional is responsible for a caseload of up to 100 patients.

PACT/ACT teams are effective for reducing the length of inpatient stays, for increasing community involvement, and for working with housing to reduce homelessness. PACT/ACT teams are also actively involved with individual and group programs, including dual-diagnosis groups (Salyers

---

> ### CASE STUDY #1
>
> Mark is a 45-year-old man with a long history of chronic paranoid schizophrenia. He lives in a government-subsidized apartment, and attends the local clubhouse model of treatment 5 days a week. At the clubhouse, his primary job is washing dishes and serving food in the cafe. Within the clubhouse setting, Mark is socially appropriate and friendly. He exhibits no positive symptoms of hallucinations or delusions, but he has some negative symptoms of blunted affect, apathy, and compromised hygiene and daily living skills. Mark had expressed a desire to ride the bus, and the nurse offered to come to his apartment to teach him the bus route from his apartment to the clubhouse.
>
> When the nurse arrives at Mark's apartment, she sees that it is a health hazard. Mark's kitchen counters are covered with moldy dishes and cockroaches. Dirty laundry is piled throughout the house, and there is a bad odor. Mark has hidden salami under his couch, because he is afraid that the neighbors will steal it out of his refrigerator. There are cigarette burns on both the couch and the bed. There are no towels in the bathroom, because Mark says that he does not bathe or wash his hands after using the toilet.
>
> **Critical Thinking**
> 1 What is the nurse' primary concern?
> 2 How will this affect Mark' treatment plan? Rank the concerns from highest to lowest priority.
> 3 What resources discussed in this chapter will be useful in Mark' treatment?
> 4 How will the nurse discuss this with Mark?
> 5 Knowing the extent of Mark' compromised hygiene, what is the nurse's role in his selection of clubhouse jobs?
> 6 What can the nurse do to protect the health of other clubhouse members?
> 7 What are some interventions that the nurse can develop to help Mark work on this issue without embarrassing him in front of the clubhouse members, while still protecting others?
> 8 What symptoms of schizophrenia in particular will interfere with Mark' ability to understand the connection between his poor hygiene and his work at the clubhouse?

---

and Tsemberis, 2007). These programs are available in many cities throughout the United States (Community Mental Health Services, 2006) and have been effective according to evidence-based research.

Clubhouse Model

The **clubhouse model**, which was developed during the late 1940s, is a credentialed international program that provides a place where persons with severe and persistent mental illness can go to rebuild their lives. The participants are viewed as members rather than patients, and the emphasis is on the members' strengths rather than their weaknesses. Members and staff work as partners to help promote the members' independence. Members receive assistance with securing housing, medical care, entitlements, and psychiatric treatment. The focus in clubhouse programs is psychosocial rehabilitation, empowerment, support, and assistance with problem-solving behavior. Services available include laundry, clothing, telephones, and help with locating jobs and housing (Mowbray et al, 2006). The clubhouse model provides consistent and high-quality programs that are available during the evenings and weekends. The programs they offer include recreational, social, exercise, nutrition, weight loss, and individual support for each member according to his or her need (Fountain House, 2006; International Center for Clubhouse Development, 2006; Pelletier et al, 2005) (see Case Study #1).

Case Management

Case management is a system that coordinates care and reduces fragmented treatment for patients with severe and persistent mental illness. Psychiatric nurses often direct the case management multidisciplinary team that includes nurses, physicians, and social workers. The team members work together to manage cases, develop a plan of care for a specific patient population, and make appropriate referrals. The focus of case management is to support individuals and their families by combining and coordinating care or multiple services. Goals for case management are as follows:

- Identification and outreach
- Assessment
- Improving patient activities of daily living
- Service plan
- Monitoring

Case managers often identify patients during hospitalization. The work of the case manager includes monitoring the patient's symptoms, adherence to medication, and ability to function on a day-to-day basis. Case managers assess all aspects of a person's life to determine the patient's needs and his or her ability to meet those needs. Nurse case managers generally have caseloads that range from 10 to 25 patients, but they may manage up to 70 individuals. Case managers who are responsible for fewer patients are likely to see more effective outcomes from their interventions (Dube and Davis, n.d.).

Bradshaw and colleagues (2006) conducted a qualitative study of persons who were patients in mental health treatment and noted that these patients were discouraged by changes in their care providers. Participants reported that their relationships with their case managers were very important. and that they relied on their case managers to help them with life situations and crises.

The case manager advocates for the patient and the family by coordinating or providing services along the continuum of care. Effective case management minimizes health care costs to the patient, the family, and society (Box 30-1). The recommended minimum preparation for a nurse case manager is a baccalaureate degree in nursing with 3 years of clinical experience. Community psychiatric case management nurses are affected by their employing agency, public policy issues, and health care reimbursement (Cohen and Cesta, 2004).

| BOX 30-1 | **WHY CASE MANAGEMENT?** |

- Case management focuses on the full spectrum of the needs of patients, families, and significant others. Patient and family satisfaction within case management systems is generally high.
- A strong component of case management is the outcome orientation to care. The goal is to move the patient and family toward optimal care outcomes.
- Case management facilitates and promotes the coordination of patient care, thereby minimizing the fragmentation of treatment.
- Case management promotes cost-effective care by minimizing fragmentation, maximizing coordination, and facilitating the movement of the patient and family through the health care system.
- Case management maximizes and coordinates the contributions of all disciplines within the health care team.
- Case management responds to the needs of insurers and other third-party payers, specifically those related to outcome-based, cost-effective care.
- The needs of patients, providers, and payers all receive attention within a case management system. Case management represents a joining of clinical and financial interests, systems, and outcomes.
- Case management can be included in the marketing strategies of hospitals and other institutions to target patients, families, insurers, and employers.

Modified from the American Nurses Association: *Case management by nurses*, Washington, DC, 1992, American Nurses Association.

LEVELS OF ASSISTED LIVING

The most important aspect of the patient's adjustment is having a place to live within the community. Maslow's hierarchy of needs identifies food, shelter, and clothing as basic necessities that people must satisfy before they are able to progress to higher needs and levels of development (Maslow, 1954) (see Figure 1-1). People with psychiatric disorders are more likely than the average population to live in poor housing, to live in high-crime neighborhoods, and to pay a higher percentage of their income on housing (Gonzalez et al, 2001). Since the 1980s, communities have developed options along the continuum of community living arrangements to meet the needs of persons with psychiatric disabilities. Persons with severe mental illness who live in an adult family homes experience lower rehospitalization rates. Table 30-1 represents living arrangements along the continuum of care.

There are two basic types of residential treatment programs in which staff supervises patients 24 hours a day: (1) programs that are supported through foster care or (2) independent living programs. Supervised adult residential treatment programs provide onsite staff 24 hours a day for 4 to 16 residents. These programs are usually in group homes, halfway houses, respite programs, or intermediate care facilities. The patients benefit from both staff and peer support. The staff monitors patients' symptoms and manages their

TABLE 30-1	COMMUNITY LIVING ARRANGEMENTS			STRUCTURED LIVING FACILITIES		
	INDEPENDENT	SEMI INDEPENDENT	ADULT FAMILY HOME	BOARD-AND-CARE HOMES AND CONGREGATE CARE FACILITIES	SKILLED NURSING FACILITIES	INTENSIVE RESIDENTIAL TREATMENT FACILITIES
Description of Function	Lives on his or her own or with others, with no need for supervision	Shares responsibilities with two to four others	Family-type living situation	Structured living facility	Structured living facility	Need for highly structured, treatment-oriented residential living facility
	Has freedom to do as he or she wishes	Has a need for minimal structure and supervision	Does not require as much structure as structured living facilities and intensive residential care	Does not require as much structure as intensive residential care	Highly supervised 24-hour care	24-hour supervision
	Exhibits responsible behavior	Works toward independent living by concentrating on needed skills	Requires 24-hour supervision	24-hour care		Different levels of need and care
	Handles responsibilities and duties appropriately	Needs to live with others for ongoing support	Has some freedom and independence, as appropriate to individual abilities			
Patient criteria	Stable	Able to demonstrate most skills needed to live independently satisfactorily	Demonstrates ability to get along with others	Able to cooperate with others	Functioning level warrants needed care	Poor history of compliance with treatment and community living
	Able to demonstrate most skills needed to live independently satisfactorily	Able to cooperate with others	Follows house rules and treatment plan (if appropriate)	Follows house rules and structure	Unable to provide for himself or herself independently	Need for 24-hour supervision
	Demonstrates satisfactory performance of activities of daily living	Demonstrates satisfactory performance of activities of daily living	Able to structure his or her own time adequately		Follows facility rules and treatment plan	Follows facility rules and treatment plan
	Able to take medications on his or her own responsibly	Able to take medications on his or her own responsibly	Demonstrates satisfactory performance of activities of daily living			
	Structures his or her own time adequately	Structures his or her own time adequately	Able to take his or her own medications appropriately			

medical regimen. There is an emphasis on interpersonal relationships between patients and staff and between patients and their peers. The residents participate in communication, prevocational preparation, and life within the facility (Platt et al, 2002). The staff helps patients to qualify for health care and teaches them the basic self-care skills such as how to take medication as prescribed, how to describe medication side effects to their doctors, grooming and hygiene, and appropriate interpersonal behavior. Studies indicate that persons with severe mental illness want normalcy and work to participate in society. They want to be like others and to be independent members of the community. Social support and empowerment are important parts of these living arrangements (see Self-care deficit nursing care plan in Chapter 16). Congregate care facilities, or board-and-care homes, are group homes for persons with psychiatric illnesses that usually house 6 to 15 residents. Congregate care facilities have 24-hour supervision; they provide residents with food, housing, and daily living skills, and they supervise medication routines. Residents of these facilities often receive outpatient care at the local community mental health center, where they often receive free consultation to the congregate care facility.

Adult family homes (supportive housing programs) provide a quieter and more personal living arrangement for patients who need supervision. They are also called *adult foster homes*, because families agree to "adopt" one or two persons into their home and care for them. The patient becomes a part of the family structure and is expected to fit into the normal routines of the household. The adult family home provider supervises medication schedules if necessary and expects the patient to perform routine tasks of daily living. Adult family homes also assist the patient with acquiring the services and skills needed to live independently in the community. This type of home is beneficial to the patient who is not able to tolerate the larger numbers of persons in congregate care facilities; however, this structure is more difficult for patients who do not like the intimacy involved in being part of a family. A study of patients who lived in a homelike setting after discharge from a psychiatric facility described the problems that they experienced when trying to conform to a family setting. Nevertheless, the patients struggled to make it work, and they believed that their competence and confidence increased because of their efforts.

Semi-independent living is for persons who live with two to four other individuals in the community with minimal supervision. An independent living skills staff usually teaches residents life skills, such as cooking and budgeting. Although these individuals may prefer independent living, they express satisfaction with supportive housing arrangements (Hanrahan et al, 2001).

HOME VISITS

Many home health agencies provide psychiatric home health care. Home health nurses assess patients, their responses to treatment, and the safety of their living arrangements. The nurses also assess potential risk for emotional or physical harm from other household members.

Some studies estimate that 70% of mentally ill individuals live in the community, and in 1979, The Health Care Financing Administration determined that Medicare and Medicaid could reimburse psychiatric home health care. To be eligible for home care, patients are unable to leave their homes, they need to demonstrate a medical necessity, and they require occasional care. For example, a woman with schizophrenia lives alone in a small apartment. Her auditory, visual, and tactile hallucinations are controlled with bimonthly injections of the antipsychotic medication haloperidol (Haldol). Without the periodic home visits for the supervision and monitoring of her medical regimen, this patient's symptoms would become so disabling that she would require hospitalization.

A broad range of psychiatric home visits are reimbursed by third-party payers, with each payer having specific criteria for reimbursement. For example, the requirement for reimbursement by Medicare is that the primary care provider is a psychiatrist.

Safety

Psychiatric home visits vary with regard to focus, time spent, intensity, and outcome. It is crucial that the nurse who is planning a home visit evaluate the potential risks of that visit before beginning the actual interventions. Risk evaluation always includes the patient's history, relationship with the nurse, current mental status, and living situation. Visiting nurse programs and community mental health programs have specific guidelines that are designed to protect nurses. The nurse is a visitor in the patient's home and needs to maintain boundaries between self and patient and self and family members. Nurses have an understanding of the patient's history, the number of people in the residence, and the type of intervention required. The nurse calls in advance and arrives and departs as scheduled. It is important to evaluate the safety of the immediate neighborhood or any potential risk. Visits are cancelled if there are animals that appear to be out of control or any evidence of drug or criminal activity. Security personnel can be available to escort nurses in high-risk areas. The nurse should leave at once if there is a change in the patient's behavior, or if family members exhibit threatening behavior. Each visit requires careful documentation (Clevenger, 2008; Sheehan, 2000). Patients in the community who are in need of treatment are often resistant to inpatient settings. In these cases, the goal of the home visit is to connect the patient with the care system through contact with the nurse or case manager. Some patients are seen in their homes for several months before they enter a mental health center for treatment. Assertive outreach is helpful for patients who generally resist traditional office-based treatment (Salyers and Tsemberis, 2007) (see Case Study #2).

A home visit gives the nurse a broader understanding of the patient's functional abilities and endurance (e.g., with activities of daily living and independent living skills). It

CASE STUDY #2

Ken is a 19-year-old college student who was discharged from inpatient psychiatric services to independent living 2 weeks ago. He was originally brought to the hospital by four of his friends when he became drunk, belligerent, and threatening at a party. His friends reported that Ken's behavior had changed during the previous month. Before he was hospitalized, Ken began staying up all night, consuming large quantities of alcohol, and fighting with other dorm residents. He also got two speeding tickets in the previous week. In the hospital, Ken was diagnosed with bipolar I disorder, single manic episode. He was treated with lithium carbonate 300 mg three times a day and clonazepam (Klonopin) 2 mg at bedtime, and he was discharged with a week's supply of medication. Today, the nurse case manager received a call from Ken's apartment manager, who was concerned because Ken had sarcastically said that he would just go kill himself when he was asked to turn his music down. The manager reported that other tenants are complaining that Ken makes noise at all hours of the night. The nurse has not seen Ken since his discharge 2 weeks ago and is unable to reach him by telephone.

Nursing Diagnoses

1 Risk for self-directed violence/risk for other-directed violence. Risk factors: verbal suicidal threat, manic excitement, increased motor activity, and provocative behaviors (consumes large amounts of alcohol, speeding tickets, fighting)

2 Risk for injury. Risk factors: destructive behaviors and hyperactivity, increased agitation, and potentially injurious behavior (drinking alcohol, speeding, fighting)

3 Insomnia related to manic excitement as evidenced by staying up all night, hyperactivity, and agitation

4 Impaired social interaction related to manic excitement as evidenced by dysfunctional interaction with peers and others (exhibits belligerent behavior with peers, threatens others, plays loud music, makes noise all night)

Critical Thinking

1 What factors should the nurse consider when making a decision about a home visit?

2 What assessments need to be performed when the nurse sees Ken? How should they be prioritized?

3 How will the nurse assess Ken's personal safety? What about the safety of others?

4 What other information is needed to complete the nursing assessment?

5 What other diagnoses from the *Diagnostic and Statistical Manual of Mental Disorders*, fourth edition, text revision, need to be explored at this point?

6 If Ken refuses to be seen or responds defensively or with denial, how should the nurse respond?

7 How should the nurse proceed with getting help for Ken while also protecting himself or herself?

PATIENT AND FAMILY TEACHING GUIDELINES

*Schizophrenia**

Teach the Patient

- Schizophrenia is a brain disorder that requires both medication and psychosocial therapy.
- Withdrawal is a common symptom, and it is important to communicate with health care providers when beginning to feel more reluctant or afraid to interact with people.
- It sometimes takes months to get the symptoms under control. Increased involvement in therapy leads to a better outcome.

Teach the Patient's Family

- Schizophrenia is a brain disease that affects 1% of the world' population. The brain disease has nothing to do with how the patient was raised. Chronic brain diseases put special stressors on the family. The National Alliance on Mental Illness, and other organizations, assist families

with the emotional burden; decrease isolation; and provide education, support, and other resources.

- High levels of expressed negative emotion within the family system sometimes worsen the symptoms of schizophrenia. It is important for all family members to find appropriate ways to express their grief and to deal with conflict.
- Prescribed medications for the patient are important and require supervision and monitoring by the family to ensure effectiveness and to evaluate symptoms.
- Local mental health centers and some school districts sometimes provide support groups to the parents and siblings of persons with mental disorders.

*See Chapter 13.

expands the nurse's knowledge of how the patient manages basic tasks in his or her own environment, on a daily basis (see the Patient and Family Teaching Guidelines box).

Neurocognitive deficits associated with mental illnesses frequently interfere with patient learning and, some patients are unable to perform a learned skill when the setting changes. A home visit is an effective approach for teaching

basic independent living skills to patients who experience transfer-of-learning deficits. During home learning, a patient has the opportunity to use his or her own equipment in a familiar setting, which increases the potential for task retention. The nurse can work with the patient and family to develop a plan to prevent and manage a relapse and teach them about the signs and symptoms of relapse.

THE HOMELESS MENTALLY ILL POPULATION

Homelessness is a major problem throughout the country as a result of poverty, unemployment, underemployment, substance abuse, and mental illness. Men are more likely to be homeless, as are the racial and ethnic populations in specific areas of the country. There have been numerous studies to determine the number of homeless persons in each state and major city.

In his extensive study on homeless persons in the Chicago area, Rossi (1991) reported that the leading cause of homelessness is the failure of the person's social network. The family support was most likely to fail when a dependent male drained the emotional and financial support of the household. This was more apparent when the family was poor and struggling for survival.

It has been reported that 20% to 25% of the homeless population has a severe mental illness that interferes with an individual's ability to form relationships with family or care providers. Persons with severe mental illness are noncompliant with medication as a result of a lack of finances, a lack of stability, and the inability to trust others to help them. In addition to uncontrolled mental illness, the homeless mentally ill population has poor hygiene and multiple health problems. It is expected that 40% of mentally ill patients are also substance abusers (Coalition for the Homeless Mentally Ill, 2003; National Coalition of Homelessness, 2009).

Racial and ethnic differences play a significant role in the family's response to mentally ill members. Some cultural groups are protective of the ill individual, whereas others soon become exhausted and emotionally drained with the care, dependency needs, and symptoms of the ill person.

Severely mentally ill persons move in and out of homelessness because of their symptoms or because they have stopped taking their medications. Attempting to live a homeless existence and struggling to acquire food, shelter, and protection every day is difficult even for a healthy person. Some patients seek shelter in places that they believe to be safe, such as in tunnels, caves, secluded parks, or under bridges. If they were to become ill or injured, they would be unable to help themselves and might even die without being found for days or weeks.

The more disengaged these individuals are from society, the more difficult it is to offer them the services that they need.

The number of homeless women has increased with the increase in poverty and inadequate housing, yet only 15% of all homeless persons are female. Homeless women tend to be young mothers with young children, single adults, or older women with psychopathology.

It is estimated that 25% of homeless women have serious mental health problems. One study reported that 41% of these women had major mental disorders (e.g., schizophrenia, mood disorders) and that another 44% of the same group demonstrated severe anxiety disorders. Unmarried adult homeless women with serious mental illness tend to have a history that is similar to that of men with serious mental illness. These women have a high rate of alcoholism or substance abuse that coexists with personality disorders or other mental disorders. They associate with one or more men for companionship and safety, or they live a solitary existence, living in fear of assault and rape. Older homeless women with serious mental illness are disaffiliated (i.e., they do not associate with family, friends, or service providers). They are more likely to have psychotic disorders that are also associated with alcoholism. The more that the person is disaffiliated from normal society, the greater his or her distance is from care providers.

> ### ❖ CLINICAL ALERT #1
>
> Women with severe and persistent mental disorders are of great risk for victimization, and children with mentally ill parents are at a significant risk for physical or mental problems or disorders (Scholler-Jaquish, 2000).

Contrary to public opinion, homeless persons are not all alike. Unfortunately, public policies and treatment programs service the "typical" homeless person. The Scholler-Jaquish intervention model for homeless persons (Scholler-Jaquish, 2008) provides a way to plan care and services for the severely mentally ill homeless population in accordance with identifiable needs (Table 30-2). The model is organized into three stages of homelessness and three levels of public health prevention. The levels of prevention include primary, secondary, and tertiary prevention. Primary prevention addresses prevention, health promotion, and education. Secondary prevention includes screening, the treatment of illness, and the reduction of disability. Tertiary prevention includes rehabilitation and palliative care (i.e., care that relieves pain or discomfort).

In stage 1, the homeless mentally ill persons are newly diagnosed and they maintain contact with service providers and family members. These individuals are the most likely to secure a place to sleep and eat, and they are the most open to outreach services and treatment.

In stage 2, the homeless mentally ill persons have few connections with conventional society and are more likely to be admitted when their psychiatric symptoms increase. They are likely to rely on alcohol or drugs to control their psychiatric symptoms. Individuals with bipolar mania are more likely to use alcohol for symptom control. Persons with schizophrenia also use alcohol to reduce the intensity of their hallucinations. Individuals who are depressed are more likely to rely on opiates for relief. These individuals may be helped if assistance is readily available, but they may not be able to approach care providers on their own. Sometimes, they are in such a state of distress that they appear frightening to emergency health care workers and are therefore rejected.

In stage 3, the homeless mentally ill persons are unconnected with society. They have no access to medications, but they sometimes respond to outreach workers who provide food or first-aid measures. This vulnerable population has

TABLE 30-2	NURSING INTERVENTION MODEL FOR HOMELESS PERSONS		
	STAGE 1	**STAGE 2**	**STAGE 3**
Primary prevention	Advocacy Promotion of low-income housing and increase in minimum wage Drug and alcohol education and treatment programs Access to health care Coping skills Job training AIDS prevention Aggression management Community mental health centers Mental health programs for ethnic and racial minorities Promoting legislation for the homeless mentally ill population	Advocacy Self-advocacy Preventing violence Interpersonal skills training Anger management Immunizations (e.g., influenza, pneumonia) Legal assistance programs Access to health care Access to mental health care Drug and alcohol treatment programs at service centers	Advocacy Multiservice outreach centers Wet detoxification* programs
Secondary prevention	Diagnostic services Mental health screenings Treatment programs for drugs, alcohol, and mental illness Illness prevention	Monitor psychiatric status Monitor compliance with medical regimens for tuberculosis and AIDS Wet detoxification	Mobile treatment programs (i.e., provide care for patient where they are or in walk-in clinics) Monitor changes in physical or mental status Monthly antipsychotic medications, if accepted Treatment for tuberculosis Access to basic nutrition
Tertiary prevention	Treatment of chronic mental illness Drug and alcohol treatment programs Case management Symptom management	Treatment for mental illness Treatment for major health problems Wet and dry detoxification programs	Wet detoxification Nutrition Outreach mental health services

*Wet detoxification refers to a controversial method that allows homeless persons who are powerless to overcome their alcohol addiction a place to live and to continue drinking during treatment.

little or no relief from their psychiatric symptoms and providing health care to them requires caregivers who are willing and able to manage their multiple and complex problems (Scholler-Jaquish, 2008).

VIOLENCE AND THE MENTALLY ILL POPULATION

Seriously mentally ill persons are more likely to harm themselves than others and have a 16% likelihood of being assaultive as compared with a 7% likelihood among the general population. It is important to remember that the rate of serious mental illness in the general population is estimated to be 3% to 5% (Friedman, 2006). Individuals who experience symptoms of visual, auditory, or tactile hallucinations often injure themselves or others during their hallucinatory experiences.

Some persons with severe and persistent mental illness have command hallucinations that instruct them to hurt or kill themselves or others. These individuals require careful monitoring by mental health professionals and family members. Even mental health workers are unable to protect themselves from violent assaults. For example, there was a case that involved a patient with schizophrenia who beat his

psychiatrist to death in the psychiatrist's office (Friedman, 2006). Unfortunately, a child or parent with mental illness may kill family members who mistakenly believe that they are able to manage the mentally ill person. Sometimes family members deny or miss threats or behaviors that are indicative of violence. Unfortunately, since the 1990s, there has been an increase in the number of mass murders by mentally ill persons, such as the 2007 incident at Virginia Tech and the 2011 shooting at a Tucson, Arizona, political event. Both young men involved in those situations had an extensive history of unusual behavior, and one of them had received some treatment for mental illness. Current laws do not go far enough to prevent mentally ill persons from purchasing guns, including automatic weapons, which can shoot many bullets in succession, resulting in more victims (Norris and Price, 2009). These incidents highlight the need for greater access to mental health care and changes in gun laws. Community mental health nurses are responsible for protecting themselves, the patient, the patient's family, and other individuals from a patient with command hallucinations that are instructing the patient to kill his or her classmates, employees, coworkers, political figures, health care givers, or family members. Angry employees, former employees, or patients have committed violent acts and killed people associated with the organizations or employers that they have come to hate or fear. Some of these individuals have been identified as persons with known psychiatric histories, or persons whose behaviors were described as "odd" or "unusual" for a long period of time as noted in the above examples.

A study of violence among severe and persistent mentally ill persons reported that noncompliance with psychotropic medications, substance abuse, and poor insight are significant factors that work together to increase the risk of violence. In addition, being a member of an ethnic minority and being victimized add to the risk for violent acts (Busko, 2009) (see Chapter 23).

The predictors of violence include the following:
- History of violence
- Noncompliance with medications
- Drug and alcohol abuse
- Serious mental illness in combination with a failure to take medication
- Neurologic impairment
- Paranoid delusions
- Command hallucinations

Severely mentally ill persons with negative symptoms are sometimes victims of abuse by others. including, family members or care providers. Physically, sexually, or emotionally abused mentally disabled persons are reluctant to tell others for fear of losing the security that they have. At other times, patients have tried to tell mental health workers, but the health care providers have not understood or believed them.

Police officers often have to deal with mentally or emotionally disturbed persons and some officers are specially trained to respond to psychiatric emergencies; however, there have been incidents in which police officers have used excessive or deadly force when dealing with mentally ill persons including killing persons who were attempting suicide. Some reports also state that emotionally troubled people carrying weapons or other lethal objects have been shot multiple times by police officers, sometimes resulting in death. In one instance, a woman with psychosis who refused to leave her home for several days was killed by the local police officers when she stepped outside of the house (Amnesty International, 2002).

Community mental health nurses need to engage in community education for law enforcement agencies and other emergency responders. The most effective intervention plan is the Memphis Plan, in which teams of police officers receive special training in crisis intervention. After the situation is resolved, the disturbed person is taken to a psychiatric facility instead of to a police department (Amnesty International, 2002).

MENTALLY ILL PERSONS IN THE CRIMINAL JUSTICE SYSTEM

The incarceration of mentally ill persons is an urgent national problem. As many as 300,000 to 400,000 mentally ill individuals are in prison (Leifman, 2004). These mentally ill

---

❖ CLINICAL ALERT #2

Be constantly alert for suicidal ideation and intent in persons with mental illness. The period of highest risk is often during the first month out of the hospital after the patient has been discharged. Patients with schizophrenia who hear voices (i.e., auditory command hallucinations) that instruct them to harm themselves are at equal or greater risk for suicide than patients with depression. One predictor of suicidal risk is a history of previous attempts and the lethality of those attempts (Fortinash and Holoday Worret, 2008).

---

persons make up 15% of the total prison population as compared with 5% of the general population. A prevalence study of mentally ill inmates reported a rate of 9% to 16% for men and from 10% to 20% for women (Steadman et al, 2009). Inmates with diagnoses of schizophrenia, major depressive disorders, bipolar disorder, and nonpsychotic disorders were most likely to have recurrent disorders (Baillargeon et al, 2009). A study supported by the American Psychiatric Association indicates that as many as 70% of persons who are in prison for nonviolent offenses have a co-occurring substance abuse problem and that there are more nonwhites in the prison system (Goin, 2004).

Some individuals are arrested for minor offenses and are held in the local jail. Mentally ill persons are sometimes arrested because no treatment facilities are available. They are often arrested for minor offenses, such as vagrancy, trespassing, disorderly conduct, or failure to pay for a meal. Jails are inadequately prepared to care for the severely mentally ill offender who is able to refuse to take psychotropic medications. The suicide rate among mentally ill offenders is higher than it is for any other group of offenders (Open Society Institute, 2002; www.ocpp.org/2003/issue031211-2.pdf).

Family members often find it necessary to have a relative with severe and persistent mental illness arrested for violent or threatening behavior. In some situations, emergency involuntary admissions require that the person who is making the arrest or signing the commitment orders also has to witness the violent behavior. If that does not happen, the individual is jailed for his or her mental illness rather than admitted to a psychiatric facility. Many persons with severe mental illness serve long-term prison sentences with a minimal amount of psychiatric treatment. There is a concern that prison facilities are becoming like the asylums of the past. Factors involved in the incarceration of mentally ill persons include the following:
- Homelessness
- Attitude of the community
- Attitude of the police force
- More strict commitment criteria
- Lack of adequate community support

Prisons usually direct the treatment of mentally ill prisoners toward symptom management rather than illness management, which results in disciplinary treatment. Severely mentally ill inmates are likely to remain in prison for longer periods of time than other prisoners with similar offenses;

when they are finally released into an unstructured life with no prospect of rehabilitation, they are often unable to control their behavior, and they are likely to return to prison.

Nursing responsibilities in correctional institutions vary and include the following:

- Assessing suicide risk
- Evaluating mental status
- Monitoring the effectiveness of medications
- Providing a link between prisoners and community caregivers
- Generating care when needed
- Providing general mental health treatment
- Educating prisoners and prison staff about mental illness

Laws concerning the administration of psychotropic medications often frustrate nurses who are working with mentally ill prisoners. The medications are often necessary to contain patients' aggressive or violent behaviors. However, the law protects a prisoner's right to refuse psychotropic medication. Unfortunately, when persons who are unable to think clearly because of mental illness refuse psychotropic medication, the result is both dangerous and tragic. Dorothea Dix (1802-1887), a historic pioneer and advocate in mental health nursing, would be stunned to find mentally ill prisoners with out-of-control behavior confined to their cells and living in subhuman conditions because of a lack of appropriate medications and other critical treatments for their illnesses.

MENTALLY ILL PERSONS WITH HUMAN IMMUNODEFICIENCY VIRUS

Persons with severe and persistent mental illness who are living in the community are likely to be sexually active and to exhibit high-risk sexual behaviors that put them at risk for HIV disease. It is the role of the mental health nurse and the interdisciplinary team to develop HIV prevention programs for their patients and significant others and to strongly encourage the development of safe, healthy, long-term relationships for their patients (Community Mental Health Service, 2006). Severely mentally ill persons who abuse substances have a greater risk of developing HIV disease, including those with diagnoses of depression, mania impulsivity, cognitive impairment, and substance abuse (Devieux et al, 2007; Hammond and Treisman, 2007). It is important that nurses set aside their own personal values about sex and recognize that mentally ill persons have the same sexual needs and desires as the general population. When sexuality is accepted as a basic human condition, then the nurse can begin to ask relevant and nonjudgmental questions about the patient's sexual activity. Some registered nurses who were assigned to work in a homeless health care clinic avoided asking homeless men about their sexual activity because it was against their personal values for people to have sex outside of marriage (Scholler-Jaquish, 1993). Substance abuse increases the probability of high-risk sexual behavior. Some nurses feel uncomfortable asking their patients about sexual activity, but it is an important element of health care for individual patients and for the health of the community at large (see Chapter 20).

OTHER COMPONENTS OF COMMUNITY PSYCHIATRIC MENTAL HEALTH NURSING

Community psychiatric mental health nursing typically involves crisis intervention with both individuals and groups. Many communities have special multidisciplinary teams of mental health professionals who provide psychiatric care as a component of disaster relief (see Chapter 21).

The natural disasters Hurricanes Katrina and Rita, which made landfall along Louisiana within a month of each other in 2005, resulted in the displacement of tens of thousands of human beings. The evacuees included severe and persistently mentally ill persons who experienced the loss of homes and loved ones as well as the emotional confusion of being subjected to multiple stressors. These mentally ill persons had no medication or support systems. Persons with psychotic symptoms were referred to mental health programs throughout the Southern and Midwestern states. Representatives from community health systems screened evacuees as they arrived by bus or train to identify persons who needed immediate attention. Mental health professionals and other relief responders faced challenges that exceeded all available emergency preparations. In such situations, providing antipsychotic medications to patients in need as quickly as possible reduces the risk of injury to patients or others.

Patients who have severe psychiatric symptoms during a community disaster need to be held in a psychiatric hospital against their will for their own safety or for the safety of the community. Community psychiatric mental health nurses need to be knowledgeable about involuntary psychiatric treatment (see Chapter 9). In addition, a comprehensive understanding of nursing interventions and other treatment methods are essential. Medication management is a fundamental role of the community psychiatric mental health nurse regardless of the care setting. Knowledge of psychopharmacology, therapeutic effects and side effects of psychotropic medications are mandatory requirements (see Chapter 25).

⊚ NURSING CARE PLAN

Bentley, a 32-year-old man with a history of psychosis, was brought to the emergency department by the police for violent behavior. He was admitted to the behavioral health unit in the hospital for psychiatric care. He had been treated in the same hospital in the past, and he had also been committed to a state psychiatric hospital three times in the past 10 years.

Bentley was the third of six children, and he appeared to behave normally until he had an onset of psychosis at the age of 16 years, with episodes of hallucinations and aggression and intermittent periods of mutism (i.e., not speaking) for long periods of time. He was placed on antipsychotic medication, and he continued to live at home until he was 26 years old, when his parents thought he would do better in a residential supervised treatment facility so that his medications could be administered on a regular basis. During the past 6 years, Bentley has lived in several different treatment facilities, and he continued to have problems with medication compliance.

When Bentley ran out of his antipsychotic medication 4 weeks ago, he became aggressive and threatened another

resident, and he accused that resident of stealing his money. When the resident manager tried to intervene, Bentley became upset and ran away. His family was unable to find him until they were notified that he was in the emergency department.

Bentley had been living on the street and in missions for the homeless since he ran away. The police had been called to a soup kitchen because of Bentley's paranoid and aggressive behavior. He was uncooperative and aggressive toward the staff and others, and he became violent when approached. Bentley also fought with the police until they were able to restrain him and take him to the hospital. He had been without antipsychotic drugs for almost 1 month.

On admission to the unit, Bentley was actively hallucinating and talking to an unseen presence. His affect was flat, and his movements were slow. When approached by the staff or other patients, Bentley either ignored them or spoke in a rude tone of voice. He has no history of drug or alcohol abuse. He was unkempt, and his clothing was soiled.

DSM-IV-TR Diagnoses

Axis I   Schizophrenia, undifferentiated, chronic, with acute exacerbation

Axis II   Deferred

Axis III   Deferred

Axis IV   Severity of psychologic stress: chronic as a result of severe mental illness, noncompliance with medications, unable to maintain stable living environment

Axis V   GAF = 30 (current); GAF = 50 (past year)

Nursing Diagnosis   *Risk for other-directed violence. Risk factors: patient's paranoid, aggressive, and belligerent behavior; auditory hallucinations that could be command type (i.e., telling the patient to harm others); stopping antipsychotic medications for 1 month; history of psychosis (unreality); unable to get along with family and caregivers*

NOC Aggression self-control; Stress level; Impulse self-control; Risk detection; Community risk control: violence; Distorted thought self-control

NIC Anger control assistance; Anxiety reduction; Environmental management: violence prevention; Distraction; Reality orientation; Medication management

PATIENT OUTCOMES	NURSING INTERVENTIONS	EVALUATION
Bentley will not act out in aggressive or violent behavior toward others in the unit.	Prevent Bentley from acting out in an aggressive or violent manner with the use of the following: 1. Close observation by staff 2. Therapeutic communication that builds trust and reduces anxiety 3. Administration of prescribed medication *This is done to maintain the safety of everyone on the unit, which is the first nursing priority.*	Bentley has not demonstrated violence or aggression toward others on the unit. He is open to communication strategies, and he accepts staff direction and prescribed medications.
Bentley will seek staff when feeling anxious or when hallucinations begin.	Make Bentley continuously familiar with the nursing unit and with the events and activities that are going on *to present reality in a nonthreatening way.*	Bentley tells staff when he is feeling anxious or when his hallucinations begin.
Bentley will understand the staff's communication and will ask them to explain words that are not clear to him.	Use clear, concrete statements and avoid abstract concepts when speaking *to help Bentley to understand the message, because persons with schizophrenia lose the ability to understand concepts.*	Bentley is trying his best to understand the nursing staff and asks them to explain words that are not clear to him.

NURSING CARE PLAN—cont'd

PATIENT OUTCOMES	NURSING INTERVENTIONS	EVALUATION
Bentley will feel safe and worthwhile in the mental health environment.	Reassure Bentley that he is safe and that he will not be harmed *to help him begin to trust the staff and the environment and to increase his self-esteem.*	Bentley states to the nurses that he feels safe and wanted on the unit and that he is sure no one will harm him.
Bentley is aware of the behavior brought on by his hallucinations versus the behavior that occurs with treatment, including his antipsychotic medications.	Help Bentley see the differences between his hallucinatory behavior and his behavior after treatment, including with his antipsychotic medications, *to help him see the importance of medication and other treatments for the management of his hallucinations.*	Bentley says that he has noticed an improvement in his behavior when he follows the treatment program. He joins in unit activities, and he takes his medication every day.
Bentley will be able to hold most conversations with staff, other patients, and family members without interference from hallucinations.	Help Bentley to focus on real events or activities *to reinforce reality and to divert Bentley's attention from his hallucinations.*	Bentley holds several conversations with staff, other patients, and family members without evidence of hallucinations.
Bentley will name the stressors that trigger the hallucinations, and he will try to avoid or reduce them.	Help Bentley to identify stressors that trigger his hallucinations *to teach Bentley, his family, and his residential supervisors how to avoid or reduce his hallucinations.*	Bentley lists two stressors that provoke his hallucinations: (1) stopping his medication and (2) too much stimulation, especially loud noises.
Bentley will state that he feels calmer knowing that he is accepted as a person with real feelings and not just as "someone who is hearing voices."	Encourage Bentley to discuss his feelings as well as his hallucinations *to demonstrate an understanding and acceptance of him as a person and to reduce his anxiety, which will help to reduce his hallucinations.*	Bentley is able to identify three feelings: anxiety, frustration, and anger. He says that he feels calmer when he expresses his feelings to the nursing staff.
Bentley shows a reduction in anxiety and hallucinations after using the techniques and strategies recommended by the nursing team and his physician.	Teach Bentley anxiety-reducing techniques and strategies such as exercising, joining an activity, listening to music, watching a favorite video, clapping, whistling, or telling the voices to "go away" when the hallucinations are too intrusive *to help reduce his anxiety and hallucinations and to get him involved in more positive and rewarding activities.*	Bentley demonstrates the effective use of techniques, activities, and strategies to manage his feelings of anxiety and his hallucinations before discharge.
Bentley will demonstrate trust in the staff and the treatment program, and he will continue to take his medication as an outpatient. He will return to his residential treatment facility and visit his parents.	Provide a consistent and structured setting that encourages the patient to join activities and to continue taking his medication and completing his other treatments in a safe and accepting setting *to promote the patient's trust, safety, sense of well-being, and desire to continue treatment after discharge.*	Bentley expresses relief that his "voices" were significantly reduced and nearly eliminated at times. He credits the staff's treatment of him as a human being with real feelings as well as the structured treatment program and medication.
Bentley will continue to attend groups and activities as an outpatient, and he will continue to take medication. He will notify support persons at the first sign of returning symptoms.	Have the nurse case manager help Bentley to make the transition to outpatient care and to continue his treatment and medication *to reduce the risk of symptoms returning.*	Bentley is making a successful transition to outpatient care; he continues to attend groups and activities of daily living classes, and he takes his medication every day with supervision. He says that he will call support persons at the first sign of hallucinations.

Nursing Diagnosis *Social isolation related to negative experiences of aloneness, auditory hallucinations, withdrawal from the community, and defensive behaviors as evidenced by living apart from family; running away from the residential facility, care providers, and the environment; talking to "internal voices"; noncommunicative and belligerent behaviors; flat affect; and minimal or absent eye contact*

Continued

⊚ NURSING CARE PLAN—cont'd

NOC Loneliness severity; Aggression self-control; Social support; Social involvement; Family social climate; Communication; Leisure participation; Social interaction skills

NIC Socialization enhancement; Support system enhancement; Activity therapy; Family therapy; Environmental management; Self-esteem enhancement

PATIENT OUTCOMES	NURSING INTERVENTIONS	EVALUATION
Bentley will interact socially with nursing staff, therapists, and other patients.	Engage Bentley in meaningful and nonthreatening individual and group interactions every day *to let the patient know that participation is expected and that he is a worthwhile member of the community.*	Bentley says that he is willing to participate in social interactions on the unit.
Bentley will demonstrate appropriate social behaviors in one-to-one and group interactions.	Role-model individual and group social behaviors for Bentley *to help Bentley to learn appropriate social skills.*	Bentley has successfully interacted socially in both individual and group settings.
Bentley will participate in social activities such as meals and games with family members and other patients as well as therapeutic activities such as exercise, arts, and crafts.	Help Bentley to socialize with trusted family members and to seek out other patients who have similar interests *to promote more comfortable and enjoyable socialization and therapeutic activities.*	Bentley participates in social and therapeutic activities on the unit and has social contact with his family.
Bentley will continue to seek out others to socialize with who have interests that are similar to his own.	Praise Bentley for his attempts to seek out others with similar interests *to promote continued positive socialization.*	Bentley continuously seeks out other patients with similar interests for social interactions and unit activities.
Bentley's family will have more contact with him.	Encourage Bentley's family to call him on the telephone and to visit him on the unit. *A strong family network will increase Bentley's social contacts and promote self-esteem.*	Bentley's family calls and visits him frequently.
Bentley will express pleasure from social conversations with other patients, staff, and family members.	Provide Bentley with social activities according to his level of tolerance *to gradually expose him to more complex social interactions.*	Bentley expresses pleasure when participating in social activities before discharge.
Bentley will attend unit outings with other patients.	Provide opportunities for Bentley to go on outings *to encourage a variety of more complex social experiences.*	Bentley engages in social conversations and activities during outings with other patients.
Bentley will participate in social activities within his overall capabilities.	Encourage Bentley to engage in social activities that are within his physical and mental capabilities *to provide him with successful social experiences.*	Bentley participates in social activities that he is able to effectively accomplish and enjoy.

Nursing Diagnosis *Impaired verbal communication related to disturbed thought processes (paranoia), disturbed sensory perceptions (hallucinations), and the inability to process and use language effectively when interacting with others (all secondary to chronic schizophrenia) as evidenced by speaking minimally or not speaking for long periods of time, defensive communications, flat affect, and lack of eye contact*

NOC Distorted thought self-control; Sensory function status; Cognitive orientation; Information processing; Communication; Patient satisfaction: communication

NIC Anxiety reduction; Active listening; Communication enhancement: speech deficit; Art therapy; Learning facilitation; Support system enhancement

PATIENT OUTCOMES	NURSING INTERVENTIONS	EVALUATION
Bentley will communicate his thoughts in a coherent and goal-directed manner with reduced anxiety.	Demonstrate a calm, quiet appearance rather than attempting to force Bentley to speak *to show acceptance and to reduce anxiety.*	Bentley communicates his thoughts and feelings in a goal-directed and calm manner.

⊚ NURSING CARE PLAN—cont'd

PATIENT OUTCOMES	NURSING INTERVENTIONS	EVALUATION
Bentley will respond positively to the nursing staff's active listening and the close attention that they pay to his communication style.	Actively listen and observe Bentley's verbal and nonverbal cues during the communication process *to show interest in meeting his needs and to indicate his self-worth.*	Bentley tries hard to use effective verbal and nonverbal methods to express his needs to the staff. He states, "I feel good that they care enough to try to understand me."
Bentley will express satisfaction with having his needs met, even if he has difficulty communicating those needs.	Anticipate Bentley's needs until he is able to communicate them effectively *to provide for Bentley's safety and comfort.*	Bentley is verbalizing his satisfaction that staff members are able to meet his needs for safety and comfort.
Bentley will demonstrate reality-based thoughts in brief 3- to 5-minute verbal conversations with others, beginning with his peers.	Teach Bentley to approach other patients for conversations about basic subjects that they all have in common, such as how their day is going or what activities they like *to allow Bentley to practice simple and realistic communication skills with his own peers in a safe setting.*	Bentley is able to maintain reality-based verbal conversations with his peers for 5 minutes.
Bentley will actively listen and give realistic responses to staff and other patients during individual and group activities.	Instruct Bentley to listen and respond to the specific topics of discussion with staff and other patients in individual and group activities *to encourage Bentley to respond to reality rather than listen to his own thoughts.*	Bentley is able to listen and respond realistically to topics of discussion with staff and other patients during individual and group activities.
Bentley will use strategies to decrease anxiety to help him to focus on realistic thoughts and meaningful verbal communication.	Teach Bentley anxiety-reducing strategies such as deep breathing, replacing irrational or negative thoughts with realistic ones (cognitive therapy), and seeking out a supportive person to help guide him when he first experiences impaired verbal communication *to decrease anxiety, which will promote more functional speech patterns.*	Bentley is able to identify and use effective strategies to control his anxiety. He uses effective verbal communication skills without signs of problematic thinking before discharge.
Bentley will continue to engage in realistic and meaningful conversations with others.	Praise Bentley for his realistic and meaningful conversations with others *to increase his self-esteem and to promote continued functional speech patterns.*	Bentley continues to use meaningful and logical speech in his conversations with others. He says, "Positive feedback makes me feel proud."

Nursing Diagnosis *Self-care deficit (bathing/hygiene, dressing/grooming) related to disturbed sensory perceptions and disturbed thought processes (secondary to schizophrenia) as evidenced by withdrawal from reality (hallucinations, isolation, paranoia) and the impaired ability to perform functions of hygiene, dressing, or grooming (i.e., he appears unbathed and disheveled)*

NOC Self care: bathing; Self-care: hygiene; Self-care: dressing; Anxiety self-control; Cognition; Self-direction of care; Comfort level; Patient satisfaction: physical care

NIC Self-care assistance: bathing/hygiene; Self-care assistance: dressing/grooming; Teaching: individual; Self-responsibility facilitation; Body image enhancement

PATIENT OUTCOMES	NURSING INTERVENTIONS	EVALUATION
Bentley will consistently perform adequate personal hygiene and grooming and dressing functions.	Assist Bentley with personal hygiene, grooming, dressing, and other activities of daily living skills until he can function independently *to preserve Bentley's dignity and self-esteem and to help him to avoid the negative responses of other patients.*	Bentley performs all self-care activities of hygiene, dressing, and grooming in an appropriate manner before discharge.

Continued

◎ NURSING CARE PLAN—cont'd

PATIENT OUTCOMES	NURSING INTERVENTIONS	EVALUATION
Bentley will perform daily routines of self-care, beginning with simple tasks and progressing to more complex functions.	Establish daily routines for Bentley's self-care functions and add more complex tasks as his condition improves *to help Bentley to organize his chaotic world and to promote his successful self-care.*	Bentley is able to complete all self-care functions before discharge.
Bentley will be able to verbalize the positive feelings that result from his self-care task performance.	Praise Bentley for his attempts at self-care and each completed task *to increase his feelings of self-worth and to promote continued self-care.*	Bentley expresses feelings of pride and self-respect after successfully performing self-care tasks. He states, "I feel like a worthwhile person now that I can do my own personal care."

GAF, Global Assessment of Functioning; NIC, Nursing Interventions Classification; NOC, Nursing Outcomes Classification.

CHAPTER SUMMARY

- Community psychiatric mental health services have greatly increased since the 1960s.
- Community psychiatric mental health programming is an essential element of the treatment of persons with severe and persistent mental illness.
- Case management is an important role for the community psychiatric mental health nurse.
- Community psychiatric mental health nurses frequently work with or participate in multidisciplinary teams.
- Partial hospitalization programs help the patient to join society.
- The purposes of a psychiatric home visit are as follows: (1) to begin the patient's treatment; (2) to assess the patient's needs; and (3) to teach the patient community-based skills.
- Managed care has a strong influence on the delivery of community psychiatric mental health treatment.
- A total of 20% to 25% of the homeless population has severe and persistent mental illness.
- Obesity is a major health problem for mentally ill persons as a side effect of medications or as a result of negative symptoms (e.g., apathy, withdrawal, lack of motivation).
- The intervention model for homelessness provides a guide for working with mentally ill homeless persons.
- As many as 16% of prison inmates are severely and persistently mentally ill.
- Severely and persistently mentally ill persons sometimes commit acts of violence associated with a failure to take medications, a history of violence, paranoid delusions, or command hallucinations.
- Family, care providers, or law enforcement officers sometimes abuse mentally ill persons.
- Mentally ill persons may exhibit high-risk sexual behaviors that put them at risk for HIV and other infectious diseases.
- Community mental health nurses play a major role in crisis situations (e.g., natural disasters).

REVIEW QUESTIONS

1. A patient with undifferentiated schizophrenia lives in a community care home and takes olanzapine (Zyprexa) daily with supervision. During the patient's monthly outpatient visits with a psychiatric nurse, which assessment parameter takes priority?
   1. Height
   2. Weight
   3. Integrity of mucous membranes
   4. Pupillary response to light

2. A community psychiatric nurse counsels a patient who was recently approved for Social Security Disability and Medicare benefits. The patient has schizoaffective disorder and takes 80 mg of ziprasidone (Geodon) orally twice daily. The nurse should first assist the patient with which aspect of case management?
   1. Determining how Medicare Plan D applies to the patient's case
   2. Applying for housing assistance through Medicaid
   3. Coaching the patient about how to obtain a driver's license
   4. Referring the patient to vocational rehabilitation for employment

3. A patient with bipolar disorder tells a nurse in the local mental health clinic, "I want to tell you about something I did that was bad, but you've got to promise me that you won't write it in my chart or tell anyone about it." Select the nurse's best response.
   1. "I'm here for you and want to be supportive. I understand how important it is to keep everything you tell me confidential."
   2. "Your privacy is guaranteed by the Health Insurance Portability and Accountability Act and state regulations. You've signed forms that state that you understand this protection."

REVIEW QUESTIONS—cont'd

3. "Tell me about what happened; then you and I can decide what the best course of action will be."

4. "I will protect your confidentiality to the extent the law allows, but I cannot keep secrets from the treatment team; we are all here to help you."

4. A nurse plans care for the following five patients. Which patients would most likely benefit from a psychiatric partial hospitalization program? You may select more than one answer.

   1. A patient who was recently discharged from an acute psychiatric facility
   2. A patient who has been diagnosed with a borderline personality disorder
   3. A patient who is actively abusing alcohol and cocaine
   4. A patient with acute, disabling, new-onset panic attacks
   5. A patient who is homeless

5. A psychiatric nurse visits a patient in the community. The patient has paranoid schizophrenia and takes 2 mg of risperidone (Risperdal) twice daily. The nurse determines that this patient needs medication education on the basis of which observation?

   1. The patient consumes a soft drink that contains caffeine.
   2. The patient eats a hamburger that has aged cheese on it.
   3. The patient gains 4 pounds over a 2-month period.
   4. The patient has a sunburn after an outing at a local swimming pool.

REFERENCES

Accordino MP et al: Deinstitutionalization of persons with severe mental illness: context and consequences, *J Rehabil* April-June, 32(6): 102-105, 2001.

Adair CE et al: Continuity of care and health outcomes among persons with severe mental illness, *Psychiatr Serv* 56:1061-1069, 2005.

American Psychiatric Association: *News release 09-04*: Mental illness does not discriminate: APA recognizes Black History Month, January 28, 2009. Available at www.psych.org.

Amnesty International: *Mentally ill or homeless: vulnerable to police abuse* (website): www.connix.com/~marpa/amnesty%20 international.htm. Accessed September 30, 2002.

Applebaum P: Law & psychiatry: least restrictive alternatives revisited: Olmstead's uncertain mandate for community-based care, *Psychiatry Serv* 50:1271-1272, 1280, 1999.

Arab-American Chaldean Council: *Arab-American and Chaldean behavioral health programs* (website): www.arabacc.org/ behavioral.htm. Accessed September 28, 2002.

Baillargeon J et al: Psychiatric disorders and repeat incarcerations: the revolving prison door, *Am J Psychiatry* 166:103-111, 2009.

Balon R: Managing compliance, *Psychiatr Times* 19(5):1-2, 2002.

Barclay L, Vega C: Sibutramine may help control weight gain associated with Olanzapine treatment, *Am J Psychiatr* 162:954-962, 2005.

Basok T et al: Counter-hegemonic Human Rights Discourses and Migrant Rights Activism in the U.S. and Canada, *Int J Comp Sociol* 50(2):183-205, 2009.

Bradshaw W et al: Recovery from severe mental illness: the lived experience of the initial phase of treatment, *Int J Psychosocial Rehab* 10(1):123-131, 2006.

Breen J, Breen P: *Mental health court: 8th judicial system, 2nd judicial system*, Las Vegas, NV, 2008, Advisory Commission on Administration of Justice.

Brekke JA et al: Neurocognitive change, functional change and service intensity during community-based psychosocial rehabilitation for schizophrenia, *Psychol Med* 39:1637-1647, 2009.

Busko M: Severe mental illness alone does not predict violent crime, *Arch Gen Psychiatry* 66:152-161, 2009.

Chou CC et al: Stages of change among Chinese people with mental illness: a preliminary study, *Rehabil Psychol* 49:39-47, 2004.

Clevenger K: Care of populations in the home setting. In Clark MJ, *Community health nursing: advocacy in population health*, ed 5, Upper Saddle River, NJ, 2009, Pearson Education, Inc.

Coalition for the Homeless Mentally Ill: *Information about mental illness and homelessness*, 2003 (website): www.homeles smentallyill.org/assisted.htm. Accessed January 17, 2011.

Cohen EL, Cesta T: *Nursing case management: from essentials to advanced practice applications*, ed 4, St. Louis, 2004, Mosby.

Community Mental Health Service: *Assertive community treatment* (website): www.mentalhealth.samhsa.gov/cmhs/ communitysupport/toolkits/community/. Accessed March 31, 2006.

Coursey RD: Competencies for direct service staff members who work with adults with severe mental illness in outpatient public mental health/managed care systems, *Psychiatr Rehabil J* 23(4):370-377, 2000.

Cutler DL et al: Four decades of community mental health: a symphony in four movements, *Community Mental Health Journal*, 39(5):381-398, 2003.

Devieux JG et al: Triple jeopardy for HIV: substance using severely mentally ill adults, *J Prev Interv Community* 33:5-18, 2007.

Dube R, Davis R: *Caseload management for CMHNS, Mental Health Nurses Association* (website): www.amicus-mhna.org/ guidecaseloadmgt.htm.

Edwards D et al: Factors influencing the effectiveness of clinical supervision, *J Psychiatr Ment Health Nurs* 12(4):405-414, 2005.

Fortinash KM and Holoday Worret PA: *Psychiatric mental health nursing*, ed 4, St. Louis, 2008, Mosby/Elsevier.

Fountain House: *Linking lives for mental health* (website): www.fountainhouse.org/moxie/resources/resources_statistics/ index.shtml. Accessed March 31, 2006.

Friedman RA: Violence and mental illness: how strong is the link? *New Engl J Med* 355:2064-2066, 2006.

Gilmer T et al: D. Adherence to treatment with antipsychotic medication and health care costs among Medicaid beneficiaries with schizophrenia, *Am J Psychiatr* 161:692-699, 2004.

Gilmer TP et al: Initiation and use of public mental health services by persons with severe mental illness and limited English proficiency, *Psychiatr Serv* 58(12):1555-1562, 2007.

Goin MK: *Mental illness and the criminal justice system: redirecting resources toward treatment, not containment,* Arlington, Va, 2004, American Psychiatric Association.

Gonzalez AR et al: Rehabilitation and social insertion of the homeless chronically mentally ill, *Int J Psychosocial Rehab* 5:79-100, 2001.

Hammond E, Treisman GJ: HIV and psychiatric illness, *Psychiatr Times* 24(14):1-2 2007.

Hampton MD, White MC, Chafetz L: Eligibility, Recruitment, and Retention of African Americans with Severe Mental Illness in Community Research, *Community Ment Health J* 45(2):137-143, 2007.

Hanrahan P et al: Housing satisfaction and service use by mentally ill persons in community integrated living arrangements, *Psychiatr Serv* 52:1206-1209, 2001.

Huggins M: Culture. In Mohr WK, editor: *Johnson's psychiatric-mental health nursing,* ed 5, Philadelphia, 2003, Lippincott Williams & Wilkins.

International Center for Clubhouse Development: *Mission* (website): www.iccd.org/mission.html. Accessed January 17, 2011.

Jampel B: Combating a stigma: mental illness in a Jewish world, *New Jersey Jewish News* January 1, 2009.

Kohen D: Diabetes mellitus and schizophrenia: historical perspective, *Br J Psychiatry* 184(Suppl 47):s64-s66, 2005.

Koller EA et al: Risperidone-associated diabetes mellitus: a pharmacovigilance study, *Pharmacotherapy* 23(6):735-744, 2003.

Laskowski C: The mental health clinical nurse specialist and the "difficult" patient: evolving meaning, *Issues Ment Health Nurs* 22(1):5-22, 2001.

Leifman S: Correctional health: aid sought for prisons overwhelmed with mentally ill, *Obesity, Fitness & Wellness Week* p. 256, July 17, 2004.

Maslow AH: *Motivation and personality,* New York, 1954, Harper & Row.

Mental Health America: *Position statement 53: mental health courts* (website): www.mentalhealthamerica.net/go/position-statements/53. Accessed January 17, 2011.

Mowbray CT et al: The clubhouse as an empowering setting, *Health Soc Work* 31(3):167-179, 2006.

Murer CG: *Psychiatric partial hospitalization: an overview* (website): www.rehabpub.com/issues/articles/2007-10_08.asp. Accessed January 17, 2011.

National Alliance on Mental Illness: *African American community mental health fact sheet,* 2004, NAMI Multicultural Action Center.

National Coalition of Homelessness: *Mental illness and homelessness, 2009* (website): www.nationalhomeless.org/factsheets/Mental_Illness.html

Norris DM, Price M: Firearms and mental illness, *Psychiatr Times* 26(11) 24-27, 2009.

O'Connell KL: Needs of families affected by mental illness, *J Psychiatr Nurs* 44(2):40-48, 2006.

Pelletier JR et al: A study of a structured exercise program with members of an ICCD certified clubhouse: structured design, benefits, and implications for feasibility, *Psychiatr Rehabil J* 29(2):89-96, 2005.

Pinto-Foltz MD, Logsdon MC: Reducing stigma related to mental disorders: initiative, interventions, and recommendations for nursing, *Archives of Psychiatric Nursing,* 2009, 23(1):32-40. Available at: www.sciencedirect.com.

Platt M et al: Developing housing for persons with severe mental illness: an innovative community foster home, *Int J Psychosoc Rehabil* 7:43-51, 2002.

Puskar R, Bernardo L: Trends in mental health: implications for advanced practice nurses, *J Am Acad Nurse Pract* 14:214-218, 2002.

Reutsch O et al: Psychotropic drugs induced weight gain: a review of the literature concerning epidemiological data, mechanisms and management, *Encephale* 31:507-516, 2005.

Rossi PH: *Down and out in America: the origins of homelessness in America,* Chicago, 1991, University of Chicago Press.

Salyers MP, Tsemberis S: ACT and recovery: integrating evidenced-based practice and recovery orientation on assertive community treatment teams, *Community Ment Health J* 43:619-641, 2007.

Sanchez F, Gaw A: Mental Health Care of Filipino Americans, Psychiatric Services, *Am Psychiatr Assoc* 58:810-815, 2007.

Sato M: Renaming schizophrenia: a Japanese perspective, *World Psychiatry* 5:53-55, 2006.

Scholler-Jaquish A: RN to BSN students in a walk-in health clinic for the homeless, *N HC Perspect Community* 17:118-123, 1993.

Scholler-Jaquish A: Homelessness in America. In Smith CM, Maurer FA, editors: *Community health nursing: theory and practice,* ed 2, Philadelphia, 2000, Saunders.

Sheehan JP: Protect your staff from workplace violence, *Nurs Manage* 31(3):24-25, 2000.

Shore JH, Manson SM: A developmental model for rural telepsychiatry, *Psychiatr Serv* 56:976-980, 2005.

Steadman HC et al: Prevalence of serious mental illness among jail inmates, *Psychiatr Serv* 60:761-765, 2009.

Substance Abuse and Mental Health Services Administration: *Home page* (website): www.samhsa.gov.

Wheeler K, Greiner L: Integrating education and research in an APRN mental health services program, *J Community Health Nurs* 21:141-152, 2002.

Wilkie D: Clinic called vital for 'urban Indians': director has fought to keep federal funding, *The San Diego Union-Tribune* p. B1, June 1, 2008.

Yamashita M: Nurse case management: negotiating care together within a developing relationship, *Perspect Psychiatr Care* 41:62-70, 2005.

Yanos PT et al: Partial hospitalization: compatible with evidenced-based and recovery-oriented treatment? *J Psychiatr Nurs* 47(2):41-47, 2009.

Zauszniewski JA, Suresky J: Evidence for psychiatric nursing practice: an analysis of three years of published research, *Online J Issues Nurs* 9(1):13, 2004.

Answers to Review Questions

Chapter 1: Psychiatric Nursing: Theory, Principles, and Trends
1. 4
2. 3
3. 3
4. 1, 2
5. 1

Chapter 2: Nursing Practice in the Clinical Setting
1. 4, 5
2. 4, 1, 2, 3
3. 3
4. 2
5. 1

Chapter 3: The Nursing Process and Standards of Care
1. 3
2. 3
3. 1
4. 4
5. 4

Chapter 4: Therapeutic Communication: Interviews and Interventions
1. 4
2. 4
3. 4
4. 2
5. 2

Chapter 5: Adaptation to Stress
1. 1
2. 2
3. 4
4. 1
5. 3

Chapter 6: Neurobiology in Mental Health and Mental Disorder
1. 1
2. 4
3. 1, 3, 5
4. 4
5. 1

Chapter 7: Human Development Across the Life Span
1. 4
2. 1
3. 3
4. 1, 3, 4
5. 1, 2, 4

Chapter 8: Culture, Ethnicity, and Spirituality
1. 1, 2
2. 4
3. 4
4. 1
5. 1

Chapter 9: Legal and Ethical Aspects in Clinical Practice
1. 4
2. 1
3. 2
4. 1
5. 1, 2, 5
6. 2

Chapter 10: Anxiety and Anxiety Disorders
1. 1
2. 2
3. 1
4. 4, 1, 3, 2
5. 3

Chapter 11: Somatoform, Factitious, and Dissociative Disorders
1. 2, 4, 5, 6
2. 1
3. 3
4. 4
5. 1

Chapter 12: Mood Disorders: Depression, Bipolar, and Adjustment Disorders
1. 4
2. 3
3. 1
4. 2, 3, 5
5. 2
6. 3, 1, 2

Chapter 13: Schizophrenia and Other Psychotic Disorders
1. 2
2. 1
3. 4
4. 1
5. 1
6. 4

Chapter 14: Personality Disorders
1. 3
2. 4
3. 1
4. 4
5. 1, 2, 5

Chapter 15: Substance-Related Disorders and Addictive Behaviors
1. 4
2. 1, 5
3. 1, 5
4. 2
5. 1

Chapter 16: Cognitive Disorders: Delirium, Dementia, and Amnestic Disorders
1. 1
2. 2, 3, 1
3. 2
4. 1, 3, 4
5. 4

Chapter 17: Disorders of Infancy, Childhood, and Adolescence
1. 3
2. 2, 4, 5
3. 1
4. 2
5. 4

Chapter 18: Eating Disorders: Anorexia Nervosa and Bulimia Nervosa
1. 1, 2, 5
2. 1
3. 2, 3, 4, 5
4. 4, 1, 2, 3
5. 4

Chapter 19: Sleep Disorders: Dyssomnias and Parasomnias
1. 1
2. 2, 4
3. 2
4. 1, 5
5. 2

Chapter 20: Sexual Disorders: Sexual Dysfunctions and Paraphilias
1. 4
2. 2
3. 3
4. 1
5. 1, 4, 5

Chapter 21: Crisis: Theory and Intervention
1. 2, 3, 1, 4
2. 3, 4, 5
3. 1
4. 4
5. 2
6. 1

Chapter 22: Suicide: Prevention and Intervention
1. 1, 4, 5
2. 2
3. 4
4. 1
5. 2

Chapter 23: Violence: Anger, Abuse, and Aggression
1. 2
2. 2
3. 1
4. 4
5. 3

Chapter 24: Forensic Nursing
1. 2
2. 1
3. 1
4. 4
5. 2

Chapter 25: Psychopharmacology
1. 1
2. 2
3. 4
4. 2, 3
5. 4

Chapter 26: Therapies: Theory and Clinical Practice
1. 4
2. 2
3. 1
4. 4
5. 2

Chapter 27: Complementary and Alternative Therapies
1. 1
2. 2
3. 1, 2
4. 4, 5
5. 3

Chapter 28: Grief: In Loss and Death
1. 4
2. 4
3. 3
4. 1
5. 4

Chapter 29: Mental and Emotional Responses to Medical Illness
1. 1, 3, 4
2. 2
3. 1
4. 2
5. 3

Chapter 30: Community Mental Health Nursing for Patients with Severe and Persistent Mental Illness
1. 2
2. 1
3. 4
4. 1, 4
5. 4

A

abstinence   The voluntary act of refraining from a behavior or from the use of a substance (e.g., alcohol, drugs, food, gambling, spending, sex) that has caused problems in the psychosocial, physical, cognitive/perceptual, or spiritual/belief dimensions of an individual's life.

abstract reasoning   The ability to think conceptually, which is reduced, impaired, or absent in patients with schizophrenia and other mental illnesses.

abuse   (1) A maladaptive pattern of substance use that may lead to problems in the psychosocial, physical, cognitive/perceptual, or spiritual/belief dimensions of an individual's life. (2) Any type of harm or injury (e.g., physical, psychologic, emotional, sexual) to a child, adult, or elderly individual.

acculturation   The adapting or modifying of cultural values and beliefs to accommodate life in a new culture.

acquired immunodeficiency syndrome (AIDS)   A late-stage infection with one of the human immunodeficiency viruses (i.e., HIV-1 or HIV-2).

acting out   The expression of internal affective states through external activities and behaviors that are often destructive or maladaptive.

activities of daily living (ADLs)   The actions that are performed as part of routine daily life and that include personal hygiene, grooming, eating, and recreation.

adaptive   The ability to adapt to change in response to internal or external circumstances or conditions.

addiction   A maladaptive and compulsive dependence on a substance (e.g., alcohol, drugs) or a behavior (e.g., gambling, spending).

adverse drug reaction   An unintended effect of a medication that results in severe and unwanted and sometimes severe symptoms or consequences.

affect   The outward bodily expression of emotions that range from joy to sorrow or anger. *Blunted affect:* The restricted expression of emotions. *Flat affect:* The lack of the outward expression of emotions. *Inappropriate affect:* An affect that is not congruent with the emotion being felt (e.g., laughing when sad). *Labile affect:* The rapid changing of emotional expression.

aggression   Acting-out behaviors that can lead to harm or injury to the self or others; this is seen with a wide range of disorders and conditions.

agnosia   The loss of comprehension of auditory, visual, or other sensations, although the senses are intact.

agraphia   The loss of the ability to write.

akathisia   A syndrome that is caused by dopamine-blocking drugs and that is characterized by both motor restlessness and a subjective feeling of inner restlessness. Literally means "not sitting."

alcoholic blackout   An episode of forgetting all or part of what occurred during or after the intake of alcohol.

alcoholism   A chronic, progressive, and potentially fatal biogenic and psychosocial disease that is characterized by impaired control over drinking alcohol. Eventual tolerance and physical dependence lead to loss of control, distorted thinking, and other physical and social consequences.

alexia   The inability to read caused by a lesion or dysfunction of the central nervous system.

alexithymia   A condition that causes individuals to have difficulty identifying and describing their emotions. The term literally means "no words for feelings." Individuals with eating disorders often have a restricted emotional life and thus exhibit this condition.

allopathic   The health beliefs and practices that are derived from the scientific models of the present time and that involve the use of technology and other modalities of modern medical health care, such as immunization and resuscitation.

altruism   The principle or practice of unselfish concern for others' welfare.

Alzheimer's disease   A neurodegenerative disease that is characterized by progressive, irreversible, and lethal structural damage to the brain that results from the presence of β-amyloid proteins and that leads to a loss of cognitive functions and occurrence of symptoms of progressive dementia.

ambivalence   Simultaneously holding two different attitudes, emotions, thoughts, or feelings about a person, object, or situation. (Examples: love and hate; admiration and envy)

amnestic disorders   Impairments of memory that occur without delirium and dementia.

amyloid plaques   Abnormal areas in the brain that are made of amyloid proteins and that surround affected neuronal cells. The amount of plaques is related to the degree of mental deterioration. Amyloid plaques interfere with cell-to-cell communication, thereby resulting in the decreased availability of acetylcholine. Also called *senile plaques* or *neuritic plaques.*

anger   A strong emotion of displeasure; common feeling during grief that is often directed toward the deceased, family members, health care providers, or a higher power. Anger is inappropriate when it involves the intent to harm or injure others. It is discussed in several chapters throughout the text.

anhedonia   The loss of pleasure and interest in activities that were previously enjoyed or in life itself.

anorexia nervosa   An eating disorder in which one is preoccupied with food and eating and may suppress the desire for food to control eating, thereby compromising nutritional intake; not necessarily a loss of appetite, as the medical term implies.

anticipatory grief   Grief that is experienced before death or loss occurs (e.g., when a loved one has a terminal illness).

anxiety   A vague and nonspecific feeling of uneasiness, tension, apprehension, and sometimes dread or pending doom. Anxiety occurs as a result of a threat to one's biologic, physiologic, or social integrity that arises from external influences. It is a universal experience and an integral part of human existence.

apathy   Indifference, disinterest, or dull attitude; this manifests as a negative symptom of schizophrenia.

aphasia   *Expressive aphasia:* The inability to speak or write. *Receptive aphasia:* The inability to comprehend what is being said or written; may progress to babbling or mutism.

apraxia   The loss of the abilities to carry out purposeful and complex movements and to use objects properly.

assent   To agree or concur to a proposal. An example is that minors cannot give legal consent to treatment in medical facilities, but can accept treatment.

autism   A pervasive developmental disorder that is characterized by the marked impairment of social and cognitive abilities.

autistic thinking   Disturbances in thought that result from the intrusion of a private fantasy world that is internally stimulated; this type of thinking results in abnormal responses to people and events in the real world.

autodiagnosis   The self-examination of one's own thoughts, feelings, perceptions, and attitudes about a particular patient or situation.

avolition   A lack of motivation or will; it is noted in patients with schizophrenia or other mental illnesses.

B

basal ganglia (nuclei)   An area of the central nervous system that is made up of cell bodies and that is responsible for motor functions and association.

battering   Physical or sexual abuse of a person by intimate partners or by those with whom they have been intimate.

behavior modification   A type of therapy that focuses on modifying observable behavior by manipulating the environment, the behavior, or the consequences of the behavior.

bereavement   The objective state that occurs after loss, especially of a loved one; the state of grieving.

binge eating disorder (BED)   A pattern of binge eating without the purging characteristic of bulimia nervosa. BED is more commonly known as *compulsive overeating.*

biofeedback   A technique that makes use of electrical equipment to help persons gain conscious control over involuntary body processes.

blackout   The loss of the memory of events that occur after the onset of the causative agent or condition (e.g., the ingestion of alcohol or drugs).

body dysmorphic disorder A somatization disorder in which one becomes obsessed with an imagined defect in one's body or body parts.

boundary The distinguishing and separating of the self from others by clarifying the limits and extent of the nurse's responsibilities and duties in relationship to the patient and others.

breach of duty The failure to perform by act of commission or omission within the scope of practice or the failure to adhere to defined standards of care.

bulimia nervosa An obsession with thinness, dieting, and a compulsive cycle of bingeing and purging. This syndrome was previously labeled *bulimarexia.*

C

case management The clinical coordination of inpatient and outpatient care designed to support the patient's highest level of functioning. Services include crisis intervention; supportive counseling; consultation and collaboration with multidisciplinary treatment providers; and medication and mental status monitoring.

cataplexy The sudden loss of muscle tone and voluntary muscle movement.

catastrophic reaction A sudden or gradual negative change in the behavior of patients with dementia that is caused by their inability to understand and cope with stimuli in the environment.

central nervous system The part of the human nervous system that contains the brain and the spinal cord.

chemical restraint The use of psychotropic drugs and sedatives to reduce or eliminate psychiatric symptoms. Symptom management through medication.

chronic mental illness A psychiatric disorder that persists over time with remissions and recurrence of severe and disabling symptoms.

chronic sorrow Grief in response to an ongoing loss, such as a long chronic illness in a loved one.

circadian rhythm The cycle of sleep and wakefulness and the fluctuation of various physiologic and behavioral parameters over a 24-hour cycle.

circumstantiality A type of speech that is characterized by unnecessary details and indirectness before the point or intent is reached; may be noted in patients with schizophrenia or other mental illnesses.

classical conditioning A theory developed by Ivan Pavlov that involves the pairing of a neutral stimulus with another stimulus.

clinical pathway A standardized format that is used to provide and monitor patient care and progress by way of the case management and interdisciplinary health care delivery system. Also known as a *critical pathway, care path,* or *care map.*

clubhouse model A system that involves a place where persons with severe and persistent mental illness go to rebuild their lives. The participants are viewed as members rather than patients, and the emphasis is on the members' strengths rather than on their weaknesses.

codependence A relationship in which the actions of a member of the family, a close friend, or a colleague of an alcohol- or drug-dependent person tend to perpetuate the person's dependence and thereby retard the process of recovery. The term is also now used figuratively to describe the way in which the community or society acts as an enabler of alcohol or drug dependence or of other areas of dysfunction (e.g., family, gambling, spending).

cognition The process of being aware, thinking, knowing, and reasoning.

cognitive behavioral therapy Therapy that is focused on changing irrational or self-defeating thoughts and behaviors into realistic ones; used to treat a variety of mental disorders.

commitment A court-ordered evaluation to certify that an individual is to be confined to a mental health facility for treatment.

communication A reciprocal process of sending and receiving messages between two or more people and their environment; the vehicle for establishing a therapeutic relationship.

community mental health center An outpatient facility that provides multiple mental health treatments and programs for people in a specified area.

Comorbid The coexistence of two or more disease processes or disorders at the same time (e.g., substance dependence and major depression).

competency to stand trial The ability of an individual to understand legal charges and their consequences, to understand the nature and object of the legal proceedings in which he or she is involved, and to advise an attorney to assist with his or her defense.

complementary and alternative medicine (CAM) CAM covers a broad range of healing philosophies, approaches, and therapies. It generally is defined as those treatments and health care practices that are not taught widely in medical schools, not generally used in hospitals, and not usually reimbursed by medical insurance companies (this is the definition that is used by the National Center for Complementary and Alternative Medicine). Additional related terms include *holistic therapies* and *integrative medicine.*

complicated grief Grief that is expressed with a significantly greater or lesser intensity over a longer or shorter period of time than is culturally expected. This may manifest itself as serious physical or emotional disabilities. Also called *traumatic, pathologic,* or *dysfunctional grief.*

compulsion An unremitting and repetitive impulse to perform a behavior (e.g., hand washing, checking, cleaning, putting things in order) or a mental act (e.g., praying, counting, repeating words silently). The object of the compulsion is to prevent or reduce anxiety or distress. Compulsive acts often occur to reduce the distress that accompanies an obsession.

concept map A critical problem-solving plan that promotes the student's understanding of the relationships between ideas, concepts, or topics.

concrete thinking The literal interpretation of information; the person is unable to think abstractly. This is often noted in patients with schizophrenia and other mental illnesses.

confabulation The fabricating of stories to fill in memory gaps; often seen in patients with Alzheimer's disease or other types of dementias; may be an attempt to preserve self-esteem; should not be mistaken for lying.

confidentiality The right of the psychiatric patient to keep information from people outside of the health care team.

congruence The consistency of agreement between verbal and nonverbal behavior.

contraband Any objects that are prohibited by law or by the rules of a facility. On an acute care psychiatric unit, this includes illegal drugs and dangerous objects such as knives, guns, or anything that may prove harmful to patients on the unit.

conventional or traditional medicine The primary type of medicine that is practiced in the United States. The major focus is on the biologic mechanisms of disease, ruling out potential causes, and then forming a diagnosis and treatment plan for a specific disease. Also known as *Western medicine, mainstream medicine, orthodox medicine, allopathic medicine,* and *biomedicine.*

conversion disorder A disorder in which one perceives deficits that affect sensory or motor function that are unrelated to a medical condition.

co-occurrence More than one psychiatric diagnosis occurring at the same time in the same individual. Also known as *comorbid* or *coexisting.*

cope The ability to adapt to a threat to one's integrity or well-being with the use of a variety of tools, including adaptive (useful) and maladaptive (ineffective) maneuvers. One can cope internally via changes in thinking or psychologic defense mechanisms or externally via actions.

countertransference The nurse's feelings toward and responses to a patient that are associated with a significant person in the nurse's life. Although countertransference may be a natural part of therapy, the nurse needs to be aware of it and manage it to avoid behaving inappropriately toward the patient.

crisis (1) An event that threatens one's well-being, such as a sudden death in the family or an earthquake, and that exceeds the person's ability to cope with the threat.

crisis intervention Therapeutic techniques for helping individuals who are experiencing a crisis.

critical thinking An intellectual and disciplined process of actively and skillfully conceptualizing, applying, analyzing, synthesizing, and evaluating information through observation, experience, reasoning, and communication as a guide for belief or action.

cultural competence A standard of practice that ensures that the caregiver accepts and recognizes multiple aspects of cultural diversity among individuals and helps patients to receive information that they understand.

culture The collective process of acquiring shared beliefs, dominant patterns of behavior, values, and attitudes that are learned through socialization.

curative factors Eleven factors as determined by Irvin Yalom that make up the dynamic of every group and that facilitate change by assisting members to understand their patterns of interacting within the group.

D

defense A means or method of protecting oneself; an unconscious mental activity or mental structure (e.g., a defense mechanism) that protects the ego from anxiety.

defense mechanisms Mental processes to protect the ego (person) from anxiety that results from feelings and impulses that threaten psychologic harm, conflict, or exposure (e.g., denial, repression). Also known as *ego defenses.*

deinstitutionalization The discharge of a patient from the psychiatric institution or hospital into the community. Specifically refers to the discharge of severely mentally ill patients with long-term hospitalizations into less-structured care during the 1960s.

delirium A disturbance of consciousness and a change in cognition that develop over a short period of time and that tend to fluctuate during the course of the day. Delirium is characterized by disorientation to time and place; reduced ability to focus, sustain, or shift attention; incoherent speech; and continual aimless physical activity.

delusions False beliefs that are fixed and resistant to reasoning.

dementia A global impairment of intellectual (cognitive) functions (e.g., thinking, remembering, reasoning) that usually is progressive and of sufficient severity to interfere with a person's normal social and occupational functioning.

denial The avoidance of reality that threatens an individual's self-concept. Denial is demonstrated by ignoring or de-emphasizing the importance of an event, observation, or feeling. At times, denial may help one to survive life stressors.

depersonalization Feelings of unreality or personal dissociation. Individuals who are experiencing depersonalization have difficulty distinguishing themselves from others. Depersonalization may occur in patients with extreme anxiety.

depression A dysphoric or depressed mood state. The relatively normal symptom of feeling somewhat depressed, sad, or blue must be distinguished from the diagnosis of major depression, which is more severe; in addition to depressed mood, it includes several other symptoms, including changes in appetite, weight, sleep, activity, libido, and energy as well as thoughts of death or suicide.

derealization The perception that the surrounding world is not real or is distorted.

dereism A loss of connection with reality and logic that occurs before the autistic thinking that is noted in patients with schizophrenia. The individual's thoughts become private and idiosyncratic.

designer drugs Illegal drugs used at all-night parties called *raves* or *trances.* Designer drugs include γ-hydroxybutyrate, ketamine, ecstasy, and Rohypnol.

detoxification The removal of toxins or poisons from a person; treatment that assists the individual with withdrawal from the physical effects of substances.

devaluation A method of coping in which a person deals with emotional conflict or stressors by attributing exaggerated negative qualities to oneself or others.

disease A term that is used to describe altered body functions and a condition that places limitations on daily activities in the presence of recognizable symptoms.

disorientation A loss of familiarity with place, time, and person, and situation.

dissociation The disruption of one's integrated personality or separation of an overwhelming event from one's conscious awareness; a prominent defense mechanism in dissociative identity disorder.

dissociative amnesia The inability to recall important personal information that is generally of a traumatic or stressful nature.

dissociative fugue A sudden or unexpected travel away from one's home or workplace with an inability to recall one's past or where one has been.

distress A subjective response to internal or external stimuli that are threatening or perceived as threatening to the self.

diurnal variation Feeling worse or more depressed in the morning and better in the evening.

domestic violence Learned behaviors used by one or more persons in an intimate or family relationship for the purpose of controlling the behavior of others. Violence may take the form of physical, psychologic, sexual, or emotional abuse; intimidation; threats; isolation; economic control; or stalking.

double-bind A situation in which contradictory messages are given to one person by another and a response or a choice between two opposing alternatives is demanded.

dual diagnosis A term that is used when the individual has two identified primary psychiatric diagnoses; it is most commonly used when one diagnosis is drug or alcohol related. For example, a patient may have both a substance-related disorder and a mood disorder.

duty to warn The legal obligation of a mental health professional to warn an intended victim of potential harm from a patient with mental illness.

dynamic An active and energetic state; the capacity or ability to change as opposed to being static, fixed, or stationary.

dysarthria Difficulty with articulating words. Dysarthria is more commonly found in patients with vascular dementias and strokes and major head injuries.

dyspareunia Painful sexual intercourse that does not result from a general medical condition.

dysphoria A depressed and sad mood.

dysthymia Chronic low-level depression that lasts more than 2 years and that may lead to more severe depression if untreated.

dystonic Abnormal muscle tonicity and spasms of the face, head, neck, and back; it is a side effect of some antipsychotic medications.

E

echolalia The involuntary repetition of words spoken by another person.

echopraxia The spontaneous imitation of movements made by another person.

eclectic approach Selecting or choosing from various sources and not following any one system. In therapy, this term refers to the use of several different modalities together when treating a patient.

ego Freud's word for the self; major role of the ego is to find safe and appropriate ways for needs (instincts) to be met (gratified) in the external world. The ego lies mostly in the conscious mind.

ego defenses Automatic psychologic processes that keep out the threat of internal and external stressors and dangers or that deny awareness to protect the self. Also known as *defense mechanisms* or *mental mechanisms.*

ego dystonic A sense of general discomfort with one's own feelings, thoughts, or behaviors that can be a catalyst toward health-seeking behaviors.

ego syntonic A sense of comfort with feelings, thoughts, or behaviors that can inhibit one toward seeking help; may be noted in patients with sexual paraphilic disorders.

electroconvulsive therapy (ECT) A type of biologic therapy in which a brief electrical stimulus is applied to the brain to produce a seizure. ECT is performed with the patient under general anesthesia, and it is most often used to treat major depression.

empathy The projecting of sensitivity and an understanding of another's feelings; communicating that understanding in a way that the patient comprehends.

enabler One who supports an undesirable behavior of another person. Example: to continue on a path of substance abuse by providing excuses for the person or helping the affected individual to avoid the consequences of his or her behavior.

encopresis The repeated passage of feces into inappropriate places (e.g., clothing, floor), whether involuntary or intentional.

enmeshed A pattern that is frequently seen in dysfunctional families in which members have diffuse rather than clear boundaries, lack clear role definitions, and are excessively involved in each other's lives. This makes it difficult to individuate and separate, which is a necessity for healthy functioning.

enuresis The repeated voiding of urine into the bed or clothing, whether involuntary or intentional.

ethnicity A specific cultural group's sense of identification associated with its common social and cultural heritage.

ethnocentrism The tendency of members of one cultural group to view the members of other cultural groups in terms of the standards of behavior, attitudes, and values of their own group; a belief in the superiority of one's own group.

eustress A nonspecific stress response associated with desirable events such as marriage, the birth of a child, or a job promotion; from the Greek word *eu*, which means "good."

euthymia A mood that is normal and level.

evidence-based practice A nursing practice that has been proven effective by virtue of having undergone research versus being accepted merely on opinions or because of a history of having been done a certain way for a long time.

executive functioning A function of the prefrontal cortex of the brain that includes the abilities to plan, organize, reason, and problem solve. This type of functioning is diminished or lost in patients with schizophrenia and other mental illnesses.

extrapyramidal symptoms (EPS) The collective term that is used to describe the troubling motor side effects of dopamine-blocking medications. EPS include acute dystonia, akathisia, parkinsonism, and tardive dyskinesia.

F

factitious disorder The intentional production of symptoms of illness so that one can assume a sick role.

faith The belief, confidence, or trust in anything that is not necessarily based on proof or substantiated by actual fact. This term may be used to refer to religious or spiritual beliefs.

feedback The measure by which the effectiveness of a message is gauged.

fetal alcohol syndrome (FAS) A set of congenital psychologic, behavioral, and physical abnormalities that occur in infants whose mothers consumed large amounts of alcohol during pregnancy.

flight of ideas The shifting from one idea to another without completing the previous idea or an abrupt change of topics expressed in a rapid flow of speech. Although this is most commonly seen during the manic phase of bipolar disorder, it may be noted in patients with schizophrenia, and it is often confused with the looseness of associations that is most often manifested in patients with schizophrenia, in which thoughts are more fragmented.

folie a deux A phenomenon in which a person takes on the delusion of another person and often manifests similar characteristics of the delusion; it may be noted in patients with schizophrenia. Also known as a *shared delusion.*

forensic nursing A branch of nursing that focuses on the clinical observation and treatment of individuals who are victims of crimes or who have mental health problems and who are charged with or convicted of crimes.

G

gateway drugs Substances that have been implicated as forerunners to polysubstance use or drug dependence (e.g., tobacco, alcohol, marijuana).

general adaptation syndrome (GAS) The syndrome described by Hans Selye as the body's response to stress. The GAS occurs in three stages: (1) alarm (fight-or-flight stage); (2) adaptation; and (3) exhaustion.

generativity In Erik Erikson's personality theory, this is the positive outcome of one of the stages of adult personality development. Generativity involves the ability to do creative work or to contribute to the raising of one's children or to society; it is the opposite of stagnation.

genuineness A quality of an effective nurse that encompasses openness, honesty, and sincerity.

gerontology The scientific study of the aging process that involves multiple disciplines and settings.

Global Assessment of Functioning (GAF) score The fifth axis (assessment category) of the *Diagnostic and Statistical Manual of Mental Disorders,* fourth edition, text revision, which describes a person's overall functioning in society; a measure of precrisis functioning and the current level of functioning.

grandiosity A characteristic that is noted in patients with mania in which the individual experiences a sense of inflated self-esteem or exaggerated confidence in his or her feats and achievements. Also known as *self-aggrandizement.*

grief The dynamic natural response to loss. Grief affects physical, cognitive, behavioral, emotional, social, and spiritual aspects of the individual.

grief work The intense psychologic effort to do the following: (1) fully express the feelings associated with grief; (2) understand the relationship with the deceased; and (3) carry on with essential activities of daily living.

guilt A pervasive theme in grief for individuals of all ages. This is especially troublesome for survivors who experienced difficult or ambivalent relationships with the deceased. Overwhelming guilt can be self-destructive.

H

hallucination A perceptual disturbance of one or more of the five senses in the absence of external stimuli.

health The absence of disease; a state of total well-being. The various definitions imply that health is dynamic, with a focus on a healthy lifestyle. Health has been referred to as a condition of adjustment or adaptation to physical, psychologic, social, and environmental changes.

holistic Of or pertaining to holism, which is a philosophy that states that, in nature, individuals function as complete units that cannot be reduced to the sum of their parts. The term *holistic medicine* refers to the comprehensive and total care of each patient in which all needs—physical, emotional, social, spiritual, and economic—are considered and treated.

homeopathic A type of therapy that use minute doses of drugs that produce the same symptoms of a targeted disease; thought to stimulate the person's own immune response.

homeostasis The way that the body, with the use of its own feedback mechanisms, maintains a stable internal environment despite changes in the external environment.

human genome All of the genes carried on human chromosomes.

hyperreligiosity A preoccupation or obsession with religion, God, or another deity.

hypertensive crisis Any severe elevation of blood pressure that is a medical emergency; may occur as a result of food or drug admixtures with some psychotropic medications.

hypervigilance An excessive watchfulness and scanning of the environment that is generally manifested in patients who are experiencing delusions or hallucinations and that may preclude acts of aggression or violence.

hypochondriasis A longstanding dependency and a preoccupation with the sick role; a fear or belief that one has serious illness despite medical reassurance to the contrary.

hypomania A mood of elation with higher-than-usual activity and social interaction; not as expansive as full mania.

I

id The basic level of the personality that lies in the unconscious and that consists of primitive drives and instincts that are aimed at self-preservation and gratification.

idealization The tendency of a patient with borderline personality disorder to idealize others beyond the capabilities of those others when they are meeting the patient's needs.

ideas of reference Incorrect interpretations of external incidents and events as having a particular or special meaning specific to the person.

identified patient In family or group therapy, the member of the family or group whose behavior is seen as causing the problem for the family or group.

illness A sickness, disease, or ailment. Illness has been labeled as an unexpected stressful event in an individual's life that can interrupt him or her from fulfilling his or her usual tasks or roles. Illness is often perceived to be a crisis event. The terms *illness* and *disease* are often used synonymously; however, the disease process may be present without the person feeling ill (e.g., a lump in the breast that has not yet been detected).

incest Sexual intercourse between blood relatives.

incidence The frequency of occurrence of a specific disorder within a designated time period; the number of new cases.

independent activities of daily living (IADLs) The activities that an individual must perform to function in the community (e.g., shopping, preparing meals, obtaining transportation).

indifference The nurse's disconnectedness or aloof lack of concern; a separation from the patient's needs or situation.

inference The interpretation of behavior, the assumption of motive, and the formation of a conclusion before having all of the relevant information.

insight The ability to perceive oneself realistically and to understand oneself and the motives behind one's behavior.

institutionalization The placement or confining of persons with mental disorders in state-run facilities or residential treatment programs designed to treat such disorders.

interpersonal communication The communication that takes place between two or more persons and that contains both verbal and nonverbal messages.

intoxication The physiologic state of being poisoned by a drug or another toxic substance.

intrapersonal communication The communication occurring within oneself and that can be functional or dysfunctional.

intrapsychic Pertaining to the mind or the mental processes.

intuition Knowing or sensing without the use of rational processes such as reasoning.

isolation A feeling of aloneness with perceived social rejection or lack of support from others.

J

Johari window A model of communication that helps the nurse to look at self-awareness through interpersonal learning styles.

judgment An opinion or a conclusion that may affect or influence another person's life circumstances or situations; the ability to make logical decisions.

K

kindling The creation of electrophysiologic sensitivity in the brain as a result of stress that results in the alteration of neural functioning.

L

la belle indifference A somatic symptom that is manifested as a general lack of concern in a patient who perceives the existence of physical symptoms or dysfunction; it is a hallmark symptom of conversion disorder.

label A word or phrase that describes a person or group. It usually has a negative connotation for patients with psychiatric disorders, and it signifies a stereotype that is detrimental for the individual.

learned helplessness The perception that events are uncontrollable, which leads to apathy, helplessness, powerlessness, and depression.

least restrictive A therapeutic intervention or treatment that is applied when all other less-intrusive methods have been tried and were unsuccessful. For example, seclusion and restraint may be initiated because talking to the patient and reducing environmental stimuli did not prevent the patient's behavior from escalating to a point of self-harm or harm to others.

legal duty Something that an individual is required by law to do.

lethality The potential for causing death related to the level of danger associated with the suicidal plan along a continuum from low to high probability (e.g., a cut on both wrists as compared with a gunshot wound to the head).

libido The energy of the instincts held in the id; the sexual drive.

life stages The framework for several theories of adult development that divide the lifespan into a series of sequential transitions.

locus of control An aspect of personality that deals with the degree of control that one perceives over one's own destiny. *Internal locus of control* refers to the ability to actively control one's own destiny. *External locus of control* refers to the inability to control one's own destiny.

looseness of associations (LOA) A thought disturbance in which the speaker rapidly shifts his or her expression of ideas from one subject to another in an unrelated and fragmented manner. This is most commonly noted in patients with schizophrenia.

loss The process of losing or being deprived of someone or something that is characterized by a series of overlapping stages that include psychologic and behavioral manifestations of acceptance, adjustment, and resolution. Most often accompanied by common grief responses.

lovemap A term coined by John Money in 1986 to describe one's idealized picture of who and what types of behaviors make up one's patterns of sexual arousal.

M

maladaptive The opposite of adaptive; the term signifies a response that may result in unfavorable circumstances, situations, or conditions for an individual who is unable or unwilling to adapt to meet standards that are accepted by the medical or social community.

mania An elevated, expansive, or irritable mood that is accompanied by hyperactivity, grandiosity, and loss of reality. It is most commonly noted in patients with bipolar disorder.

mental status examination An organized collection of data that reflects an individual's functioning at the time of the interview. Mood, affect, thoughts, and perceptions are a few components that make up the examination, and it also includes psychosocial criteria (e.g., coping).

mild cognitive impairment A level of cognitive functioning that is below the functioning that is associated with normal aging but that does not meet the criteria for dementia.

milieu therapy A type of therapy that recreates a community atmosphere in an inpatient hospital unit, a partial hospitalization unit, or a day-treatment setting to facilitate interaction among patient peers to identify and problem-solve issues that occur when relating to others.

mindfulness meditation A method of reducing stress by concentrating on one's body, breathing, and intrusive thoughts.

mirroring A technique that is used in psychodrama and movement/dance therapy in which one individual imitates the behavior patterns of another to show the person how other people perceive and react to him or her.

modeling A principle that argues that behavioral change occurs as a result of observing behaviors in others that bring positive or negative consequences.

mood A subjective feeling state that is reported by the patient and that can vary with external and internal changes.

moral development A process that encompasses the development of moral judgment and reasoning and that involves making decisions about right or wrong actions in a particular situation.

mourning The social and psychologic expression of grief.

N

NANDA-I diagnoses The North American Nursing Diagnosis Association International (NANDA-I) defines a nursing diagnosis as "a clinical judgment about an individual, family or community response to actual or potential health problems/life processes which provide the basis for definitive therapy toward achievement of outcomes for which the nurse is accountable."

narcissistic personality disorder A disorder in which one manifests a grandiose view of self, a lack of empathy toward others, and an insatiable need for admiration and love.

negative symptoms Symptoms that include flat affect, poverty of speech, poor grooming, withdrawal, and disturbances in volition and that are often seen in patients with schizophrenia.

neglect   The intentional avoidance of attending to or caring for the physical, emotional, or psychologic needs of another (usually a child or an elderly individual).

neologisms   Invented words to which meanings are attached. Seen most often in patients with schizophrenia.

neuritic plaques   Insoluble deposits of protein and cellular material outside of the neuron and that are associated with Alzheimer's disease.

neurofibrillary tangle   Insoluble twisted filaments that accumulate inside of the neuron and that are associated with Alzheimer's disease.

neuroleptic   Literally means "to clasp the neuron"; a term that is used to describe antipsychotic medications.

neuroleptic malignant syndrome (NMS)   A rare but potentially lethal toxic reaction to dopamine-blocking drugs that presents with a constellation of symptoms, including fever, autonomic instability, increased muscular rigidity, and altered mental status.

neuroplasticity   Capacity of neurons and neural networks in the brain to change connections and reorganize throughout life.   Examples can be found in people who recover function after a major head injuries or strokes.

neurotransmitter   A chemical substance that is released by stimulated presynaptic cells that functions to activate postsynaptic cells and thus cause them to act as messengers in the central nervous system. Common neurotransmitters are acetylcholine, dopamine, norepinephrine, serotonin, and γ-aminobutyric acid.

nihilism   The belief that existence is senseless and useless. Patients with schizophrenia may experience nihilistic delusions in which they believe the world is nonexistent.

nonverbal communication   Nonverbal behaviors displayed by individuals during the process of an interaction, such as eye movements, facial expressions, posture, and gestures.

norms   The standards of behavior, attitudes, and perceptions that a group has for its members. Norms represent the shared expectations of appropriate behavior.

nuclear family   A family that is made up of the parental dyad and the individual's siblings.

nurse–patient relationship   A professional (not a social) relationship with specific objectives to facilitate the patient's process of achieving a state of well-being.

nursing   Nursing has many definitions. The American Nurses Association Social Policy Statement issued in 1995 defines nursing as the diagnosis and treatment of human responses to actual and potential health problems. The statement emphasizes the nurse's role in addressing a wide range of human experiences and responses to health and disease and the provision of a caring relationship that promotes healing and health maintenance. It is the application of nursing science and theory and the integration of the art of nursing that create environments that facilitate healing. The goal of holistic nursing is nursing practice that enhances the healing of the whole person from birth to death.

Nursing Interventions Classification (NIC)   The first comprehensive standardized classification of treatments performed by nurses; it was developed in 1987 by members of the Iowa Intervention Project research team.

Nursing Outcomes Classification (NOC)   The first comprehensive standardized classification used to describe patient outcomes that are influenced by nursing; it was developed in 1991 by the Iowa Outcomes Project research team. Outcomes include indicators such as patient states, behaviors, and self-reported perceptions.

O

object constancy   The ability to maintain a relationship regardless of frustration and changes in the relationship. A phase of growth and development in which the child can maintain the image of a person or an object even when the person or object is out of sight.

object relations   The stability and depth of an individual's relationships with significant others as manifested by warmth, dedication, concern, and tactfulness.

objectivity   The state of remaining free from bias, prejudice, and personal identification during an interaction with another person.

obsessions   Persistent ideas, thoughts, impulses, or images that involve death, sexual matters, religion, or any themes that lead to the person's efforts to resist them. Obsessions result in marked anxiety or distress.

omnipotence   The feeling of invincibility and self-aggrandizement that is often seen during the manic phase of bipolar disorder.

operant conditioning   A term coined by B.F. Skinner to describe his method of modifying behavior in animals, which he later also applied to humans.

P

pain   A subjective feeling of discomfort as indicated by the patient, generally on a scale of 1 to 10, where 1 to 3 is mild, 4 to 6 is moderate, and 7 to 10 is severe. Pain is considered a fifth vital sign by the accrediting bodies of The Joint Commission and the Board of Registered Nursing.

panic   A circumscribed period of extreme anxiety. During panic, one's perceptions are distorted, and the ability to integrate and separate environmental stimuli is impaired.

paradigm   A model, pattern, example, or overall concept accepted by persons in an intellectual community as a science due to its effectiveness in explaining a complex process, idea, or set of data.

paranoia   A mental disorder that is characterized by persecutory thoughts or delusions.

paraphilias   Sexual deviations and disorders that present with inappropriate sexual fantasies that involve deviant sexual acts, inappropriate sexual urges, and the acting out of these fantasies and urges.

perseveration   The excessive and persistent repetition of the same ideas in response to different questions. This condition is noted in patients with schizophrenia and in those with cognitive disorders such as Alzheimer's disease.

personality traits   Behaviors and enduring patterns of perceiving, relating to, and thinking about the environment and oneself that are exhibited in a wide range of social and personal contexts.

pervasive developmental disorders   A collection of disorders in which the child experiences deficits in a broad range of developmental areas.

pheromones   Airborne odorous chemicals that are often unconsciously perceived and that may influence bonding and sexual attraction.

phobias   A group of disorders that are primarily characterized by the avoidance of a specific situation or escaping if the situation is unexpectedly encountered.

physical dependence   A physiologic state of adaptation to a drug or alcohol that is usually characterized by the development of tolerance to the substance's effects.

pleasure principle   The goal of experiencing pleasure while avoiding pain. This principle represents the id's goal in the personality to satisfy a person's innate needs and instincts.

plethysmography   The use of a strain gauge that fits around the penis to detect erection; a medical intervention for male sexual dysfunction.

positive affirmation   A self-supporting message that reinforces confidence and enhances performance.

positive regard   The acceptance of and respect for a patient.

positive symptoms   Symptoms that include hallucinations, delusions, increased speech production with loose associations, and bizarre behavior and that are often seen in patients with schizophrenia.

positron emission tomography (PET)   A test that illustrates brain activity and function with the use of an injected radioactive substance that travels to the brain and that appears as a bright image on a screen. PET scans are used to show a variety of anomalies in brain structure and function.

poverty of thought   A psychopathologic thought disturbance seen in patients with schizophrenia. The patient's inability to think logically and sequentially is reflected in the poverty of content of his or her speech, which is vague, repetitious, and disconnected.

premorbid   The period just before the onset of a mental illness. The characteristics of the individual's personality may indicate the type of disorder that will occur.

pressured speech   Rapid speech with an urgent quality. Often noted in patients with mania.

prevalence   The number of cases of a specific disorder in a normal population at a given point in time; the number of existing cases.

priapism   A painful, persistent, and abnormal penile erection that is unaccompanied by sexual stimulation and that may lead to permanent impotence. It may be a rare side effect of the selective serotonin reuptake inhibitor and antidepressant trazodone. Priapism is a medical emergency that is treated with epinephrine injections or surgical intervention.

primary prevention   Prevention efforts that focus on the reduction of the incidence of mental disorders within the community. It is directed toward the occurrence of mental health problems with an emphasis on health promotion and the prevention of disorders.

primary process thinking   Prelogical thought that aims for wish fulfillment. This type of thinking is associated with the pleasure principle characteristic of the id portion of the personality.

privileged communication   Communication that occurs between a professional and a patient that is confidential and that is protected from forced disclosure in court unless such disclosure is authorized by the patient. The privilege is delegated by statutes in the various states.

problem solving   The process that is involved in discovering the correct sequence of alternatives to lead to a goal or to an ideational solution.

process recording   A written account of an interaction between a nurse and a patient that helps the nurse to examine the relationship. This was first introduced by Hildegard Peplau, a nurse educator and theorist.

prodromal symptoms   Early symptoms, such as a deterioration in functioning, that may mark the onset of a mental illness.

projection   The process whereby a person deals with his or her internal and external emotional conflicts and stressors by unconsciously and falsely attributing to another person his or her own unacceptable feelings, impulses, or thoughts.

projective identification   Projecting one's emotional conflicts and stressors onto another who does not fully disavow what is projected. The individual remains aware of his or her own affects or impulses but misattributes them as justifiable reactions to the other person.

psychoanalytic theory   A theory introduced by Sigmund Freud that explores the relationship between the ego and the unconscious; this is also the basis for psychoanalysis.

psychologic dependence   The compulsive use of substances that leads to a state of craving a drug or alcohol for its positive effect or to avoid the negative effects associated with its absence.

psychomotor agitation   Agitated motor activity. such as restlessness, pacing, and irritability, often noted in patients with mental illness.

psychomotor retardation   The slowing of physiologic processes that results in slowed movement, speech, and reaction time. Often noted in patients with severe depression and other mental disorders.

psychosis   The inability to recognize reality, the displaying of bizarre behaviors, or the inability to deal with life's demands. A symptom noted in schizophrenia and other mental illnesses.

psychosocial theory   Erik Erikson's theory that involves eight stages of a person's social development. Each stage is marked by a particular type of crisis that results from the ego's attempt to meet the demands of social reality.

psychosomatic illness   A physical disorder that is notably influenced or caused by emotional or mental factors that involve the mind and the body.

psychotropic   Literally means "mind nutrition." This term is used to describe drugs that affect the central nervous system.

purging   The use of self-induced vomiting or the abuse of laxatives, diuretics, syrup of ipecac, diet pills, or enemas to avoid weight gain after a binge. One or more of these behaviors as well as periods of fasting and excessive exercise during an episode of bulimia nervosa may be used.

R

rape   The act of physically forcing sexual intercourse. Rape is considered an act of violence for the purpose of exerting power and dominance over an individual.

rapid eye movement (REM) sleep   An active cerebral sleep state in which in there is an increase in cerebral metabolism with brain wave activity paralleling that seen during an awake state. Dreams have been reported by patients during the REM state.

rave   Raves and trance events are generally all-night dances that are often held in warehouses. Club drugs, which are sometimes referred to as *designer drugs,* are often used by teens and young adults who participate in nightclub, bar, rave, or trance scenes.

reality principle   The goal of postponing immediate gratification until a suitable object for this satisfaction is found. The ego is ruled by this principle.

receptors   Protein molecules located in the cell walls of tissues that receive chemical stimulation and that result in the stimulation or inhibition of the activity of the target cell.

refractory   Refers to the condition of an individual who is not responsive to medication or other types of treatment and who generally requires new or different therapeutic measures.

reframing   A technique of changing the viewpoint of a situation and replacing it with another viewpoint that fits the facts equally well but that changes the entire meaning.

relapse   The resumption of a pattern of substance use or dependency after a period of sobriety or abstinence.

relapse prevention   A means of helping the chemically dependent individual to maintain behavioral changes over a prolonged period of time.

religion   An organized system of beliefs regarding the cause, nature, and purpose of life that is often expressed through the belief in or worship of divine beings.

repression   The involuntary exclusion of a painful or threatening experience. Repression can begin during infancy and continue throughout life. It underlies all other defense mechanisms, but it also operates as its own defense mechanism.

residual symptoms   Minor disturbances that may remain after an episode of schizophrenia but that do not include delusions, hallucinations, incoherence, or gross disorganization.

resilience   An internal protective factor that plays a critical role in determining an individual's wellness outcomes and his or her ability to withstand physical, emotional, and psychologic stress.

resistance   The inability—whether conscious or unconscious—to accept change; the denial of new problems.

restrictive environment   An environment that restricts the activity of a patient to help the patient regain control of his or her behavior. The individual may be placed in open-door or closed-door seclusion during periods of extreme agitation, suicidal ideations, or threats of violence to the self or others.

risk factors   Certain identified internal characteristics or external influences that are present before a disorder occurs. An individual is more vulnerable to develop a disorder when these factors are present.

rites of passage   Rituals such as puberty, marriage, birth, and death that facilitate maturational development and that are associated with life transition. These rites commonly consist of three stages: (1) separation; (2) transition; and (3) incorporation.

roles   Expected social behavior patterns that are generally determined by an individual's status in a particular group. Hildegard Peplau identified four roles for the psychiatric mental health nurse: (1) resource person; (2) counselor; (3) surrogate; and (4) technical expert.

S

safety   The sense of security that is developed within the therapeutic relationship when the responsibilities and expectations of each party are clearly defined. Safety develops from knowing the boundaries of a relationship and acting within them.

schemata   Internal representations of the self and the world that are used by the mind to understand, code, and recall information. Aaron Beck proposed that negative schemata may lead to depression.

seasonal affective disorder (SAD)   A depressive disorder that is experienced by persons who are deprived of light during the winter months; light therapy is one treatment for this condition.

secondary gain   Any benefit that results from illness, such as personal attention, sympathy from others, or escape from unwanted responsibilities. Individuals with eating disorders may experience secondary gain when family or friends pay a great deal of attention to their eating behavior by preparing special meals or making special arrangements in an attempt to encourage them to eat.

secondary prevention Prevention efforts directed toward reducing the prevalence of mental disorders through the early identification and treatment of problems. This stage occurs after the problem arises and aims at shortening the course or duration of the episode.

selective attention The act of focusing on only part of incoming stimuli or information.

self-actualization A concept developed by Abraham Maslow to address the idea of an ongoing actualization of potentials, capacities, and talents for the fulfillment of perceived mission and for the greater knowledge and acceptance of one's own intrinsic nature.

self-system Harry Stack Sullivan's term for the system that infants develop to cope with the anxiety that is associated with the interpersonal process of need satisfaction and security. The individual develops self-appraisal as a result of significant others' responses to the actions of the individual. Actions that cause anxiety result in "bad-me" self-appraisals. Actions that cause no anxiety result in "good-me" self-appraisals. Actions of disapproval cause severe anxiety, emotional withdrawal, and "not-me" self-appraisals.

serotonin syndrome An adverse drug reaction that results in excessive production of serotonin in the brain; it may be life threatening.

severe and persistent This term is currently widely accepted as a replacement for the term *chronic* when referring to unremitting or frequently recurring symptoms of certain psychiatric disorders (e.g., schizophrenia) that continue to distress an individual and to interfere with his or her function throughout life.

severe and persistent mental illness A psychiatric disorder that persists over time and that involves multiple recurrences of severe and disabling symptoms.

sexting The transmission of a sexually explicit message or image via a cell phone or the Internet.

sexual recidivism The chronic and repetitive acting out of sexual behaviors that are considered to be unacceptable and that have or have not resulted in criminal conviction.

sexual response cycle The cycle that involves the stages of desire, arousal, and orgasm.

sexual victimization The act of being sexually aggressive toward another person with the use of deceitfulness or power that causes physical, emotional, psychologic, or spiritual injury.

sick role A set of social expectations that an ill person meets, including the following: (1) being exempt from usual social role responsibilities; (2) not being morally responsible for being ill; (3) being obligated to "want to get well"; and (4) being obligated to seek competent help.

side effect An undesired, nontherapeutic, and often predictable consequence of medication that frequently diminishes with time. This is in contrast with an adverse drug reaction, which is always negative.

sleep apnea syndrome The temporary cessation or absence of breathing during sleep that is often obstructive and that requires treatment with a continuous positive airway pressure unit or surgery.

SOAP note A problem-solving method that nurses commonly use in health care settings to analyze relevant patient problems and to reduce lengthy charting. The acronym *SOAP* stands for the following: *s*ubjective, *o*bjective, *a*ssessment, and *p*lanning.

sobriety The state of complete abstinence from alcohol or other drugs of abuse.

social learning The process by which children acquire the behaviors that they need to survive and function in society. These behaviors result from repeated interactions in their environments.

social support The presence of other individuals who are able to provide understanding, encouragement, and other assistance throughout life, especially during difficult times.

socialization The process of being raised within a culture and acquiring the characteristics of the given group.

somatic complaints Expressions of grief, depression, resentment, or other internal feelings that are manifested instead as bodily pain and discomfort. Often children, adolescents, and adults describe biologic symptoms of what are actually psychiatric disorders or dysfunctional responses to life crises.

somatization The conversion of mental states or experiences into bodily symptoms that are associated with anxiety.

spectatoring A term created by William Masters and Virginia Johnson in 1970 to refer to a physiologic phenomenon that involves the tendency to observe, monitor, and critique one's own sexual experience; it may be related to early sexual trauma or depression.

spirituality The effort to find purpose and meaning in life through a search for the sacred that may or may not be based on a specific religion.

splitting Keeping the positive and negative aspects of oneself or others separate from each other. An individual who uses the unconscious defense mechanism of splitting cannot tolerate ambiguity; therefore, people, events, or ideas are either good or bad, right or wrong, and black or white—there are no shades of gray. Often noted in the borderline personality disorder.

stalking The act of stealthily pursuing another person that is usually the result of a compulsion.

Standards of Practice The professional activities that the nurse performs during the six-step nursing process of assessment, diagnosis, outcomes, planning, implementation, and evaluation; developed by the American Nurses Association.

static Fixed, stationary, and unchanging; the opposite of dynamic.

stem cells Cells that have the complete genome intact but that have not yet differentiated.

stereotype An oversimplified and standardized opinion of a person or a group of people that is often made without adequate information.

stigma Social reproach; the attitudinal devaluation and demeaning by society of an individual or group of people with disabilities or disorders who are judged, labeled, alienated, and thought to be incapable of fulfilling valued social roles or of contributing to society.

stress (1) A term that refers to both a stimulus and a response. It can denote a nonspecific response of the body to any demand placed on it, whether the causal event is negative (i.e., a painful experience) or positive (i.e., a happy occasion). (2) A state produced by a change in the environment that is perceived as challenging, threatening, or damaging to the person's dynamic equilibrium. (3) The wear and tear on the body over time. (4) Psychologic stress has been defined as all processes, whether originating in the external environment or within the person, that demand a mental appraisal of the event before the involvement or activation of any other system.

stress response The body's reaction to a significant physical, emotional, or psychologic stressor. The response is an attempt to adapt as described in Hans Selye's General Adaptation Syndrome.

subjectivity Emphasizing one's own moods, attitudes, and opinions during an interaction with another person.

substance A chemical or drug.

suicidal ideation The experience of suicidal thinking on a consistent basis, which is a risk factor for suicide and warrants close supervision in a secured environment.

suicide The act of taking one's own life.

suicidology The scientific and humane study of suicide and self-destruction.

sundowner's syndrome The confusion and irritation that are common among patients with dementia at the end of the day, probably as a result of general tiredness and an inability to process any more information after a long day of struggling to interpret their environment correctly.

superego The portion of the mind that is differentiated from the ego and that contains the traditional values and taboos of society as interpreted by the child's parents and that becomes part of the self; the superego lies in the preconscious mind.

synapse An electrical or chemical function that allows neurotransmitters to travel across cell membranes; the failure of a synapse to function effectively can lead to depression and other disorders.

T

tangentiality Responding in a manner that is irrelevant to the topic at hand; a thought disturbance that is noted in patients with schizophrenia and other mental illnesses.

tardive dyskinesia (TD) A syndrome of abnormal involuntary movements that occurs after months or years of treatment with neuroleptic drugs that block dopamine type 2 receptors. These movements are often described as oral, buccal, lingual, or masticatory, but they can occur throughout the body.

tasks in grief Activities that are common to the psychosocial experience of grieving. Accomplishing these tasks helps the individual to resolve grief.

taxonomy A classification of known phenomena under a hierarchic structure.

tertiary prevention Prevention efforts that have the dual focus of reducing residual effects of a mental disorder and rehabilitating the individual who experienced the disorder.

themes Repeated patterns of interactions that the patient experiences in relationships with the self or others.

therapeutic alliance A goal-oriented and purposeful relationship between a professional member of a treatment team and a patient in which each agrees to work together to help the patient resolve problematic areas in the patient's life. In nursing, this is the nurse–patient relationship.

therapeutic communication Verbal and nonverbal communication that takes place between the nurse and the patient. The content signifies what is being discussed; it has meaning and focuses primarily on the patient's concerns. The therapeutic communication process refers to all aspects of meta-communication or how the patient and nurse communicate and the intent of each message.

therapeutic milieu An environment that has been designed to promote emotional health and that is based on the assumption that the patients are active participants in their own lives and therefore need to be involved in the management of their behavior and environment.

therapeutic play Age-appropriate play activities that the nurse uses purposefully for the assessment, intervention, and promotion of normal growth and development in children.

therapeutic relationship A personal relationship that is established to help one of the participants deal more effectively and maturely with some difficulty in life. It is a goal-directed, patient-centered, and objective relationship.

thought blocking An abrupt interruption in the flow of thoughts or ideas that results from a disturbance in the speed of associations.

tic A sudden, rapid, recurrent, nonrhythmic, and stereotyped movement or vocalization that is considered irresistible but that is often suppressible for short periods.

titration An incremental adjustment of a medication dose to allow for tolerance to side effects. For example, many medications are administered in low doses that may be slowly titrated to higher doses to avoid any untoward effects of the drug. Titration is also used to designate the incremental release of a patient from a locked unit to see whether the patient is able to tolerate specified activities on the unlocked unit or to go to dinner in the dining room off of the locked unit and then return.

tolerance The need for greatly increased amounts of a substance used to achieve intoxication or the desired mind-altering effects or markedly decreased effects with the continued use of the same amount of the substance.

transference The feelings or responses that a patient has toward the nurse that are associated with someone significant in the patient's life. Although transference may be a natural part of therapy, the nurse needs to be aware of it and to manage it to avoid the inappropriate behavior of the patient toward the nurse.

transitional objects Objects that remind one of a significant person. For example, a man keeps a picture of his wife on his desk to remind him of her during work hours, or a child keeps pieces of a blanket that he or she had as a baby to bring comfort during stressful moments.

triggers Any stimulus that evokes a response.

trust The reliance on the truthfulness or accuracy of the therapeutic relationship that is developed through the consistency of the nurse's words and actions.

U

unconditional positive regard The stance of the therapist who is modeling the unconditional acceptance of the patient and that is based on the belief that the patient is competent to direct himself or herself in his or her natural tendency to move forward toward integration.

unconscious suicidal intention A state that is outside of conscious awareness during which individuals engage in risk-taking behaviors that have a high likelihood of causing their deaths.

V

verbal communication Spoken or written words that compose the symbols of language.

vicarious learning Learning through imagining the experiences of others as if they are one's own.

victimization An act directed toward a stranger or an individual to establish a relationship for the primary purpose of victimization; may refer to acts of sexual aggression or other types of violence.

victimizer Another term used to define a sex offender; may be used when discussing the familial transmission of a paraphilia.

vigilance The ability to sustain attention over long periods of time.

violence Behavior that is physically, psychologically, or sexually harmful, injurious, or assaultive (e.g., child abuse, domestic violence, elder abuse, family violence).

voyeurism The act of observing unsuspecting persons in the act of disrobing or engaging in sexual activity so that the observer can obtain sexual arousal. Also known as *peeping Tom behavior*.

W

Wernicke's center An area of the brain's dominant hemisphere that recognizes, recalls, and interprets words. It may be affected in patients with chronic alcoholism or severe malnutrition.

X

xenophobia A morbid fear of strangers and of those who are not members of one's own ethnic group.

INDEX

Page numbers followed by "f" indicate figures, "t" indicate tables, and "b" indicate boxes.

NANDA INTERNATIONAL-APPROVED NURSING DIAGNOSES

Activity intolerance
Activity intolerance, Risk for
Activity planning, Ineffective
Airway clearance, Ineffective
Allergy response, Latex
Allergy response, Risk for latex
Anxiety
Anxiety, Death
Aspiration, Risk for
Attachment, Risk for impaired parent/infant/child
Autonomic dysreflexia
Autonomic dysreflexia, Risk for

Behavior, Risk-prone health
Bleeding, Risk for
Body image, Disturbed
Body temperature, Risk for imbalanced
Bowel incontinence
Breastfeeding, Effective
Breastfeeding, Ineffective
Breastfeeding, Interrupted
Breathing pattern, Ineffective

Cardiac output, Decreased
Cardiac perfusion, Risk for decreased
Cardiac tissue perfusion, Risk for ineffective
Caregiver role strain
Caregiver role strain, Risk for
Cerebral tissue perfusion, Risk for ineffective
Childbearing process, Readiness for enhanced
Comfort, Impaired
Comfort, Readiness for enhanced
Communication, Impaired verbal
Communication, Readiness for enhanced
Conflict, Decisional
Conflict, Parental role
Confusion, Acute
Confusion, Chronic
Confusion, Risk for acute
Constipation
Constipation, Perceived
Constipation, Risk for
Contamination
Contamination, Risk for
Coping, Compromised family
Coping, Defensive
Coping, Disabled family
Coping, Ineffective
Coping, Ineffective community
Coping, Readiness for enhanced
Coping, Readiness for enhanced community
Coping, Readiness for enhanced family

Death syndrome, Risk for sudden infant
Decision making, Readiness for enhanced
Denial, Ineffective
Dentition, Impaired
Development, Risk for delayed
Diarrhea
Dignity, Risk for compromised human
Distress, Moral
Disuse syndrome, Risk for
Diversional activity, Deficient

Electrolyte imbalance, Risk for
Energy field, Disturbed
Environmental interpretation syndrome, Impaired

Failure to thrive, Adult
Falls, Risk for
Family processes: alcoholism, Dysfunctional
Family processes, Interrupted
Family processes, Readiness for enhanced
Fatigue
Fear
Fluid balance, Readiness for enhanced
Fluid volume, Deficient
Fluid volume, Excess
Fluid volume, Risk for deficient
Fluid volume, Risk for imbalanced

Gas exchange, Impaired
Gastrointestinal motility, Dysfunctional

Gastrointestinal motility, Risk for dysfunctional
Gastrointestinal tissue perfusion, Risk for ineffective
Glucose level, Risk for unstable
Grieving
Grieving, Complicated
Grieving, Risk for complicated
Growth and development, Delayed

Health maintenance, Ineffective
Health management, Ineffective self
Health management, Readiness for enhanced self
Health-seeking behaviors
Home maintenance, Impaired
Hope, Readiness for enhanced
Hopelessness
Hyperthermia
Hypothermia

Identity, Disturbed personal
Immunization status, Readiness for enhanced
Incontinence, Functional urinary
Incontinence, Overflow urinary
Incontinence, Reflex urinary
Incontinence, Risk for urge urinary
Incontinence, Stress urinary
Incontinence, Total urinary*
Incontinence, Urge urinary
Infant behavior, Disorganized
Infant behavior, Readiness for enhanced organized
Infant behavior, Risk for disorganized
Infant feeding pattern, Ineffective
Infection, Risk for
Injury, Risk for
Injury, Risk for perioperative-positioning
Insomnia
Intracranial adaptive capacity, Decreased

Jaundice, Neonatal

Knowledge, Deficient
Knowledge, Readiness for enhanced

Lifestyle, Sedentary
Liver function, Risk for impaired
Loneliness, Risk for

Maternal/fetal dyad, Risk for disturbed
Memory, Impaired
Mobility, Impaired bed
Mobility, Impaired physical
Mobility, Impaired wheelchair

Nausea
Neglect, Self
Neglect, Unilateral
Noncompliance
Nutrition: less than body requirements, Imbalanced
Nutrition: more than body requirements, Imbalanced
Nutrition: more than body requirements, Risk for imbalanced
Nutrition, Readiness for enhanced

Oral mucous membrane, Impaired

Pain, Acute
Pain, Chronic
Parenting, Impaired
Parenting, Readiness for enhanced
Parenting, Risk for impaired
Peripheral neurovascular dysfunction, Risk for
Peripheral tissue perfusion, Ineffective
Poisoning, Risk for
Post-trauma syndrome
Post-trauma syndrome, Risk for
Power, Readiness for enhanced
Powerlessness
Powerlessness, Risk for
Protection, Ineffective

Rape-trauma syndrome
Rape-trauma syndrome: compound reaction*

Rape-trauma syndrome: silent reaction*
Relationship, Readiness for enhanced
Religiosity, Impaired
Religiosity, Readiness for enhanced
Religiosity, Risk for impaired
Relocation stress syndrome
Relocation stress syndrome, Risk for
Renal perfusion, Risk for ineffective
Resilience, Impaired individual
Resilience, Readiness for enhanced
Resilience, Risk for compromised
Role performance, Ineffective

Self-care, Readiness for enhanced
Self-care deficit, Bathing/hygiene
Self-care deficit, Dressing/grooming
Self-care deficit, Feeding
Self-care deficit, Toileting
Self-concept, Readiness for enhanced
Self-esteem, Chronic low
Self-esteem, Risk for situational low
Self-esteem, Situational low
Self-mutilation
Self-mutilation, Risk for
Sensory perception, Disturbed
Sexual dysfunction
Sexuality pattern, Ineffective
Shock, Risk for
Skin integrity, Impaired
Skin integrity, Risk for impaired
Sleep deprivation
Sleep, Readiness for enhanced
Sleep pattern, Disturbed
Social isolation
Social interaction, Impaired
Sorrow, Chronic
Spiritual distress
Spiritual distress, Risk for
Spiritual well-being, Readiness for enhanced
Stress overload
Suffocation, Risk for
Suicide, Risk for
Surgical recovery, Delayed
Swallowing, Impaired

Therapeutic regimen management, Effective*
Therapeutic regimen management, Ineffective community*
Therapeutic regimen management, Ineffective family
Thermoregulation, Ineffective
Thought processes, Disturbed*
Tissue integrity, Impaired
Tissue perfusion, Ineffective
Transfer ability, Impaired
Trauma, Risk for

Urinary elimination, Impaired
Urinary elimination, Readiness for enhanced
Urinary retention

Vascular trauma, Risk for
Ventilation, Impaired spontaneous
Ventilatory weaning response, Dysfunctional
Violence, Risk for other-directed
Violence, Risk for self-directed

Walking, Impaired
Wandering

From the North American Nursing Diagnosis Association International: *NANDA-I nursing diagnoses: definitions and classification 2009–2011*, Oxford, United Kingdom, 2009, North American Nursing Diagnosis Association International.
*Retired diagnoses from the North American Nursing Diagnosis Association International: *NANDA-I nursing diagnoses: definitions and classification 2007–2008*, Philadelphia, 2007, North American Nursing Diagnosis Association International.